RC 683.5 .U5 O87 2018
Otto, Catherine M.
Textbook of clinical
echocardiography

NORTHAMPTON COMMUNITY COLLEGE
Paul & Harriett Mack Library
3835 Green Pond Road
Bethlehem, PA 18020

TEXTBOOK of
CLINICAL
ECHOCARDIOGRAPHY

SIXTH EDITION

TEXTBOOK of CLINICAL ECHOCARDIOGRAPHY

Catherine M. Otto, MD

J. Ward Kennedy-Hamilton Endowed Chair in Cardiology
Professor of Medicine
University of Washington School of Medicine;
Director, Heart Valve Disease Clinic;
Associate Director, Echocardiography Laboratory
University of Washington Medical Center
Seattle, Washington

ELSEVIER

ELSEVIER

1600 John F. Kennedy Blvd.
Ste 1800
Philadelphia, PA 19103-2899

TEXTBOOK OF CLINICAL ECHOCARDIOGRAPHY: SIXTH EDITION   ISBN: 978-0-323-48048-2

Copyright © 2018 by Elsevier, Inc. All rights reserved.

No part of this publication may be reproduced or transmitted in any form or by any means, electronic or mechanical, including photocopying, recording, or any information storage and retrieval system, without permission in writing from the Publisher. Details on how to seek permission, further information about the Publisher's permissions policies, and our arrangements with organizations such as the Copyright Clearance Center and the Copyright Licensing Agency can be found at our website: www.elsevier.com/permissions.

This book and the individual contributions contained in it are protected under copyright by the Publisher (other than as may be noted herein).

Notices

Knowledge and best practice in this field are constantly changing. As new research and experience broaden our understanding, changes in research methods, professional practices, or medical treatment may become necessary.

Practitioners and researchers must always rely on their own experience and knowledge in evaluating and using any information, methods, compounds, or experiments described herein. In using such information or methods, they should be mindful of their own safety and the safety of others, including parties for whom they have a professional responsibility.

With respect to any drug or pharmaceutical products identified, readers are advised to check the most current information provided (i) on procedures featured or (ii) by the manufacturer of each product to be administered, to verify the recommended dose or formula, the method and duration of administration, and contraindications. It is the responsibility of practitioners, relying on their own experience and knowledge of their patients, to make diagnoses, to determine dosages and the best treatment for each individual patient, and to take all appropriate safety precautions.

To the fullest extent of the law, neither the Publisher nor the authors, contributors, or editors assume any liability for any injury and/or damage to persons or property as a matter of products liability, negligence, or otherwise or from any use or operation of any methods, products, instructions, or ideas contained in the material herein.

Previous editions copyrighted 2013, 2009, 2004, 2000, 1995

ISBN: 978-0-323-48048-2

Executive Content Strategist: Dolores Meloni
Senior Content Development Specialist: Jennifer Ehlers
Publishing Services Manager: Catherine Albright Jackson
Senior Project Manager: Doug Turner
Designer: Margaret Reid

Printed in China

Last digit is the print number: 9 8 7 6 5 4 3 2 1

Working together
to grow libraries in
developing countries

www.elsevier.com • www.bookaid.org

PREFACE

Echocardiography is an integral part of clinical cardiology, with important applications in diagnosis, clinical management, and decision making for patients with a wide range of cardiovascular diseases. In addition to examinations performed in the echocardiography laboratory, ultrasound imaging is now used in many other clinical settings, including the emergency department, coronary care unit, intensive care unit, operating room, catheterization laboratory, and electrophysiology laboratory, both for diagnosis and for monitoring the effects of therapeutic interventions. Echocardiographic applications continue to expand because of the detailed and precise anatomic and physiologic information that can be obtained at the bedside with this technique at a relatively low cost and with minimal risk to the patient.

This textbook on general clinical echocardiography is intended to be read by individuals new to echocardiography and by those interested in updating their knowledge in this area. Thus, this book is aimed primarily at cardiology fellows on their basic echocardiography rotation but also will be of value to residents and fellows in general internal medicine, radiology, anesthesiology, and emergency medicine, as well as to cardiac sonography students. For physicians in practice, this textbook provides a concise and practical update.

Textbook of Clinical Echocardiography is structured around a clinical approach to echocardiographic diagnosis. First, a framework of basic principles is provided with chapters on ultrasound physics, normal tomographic transthoracic and transesophageal views, intracardiac flow patterns, indications for echocardiography, and evaluation of left ventricular systolic and diastolic function. A chapter on advanced echocardiographic modalities summarizes basic concepts for 3D echocardiography, myocardial mechanics, contrast echocardiography, and intracardiac echocardiography. Clinical use of these modalities is fully integrated into subsequent chapters, organized by disease categories aligned with the current practice of clinical cardiology.

Each of these chapters summarizes basic principles, the echocardiographic approach, differential diagnosis, technical considerations, and alternate diagnostic approaches. Schematic diagrams illustrate core concepts; echocardiographic images and Doppler recordings show typical findings for each disease process. Transthoracic and transesophageal images, Doppler data, 3D imaging, and other advanced imaging modalities are used throughout the text, reflecting their use in clinical practice. Tables are used frequently to summarize studies validating quantitative echocardiographic methods and to highlight the clinical correlates for each echocardiographic finding. A selected list of annotated references is included at the end of each chapter for those interested in reading more about a particular subject.

Some special features of this book that grew out of my experience teaching physicians and sonographers include The Echo Exam and Echo Math boxes. The Echo Exam consists of concise tables that summarize key concepts at the end of each chapter. Echo Math boxes provide examples of the quantitative calculations used in the day-to-day clinical practice of echocardiography. My hope is that The Echo Exam and Echo Math boxes will serve as quick reference guides in daily practice.

In this sixth edition, each chapter has been revised to reflect advances in the field, suggested readings have been updated, and the majority of the figures have been replaced with recent examples that more clearly illustrate the disease process. Most figures now have a linked video; on your smart device, simply click the video icon to see the echo images in motion. Detailed tables for normal reference values and evidence tables summarizing validation of quantitative echocardiographic methods are provided in Appendices at the end of the book.

A more advanced discussion of the impact of echocardiographic data in clinical medicine is available in a larger reference book, *The Practice of Clinical Echocardiography*, fifth edition (CM Otto [ed], 2017), also published by Elsevier. Additional clinical examples, practical tips for data acquisition, and multiple-choice self-assessment questions with detailed answers can be found in *Echocardiography Review Guide*, fourth edition, by Freeman, Schwaegler, Linefsky, and Otto (Elsevier, 2018), which exactly parallels the chapters in this textbook.

It should be emphasized that this textbook (or any book) is only a starting point or frame of reference for learning echocardiography. Appropriate training includes competency in the acquisition and interpretation of echocardiographic and Doppler data in real time. Additional training is needed for performance of stress and transesophageal examinations. As echocardiography continues to evolve and new techniques become practical and widely available, practitioners need to update their knowledge. Obviously, a textbook cannot replace the experience gained from performing studies on patients with a range of disease processes, and selected figures with videos do not replace the need for acquisition and review of complete patient examinations. Guidelines for training in echocardiography have been published, as referenced in Chapter 5, and include recommendations for determining clinical competency. Although this textbook is not a substitute for appropriate training and experience, my hope is that it will enhance the learning experience of those new to the field and provide a review for those currently engaged in the acquisition and interpretation of echocardiography. Every patient deserves a clinically appropriate and diagnostically accurate echocardiographic examination; each of us needs to continuously strive toward that goal.

Catherine M. Otto, MD

ACKNOWLEDGMENTS

Many people have provided input to each edition of the *Textbook of Clinical Echocardiography*, and the book is immeasurably enhanced by their contributions—not all can be individually thanked here. First, my special thanks go to the cardiac sonographers at the University of Washington for the outstanding quality of their echocardiographic examinations and for our frequent discussions of the details of image acquisition and the optimal echocardiography examination. Their skill in obtaining superb images provides the basis of many of the figures in this book. My thanks to Pamela Clark, RDCS; Sarah Curtis, RDCS; Maurizio Corona, RDCS; Caryn D'Jang, RDCS; Margaret Falkenreck, RDCS; Michelle Fujioka, RDCS; Carolyn Gardner, RDCS; Deanna Knox, RDCS; Yelena Kovolenko, RDCS; Carol Kraft, RDCS; Carin Lodell, RDCS; Chris McKenzie, RDCS; Irina Nesterova, RDCS; Amy Owens, RDCS; Becky Schwaegler, RDCS; Joanna Shephard, RDCS; Karl Skinner, RDCS; Hoang Tran, RDCS; Yu Wang, RDCS; and Todd Zwink, RDCS.

My gratitude extends to my colleagues at the University of Washington who shared their expertise and helped identify images for the book, with special thanks to Rosario Freeman, MD; Jim Kirkpatrick, MD; Don Oxorn, MD; and G. Burkhard Mackensen, MD. The University of Washington Cardiology Fellows also provided thoughtful (and sometimes humbling) insights and helped identify cases with teaching quality images; particular recognition goes to James C. Lee. In addition, my gratitude is extended to those individuals who kindly gave permission for reproduction of previously published figures. Joe Chovan and Starr Kaplan are to be commended for their skills as medical illustrators and for providing such clear and detailed anatomic drawings.

My most sincere appreciation extends to the many readers who provided suggestions for improvement, with particular thanks to Jason Linefsky, MD, and Rosario Freeman, MD.

Many thanks to my editor, Delores Meloni, at Elsevier for providing the support needed to write this edition and to Jennifer Ehlers and the production team for all the detail-oriented hard work that went into making this book a reality.

Finally, my most appreciative thanks to my husband, daughter, and granddaughter for their unwavering support in every aspect of life.

Catherine M. Otto, MD

CONTENTS

Glossary, *xi*

Key Equations, *xiv*

1 Principles of Echocardiographic Image Acquisition and Doppler Analysis, *1*
  Ultrasound Waves, 1
  Ultrasound Tissue Interaction, 4
  Transducers, 6
  Ultrasound Imaging Modalities, 10
  Doppler Echocardiography, 16
  Bioeffects and Safety, 27
  The Echo Exam, 30
  Suggested Reading, 31

2 Normal Anatomy and Flow Patterns on Transthoracic Echocardiography, *33*
  Basic Imaging Principles, 33
  Transthoracic Tomographic Views, 36
  M-Mode Recordings, 49
  Normal Intracardiac Flow Patterns, 52
  Aging Changes on Echocardiography, 61
  The Diagnostic Echocardiogram, 61
  The Echo Exam, 64
  Suggested Reading, 65

3 Transesophageal Echocardiography, *67*
  Protocols and Risks, 67
  Tomographic Views, 68
  Valve Anatomy and Function, 80
  Chamber Anatomy and Filling Patterns, 87
  Imaging Sequence, 90
  The Echo Exam, 92
  Suggested Reading, 94

4 Specialized Echocardiography Applications, *96*
  Three-Dimensional Echocardiography, 96
  Myocardial Mechanics, 106
  Contrast Echocardiography, 112
  Intracardiac Echocardiography, 115
  The Echo Exam, 118
  Suggested Reading, 118

5 Clinical Indications and Quality Assurance, *120*
  Types of Echocardiographic Studies, 120
  Basic Principles of Diagnostic Testing, 122
  Indications and Appropriateness Criteria, 126
  Indications for Diagnostic Echocardiography, 127
  Point of Care Cardiac Ultrasound Studies, 133
  Quality Assurance in Echocardiography, 135
  The Echo Exam, 139
  Suggested Reading, 141

6 Left and Right Ventricular Systolic Function, *144*
  Basic Principles, 144
  Imaging the Left Ventricle, 147
  Doppler Evaluation of Left Ventricular Systolic Function, 158
  Echo Approach to Right Ventricular Systolic Function, 163
  Pulmonary Vasculature, 168
  The Echo Exam, 175
  Suggested Reading, 176

7 Ventricular Diastolic Filling and Function, *178*
  Basic Principles, 179
  Anatomic Parameters, 182
  Doppler Evaluation of LV Filling, 183
  Tissue Doppler Myocardial Imaging, 185
  Left Atrial Filling, 187
  Other Approaches, 189
  Confounding Factors, 190
  Clinical Classification of Diastolic Dysfunction, 194
  Right Ventricular Diastolic Function, 198
  Alternate Approaches, 200
  Diastolic Function Reporting, 200
  The Echo Exam, 202
  Suggested Reading, 202

8 Coronary Artery Disease, *204*
  Basic Principles, 204
  Myocardial Ischemia, 211
  Myocardial Infarction, 221
  End-Stage Ischemic Cardiac Disease, 228
  The Echo Exam, 230
  Suggested Reading, 232

9 Cardiomyopathies, Hypertensive and Pulmonary Heart Disease, *235*
  Dilated Cardiomyopathy, 236
  Hypertrophic Cardiomyopathy, 245
  Restrictive Cardiomyopathy, 252

Other Cardiomyopathies, 256
Advanced Heart Failure Therapies, 257
Hypertensive Heart Disease, 260
Pulmonary Heart Disease, 262
The Echo Exam, 265
Suggested Reading, 266

10 Pericardial Disease, *268*

Pericardial Anatomy and Physiology, 268
Pericarditis, 268
Pericardial Effusion, 271
Pericardial Tamponade, 275
Pericardial Constriction, 278
The Echo Exam, 285
Suggested Reading, 285

11 Valvular Stenosis, *288*

Basic Principles, 288
Aortic Stenosis, 291
Mitral Stenosis, 305
Tricuspid Stenosis, 315
Pulmonic Stenosis, 316
The Echo Exam, 320
Suggested Reading, 322

12 Valvular Regurgitation, *324*

Basic Principles, 324
Approaches to Quantitation of Regurgitant Severity, 327
Aortic Regurgitation, 336
Mitral Regurgitation, 345
Tricuspid Regurgitation, 359
Pulmonic Regurgitation, 363
The Echo Exam: Valve Regurgitation, 365
Suggested Reading, 367

13 Prosthetic Valves, *370*

Basic Principles, 370
Echocardiographic Approach, 375
Limitations and Alternate Approaches, 387
Clinical Utility, 387
The Echo Exam, 397
Suggested Reading, 398

14 Endocarditis, *400*

Basic Principles, 400
Echocardiographic Approach, 402
Limitations and Technical Considerations, 413
Clinical Utility, 415
The Echo Exam, 419
Suggested Reading, 419

15 Cardiac Masses and Potential Cardiac Source of Embolus, *422*

Basic Principles, 422
Valve Vegetations, 425

Cardiac Tumors, 425
Left Ventricular Thrombus, 431
Left Atrial Thrombus, 434
Right-Sided Heart Thrombi, 436
Cardiac Source of Embolus, 437
The Echo Exam, 444
Suggested Reading, 445

16 Diseases of the Great Arteries, *447*

Basic Principles, 447
Echocardiographic Approach, 449
Aortic Dilation and Aneurysm, 455
Aortic Dissection, 458
Aortic Intramural Hematoma, 463
Aortic Pseudoaneurysm, 463
Traumatic Aortic Disease, 464
Sinus of Valsalva Aneurysm, 464
Atherosclerotic Aortic Disease, 465
Pulmonary Artery Abnormalities, 465
Alternate Approaches, 466
The Echo Exam, 469
Suggested Reading, 470

17 The Adult With Congenital Heart Disease, *473*

Basic Principles, 474
Congenital Stenotic Lesions, 480
Congenital Abnormalities of the Aorta and Coronary Arteries, 482
Congenital Regurgitant Lesions, 483
Intracardiac Shunts, 484
Other Conditions Manifesting in Adulthood, 491
Common Types of Palliated Adult Congenital Heart Disease, 494
Limitations of Echocardiography and Alternate Approaches, 500
Integrating the Diagnostic Approach, 503
The Echo Exam, 504
Suggested Reading, 505

18 Intraoperative and Interventional Echocardiography, *507*

Basic Principles, 508
Echocardiographic Approach, 512
Limitations and Technical Considerations, 516
Clinical Utility of Intraoperative TEE, 519
Clinical Utility in Transcatheter and Hybrid Procedures, 530
The Echo Exam, 538
Suggested Reading, 539

Appendix A: Normal Values for Echocardiographic Measurements, *542*

Appendix B: Evidence Tables, *549*

GLOSSARY: Abbreviations Used in Figures, Tables, and Equations

2D = two-dimensional
3D = three-dimensional

A = late diastolic ventricular filling velocity with atrial contraction
A' = diastolic tissue Doppler velocity with atrial contraction
A2C = apical two-chamber
A4C = apical four-chamber
AcT = acceleration time
a_{dur} = pulmonary vein a-velocity duration
A_{dur} = transmitral A-velocity duration
AF = atrial fibrillation
A-long = apical long-axis
A-mode = amplitude mode (amplitude versus depth)
AMVL = anterior mitral valve leaflet
ant = anterior
Ao = aortic or aorta
AR = aortic regurgitation
AS = aortic stenosis
ASD = atrial septal defect
ATVL = anterior tricuspid valve leaflet
AV = atrioventricular
AVA = aortic valve area
AVR = aortic valve replacement

BAV = bicuspid aortic valve
BP = blood pressure
BSA = body surface area

c = propagation velocity of sound in tissue
CAD = coronary artery disease
cath = cardiac catheterization
cm = centimeters
Cm = specific heat of tissue
cm/s = centimeters per second
CMR = cardiac magnetic resonance imaging
CO = cardiac output
cos = cosine
CPB = cardiopulmonary bypass
CS = coronary sinus
CSA = cross-sectional area
CT = computed tomography
CW = continuous-wave
Cx = circumflex coronary artery

D = diameter
DA = descending aorta
dB = decibels
dP/dt = rate of change in pressure over time
DT = deceleration time
dT/dt = rate of increase in temperature over time
D-TGA = complete transposition of the great arteries
dyne • s • cm^{-5} = units of resistance

E = early diastolic peak velocity
E' = early diastolic tissue Doppler velocity
ECG = electrocardiogram
echo = echocardiography
ED = end-diastole
EDD = end-diastolic dimension
EDV = end-diastolic volume
EF = ejection fraction
endo = endocardium
epi = epicardium
EPSS = E-point septal separation
ES = end-systole
ESD = end-systolic dimension
ESV = end-systolic volume
ETT = exercise treadmill test

Δf = frequency shift
f = frequency
FL = false lumen
F_n = near field
F_o = resonance frequency
F_s = scattered frequency
FSV = forward stroke volume
F_T = transmitted frequency

HCM = hypertrophic cardiomyopathy
HPRF = high-pulse repetition frequency
HR = heart rate
HV = hepatic vein
Hz = Hertz (cycles per second)

I = intensity of ultrasound exposure
IAS = interatrial septum
inf = inferior
IV = intravenous
IVC = inferior vena cava

IVCT = isovolumic contraction time
IVRT = isovolumic relaxation time

kHz = kilohertz

l = length
LA = left atrium
LAA = left atrial appendage
LAD = left anterior descending coronary artery
LAE = left atrial enlargement
lat = lateral
LCC = left coronary cusp
LMCA = left main coronary artery
LPA = left pulmonary artery
LSPV = left superior pulmonary vein
L-TGA = corrected transposition of the great arteries
LV = left ventricle
LV-EDP = left ventricular end-diastolic pressure
LVH = left ventricular hypertrophy
LVID = left ventricular internal dimension
LVOT = left ventricular outflow tract

MAC = mitral annular calcification
MI = myocardial infarction
M-mode = motion display (depth versus time)
MR = mitral regurgitation
MS = mitral stenosis
MV = mitral valve
MVA = mitral valve area
MVL = mitral valve leaflet
MVR = mitral valve replacement

n = number of subjects
NBTE = nonbacterial thrombotic endocarditis
NCC = noncoronary cusp

ΔP = pressure gradient
P = pressure
PA = pulmonary artery
PAP = pulmonary artery pressure
PCI = percutaneous coronary intervention
PDA = patent ductus arteriosus or posterior descending artery (depends on context)
PE = pericardial effusion
PEP = preejection period
PET = positron emission tomography
PISA = proximal isovelocity surface area
PLAX = parasternal long-axis
PM = papillary muscle
PMVL = posterior mitral valve leaflet
post = posterior (or inferior-lateral) ventricular wall
PR = pulmonic regurgitation
PRF = pulse repetition frequency
PRFR = peak rapid filling rate
PS = pulmonic stenosis
PSAX = parasternal short-axis
PV = pulmonary vein

PVC = premature ventricular contraction
PV_D = pulmonary vein diastolic velocity
PVR = pulmonary vascular resistance
PWT = posterior wall thickness

Q = volume flow rate
Q_p = pulmonic volume flow rate
Q_s = systemic volume flow rate

r = correlation coefficient
R = ventricular radius
RA = right atrium
RAE = right atrial enlargement
RAO = right anterior oblique
RAP = right atrial pressure
RCA = right coronary artery
RCC = right coronary cusp
R_e = Reynolds number
RF = regurgitant fraction
RFR = regurgitant instantaneous flow rate
RJ = regurgitant jet
R_o = radius of microbubble
ROA = regurgitant orifice area
RPA = right pulmonary artery
RSPV = right superior pulmonary vein
RSV = regurgitant stroke volume
RV = right ventricle
RVE = right ventricular enlargement
RVH = right ventricular hypertrophy
RVol = regurgitant volume
RVOT = right ventricular outflow tract

s = second
SAM = systolic anterior motion
SC = subcostal
SEE = standard error of the estimate
SPPA = spatial peak pulse average
SPTA = spatial peak temporal average
SSN = suprasternal notch
ST = septal thickness
STJ = sinotubular junction
STVL = septal tricuspid valve leaflet
SV = stroke volume or sample volume (depends on context)
SVC = superior vena cava

$T\frac{1}{2}$ = pressure half-time
TD = thermodilution
TEE = transesophageal echocardiography
TGA = transposition of the great arteries
TGC = time-gain compensation
Th = wall thickness
TL = true lumen
TN = true negatives
TOF = tetralogy of Fallot
TP = true positives
TPV = time to peak velocity
TR = tricuspid regurgitation

TS = tricuspid stenosis
TSV = total stroke volume
TTE = transthoracic echocardiography
TV = tricuspid valve

v = velocity
V = volume or velocity (depends on context)
VAS = ventriculo-atrial septum
Veg = vegetation
V_{max} = maximum velocity
VSD = ventricular septal defect
VTI = velocity-time integral

WPW = Wolff-Parkinson-White syndrome

Z = acoustic impedance

Symbols	Greek Name	Used for
α	alpha	Frequency
γ	gamma	Viscosity
Δ	delta	Difference
θ	theta	Angle
λ	lambda	Wavelength
μ	mu	Micro-
π	pi	Mathematical constant (approx. 3.14)
ρ	rho	Tissue density
σ	sigma	Wall stress
τ	tau	Time constant of ventricular relaxation

Units of Measure

Variable	Unit	Definition
Amplitude	dB	Decibels = a logarithmic scale describing the amplitude ("loudness") of the sound wave
Angle	degrees	Degree = $(\pi/180)$rad. Example: intercept angle
Area	cm^2	Square centimeters. A 2D measurement (e.g., end-systolic area) or a calculated value (e.g., continuity equation valve area)
Frequency (f)	Hz kHz MHz	Hertz (cycles per second) Kilohertz = 1000 Hz Megahertz = 1,000,000 Hz
Length	cm mm	Centimeter (1/100 m) Millimeter (1/1000 m or 1/10 cm)
Mass	g	Grams. Example: LV mass
Pressure	mmHg	Millimeters of mercury, 1 mmHg = 1333.2 dyne/cm^2, where dyne measures force in cm-mg-s^2
Resistance	dyne • s • cm^{-5}	Measure of vascular resistance
Time	s ms μs	Second Millisecond (1/1000 s) Microsecond
Ultrasound intensity	W/cm^2 mW/cm^2	Where watt (W) = joule per second and joule = m^2 • kg • s^{-2} (unit of energy)
Velocity (v)	m/s cm/s	Meters per second Centimeters per second
Velocity-time integral (VTI)	cm	Integral of the Doppler velocity curve (cm/s) over time (s), in units of cm
Volume	cm^3 mL L	Cubic centimeters Milliliter, 1 mL = 1 cm^3 Liter = 1000 mL
Volume flow rate (Q)	L/min mL/s	Rate of volume flow across a valve or in cardiac output L/min = liters per minute mL/s = milliliters per second
Wall stress	dyne/cm^2 kdyn/cm^2 kPa	Units of meridional or circumferential wall stress Kilodynes per cm^2 Kilopascals where 1 kPa = 10 kdyn/cm^2

KEY EQUATIONS

Ultrasound Physics
Frequency $\quad f = \text{cycles/s} = \text{Hz}$
Wavelength $\quad \lambda = c / f = 1.54 / f \, (\text{MHz})$
Doppler equation $\quad v = c \times \Delta f / [2F_T (\cos\theta)]$
Bernoulli equation $\quad \Delta P = 4V^2$

LV Imaging
Stroke volume
Ejection fraction $\quad \text{EF}(\%) = (\text{SV} / \text{EDV}) \times 100\%$
Wall stress $\quad \sigma = \text{PR} / 2\text{Th}$

Doppler Ventricular Function
Stroke volume $\quad \text{SV} = \text{CSA} \times \text{VTI}$
Rate of pressure rise $\quad dP/dt = 32 \text{ mmHg} / \text{Time from 1 to 3 m/s of MR CW jet(sec)}$
Myocardial performance index $\quad \text{MPI} = (\text{IVRT} + \text{IVCT}) / \text{SEP}$

Pulmonary Pressures and Resistance
Pulmonary systolic pressure $\quad \text{PAP}_{\text{systolic}} = 4(V_{\text{TR}})2 + \text{RAP}$
PAP (when PS is present) $\quad \text{PAP}_{\text{systolic}} = [4(V_{\text{TR}})2 + \text{RAP}] - \Delta P_{\text{RV-PA}}$
Mean PA pressure $\quad \text{PAP}_{\text{mean}} = \text{Mean } \Delta P_{\text{RV-RA}} + \text{RAP}$
Diastolic PA pressure $\quad \text{PAP}_{\text{diastolic}} = 4(V_{\text{PR}})^2 + \text{RAP}$
Pulmonary vascular resistance $\quad \text{PVR} \approx 10(V_{\text{TR}}) / \text{VTI}_{\text{RVOT}}$

Aortic Stenosis
Maximum pressure gradient (integrate over ejection period for mean gradient) $\quad \Delta P_{\text{max}} = 4(V_{\text{max}})^2$
Continuity equation valve area $\quad \text{AVA}(\text{cm}^2) = [\pi(\text{LVOT}_D / 2)^2 \times \text{VTI}_{\text{LVOT}}] / \text{VTI}_{\text{AS-Jet}}$
Simplified continuity equation $\quad \text{AVA}(\text{cm}^2) = [\pi(\text{LVOT}_D / 2)^2 \times V_{\text{LVOT}}] / V_{\text{AS-Jet}}$
Velocity ratio $\quad \text{Velocity ratio} = V_{\text{LVOT}} / V_{\text{AS-Jet}}$

Mitral Stenosis
Pressure half-time valve area $\quad \text{MVA}_{\text{Doppler}} = 220 / T_{1/2}$

Aortic Regurgitation
Total stroke volume $\quad \text{TSV} = \text{SV}_{\text{LVOT}} = (\text{CSA}_{\text{LVOT}} \times \text{VTI}_{\text{LVOT}})$
Forward stroke volume $\quad \text{FSV} = \text{SV}_{\text{MA}} = (\text{CSA}_{\text{MA}} \times \text{VTI}_{\text{MA}})$
Regurgitant volume $\quad \text{RVol} = \text{TSV} - \text{FSV}$
Regurgitant orifice area $\quad \text{ROA} = \text{RSV} / \text{VTI}_{\text{AR}}$

Mitral Regurgitation
Total stroke volume (or 2D or 3D LV stroke volume) $\quad \text{TSV} = \text{SV}_{\text{MA}} = (\text{CSA}_{\text{MA}} \times \text{VTI}_{\text{MA}})$
Forward stroke volume $\quad \text{FSV} = \text{SV}_{\text{LVOT}} = (\text{CSA}_{\text{LVOT}} \times \text{VTI}_{\text{LVOT}})$
Regurgitant volume $\quad \text{RVol} = \text{TSV} - \text{FSV}$
Regurgitant orifice area $\quad \text{ROA} = \text{RSV} / \text{VTI}_{\text{AR}}$

PISA Method
Regurgitant flow rate $\quad R_{\text{FR}} = 2\pi r^2 \times V_{\text{aliasing}}$
Orifice area (maximum) $\quad \text{ROA}_{\text{max}} = R_{\text{FR}} / V_{\text{MR}}$
Regurgitant volume $\quad \text{RV} = \text{ROA} \times \text{VTI}_{\text{MR}}$

Aortic Dilation
Predicted sinus diameter
   Children (<18 years): Predicted sinus dimension = 1.02 + (0.98 BSA)
   Adults (18–40 years): Predicted sinus dimension = 0.97 + (1.12 BSA)
   Adults (>40 years): Predicted sinus dimension = 1.92 + (0.74 BSA)
   Ratio = Measured maximum diameter / Predicted maximum diameter

Pulmonary (Q_p) to Systemic (Q_s) Shunt Ratio
$Q_p:Q_s = [\text{CSA}_{\text{PA}} \times \text{VTI}_{\text{PA}}] / [\text{CSA}_{\text{LVOT}} \times \text{VTI}_{\text{LVOT}}]$

1 Principles of Echocardiographic Image Acquisition and Doppler Analysis

ULTRASOUND WAVES
ULTRASOUND TISSUE INTERACTION
   Reflection
   Scattering
   Refraction
   Attenuation
TRANSDUCERS
   Piezoelectric Crystal
   Types of Transducers
   Beam Shape and Focusing
   Resolution
ULTRASOUND IMAGING MODALITIES
   M-Mode
   Two-Dimensional Echocardiography
      Image Production
      Instrument Settings
      Imaging Artifacts
   Three-Dimensional Echocardiography
   Echocardiographic Imaging Measurements

DOPPLER ECHOCARDIOGRAPHY
   Doppler Velocity Data
      Doppler Equation
      Spectral Analysis
      Continuous-Wave Doppler Ultrasound
      Pulsed Doppler Ultrasound
      Doppler Velocity Instrument Controls
      Doppler Velocity Data Artifacts
   Color Doppler Flow Imaging
      Principles
      Color Doppler Instrument Controls
      Color Doppler Imaging Artifacts
   Tissue Doppler
BIOEFFECTS AND SAFETY
   Bioeffects
   Safety
THE ECHO EXAM
SUGGESTED READING

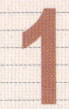n understanding of the basic principles of ultrasound imaging and Doppler echocardiography is essential both during data acquisition and for correct interpretation of the ultrasound information. Although, at times, current instruments provide instantaneous images so clear and detailed that it seems as if we can "see" the heart and blood flow directly, in actuality we always are looking at images and flow data generated by complex analyses of ultrasound waves reflected and backscattered from the patient's body. Knowledge of the strengths, and more importantly the limitations, of this technique is critical for correct clinical diagnosis and patient management. On the one hand, echocardiography can be used for decision making with a high degree of accuracy in a variety of clinical settings. On the other hand, if an ultrasound artifact is mistaken for an anatomic abnormality, a patient could undergo other needless, expensive, and potentially risky diagnostic tests or therapeutic interventions.

In this chapter, a brief (and necessarily simplified) overview of the basic principles of cardiac ultrasound imaging and flow analysis is presented. The reader is referred to the Suggested Reading at the end of the chapter for more information on these subjects. Because the details of image processing, artifact formation, and Doppler physics become more meaningful with experience, some readers may choose to return to this chapter after reading other sections of this book and after participating in some echocardiographic examinations.

ULTRASOUND WAVES

Sound waves are mechanical vibrations that induce alternate refraction and compression of any physical medium through which they pass (Fig. 1.1). Like other waves, sound waves are described in terms of (Table 1.1):

- Frequency: cycles per second, or hertz (Hz)
- Velocity of propagation
- Wavelength: millimeters (mm)
- Amplitude: decibels (dB)

Frequency (f) is the number of ultrasound waves in a 1-second interval. The units of measurement are hertz, abbreviated Hz, which simply means cycles per second. A frequency of 1000 cycles/s is 1 kilohertz (kHz), and 1 million cycles/s is 1 megahertz (MHz). Humans can hear sound waves with frequencies between 20 Hz and 20 kHz; frequencies higher than this range are termed *ultrasound*. Diagnostic medical ultrasound typically uses transducers with a frequency between 1 and 20 MHz.

The speed that a sound wave moves through the body, called the *velocity of propagation (c)*, is different for each type of tissue. For example, the velocity of propagation in bone is much faster (about 3000 m/s) than in lung tissue (about 700 m/s). However, the velocity of propagation in soft tissues, including myocardium, valves, blood vessels, and blood, is relatively uniform, averaging about 1540 m/s.

ECHO MATH: Wavelength

Wavelength (λ) is the distance from peak to peak of an ultrasound wave. Wavelength can be calculated by dividing the frequency (*f* in Hz) by the propagation velocity (*c* in m/s):

$$\lambda = c/f \qquad \text{(Eq. 1.1)}$$

Because the propagation velocity in the heart is constant at 1540 m/s, the wavelength for any transducer frequency can be calculated (Fig. 1.2) as:

$$\lambda \text{ (mm)} = [1540 \text{ m/s}/f(\text{Hz})]/1000 \text{ mm/m}$$

or

$$\lambda \text{ (mm)} = 1.54/f$$

For example, the wavelength emitted by a 5-MHz transducer can be calculated as:

$$\lambda = 1540 \text{ m/s}/5{,}000{,}000 \text{ cycle/s} = 0.000308$$
$$m = 0.308 \text{ mm}$$

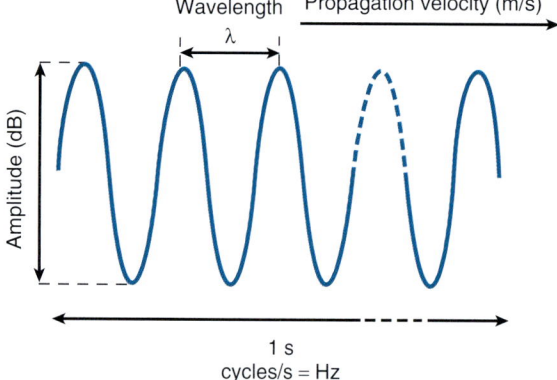

Fig. 1.1 Schematic diagram of an ultrasound wave.

TABLE 1.1　Ultrasound Waves

	Definition	Examples	Clinical Implications
Frequency (*f*)	The number of cycles per second in an ultrasound wave *f* = cycles/s = Hz	Transducer frequencies are measured in MHz (1,000,000 cycles/s). Doppler signal frequencies are measured in kHz (1000 cycles/s).	Different transducer frequencies are used for specific clinical applications because the transmitted frequency affects ultrasound tissue penetration, image resolution, and the Doppler signal.
Velocity of propagation (*c*)	The speed that ultrasound travels through tissue	The average velocity of ultrasound in soft tissue is ≈1540 m/s.	The velocity of propagation is similar in different soft tissues (e.g., blood, myocardium, liver, fat) but is much lower in lung and much higher in bone.
Wavelength (λ)	The distance between ultrasound waves: λ = c/f = 1.54 / f (MHz)	Wavelength is shorter with a higher-frequency transducer and longer with a lower-frequency transducer.	Image resolution is greatest (≈1 mm) with a shorter wavelength (higher frequency). Depth of tissue penetration is greatest with a longer wavelength (lower frequency).
Amplitude (dB)	Height of the ultrasound wave or "loudness" measured in decibels (dB)	A log scale is used for dB. On the dB scale, 80 dB represents a 10,000-fold and 40 dB indicates a 100-fold increase in amplitude.	A very wide range of amplitudes can be displayed using a gray-scale display for both imaging and spectral Doppler.

Wavelength is important in diagnostic applications for at least two reasons:

- Image resolution is no greater than 1 to 2 wavelengths (typically about 1 mm).
- The depth of penetration of the ultrasound wave into the body is directly related to wavelength; shorter wavelengths penetrate a shorter distance than longer wavelengths.

Thus there is an obvious trade-off between image resolution (shorter wavelength or higher frequency preferable) and depth penetration (longer wavelength or lower frequency preferable).

The acoustic pressure, or amplitude, of an ultrasound wave indicates the energy of the ultrasound signal. Power is the amount of energy per unit time. Intensity (I) is the amount of power per unit area:

$$\text{Intensity (I)} = \text{Power}^2 \qquad \text{(Eq. 1.2)}$$

This relationship shows that if ultrasound power is doubled, intensity is quadruped. Instead of using direct measures of pressure energy, ultrasound amplitude is described relative to a reference value using the decibel scale. Decibels (dB) are familiar to all of us as the standard description of the loudness of a sound.

ECHO MATH: Decibels

Decibels are logarithmic units based on a ratio of the measured amplitude (A_2) to a reference amplitude (A_1) such that:

$$dB = 20 \log(A_2/A_1) \qquad \text{(Eq. 1.3)}$$

Thus a ratio of 1000 to 1 is

$$20 \times \log(1000) = 20 \times 3 = 60 \text{ dB}$$

a ratio of 100 to 1 is

$$20 \times \log(100) = 20 \times 2 = 40 \text{ dB}$$

and a ratio of 2 to 1 is

$$20 \times \log(2) = 20 \times 0.3 = 6 \text{ dB}$$

A simple rule to remember is that a 6-dB change represents a doubling or halving of the signal amplitude or that a 40-dB change represents a 100 times difference in amplitude (Fig. 1.3).

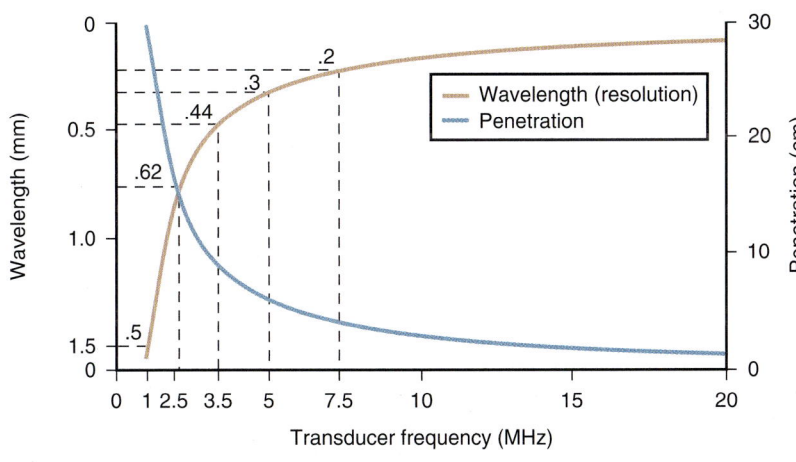

Fig. 1.2 Transducer frequency versus wavelength and penetration of the ultrasound signal in soft tissue. Wavelength has been plotted inversely to show that resolution increases with increasing transducer frequency while penetration decreases. The specific wavelengths for transducer frequencies of 1, 2.5, 3.5, 5, and 7.5 MHz are shown.

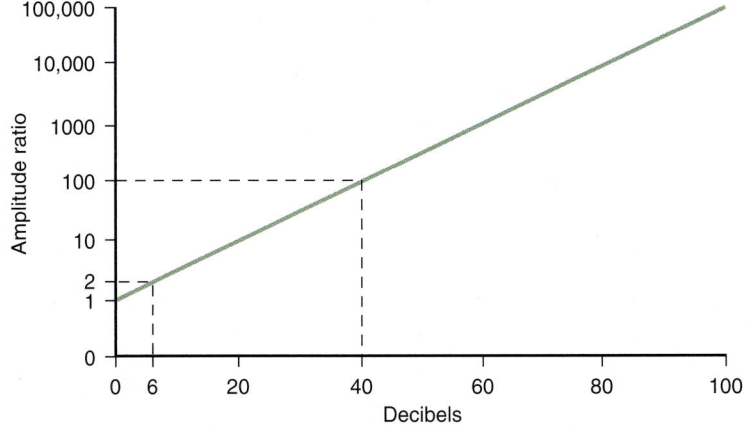

Fig. 1.3 Graph of the decibel scale. The logarithmic relationship between the decibel scale (horizontal axis) and the amplitude ratio (vertical axis) is seen. A doubling or halving of the amplitude ratio corresponds to a 6-dB change, and a 100-fold difference in amplitude corresponds to a 20-dB change.

If acoustic intensity is used instead of amplitude, the constant 10 replaces 20 in the equation so that a 3-dB change represents doubling, and a 20-dB change indicates a 100-fold difference in amplitude. Both these decibel scales are used to refer to transmitted or received ultrasound waves or to describe attenuation effects. The advantages of the decibel scale are that a very large range can be compressed into a smaller number of values and that low-amplitude (weak) signals can be displayed alongside very high-amplitude (strong) signals. In an echocardiographic image, amplitudes typically range from 1 to 120 dB. The decibel scale is the standard format both for echocardiographic image display and for the Doppler spectral display, although other amplitude scales are sometimes available.

ULTRASOUND TISSUE INTERACTION

Propagation of ultrasound waves in the body to generate ultrasound images and Doppler data depends on a tissue property called *acoustic impedance* (Table 1.2).

Acoustic impedance (Z) depends on tissue density (ρ) and on the propagation velocity in that tissue (c):

$$Z = \rho c \qquad \text{(Eq. 1.4)}$$

Although the velocity of propagation differs among tissues, tissue density is the primary determinant of acoustic impedance for diagnostic ultrasound. Lung tissue has a very low density compared with bone, which has a very high density. Soft tissues, such as blood and myocardium, have much smaller differences in tissue density and acoustic impedance. Acoustic impedance determines the transmission of ultrasound waves through a tissue; *differences* in acoustic impedance result in reflection of ultrasound waves at tissue boundaries.

The interaction of ultrasound waves with the organs and tissues of the body can be described in terms of (Fig. 1.4):

- Reflection
- Scattering
- Refraction
- Attenuation

TABLE 1.2 Ultrasound Tissue Interaction

	Definition	Examples	Clinical Implications
Acoustic impedance (Z)	A characteristic of each tissue defined by tissue density (ρ) and propagation of velocity (c) as: $Z = \rho \times c$	Lung has a low density and slow propagation velocity, whereas bone has a high density and fast propagation velocity. Soft tissues have smaller differences in tissue density and acoustic impedance.	Ultrasound is reflected from boundaries between tissues with differences in acoustic impedance (e.g., blood vs. myocardium).
Reflection	Return of ultrasound signal to the transducer from a smooth tissue boundary	Reflection is used to generate 2D cardiac images.	Reflection is greatest with the ultrasound beam in perpendicular to the tissue interface.
Scattering	Radiation of ultrasound in multiple directions from a small structure (e.g., blood cells)	The change in frequency of signals scattered from moving blood cells is the basis of Doppler ultrasound.	The amplitude of scattered signals is 100 to 1000 times less than reflected signals.
Refraction	Deflection of ultrasound waves from a straight path due to differences in acoustic impedance	Refraction is used in transducer design to focus the ultrasound beam.	Refraction in tissues results in double image artifacts.
Attenuation	Loss in signal strength due to absorption of ultrasound energy by tissues	Attenuation is frequency dependent with greater attenuation (less penetration) at higher frequencies.	A lower-frequency transducer is needed for apical views or in larger patients on transthoracic imaging.
Resolution	The smallest resolvable distance between two specular reflectors on an ultrasound image	Resolution has three dimensions: along the length of the beam (axial), lateral across the image (azimuthal), and in the elevational plane.	Axial resolution is most precise (as small as 1 mm), so imaging measurements are best made along the length of the ultrasound beam.

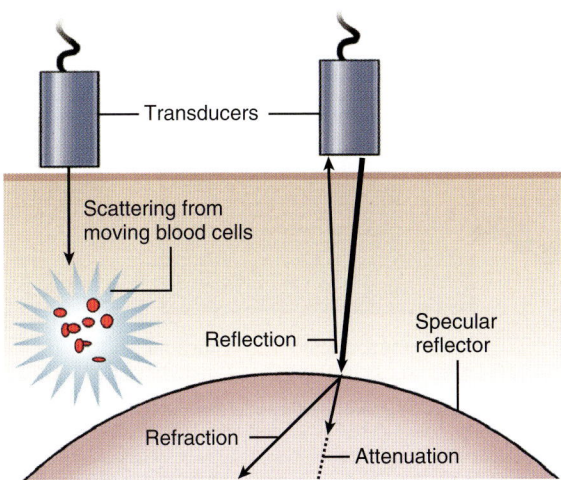

Fig. 1.4 Diagram of the interaction between ultrasound and body tissues. Doppler analysis is based on the scattering of ultrasound in all directions from moving blood cells with a resulting change in frequency of the ultrasound received at the transducer. 2D imaging is based on reflection of ultrasound from tissue interfaces (specular reflectors). Attenuation limits the depth of ultrasound penetration. Refraction, a change in direction of the ultrasound wave, results in imaging artifacts.

Reflection

The basis of ultrasound imaging is *reflection* of the transmitted ultrasound signal from internal structures. Ultrasound is reflected at tissue boundaries and interfaces, with the amount of ultrasound reflected dependent on the:

- Difference in acoustic impedance between the two tissues
- Angle of reflection

Smooth tissue boundaries with a lateral dimension greater than the wavelength of the ultrasound beam act as specular, or "mirror-like," reflectors. The amount of ultrasound reflected is constant for a given interface, although the amount received back at the transducer varies with angle because (like light reflected from a mirror) the angle of incidence and reflection is equal. Thus optimal return of reflected ultrasound occurs at a perpendicular angle (90°). Remembering this fact is crucial for obtaining diagnostic ultrasound images. It also accounts for ultrasound "dropout" in a two-dimensional (2D) or three-dimensional (3D) image when too little or no reflected ultrasound reaches the transducer resulting from a parallel alignment between the ultrasound beam and tissue interface.

Scattering

Scattering of the ultrasound signal, instead of reflection, occurs with small structures, such as red blood cells suspended in fluid, because the radius of the cell (about 4 μm) is smaller than the wavelength of the ultrasound signal. Unlike a reflected beam, scattered ultrasound energy radiates in all directions. Only a small amount of the scattered signal reaches the receiving transducer, and the amplitude of a scattered signal is 100 to 1000 times (40–60 dB) less than the amplitude of the returned signal from a specular reflector. Scattering of ultrasound from moving blood cells is the basis of Doppler echocardiography.

The *extent* of scattering depends on:

- Particle size (red blood cells)
- Number of particles (hematocrit)
- Ultrasound transducer frequency
- Compressibility of blood cells and plasma

Although experimental studies show differences in backscattering with changes in hematocrit, variation over the clinical range has little effect on the Doppler signal. Similarly, the size of red blood cells and the compressibility of blood cells and plasma do not change significantly. Thus the primary determinant of scattering is transducer frequency.

Scattering also occurs within tissues, such as the myocardium, from interference of backscattered signals from tissue interfaces smaller than the ultrasound wavelength. Tissue scattering results in a pattern of *speckles*; tissue motion can be measured by tracking these speckles from frame to frame, as discussed in Chapter 4.

Refraction

Ultrasound waves can be *refracted*—deflected from a straight path—as they pass through a medium with a different acoustic impedance. Refraction of an ultrasound beam is analogous to refraction of light waves as they pass through a curved glass lens (e.g., prescription eyeglasses). Refraction allows enhanced image quality by using acoustic "lenses" to focus the ultrasound beam. However, refraction also occurs in unplanned ways during image formation, with resulting ultrasound artifacts, most notably the "double-image" artifact.

Attenuation

Attenuation is the loss of signal strength as ultrasound interacts with tissue. As ultrasound penetrates into the body, signal strength is progressively *attenuated* because of absorption of the ultrasound energy by conversion to heat, as well as by reflection and scattering. The degree of attenuation is related to several factors, including the:

- Attenuation coefficient of the tissue
- Transducer frequency
- Distance from the transducer
- Ultrasound intensity (or power)

The attenuation coefficient (α) for each tissue is related the decrease in ultrasound intensity (measured in dB) from one point (I_1) to a second point (I_2) separated by a distance *(l)* as described by the equation:

$$I_2 = I_1 e^{-2\alpha l} \quad \text{(Eq. 1.5)}$$

The attenuation coefficient for air is very high (about 1000×) compared with soft tissue so that any air between the transducer and heart results in substantial signal attenuation. This is avoided on transthoracic examinations by use of a water-soluble gel to form an airless contact between the transducer and the skin; on transesophageal echocardiography (TEE) examination, attenuation is avoided by maintaining close contact between the transducer and esophageal wall. The air-filled lungs are avoided by careful patient positioning and the use of acoustic "windows" that allow access of the ultrasound beam to the cardiac structures without intervening lung tissue. Other intrathoracic air (e.g., pneumomediastinum, residual air after cardiac surgery) also results in poor ultrasound tissue penetration because of attenuation, resulting in suboptimal image quality.

The power output of the transducer is directly related to the overall degree of attenuation. However, an increase in power output causes thermal and mechanical bioeffects as discussed in "Bioeffects and Safety," p. 27.

Overall attenuation is frequency dependent such that lower ultrasound frequencies penetrate deeper into the body than higher frequencies. The depth of penetration for adequate imaging tends to be limited to approximately 200 wavelengths. This translates roughly into a penetration depth of 30 cm for a 1-MHz transducer, 6 cm for a 5-MHz transducer, and 1.5 cm for a 20-MHz transducer, although diagnostic images at depths greater than these postulated limits can be obtained with state-of-the-art equipment. Thus attenuation, as much as resolution, dictates the need for a particular transducer frequency in a specific clinical setting. For example, visualization of distal structures from the apical approach in a large adult patient often requires a low-frequency transducer. From a TEE approach, the same structures can be imaged (at better resolution) with a higher-frequency transducer. The effects of attenuation are minimized on displayed images by using different gain settings at each depth, an instrument control called time-gain (or depth-gain) compensation.

TRANSDUCERS

Piezoelectric Crystal

Ultrasound transducers use a piezoelectric crystal both to generate and to receive ultrasound waves (Fig. 1.5). A piezoelectric crystal is a material (e.g., quartz or a titanate ceramic) with the property that an applied electric current results in alignment of polarized

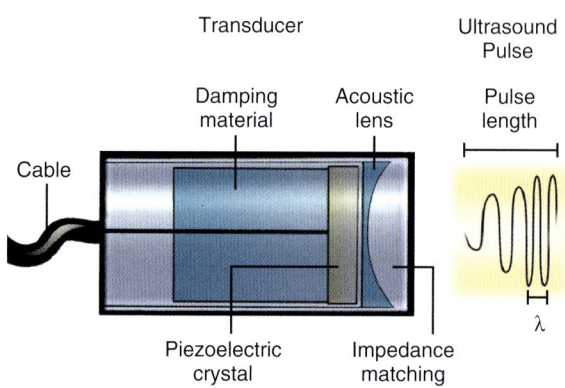

Fig. 1.5 Schematic diagram of an ultrasound transducer. The piezoelectric crystal both produces and receives ultrasound signals, with the electric input-output transmitted to the instrument via the cable. Damping material allows a short pulse length (improved resolution). The shape of the piezoelectric crystal, an acoustic lens, or electronic focusing (with a phased-array transducer) is used to modify beam geometry. The material of the transducer surface provides impedance matching with the skin. The ultrasound pulse length for 2D imaging is short (1–6 ms), typically consisting of two wavelengths (λ). "Ring down"—the decrease in frequency and amplitude in the pulse—depends on damping and determines bandwidth (the range of frequencies in the signal).

particles perpendicular to the face of the crystal with consequent expansion of crystal size. When an alternating electric current is applied, the crystal alternately compresses and expands, generating an ultrasound wave. The frequency that a transducer emits depends on the nature and thickness of the piezoelectric material.

Conversely, when an ultrasound wave strikes the piezoelectric crystal, an electric current is generated. Thus the crystal can serve both as a "receiver" and as a "transmitter." Basically, the ultrasound transducer transmits a brief burst of ultrasound and then switches to the "receive mode" to await the reflected ultrasound signals from the intracardiac acoustic interfaces. This cycle is repeated temporally and spatially to generate ultrasound images. Image formation is based on the *time delay* between ultrasound transmission and return of the reflected signal. Deeper structures have a longer time of flight than shallower structures, with the exact depth calculated based on the speed of sound in blood and the time interval between the transmitted burst of ultrasound and return of the reflected signal.

The burst, or pulse, of ultrasound generated by the piezoelectric crystal is very brief, typically 1 to 6 μs, because a short pulse length results in improved axial (along the length of the beam) resolution. Damping material is used to control the ring-down time of the crystal and hence the pulse length. Pulse length also is determined by frequency because a shorter time is needed for the same number of cycles at higher frequencies. The number of ultrasound pulses per second is called the *pulse repetition frequency*

(PRF). The total time interval from pulse to pulse is called the *cycle length*, with the percentage of the cycle length used for ultrasound transmission called the *duty factor*. Ultrasound imaging has a duty factor of about 1% compared with 5% for pulsed Doppler and 100% for continuous-wave (CW) Doppler. The duty factor is a key element in the patient's total ultrasound exposure.

The range of frequencies contained in the pulse is described as its *frequency bandwidth*. A wider bandwidth allows better axial resolution because of the ability of the system to produce a narrow pulse. Transducer bandwidth also affects the range of frequencies that can be detected by the system with a wider bandwidth, which allows better resolution of structures distant from the transducer. The stated frequency of a transducer represents the center frequency of the pulse.

Types of Transducers

The simplest type of ultrasound transducer is based on a single piezoelectric crystal (Table 1.3). Alternate pulsed transmission and reception periods allow repeated sampling along a single line, with the sampling rate limited only by the time delay needed for return of the reflected ultrasound wave from the depth of interest. An example of using the transducer for simple transmission and reception along a single line is an A-mode (amplitude vs. depth) or M-mode (depth vs. time) cardiac recording when a high sampling rate is desirable.

Formation of more complex images uses an array of ultrasound crystals arranged to provide a 2D tomographic or 3D volumetric data set of signals. Each element in the transducer array can be controlled electronically both to direct the ultrasound beam across the region of interest and to focus the transmitted and received signals. Echocardiographic imaging uses a *sector scanning* format with the ultrasound signal originating from a single location (the narrow end of the sector), thus resulting in a fanlike shape of the image. Sector scanning is optimal for cardiac applications because it allows a fast frame rate to show cardiac motion and a small transducer size (aperture or "footprint") to fit into the narrow acoustic windows used for echocardiography. 3D imaging transducers are discussed in Chapter 4.

Most transducers can provide simultaneous imaging and Doppler analysis, for example, 2D imaging and a superimposed color Doppler display. Quantitative Doppler velocity data are recorded with the image "frozen" or with only intermittent image updates, with the ultrasound crystals used to optimize the Doppler signal. Although CW Doppler signals can be obtained using two elements of combined transducer, use of a dedicated nonimaging transducer with two separate crystals (with one crystal continuously transmitting and the other continuously receiving ultrasound waves) is recommended when accurate high-velocity recordings are needed. The final configuration of a transducer depends on transducer frequency (higher-frequency transducers are smaller) and beam focusing, as well as the intended clinical use, for example, transthoracic versus TEE imaging.

Beam Shape and Focusing

An unfocused ultrasound beam is shaped like the light from a flashlight, with a tubular beam for a short distance that then diverges into a broad cone of light (Fig. 1.6). Even with current focused transducers, ultrasound beams have a 3D shape that affects measurement accuracy and contributes to imaging artifacts. Beam shape and size depend on several factors, including:

- Transducer frequency
- Distance from the transducer
- Aperture size and shape
- Beam focusing

Aperture size and shape and beam focusing can be manipulated in the design of the transducer, but the effects of frequency and depth are inherent to ultrasound physics. For an unfocused beam, the initial segment of the beam is columnar in shape (near-field F_n) with a length dependent on the diameter (D) of the transducer face and wavelength (λ):

$$F_n = D^2/4\lambda \qquad \text{(Eq. 1.6)}$$

For a 3.5-MHz transducer with a 5-mm diameter aperture, this corresponds to a columnar length of 1.4 cm. Beyond this region, the ultrasound beam diverges (far field), with the angle of divergence θ determined as:

$$\sin\theta = 1.22\lambda/D \qquad \text{(Eq. 1.7)}$$

This equation indicates a divergence angle of 6° beyond the near field, resulting in an ultrasound beam width of about 4.4 cm at a depth of 20 cm for this 3.5-MHz transducer. With a 10-mm diameter aperture, F_n would be 5.7 cm, and beam width at 20 cm would be about 2.5 cm (Fig. 1.7).

The shape and focal depth (narrowest point) of the primary beam can be altered by making the surface of the piezoelectric crystal concave or by the addition of an acoustic lens. This allows generation of a beam with optimal characteristics at the depth of most cardiac structures, but again, divergence of the beam beyond the focal zone occurs. Some transducers allow manipulation of the focal zone during the examination. Even with focusing, the ultrasound beam generated by each transducer has a lateral and an elevational dimension that depends on the transducer aperture, frequency, and focusing. Beam geometry for phased-array transducers also depends

TABLE 1.3 Ultrasound Transducers

	Definition	Examples	Clinical Implications
Type	Transducer characteristics and configuration. Most cardiac transducers use a phased array of piezoelectric crystals.	TTE (adult and pediatric) Nonimaging CW Doppler 3D echocardiography TEE Intracardiac	Each transducer type is optimized for a specific clinical application. More than one transducer may be needed for a full examination.
Transmission frequency	The central frequency emitted by the transducer	Transducer frequencies vary from 2.5 MHz for TTE to 20 MHz for intravascular imaging.	A higher-frequency transducer provides improved resolution but less penetration. Doppler signals are optimal at a lower transducer frequency than used for imaging.
Power output	The amount of ultrasound energy emitted by the transducer	An increase in transmitted power increases the amplitude of the reflected ultrasound signals.	Excessive power output may result in bioeffects measured by the mechanical and thermal indexes.
Bandwidth	The range of frequencies in the ultrasound pulse	Bandwidth is determined by transducer design.	A wider bandwidth allows improved axial resolution for structure distant from the transducer.
Pulse (or burst) length	The length of the transmitted ultrasound signal	A higher-frequency signal can be transmitted in a shorted pulse length compared with a lower-frequency signal.	A shorter pulse length improves axial resolution.
Pulse repetition frequency (PRF)	The number of transmission-receive cycles per second	The PRF decreases as imaging (or Doppler) depth increases because of the time needed for the signal to travel from and to the transducer.	Pulse repetition frequency affects image resolution and frame rate (particularly with color Doppler).
Duty factor	The percentage to time that ultrasound is transmitted	It ranges from ≈1% for 2D imaging, to 5% for pulsed Doppler, and 100% for CW Doppler.	A higher duty factor means more tissue exposure to ultrasound.
Focal depth	Beam shape and focusing are used to optimize ultrasound resolutions at a specific distance from the transducer	Structures close to the transducer are best visualized with a short focal depth, and distant structures are best visualized with a long focal depth.	The length and site of a transducer's focal zone are primarily determined by transducer design but are adjustable during the examination.
Aperture	The surface of the transducer face where ultrasound is transmitted and received	A small nonimaging CW Doppler transducer allows optimal positioning and angulation of the ultrasound beam.	A larger aperture allows a more focused beam A smaller aperture allows improved transducer angulation on TTE imaging.

on the size, spacing, and arrangement of the piezoelectric crystals in the array.

In addition to the main ultrasound beam, dispersion of ultrasound energy laterally from a single-crystal transducer results in formation of *side lobes* at an angle θ from the central beam where $\sin\theta = m\lambda/D$, and m is an integer describing sequential side lobes (i.e., 1, 2, 3, and so on) (Fig. 1.8). Reflected or backscattered signals from these side lobes are received by the transducer, resulting in image or flow artifacts. With phased-array transducers, additional accessory beams at an even greater angle from the primary beam, termed *grating lobes*, also occur as a result of constructive interference of ultrasound wave fronts. Both the side lobes and the grating lobes affect the lateral and elevational resolution of the transducer.

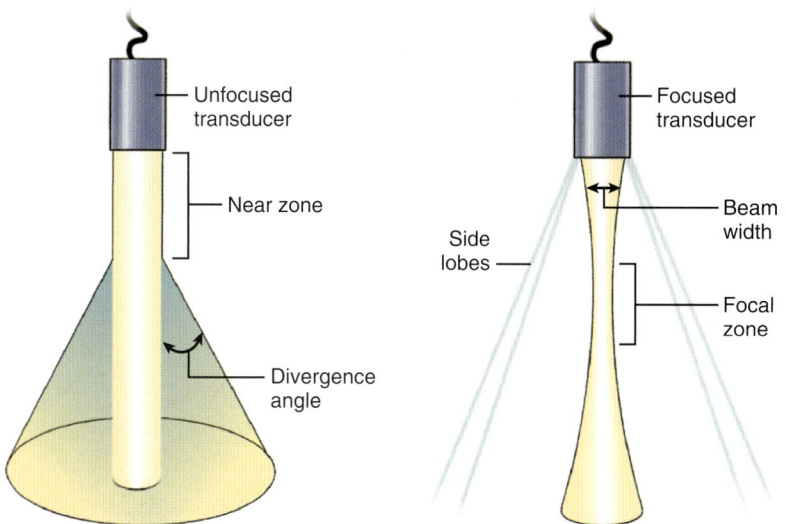

Fig. 1.6 Schematic diagram of beam geometry for an unfocused *(left)* and focused *(right)* transducer. The length of the near zone and the divergence angle in the far field depend on transducer frequency and aperture. The focal zone of a focused transducer can be adjusted, but beam width still depends on depth. Side lobes (and grating lobes with phased-array transducers) occur with both focused and unfocused transducers and, like the central beam, are 3D.

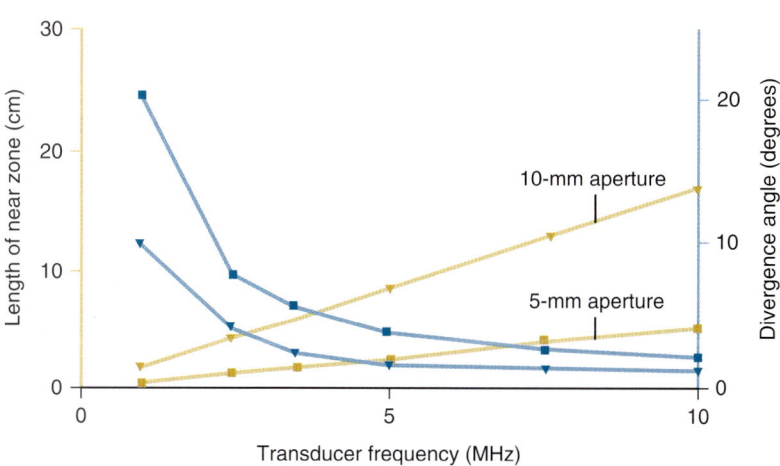

Fig. 1.7 Transducer frequency versus near zone length and divergence angle. Transducer frequency is shown on the horizontal axis with the length of the near zone shown in yellow and divergence angle in blue for unfocused 5-mm *(squares)* and 10-mm *(triangles)* diameter aperture transducers. Eqs. 1.6 and 1.7 were used to generate these curves.

Resolution

Image resolution occurs for each of three dimensions (Fig. 1.9):

- *Axial resolution* along the length of the ultrasound beam
- *Lateral resolution* side to side across the 2D image
- *Elevational resolution* or thickness of the tomographic slice

Of these three, axial resolution is most precise, so quantitative measurements are made most reliably using data derived from a perpendicular alignment between the ultrasound beam and structure of interest. Axial resolution depends on the transducer frequency, bandwidth, and pulse length but is independent of depth (Table 1.4). Determination of the smallest resolvable distance between two specular reflectors with ultrasound is complex but is typically about twice the transmitted wavelength; higher-frequency (shorter-wavelength) transducers have greater axial resolution. For example, with a 3.5-MHz transducer, axial resolution is about 1 mm, versus 0.5 mm with a 7.5-MHz transducer. A wider bandwidth also improves resolution by allowing a shorter pulse, thus avoiding overlap between the reflected ultrasound signals from two adjacent reflectors.

Lateral resolution varies with the depth of the specular reflector from the transducer, primarily related to beam width at each depth. In the focal region where beam width is narrow, lateral resolution approaches axial resolution, and a point target will appear as a point on the 2D image. At greater depths, beam width diverges so a point target results in a reflected signal as wide as the width of the beam and accounts for "blurring" of images in the far field. If the 2D image is examined carefully, progressive widening of the echo signals from similar targets along the length of the ultrasound beam can be appreciated (Fig. 1.10). Erroneous interpretations occur when the effects of beam width are not recognized. For example, beam width artifact from a strong

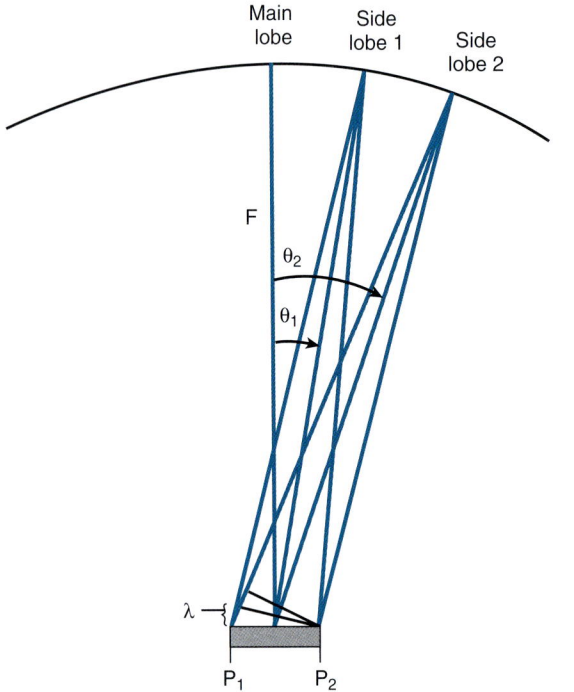

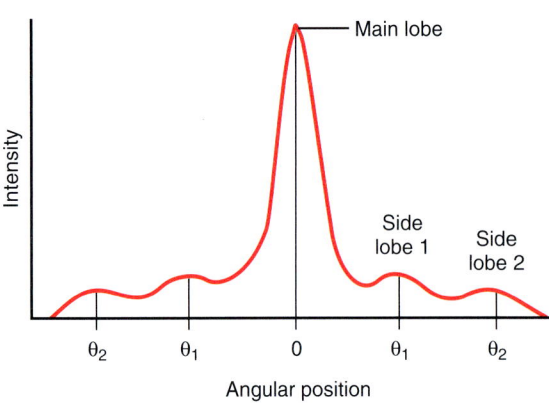

Fig. 1.8 Transducer beam side lobes. *(Top)* This diagram shows that side lobes occur at the points where the distances traversed by the ultrasound pulse from each edge of the crystal face differ by exactly one wavelength. The distance from the left edge of the crystal (P_1) to the position of side lobe 1 is exactly one wavelength (λ) longer than the distance from the extreme right edge of the crystal (P_2) to the position of side lobe 1. *(Bottom)* The beam intensity plot formed by sweeping along an arc at focal length F. *(From Geiser EA: Echocardiography: physics and instrumentation. In Skorton DJ, Schelbert AR, et al, editors:* Marcus Cardiac Imaging, *ed 2, Philadelphia, 1996, Saunders, p 280. Used with permission.)*

TABLE 1.4	Determinants of Resolution in Ultrasound Imaging
Axial Resolution	
Transducer frequency	
Transducer bandwidth	
Pulse length	
Lateral Resolution	
Transducer frequency	
Beam width (focusing) at each depth*	
Aperture (width) of transducer	
Bandwidth	
Side and grating lobe levels	
Elevational Resolution	
Transducer frequency	
Beam width in elevational plane	

*Most important.

depending on transducer design and focusing, both of which affect beam width in the elevational plane at each depth. In general, cardiac ultrasound images have a "thickness" of approximately 3 to 10 mm depending on depth and the specific transducer used. The tomographic image generated by the instrument, in effect, includes reflected and backscattered signals from this entire thickness. Strong reflectors adjacent to the image plane can appear to be "in" the image plane because of elevational beam width. Even more distant strong reflectors sometimes appear superimposed on the tomographic plane because of side lobes in the elevational plane. For example, a linear echo in the aortic lumen from an adjacent calcified atheroma may look like a dissection flap. These principles of ultrasound imaging also apply to 3D echocardiography.

ULTRASOUND IMAGING MODALITIES

M-Mode

Historically, cardiac ultrasound began with a single-crystal transducer display of the amplitude *(A)* of reflected ultrasound versus depth on an oscilloscope screen. This A-mode display used to be shown on the 2D image screen to aid the examiner in optimal adjustment of the instrument controls. Repeated pulse transmission-and-receive cycles allow rapid updating of the amplitude-versus-depth information so that rapidly moving structures, such as the aortic or mitral valve leaflets, can be identified by their characteristic timing and pattern of motion (Fig. 1.11).

With the time dimension shown explicitly on the horizontal axis and each amplitude signal along the length of the ultrasound beam converted to a corresponding gray-scale level, a *motion (M) mode display*

specular reflector often appears to be an abnormal linear structure. Other factors that affect lateral resolution are transducer frequency, aperture, bandwidth, and side and grating lobe levels.

Resolution in the elevational plane is more difficult to recognize on the 2D image but is equally important in clinical diagnosis. The thickness of the tomographic plane varies across the 2D image,

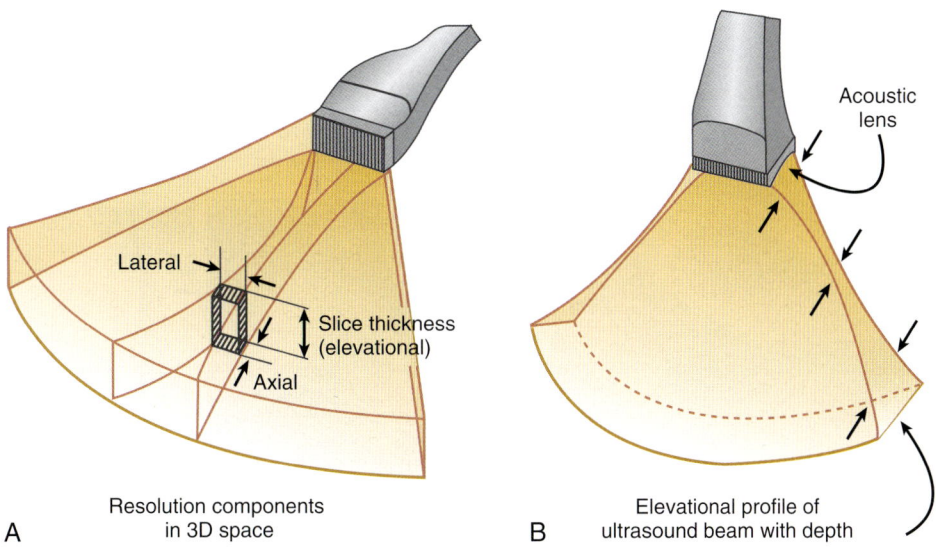

Fig. 1.9 Axial, lateral, and elevational slice thickness in 3D for a phased-array transducer ultrasound beam. (A) Axial resolution along the direction of the beam is independent of depth; lateral resolution and elevational resolution are strongly depth dependent. Lateral resolution is determined by transmit and receive focus electronics; elevational resolution is determined by the height of the transducer elements. At the focal distance, axial is better than lateral and is better than elevational resolution. (B) Elevational resolution profile with an acoustic lens across the transducer array produces a focal zone in the slice thickness direction. *(Adapted from Bushberg JT, Seibert JA, Leidholdt EH, et al:* The essential physics of medical imaging, *2 ed, Philadelphia, 2002, Lippincott Williams & Wilkins, Fig. 16.21).*

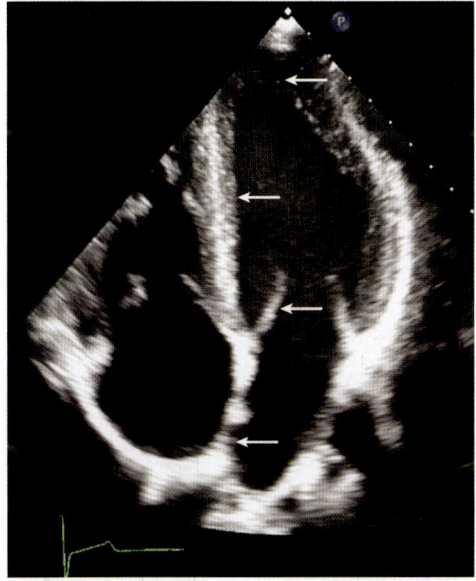

Fig. 1.10 ▶ **Beam width effect on 2D imaging.** 2D echocardiographic view of the LV from an apical approach. The effect of beam width can be appreciated by comparing the length of reflections from point targets near and at greater distances from the transducer as shown by the *arrows*.

Because only a single "line of sight" is included in an M-mode tracing, the PRF of the transmission-and-receive cycle is limited only by the time needed for the ultrasound beam to travel to the maximum depth of interest and back to the transducer. Even a depth of 20 cm requires only 0.26 ms (given a speed of propagation of 1540 m/s), thus allowing a PRF up to 3850 times/s. In actual practice, sampling rates of about 1800 times/s are used. This extremely high sampling rate is valuable for accurate evaluation of rapid normal intracardiac motion such as valve opening and closing. In addition, continuously moving structures, such as the ventricular endocardium, are identified more accurately when motion versus time, as well as depth, is displayed clearly on the M-mode recording. Other examples of rapid intracardiac motion best demonstrated with M-mode imaging include the high-frequency fluttering of the anterior mitral leaflet in patients with aortic regurgitation and the rapid oscillating motion of valvular vegetations.

Two-Dimensional Echocardiography

Image Production

A 2D echocardiographic image is generated from the data obtained by electronically "sweeping" the ultrasound beam across the tomographic plane. For each scan line, short pulses (or bursts of ultrasound) are emitted at a PRF determined by the time needed for ultrasound to travel to and from the maximum image depth. The pulse repetition period is the total time is produced. M-mode data are shown on the video monitor either "scrolling" or "sweeping" across the screen at 50 to 100 mm/s. The 2D imaging allows guidance of the M-mode beam to ensure an appropriate angle between the M line and the structures of interest.

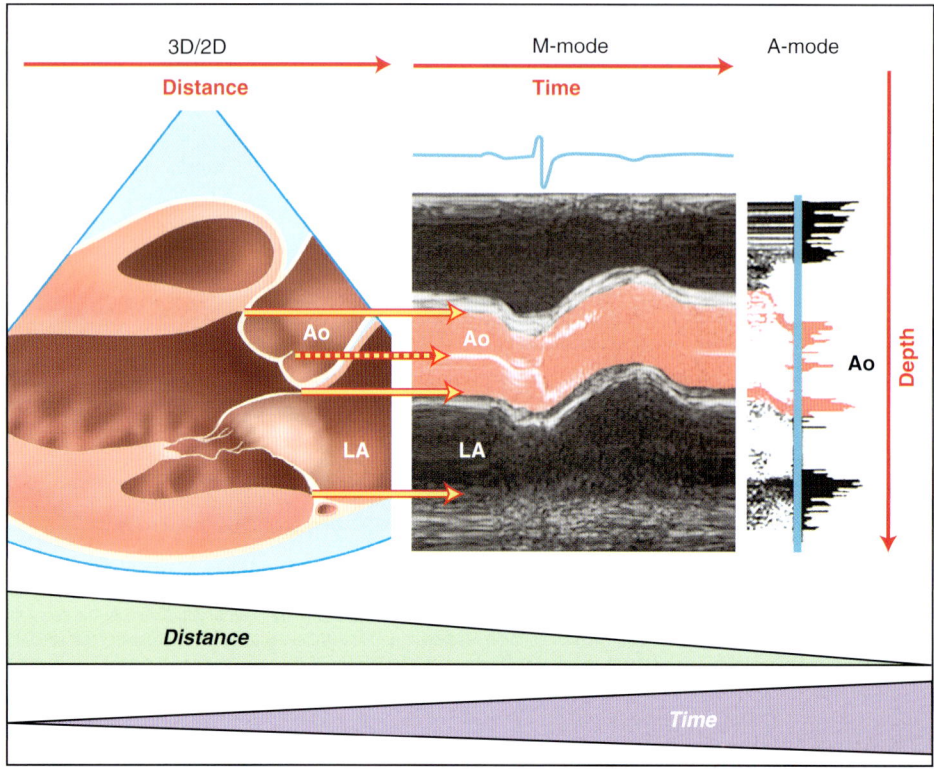

Fig. 1.11 3D, 2D, M-mode, and A-mode recordings of aortic valve motion. This illustration shows the following: the relationship between the 3D and 2D long-axis image of the aortic valve *(left)*, which shows distance in both the vertical and horizontal direction; M-mode recording of aortic root *(Ao)*, LA, and aortic valve motion, which shows depth-versus-time *(middle);* and A-mode recording *(right)*, which shows depth only (with motion seen on the video screen). Spatial relationships are best shown with 3D or 2D imaging, but temporal resolution is higher with M-mode and A-mode imaging.

from pulse to pulse, including the length of the ultrasound signal plus the time interval between signals.

Because a finite time is needed for each scan line of data (depending on the depth of interest), the time needed to acquire all the data for one image frame is directly related to the number of scan lines and the imaging depth. Thus PRF is lower at greater imaging depths and higher at shallow depths. In addition, a trade-off exists between scan line density and image frame rate (the number of images per second). For cardiac applications, a high frame rate (≥30 frames per second) is desirable for accurate display of cardiac motion. This frame rate allows 33 ms per frame or 128 scan lines per 2D image at a displayed depth of 20 cm.

The reflected ultrasound signals for each scan line are received by the piezoelectric crystal and a small electric signal generated with:

- Amplitude proportional to incident angle and acoustic impedance
- Timing proportional to distance from the transducer

This signal undergoes complex manipulation to form the final image displayed on the monitor. Typical processing includes signal amplification, time-gain compensation (TGC), filtering (to reduce noise), compression, and rectification. Envelope detection generates a bright spot for each signal along the scan line, which then undergoes analog-to-digital scan conversion because the original polar coordinate data must be fit to a rectangular matrix with appropriate interpolation for missing matrix elements. This image is subject to further "postprocessing" to enhance the visual appreciation of tomographic anatomy and is displayed in "real time" (nearly simultaneous with data acquisition) on the monitor screen.

Although standard ultrasound imaging is based on reflection of the fundamental transmitted frequency from tissue interfaces, *tissue harmonic imaging (THI)* instead is based on the harmonic frequency energy generated as the ultrasound signal propagates through the tissues. These harmonic frequencies result from the nonlinear effects of the interaction of ultrasound with tissue and with the key properties:

- Harmonic signal strength increases with depth of propagation.
- Harmonic frequencies are maximal at typical cardiac imaging depths.
- Stronger fundamental frequencies produce stronger harmonics.

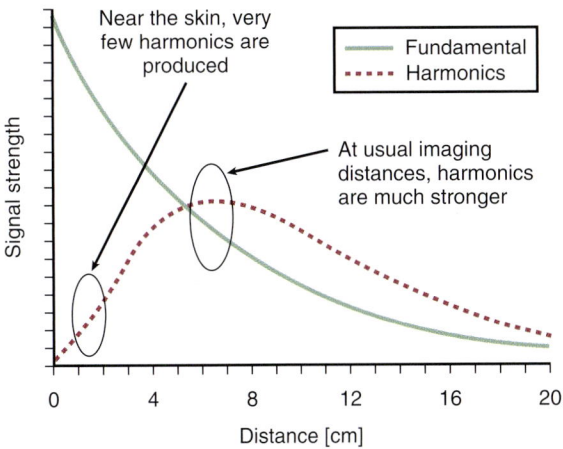

Fig. 1.12 Relation between imaging distance and strength of fundamental and harmonic frequencies. As ultrasound pulse propagates, strength of fundamental frequency declines while strength of harmonic frequency increases. At usual imaging distances for cardiac structures, strength of harmonic frequency is maximized. In this schematic, harmonic frequency strength is exaggerated; harmonic frequency signal strength is much lower than fundamental frequency signal strength. *(From Thomas JD, Rubin DN: Tissue harmonic imaging: why does it work? J Am Soc Echocardiogr 11:803–808, 1998.)*

Thus harmonic imaging reduces near-field and side-lobe artifacts and improves endocardial definition, particularly in patients with poor fundamental frequency images (Fig. 1.12). THI improves visualization of the left ventricular (LV) endocardium, which allows border tracing for calculation of ejection fraction, reduces measurement variability, and results in visualization of more myocardial segments during stress echocardiography. However, although THI improves lateral resolution by 20% to 50%, it reduces axial resolution by 40% to 100%. Valves and other planar objects therefore appear thicker with harmonic, compared with fundamental, frequency imaging, so that caution is needed when diagnosing valve abnormalities or making measurements of chamber or vessel size.

Instrument Settings

Many of the elements in the process of image formation are features of a particular transducer and instrument that cannot be modified by the operator. However, for each patient and echocardiographic view, optimal image quality depends on transducer selection and instrument settings. Standard imaging controls available in most ultrasound systems include:

- *Power output:* This control adjusts the total ultrasound energy delivered by the transducer in the transmitted bursts; higher power outputs result in higher-amplitude reflected signals.
- *Gain:* The control adjusts the displayed amplitude of the received signals, similar to the volume control in an audio system.
- *TGC:* This control allows differential adjustment of gain along the length of the ultrasound beam to compensate for the effects of attenuation. Near-field gain can be set lower (because reflected signals are stronger) with a gradually increased gain over the midfield ("ramp" or "slope") and a higher gain in the far field (because reflected signals are weaker). On some instruments, near-field gain and far-field gain beyond the range of the TGC are adjusted separately.
- *Depth:* Displayed depth affects the PRF and frame rate of the image and also allows maximal display of the area of interest on the screen. Standard depth settings show the entire plane (from the transducer down), whereas "resolution," "zoom," or "magnification" modes focus on a specific depth range of interest.
- *Dynamic range or compression:* The amplitude range (in dB) of the reflected signal is greater than the display capacity of ultrasound systems so the signal is compressed into a range of values from white to black, or gray scale. The number of levels of gray in the image, or *dynamic range*, can be adjusted to provide an image with marked contrast between light and dark areas or a gradation of gray levels between the lightest and darkest areas. A variation of standard gray scale is to use color intensity for each amplitude value.

Other typical instrument controls include preprocessing and postprocessing settings that change the appearance of the displayed image. Image quality and resolution also depend on scan-line density and other factors (see Table 1.4). Scan-line density (or frame rate or both) can be increased by using a lower depth setting or by narrowing the sector to less than the standard 60° wide image.

Imaging Artifacts

Imaging artifacts include (1) extraneous ultrasound signals that result in the appearance of "structures" that are not actually present (at least at that location), (2) failure to visualize structures that are present, and (3) an image of a structure that differs in size or shape or both from its actual appearance. Obviously, recognition of image artifacts is important for both the individual performing the study and the individual interpreting the echocardiographic data (Table 1.5).

The most common image "artifact" is *suboptimal image quality* resulting from poor ultrasound tissue penetration related to the patient's body habitus with interposition of high-attenuation tissues (e.g., lung or bone) or an increased distance (e.g., adipose tissue) between the transducer and cardiac structures. Although, strictly speaking, poor image quality is not

TABLE 1.5 Ultrasound Imaging Artifacts

Artifact	Mechanism	Example(s)
Suboptimal image quality	Poor ultrasound tissue penetration	Body habitus (obesity, lung disease) Postcardiac surgery status
Acoustic shadowing	Reflection of all the ultrasound signal by a strong specular reflector	Prosthetic valve Calcification
Reverberations	Reverberation between two strong parallel reflectors	Prosthetic valve
Beam width	Superimposition of structures within the beam profile (including side lobes) into a single tomographic image	Aortic valve "in" left atrium Atheroma "in" aortic lumen
Lateral resolution	Displayed width of a point target varies with depth	Excessive width of calcified mass or prosthetic valve
Refraction	Deviation of ultrasound signal from a straight path along the scan line	Double aortic valve or LV image in short-axis view
Range ambiguity	Echo from previous pulse reaches transducer on next cycle	Second, deeper, heart image
Electronic processing	Instrument specific	Variable

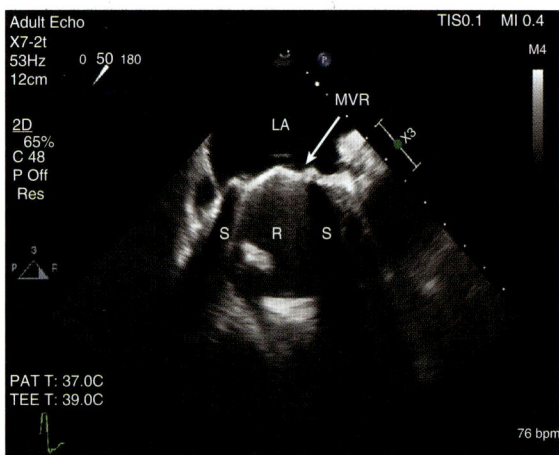

Fig. 1.13 ▶ **Example of acoustic shadowing and reverberations.** TEE view in a patient with a valve replacement *(MVR)* shows shadowing *(S)* by the sewing ring with reverberations *(R)* from the valve occluders further obscuring the ventricle.

an "artifact," a low signal-to-noise ratio makes accurate diagnosis difficult and precludes quantitative measurements. In many patients with suboptimal ultrasound penetration, image quality is improved by use of tissue harmonic imaging. In some cases, TEE imaging is needed to make an accurate diagnosis.

Acoustic shadowing (Fig. 1.13) occurs when a structure with a marked difference in acoustic impedance (e.g., prosthetic valve, calcium) blocks transmission of the ultrasound wave beyond that point. The image appears devoid of reflected signals distal to this structure because no signal penetrates beyond the shadowing structure. The shape of the shadow (like a light shadow) follows the ultrasound path, so a small structure near the transducer casts a large shadow. When shadowing occurs, an alternate acoustic window is needed for evaluation of the area of interest. In some cases, a different transthoracic view will suffice. In other cases (e.g., prosthetic mitral valve), TEE imaging is necessary.

Reverberations (Fig. 1.14) are multiple, linear, high-amplitude echo signals originating from two strong specular reflectors resulting in back-and-forth reflection of the ultrasound signal before it returns to the transducer. On the image, reverberations appear as relatively parallel, irregular, dense lines extending from the structure into the far field. Like acoustic shadowing, prominent reverberations limit evaluation of structures in the far field. In less dramatic cases, reverberations appear to represent abnormal structures. For example, in the parasternal long-axis view, a linear echo in the aortic root that originates as a reverberation from anterior structures (e.g., ribs) may be mistaken for a dissection flap.

The term *beam width artifact* is applied to two separate sources of image artifacts. First, remember that all the structures within the 3D volume of the ultrasound beam are displayed in a single tomographic plane. In the focal zone of the beam, the 3D volume is quite small, and the tomographic "slice" is narrow. In the far zone, however, strong reflectors at the edge of a larger beam are superimposed on structures in the central zone of the beam even though signal intensity falls off at the edges of the beam. In addition, strong reflectors in side lobes of the beam are displayed in the tomographic section corresponding to the main beam (Fig. 1.15).

Principles of Echocardiographic Image Acquisition and Doppler Analysis | Chapter 1

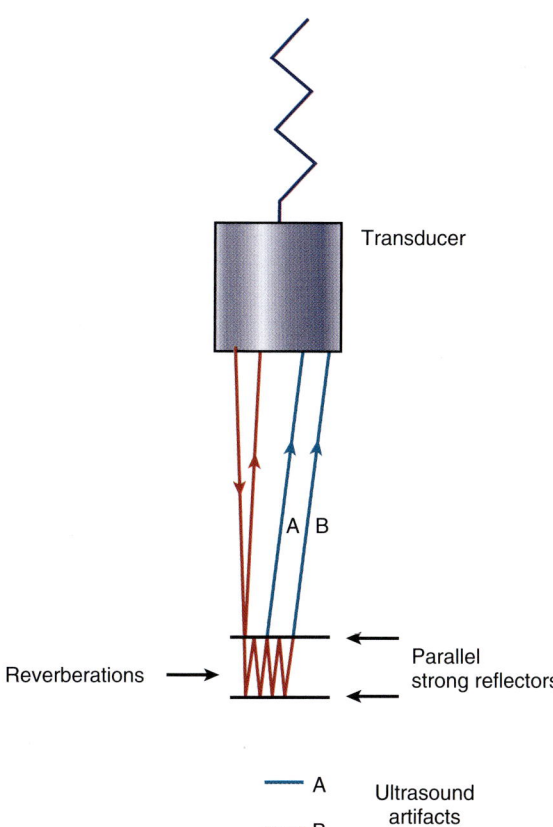

Fig. 1.14 Reverberation artifacts result from the interaction of ultrasound with two parallel strong reflectors. The transmitted ultrasound beam *(red with downward arrow)* is reflected from the first reflector and returns to the transducer *(red with upward arrow),* thus resulting in an ultrasound signal that corresponds to the correct depth of the reflector. However, ultrasound signals also reflect back and forth between the two strong reflectors, with some signals returning to the transducer after two *(A),* three *(B),* or more reverberation cycles. The longer time from transmission to reception of these late-returning signals results in their display on the ultrasound image at points distal to the actual reflector. In clinical imaging, reverberation artifacts can appear either as a single linear signal distal to the actual object or as a band of signals obscuring distal structures (see Fig. 1.13) because of multiple parallel reflectors.

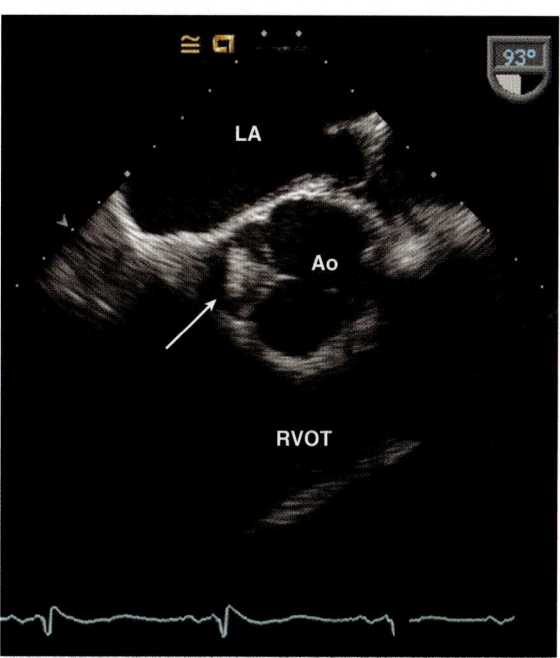

Fig. 1.15 Example of beam width artifact. Apparent "mass" *(arrow)* attached to the aortic valve on this off-axis TEE view is the noncoronary cusp of the aortic valve seen en face. Imaging in other planes demonstrated a normal trileaflet aortic valve. *Ao,* Aorta; *RVOT,* right ventricular outflow tract.

The second type of beam width artifact is a consequence of varying lateral resolution at different imaging depths. A point target appears as a line whose length depends on the beam characteristics at that depth and the amplitude of the reflected signal. For example, the struts on a prosthetic valve can appear much longer than their actual dimension because of poor lateral resolution. Sometimes beam width artifacts can be mistaken for abnormal structures such as a valvular vegetation, an intracardiac mass, or an aortic dissection flap.

The appearance of a side-by-side double image results from ultrasound *refraction* as it passes through a tissue proximal to the structure of interest. This artifact often is seen in parasternal short-axis views of the aortic valve or LV, where a second valve or LV is "seen" medial to and partly overlapping the actual valve or LV. The explanation for this appearance is that the transmitted ultrasound beam is deviated from a straight path (the scan line) by refraction as it passes through a tissue near the transducer. When this refracted beam is reflected back to the transducer by a tissue interface, the reflected signal is assumed to have originated from the scan line of the transmitted pulse (Fig. 1.16) and thus is displayed on the image in the wrong location.

Range ambiguity occurs when echo signals from an earlier pulse cycle reach the transducer on the next "listen cycle" for that scan line; as a result, deep structures appear closer to the transducer than their actual location. The appearance of an anatomically unexpected echo within a cardiac chamber often is due to range ambiguity, as can be demonstrated by the disappearance or a change in position of this artifact when the depth setting (and *PRF*) is changed. Another type of range ambiguity is the appearance of an apparent second heart, deeper than the actual heart—a double image on the vertical axis. This type of range ambiguity results from echoes being re-reflected by a structure close to the transducer (e.g., a rib), being re-reflected by the cardiac structures, and thus received at the transducer at a time *twice* normal. This artifact can be eliminated (or obscured) by decreasing the depth setting or adjusting the transducer position to a better acoustic window.

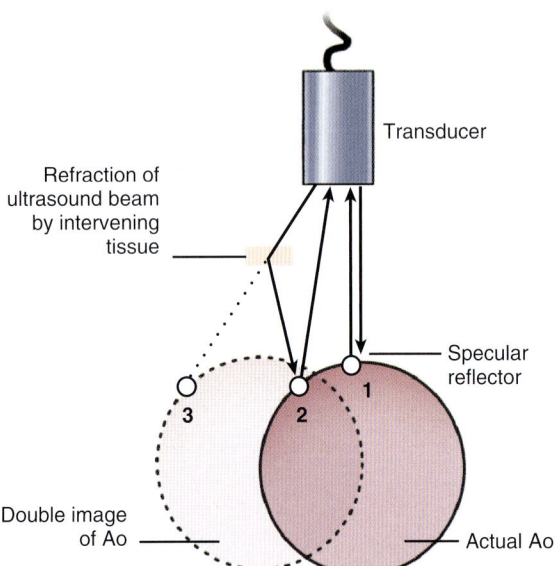

Fig. 1.16 Mechanism of a double-image artifact on 2D echocardiography. An ultrasound pulse reflected from *point 1* of the LV endocardium returns to the transducer and is shown appropriately as a bright spot in the correct position on the 2D image. Later in the scan, an ultrasound pulse is refracted by an intervening tissue so that the beam is reflected back to the transducer from *point 2*. However, this reflected signal is shown along the transmission scan line *(point 3)* because this is the presumed origin of the reflected signal. *Ao,* Aorta in cross section.

Electronic processing artifacts can be difficult to identify and vary from instrument to instrument. In addition, types of artifacts other than those listed have been described.

Three-Dimensional Echocardiography

Three-dimensional echocardiographic imaging is based on the same ultrasound principles used in 2D imaging with more complex acquisition of a volume of ultrasound data and more complex display options. (See Chapter 4 for details.) The physics of 3D imaging is very similar to that of 2D imaging, and issues such as beam width, resolution, and frame rate affect both approaches. The 3D echocardiographic displays currently used in clinical practice provide perspective-type anatomic images from different points of view, for example, a view of the left atrial (LA) side of the mitral valve. The same imaging artifacts seen on 2D images also can be seen with 3D imaging.

Echocardiographic Imaging Measurements

Echocardiographic measurements are most accurate using axial resolution (i.e., along the length of the ultrasound beam). Measurements can be made using the *leading edge–to–leading edge* convention or at the white-black interface between tissues. The rationale for measuring from the leading edge is that the first reflection detected from the tissue interface is the best measure of its actual location, with other signals arriving slightly later because of reflections from within the tissue, reverberations, and ring-down artifact. The leading edge convention is used for M-mode studies, and much of the literature validating echocardiographic measurements for clinical decision making is based on this measurement approach.

On 2D images, identification of the leading edge is challenging—for example, in a parasternal long-axis view, separating the leading edge of the LV septal endocardium from signals originating within the septal myocardium. Instead, 2D measurements of cardiac chambers and great vessels are made using the white-black interface; LV internal dimensions are measured from the white-black interface of the septum to the white-black interface of the posterior wall. With current image quality, the white-black interface is a reasonable representation of the actual tissue-blood interface because the leading edge of the endocardial echo and the white-black interface are nearly identical. For measurements of great vessels, such as the aorta, the white-black interface convention is more reproducible than attempts to identify a leading edge on 2D images. Measurement of small solid or planar structures is problematic, so direct measurements of valve thickness, for example, are not routine.

Quantitative measurements are problematic because the 3D data are viewed as a 2D image, so measurements are made on 2D images within the 3D dataset. Using this approach, 3D echocardiographic LV volumes are more accurate than those obtained by 2D imaging, as discussed in Chapter 4.

DOPPLER ECHOCARDIOGRAPHY

Doppler Velocity Data
Doppler Equation

Doppler echocardiography is based on the change in frequency of the backscattered signal from small moving structures (e.g., red blood cells) intercepted by the ultrasound beam (Table 1.6). A visual analogy is that Doppler scattering from blood is similar to scattering of light in fog, whereas imaging is similar to reflections from a mirror. A stationary target, if much smaller than the wavelength, will scatter ultrasound in all directions, with the frequency of the scattered signal being the same as the transmitted frequency when observed from any direction. A moving target, however, will backscatter ultrasound to the transducer so that the frequency observed when the target is moving *toward* the transducer is higher and the frequency observed when the target is moving *away* from the transducer is lower than the original transmitted frequency (Fig. 1.17). This Doppler effect

TABLE 1.6 Doppler Physics

	Definition	Examples	Clinical Implications
Doppler effect	The change in frequency of ultrasound scattered from a moving target: $v = c \times \Delta F / [2 F_T (\cos \theta)]$	A higher velocity corresponds to a higher Doppler frequency shift, ranging from 1 to 20 kHz for intracardiac flow velocities.	Ultrasound systems display velocity, which is calculated using the Doppler equation, based on transducer frequency and the Doppler shift, assuming cos θ equals 1.
Intercept angle	The angle (θ) between the direction of blood flow and the ultrasound beam	When the ultrasound beam is parallel to the direction of blood flow (0° or 180°), cos θ is 1 and can be ignored in the Doppler equation.	Velocity is underestimated when the intercept angle is not parallel; this can lead to errors in hemodynamic measurements.
CW Doppler	Continuous ultrasound transmission with reception of Doppler signals from the entire length of the ultrasound beam	CW Doppler allows measurements of high-velocity signals but does not localize the depth of origin of the signal.	CW Doppler is used to measure high velocities in valve stenosis and regurgitation.
Pulsed Doppler	Pulsed ultrasound transmission with timing of reception determining depth of the backscattered signal	Pulsed Doppler samples velocities from a specific site but can measure velocity only over a limited range.	Pulsed Doppler is used to record low velocity signals at a specific site, such as LV outflow velocity or LV inflow velocity.
Pulse repetition frequency (PRF)	The number of pulsed transmitted per second	The PRF is limited by the time needed for ultrasound to reach and return from the depth of interest. PRF determines the maximum velocity that can be unambiguously measured.	The maximum velocity measurable with pulsed Doppler is ≈1 m/s at 6 cm depth.
Nyquist limit	The maximum frequency shift (or velocity) measurable with pulsed Doppler equal to ½ PRF	The Nyquist limit is displayed as the top and bottom of the velocity range with the baseline centered.	The greater the depth, the lower the maximum velocity measurable with pulsed Doppler.
Signal aliasing	The phenomenon that the direction of flow for frequency shifts greater than the Nyquist limit cannot be determined	With aliasing of the LV outflow signal, the peak of the velocity curve is "cut off" and appears as flow in the opposite direction.	Aliasing can result in inaccurate velocity measurements, if not recognized.
Sample volume	The intracardiac location where the pulsed Doppler signal originated	Sample volume depth is determined by the time interval between transmission and reception. Sample volume length is determined by the duration of the receive cycle	Sample volume depth and length are adjusted to record the flow of interest.
Spectral analysis	Method used to display Doppler velocity data versus time, with gray scale indicating amplitude	Spectral analysis is used for both pulsed and CW Doppler.	The velocity scale, baseline position, and time scale of the spectral display are adjusted for each Doppler velocity signal.

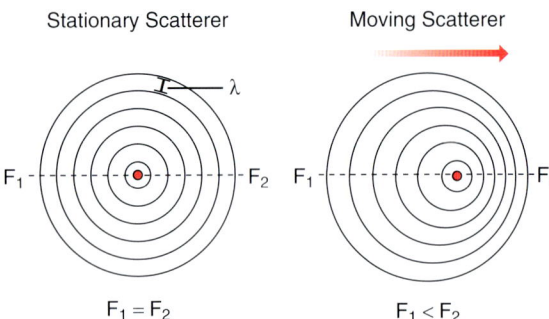

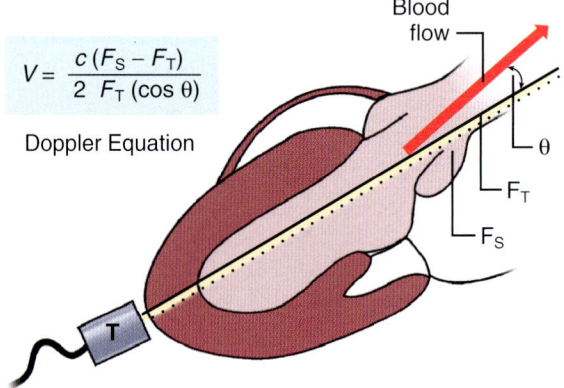

Fig. 1.17 The Doppler effect. *(Left)* A stationary scatterer scatters ultrasound symmetrically in all directions with a wavelength identical to the transmitted wavelength and with the same frequency in all directions (no Doppler shift). *(Right)* A moving scatterer also scatters ultrasound symmetrically in all directions. However, the frequency will be higher when the scatterer is moving toward the transducer (F_2) than when it is moving away from the transducer (F_1) because of the movement of the scatterer resulting in waves closer together in advance of and farther apart behind the moving object.

Fig. 1.18 The Doppler equation. The velocity V of blood flow can be calculated from the speed of sound in blood c, transducer frequency F_T, backscattered frequency F_S, and the cosine of the angle θ between the ultrasound beam and direction of blood flow. T, Transducer.

is known to all of us from audio examples of the change in sound of a car horn, siren, or train whistle as it moves toward (higher pitch) and then away (lower pitch) from the observer.

The difference in frequency between the transmitted frequency (F_T) and the scattered signal received back at the transducer (F_s) is the Doppler shift:

$$\text{Doppler shift} = (F_s - F_T) \quad \text{(Eq. 1.8)}$$

Doppler shifts are in the audible range (0–20 kHz) for intracardiac velocities using diagnostic ultrasound transducer frequencies. The relationship between the Doppler shift and blood flow velocity (v, in m/s) is expressed in the Doppler equation:

$$v = c\,(F_s - F_T)/[2\,F_T(\cos\theta)] \quad \text{(Eq. 1.9)}$$

where c is the speed of sound in blood (1540 m/s), θ is the intercept angle between the ultrasound beam and the direction of blood flow, and 2 is a factor to correct for the transit time both *to* and *from* the scattering source (Fig. 1.18).

Note that the intercept angle is critically important in calculation of blood flow velocity. The cosine of an angle of 0° or 180° (parallel toward or away from the transducer) is 1, allowing this term to be ignored when the ultrasound beam is aligned parallel to the direction of blood flow. In contrast, the cosine of 90° is *zero*, indicating that no Doppler shift will be recorded if the ultrasound beam is perpendicular to blood flow.

In cardiac Doppler applications, the ultrasound beam is aligned as close as possible to parallel with the direction of blood flow so that the $\cos\theta$ can be assumed to be 1. Because the direction of intracardiac blood flow can be difficult to ascertain and is not predictable from the 2D image, especially with abnormal flow patterns, attempts to "correct" for intercept angle usually result in significant errors in velocity calculation. Even when blood flow direction is apparent in a 2D plane, direction in the elevational plane remains unknown. Deviation up to 20° from a parallel intercept angle results a calculated velocity only 6% less than the actual blood flow velocity. However, a 60° intercept angle results in a calculated velocity that is only one-half the actual velocity. The importance of the intercept angle is particularly underlined in the setting of abnormal blood flow with high-velocity jets, such as in valvular stenosis. Although angle correction for the presumed direction of blood flow is used in some peripheral vascular applications, this approach is not acceptable for cardiac applications because of the likelihood that the "correction" will be erroneous.

Spectral Analysis

When the backscattered signal is received at the transducer, the difference between the transmitted and backscattered signals is determined by "comparing" the two waveforms. This is a complex process because multiple frequencies are present in the backscattered signal. Typically, the frequency content of the signal is analyzed by a process known as a *fast Fourier transform* (FFT) that derives the component frequencies of a complex signal. Alternate methods of frequency analysis include the analog Chirp-Z method.

The display generated by this frequency analysis is termed *spectral analysis* (Fig. 1.19). By convention, this display shows time on the horizontal axis, the zero baseline in the center, and frequency shifts toward the transducer above and frequency shifts away from the transducer below the baseline. Because multiple frequencies exist at any time point, each frequency signal is displayed as a pixel on the vertical axis, with the gray scale indicating the amplitude (or loudness) and the position on the vertical axis

Each of these components is displayed at 4-ms intervals (or 250 times/s) simultaneous with data acquisition.

Continuous-Wave Doppler Ultrasound

CW Doppler uses two ultrasound crystals; one continuously transmits and one continuously receives the ultrasound signal. The major advantage of CW Doppler is that very high-frequency shifts (velocities) can be measured accurately because sampling is continuous. The potential disadvantage of CW Doppler is that signals from the entire length of the ultrasound beam are recorded simultaneously. However, even with overlap of flow data, a given signal often is characteristic in timing, shape, and direction, thus allowing correct identification of the origin of the signal. In some cases, other methods (e.g., 2D, color, pulsed Doppler) must be used to determine the depth of origin of the Doppler signal.

CW Doppler optimally is performed with a dedicated, nonimaging transducer with two crystals. This type of transducer has a high signal-to-noise ratio and a small footprint, allowing it to fit into small acoustic windows (e.g., between ribs) and to be angled to obtain a parallel intercept angle between the ultrasound beam and the direction of blood flow. Use of a simultaneous imaging transducer is helpful in some cases, but signal quality is poorer, angulation is more difficult, and the 2D image distracts the operator from optimizing the *flow* signal instead of the anatomic image (which often do not coincide).

Careful technique yields a Doppler spectral signal that has a smooth contour with a well-defined edge and maximum velocity, as well as with clearly defined onset and end of flow. The audible signal is tonal and smooth. A CW Doppler velocity curve is "filled in" because lower-velocity signals proximal and distal to the point of maximum velocity also are recorded. Although the maximum frequency shift depends on the intercept angle between the Doppler beam and the flow of interest, amplitude (gray-scale intensity), shape, and audible quality are less dependent on intercept angle. Thus a "good-quality" Doppler signal recorded at a nonparallel intercept angle results in underestimation of flow velocity. The empirical method to ensure a parallel intercept angle is to examine the flow of interest from multiple windows with transducer angulation both in the plane of view and in the elevational plane to discover the highest-frequency shift. The highest value found is then assumed to represent a parallel intercept angle.

Pulsed-Wave Doppler Ultrasound

Pulsed Doppler echocardiography allows sampling of blood flow velocities from a specific intracardiac depth. A pulse of ultrasound is transmitted, and then, after

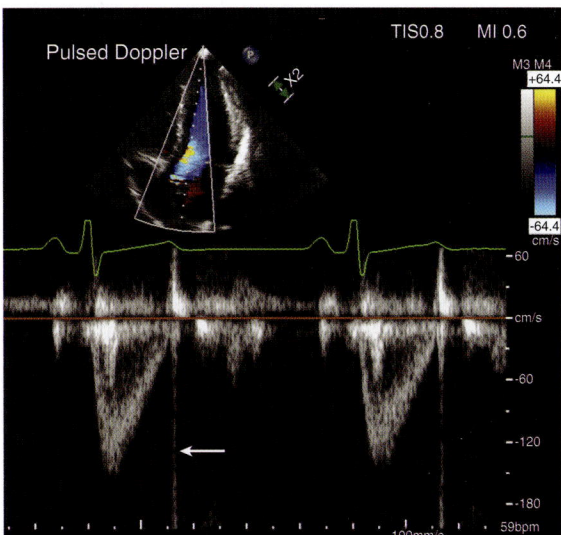
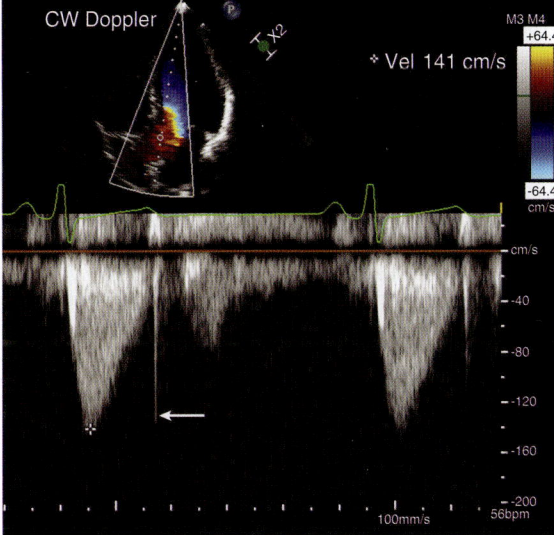

Fig. 1.19 Examples of *(top)* **pulsed and** *(bottom)* **CW spectral Doppler displays.** LV outflow recorded from an apical approach is shown in the standard format. The baseline has been moved from the middle of the vertical axis to display the antegrade flow signal. Velocities *(Vel)* toward the transducer are shown above and velocities away from the transducer below the baseline. The velocity range is determined by the Nyquist limit (½ pulse-repetition frequency) with pulsed Doppler echocardiography. Velocities are shown in shades of gray corresponding to the amplitude (dB) of the signal. Note the "envelope" of flow with pulsed Doppler because flow is sampled at a specific intracardiac location with relatively uniform blood flow velocities. With CW Doppler, the curve is "filled in" due to multiple blood flow velocities along the entire length of the ultrasound beam. *Arrows* indicate aortic valve closing click.

indicating the blood flow velocity (or frequency shift) component. Thus, each time point on the spectral display shows:

- Blood flow direction
- Velocity (or frequency shift)
- Signal amplitude

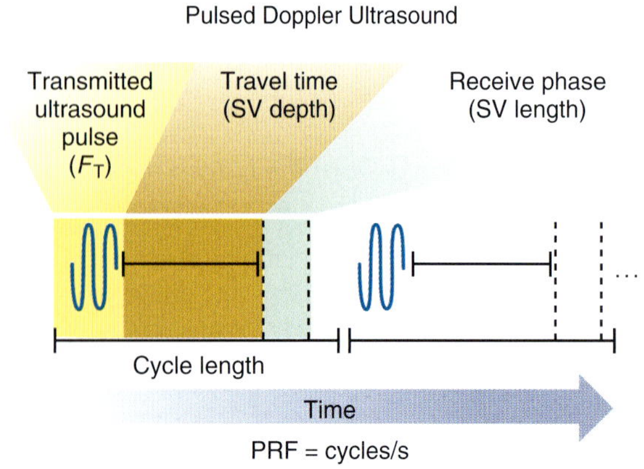

Fig. 1.20 Pulsed Doppler ultrasound. The pulsed Doppler transducer goes through a repetitive cycle of transmission of an ultrasound pulse at the transducer frequency (F_T), a waiting period determined by the time needed for the signal to travel to and from the depth of interest, and a receive phase when the backscattered signals are sampled. The travel-time duration determines sample volume *(SV)* depth. The duration of the receive phase determines sample volume. *PFR,* Pulse-repetition frequency.

a time interval determined by the depth of interest, the transducer briefly "samples" the backscattered signals. This transducer cycle of transmit-wait-receive is repeated at an interval termed the *pulse repetition frequency* (Fig. 1.20). Because the "wait" interval is determined by the depth of interest—the time it takes ultrasound to travel to and from this depth—each transducer cycle is longer for increasing depths. Thus the PRF also is depth dependent, being high at shallow depths and low for more distant sites.

The pulsed Doppler depth of interest is called the *sample volume* because signals from a small volume of blood are sampled, with the width and height of this volume dependent on beam geometry. The length of the sample volume can be varied by adjusting the length of the transducer "receive" interval. Typically, a sample volume length of 3 mm is used to balance range resolution and signal quality, but a longer (5–10 mm) or shorter (1–2 mm) sample volume is useful in specific cases.

Because pulsed Doppler echocardiography repeatedly samples the returning signal, a maximum limit to the frequency shift (or velocity) can be measured unambiguously. A waveform must be sampled at least twice in each cycle for accurate determination of wavelength. This phenomenon of ambiguity in the speed, direction, or speed and direction of the sampled signal is known as *signal aliasing* (Fig. 1.21). For the frequency of an ultrasound waveform to be correctly identified, it must be sampled at least twice per wavelength. Thus the maximum detectable frequency shift (the *Nyquist limit*) is one-half the PRF.

If the velocity of interest exceeds the Nyquist limit by a small degree, signal aliasing is seen with the signal cut off at the edge of the display and the "top" of the waveform appearing in the reverse channel

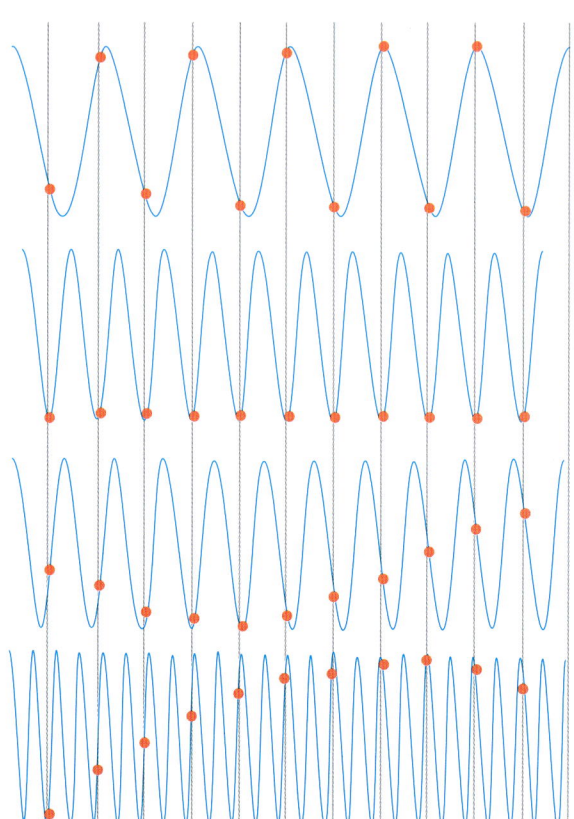

Fig. 1.21 Principle of signal aliasing. This schematic diagram shows how sampling at a constant interval (shown by vertical gray lines with a red dot where the waveform is sampled) results in ambiguity in the measured sound wave frequency. Sampling at twice the frequency of the wavelength, as shown at the top, correctly measures the sound wave frequency. As the sound wave frequency increases from top to bottom, intermittent sampling results in apparent frequencies that are lower and in the opposite direction of the actual sound waveform.

(Fig. 1.22). In these cases, baseline shift (in effect, an electronic "cut and paste") restores the expected velocity curve and allows calculation of maximum velocity. When velocities further exceed the Nyquist limit, repeat "wraparound" of the signal occurs first into the reverse channel, then back to the forward channel, and so on. Occasionally, the shape of the waveform can be discerned, but more often only an undifferentiated band of velocity signals can be appreciated. Both nonlaminar disturbed flow and aliased laminar high-velocity flow appear (and sound) similar on spectral analysis. Methods that can be used to resolve aliasing include:

- Using CW Doppler ultrasound
- Increasing the PRF to the maximum for that depth (the Nyquist limit)
- Increasing the number of sample volumes (high-PRF Doppler)
- Using a lower-frequency transducer
- Shifting the baseline to the edge of the display

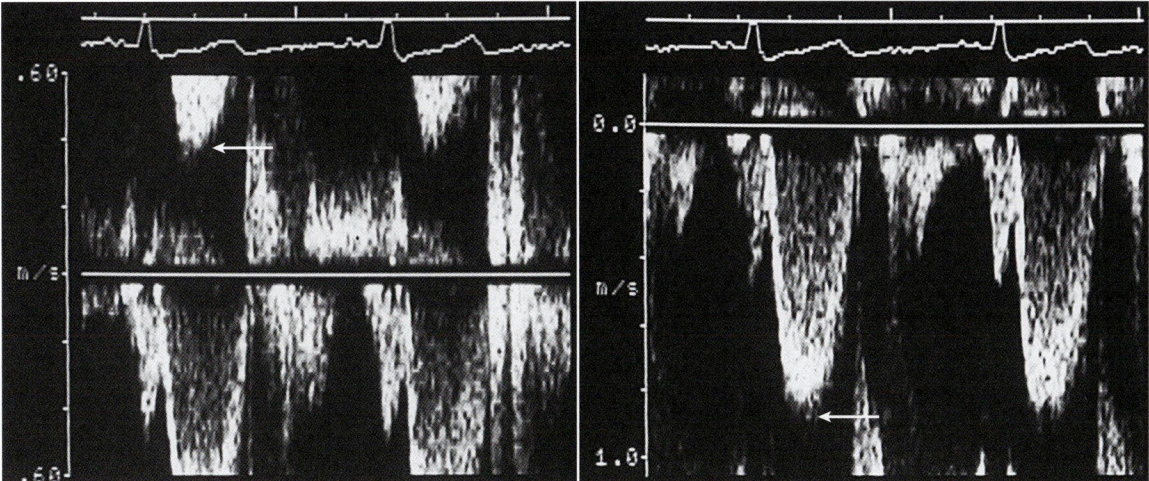

Fig. 1.22 Pulsed Doppler signal aliasing. The velocity of LV outflow recorded from an apical approach exceeds the Nyquist limit so that aliasing occurs *(left)* with the appearance of the peak of the outflow curve in the reverse channel *(arrow)*. This degree of aliasing can be resolved by shifting the baseline *(right)*, in effect an electronic "cut and paste" of the spectral display.

CW Doppler is the most reliable approach to resolving aliasing for very high velocities. The other approaches are useful when the aliased velocity exceeds the Nyquist limit by a modest degree (e.g., up to twice the Nyquist limit).

High-PRF Doppler is the deliberate use of range ambiguity to increase the maximum velocity that can be measured with pulsed Doppler echocardiography (Fig. 1.23). When the transducer sends out a pulse, backscattered signals from the entire length of the ultrasound beam return to the transducer. Range resolution is achieved by sampling only those signals in the short time interval corresponding to the depth of interest. However, signals from exactly twice as far away as the sample volume will reach the transducer during the "receive" phase of the next cycle. Thus signals from "harmonics" at 2×, 3×, 4×, and so on from the sample volume depth have the potential of being analyzed. Usually signal strength is low, and few moving scatterers are present at these depths, so this range ambiguity can be ignored. If, instead, the sample volume is placed purposely at one-half the depth of interest, backscattered signals from this sample volume (SV_1) and a second sample volume (SV_2) twice as far away (i.e., the depth of interest) will return to the transducer during the "receive" phase (albeit one cycle later). This recording of the signal of interest at a higher PRF allows measurement of higher velocities without signal aliasing (Fig. 1.24). An even higher PRF can be achieved by using additional (three or four) proximal sample volumes. Of course, the limitation of this approach is range ambiguity. The spectral analysis now includes signals from each of the sample volume depths and, as with CW Doppler, the origin of the signal of interest must be determined based on ancillary data. However, high-PRF Doppler is useful for evaluation of

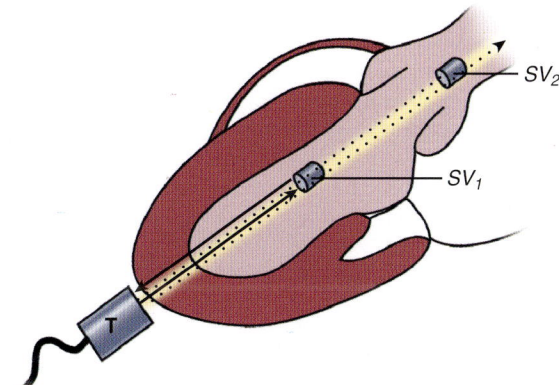

Fig. 1.23 High–pulserepetition frequency Doppler ultrasound. This technique is based on the concept that with a given sample volume depth (SV_1), some ultrasound will penetrate beyond that depth. Backscattered signals from exactly twice the set depth (SV_2) will return to the transducer (T) during the receive phase of the next cycle. Thus signals from both sample volume depths are recorded simultaneously.

velocities just above the aliasing limit of conventional pulsed Doppler. Often, the high PRF mode is automatically enabled when the Doppler velocity range is increased.

Doppler Velocity Instrument Controls

Pulsed and CW Doppler instrument controls typically include:

- Power output—adjusts the amount of electrical energy transmitted to the transducer
- Receiver gain—changes the degree of amplification of returning signals
- "Wall" or high-pass filters—eliminate low-frequency Doppler shifts that result from motion

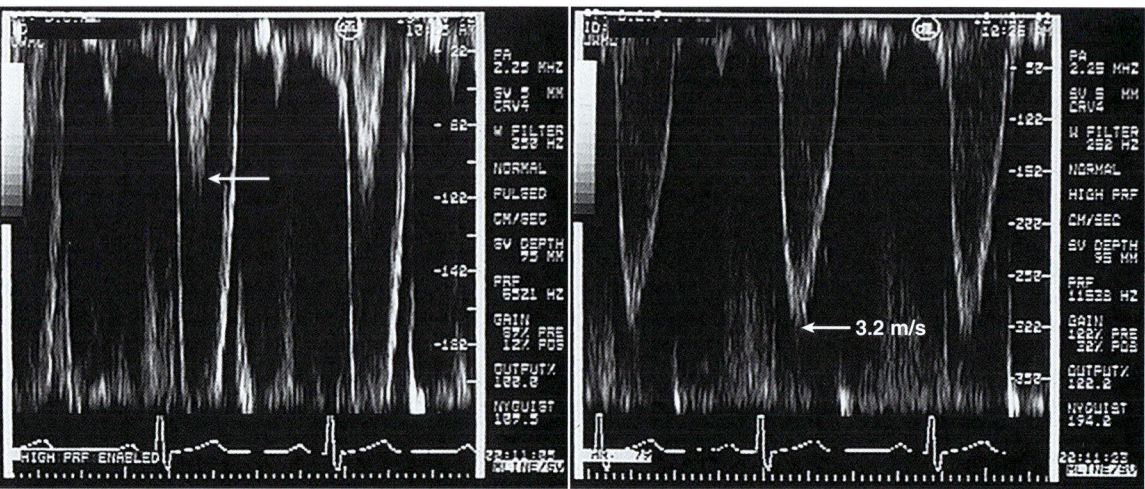

Fig. 1.24 Example of high–pulse repetition frequency Doppler. In this case, LV outflow velocity exceeds twice the Nyquist limit so that aliasing persists even after baseline shift *(left)*. The "wrapped around" peak velocity is clearly seen *(arrow)*. With this Doppler technique, the maximum velocity is resolved in this patient with a subaortic membrane *(right)*.

of myocardium and valves (allowing only the higher frequencies to pass the filter)
- Baseline shift—moves the zero line toward the top or bottom of the display
- Velocity range—increases or decreases the scale (within the limits for each Doppler modality)
- Dynamic range—compresses the signal amplitude into shades of gray

In addition, pulsed Doppler controls include:

- Sample volume depth
- Sample volume length
- The number of sample volumes (high-PRF Doppler echocardiography)

Each of the three major Doppler modalities may be integrated with 2D imaging. However, although color Doppler flow imaging is nearly always conjoined with 2D imaging, pulsed Doppler signal quality is optimized when the 2D image is "frozen," and CW Doppler is optimized using a dedicated, small-footprint transducer with no 2D imaging.

Doppler Velocity Data Artifacts

Many Doppler artifacts are related to ultrasound physics and beam geometry, analogous to those seen with 2D imaging. Others are specific to Doppler echocardiography (Table 1.7).

Clinically, the most important potential artifact is *velocity underestimation* resulting from a nonparallel intercept angle between the ultrasound beam and the direction of blood flow (Fig. 1.25). Velocity underestimation can occur with either pulsed or CW Doppler techniques and is of most concern when measuring high-velocity jets due to valve stenosis, regurgitation, or other intracardiac abnormalities.

TABLE 1.7	Doppler Ultrasound Artifacts
Artifact	**Result**
Nonparallel intercept angle	Underestimation of velocity
Aliasing	Inability to measure maximum velocity
Range ambiguity	Recording of Doppler signals from more than one depth along the ultrasound beam
Beam width	Overlap of Doppler signals from adjacent flows
Mirror image	Spectral display showing unidirectional flow both above and below the baseline
Electronic interference	Band-like interference signal obscuring Doppler flow
Transit-time effect	Change in the velocity of the ultrasound wave as it passes through a moving media resulting in slight overestimation of Doppler shifts

With pulsed Doppler echocardiography, *signal aliasing* limits the maximum measurable velocity. If the examiner recognizes that aliasing has occurred, appropriate steps can be taken to resolve the velocity data if needed. Aliasing can be due to nonlaminar disturbed flow, as well as high-velocity laminar flow.

Range ambiguity is inherent to CW Doppler but can occur with pulsed Doppler as well. With a sample volume positioned close to the transducer, strong signals from twice (or three times) the depth of the sample volume will be received in the next "receive"

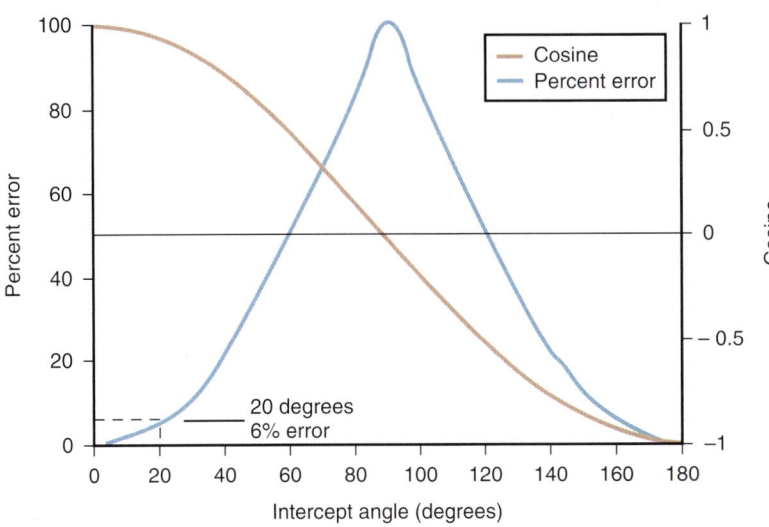

Fig. 1.25 **Effect of intercept angle on velocity calculations.** The importance of a parallel intercept angle between the ultrasound beam and direction of blood flow is shown. The cosine function versus intercept angle (horizontal axis) varies from 1 at a parallel angle (0° and 180°) to 0 at a perpendicular angle (90°). The error with a nonparallel intercept angle varies from only 6% at a 20° angle to 50% at a 60° angle. At a perpendicular (90°) intercept angle, no blood flow velocities are recorded.

phase and may be misinterpreted as originating from the set sample volume depth. For example, in an apical four-chamber view, placement of a sample volume in the LV apex at one-half the distance to the mitral annulus results in a spectral display showing the inflow signal across the mitral valve from the "second" sample volume depth. This phenomenon of range ambiguity is used constructively in the high-PRF Doppler mode.

Beam width (and side or grating lobes) affects the Doppler signal, as occurs with 2D imaging, and results in superimposition of spatially adjacent flow signals on the spectral display. For example, LV outflow and inflow often are seen on the same recording, especially with CW Doppler. Similarly, the LV inflow signal can be superimposed on the aortic regurgitant jet (Fig. 1.26).

A *mirror-image artifact* is common with spectral analysis, appearing as a symmetric signal of somewhat less intensity than the actual flow signal in the opposite flow direction (Fig. 1.27). Mirroring often can be reduced or eliminated by decreasing the power output or gain of the instrument. Interrogation of a flow signal from a near-perpendicular angle also can result in flow signals on both sides of the baseline.

Electronic interference appears as a band of signals across the spectral display that partially obscure the flow signals. These artifacts are the result of inadequate shielding of other electric instruments in the examination environment and are particularly common during studies in the intensive care unit, interventional procedure areas, or operating room.

The *transit time effect* is the change in propagation speed that occurs as an ultrasound wave passes through a moving medium, such as blood. This phenomenon is separate from the Doppler effect (which affects the backscattered signal) and is the basis of volume flow measurement with a transit-time flow probe. On the

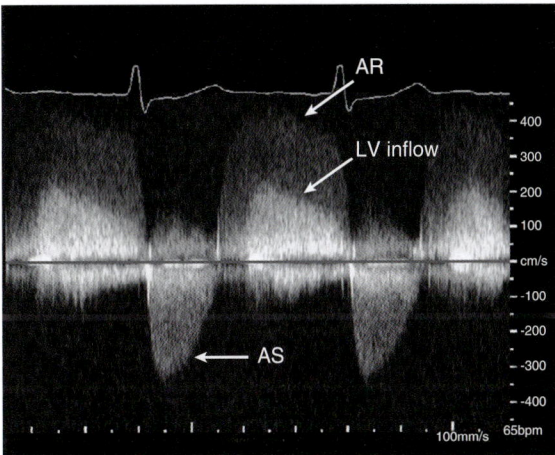

Fig. 1.26 **Doppler beam width artifact.** This CW Doppler recording from an apical window shows superimposed signals of aortic regurgitation (AR) and LV inflow in diastole because the width of the ultrasound beam encompasses both flows. Bright lines caused by motion of prosthetic mitral valve disks also are seen *(short arrow)*. *AS,* Aortic stenosis.

spectral display, the transit-time effect results in a slight broadening of the velocity range at a given time point ("blurring" on the vertical axis), which potentially can result in slight overestimation of velocity.

Color Doppler Flow Imaging
Principles

Doppler color flow imaging is based on the principles of pulsed Doppler echocardiography. However, rather than one sample volume depth along the ultrasound beam, multiple sample volumes are evaluated along each sampling line (Fig. 1.28). By combining data from adjacent lines, a 2D image of intracardiac flow is generated.

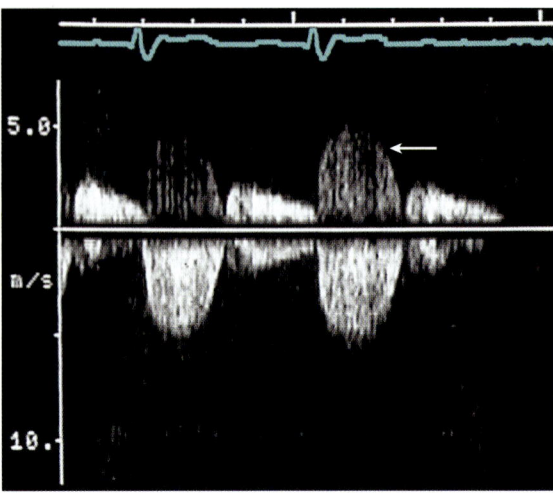

Fig. 1.27 Mirror-image Doppler artifact. A mirror-image Doppler artifact with apparent weaker flow signals in the reverse channel *(arrow)*.

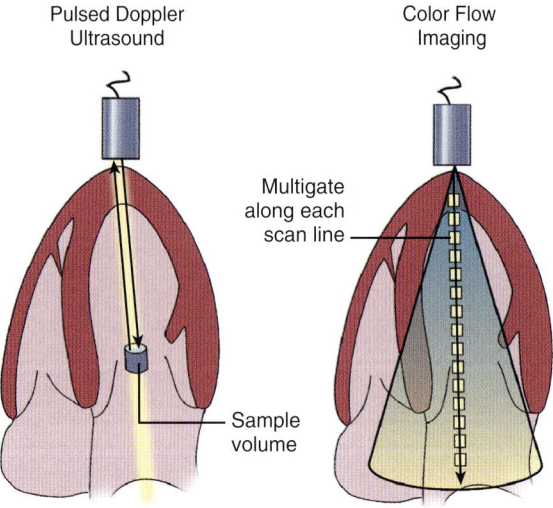

Fig. 1.28 Color Doppler flow imaging. *(Left)* With pulsed Doppler, the sample volume depth is determined by the time needed for ultrasound to travel to and from the depth of interest. *(Right)* With color flow imaging, multiple sample volume "gates" along each scan line are interrogated, with this process repeated for scan lines across the 2D image.

Along each scan line, a pulse of ultrasound is transmitted, and then the backscattered signals are received from each depth along that scan line (Table 1.8). To calculate accurate velocity data, several bursts along each scan line are used—typically eight—which is known as the *burst length* (Fig. 1.29). The PRF, as for conventional pulsed Doppler, is determined by the maximum depth of the Doppler signals. Signals from the eight sampling bursts at each position are analyzed to obtain mean velocity estimates for each depth along the scan line. Velocities are displayed using a color scale showing flow toward the transducer in red and flow away from the transducer in blue, with the shade of color indicating velocity up to the Nyquist limit. The option of displaying "variance" allows an additional color (usually green) to be added to indicate variability in the estimated mean velocity for the eight bursts along that sample line, thus indicating either a flow disturbance or aliasing of a high-velocity signal. This process is repeated for each adjacent scan line across the image plane. Because each of these processes takes a finite amount of time depending on the speed of sound in tissue, the rapidity with which this image can be updated (the frame rate) depends on a combination of these factors.

Color Doppler Instrument Controls

The color flow display depends on each specific ultrasound instrument to some extent. However, many parameters are adjustable by the operator, so an optimal examination requires careful attention to instrument settings.

The *color flow map* usually can be varied in terms of:

- Color scale (assignment of colors to direction and velocity)
- Velocity range (within the Nyquist limit at that depth)
- Zero baseline position on the color scale
- Addition of variance to the color scale

The specific color scale used is a matter of personal preference, with the diagnostic goal being to optimize the display and recognition of abnormal flow patterns.

The *velocity range* of the color flow map is determined by the Nyquist limit, and as for conventional pulsed Doppler, the range can be altered by shifting the zero baseline, changing the pulse repetition frequency, or altering the depth of the displayed image. In addition, the velocity range can be set at a value lower than the Nyquist limit to enhance visualization of low-velocity flows, such as pulmonary venous inflow.

Color Doppler *power output* and *gain* are adjusted so that gain is just below the level at which random background noise appears. "Wall filters" can be varied to exclude low-velocity signals from the color flow display. In addition, many instruments allow variation in the assignment of a returning signal to 2D or Doppler display (depending on signal strength). One approach to optimizing the color flow display is to reduce the 2D gain because the instrument does not display flow data on top of "structures," even when the 2D signal is due to excessive gain.

Perhaps the most important technical factor in color flow imaging is optimization of *frame rate*. Color flow frame rate depends on sector width, depth, pulse repetition frequency, and the number of samples per sector line. The examiner optimizes frame rate by

TABLE 1.8 Color Doppler Flow Imaging

	Definition	Examples	Clinical Implications
Sampling line	Doppler data displayed from multiple sampling lines across the 2D image	Instead of sampling backscattered signals from one depth (as in pulsed Doppler), signals from multiple depths along the beam are analyzed.	A greater number of sampling lines results in denser Doppler data, but a slower frame rate.
Burst length	The number of ultrasound bursts along each sampling line	Mean velocity is estimated from the average of the backscattered signals from each burst.	A greater number of bursts results in more accurate mean velocity estimates but a slower frame rate.
Sector scan width	The width of the displayed 2D and color image	A greater sector width requires more sampling lines or less dense velocity data.	A narrower sector scan allows a greater sampling line density and faster frame rate.
Sector scan depth	The depth of the displayed color Doppler image	The maximum depth of the sector scan determines PRF (as with pulsed Doppler) and the Nyquist limit.	The minimum depth needed to display the flow of interest provides the optimal color display.
Color scale	Color display of Doppler velocity and flow direction	Most systems use shades of red for flow toward the transducer and blue for flow away from the transducer.	The color scale can be adjusted by shifting the baseline and adjusting the maximum velocity displayed (within the Nyquist limit
Variance	The degree of variability in the mean velocity estimate at each depth along a sampling line	Variance typically is displayed as a green scale superimposed on the red-blue velocity scale. Variance can be turned on or off.	A variance display highlights flow disturbances and high velocity flow, but even normal flows will be displayed as showing variance if velocity exceeds the Nyquist limit.

PRF, Pulse repetition frequency.

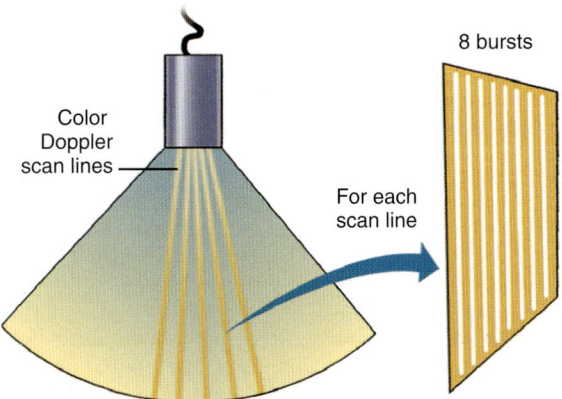

Fig. 1.29 Color Doppler flow imaging burst length. Along each color Doppler scan line, several (typically eight) bursts of ultrasound are transmitted and received to allow adequate velocity resolution.

focusing on the flow of interest, narrowing the sector, and decreasing the depth as much as possible (Fig. 1.30). When frame rate remains inadequate for timing flow abnormalities, a color M-line through the area of interest often is helpful (e.g., in assessment of aortic regurgitation).

Color Doppler Imaging Artifacts

Color flow artifacts again relate to the physics of 2D and Doppler flow image generation (Table 1.9). *Shadowing* is prominent distal to strong reflectors with absence of both 2D and flow data within the acoustic shadow.

Ghosting is the appearance of brief (usually one or two frames), large color patterns that overlie anatomic structures and do not correspond to underlying flow patterns. This artifact is caused by strong moving reflectors (e.g., prosthetic valve disks). Typically, this artifact is solid red or blue and is inconsistent from beat to beat.

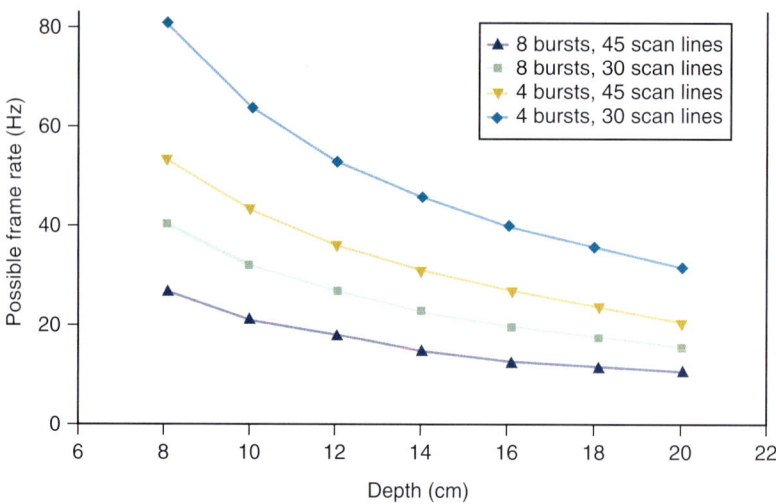

Fig. 1.30 Color Doppler frame rate. Graph of the maximum possible color Doppler frame rate (vertical axis) versus depth (horizontal axis) for 8 or 4 bursts per scan line and 30 or 45 scan lines per frame. Note that at a depth of 16 cm, a frame rate 20 or greater can be achieved only by decreasing the burst length to 4 or narrowing the sector to 30 scan lines.

TABLE 1.9	Color Doppler Artifacts
Artifact	**Appearance**
Shadowing	Absence of flow signal distal to strong reflector
Ghosting	Brief flashes of color that overlie anatomic structures and do not correlate with flow patterns
Background noise	Speckled color pattern over 2D sector due to excessive gain
Underestimation of flow signal	Loss of true flow signals due to inadequate gain
Intercept angle	Change in color (or absence at 90°) due to the angle between the flowstream and ultrasound beam across the image plane
Aliasing	"Wraparound" of color display resulting in a "variance" display even for laminar flow.
Electronic interference	Linear or complex color patterns across the 2D image

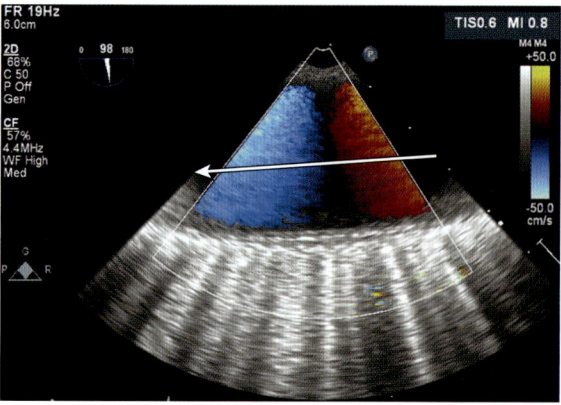

Fig. 1.31 **Effect of intercept angle on the color Doppler flow display.** In this TEE long-axis image of the descending thoracic aorta, flow in systole goes from right to left across the image plane as shown by the *arrow*. However, flow on the right side of the image appears red (because flow is directed toward the transducer), and flow on the left side of the image appears blue (because flow is directed away from the transducer), with a black area in the center of the image where the ultrasound beam is perpendicular to flow.

Color Doppler gain settings have a dramatic effect on the color flow image. Extensive gain settings result in a uniform speckled pattern across the 2D image plane resulting from random *background noise*. Conversely, too low a gain setting results in a smaller displayed flow area than is actually present, an effect colloquially known as "dial-a-jet." Most experienced echocardiographers recommend setting the gain level just below the level of random background noise to optimize the flow signal.

As for any Doppler technique, the *intercept angle* between the ultrasound beam and direction of blood flow *for each scan line* affects the color display in terms of both direction and velocity. Thus a uniform flow velocity traversing the image plane appears red (toward the transducer) at one side of the sector and blue (away from the transducer) at the other edge of the sector, with a black area in the center where the flow direction is perpendicular to the ultrasound beam (Fig. 1.31).

Flow velocities that exceed the Nyquist limit at any given depth result in *signal aliasing*. Aliasing on color flow results in "wraparound" of the velocity signal, similar to that seen on a spectral display, so

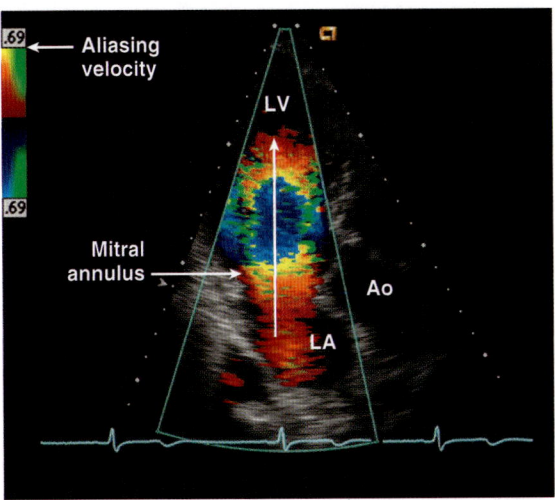

Fig. 1.32 Signal aliasing with color Doppler flow imaging. A normal LV inflow signal *(top)* shows aliasing from red to blue at the mitral annulus level because the velocity exceeds the Nyquist limit of 69 cm/s. *Ao,* Aorta.

an aliased velocity toward the transducer (should be red) appears to be traveling away from the transducer (displayed in blue). Aliasing on color flow images is very common; for example, the LV inflow stream appears red and then blue (due to aliasing) in the apical view (Fig. 1.32). Color aliasing can be used to advantage to quantitate flow based on the proximal isovelocity surface area method described in Chapter 12. In some cases, aliasing results in a variance display (due to an apparent range of velocities at that site), a finding emphasizing that a variance display does not always indicate disturbed flow.

Electronic interference on color flow displays is instrument dependent. As with other electric interference artifacts, it is most likely to occur in settings where numerous other instruments or devices are in use (e.g., operating room, intensive care unit). Sometimes it appears as a linear multicolored band on the image along a few scan lines; sometimes more complex patterns are seen. Caution is needed because sometimes electronic interference results in suppression of the color flow signal. This artifact can be recognized by the absence of normal antegrade flow patterns.

Tissue Doppler

The Doppler principle also can be used to measure motion of the myocardium using either pulsed Doppler with a sample volume at a specific site in the myocardium or color Doppler to display myocardium motion in the entire image plane. The basic principles of Doppler ultrasound also apply to tissue Doppler. Tissue Doppler signals are very high amplitude, so power output and gain settings are low, whereas tissue Doppler velocities are very low, so the velocity range is small. (See Chapter 4 for details).

Both pulsed and color tissue Doppler velocities are angle dependent, showing motion toward and away from the transducer. Pulsed tissue Doppler uses a spectral display, allowing accurate measurement of velocity data. The color tissue Doppler display, like other color Doppler images, displays mean velocities for the component of motion toward and away from the transducer. The derivation of strain rate and strain from tissue Doppler data is discussed in Chapter 4.

BIOEFFECTS AND SAFETY

The use of ultrasound for diagnostic cardiac imaging has no known adverse biologic effects. However, ultrasound waves do have the potential to cause significant bioeffects depending on the intensity of exposure. Thus the physician and the cardiac sonographer must be aware of potential bioeffects in assessing the overall safety of the procedure.

Bioeffects

Ultrasound bioeffects (Table 1.10) can be divided into three basic categories:

- Thermal effects
- Cavitation
- Other (such as torque forces and micro streaming)

Thermal effects predominate with diagnostic ultrasound examinations. As the ultrasound wave passes through a tissue, heating occurs because of absorption of the mechanical energy of the sound wave. The rate of increase in temperature dT/dt depends on the absorption coefficient of the tissue for a given frequency α, the density ρ, and specific heat C_m of the tissue and the intensity I of ultrasound exposure:

$$dT/dt = 2\alpha I/\rho C_m \quad \text{(Eq. 1.10)}$$

Increases in temperature as a result of ultrasound exposure are offset by heat loss because of blood flow through the tissue (convective loss) and heat diffusion. Denser tissues (e.g., bone) heat more rapidly than less dense tissue (e.g., fat). However, the actual elevation in temperature for a specific tissue is difficult to predict both because of the complexity of the entire biologic system and because it is difficult to assess the intensity of exposure accurately. In addition, the actual degree of tissue heating depends on transducer frequency, focus, power output, depth, perfusion, and tissue density.

Cavitation is the creation or vibration of small, gas-filled bodies by the ultrasound beam. Cavitation tends to occur only with higher-intensity exposures.

TABLE 1.10 Ultrasound Terminology: Safety

	Definition	Examples	Clinical Implications
Exposure Intensity (I)	Ultrasound exposure depends on power and area: $I = \text{power/area} = \text{W/cm}^2$	Common measures of intensity are the SPTA or the SPPA.	Transducer output and tissue exposure affect the total ultrasound exposure of the patient.
Thermal bioeffects	Heating of tissue due to absorption of ultrasound energy described by the thermal index (TI)	The degree of tissue heating is affected by tissue density and blood flow. TI is the ratio of transmitted acoustic power to the power needed to increase temperature by 1°C. TI is most important with Doppler and color flow imaging.	Total ultrasound exposure depends on transducer frequency, power output, focus, depth, and examination duration. When the TI exceeds 1, the benefits of the study should be balanced against potential biologic effects.
Cavitation	Creation or vibration of small gas-filled bodies by the ultrasound wave	Mechanical index (MI) is the ratio of peak rarefactional pressure to the square root of the transducer frequency. MI is most important with 2D imaging.	Cavitation or vibration of microbubbles occurs with higher-intensity exposure. Power output and exposure time should be monitored.

SPPA, Spatial peak pulse average; *SPTA*, spatial peak temporal average.

Microbubbles resonate (expand and decrease in size) depending on their dimension in relation to the sound wave, with a resonance frequency F_0 defined by the radius of the microbubble (R_0 in microns):

$$F_0 = 3260/R_0 \quad \text{(Eq. 1.11)}$$

Microbubbles also can be created by ultrasound by expansion of small cavitation nuclei. Cavitation has not been shown to occur with ultrasound exposure because of diagnostic ultrasound systems. However, this effect is more important when gas-filled bodies are introduced into the ultrasound field, such as with the use of contrast echocardiography.

Other ultrasound bioeffects occur only with much higher exposures than occur with diagnostic ultrasound. These effects include micro streaming, torque forces, and other complex biologic effects.

Safety

The intensity *(I)* of ultrasound exposure can be expressed in several ways. The most commonly used unit of measure of intensity is power per area, where power is energy over a specific time interval:

$$I = \text{power/area} = \text{watt/cm}^2 \quad \text{(Eq. 1.12)}$$

The maximum overall intensity is then described as the highest exposure within the beam (spatial peak) averaged over the period of exposure (temporal average) and is known as the *spatial peak temporal average* *(SPTA) intensity*. Another common measure is the *spatial peak pulse average (SPPA)*, defined as the average pulse intensity at the spatial location where the pulse intensity is maximum. The Food and Drug Administration provides two maximum allowed limits for I_{SPTA} for cardiac applications: a regulated application-specific limit of 430 mW/cm².

A major limitation of measuring the intensity of ultrasound exposure is that although measuring the *output* of the transducer is straightforward (e.g., in a water bath), estimating the actual tissue *exposure* is more difficult due to attenuation and other interactions with the tissue. Furthermore, tissue exposure is limited only to transmission periods, as reflected in the duty factor, and the time the ultrasound beam dwells at a specific point, both of which are considerably shorter than the total examination time. Other indices that incorporate these factors have been developed to define the exposure levels with diagnostic ultrasound more clearly. These measures include the thermal index (TI) and the mechanical index (MI).

The soft tissue TI is based on the ratio of transmitted acoustic power to the power needed to raise tissue temperature by 1°C:

$$\text{TI} = W_p/W_{\text{deg}} \quad \text{(Eq. 1.13)}$$

where W_p is a power parameter calculated from output power and acoustic attenuation, and W_{deg} is the estimated power needed to increase the tissue temperature by 1°C. Different TIs used for bone and cranial bone are less relevant for cardiac ultrasound.

The MI describes the nonthermal effects of ultrasound (cavitation and other effects) as the ratio of peak rarefactional pressure and the square root of transducer frequency, with the specific definition:

$$MI = [\rho_{r.3}/(f_c^{1/2})]/C_{MI} \qquad (Eq.\ 1.14)$$

Where C_{MI} equals 1 Mpa MHz$^{-1/2}$, $\rho_{r.3}$ is the attenuated peak-rarefactional pressure in megapascals, and f_c is the center frequency of the transducer in MHz.

An MI or TI less than 1 is generally considered safe; higher numbers indicate a higher probability of a biologic effect. These indexes are displayed only on instruments capable of exceeding an MI or TI of 1. With a higher index, the potential risks of ultrasound exposure must be balanced against the benefits of the diagnostic examination (Fig. 1.33). The thermal index is most important with Doppler and color flow imaging, whereas the MI is most important with 2D imaging.

Although no known risks are associated with the diagnostic use of cardiac ultrasound imaging in adults, a prudent approach is to:

- Perform echocardiography only when indicated clinically (see Chapter 5), as part of an approved research protocol, or in appropriate teaching settings.
- Know the power output and exposure intensity of different modalities (imaging and Doppler) of each instrument.
- Limit the power output and exposure time as much as possible within the constraints of acquiring the necessary information.
- Keep up to date on any new scientific findings or data relating to possible adverse effects.

These principles are summarized by the acronym ALARA (As Low As Reasonably Achievable) with the core concepts of using ultrasound only when indicated and minimizing both exposure time and intensity.

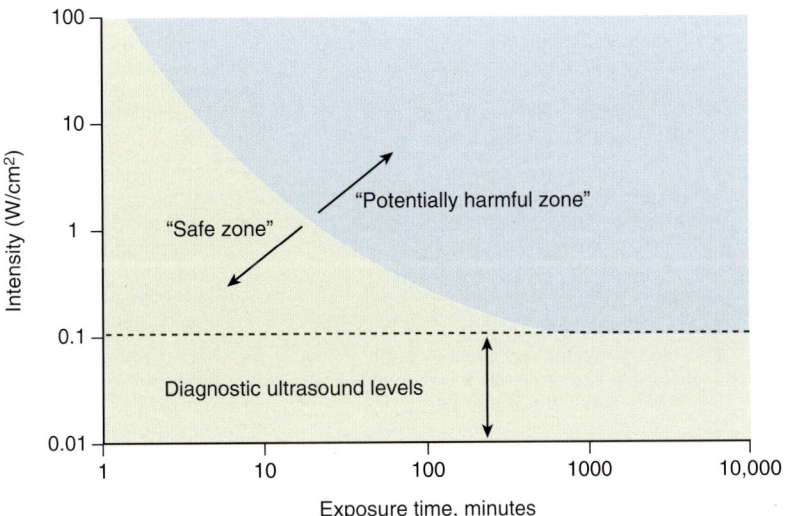

Fig. 1.33 Potential bioeffects from ultrasound. Safe and potentially harmful regions are delineated according to ultrasound intensity levels and exposure time. The *dashed line* shows the upper limit of intensities typically encountered in diagnostic ultrasound applications. *(Adapted from Bushberg JT, Seibert JA, Leidholdt EH, et al: The essential physics of medical imaging, ed 2, Philadelphia, 2002, Lippincott Williams & Wilkins, 2002, Fig. 16.21.)*

THE ECHO EXAM

Basic Principles

OPTIMIZATION OF ECHOCARDIOGRAPHIC IMAGES

Instrument Control	Data Optimization	Clinical Issues
Transducer	• Different transducer types and transmission frequencies are needed for specific clinical. • Transmission frequency is adjusted for tissue penetration in each patient and for ultrasound modality (Doppler vs. imaging).	• A higher transducer frequency provides improved resolution but less penetration • A larger aperture provides a more focused beam.
Power output	• Power output reflects the amount of ultrasound energy transmitted to the tissue. • Higher power output results in greater tissue penetration.	• Potential bioeffects must be considered. • Exam time and mechanical and thermal indexes should be monitored.
Imaging mode	• 2D imaging is the clinical standard for most indications. • M-mode provides high time resolution along a single scan line. • 3D imaging provides improved appreciation of spatial relationships.	• Optimal measurement of cardiac chambers and vessels may require a combination of imaging modes.
Transducer position	• Acoustic windows allow ultrasound tissue penetration without intervening lung or bone tissue. • Transthoracic acoustic windows include parasternal, apical subcostal, and suprasternal • TEE acoustic windows include high esophageal and transgastric.	• Optimal patient positioning is essential for acoustic access to the heart. • Imaging resolution is optimal when the ultrasound beam is reflected perpendicular to the tissue interface. • Doppler signals are optimal with the ultrasound beam is aligned parallel to flow.
Depth	• Depth is adjusted to show the structure of interest. • PRF depends on maximum image depth.	• PRF is higher at shallow depths and contributes to improved image resolution. • Axial resolution is the same along the entire length of the ultrasound beam. • Lateral and elevations resolution depend on the 3D shape of the ultrasound beam at each depth.
Sector width	• Standard sector width is 60°, but a narrower sector allows a higher scan-line density and faster frame rate.	• Sector width should be adjusted as needed to optimize the image. • Too narrow a sector may miss important anatomic or Doppler findings.
Gain	• Overall gain affects the display of the reflected ultrasound signals.	• Excessive gain obscures border identification. • Inadequate gain results in failure to display reflections from tissue interfaces.
TCG	• TGC adjusts gain differentially along the length of the ultrasound bean to compensate for the effects of attenuation.	• An appropriate TCG curve results in an image with similar brightness proximally and distally in the sector image.
Gray-scale or dynamic range	• Ultrasound amplitude is displayed using a decibel scale in shades of gray.	• The range of displayed amplitudes is adjusted to optimize the image using the dynamic range or compression controls.
Harmonic imaging	• Harmonic frequencies are proportional to the strength of the fundament frequency but increase with depth of propagation.	• Harmonic imaging improves endocardial definition and decreased near-field and side-lobe artifacts. • Flat structures, such as valves, appear thicker with harmonic than with fundamental imaging. • Axial resolution is reduced.
Focal depth	• Transducer design parameters that affect focal depth include array pattern, aperture size, and acoustic focusing.	• The ultrasound beam is most focused at the junction between the near zone and far field of the beam pattern. • Transducer design allows a longer focal zone. In some cases, focal zone can be adjusted during the examination.

Basic Principles—cont'd

OPTIMIZATION OF ECHOCARDIOGRAPHIC IMAGES

Instrument Control	Data Optimization	Clinical Issues
Zoom mode	• The ultrasound image can be restricted to a smaller depth range and narrow section. The maximum depth still determines PRF, but scan line density and frame rate can be optimized in the region of interest.	• Zoom mode is used to examine areas on interest identified on standard views.
ECG	• The ECG signal is essential for triggering digital cine loop acquisition.	• A noisy signal or low amplitude ECG results in incorrect triggering or inadvertent recording of an incomplete cardiac cycle.

2D, Two-dimensional; *3D*, three-dimensional; *ECG*, electrocardiogram; *PRF*, pulse repetition frequency; *TEE*, transesophageal echocardiography; *TGC*, time-gain compensation.

Optimization of Doppler Recordings

Modality	Data Optimization	Common Artifacts
Pulsed	• 2D guided with "frozen" image • Parallel to flow • Small sample volume • Velocity scale at Nyquist limit • Adjust baseline for aliasing • Use low wall filters • Adjust gain and dynamic range	• Nonparallel angle with underestimation of velocity • Signal aliasing; Nyquist limit = ½ pulse repetition frequency (PRF) • Signal strength or noise
Continuous wave	• Dedicated nonimaging transducer • Parallel to flow • Adjust velocity scale so flow fits and fills displayed range • Use high wall filters • Adjust gain and dynamic range	• Nonparallel angle with underestimation of velocity • Range ambiguity • Beam width • Transit time effect
Color flow	• Use minimal depth and sector width for flow of interest (best frame rate) • Adjust gain just below random noise • Color scale at Nyquist limit • Decrease 2D gain to optimize Doppler signal • 3D color imaging allows better visualization of the size and shape of jet geometry proximal to a restrictive orifice (e.g., valve regurgitation)	• Shadowing • Ghosting • Electronic interference

SUGGESTED READING

1. Kremkau FW: *Sonography Principles and Instruments*, 9th ed, Philadelphia, 2015, Saunders.
   Basic textbook with concise clear text and informative illustrations In addition to the physics of ultrasound, detailed chapters address ultrasound transducers, imaging instruments, Doppler principles, artifacts, and safety. Each chapter has a review section with multiple-choice questions. A comprehensive examination (with answers) is included. Highly recommended for physicians and sonographers who perform or interpret echocardiograms.
2. Bushberg JT, Seibert JA, Leidholdt JR, et al: Ultrasound. *The Essential Physics of Medical Imaging*, 3rd ed, Philadelphia, 2011, Lippincott Williams & Wilkins.
   Concise but detailed summary of ultrasound physics for the physician. Sections include characteristics of sound, interaction with tissue, transducer design and beam properties, resolution, image acquisition, artifacts, Doppler ultrasound, and bioeffects.
3. Owens CA, Zagzebski JA: *Ultrasound Physics Review*, Pasadena, CA, 2009, Davies.
   Review of ultrasound physics for the beginning student. Concise text with clear schematic illustrations and tables. Topics covered include physics of diagnostic ultrasound, image storage and display, Doppler instrumentation, and bioeffects. Questions for review included with each chapter. Additional suggested readings.
4. O'Brien WD, Jr: Ultrasound-biophysics mechanisms, *Prog Biophys Mol Biol* 93:212–255, 2007.
   A detailed discussion, including mathematical principles, of ultrasound bioeffects including ultrasound waves, acoustic propagation, impedance and attenuation, interactions with tissues, and the mechanisms and magnitude of thermal and nonthermal bioeffects. 285 references.
5. Barnett SB, Haar GR, Ziskin MC, et al: International recommendations and guidelines for the safe use of diagnostic ultrasound in medicine, *Ultrasound in Med & Biol* 26:355–366, 2000.
   Review article based on symposium sponsored by the World Federation for Ultrasound in

Medicine and Biology (WFUMB) comparing national and international recommendations on the safe use of diagnostic ultrasound. Includes a summary of U.S. Food and Drug Administration (FDA) regulation by application-specific limits on acoustic power and the newer approach of user responsibility for appropriate use based on real-time display of safety indices.

6. American Institute of Ultrasound, Medical Ultrasound Safety, 3rd Ed. 2014. ISBN 1-932962-30-1 http://www.aium.org/officialStatements/39 (Accessed 24 May 2016).

   This book includes sections on bioeffects and biophysics, prudent use and implementing ALARA.

7. Fowlkes JB: American Institute of Ultrasound in Medicine consensus report on potential bioeffects of diagnostic ultrasound: executive summary, *J Ultrasound Med* 27:503–515, 2008.

   American Institute of Ultrasound in Medicine (AIUM) Consensus Development Conferences on ultrasound safety and bioeffects including contrast agents and thermal and nonthermal effects. This issue of the Journal of Ultrasound Medicine includes five additional papers on each aspect of ultrasound safety.

8. Shankar H, Pagel PS: Potential adverse ultrasound-related biological effects: a critical review, *Anesthesiology* 115(5):1109–1124, 2011.

   Detailed review of the biologic effects of ultrasound including a table with definitions of terminology and sections on thermal effects, mechanical effects, safety standards, and known biologic effects of ultrasound. The authors conclude that, although ultrasound has the potential to cause adverse effects, there have been no major reports of harm in humans.

9. Bigelow TA, Church CC, Sandstrom K, et al: The thermal index: its strengths, weaknesses, and proposed improvements, *J Ultrasound Med* 30(5):714–734, 2011.

   Review of the TI as a measure of diagnostic ultrasound exposure, with a discussion of possible limitations including focusing, time dependence, temperature, and nonlinear propagation. The AIUM Output Standards Subcommittee recommends resolution of inconsistencies in the current TI calculations and that efforts continue to develop a new indicator of thermal risk. 40 references.

2 Normal Anatomy and Flow Patterns on Transthoracic Echocardiography

BASIC IMAGING PRINCIPLES
    Tomographic Imaging
    Nomenclature of Standard Views
    Image Orientation
    Examination Technique
    Technical Quality
    Echocardiographic Image Interpretation

TRANSTHORACIC TOMOGRAPHIC VIEWS
    Parasternal Window
        Long-Axis Views
        Right Ventricular Inflow and Outflow Views
        Short-Axis Views
    Apical Window
        Four-Chamber View
        Two-Chamber View
        Long-Axis View
        Other Apical Views
    Subcostal Window
    Suprasternal Notch Window
    Other Acoustic Windows

M-MODE RECORDINGS
    Aortic Valve and Left Atrium
    Mitral Valve
    Left Ventricle
    Other M-Mode Recordings

NORMAL INTRACARDIAC FLOW PATTERNS
    Basic Principles
        Laminar Versus Disturbed Flow
        Flow-Velocity Profiles
    Clinical Quantitative Doppler Methods
        Measurement of Volume Flow
        Velocity-Pressure Relationships
        Spatial Pattern of Flow
    Normal Antegrade Intracardiac Flows
        Left Ventricular Outflow
        Right Ventricular Outflow
        Left Ventricular Inflow
        Right Ventricular Inflow
        Left Atrial Filling
        Right Atrial Filling
        Descending Aorta
    Normal Color Doppler Flow Patterns
        Impact of Color Doppler Physics
        Normal Ventricular Outflow Patterns
        Normal Ventricular Inflow Patterns
        Normal Atrial Inflow Patterns
        Physiologic Valvular Regurgitation

AGING CHANGES ON ECHOCARDIOGRAPHY

THE DIAGNOSTIC ECHOCARDIOGRAM
    Core Elements
    Additional Components

THE ECHO EXAM

SUGGESTED READING

BASIC IMAGING PRINCIPLES

Tomographic Imaging

Echocardiography provides tomographic images of cardiac structures and blood flow, analogous to a thin "slice" through the heart. Two-dimensional (2D) echocardiographic images provide detailed anatomic data in a given image plane, but complete evaluation of the cardiac chambers and valves requires integration of information from multiple image planes. Small structures that traverse numerous tomographic planes (e.g., the coronary arteries) are difficult to evaluate fully. In addition, structures move in and out of the imaging plane as a result of motion caused by cardiac contraction or respiratory movement of the heart within the chest. Respiratory variation in cardiac location is recognized easily by its timing, but any movement of the heart during the cardiac cycle is more problematic because it is not obvious on the 2D image. Cardiac motion relative to surrounding structures is described in three dimensions as:

- Translation (movement of the heart as a whole in the chest)
- Rotation (circular motion around the long axis of the left ventricle [LV])
- Torsion (unequal rotational motion at the apex versus the base of the LV)

Even if the 2D image plane is fixed in position, the location of underlying structures varies between systole and diastole. For example, in the apical four-chamber view, adjacent segments of the LV (often supplied by different coronary arteries) might be seen in systole versus diastole. Compared with tomographic imaging, three-dimensional (3D) imaging provides a wider field of view that provides more intuitive cardiac images, but it has poorer resolution and a slower frame rate and is affected by respiratory and cardiac motion, as is 2D imaging (see Chapter 4). Thus, both modalities are used together as appropriate during the echocardiographic study.

Nomenclature of Standard Views

Each tomographic image is defined by its acoustic *window* (the position of the transducer) and *view* (the image plane) (Table 2.1). The standard three orthogonal echocardiographic image planes are determined by the axis of the heart itself (with the LV as the major point of reference), rather than by skeletal or external body landmarks (Fig. 2.1). The primary reference points on the heart are the apex, defined

TABLE 2.1	Transthoracic Echo Image Orientation Nomenclature
Window (Transducer Location)	
Parasternal	
Apical	
Subcostal	
Suprasternal	
Image Planes	
Short-axis	
Long-axis	
4-chamber	
2-chamber	
Reference Points	
Apex versus base	
Lateral versus medial	
Anterior versus posterior	

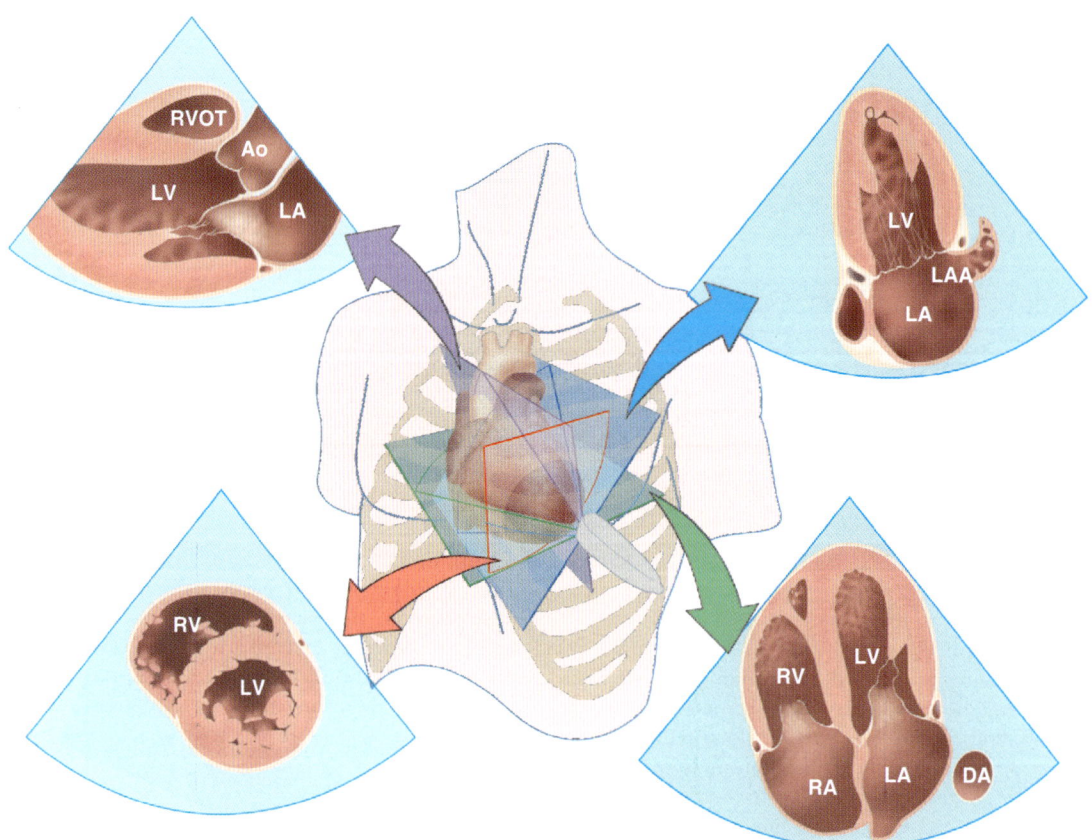

Fig. 2.1 Basic image planes used in transthoracic echocardiography. The long-axis view *(purple arrow)* extends from the LV apex through the aortic valve plane. The short-axis view *(red arrow)* is perpendicular to the long-axis view, thus resulting in a circular view of the LV. The two-chamber *(blue arrows)* and four-chamber *(green arrow)* views are each about 60° rotation from the long-axis view, and both are perpendicular to the short-axis view. The four-chamber view includes both ventricles and both atria. The two-chamber view includes the LV and LA. *Ao,* Aorta; *DA,* descending thoracic aorta; *LAA,* LA appendage; *RVOT,* RV outflow tract.

as the tip of the LV, and the base, defined by the plane of the atrioventricular (e.g., mitral and tricuspid) valves. The four standard image planes are:

- *Long-axis plane:* Parallel to the long axis of the LV, with the image plane intersecting the LV apex and center of the aortic valve, aligned with the anterior-posterior diameter of the mitral annulus
- *Short-axis planes:* A series of image planes perpendicular to the long axis of the ventricle and resulting in circular cross-sectional views of the LV, mitral valve, and aortic valve
- *Four-chamber plane:* An image plane from apex to base, perpendicular to the short-axis view, that includes both ventricles and atria, aligned with the medial-lateral diameter of both the mitral and tricuspid annulus
- *Two-chamber plane:* An image plane from apex to base that includes the LV and left atrium (LA), perpendicular to the short-axis view, and rotated to be midway between the long-axis and four-chamber views

In addition to apical versus basal, other standard directional terms are medial versus lateral (the horizontal axis in a short-axis or four-chamber view) and anterior versus posterior (the vertical axis in a short-axis or long-axis view). This standard terminology also applies to visualization of cardiac anatomy with 3D echocardiography.

Acoustic windows are transducer positions that allow ultrasound access to the heart. The bony thoracic cage and adjacent air-filled lung limit acoustic access, thereby making patient positioning and sonographer experience critical factors in obtaining diagnostic images. Transthoracic images typically are obtained from parasternal, apical, subcostal, and suprasternal notch acoustic windows. The transducer motions used to obtain the desired view are described as follows (Fig. 2.2):

- *Move* the transducer to a different position on the chest.
- *Tilt or point* the transducer tip with a rocking motion to image different structures in the same tomographic plane.
- *Angle* the transducer from side to side to obtain different tomographic planes somewhat parallel to the original image plane.
- *Rotate* the image plane at a single position to obtain intersecting tomographic planes.

Image Orientation

Most laboratories follow the American Society of Echocardiography (ASE) guidelines for image orientation in adults, although some pediatric cardiologists use alternate formats. The recommended orientation

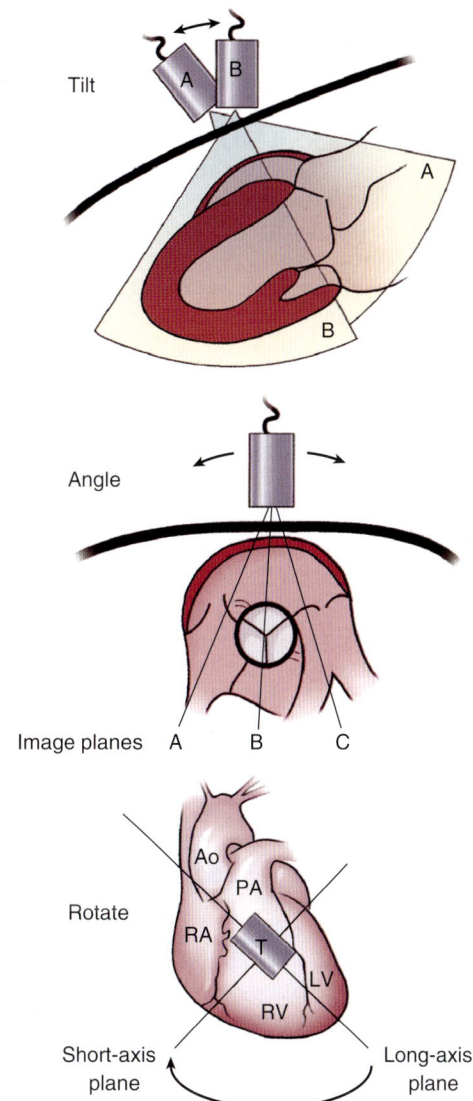

Fig. 2.2 Transducer motion. This example, using a left parasternal transducer (T) position, demonstrates: *Tilt:* The transducer is "rocked" to provide images (*A* or *B*) in the same tomographic plane. *Angle:* Different image planes (perpendicular to the plane of the figure at lines *A*, *B*, and *C*) are obtained by angulation of the transducer. *Rotation:* The transducer is "twisted" with a circular motion to provide a different image plane while maintaining the same orientation between the transducer itself and the chest wall. *Ao,* Aorta; *PA,* pulmonary artery.

is with the transducer position (narrowest portion of the sector scan) at the top of the screen so that structures closer to the transducer are at the top of the image and structures farther from the transducer are at the bottom of the image. Thus, a transthoracic four-chamber view is displayed with the apex at the top of the image (because it is closest to the transducer), whereas a transesophageal echocardiographic (TEE) four-chamber view is displayed with the apex at the bottom of the image (because it is most distant from the transducer). This orientation aids in prompt recognition of ultrasound artifacts, shadowing, and reverberations because the display of the origin of the ultrasound signal is the same for all acoustic windows and image planes.

In short-axis views, lateral cardiac structures are displayed on the right side of the screen, with medial structures on the left side, as if the viewer is looking from the apex toward the cardiac base. In long-axis views, basal structures (e.g., the aortic valve) are shown on the right and apical structures on the left, as if the viewer is looking from the patient's left side. The four-chamber plane is displayed with lateral structures on the right side of the screen and medial structures on the left side (as for the short-axis view); thus with normal cardiac anatomy the LV is on the right side of the screen and the right ventricle (RV) is on the left side.

Examination Technique

A diagnostic echocardiographic examination is performed by a physician or by a trained cardiac sonographer under the supervision of a qualified physician. Point of care ultrasound studies also are performed by other health care providers within a defined scope of practice. Guidelines and recommendations for education and training in echocardiography for cardiologists, anesthesiologists, sonographers, and other health care providers have been published, as referenced in Chapter 5.

At the time of a transthoracic echocardiography (TTE) examination, relevant clinical data, prior imaging studies, and the indications for the study are reviewed. Blood pressure is recorded along with age, height, and weight. The patient is positioned comfortably for each view in either a left lateral decubitus or supine position. Electrocardiographic (ECG) electrodes are attached for display of a single lead (usually lead II) to aid in timing cardiac events. Specially designed echocardiographic examination stretchers provide apical cutouts for optimal transducer positioning at the apex. The transducer is applied to the chest and upper abdomen by using a water-soluble gel to obtain good contact without intervening air. The time needed to perform an echocardiographic examination depends on the specific clinical situation—from a few minutes in a critically ill patient to document cardiac tamponade to more than 1 hour to quantitate multiple lesions in a patient with complex valvular or congenital heart disease.

Technical Quality

Image quality depends on the degree of ultrasound tissue penetration, transducer frequency, instrument settings, and the sonographer's skill. Ultrasound tissue penetration or "acoustic access" to the cardiac structures is largely determined by body habitus, specifically how the heart is positioned relative to the lungs and chest wall. Conditions that increase transducer distance from the heart (e.g., adipose tissue), decrease ultrasound penetration (e.g., scar tissue), or interpose air-containing tissues between the transducer and the heart (e.g., chronic lung disease, recent cardiac surgery) all lead to poor image quality. TEE images tend to show better definition of cardiac structures given the shorter distance between the transducer and the heart, the absence of interposed lung, and the use of a higher transducer frequency. On transthoracic studies, optimal patient positioning for each acoustic window brings the cardiac structures against the chest wall. In addition, respiratory variation can be used to the sonographer's advantage by having the patient suspend breathing briefly in whichever phase of the respiratory cycle yields the best image quality. Unfortunately, even with careful attention to examination technique, echocardiographic images remain suboptimal in some patients.

Echocardiographic Image Interpretation

The physician uses the tomographic 2D echocardiographic images to build a mental 3D reconstruction of the cardiac chambers and valves or uses a 3D echocardiographic data set to examine anatomy in specific image planes (see Chapter 4). To do this, an understanding of image planes and orientation and the technical aspects of image acquisition (e.g., in recognizing artifacts) is needed, along with a detailed knowledge of cardiac anatomy (Table 2.2). Recording images as the tomographic plane is moved between standard image planes is important for this analysis and ensures that abnormalities lying outside or between our arbitrary "standard" views are not missed. 3D imaging is helpful for elucidating anatomic relationships in complex cases and aids in identifying the optimal 2D image planes for display of abnormal findings. Information obtained from anatomic imaging then is integrated with physiologic Doppler data and clinical information in the final echocardiographic interpretation.

TRANSTHORACIC TOMOGRAPHIC VIEWS

Normal echocardiographic anatomy is described in this section for each tomographic view. The best views for specific cardiac structures are indicated in Table 2.3.

Parasternal Window
Long-Axis Views

With the patient in a left lateral decubitus position and the transducer in the left third or fourth intercostal

TABLE 2.2	Terminology for Normal Echocardiographic Anatomy
Aortic root	Sinuses of Valsalva Sinotubular junction Coronary ostia
Aortic valve	Right, left, and noncoronary cusps Nodules of Arantius Lamb1 excrescence
Mitral valve	Anterior and posterior leaflets Posterior leaflet scallops (lateral, central, medial) Chordae (primary, secondary, tertiary; basal and marginal) Commissures (medial and lateral)
Left ventricle	Wall segments (see Chapter 8) Septum, free wall Base, apex Medial and lateral papillary muscles
Right ventricle	Inflow segment Moderator band Outflow tract (conus) Supraventricular crest Anterior, posterior, and conus papillary muscles
Tricuspid value	Anterior, septal, and posterior leaflets Chordae Commissures
Right atrium	Right atrial appendage SVC, IVC junctions Valve of IVC (Chiari network) Crista terminalis Fossa ovalis Patent foramen ovale
Left atrium	Left atrial appendage Superior and inferior left pulmonary veins Superior and inferior right pulmonary veins Ridge at junction of left atrial appendage and left superior pulmonary vein
Pericardium	Oblique sinus Transverse sinus

IVC, Inferior vena cava; *SVC*, superior vena cava.

TABLE 2.3	Transthoracic Echo: Views for Specific Cardiac Structures
Anatomic Structures	**Best Views**
Aortic valve	PLAX PSAX Apical long-axis Anteriorly angulated apical 4-chamber
Mitral valve	PLAX PSAX-mitral valve level Apical 4-chamber Apical long-axis
Pulmonic valve	PSAX (aortic valve level) RV outflow Subcostal short-axis (aortic valve level)
Tricuspid valve	RV inflow Apical 4-chamber Subcostal 4-chamber and short-axis
Left ventricle	PLAX PSAX Apical 4-chamber, 2-chamber, long-axis Subcostal 4-chamber and short-axis
Right ventricle	PLAX (RV outflow tract only) RV inflow PSAX (MV and LV levels) Apical 4-chamber Subcostal 4-chamber
Left atrium	PLAX PSAX Apical 4-chamber, 2-chamber, long-axis Subcostal 4-chamber
Right atrium	PSAX (aortic valve level) Apical 4-chamber Subcostal 4-chamber and short-axis
Aorta • Ascending • Arch • Descending thoracic	PLAX (standard and up an interspace) Suprasternal notch Suprasternal notch Parasternal with angulation Modified apical 2-chamber Subcostal
Interatrial septum	PSAX Subcostal 4-chamber
Coronary sinus	PLAX to RV inflow view (sweep) Posterior angulation from apical 4-chamber

PSAX, Parasternal long axis; *PLAX*, parasternal short axis.

space, adjacent to the sternum, a long-axis view of the heart is obtained that bisects the long axis of both aortic and mitral valves (Figs. 2.3 and 2.4). In this standard view, the *aortic sinuses*, sinotubular junction, and proximal 3 to 4 cm of the ascending aorta are seen; further segments of the ascending aorta are visualized by moving the transducer cephalad one or two interspaces. The term "aortic root" often is used to refer to the entire proximal aorta including the annulus, sinuses, sinotubular junction, and ascending aorta. The upper limit of normal for aortic end-diastolic dimension in adults is 1.6 cm/m^2 at the annulus and 2.1 cm/m^2 at the sinuses.

Fig. 2.3 Cardiac anatomy in the long-axis view. The parasternal long-axis view in diastole shows: the closed right and noncoronary cusps of the aortic valve; the aortic sinuses, sinotubular junction, and proximal ascending aorta; the open anterior and posterior mitral valve leaflets; the basal and mid-ventricular segments of the anterior septum and posterior LV wall; the RV outflow tract anteriorly, and the coronary sinus in the atrioventricular groove. The medial papillary muscle is shown for reference, although slight medial angulation typically is needed to visualize this structure in the long-axis view. *Asterisk,* Intervalvular fibrosa. *(From Otto CM: Echocardiographic evaluation of valvular heart disease. In Otto CM, Bonow R, editors:* Valvular Heart Disease: A Companion to Braunwald's Heart Disease, *ed 3, Philadelphia, 2009, Saunders.)*

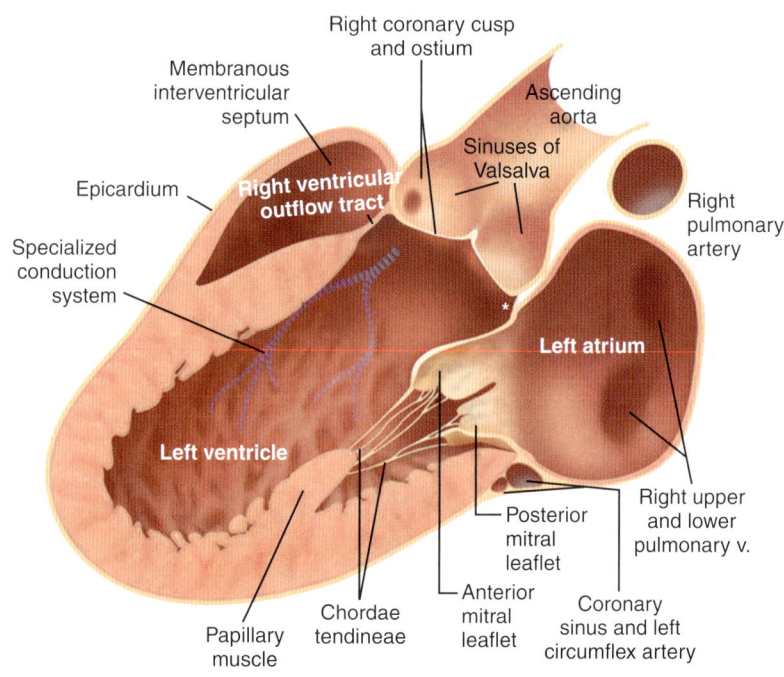

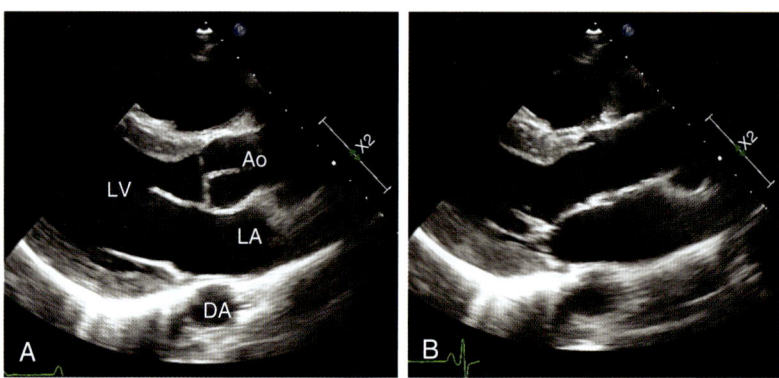

Fig. 2.4 ▶ **Normal parasternal long-axis 2D echo images.** (A) End-diastolic and (B) end-systolic images show the anatomic features seen in Fig. 2.3. In addition, the descending thoracic aorta *(DA)* is seen posterior to the LA. *Ao,* Aorta.

In the long-axis view, the right coronary cusp of the *aortic valve* is anterior and the noncoronary cusp is posterior (the left coronary cusp is lateral to the image plane). In systole, the thin aortic leaflets open widely, assuming a parallel orientation to the aortic walls. In diastole, the leaflets are closed, with a small obtuse closure angle between the two leaflets. The leaflets appear linear from the closure line to the aortic annulus because of the hemicylindrical shape of the closed leaflets (linear along the length of the cylinder, curved along its short axis). In normal young individuals, the leaflets are so thin that only the apposed portions at the leaflets' closure line may be seen. The 3D anatomy of the attachment line of the aortic leaflets to the aortic root is shaped like a crown with the three commissures attached near the tops of the sinuses of Valsalva and the mid-portion of each leaflet attached near the base of each sinus (Fig. 2.5). The fibrous continuity between the aortic root and the anterior mitral leaflet (absence of intervening myocardium) helps identify the anatomic LV in complex congenital disease.

The anterior and posterior *mitral valve* leaflets appear thin and uniform in echogenicity, with chordal attachments leading toward the medial (or posteromedial) papillary muscle seen in the long-axis view, although the papillary muscle itself is slightly medial to the long-axis plane. The anterior mitral leaflet is longer than the posterior leaflet but has a smaller annular length so that the surface areas of the two leaflets are similar (Fig. 2.6). As the mitral leaflets open in diastole, the tips separate, and the anterior leaflet touches or comes very close to the ventricular septum. In systole, the leaflets coapt, with some overlap between the leaflets (apposition zone) and a slightly obtuse (>180°) angle relative to the mitral annulus plane.

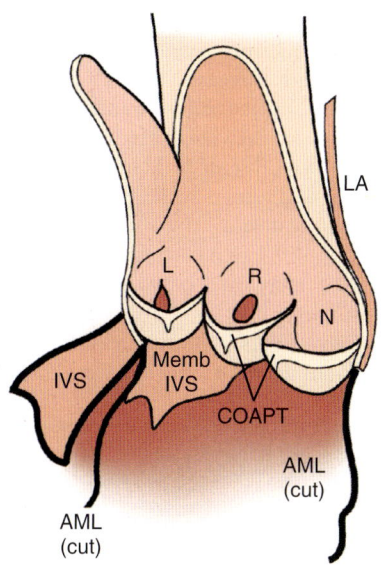

Fig. 2.5 Aortic valve anatomy. Schematic diagram in a frontal view with the aortic root "opened" between the left *(L)* and noncoronary *(N)* cusps by cutting through the anterior mitral leaflet *(AML)* to demonstrate the crown-shaped "annulus." The commissures are near the top of each sinus, and each leaflet has a hemicylindrical shape so that the closed leaflets appear as a straight line in the long-axis view. Each aortic leaflet has a coaptation *(COAPT)* zone, with overlap between adjacent leaflets and a thicker region, the nodule of Arantius, at the center of each cusp. The close anatomic relationships of the aortic valve with the interventricular septum *(IVS)*, membranous septum, mitral valve, and LA can be appreciated. *R*, Right coronary cusp.

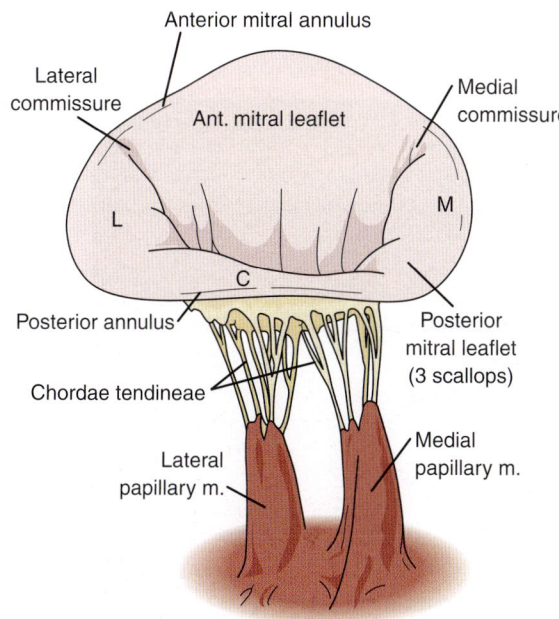

Fig. 2.6 Mitral valve anatomy. The mitral valve apparatus includes the leaflet, annulus, chordae, and papillary muscles *(m.)*. The anterior mitral leaflet attaches to a smaller portion of the circumference of the annulus than the posterior mitral leaflet, but the anterior leaflet is longer. The posterior leaflet consists of three segments designated the medial *(M)*, central *(C)*, and lateral *(L)* scallops. Both leaflets attach to both the medial and lateral papillary muscle.

The chordae normally remain posterior to the plane of leaflet coaptation in systole. Some normal individuals have systolic anterior motion of the chordae resulting from mild redundancy of chordal tissue that is not associated with hemodynamic abnormalities. This must be distinguished from the pathologic systolic anterior motion of the mitral leaflets seen in hypertrophic cardiomyopathy. The mitral annulus (the attachment between the mitral leaflets, LA, and LV) is an anatomically well-defined fibrous structure shaped like a bent ellipse, with the more apical major axis bisected in the four-chamber view and the more basal minor axis bisected in the long-axis view.

The *left atrium* is seen posterior to the aorta and has an anteroposterior diameter similar to that of the aortic sinuses in normal adults. The *right pulmonary artery* lies between the proximal ascending aorta and the superior aspect of the LA but usually is not well seen on transthoracic images in adults. The *coronary sinus* is seen in the atrioventricular groove posterior to the mitral annulus. Dilation of the coronary sinus resulting from a persistent left superior vena cava (which can be confirmed by echo-contrast injection in a left arm vein if needed) is seen in about 0.4% of studies; it is an isolated incidental finding in about half of these cases and is associated with congenital heart disease in the remainder.

Posterior to the LA, the *descending thoracic aorta* is seen in cross section. A long-axis view of the descending thoracic aorta can be obtained by rotating the transducer counterclockwise. The oblique sinus of the pericardium lies between the LA and the descending thoracic aorta so that a pericardial effusion can be seen between these two structures, whereas a pleural effusion is seen only posterior to the descending thoracic aorta.

The *left ventricle* septum and posterior wall are seen at the base and mid-ventricular level in the long-axis view, thus allowing assessment of wall thickness, chamber dimensions, endocardial motion, and wall thickening of these myocardial segments. LV end-diastolic and end-systolic measurements of wall thickness and internal dimensions are made in the long-axis view on 2D images from the septal to posterior wall tissue-blood interface or using a 2D-guided M-mode recording when a perpendicular alignment can be obtained (see Chapter 6). From the parasternal window, the LV apex is not seen; the apparent "apex" usually is an oblique image plane through the anterolateral wall.

A portion of the muscular *right ventricular outflow tract* is seen anteriorly. Unlike the symmetric prolate ellipsoid shape of the LV, the RV does not have an easily defined long or short axis. In effect, the RV is "wrapped around" the LV, with an inflow region, an apical region, and an outflow region forming a somewhat anteroposteriorly flattened U-shaped structure. Most standard image planes result in oblique tomographic sections of the RV, so right ventricular size and systolic function are best evaluated from multiple views or with 3D imaging, as discussed more fully in Chapter 6.

Right Ventricular Inflow and Outflow Views

In the long-axis plane, the transducer is moved apically and then angulated medially to obtain a view of the *right atrium, tricuspid valve,* and *right ventricle* (Fig. 2.7). In this RV inflow view, the septal and anterior leaflets of the tricuspid valve are well seen. The RV apex is heavily trabeculated, whereas the outflow tract (supracristal region) has a smoother endocardial surface. The moderator band, a prominent muscle trabeculation that traverses the RV apex obliquely and contains the right bundle branch, is seen in both parasternal and apical views (Fig. 2.8). The papillary muscles are more difficult to identify in the RV than in the LV. Typically, two principal papillary muscles (anterior and posterior) are seen, with a smaller supracristal (or conus) papillary muscle. The moderator band attaches near the base of the anterior RV papillary muscle.

The *coronary sinus* is identified as it enters the right atrium (RA) adjacent to the tricuspid annulus. By

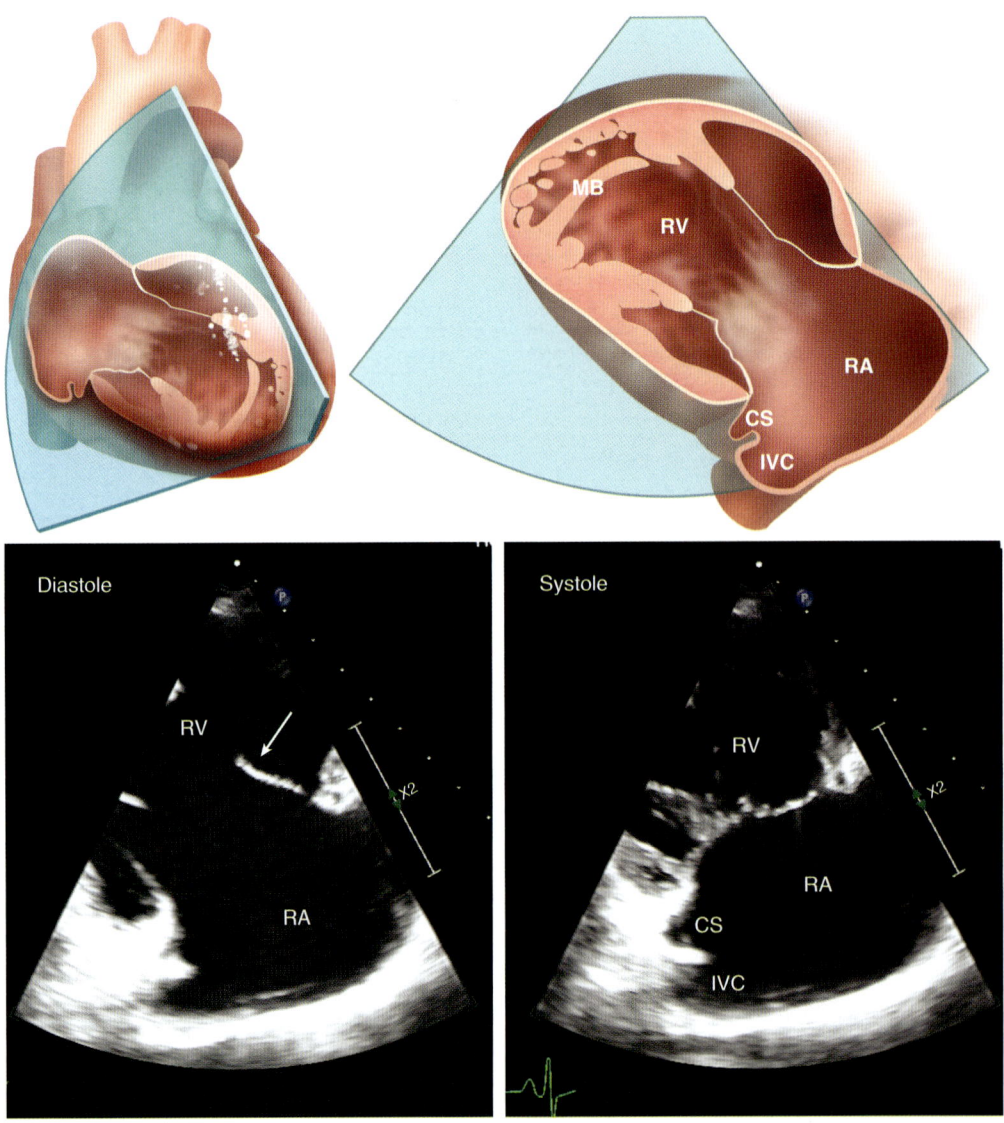

Fig. 2.7 **Right ventricular inflow view.** The position of the image plane is shown in the 3D heart *(top left)*, which is opened and rotated to the position corresponding to the echocardiographic image plane *(top right)*. 2D images in diastole *(bottom left)* and systole *(bottom right)* in the standard orientation show the RV and RA, tricuspid valve, and ostia of the coronary sinus *(CS)* and inferior vena cava *(IVC)*. In this view, two tricuspid leaflets are seen, typically the anterior *(arrow)* and septal leaflets, but the posterior leaflet may be seen depending on the exact image plane and individual variation. *MB,* Moderator band.

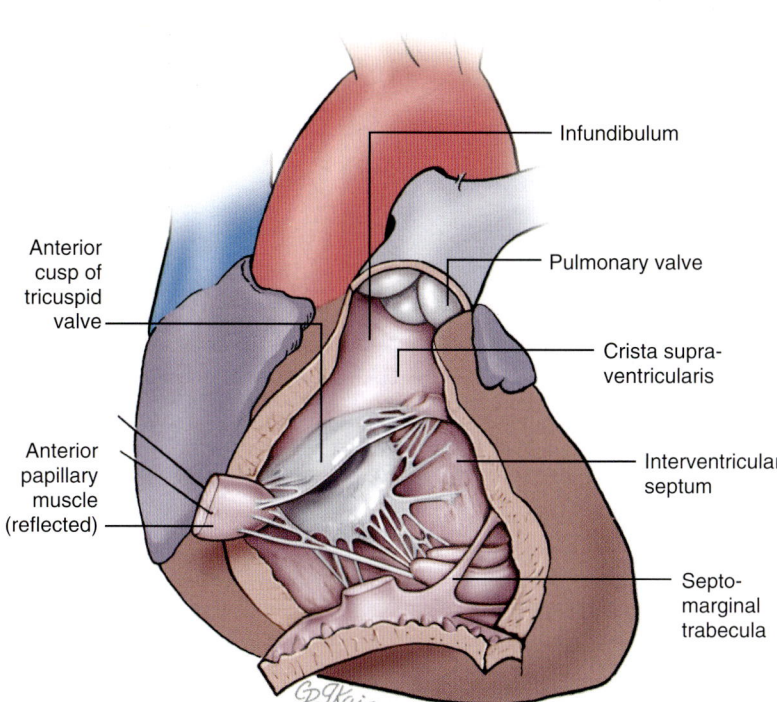

Fig. 2.8 Anatomy of the right ventricle. The crista supraventricularis separates the inflow part of the ventricle from the infundibulum, or conus arteriosus. Note the great distance between the septal leaflet of the tricuspid valve and the pulmonary valve. *(From Rosse C, Gaddum-Rosse P: Hollinshead's textbook of anatomy, ed 5, Philadelphia, 1997, Lippincott-Raven, p 473. Used with permission.)*

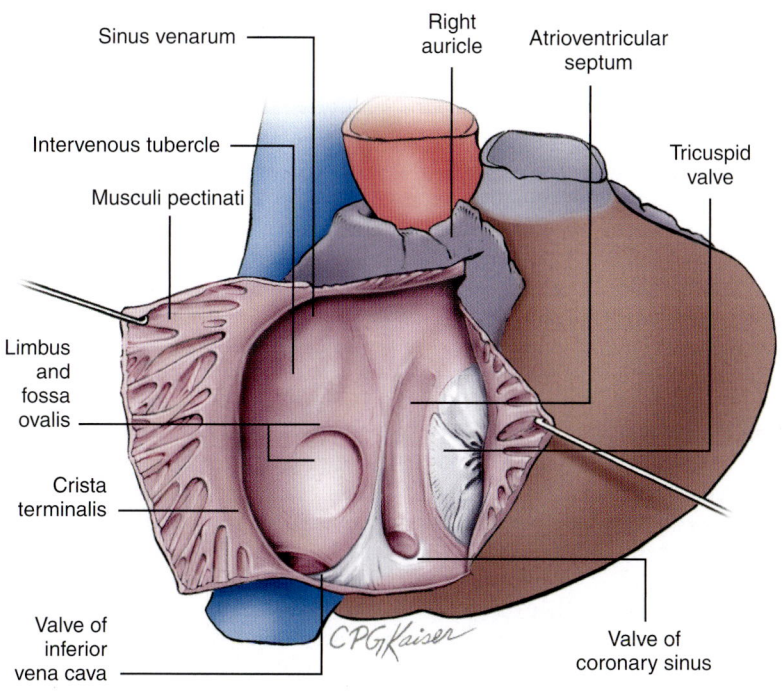

Fig. 2.9 Anatomy of the right atrium. The interior of the RA seen from the right side. The view is toward the interatrial septum. *(From Rosse C, Gaddum-Rosse P: Hollinshead's textbook of anatomy, ed 5, Philadelphia, 1997, Lippincott-Raven, p 473. Used with permission.)*

slowly scanning back to an LV long-axis view, the coronary sinus can be followed along its length.

Another normal anatomic feature of the RA (Fig. 2.9) is the *crista terminalis,* a muscular ridge that courses anteriorly from the superior vena cava to the inferior vena cava and divides the trabeculated anterior portion of the RA from the posterior, smooth-walled sinus venosus segment. The RA appendage is rarely seen on transthoracic imaging, but it is a trabeculated protrusion of the RA that extends anterior to the RA free wall and base of the aorta.

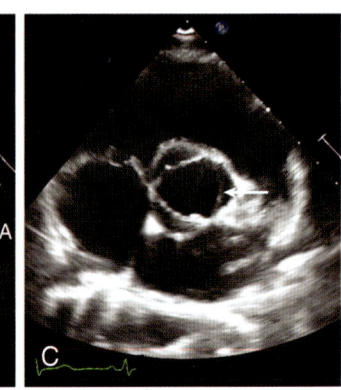

Fig. 2.10 ▶ **Aortic valve short-axis view.** (A) Parasternal short-axis view at the aortic valve level showing the relationship between the three cusps of the aortic valve—right coronary cusp *(R)*, noncoronary cusp *(N)*, left coronary cusp *(L)*—and the LA, RA, RV outflow tract *(RVOT)*, and pulmonary artery *(PA)*. The positions of the right coronary artery *(RCA)*, left main coronary artery *(LMCA)*, superior vena cava *(SVC)*, pulmonic valve *(PV)*, and tricuspid valve *(TV)* are shown. 2D echocardiographic images at the aortic valve level in (B) diastole and (C) systole. Note the three open leaflets of the aortic valve in systole. The left coronary cusp *(arrow)* can be difficult to visualize due to the parallel orientation of the open leaflet relative to the ultrasound beam. *LAA,* LA appendage.

The *inferior vena cava* is seen entering the RA inferior to the coronary sinus. In some individuals, a prominent Eustachian valve is seen at the junction of the inferior vena cava and RA both in this view and from the subcostal window. When a more extensive fenestrated valve is present, it forms a Chiari network extending from the inferior to the superior vena cava, attached to the crista terminalis posteriorly and the fossa ovalis medially, with a netlike structure that appears as bright mobile echo densities in the RA. Both these findings are considered normal variants.

The interatrial septum is not well seen in the RV inflow view, being just inferior and parallel to the image plane. However, careful angulation between the long-axis and RV inflow views allows examination of the atrial septum with recognition of the thick primum septum at its junction with the central fibrous body, the thin fossa ovalis in the central portion of the atrial septum, the ridge-like limbus located superior to the fossa, and the ridge adjacent to the junction with the coronary sinus.

Moving the transducer toward the base and then angulating laterally, a long-axis view of the RV outflow tract, *pulmonic valve,* and pulmonary artery is obtained. This view is particularly useful for recording flow velocities in the RV outflow tract and pulmonary artery.

Short-Axis Views

Short-axis views are obtained from the parasternal window by rotating the transducer clockwise 90° and then moving or angulating the transducer superiorly or inferiorly to obtain specific image planes.

At the *aortic valve* level (Fig. 2.10), the short-axis view demonstrates all three aortic valve leaflets: right, left, and noncoronary cusps. In systole, the aortic leaflets open to a near-circular orifice. In diastole, the typical Y-shaped arrangement of the coaptation lines of the leaflets is seen with three points of aortic attachment, or commissures. Identification of the number of aortic valve leaflets (or commissures) is made most accurately in systole because a bicuspid valve may appear trileaflet in diastole as a result of a raphe in the larger leaflet but the presence of only two commissures in systole. The normal valve leaflets are thin at the base with an area of thickening on the ventricular aspect in the middle of the free edge of each cusp that serves to fill the space at the center of the closed valve. These nodules normally enlarge with age (nodules of Arantius) and can have small, mobile filaments attached on the ventricular surface (Lambl excrescences). These small but normal structures may be seen when echocardiographic images are of high quality and should not be mistaken for pathologic conditions. The origins of the left main and right coronary arteries often can be identified in this view.

The aortic and pulmonic valve planes normally lie perpendicular to each other. Thus, when the aortic valve is seen in the short axis, the pulmonic valve is seen in the long axis. In adults, evaluation of the leaflets of the pulmonic valve is limited; usually only one or two leaflets are seen well, and a short-axis view often is not obtainable. The close relationship between the aortic valve and other intracardiac structures is apparent in this short-axis view (Fig. 2.11). The pulmonic valve and RV outflow tract are seen anterolaterally, adjacent to the left coronary cusp, and portions of the septal and anterior tricuspid valve leaflets are seen anteriorly and slightly medially, adjacent to the right coronary cusp. Posteriorly, the RA, interatrial septum, and LA lie in proximity to the noncoronary cusp of the aortic valve. The LA appendage can be better imaged from this view by a slight lateral angulation and a superior rotation of

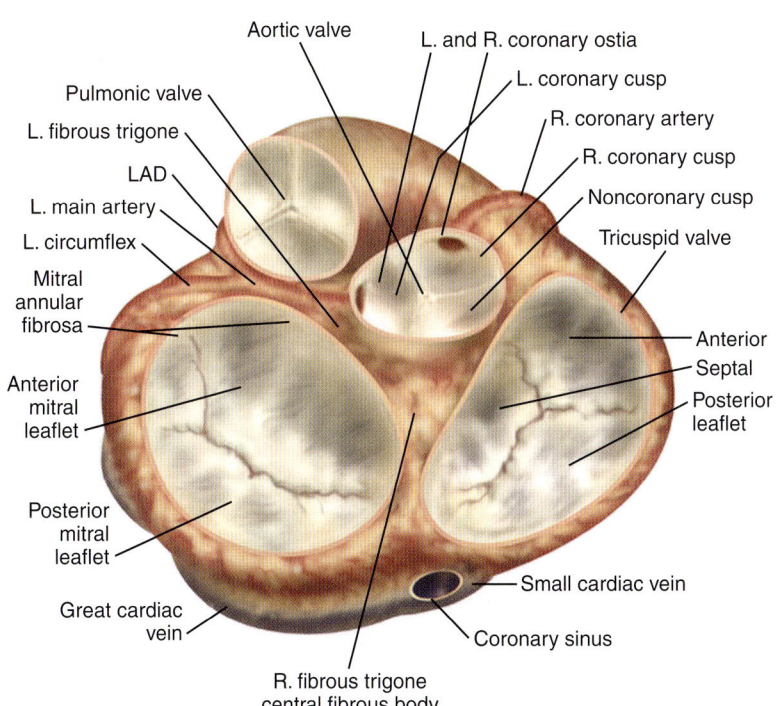

Fig. 2.11 **Anatomic valve relationships.** An anatomic view of the cardiac base looking toward the apex in a surgeon's view demonstrates the close relationships among the four cardiac valves. The aortic and pulmonic valve planes are perpendicular to each other. *L*, Left; *LAD*, left anterior descending coronary artery; *R*, right. *(From Otto CM: Echocardiographic evaluation of valvular heart disease. In Otto CM, Bonow R, editors:* Valvular Heart Disease: A Companion to Braunwald's Heart Disease, *ed 3, Philadelphia, 2009, Saunders.)*

the transducer. The central location of the aortic valve illustrates how disease processes can extend from the aortic valve or root into the RV outflow tract, RA, or LA. Extension of disease processes into the ventricular septum or anterior mitral leaflet also is possible, as evident in the long-axis view.

At the *mitral valve* short-axis level (Fig. 2.12), the thin anterior and posterior mitral leaflets are seen as they open nearly to the full cross-sectional area of the LV in diastole and close in systole. The posterior leaflet consists of three major scallops—lateral, central, and medial (also called P1, P2, and P3)—although considerable individual variability exists. The two mitral commissures (the points on the annulus where the anterior and posterior leaflets meet) are located medially and laterally. Note that this parallels the arrangement of the papillary muscles so that chordae from the medial aspects of both anterior and posterior leaflets attach to the medial (or posteromedial) papillary muscle, and chordae from the lateral aspects of both leaflets attach to the lateral (or anterolateral) papillary muscle. Chordae branch at three levels (primary, secondary, and tertiary) between the papillary muscle tip and mitral leaflet with a progressive decrease in chordal diameter and increase in the number of chordae from approximately 12 at the papillary muscle to 120 at the mitral leaflet. Most chordae attach at the free edge of the leaflets (called *marginal chordae*), but some (called *basal or strut chordae*) attach to the LV surface of the leaflet. Occasionally, aberrant chordae to the ventricular septum or other structures are seen in an otherwise normal individual.

At the mid-ventricular (or *papillary muscle*) level (Fig. 2.13), the normal LV is circular in the short-axis view. An elliptical appearance of the chamber usually is due to a nonperpendicular orientation relative to the long axis of the LV. Moving the transducer superiorly with apical angulation resolves this problem. In some normal individuals, the LV appears flattened along the diaphragm in diastole, but it has a normal circular appearance in systole. A noncircular appearance in systole is consistent with myocardial disease, such as myocardial infarction or aneurysm formation, or with abnormal septal curvature due to right heart disease. Although 2D linear measurements of LV diameter are made in the long-axis view, rotating the transducer between the long- and short-axis views at this level ensures that this measurement is both centered in the chamber and perpendicular to the long axis. Oblique measurements result in overestimation of wall thickness and ventricular dimensions.

This view also allows assessment of segmental endocardial motion and wall thickening at the mid-ventricular level. The nomenclature of LV myocardial segments is based on coronary anatomy as discussed in Chapter 8. Basically, the ventricle is divided into anterior (septum and free wall), anterolateral, inferolateral (also called posterior), and inferior (free wall and septum) segments for consistent descriptors of the location of abnormalities. The segments are further defined by their location along the length of the ventricle as basal, mid-ventricular, or apical. Ventricular septal motion reflects abnormalities other than

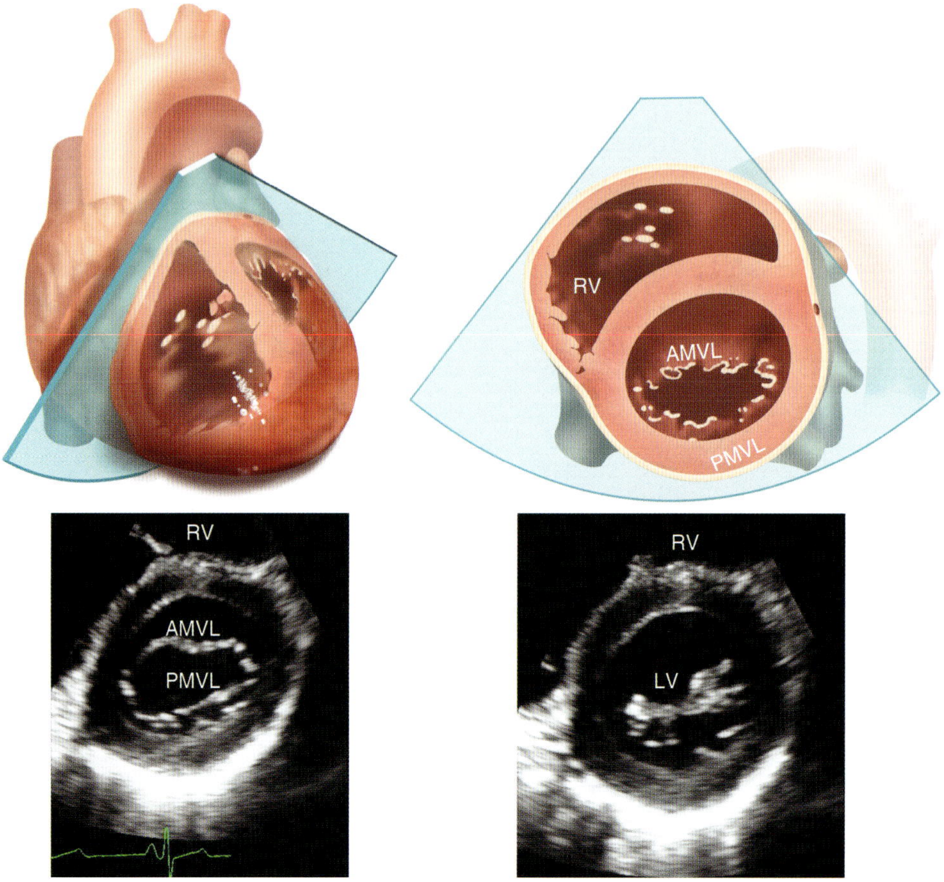

Fig. 2.12 ▶ **Short-axis plane at the mitral valve level.** The position of the image plane is shown in the 3D heart, which is opened and rotated to the position corresponding to the echocardiographic image plane. 2D images in diastole and systole in the standard orientation show the LV with the anterior and posterior mitral valve leaflets (*AMVL* and *PMVL*).

coronary disease, including RV volume overload, pressure overload, or both; conduction abnormalities; and the post–cardiac surgery state (see Fig. 6.22).

The medial and lateral papillary muscles are seen in this short-axis plane and serve as landmarks identifying the mid-ventricular level. Rarely, one of the papillary muscles is bifid, resulting in an appearance of three separate papillary muscles. Note that the apical segments of the LV myocardium are not seen in standard parasternal views. However, in some patients, a short-axis view of the LV near the apex can be obtained by moving the transducer laterally and angling medially. Alternatively, 3D volumetric imaging can be used to display multiple simultaneous short-axis views of the LV from base apex (see Chapter 4).

Apical Window

The apical window is identified initially by palpation of the LV apex with the patient in a steep left lateral decubitus position. An apical "cutout" in the examination stretcher allows optimal patient positioning and easier positioning of the transducer at the apical impulse. Transducer position then is adjusted as needed to obtain optimal images. The relationship between the three basic apical views and the short-axis plane is shown in Fig. 2.14.

Four-Chamber View

In the apical four-chamber view, the length of the *left ventricle* is seen in a plane perpendicular to both the short-axis and long-axis planes (Fig. 2.15). The anterolateral wall, apex, and inferior septum lie in this tomographic plane. The LV appears as a truncated ellipse with a longer length than width and a tapered but rounded apex. If the transducer is not positioned at the true apex, the LV will appear foreshortened, with a more spherical shape and little tapering of the apex. Foreshortening of the long-axis plane must be distinguished from disease processes, such as chronic aortic regurgitation, which result in increased sphericity of the ventricle. Although the RV is more trabeculated than the LV, prominent trabeculation also can be seen at the LV

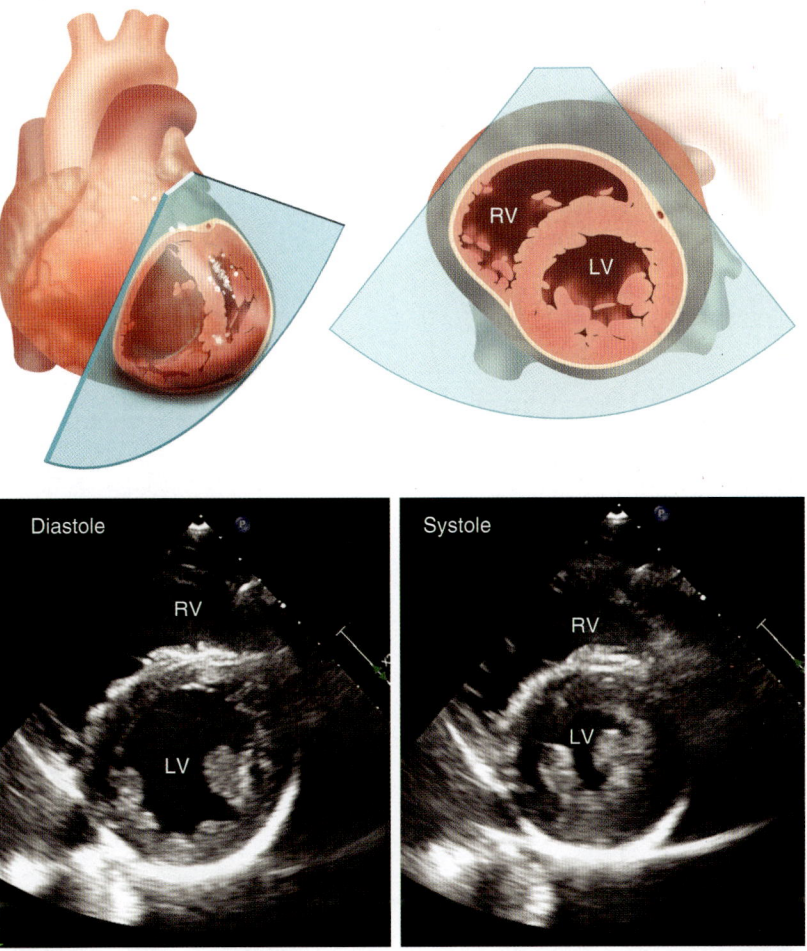

Fig. 2.13 ▶ **Short-axis plane at the papillary muscle level.** The position of the image plane is shown in the 3D heart, which is opened and rotated to the position corresponding to the echocardiographic image plane. 2D images in diastole and systole in the standard orientation demonstrate the circular shape of the LV with symmetric wall thickening and inward endocardial motion with contraction.

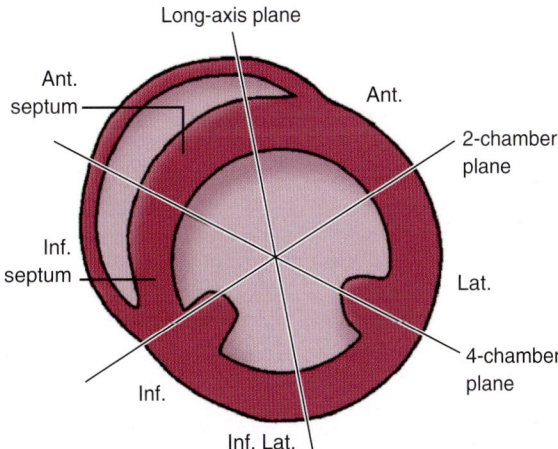

Fig. 2.14 Apical image planes. The apical image planes are perpendicular to the short-axis plane with the lines on this diagram indicating the locations of the four-chamber, two-chamber, and aortic long-axis image plane, each about 60° apart, along with the LV wall segments intersected by each image plane. *Ant.*, anterior; *Inf.*, inferior; *Lat.*, lateral.

apex and must be distinguished from apical thrombus. An aberrant LV trabecula that traverses the ventricular chamber is an incidental finding, often called an LV "chord."

Medially, the *right ventricle* is triangular with a cavity about half the area of the LV. The RV apex is less round and more basal than the LV apex, and the moderator band traverses the RV chamber near the apex. The RV can be further evaluated by moving the transducer medially over the RV apex. Considerable individual variability in the shape and wall motion of the RV, particularly at the apex, is seen in normal individuals, so caution is needed in diagnosing an abnormal RV from any single tomographic plane.

The four-chamber view also shows the mitral annulus in its major dimension and the anterior (located adjacent to the septum) and posterior (adjacent to the lateral wall) mitral valve leaflets, along with chordal attachments to the lateral papillary muscle. The mitral leaflet tips separate widely in diastole. In systole the closure plane of the leaflets may appear

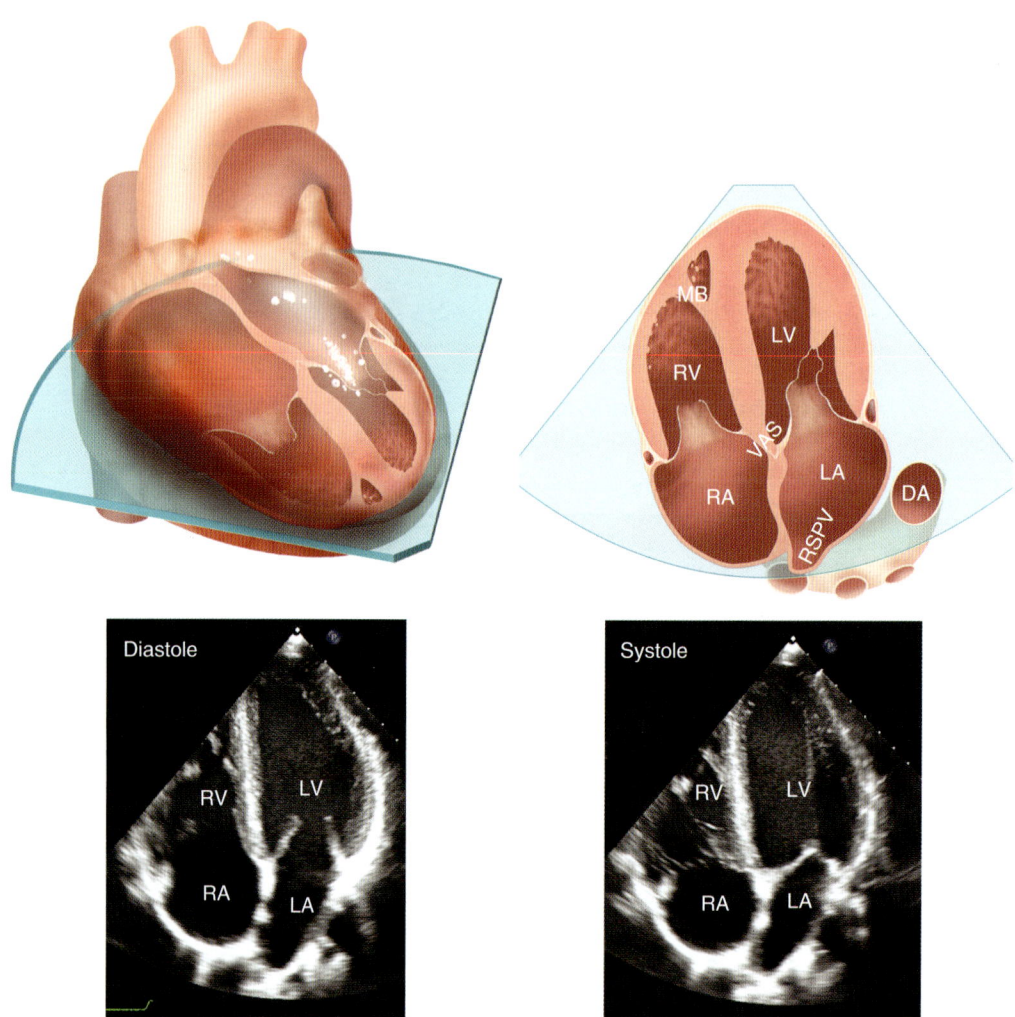

Fig. 2.15 ▶ **Apical four-chamber view.** The four-chamber view is obtained with the transducer on the LV apex and shows the relationships of the LV and RV and LA and RA in the intact heart *(upper left)*. The 2D image plane is oriented with the transducer position at the top of the image *(upper right)*. In the LV, the papillary muscle, chordae, and anterior and posterior mitral leaflets are seen. The descending aorta *(DA)* is seen in partial cross section lateral to the left atrium, and the right superior pulmonary vein *(RSPV)* drains into the LA adjacent to the interatrial septum. In the RV, the moderator band *(MB)* and the anterior and septal tricuspid valve leaflets are seen. Note the ventriculoatrial septum *(VAS)* separating the LV from the RA in association with the normal, slightly more apical position of the tricuspid compared with the mitral valve annulus. 2D echo images in an apical four-chamber view at end-diastole and end-systole are shown *(bottom)*.

"flat" (a 180° closure angle) because of the nonplanar "saddle" shape of the annulus, with the four-chamber view bisecting the annulus at its most apical position compared with the more basal annulus segments seen in a long-axis view.

The tricuspid annulus lies slightly (up to 1.0 cm) closer to the apex than the mitral annulus. The tricuspid leaflets show a wide diastolic opening; thin, uniformly echogenic, leaflets; and normal coaptation in systole. The septal leaflet is imaged adjacent to the septum. The tricuspid leaflet adjacent to the free wall may be either the anterior or posterior leaflet, depending on the exact rotation and angulation of the image plane.

The *left and right atria* are distal from the apical transducer position. Apical views are useful for measurement of LA volume (Fig. 2.16), but ultrasound resolution at this depth is poor, so detailed evaluation of atrial tumors or exclusion of thrombus typically requires TEE imaging. The interatrial septum lies parallel to the ultrasound beam in this view, so "dropout"—absence of reflected signal—from the region of the fossa ovalis is common and should not be mistaken for an atrial septal defect. The descending thoracic aorta is seen lateral to the LA. The pulmonary veins enter the LA posteriorly but are difficult to image at this depth in adults. If the transducer is angulated posteriorly from the four-chamber view, more posterior portions of the lateral and inferior septal myocardium are seen. In addition, the length of the coronary sinus comes into view in the atrioventricular groove.

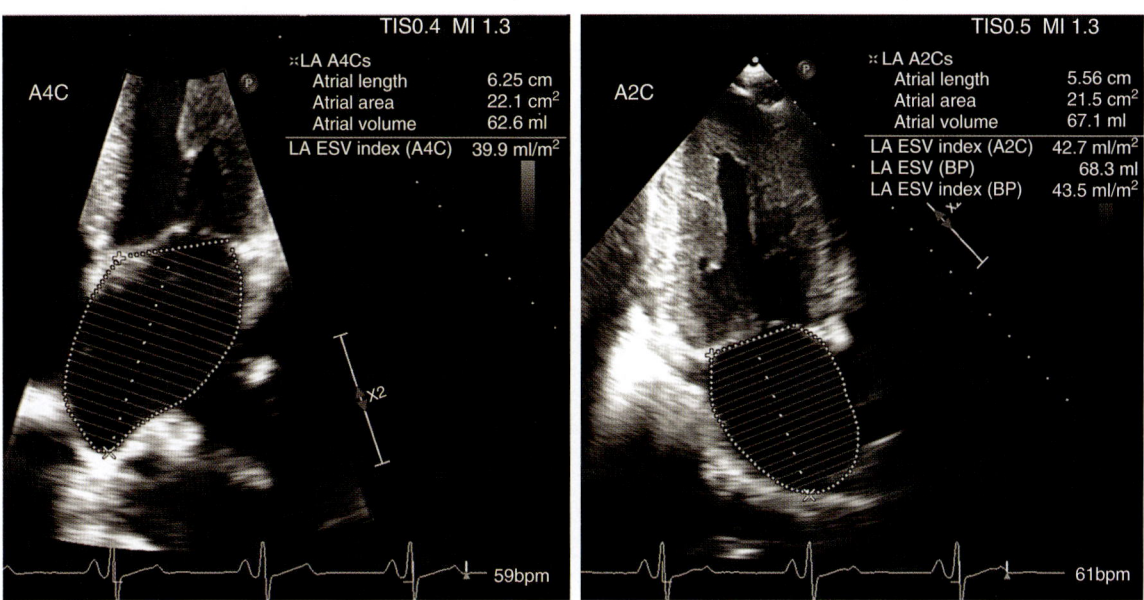

Fig. 2.16 Left atrial volume measurement. LA area is traced in systole in the apical four-chamber *(A4C)* and apical two-chamber *(A2C)* views for measurement of length, area, and volume. The biplane *(BP)* end-systolic volume *(ESV)* and indexed ESV are calculated from the two atrial tracings.

By angulating the transducer anteriorly, the aortic valve and root are seen in an oblique long view. This view is sometimes referred to as the apical "five-chamber" view. More anterior portions of the septum and lateral wall are seen, especially at the base, as the transducer is angulated anteriorly. This view of the anterior mitral leaflet, LV outflow tract, and aortic valve is at an angle approximately 60° to 90° from the long-axis view. In some adults, further anterior angulation of the transducer allows visualization of the pulmonary artery arising from the RV. A view of the pulmonic valve from the apical window is more easily obtained in young adults and children.

Two-Chamber View

From the four-chamber view, the transducer is rotated counterclockwise about 60° to obtain the two-chamber view of the LV, mitral valve, and LA (Fig. 2.17). The apical two-chamber view is used for evaluation of the anterior LV wall (seen to the right of the screen) and the inferolateral (posterior) wall (seen on the left). Fine adjustments in transducer position may be needed to visualize the anterior wall endocardium because of interference from adjacent lung tissue. To ensure that the proper rotation has been made for a two-chamber view, the transducer is angled posteriorly to intersect both papillary muscles symmetrically. Then the transducer is angled slightly anteriorly so that neither papillary muscle is seen in its long axis in this view. The anterior mitral leaflet is seen en face, so the apparent closure plane of the leaflet relative to the annulus can be misleading. The LA appendage may be visualized adjacent to the anterior wall. A long-axis view of the descending thoracic aorta can be obtained by angulating posteriorly and rotating counterclockwise from the two-chamber view.

Long-Axis View

Rotating the transducer another 60° from the two-chamber view (120° from the four-chamber view) yields a long-axis view similar to the parasternal long-axis view (Fig. 2.18). The aortic valve, LV outflow tract, and mitral valve are seen in long axis. The LV walls visualized in this view are the anterior septum (on the right side of the screen) and posterior or inferolateral wall (on the left). Compared with the parasternal long-axis view, the LV apex now is seen, but the aortic and mitral valves are at a greater image depth (with consequent poorer image resolution).

Other Apical Views

Nonstandard short-axis views of the LV apex that use a higher-frequency transducer (5 or 7.5 MHz) are helpful if an LV apical thrombus is suspected. One useful view is obtained by sliding the transducer laterally from the LV apex and then angulating medially.

Subcostal Window

With the patient supine and the legs bent at the knees (if necessary) to relax the abdominal wall

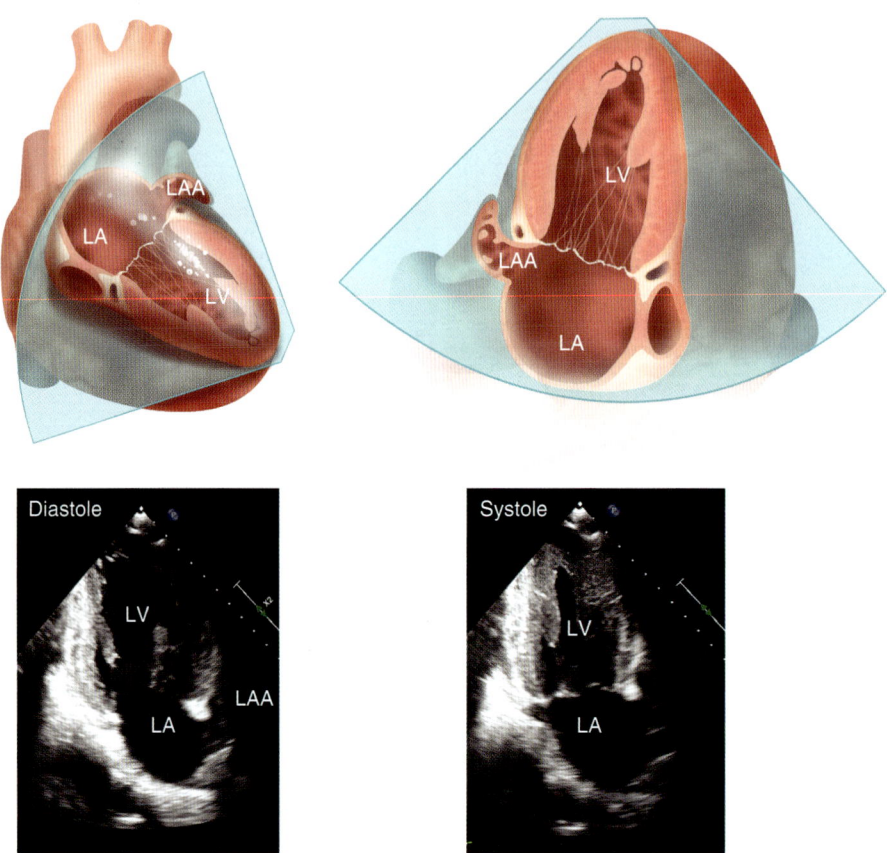

Fig. 2.17 **Apical two-chamber view.** The position of the image plane is shown in the 3D heart, which is opened and rotated to the position corresponding to the echocardiographic image plane. 2D images in diastole and systole in the standard orientation show the cross section of the LA and ventricle with the LA appendage *(LAA)*, coronary sinus in the atrioventricular groove, and mitral valve. In the two-chamber view, small portions of the posterior mitral leaflet are seen laterally and medially with the anterior leaflet filling most of the annulus area. Part of a papillary muscle has been shown for orientation, but the papillary muscles are seen located symmetrically posterior to the image plane. In this view, the inferior and anterior LV walls are seen. Corresponding 2D images in diastole and systole are shown.

musculature, subcostal images of the cardiac structures are obtained. A view of all four chambers shows the RV free wall, the mid-section of the interventricular septum, and the anterolateral LV wall (Fig. 2.19). In this view, the interatrial septum is perpendicular to the direction of the ultrasound beam, thereby allowing evaluation of atrial septal defects.

A subcostal short-axis view of the LV allows measurements of LV wall thickness and dimensions that are comparable with dimensions obtained from a parasternal short-axis view, albeit at a greater depth and through different myocardial segments. The subcostal window provides a useful alternative for qualitative and quantitative evaluation of the LV when the parasternal window is inadequate.

Rotating the transducer inferiorly from the subcostal four-chamber view, a long-axis view of the inferior vena cava is obtained as it enters the RA (see Fig. 6.26). The size of the inferior vena cava (1–2 cm from the RA junction) at rest and changes in size with respiration are used to estimate RA pressure (see Table 6.9). The hepatic veins (particularly the central hepatic vein, which courses parallel to the ultrasound beam in this view) are helpful in assessing RA pressure and for recording RA Doppler filling patterns. The proximal abdominal aorta is imaged in the long axis medial to the inferior vena cava.

Suprasternal Notch Window

With the patient supine and the neck extended, the transducer is positioned in the suprasternal notch or right supraclavicular position to obtain a view of the aortic arch in long- and short-axis views. The long-axis view (with respect to the aortic arch) shows the

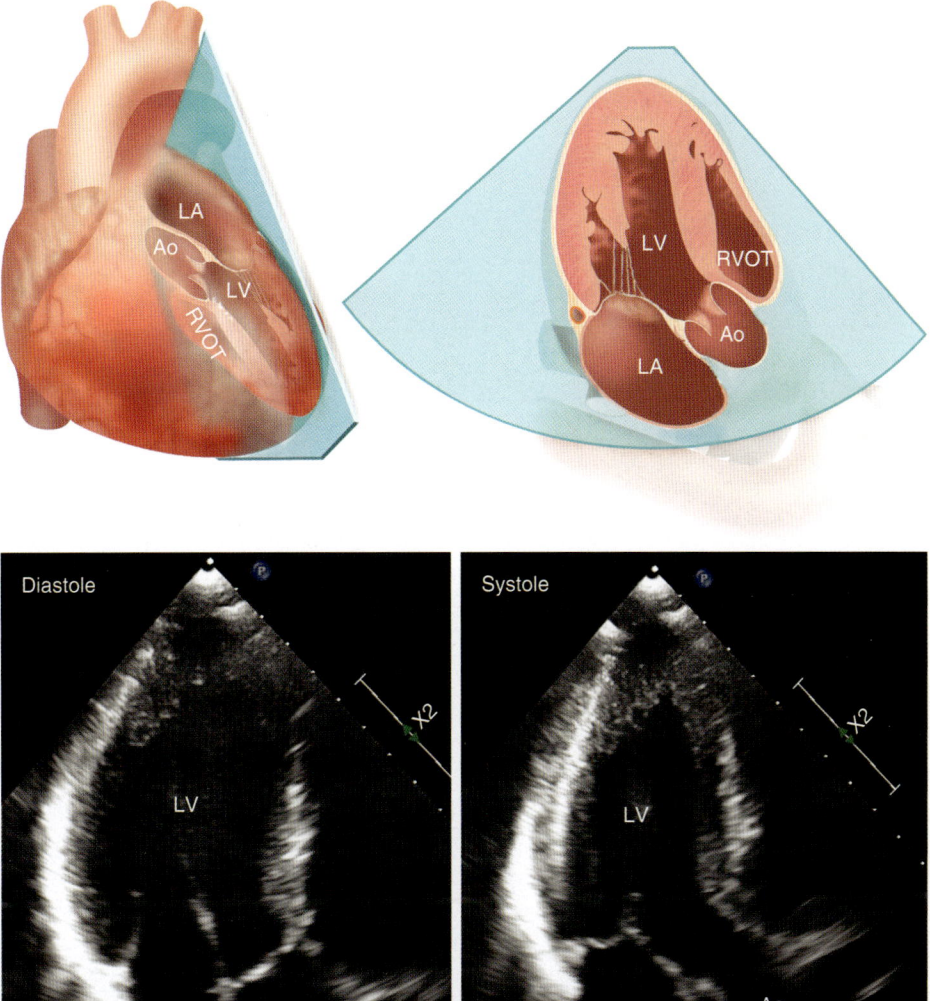

Fig. 2.18 ▶ **Apical long-axis view.** The position of the image plane is shown in the 3D heart, which is opened and rotated to the position corresponding to the echocardiographic image plane. In this view, the anterior septal and posterior (inferolateral) LV walls are seen. *Ao,* Aorta; *RVOT,* RV outflow tract.

ascending aorta, arch, proximal descending thoracic aorta, and the origins of the right brachiocephalic and left common carotid and subclavian arteries (Fig. 2.20). The corresponding veins lie superior to the aortic arch, with the superior vena cava lying adjacent to the ascending aorta. The right pulmonary artery is seen "under" the curve of the aortic arch and can be followed to its branch point by rotating the transducer medially.

The short-axis view shows the aortic arch in cross section. The left pulmonary artery can be imaged by rotating slightly laterally. The LA lies inferior to the pulmonary arteries in both long- and short-axis views, so it is occasionally possible to evaluate atrial pathology or flow disturbances from this window.

Other Acoustic Windows

In specific cases, other acoustic windows are needed. For example, a dextropositioned heart would necessitate mirror-image acoustic windows. When a large pleural effusion is present, good-quality images may be obtained in some cases by imaging from the posterior chest wall through the effusion with the patient in a sitting position.

M-MODE RECORDINGS

Although M-mode recordings have largely been replaced by 2D or 3D imaging, M-mode recordings

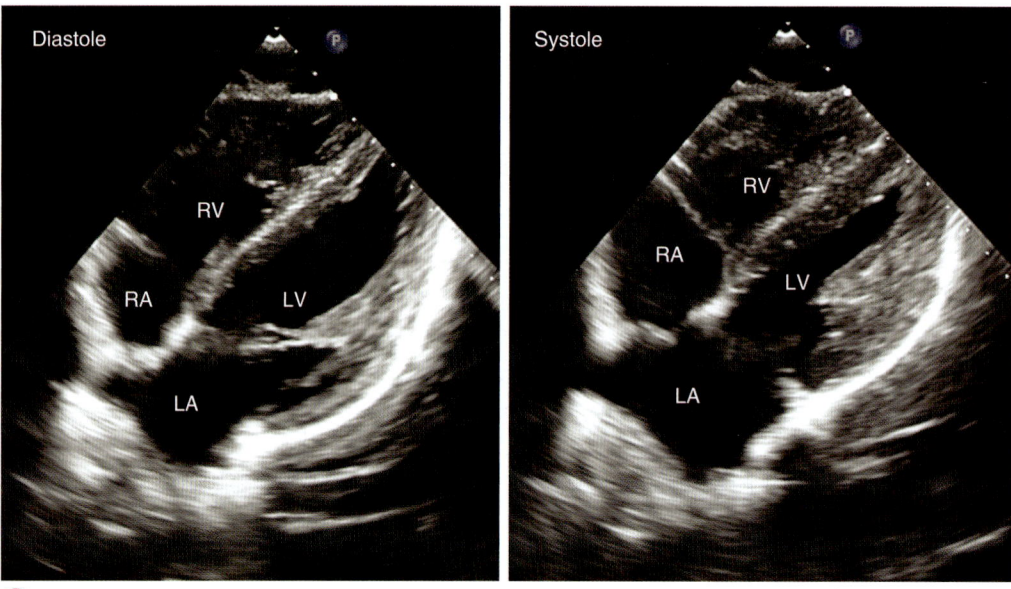

Fig. 2.19 ▶ **Subcostal four-chamber view.** The position of the image plane is shown in the 3D heart, which is opened and rotated to the position corresponding to the echocardiographic image plane. The interatrial septum is perpendicular to the ultrasound beam from this window, thus allowing evaluation for atrial septal defects.

still have an important role in evaluation of rapid motion of cardiac structures because the sampling rate is 1800 frames per second rather than the 30 to 60 frames per second used for 2D or 3D imaging. The rapid sampling rate also makes identification of thin moving structures, such as the LV endocardium, more accurate and reproducible by showing motion as well as depth of the structure of interest. The potential disadvantage of M-mode data, a nonperpendicular orientation to the structure of interest, can be avoided by using the 2D image in two orthogonal planes to position the M-mode sampling line.

Use of the M-mode feature is most helpful when guided by the 2D image and used for:

- Timing of rapid cardiac motions
- Precise measurements of cardiac dimensions
- Further evaluation of structures seen on 2D imaging (e.g., suspected vegetations) to aid in their identification

Aortic Valve and Left Atrium

An M-mode recording through the aortic root at the leaflet tip level shows the parallel walls of the aorta

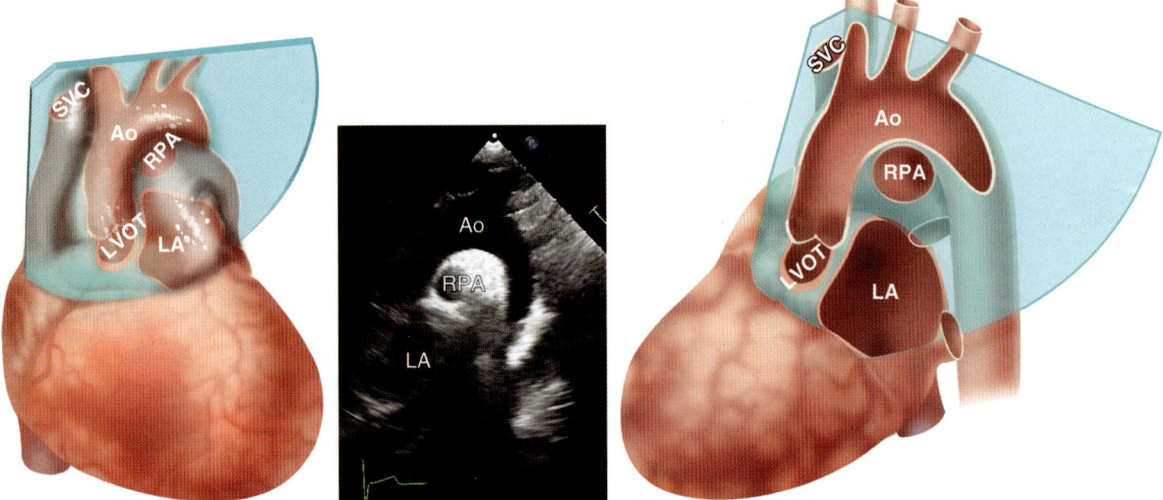

Fig. 2.20 ▶ **Suprasternal notch view.** The position of the image plane is shown in the 3D heart, which is opened and rotated to the position corresponding to the echocardiographic image plane. 2D and color Doppler views show the ascending aorta *(Ao)*, arch, and proximal descending aorta with the origins of the left carotid and subclavian arteries. The right pulmonary artery *(RPA)* lies immediately inferior to the arch, with the LA and aortic valve sometimes seen from this window. *LVOT,* LV outflow tract; *SVC,* superior vena cava.

moving anteriorly in systole and posteriorly in diastole (Fig. 2.21). The LA is posterior to the aortic root and shows filling in atrial diastole (ventricular systole) and emptying in atrial systole (ventricular diastole). LA filling is largely responsible for the anterior displacement of the aortic root, so aortic root "motion" on an M-mode recording reflects variations in LA size. Increased aortic root motion is seen with increased LA filling and emptying (e.g., with mitral regurgitation). Decreased aortic root motion is seen in low cardiac output states, with corresponding low volumes of atrial filling and emptying.

The aortic leaflet coaptation point is seen as a thin line in diastole. In systole, the leaflets separate rapidly and completely, forming a boxlike appearance on the M-mode recording. Fine systolic fluttering of the aortic valve leaflets is seen in normal individuals.

Mitral Valve

An M-mode recording at the mitral valve level intercepts the anterior RV wall and chamber, the interventricular septum, the anterior and posterior mitral leaflets, the posterior LV wall, and the pericardium (Fig. 2.22). The coaptation point of the mitral leaflets in systole is seen as a thin line that moves slightly anteriorly during systole and parallels the motion of the posterior wall. In early diastole, the leaflets separate widely, with the maximum early-diastolic motion of the anterior leaflet termed the *E-point.* Normally, only a small distance is present between the E-point and the maximal posterior motion of the ventricular septum—E-point septal separation (EPSS). In the absence of mitral stenosis, an increased EPSS indicates LV dilation, systolic dysfunction, or aortic regurgitation.

The leaflets move toward each other in mid-diastole (diastasis) and then separate again with atrial systole, thus resulting in the late-diastolic peak, the *A point.* The slope of anterior mitral leaflet closure from *A* to the closure point *(C)* is linear unless LV end-diastolic pressure is elevated, when a "*B* bump" or "*A-C* shoulder" may be seen on the M-mode recording of mitral valve motion. Fine fluttering of the anterior mitral leaflet is not seen in normal individuals and usually indicates aortic regurgitation.

Left Ventricle

A 2D-guided M-mode recording perpendicular to the long axis of and through the center of the LV at the papillary muscle level provides standard measurements of systolic and diastolic wall thickness and chamber dimensions (Fig. 2.23). These measurements are limited in that they represent only a single line through the LV and thus do not accurately describe the LV when the disease process is asymmetric, such as with prior myocardial infarction. However, many disease processes do result in symmetric changes in the LV (volume overload, hypertrophy), and the accuracy and reproducibility of these measurements make them useful in clinical trials and in patient management. Examples of their utility include sequential evaluations of LV end-systolic dimension in patients with chronic valve regurgitation and assessment of LV hypertrophy in hypertensive patients.

The posterior wall endocardium is identified as the continuous line with the steepest upslope in early systole, but care must be taken to distinguish the

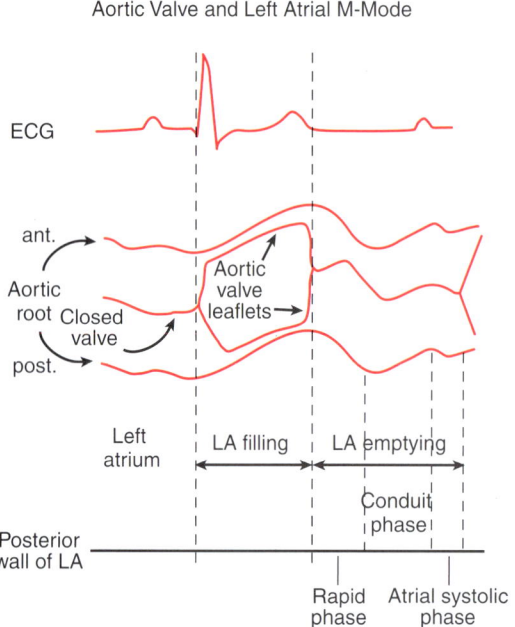

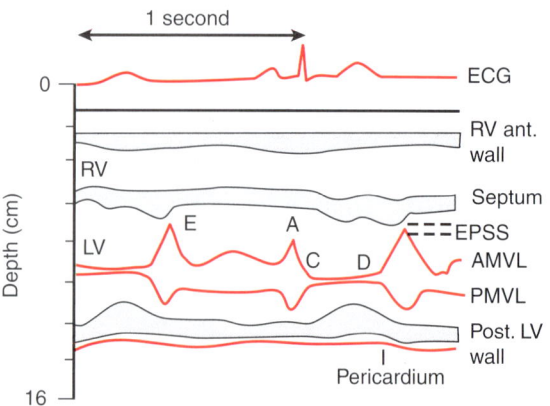

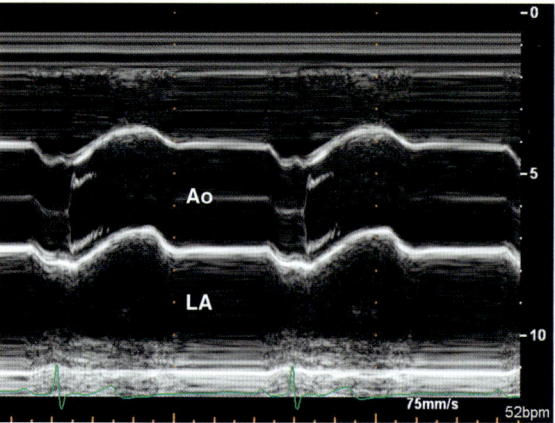

Fig. 2.21 Aortic valve M-mode recording. Schematic *(top)* and M-mode tracing *(bottom)* of a normal aortic valve and LA. *ant.,* Anterior; *Ao,* aorta; *ECG,* electrocardiogram; *post.,* posterior.

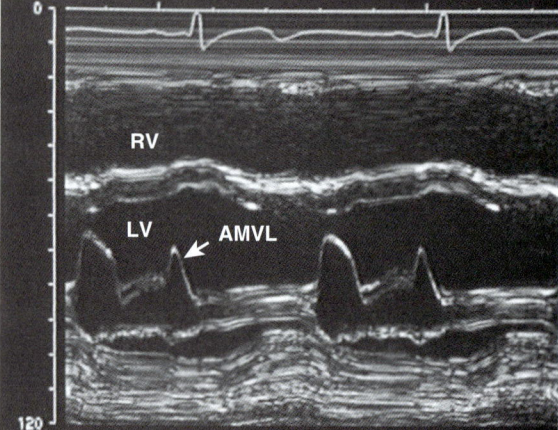

Fig. 2.22 Mitral valve M-mode recording. Schematic *(top)* and M-mode tracing *(bottom)* of a normal mitral valve. *AMVL,* anterior mitral valve leaflet; *ant.,* anterior; *ECG,* electrocardiogram; *EPSS,* E-point septal separation; *PMVL,* posterior mitral valve leaflet; *Post.,* posterior.

endocardium from reflections caused by overlying mitral chordal structures. Similarly, the endocardium of the septum is identified as a continuous line with systolic inward motion. Measurements are made from the leading edge of the septal endocardial echo to the leading edge of the posterior wall endocardium.

An M-mode recording at this level also is helpful in timing the motion of the RV free wall when cardiac tamponade is suspected or for detection of a small posterior pericardial effusion.

Other M-Mode Recordings

An M-mode recording through the pulmonic valve is similar to an aortic valve M-mode recording, except that usually only one leaflet can be recorded in adults. The slight displacement of the leaflet in diastole (after atrial contraction), called the *A*-wave, is increased (>7 mm) when pulmonic stenosis is present and is decreased (<2 mm) when pulmonary hypertension is present. Transient mid-systolic closure (or "notching") of the pulmonic valve on M-mode is seen when pulmonary hypertension is present (Fig. 2.24). Tricuspid annular plane systolic excursion (TAPSE) measured on an apical M-mode recording is useful for evaluation of RV systolic function (see Chapter 6).

NORMAL INTRACARDIAC FLOW PATTERNS

Basic Principles
Laminar Versus Disturbed Flow

Normal intracardiac flow patterns are characterized by laminar flow. *Laminar flow* is defined as movement of fluid

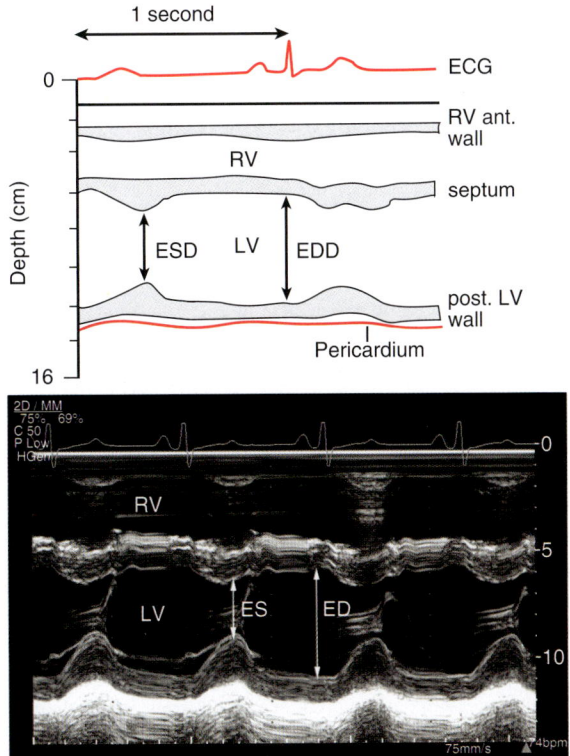

Fig. 2.23 Left ventricular M-mode recording. Schematic *(top)* and M-mode tracing *(bottom)* at the LV papillary muscle level. Accurate measurements require a perpendicular orientation between the M-line and the LV long axis, centered in the LV chamber. *ant.,* Anterior; *ED,* end-diastole; *EDD,* End-diastolic dimension; *ES,* end-systole; *ESD,* end-systolic dimension; *post.,* posterior.

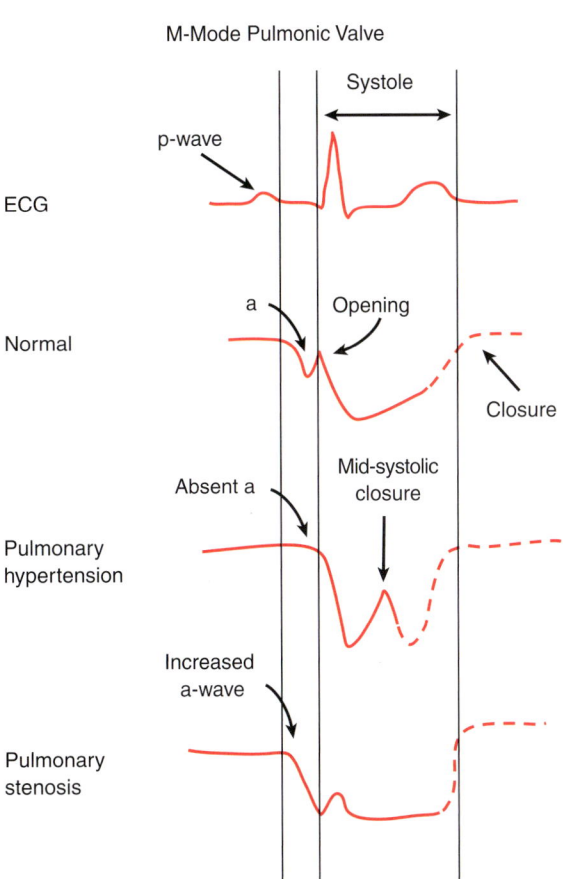

Fig. 2.24 Patterns of pulmonic valve motion. Examples of pulmonic valve M-mode tracings for several clinical conditions. Normal pulmonic valve motion is similar to aortic valve motion, but only one leaflet is seen, with slower rates of leaflet opening and closure. *ECG,* Electrocardiogram.

along well-defined parallel stream lines with uniform flow velocities (Fig. 2.25). In three dimensions, laminar flow consists of concentric layers (or lamina) of flow, each with a predictable and uniform direction and velocity.

Steady laminar flow becomes disturbed when the dimensionless Reynolds number exceeds 2000 to 2500. The Reynolds number (R_e) is directly related to blood flow velocity V, lumen diameter d, and blood density ρ and inversely related to viscosity γ:

$$Re = (Vd\rho)/\gamma \quad \text{(Eq. 2.1)}$$

When blood flow patterns are disturbed, blood cells move in multiple directions at multiple velocities, rather than along uniform, parallel stream lines. *Turbulence*, in fluid dynamic terms, refers to the specific situation in which the flow pattern of a particular fluid element is no longer predictable. Although intracardiac flow disturbances rarely exhibit true turbulence, this term is used clinically to denote nonlaminar flow.

Flow-Velocity Profiles

The spatial distribution of velocities in cross section at a specific intracardiac location and at a specific time point in the cardiac cycle is known as the *flow-velocity profile* (Fig. 2.26). If all the parallel stream lines in a laminar flow pattern have the same velocity, then the flow-velocity profile is "flat." If velocity is higher in the center of the vessel and lower at the walls of the vessel, the flow profile is "curved" (usually parabolic). Although normal flow in peripheral vessels has a curved flow-velocity profile, many intracardiac flows have a relatively flat flow-velocity profile. Factors that tend to equalize the velocity distribution across the cross-sectional area of flow include anatomic tapering of the flow area, acceleration of flow, and inlet-type geometry (e.g., an abrupt transition from a large chamber to a smaller orifice). Thus, the proximal aorta and pulmonary artery and the mitral and tricuspid annuli have reasonably flat flow-velocity profiles at their inlets. Downstream, the spatial distribution changes; for example, in the ascending aorta, the flow profile is asymmetric, with higher flow velocities along the inside curve of the aortic arch and lower velocities along the outer curve. Many Doppler quantitative methods make assumptions about

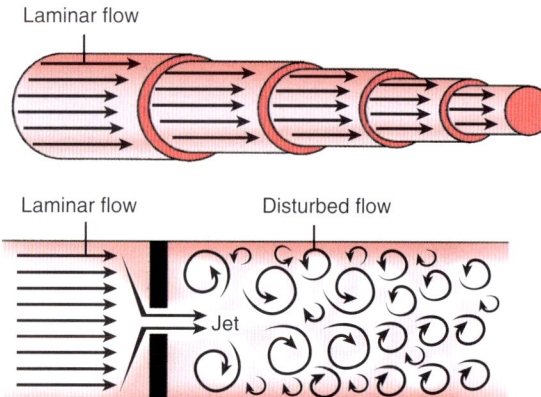

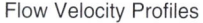

Fig. 2.25 **Intracardiac blood flow patterns.** Laminar flow is characterized by parallel stream lines at uniform velocities with concentric layers of flow, each with a predictable and uniform direction and velocity *(top)*. Disturbed flow occurs downstream from areas of narrowing (stenotic orifice, regurgitant orifice, or intracardiac shunt) with blood flow in multiple directions and velocities *(bottom)*. In the orifice itself, a laminar high-velocity jet occurs.

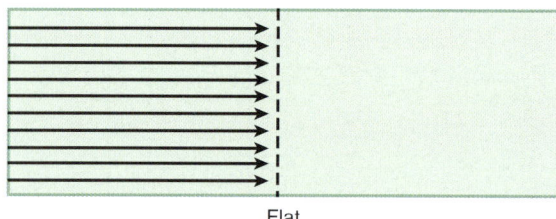

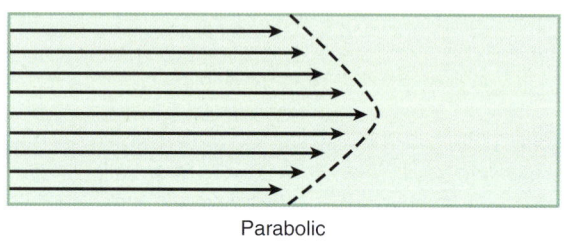

Fig. 2.26 **Flow-velocity profiles.** In a schematic longitudinal cross section of a flow stream, with the length of each arrow proportional to velocity, the difference between a flat *(top)* and a parabolic *(bottom)* flow-velocity profile is shown.

- Measurement of volume flow in Chapter 6
- The relationship between velocity and pressure gradients in Chapter 11
- The spatial flow pattern through a small orifice (e.g., regurgitant valve) in Chapter 12

Measurement of Volume Flow

Doppler echocardiography allows accurate measurement of the volume of blood ejected by the heart on each beat or of the amount of blood passing across each cardiac valve. This method is used clinically to measure stroke volume and cardiac output at rest or after physiologic or pharmacologic interventions, to evaluate the severity of valvular regurgitation, as a component in the equation for valve area calculations, and to quantitate the ratio of pulmonary to systemic blood flow in patients with intracardiac shunts.

ECHO MATH: Measurement of Volume Flow

When blood flow is laminar with a flat flow-velocity profile, it is intuitive that the instantaneous flow rate can be calculated as cross-sectional area, or CSA (in cm^2), times flow velocity (in cm/s). Thus, by integrating flow velocity over the duration of flow, stroke volume, or SV (in cm^3), can be calculated as:

$$SV\,(\text{cm}^3) = CSA\,(\text{cm}^2) \times VTI\,(\text{cm}) \quad \text{(Eq. 2.2)}$$

where VTI is the velocity-time integral (cm) of the Doppler velocity curve.

For example, if the LV outflow tract diameter is 2.4 cm and we assume a circular CSA (πr^2) and the VTI of flow at that site is 18 cm, then volume flow rate is calculated as:

$$SV = 3.14\,(1.2\,\text{cm})^2 \times 18\,\text{cm} = 81\,\text{cm}^3 = 81\,\text{mL}$$

If heart rate *(HR)* is 80 beats per minute, cardiac output *(CO)* then is:

$$CO = SV \times HR = 81\,\text{mL} \times 80 = 6480\,\text{mL/min}$$
$$= 6.48\,\text{L/min}$$

the spatial flow profile at a particular intracardiac site. In some cases, these assumptions can be verified by careful pulsed or color Doppler evaluation.

Clinical Quantitative Doppler Methods

Three basic principles are common to the clinical use of Doppler ultrasound in evaluation of cardiac disease. These are presented briefly here and in more detail, including technical aspects and potential pitfalls, in subsequent chapters, as follows:

Velocity-Pressure Relationships

At any area of significant narrowing in the flowstream—whether a stenotic valve, a ventricular septal defect, or a regurgitant orifice—flow velocity increases in relation to the degree of narrowing; the narrower the opening, the faster is the velocity for a given volume flow rate. This relationship between pressure gradient and velocity is important for quantitation of valve stenosis severity, noninvasive determination of pulmonary artery pressures, and evaluation of other intracardiac hemodynamics using continuous-wave (CW) Doppler ultrasound.

ECHO MATH: Velocity-Pressure Relationships

In most clinical situations, the velocity in a high-velocity "jet" through a narrowed orifice is related quantitatively to the pressure gradient across the narrowing, as stated in the simplified Bernoulli equation:

$$\Delta P = 4v^2 \quad \text{(Eq. 2.3)}$$

where ΔP is the instantaneous pressure gradient (mmHg) and v is the instantaneous velocity (m/s) and the number 4 converts from units of velocity (m/s) to pressure (mmHg).

For example, if the velocity across a narrowed aortic valve is 5 m/s, then the maximum pressure gradient is:

$$\Delta P = 4\,(5)^2 = 100 \text{ mmHg}$$

TABLE 2.4 Transthoracic Views for Normal Antegrade Flow Velocities

Antegrade Flow	View
LV outflow tract	Apical 4-chamber (angulated anterior) Apical long-axis
Aorta (ascending)	LV-apex SSN
Descending aorta • (Thoracic) • (Proximal abdominal)	SSN Subcostal
LV inflow (mitral)	Apical 4-chamber or long-axis
RV outflow tract	Parasternal short-axis (aortic valve level) Subcostal short-axis
RV inflow (tricuspid)	RV inflow Apical 4-chamber
LA inflow (pulmonary vein)	Apical 4-chamber
RA inflow	Subcostal (central hepatic vein) SSN (superior vena cava)

SSN, Suprasternal notch.

Spatial Pattern of Flow

Flow through a small orifice is characterized by a:

- Proximal flow convergence region
- Narrow flowstream through the orifice, called the vena contracta
- Downstream flow disturbance

Each of these components of the spatial flow pattern can be evaluated with color flow imaging, which allows real-time demonstrations of flow patterns in each tomographic plane (e.g., with valve regurgitation). The proximal flow convergence region allows calculation of volume flow rates. The vena contracta provides a simple measure of regurgitant severity. The downstream flow disturbance allows detection of valvular regurgitation and intracardiac shunts and determination of the anatomic level of RV or LV outflow obstruction. In addition, the 3D shape of the flow disturbance provides clues to the cause of regurgitation.

Normal Antegrade Intracardiac Flows

Normal antegrade intracardiac flows can be evaluated with either pulsed or CW Doppler ultrasound (Table 2.4). Accurate measurement of antegrade flow velocities is dependent on several technical factors. Most important is a parallel alignment between the ultrasound beam and the direction of blood flow. The ultrasound instrument measures Doppler frequency shifts. The displayed velocities are *calculated* with the Doppler equation based on transducer frequency, the speed of sound in blood, and the angle between the Doppler beam and flow of interest. For intracardiac flows, the 3D direction of flow is difficult to determine, particularly when flow is abnormal, and attempts to "correct" for the presumed intercept angle are likely to increase, rather than decrease, measurement error. Instead, the examiner positions the ultrasound beam as parallel as possible to the flow of interest based on obtaining the highest calculated velocity with careful transducer positioning and angulation. In the Doppler equation, $\cos\theta = 1$ (and therefore can be ignored) when flow is oriented directly away (intercept angle = 0°) or straight toward (intercept angle = 180°) the ultrasound transducer. Small deviations from a parallel intercept angle (up to 20°) result in only a small error (6%) in velocity calculations (see Fig. 1.25). Although this approach generally results in accurate velocity data, the possibility of underestimation of intracardiac velocities resulting from a nonparallel intercept angle always must be considered in all echocardiographic examinations. This potential limitation becomes significant when recording high-velocity flows in valvular stenosis, regurgitation, or intracardiac shunts.

Other technical factors pertinent to recording antegrade flow velocities include the use of an appropriate velocity scale, wall filters, and gain settings. The standard velocity format is to display flows toward the transducer above and flows away from the transducer below the zero baseline. The baseline is shifted to maximize the flow of interest and the velocity scale adjusted so that the velocity curve uses the entire displayed range. Wall filters are set as low as possible, without resulting in excessive noise, to allow accurate measurement of time intervals. Gain settings are adjusted to show the peak velocity and velocity curve clearly without excessive background noise. A sample volume length of 2 to 4 mm typically is used to record antegrade flow velocities because this length provides reasonable intracardiac localization with adequate signal strength.

Signal aliasing (as discussed in Chapter 1) occurs even with normal intracardiac flow velocities. Use of the baseline shift can resolve this problem in most cases. If aliasing persists, use of high–pulse repetition frequency or CW Doppler is needed for unambiguous display of the maximum velocity.

With appropriate instrument settings and attention to technical details, antegrade velocities with pulsed Doppler ultrasound appear as smooth envelopes with a well-defined onset and end of flow, a well-defined maximum velocity, and a thin band of velocities at each time point. The area under the velocity curve is "clear" because the flow velocities at a specific intracardiac site are relatively uniform. CW Doppler recordings differ in that the curve is "filled in" because of inclusion of lower velocities along the entire length of the ultrasound beam.

Left Ventricular Outflow

An apical or suprasternal notch window is used to obtain a parallel intercept angle between the ultrasound beam and the direction of blood flow in the LV outflow tract and ascending aorta. In general, LV outflow velocities are most accurately recorded from a transthoracic approach because it is more difficult to obtain a parallel intercept angle from the TEE approach. In some cases, a TEE transgastric "apical" approach may be useful, but potential underestimation of velocity resulting from a nonparallel intercept angle always should be considered.

With a pulsed Doppler sample volume positioned on the LV side of the aortic valve, an ejection velocity curve is recorded with a steep acceleration slope, a sharply peaked early systolic maximum velocity, and a less steep deceleration slope (Fig. 2.27). A normal LV outflow tract velocity is about 0.7 to 1.1 m/s. Note the narrow band of velocities at any instant in time during acceleration that reflects the uniformity of blood flow velocity in the outflow tract during acceleration. During deceleration, the range of flow velocities at any instant is slightly wider (spectral broadening) because instability in the flow pattern during deceleration results in slight variation in flow velocities. The aortic valve closing click is seen immediately following end-ejection. Flow recordings with pulsed Doppler on the aortic side of the valve appear similar, except that the aortic valve opening click, rather than the closing click, is seen, and the maximum velocity is slightly higher than the outflow tract velocity because of a slight narrowing of the cross-sectional area of flow at the aortic leaflet tips.

With CW Doppler interrogation of the aortic valve, both opening and closing clicks are recorded. The area under the velocity curve is filled in with lower-velocity signals because lower-velocity blood flow signals that originate in the LV along the length of the ultrasound beam are displayed as well. With a normal aortic valve, the area under the velocity curve (the velocity-time integral) reflects stroke volume, which can be calculated by multiplying by cross-sectional area. The normal antegrade maximum velocity across the valve is between 1.0 and 1.7 m/s and is the same whether measured by pulsed or CW Doppler methods.

The relationship between velocity and pressure gradients across *nonstenotic* valves is somewhat complex and is not fully described by the Bernoulli equation (which applies to areas of narrowing). The period of acceleration corresponds to a slight pressure gradient from the LV to the aorta, with the maximum pressure gradient corresponding to maximum acceleration. LV pressure falls below aortic pressure in mid-systole, and at this point, deceleration of flow occurs. Thus, for the normal valve, maximum velocity occurs at the pressure crossover point (see Fig. 6.1). During deceleration, aortic pressure remains slightly higher than LV pressure until flow decelerates to zero and the valve closes. At this point, LV pressure continues to decline rapidly.

Right Ventricular Outflow

The RV outflow tract and pulmonary artery velocities are recorded from a parasternal short-axis or an RV outflow view (Fig. 2.28). In a normal individual, the RV ejection curve is similar to the LV ejection curve, except that peak velocity is slightly lower (0.5 to 1.3 m/s), the ejection period is longer, and the velocity curve is more rounded, with the maximum velocity occurring in mid-systole. The shapes of the RV and LV ejection curves appear to relate to the downstream vascular resistance. The low-resistance pulmonary vasculature results in a slower rate of acceleration of blood flow, with the maximum velocity (and pressure crossover) occurring later in the ejection cycle. When pulmonary vascular resistance is increased, the RV ejection curve resembles LV ejection more closely with a sharper velocity curve and earlier peak velocity.

Left Ventricular Inflow

Diastolic flow across the mitral valve shows two peaks: an early-diastolic peak velocity (*E*-wave) reflecting passive early-diastolic filling and a late diastolic peak velocity as a result of atrial contraction (*A*-wave) (Fig. 2.29). The normal *E* velocity in healthy, young individuals is about 1 m/s, with an *A* velocity of 0.2 to 0.4 m/s, reflecting the normal small contribution

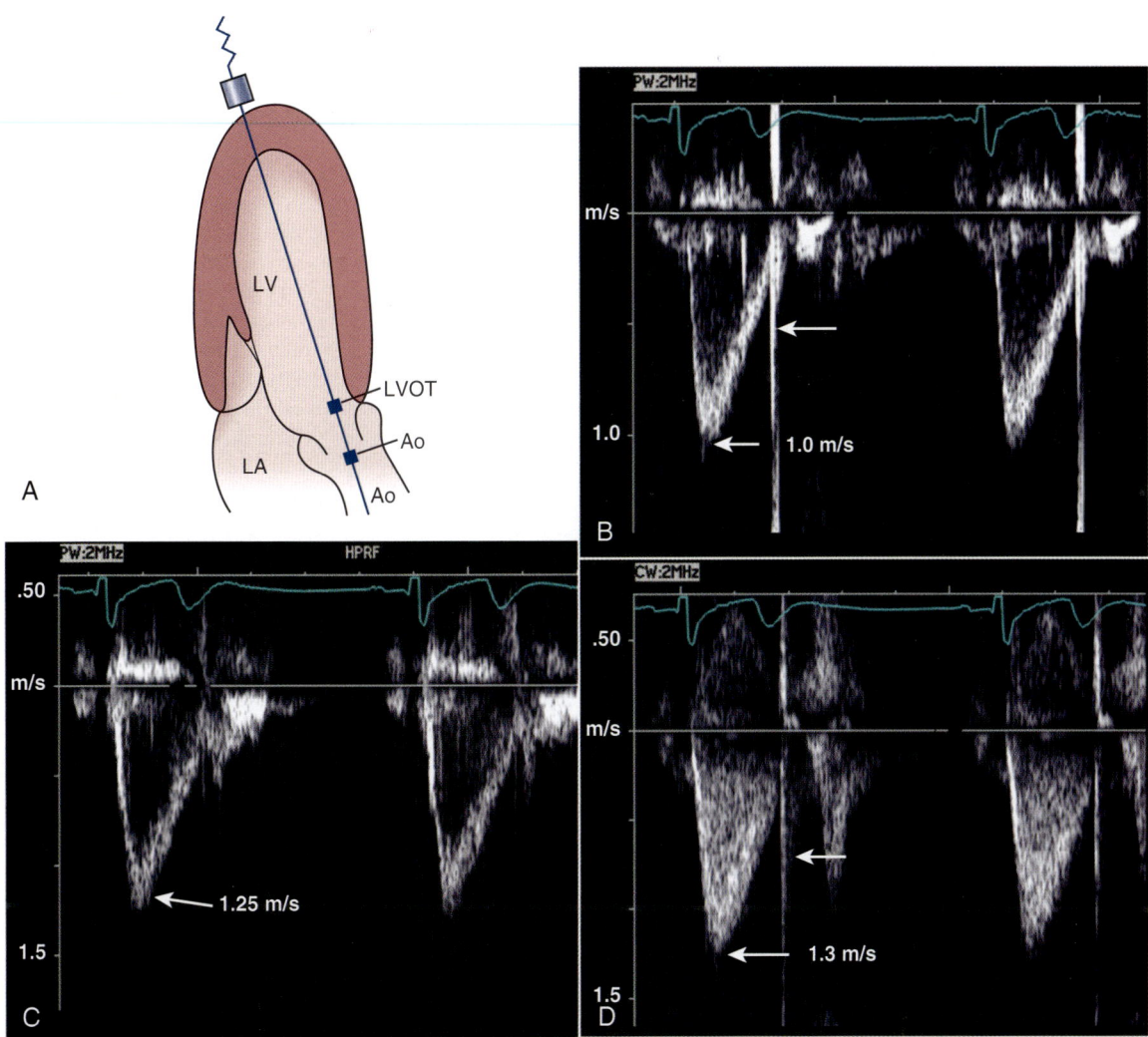

Fig. 2.27 LV outflow velocity. (A) LV outflow tract *(LVOT)* velocity is recorded with pulsed Doppler from an anteriorly angulated apical four-chamber view (as shown here) or an apical long-axis view. (B) The correct position for recording LVOT velocity is with the sample volume positioned just proximal to the aortic valve closure plane. The pulsed Doppler signal shows a smooth velocity curve with a well-defined peak between 0.8 and 1.2 m/s with a linear bright aortic valve closing click *(arrow)*. Flow velocities are uniform during acceleration but vary during deceleration, thus resulting in slight spectral broadening in the second half of systole. (C) The sample volume depth is increased to just beyond the tips of the open valve leaflets in systole for recording the higher aortic *(Ao)* flow laminar velocity curve with no visible closing click. (D) CW Doppler recording of aortic flow shows a higher velocity as blood flow crosses with valve plane, with both an opening and closing click and filling in of the velocity curve due to recording velocity along the entire length of the ultrasound beam.

of atrial contraction to LV diastolic filling. If diastole is long enough, a period of no flow, or diastasis, between the two flow curves is seen. The pattern of LV diastolic filling varies with age, loading conditions, heart rate, and pulmonic regurgitation (PR) interval. With age, a gradual reduction in E velocity, prolongation in the rate of early-diastolic deceleration, and increase in A velocity occur such that the ratio of E to A velocity changes from >1 in young individuals, to about 1 at 50 to 60 years of age, to <1 in older normal individuals (see Chapter 7).

Typically, LV diastolic filling is recorded from an apical window on transthoracic studies. In addition to the physiologic variability discussed earlier, the peak E velocity and the ratio of the E to A peaks differs depending on whether the sample volume is placed at the mitral annulus or at the mitral leaflet tips. Appropriate positioning of the sample volume depends on whether the Doppler curve is used to evaluate diastolic filling of the LV (leaflet tips are probably most useful) or transmitral stroke volume (mitral annular level is most useful). CW Doppler recordings show the highest velocities wherever they occur along the length of the ultrasound beam. LV diastolic filling is discussed in more detail in Chapter 7.

Right Ventricular Inflow

RV inflow can be recorded from an apical approach or from the parasternal RV inflow view. The pattern of RV diastolic filling is similar to LV filling, although peak flow velocities are slightly lower with a normal RV inflow E velocity of 0.3 to 0.7 m/s.

Left Atrial Filling

It is technically challenging to record LA filling from a transthoracic approach because of suboptimal signal strength at the depth of the pulmonary veins in many adults. However, with careful attention to technical details, this flow curve is obtainable in the right superior pulmonary vein in an apical four-chamber view in about 90% of patients. From a TEE approach, flow in both right and left pulmonary veins can be recorded, with the most laminar flow signals obtained from the left superior pulmonary vein (see Fig. 2.29). The venous flow signals in the pulmonary veins are low velocity, about 0.5 m/s in both systole and diastole.

Atrial contraction results in brief low-velocity (about 0.3 m/s) backflow in the pulmonary veins (*a*-wave), followed by a biphasic filling pattern with prominent filling of the atrium (*x*-descent) during ventricular systole, a second brief reversal of flow (*v*-wave) following ventricular contraction, and a second atrial filling curve (*y*-descent) during ventricular diastole (see Chapter 7). Abnormalities of LA filling can be seen in patients with mitral regurgitation (see Chapter 12), constrictive pericarditis (see Chapter 10) and restrictive cardiomyopathy (see Chapter 9).

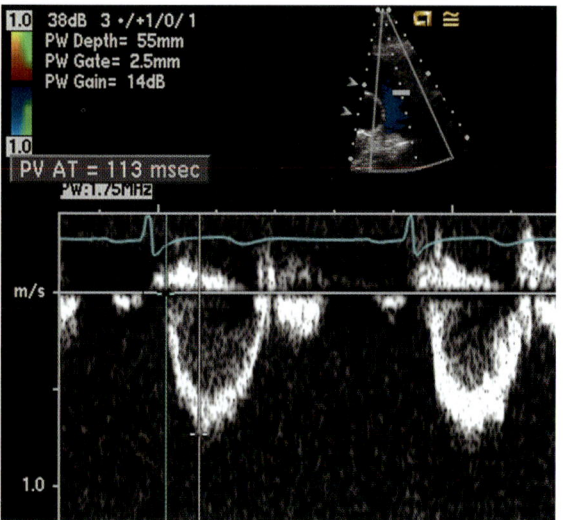

Fig. 2.28 Normal pulmonary artery velocity curve. The pulsed Doppler sample volume is positioned in the mid-pulmonary artery from a parasternal short-axis view. The velocity curve is rounded with a peak in mid-systole and a maximum velocity of about 0.8 m/s. Compare the shape of this velocity curve with the LV outflow curve seen in Fig. 2.27. *PV AT,* Pulmonic valve acceleration time.

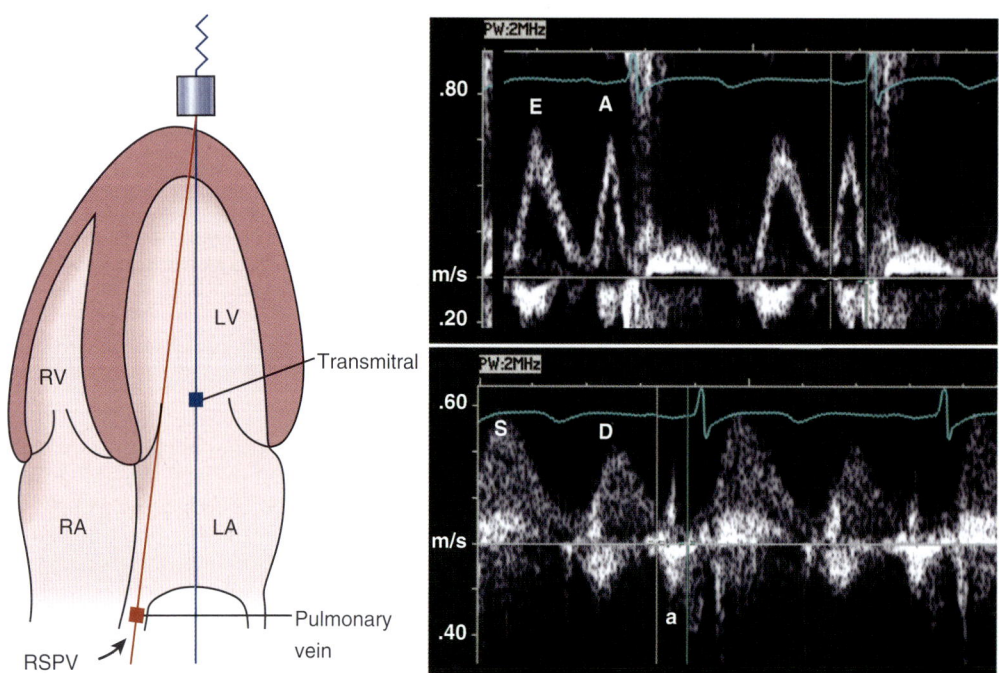

Fig. 2.29 Normal LV inflow and pulmonary vein velocity signals. *(Left)* LV inflow is recorded from the apical view, usually in a four-chamber plane, with the sample volume positioned at the mitral leaflet tips in diastole. *(Right, top)* Pulsed Doppler transmitral LV inflow shows rapid early-diastolic filling *(E)* and the small atrial *(A)* contribution to late diastolic filling in this normal young individual. *(Right, bottom)* Pulmonary vein flow is recorded in the right superior pulmonary vein *(RSPV)* in the four-chamber view with the sample volume positioned about 1 cm into the pulmonary vein. The pulsed Doppler LA filling curve shows systolic *(S)* and diastolic *(D)* filling with a small atrial *(a)* reversal of flow.

Right Atrial Filling

RA filling can be assessed from Doppler recordings of superior vena caval flow (from a suprasternal notch approach) or central hepatic vein flow (which lies parallel to the ultrasound beam from a subcostal window). The pattern of flow again is analogous to the pulsation pattern of the neck veins seen on clinical examination, with an *a*-wave, an *x*-descent reflecting systolic filling, a *v*-wave, and a *y*-descent reflecting diastolic filling of the RA (see Fig. 7.5).

Descending Aorta

Flow patterns in the descending aorta are important in the evaluation of cardiac disorders because the downstream flow pattern depends on the presence and severity of specific cardiac lesions. Examples include aortic regurgitation, patent ductus arteriosus, and aortic coarctation. Descending thoracic aorta flow can be recorded from a suprasternal notch approach and shows antegrade flow with a systolic velocity curve, a peak velocity of about 1 m/s, and brief early-diastolic flow reversal (see Fig. 16.9). The proximal abdominal aorta recorded from a subcostal approach shows a similar flow pattern (see Fig. 16.10).

Normal Color Doppler Flow Patterns
Impact of Color Doppler Physics

Although spectral Doppler (pulsed or continuous) is preferable for accurate measurement of specific intracardiac blood flow velocities, the overall pattern of intracardiac flow is better demonstrated with color flow imaging. Of course, as with any Doppler modality, color Doppler flow images are *angle dependent*. For example, flow in the LV outflow tract is a uniform red color from a parasternal long-axis view because the direction of flow is toward the transducer. The same flow is a uniform *blue* color from an apical approach because now it is directed away from the transducer (Fig. 2.30).

Angle dependence of flow patterns also can be seen in a single image plane. For example, antegrade flow in the aortic arch from a suprasternal notch view appears red (toward the transducer) in the more proximal segment and blue (away from the transducer) more distally, with a small black area in the center of the image where the ultrasound beam is perpendicular to flow. Similarly, in the abdominal aorta from a subcostal approach, antegrade flow appears alternatively red and then blue as it traverses the image plane (see Fig. 1.31). In these examples, the change in color is due to a change in intercept angle between the ultrasound beam and blood flow at the left versus right edge of the sector, rather than a change in the direction or velocity of blood flow.

Less dramatic changes in intercept angle across the 2D image also result in a complex color flow pattern for laminar normal flow. For example, evaluation of the LV outflow tract in an apical long-axis view may show an apparent higher systolic velocity along the ventricular septum than along the anterior mitral leaflet (Fig. 2.31). This appearance results from a more parallel intercept angle between the Doppler beam and blood flow along the septum than adjacent to the mitral valve. The same actual velocities across

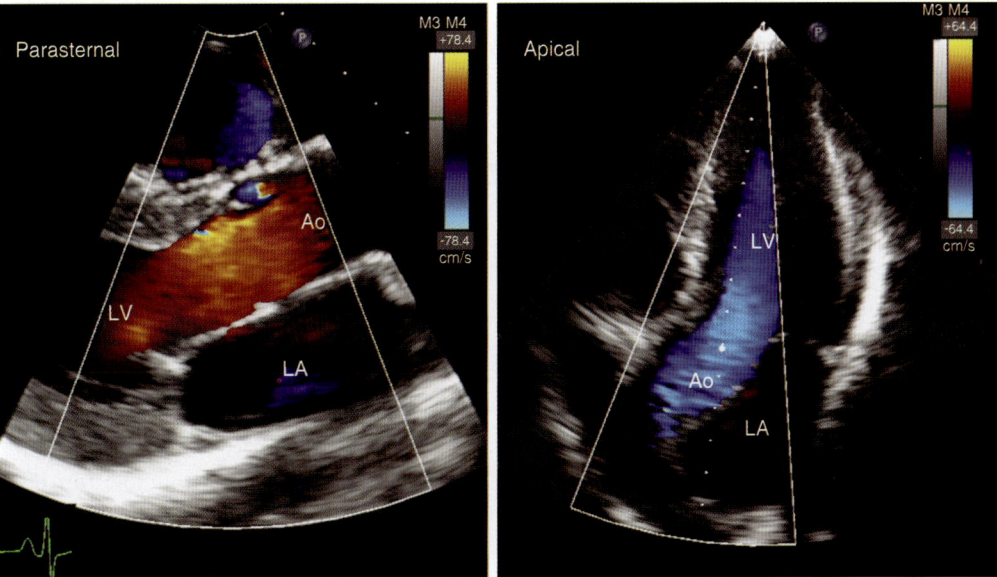

Fig. 2.30 Doppler color LV outflow patterns. Antegrade flow from the LV into the aorta *(Ao)* in systole recorded from a parasternal approach *(left)* is *red* (toward the transducer), whereas the same flow from an apical position *(right)* is *blue* (away from the transducer).

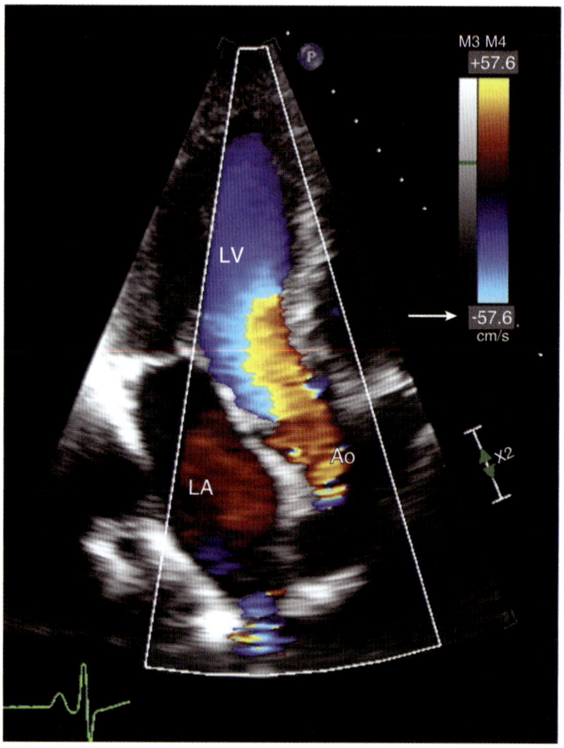

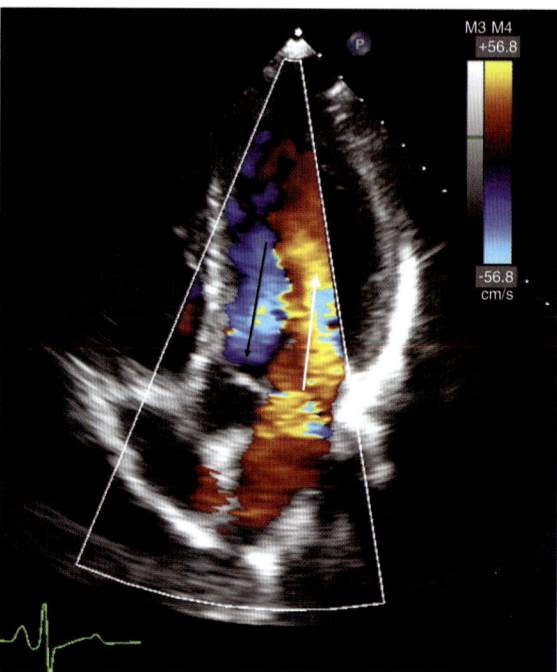

Fig. 2.31 ▶ **Color Doppler signal aliasing.** Color Doppler imaging of LV outflow from an apical long-axis view shows aliasing proximal to the aortic valve because the flow velocity (about 1 m/s) exceeds the Nyquist limit (0.67 m/s) at this depth. The color change pattern across the outflow tract is the result of a more parallel intercept angle between the ultrasound beam and flow along the septum compared with near the mitral valve. *Ao,* Aorta.

Fig. 2.32 ▶ **Color Doppler LV inflow patterns.** Normal pattern of LV filling in mid-diastole in an apical four-chamber view shows flow toward the apex along the lateral wall *(white arrow)* simultaneously with flow away from the transducer along the septum *(black arrow).*

the outflow tract result in differing Doppler frequency shifts depending on this intercept angle. Because the instrument assumes that $\cos \theta = 1$ for each signal, a falsely low velocity is calculated for nonparallel intercept angles, with the resulting image showing an apparent increase in velocity across the image plane as a result of differing intercept angles.

In addition to intercept angle, color flow images also are affected by the phenomenon of *signal aliasing.* The Nyquist limit, as displayed at the top and bottom of the color scale, typically is 60 to 80 cm/s with a 2- or 3-MHz transducer at depths used for transthoracic cardiac imaging. Because normal intracardiac flow velocities often exceed this limit, signal aliasing occurs. Flow toward the transducer is displayed in red at velocities less than the Nyquist limit, but once aliasing occurs, this same flow signal is displayed in blue. Thus, flow toward the transducer is red aliasing to blue, whereas flow away from the transducer is blue aliasing to red. In fact, multiple aliases can occur with high-velocity flows displayed sequentially as going from red to blue to red and so on. An example of normal aliasing is seen in the LV inflow pattern on the apical four-chamber view, where the red flow toward the apex turns blue as it exceeds the Nyquist limit (see Fig. 1.32). Although confusing at first, patterns of signal aliasing can be advantageous in the quantitation of intracardiac flows using the proximal isovelocity surface area approach discussed in Chapter 12.

Another color image pattern seen even with normal intracardiac flows is *variance,* which often is encoded as green on the color display. Although the concept of variance is that a single intracardiac site exhibits multiple flow velocities and directions (e.g., in a regurgitant jet), from the foregoing discussions of intercept angle and aliasing, it is apparent that a normal flow pattern might meet variance criteria. For example, in a region at the aliasing limit, the instrument sequentially measures flow toward and then away from the transducer due to aliasing and then assigns variance to that color pixel. Awareness that a color variance pattern can occur with normal intracardiac flows avoids erroneous interpretations.

Normal Ventricular Outflow Patterns

Color flow imaging of LV outflow can be recorded from an apical approach in either an anteriorly angulated four-chamber view or a long-axis view. Flow is laminar, but aliasing typically occurs at this depth, resulting in a complex color pattern. Although measurement of stroke volume proximal to the aortic valve, which assumes a flat flow-velocity profile, has been validated, it remains controversial whether the appearance of aliasing along the ventricular septum in systole is due to a skewed flow profile or to variations in intercept angle across the color sector.

RV outflow can be visualized from a parasternal short-axis view, from the RV outflow view, or from a subcostal short-axis view. Because velocities are slightly lower and the depth of interrogation is less than for LV outflow, the flow pattern away from the transducer typically shows a uniform blue color.

Normal Ventricular Inflow Patterns

In the apical four-chamber view, LV inflow appears as a broad flowstream extending laterally across the mitral annulus and lengthwise to the LV apex. If the Nyquist limit is exceeded, signal aliasing occurs with a color shift at the aliasing velocity. In real time, the separate flows of early and late diastolic filling may be seen. When ultrasound penetration is optimal, diastolic flow extends from the pulmonary veins to the LV apex. The normal spatial pattern of the LV inflow is directed along the lateral LV wall, in mid-diastole, with blue flow away from the transducer along the ventricular septum consistent with a "vortex" of flow in the LV in diastole (Fig. 2.32). This normal counterclockwise vortex often is reversed in patients after mitral valve replacement. RV inflow patterns on color flow imaging are analogous to the patterns seen in the LV.

Normal Atrial Inflow Patterns

Inflow into the LA occurs via the four pulmonary veins. On transthoracic imaging, the right superior pulmonary vein is the easiest to visualize in the apical four-chamber view. Color flow imaging showing the biphasic red inflow from this vein allows correct placement of a pulsed Doppler sample volume for recording the spectral Doppler data. TEE imaging is needed for reliable identification of all four pulmonary veins, which are rarely visualized on transthoracic imaging in adults.

Inflow into the RA occurs via the superior and inferior venae cavae and the coronary sinus. Evaluation may be complicated by some degree of tricuspid regurgitation (present in 80% to 90% of normal subjects and a higher percentage of patients), which typically is directed along the interatrial septum. Flow from the inferior vena cava and coronary sinus is seen in the RV inflow view, as well as in the short-axis view at the aortic valve level and in the apical four-chamber view. Superior vena caval flow is seen from the suprasternal notch approach. In the RA, recognition of the several normal inflow patterns is important when an atrial septal defect is suspected. About 20% to 30% of normal subjects have a patent foramen ovale (demonstrable by intravenous echo contrast during a Valsalva maneuver), but color flow evidence for a patent foramen ovale is seen on transthoracic imaging in only about 5% of normal individuals.

Physiologic Valvular Regurgitation

With careful examination techniques, a small amount of mitral and tricuspid regurgitation is detectable in 50% to 80% of normal people. In addition, mild pulmonic regurgitation, appearing as a narrow red "flame" in diastole, is an incidental finding (present in 70% to 80% of normal individuals). These physiologic degrees of regurgitation are characterized by a localized signal that often is seen only briefly during the cardiac cycle. Small amounts of mitral, tricuspid, and pulmonic valvular regurgitation are of no apparent clinical significance. In contrast, color Doppler evidence of aortic regurgitation is seen in only about 5% of otherwise normal adults.

AGING CHANGES ON ECHOCARDIOGRAPHY

Between young adulthood and age 70 years, typical echocardiographic changes include an increase in LV wall thickness by about 2 mm with little change in chamber size, LV diastolic dysfunction with *E-A* reversal at about age 50 years, and progressive mild LA enlargement. Aortic dimensions also increase slightly, with about a 6% increase between the fourth and eighth decades of life. Calcific cardiac changes also are common, particularly mild aortic valve leaflet thickening without obstruction to outflow (e.g., aortic sclerosis), which is present in about 25% of adults older than 65 years of age, and calcification of the mitral annulus, seen in up to 50% of older adults. Many older adults, particularly those with a history of hypertension, have a more acute angle between the aorta and ventricular septum, resulting in apparent basal septal thickening, or a "septal knuckle." None of these findings is strictly "normal," but they are seen in many older adults and should be interpreted in that context.

THE DIAGNOSTIC ECHOCARDIOGRAM

Core Elements

A diagnostic echocardiogram is defined as a clinical study, performed under the supervision of a physician with special expertise in echocardiography, with generation of a formal interpretation and long-term image storage. In contrast, point of care or handheld ultrasound, discussed in Chapter 4, is a focused examination performed by the physician caring for the patient; it is used to guide short-term patient management Although the diagnostic echocardiographic examination should be directed toward the specific clinical question in each individual patient, it is important to use a systematic and consistent format with the supervising physician ensuring that instrumentation and data acquisition are appropriate for the clinical indication. Additional imaging and Doppler elements may be needed to pursue the clinical question or any observed abnormalities fully.

The core diagnostic echocardiographic elements differ from laboratory to laboratory, but the concept of a standardized examination sequence is critical to ensure that abnormalities are not missed. Blood pressure and study indications are reviewed before beginning the examination. An electrocardiographic lead is recorded to assist in evaluating the timing of cardiac motion and Doppler flows. Measurements of the cardiac chambers, great vessels, and Doppler flow appropriate for the clinical indication are made using M-mode, 2D, and 3D imaging (Table 2.5; see Tables A.1 to A.4 in Appendix A).

The Core Elements of the examination allow the physician to evaluate the:

Left ventricle:
- Chamber size and wall thickness
- Segmental wall motion abnormalities
- Overall systolic function (including ejection fraction)
- Diastolic filling

Aortic valve and aorta:
- Aortic sinus dimensions and shape
- Ascending aortic diameter
- Aortic valve anatomy
- Evidence for regurgitation or stenosis

Mitral valve and left atrium:
- Mitral valve anatomy and motion
- Evidence for stenosis or regurgitation
- LA size

Right side of the heart:
- RV size and systolic function
- RA size
- Valve anatomy and function
- Estimated pulmonary artery pressure

Pericardium:
- Evidence for thickening or effusion

Additional Components

Additional imaging and Doppler data are recorded as needed based on the clinical indications for the study and any abnormalities seen on the basic examination. The combination of Core Elements and Additional Components then constitutes a complete echocardiographic examination.

An example of findings on the Core Elements leading to additional data recording is when a calcified aortic valve is present. With this finding, attention is focused first on the precise valve anatomy—bicuspid, calcific, rheumatic—and then on the function of the valve. The degree of stenosis is quantitated from the maximum aortic jet velocity and calculation of valve area (see Chapter 11), and the degree of regurgitation is evaluated with color flow and CW Doppler techniques (see Chapter 12). Next, the LV response to the pressure load imposed by the abnormal aortic valve is assessed both for systolic function (see Chapter 6) and diastolic function (see Chapter 7).

Another example is evaluation of a patient after myocardial infarction. In this case, attention is focused on the extent and distribution of LV segmental wall motion abnormalities (see Chapter 8). If apical akinesis or dyskinesis is noted, a diligent search for an apical thrombus is indicated (see Chapter 15). If the patient has a new murmur, careful evaluation is performed to assess the possibility of mitral regurgitation as a result of papillary muscle dysfunction or the possibility of a postinfarction ventricular septal defect. Overall LV systolic function is evaluated, as is RV function.

Even if no obvious abnormalities are noted during the basic examination, the study is focused toward the specific clinical question in that patient. For example, if endocarditis is suspected (see Chapter 14), more attention to valvular anatomy is needed, with careful transducer angulation and nonstandard views to optimize visualization of possible valvular vegetations. Another example of how the clinical indication affects the examination is the patient referred for symptoms of heart failure. Even if the Core Elements are unremarkable, more complete evaluation of diastolic LV function is helpful to evaluate for a cardiac cause of the patient's symptoms.

The need to focus the examination on the specific clinical question and at the same time ensure that significant abnormalities are not missed highlights the necessity for appropriate training of both the physician responsible for the examination and the sonographer performing the study, as well as for close interaction between these two individuals during the performance and interpretation of the study. Furthermore, interaction with the referring physician is recommended either before the examination is performed to clarify the differential diagnosis and clinical questions or after the examination to integrate the pretest likelihood with the echocardiographic findings and estimate the probability of any remaining diagnostic problems.

TABLE 2.5 Clinical Echocardiographic Chamber and Great Vessel Measurements*

Cardiac Structure	Basic Measurements	Additional Measurements	Technical Details
Left ventricle	ED-dimension ES dimension ED wall thickness Ejection fraction	ED volume ES volume 2D stroke volume Relative wall thickness LV mass	• 2D imaging is used to ensure measurements are centered and perpendicular to the long axis of the LV. • M-mode provides superior time resolution and more accurate identification of endocardial borders but is inaccurate if oblique. • LV ejection fraction is measured by the apical biplane approach or from 3D imaging.
Left atrium	ES AP diameter (PLAX)	LA area LA volume	• LA AP dimension provides a quick screen but may underestimate LA size. • When LA size is important for clinical decision making, measurement of LA volume from apical views is helpful.
Right ventricle	ED basal RV dimension in A4C view RV systolic function	RV wall thickness RVOT dimensions RV FAC or TAPSE	• RV dimensions are measured in apical views at ED. RVOT is measured in PLAX views. • TAPSE is measured from an apical M-mode recording of the tricuspid annulus (see Chapter 6).
Right atrium	Visual estimate of size	RA area in A4C view	• RA size is usually compared with the LA in the apical 4-chamber view.
Aorta	ED diameter at sinuses (PLAX)	ED diameter indexed to expected dimension Diameter at multiple sites in aorta	• With 2D echo, inner edge to inner edge measurements are more reproducible. • Measurements at ES about 2 mm greater than ED measurements
Pulmonary artery		ED diameter	

*2D measurements are made from the white-black interface on the image. M-mode measurements are made using the leading edge to leading edge convention.
A4C, Apical four-chamber view; *AP*, anterior-posterior; *ED*, end-diastole (onset of the QRS), end-diastolic; *ES*, end-systole (minimum LV volume), end-systolic; *FAC*, fractional area change; *PLAX*, parasternal long-axis view; *RVOT*, RV outflow tract; *TAPSE*, tricuspid annular plane systolic excursion.

THE ECHO EXAM

Diagnostic TTE: Core Elements

A COMPLETE ECHO EXAM CONSISTS OF CORE ELEMENTS + ADDITIONAL COMPONENTS

Modality	Window	View/Signal	Basic Measurements
Clinical data		Indication for echo Key history and PE findings Previous cardiac imaging data	Blood pressure at time of Echo exam
2D imaging	Parasternal	Long-axis Short-axis aortic valve Short-axis mitral valve Short-axis LV (papillary muscle level) RV inflow	LV ED and ES dimensions LV ED wall thickness Aortic ED sinus dimension LA dimension
	Apical	4-chamber Anteriorly angulated 4-chamber 2-chamber Long-axis	Visual estimate or biplane ejection fraction
	Subcostal	4-chamber IVC with respiration Proximal abdominal aorta	
	Suprasternal	Aortic arch	
Pulsed Doppler	Parasternal Apical	Pulmonary artery flow LV inflow LV outflow	PA velocity E velocity A velocity LV outflow velocity
Color flow	Parasternal	Long-axis: aortic and mitral valves Short-axis: aortic and pulmonic valves RV inflow : tricuspid valve	Color flow to identify regurgitation of all 4 valves. If more than mild, measure vena contracta
	Apical	4-chamber: mitral and tricuspid valves Long-axis: aortic and mitral valves	
CW Doppler	Parasternal	Tricuspid valve Pulmonic valve	TR-jet velocity
	Apical	Aortic valve Mitral valve Tricuspid valve	Aortic velocity TR-jet (pulmonary pressures)

ED, End-diastole; *ES*, end-systole; *IVC*, inferior vena cava; *PA*, pulmonary artery; *PE*, physical examination; *TR*, tricuspid regurgitation.

Diagnostic TTE: Additional Components

Abnormality on Core Elements	Additional Echo Exam Components (Chapter)
Reason for echo	Additional components to address specific clinical question[a]
Left ventricle • Decreased ejection fraction • Abnormal LV filling velocities • Regional wall motion abnormality • Increased wall thickness	 See Systolic Function (6) See Diastolic Function (7) See Ischemic Heart Disease (8) See Hypertrophic Cardiomyopathy, Restrictive Cardiomyopathy and Hypertensive Heart Disease (9)
Valves • Imaging evidence for stenosis or an increased antegrade transvalvular velocity • Regurgitation greater than mild on color flow imaging or CW Doppler • Prosthetic valve • Valve mass or suspected endocarditis	 See Valve Stenosis (11) See Valve Regurgitation (12) See Prosthetic Valves (13) See Endocarditis and Masses (14, 15)
Right heart • Enlarged right ventricle • Elevated TR-jet velocity	 See Pulmonary Heart Disease and Congenital Heart Disease (9, 17) See Pulmonary Pressures (6)

Normal Anatomy and Flow Patterns on Transthoracic Echocardiography | Chapter 2

Diagnostic TTE: Additional Components—cont'd	
Abnormality on Core Elements	**Additional Echo Exam Components (Chapter)**
Pericardium • Pericardial effusion • Pericardial thickening	See Pericardial Effusion (10) See Constrictive Pericarditis (10)
Great vessels • Enlarged aorta	See Aortic Disease (16)

^aThe Echo Exam should always include additional components to address the clinical indication. For example, if the indication is "heart failure," additional components to evaluate systolic and diastolic function are needed even if the Core Elements do not show obvious abnormalities. If the indication is "cardiac source of embolus," the Additional Components for that diagnosis are needed.
TR, tricuspid regurgitation

Principles of Doppler Quantitation		
Method	**Assumptions/Characteristics**	**Examples of Clinical Applications**
Volume flow Stroke volume (SV) = CSA × VTI	• Laminar flow • Flat flow profile • Cross-sectional area (CSA) and velocity time integral (VTI) measured at same site	• Cardiac output • Continuity equation for valve area • Regurgitant volume calculations • Intracardiac shunts, pulmonary to systemic flow ratio
Velocity-pressure relationship $\Delta P = 4v^2$	• Flow limiting orifice • CW Doppler signal recorded parallel to flow	• Stenotic valve gradients • Calculation of pulmonary pressures • LV dP/dt
Spatial flow patterns	• Proximal flow convergence region • Narrow flow stream in orifice (vena contracta) • Downstream flow disturbance	• Detection of valve regurgitation and intracardiac shunts • Level of obstruction • Quantitation of regurgitant severity

SUGGESTED READING

General

1. Rimington H, Chambers J: *Echocardiography: A Practical Guide for Reporting and Interpretation*, 3 ed, Boca Raton, FL, 2015, CRC Press.
   This short paperback book offers a simple approach to echocardiographic measurements and interpretation.

2. Gardin JM, Adams DB, Douglas PS, et al: Recommendations for a standardized report for adults transthoracic echocardiography: a report from the American Society of Echocardiography's Nomenclature and Standards Committee and Task Force for a Standardized Echocardiography Report, *J Am Soc Echocardiogr* 15:275–290, 2002.
   Recommendations for performing and reporting transthoracic echocardiography examinations in adults. An excellent resource for developing a standardized echocardiography examination in each laboratory.

3. Lang RM, Badano LP, Mor-Avi V, et al: Recommendations for cardiac chamber quantification by echocardiography in adults: an update from the American Society of Echocardiography and the European Association of Cardiovascular Imaging, *J Am Soc Echocardiogr* 28(1):1–39, 2015.
   Detailed discussion of methods for quantitation of LV and RV systolic function by 2D echocardiography and measurement of atrial size and aortic root dimensions. Technical details of image acquisition, diagrams illustrating quantitative methods, and tables of normal values are included in this comprehensive document.

4. Chen MA: Aging changes seen on echocardiography. In Otto CM, editor: *The Practice of Clinical Echocardiography*, 5th ed, Philadelphia, 2017, Elsevier.
   Detailed review of the normal cardiac changes with aging as assessed by echocardiography, including age-grouped tables of normal values for LV dimensions and function and Doppler flow velocities. The clinical utility of echocardiography and outcome data related to age are summarized.

5. Linefsky J: Echocardiography in nutritional and metabolic disorders. In Otto CM, editor: *The Practice of Clinical Echocardiography*, 5th ed, Philadelphia, 2017, Elsevier.
   Typical cardiac changes seen in obese patients include an increase in both LV mass and chamber dimensions, combined with a decrease in systolic function. Diastolic function parameters also often are abnormal, LA size is increased, and the aortic root may be enlarged. Evaluation of echocardiographic findings in obese patients should be made in the context of these typical changes.

Left Ventricle

6. Aurigemma GP: Left ventricular structure and systolic function: quantitative echocardiography. In Otto CM, editor: *The Practice of Clinical Echocardiography*, 5th ed, Philadelphia, 2017, Elsevier.
   This chapter provides a detailed discussion of left ventricular geometry and function. Approaches to assessment of LV systolic function include ejection fraction, fractional

shortening, stress-shortening relationships, and pressure-volume loops. Different types of LV hypertrophy are reviewed, and the clinical implications of alterations in LV geometry are discussed. 87 references.

7. De Simone G, Izzo R, Aurigemma GP, et al: Cardiovascular risk in relation to a new classification of hypertensive left ventricular geometric abnormalities, J Hypertens 33:745–754, 2015.

    In a cohort of almost 9000 hypertensive patients, the presence, severity, and type of LV hypertrophy were associated with adverse cardiovascular events. Concentric hypertrophy in association with LV dilation was associated with the greatest increase in LV mass, compared with hypertensive patients with eccentric hypertrophy or concentric remodeling.

8. Marwick TH, Gillebert TC, Aurigemma G, et al: Recommendations on the use of echocardiography in adult hypertension: a report from the European Association of Cardiovascular Imaging (EACVI) and the American Society of Echocardiography (ASE), J Am Soc Echocardiogr 28(7):727–754, 2015.

    This guideline document reviews the cardiovascular effects of primary hypertension with sections on pathophysiology; measurement of LV mass, geometry, and function; and effects of treatment on these parameters. Detailed illustrations on optimal approach for echocardiographic measurements. 203 references.

Right Ventricle

9. Vaidya A, Kirkpatrick J: Right ventricular anatomy, function and echocardiographic evaluation. In Otto CM, editor: *The Practice of Clinical Echocardiography*, 5th ed, Philadelphia, 2017, Elsevier.

    This chapter provides details of RV anatomy and function, along with the recommended approach for echocardiographic evaluation. Clinical outcomes studies are summarized. Reference values for normal RV anatomy and function are provided.

10. Shiota T: Two-dimensional and three-dimensional echocardiographic evaluation of the right ventricle. In Gillam LD, Otto CM, editors: *Advanced Approaches in Echocardiography*, Philadelphia, 2012, Saunders.

    Advanced discussion of RV anatomy with concise bulleted text, key points, and numerous illustrations. Includes a discussion of both 2D and 3D imaging of the right ventricle.

11. Sheehan F, Redington A: The right ventricle: anatomy, physiology and clinical imaging, Heart 94(11):1510–1515, 2008, doi:10.1136/hrt.2007.132779.

    The complex anatomy and physiology of the right ventricle are explored with a detailed text and with figures showing 3D anatomy, normal and abnormal pressure curves, and pressure-volume loops.

Left Atrium

12. Rosca M, Lancellotti P, Bogdan A, et al: Left atrial function: pathophysiology, echocardiographic assessment, and clinical applications, Heart 97:1982–1989, 2011.

    Comprehensive review of LA anatomy and function correlated with the echocardiographic approach to evaluation of the LA. In addition to standard imaging, Doppler flow pattern, LA strain, and speckle tracking of the LA are discussed. Changes in LA anatomy and function with aging, atrial fibrillation, heart failure, valve disease, and cardiomyopathies are summarized.

13. Vyas H, Jackson K, Chenzbraun A: Switching to volumetric left atrial measurements: impact on routine echocardiographic practice, Eur J Echocardiogr 12(2):107–111, 2011.

    In 168 consecutive adults referred for echocardiography, linear dimensions identified LA enlargement in 40%, whereas LA volumes were enlarged in 65%. This finding emphasizes that LA volume measurements have a higher sensitivity than linear dimensions for detection of atrial enlargement.

14. Sakaguchi E, Yamada A, Sugimoto K, et al: Prognostic value of left atrial volume index in patients with first acute myocardial infarction, Eur J Echocardiogr 12(6):440–444, 2011.

    In 205 consecutive patients with acute myocardial infarction, echocardiographic LA volume at discharge and the change in LA volume between hospital admission and discharge was predictive of major cardiac events (cardiac death caused by heart failure and heart failure hospitalization) during a mean follow-up of 26 months. An LA volume index greater than 32.0 mL/m^2 at discharge had a sensitivity of 93% and specificity of 69% for subsequent adverse cardiovascular outcome.

15. Marchese P, Bursi F, Delle Donne G, et al: Indexed left atrial volume predicts the recurrence of non-valvular atrial fibrillation after successful cardioversion, Eur J Echocardiogr 12(3):214–221, 2011.

    In 411 adults (mean age 64.1 ± 11.4 years, 34.5% women) who underwent successful cardioversion, atrial fibrillation recurrence occurred in 61% at a median follow-up about 1 year. On multivariate analysis, each mL/m^2 increase echocardiographic LA volume index was independently associated with a 21% increase in the risk of recurrence of atrial fibrillation (odds ratio: 1:21; confidence intervals: 1.11–1.30; P < 0.001).

Doppler Flows

16. Quinones MA, Otto CM, Stoddard M, et al: Recommendations for quantification of Doppler echocardiography: a report from the Doppler quantification task force of the nomenclature and standards committee of the American Society of Echocardiography, J Am Soc Echocardiogr 15:167–184, 2002.

    Nomenclature standards for recording, measuring, and reporting Doppler data including pulsed, continuous, and color flow Doppler. Excellent review of normal flow patterns and basic Doppler principles for calculation of volume flow rate, pressure gradients, and regurgitant valve lesions. 77 references and useful glossary of Doppler terms.

17. Sengupta PP, Pedrizzetti G, Kilner PJ, et al: Emerging trends in CV flow visualization, JACC Cardiovasc Imaging 5(3):305–316, 2012.

    An elegant discussion of normal intracardiac flow patterns with details and examples of flow visualization with cardiac magnetic resonance imaging, color Doppler echocardiography, and particle imaging velocimetry. Vortex formation in the ventricle and in blood vessels is illustrated. Clinical applications and future directions are outlined. The flow visualization images will help the echocardiographer understand normal intracardiac flow patterns and how these affect the Doppler echocardiographic data analysis.

18. Morris PD, Narracott A, von Tengg-Kobligk H, et al: Computational fluid dynamics modelling in cardiovascular medicine, Heart 102(1):18–28, 2016.

    Computational fluid dynamics modeling enables detailed analysis of flow patterns in different types of structural heart disease and with interventions, such as prosthetic valves or vascular stents. An understanding of normal flow patterns provides insight into the Doppler velocity data recorded during a clinical echocardiographic examination.

3 Transesophageal Echocardiography

PROTOCOL AND RISKS

TOMOGRAPHIC VIEWS
  Esophageal Position
    Four-Chamber Plane
    Two-Chamber Plane
    Long-Axis Plane
    Other Long-Axis Image Planes
    Short-Axis Plane
  Transgastric Position
    Short-Axis Plane
    Two-Chamber Plane
    Four-Chamber Plane
    Long-Axis Plane
  Descending Thoracic Aorta

VALVE ANATOMY AND FUNCTION
  Aortic Valve
  Mitral Valve
  Pulmonic Valve
  Tricuspid Valve

CHAMBER ANATOMY AND FILLING PATTERNS
  Left Ventricle
  Left Atrium
  Right Ventricle
  Right Atrium

IMAGING SEQUENCE

THE ECHO EXAM

SUGGESTED READING

Transesophageal echocardiography (TEE) offers the advantage of improved image quality compared with transthoracic echocardiographic images, particularly of posterior structures, such as the interatrial septum, mitral valve, left atrium (LA), and pulmonary veins. Image quality is improved both because of the decreased distance between the transducer and the structures of interest and because of the absence of intervening lung or bone tissue. A better signal-to-noise ratio and decreased image depth also allow for the use of higher-frequency (5- and 7-MHz) transducers, which further enhances image quality. Three-dimensional (3D) TEE imaging is increasingly used to evaluate mitral valve and atrial septal anatomy and to guide complex interventional procedures (see Chapter 18).

However, TEE imaging is more risky than transthoracic imaging because of the insertion of the probe in the esophagus and the need for conscious sedation in most patients. Typically, a TEE examination provides additional information but does not replace a transthoracic examination, and in some situations, transthoracic imaging provides better image quality and diagnostic Doppler data. For example, anterior structures, such as a prosthetic aortic valve, may be better imaged from the transthoracic approach. For Doppler velocity measurements, the transthoracic approach offers more acoustic windows with the ability to adjust the transducer angle freely in both the transverse and elevational planes. In contrast, transducer position and angulation are constrained with the TEE approach by the relative positions of the esophagus and heart. The inability to align the Doppler beam parallel to the flow of interest often results in substantial velocity underestimation. In addition, it often is more difficult to obtain standard anatomic measurements from the TEE approach because of oblique two-dimensional (2D) image planes. Thus, even when TEE imaging is necessary, data from the transthoracic examination are integrated into the final clinical interpretation.

In this chapter, the TEE procedure and its risks are briefly outlined, followed by a description of the standard views obtained from each acoustic window (upper esophageal, mid-esophageal, transgastric, transgastric apical, and descending aorta). Sections on the TEE imaging and Doppler evaluation of each cardiac valve and chamber are included to guide the reader to the optimal views for each anatomic structure. This chapter focuses on normal anatomy and flow patterns. Clinical indications for TEE imaging are discussed in Chapter 5, and pathologic images are integrated into subsequent chapters. The use of TEE imaging to monitor surgical and interventional procedures is discussed in Chapter 18.

PROTOCOLS AND RISKS

The TEE procedure is performed by a physician skilled in both echocardiography and the endoscopy procedure, as detailed in published guidelines for physician training. Typically, a cardiac sonographer assists the physician, by adjusting instrument settings for optimal image quality and data acquisition. Many physicians use conscious sedation for their patients, in addition to local anesthesia of the pharynx, to minimize patients' discomfort and improve tolerance of the procedure. When sedation is used, a designated, qualified individual (usually a nurse) monitors and documents the patient's blood pressure, heart rate, respiratory rate, arterial oxygen saturation, and level of consciousness throughout the procedure. The nurse also ensures patency of the airway and provides suction of oral secretions as needed. The specific protocols, medications used for sedation, and monitoring procedures are dictated by the standards of each institution.

TEE has a very low incidence of complications when performed by trained individuals with appropriate patient selection and monitoring. However, this procedure does have known risks, which must be taken into consideration in deciding whether the potential information obtained justifies use of this procedure; TEE is contraindicated in some clinical situations, as summarized in Table 3.1. The rate of complications serious enough to interrupt the procedure is less than 1%, with a reported mortality rate of less than 1 in 10,000 patients (Table 3.2). If the preprocedure history or physical examination suggests an increased risk for conscious sedation, appropriate consultation with anesthesiology is essential. If the patient has a history of esophageal disease or symptoms related to impaired swallowing, evaluation of the esophagus or a gastroenterology consultation is needed before TEE.

After sedation and local anesthesia of the pharynx, the probe is gently inserted via a bite block, positioned in the esophagus, and advanced as needed to obtain diagnostic images. In intubated patients in the intensive care unit, interventional suite, or operating room, care is needed to avoid compromise of the endotracheal tube position. Indwelling nasogastric or feeding tubes may limit probe motion or result in air between the transducer and the heart, so these tubes often need to be removed for the TEE procedure.

The risk of aspiration is minimized by: having the patient fast for several hours before the procedure, by using a left lateral decubitus position during probe insertion, and by having the patient continue to fast after the procedure until recovery from the local anesthesia of the pharynx. Esophageal trauma or perforation is unlikely in the absence of a history of esophageal disease or swallowing difficulty, both of which are ascertained by clinical history. Bleeding complications are rare and usually mild, and the procedure can be safely performed with therapeutic levels of systemic anticoagulation. Initial concern that TEE imaging could increase the risk of endocarditis has been alleviated by several studies showing the absence of bacteremia following this procedure; therefore most physicians do not routinely use antibiotic prophylaxis.

TABLE 3.1 TEE Contraindications and Clinical Features Associated With Increased Procedural Risk

Contraindications to Esophageal Ultrasound Probe Positioning

Absolute	Relative
Esophageal stricture, mass, or perforation	Esophageal diverticulum or varices
Active upper GI bleeding	Previous esophageal surgery
Recent esophageal or upper GI surgery	Dysphagia
Uncooperative patient	Coagulopathy, thrombocytopenia

Clinical Features Associated With Increased Risk of Respiratory Compromise During Moderate Conscious Sedation

Airway patency	History of airway management problems Obstructive sleep apnea Significant malocclusion Atlantoaxial joint disease or severe cervical arthritis (e.g., restricted cervical mobility)
Older adult patients	Increased sensitivity to sedatives Higher incidence of interactions of with other medications
Congestive heart failure	Severe LV systolic dysfunction Severe aortic stenosis
Underlying respiratory disease	Oxygen dependency Severe pulmonary hypertension RV systolic dysfunction
Neurologic or neuromuscular disorders	Impaired respiratory strength Impaired swallowing or aspiration risk Inability to follow commands
Nonfasting state	Increased aspiration risk

GI, Gastrointestinal.

TOMOGRAPHIC VIEWS

The exact views obtained on a TEE study vary depending on the relative positions of the heart, esophagus, and diaphragm in each patient (Fig. 3.1). Even though a multiplane probe allows full rotation of the scan plane, the fixed position of the transducer

TABLE 3.2 TEE: Risk of Complications	
Complication	Rate (%)
Death	<0.01–0.02
Esophageal perforation	<0.01
Major bleeding	<0.01
Minor bleeding	0.01–0.2
Bronchospasm	0.07
Dental injury	0.1
Arrhythmia	0.06–0.3
Dental injury	0.1
Dysphagia	1.8
Hoarseness	12
Lip injury	13

Adapted from Hilberath JN, Oakes DA, Shernan SK, et al: Safety of transesophageal echocardiography, *J Am Soc Echocardiogr* 23(11):1115–1127, 2010.

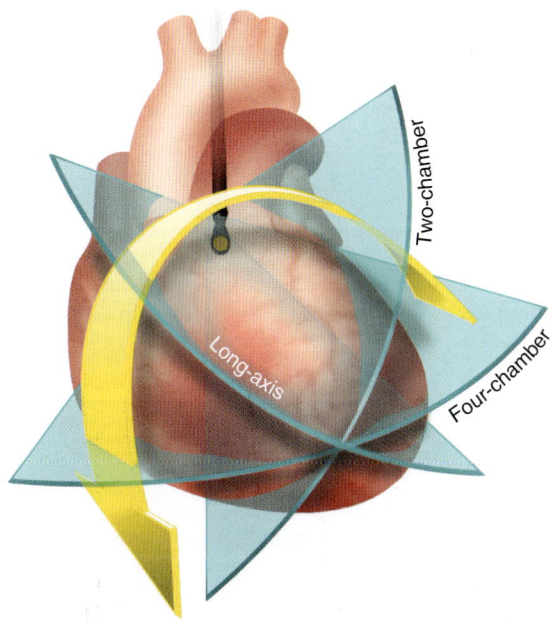

Fig. 3.1 Transesophageal echocardiography image plane rotation. Rotation of the image plane starting from the four-chamber view (see Fig. 3.3), with the LV apex centered in the image, allows a two-chamber view (see Fig. 3.7) at approximately 60° rotation and a long-axis view (see Fig. 3.9) at approximately 120° rotation. Slight repositioning and angulation of the transducer may be needed as the image plane is rotated to ensure inclusion of the LV apex in the image.

examination, using standard short-axis, long-axis, two-chamber, and four-chamber image planes whenever possible. Standard views then are supplemented with additional image planes to demonstrate the specific pathologic processes in each patient.

3D echocardiographic techniques can facilitate obtaining optimal views and display of spatial relationships, particularly for the atrial septum and mitral valve. 3D imaging is optimal when 3D acquisitions start from a standard 2D tomographic image plane. The recommended sequence of 2D images, 3D data sets, and Doppler recordings for a standard TEE study is shown in The Echo Exam summary at the end of this chapter. The following sections describe both the 2D and 3D views useful for evaluation of the valves and cardiac chambers. Often additional views or Doppler data are needed to supplement the basic examination, depending on the specific clinical question.

The position of the tip of the probe is described as esophageal or transgastric and is referenced to the cardiac structures seen in each view. The absolute distance of the transducer from the patient's mouth will vary depending on body size and cardiac position. The exact degree of rotation, tilt, and angulation needed to obtain the best short-axis, long-axis, two-chamber, and four-chamber views also varies. When standard views are obtained, the images correspond to the anatomy described for the equivalent transthoracic views, with the major difference being image orientation given the TEE transducer position.

For TEE echocardiograms, transducer motions (Fig. 3.2) are referred to as:

- *Repositioning*, defined as movement of the probe up and down in the esophagus
- *Rotation*, defined as rotating the image plane from 0° to 180° using the multiplane control knob
- *Turning*, defined as moving the entire transducer in a rotational fashion in the esophagus to show a mediolateral change in image plane
- *Angulation*, defined as bending and extending the probe so that the image plane is directed superiorly or inferiorly at an angle to the original image plane
- *Tilt*, defined as lateral motion of the transducer tip to image different structures in the same image plane (although slight superior motion occurs as well)

From the TEE position, most image planes are achieved using repositioning, rotation, and turning of the transducer. The use of angulation is particularly important on transgastric views. A key principle in using a multiplane probe is that the anatomic area of interest should be centered in the image before rotation to a new view; this ensures that the structure of interest remains in the image plane.

in the esophagus constrains the possible image planes that can be obtained, potentially resulting in oblique 2D image orientations compared with standard echocardiographic image planes. The goal of a TEE study is to perform a systematic and comprehensive

Esophageal Position

Four-Chamber Plane

As the transducer is advanced into the esophagus from the mouth toward the stomach, acoustic access is limited by interposition of the air-filled trachea until the transducer passes the level of the carina. From a high TEE position, with the probe located posterior to the LA, a standard four-chamber view is obtained in the 0° position with angulation of the transducer toward the left ventricular (LV) apex (Fig. 3.3). In the four-chamber view the lateral wall and inferior septal segments of the LV are seen, along with the central portions of both the anterior and posterior leaflets of the mitral valve.

Care is needed to include as much of the full length of the ventricle as possible in this view. Typically, even with optimal positioning and angulation, TEE views are somewhat foreshortened compared with the true long-axis of the ventricle, and the apparent apex may actually represent a more proximal segment of the anterior wall. The four-chamber view is useful for the evaluation of overall ventricular systolic function, regional wall motion (recognizing that the apex often be missed), and the pattern of septal motion. Biplane ejection fraction also can be calculated from traced endocardial borders at end-diastole and end-systole, although volumes may be underestimated because of foreshortening of the ventricular length.

From the four-chamber view, anterior angulation shows the LV outflow tract and aortic valve (the "five-chamber" view) (Figs. 3.4 and 3.5). Posterior angulation provides images of the lateral segments of the mitral valve leaflets, with the coronary sinus visualized on extreme posterior angulation. A 3D image of the mitral valve, viewed from the LA side, obtained by real-time imaging from stored full-volume data acquisition, is helpful when mitral valve pathology is present.

While examining the LA in the four-chamber plane, it is helpful to slowly advance and withdraw the transducer to visualize the full superior and inferior extent or to slowly angulate the probe tip to provide

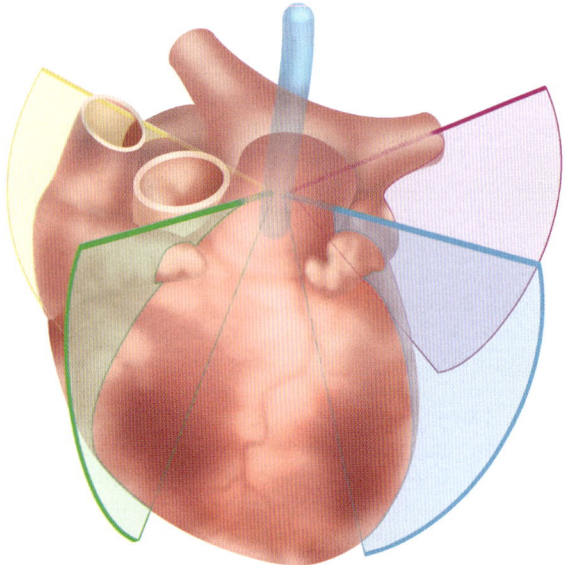

Fig. 3.2 Turning the transesophageal echocardiography image plane. From a mid-esophageal position, turning the image plane from left to right provides images of the left pulmonary veins *(purple)*, aorta and LV *(blue)*, RV *(green)*, and RA with superior and inferior vena cavae *(yellow)*.

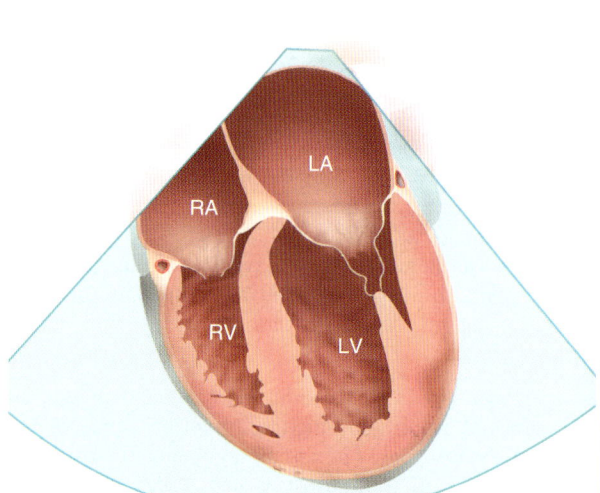
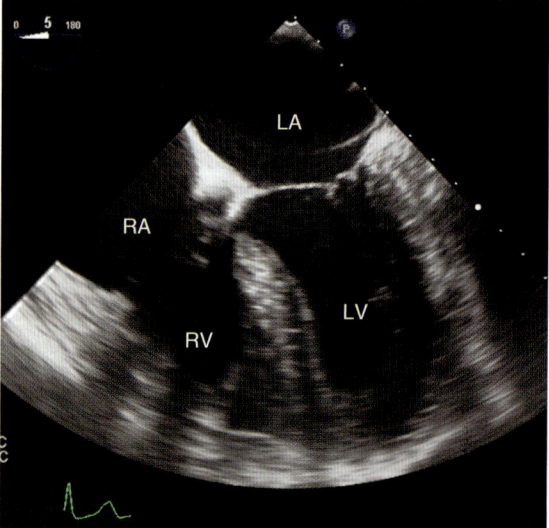

Fig. 3.3 ▶ **Transesophageal echocardiography four-chamber view.** Drawing *(left)* and echocardiographic image *(right)* obtained from an upper TEE position with the multiplane probe at 0° rotation. In this view, the apparent apex may actually represent a segment of the anterior wall because of foreshortening of the long axis of the ventricle.

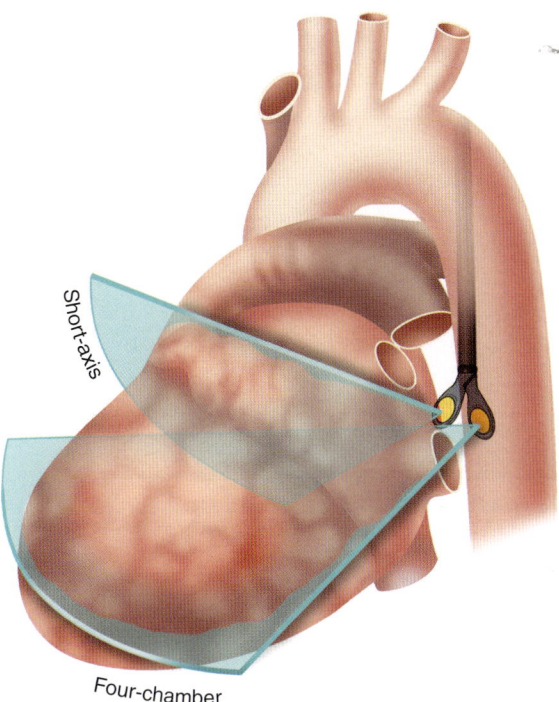

Fig. 3.4 Transesophageal echocardiography probe angulation. From an upper esophageal position with the probe at 0° rotation, the transducer tip is extended to obtain a four-chamber view (as shown in Fig. 3.3) or flexed for a short-axis view of the LA appendage (as shown in Fig. 3.8).

sequential cross sections of the LA. Because the LA is in the near field of the image, careful adjustment of imaging parameters is needed to avoid misinterpretation of near-field artifacts. For this reason, identification of a small thrombus along the posterior LA wall is problematic.

In the standard four-chamber TEE image, the size, shape, and systolic function of the right ventricle (RV) are assessed by turning the probe toward the patient's right side. This view also provides visualization of the septal and anterior leaflets of the tricuspid valve and the right atrium (RA). The interatrial septum is well visualized, with the fossa ovalis and primum septal region clearly identifiable (Fig. 3.6).

Two-Chamber Plane

After ensuring that the LV apex is in the center of the image in a four-chamber view, the image plane is rotated to about 60° to obtain a two-chamber view. Because the apex often is not exactly centered in three dimensions, the position and angulation of the transducer are adjusted to obtain a two-chamber view that includes the full length of the LV (Fig. 3.7). In this view, the inferior and anterior LV walls of the LV are seen, allowing assessment of regional function and providing the orthogonal plane (along with the four-chamber view) for calculation of ejection fraction. In the two-chamber view, typically only the anterior leaflet of the mitral valve is seen, so it is difficult to evaluate leaflet prolapse in this view.

With further rotation to about 90°, the LA appendage is visualized in a view approximately perpendicular

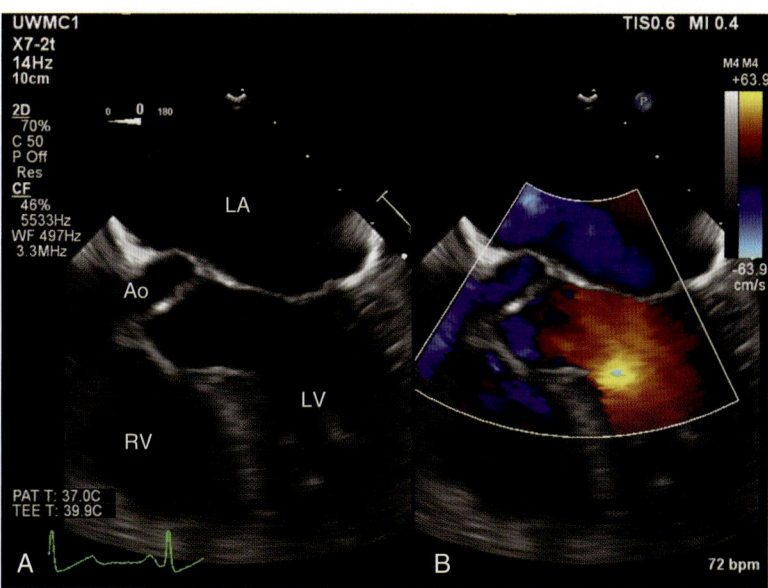

Fig. 3.5 ▶ **Left ventricular outflow view.** (A) Slight anterior angulation from the four-chamber view, midway between the image planes shown in Fig. 3.4, allows visualization of the aortic valve and LV outflow tract. (B) Color flow shows normal systolic laminar flow in the outflow tract. *Ao,* Aorta.

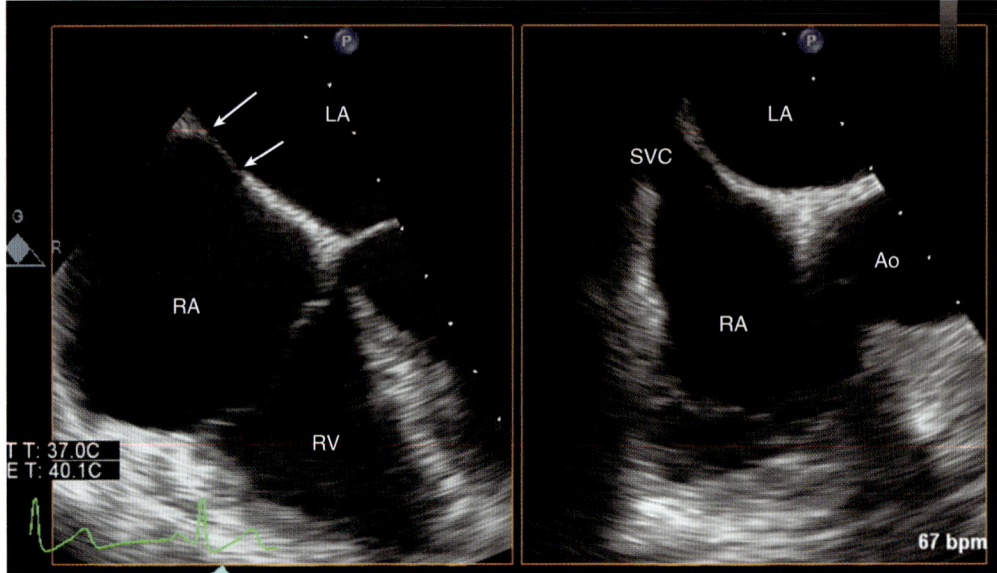

Fig. 3.6 ▶ **Interatrial septum view.** A biplane view of the interatrial septum is obtained by turning the transducer from the four-chamber view toward the patient's right side in a four-chamber view *(left)*. The thin central region of the interatrial septum known as the fossa ovalis is between the *arrows*. The biplane image at 90° shows a second view of the interatrial septum. *Ao,* Aorta; *SVC,* superior vena cava.

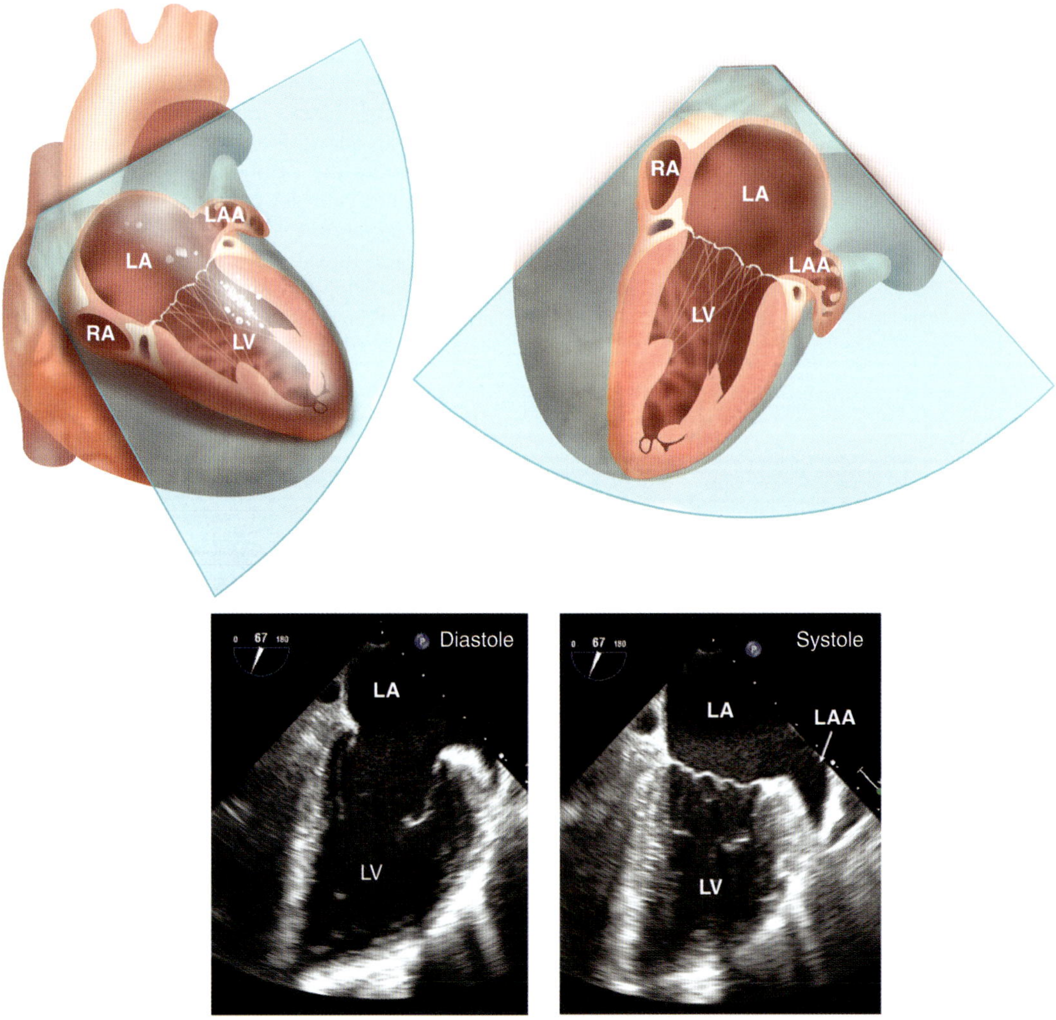

Fig. 3.7 ▶ **Transesophageal echocardiography two-chamber view.** The two-chamber, or vertical long-axis, plane is shown in the 3D heart and then rotated with the vertex of the sector at the top to correspond to the systolic and diastolic echocardiographic images. This view shows the LA and LV with the LA appendage *(LAA),* coronary sinus in the atrioventricular groove, and the mitral valve. In the two-chamber view, small portions of the posterior mitral leaflet are seen laterally and medially with the anterior leaflet filling most of the annulus area. Part of a papillary muscle has been shown for orientation, but the papillary muscles are located symmetrically posterior to the image plane.

Transesophageal Echocardiography | Chapter 3

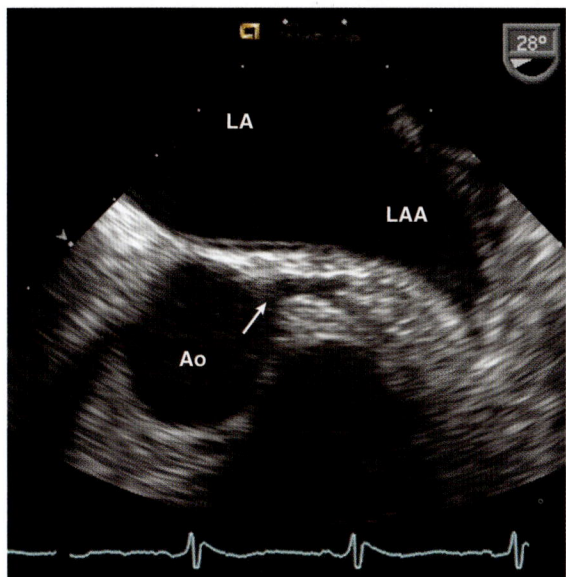

Fig. 3.8 ▶ **Left coronary artery.** LA appendage *(LAA)* and left main coronary artery seen at a rotation angle of about 30°. Starting in the four-chamber view the probe is slightly withdrawn and angulated anteriorly. Note the normal trabeculation in the LAA compared with the smooth LA wall. This image was obtained with a 7.0-MHz transducer to optimize detection of atrial appendage thrombus. *Ao,* Aorta.

to that obtained in the transverse plane (Fig. 3.8). The left superior pulmonary vein is seen entering the LA by slightly withdrawing and turning the probe laterally. The 90° view is also useful for evaluation of mitral valve anatomy.

Long-Axis Plane

From the high-TEE probe position, further rotation of the image plane to about 120° results in a long-axis view of the LV and aorta (Fig. 3.9). Again, slight adjustment of transducer position and angulation is needed to obtain a view that includes the LV apex. Similar to a transthoracic long-axis view, the proximal ascending aorta, sinuses of Valsalva, and right coronary and noncoronary leaflets of the aortic valve are well visualized. In a correctly aligned long-axis plane, the aortic valve leaflets should look linear with a closure slightly more cephalad than the leaflet attachment sites. Scanning between this view and the 90° image planes allows appreciation of the perpendicular relationship between the aortic and pulmonic valve planes and the slightly more cephalad position of the pulmonic valve. Note that in the esophageal long-axis plane, withdrawing the transducer in the esophagus results in more cephalad images of the ascending aorta, with the superior limit of imaging determined by the interposed air-filled bronchus (Fig. 3.10).

The anterior and posterior mitral leaflets are seen in a long-axis orientation, and the coronary sinus is identified in cross section in the atrioventricular groove. The right pulmonary artery is visualized posterior to the aortic root at the superior aspect of the LA. In the long-axis view, the anterior septum and posterior wall of the LV are seen. In addition, a portion of the RV outflow tract is seen anterior to the aortic valve (in the far field of the image).

Other Long-Axis Image Planes

At a rotation angle of 90°, the probe is turned from the LV long-axis view toward the patient's left side to obtain a long-axis view of the pulmonic valve and RV outflow tract (Fig. 3.11). In this view, the pulmonic valve is in the far field of the image, with shadowing by the aortic valve and root if calcification is present. Portions of the RV and tricuspid valve are seen, depending on the exact position of the heart relative to the esophagus in each patient.

At a 90° rotation with the probe turned toward the patient's right side, images of the RV and tricuspid valve in an inflow view are obtained. If the probe is turned farther to the right, the bicaval view is obtained, showing the RA and RA appendage, with the superior vena cava entering from the right side of the screen and the inferior vena cava from the left (Fig. 3.12). In some individuals, a Eustachian valve at the inferior caval-atrial junction is seen. The trabeculated RA appendage often is seen with slight medial rotation from this view.

Short-Axis Plane

A short-axis view at the aortic valve level is obtained by rotating the image plane to between 30° and 45° and withdrawing the probe in the esophagus to the level of the aortic valve. Visualization of aortic valve anatomy is excellent, showing the three leaflets and sinuses of Valsalva (Fig. 3.13). The interatrial septum is well seen, with the fossa ovalis clearly defined. The origin of the left main coronary artery is easily identified after minor adjustments in the depth and tilt of the image plane. The right coronary artery is more difficult to visualize in the short-axis view but often is seen in the long-axis view of the aortic valve and ascending aorta..

By turning the transducer laterally and angulating superiorly from the 0° esophageal position, the LA appendage and left superior pulmonary vein are seen (Fig. 3.14). Prominent features include normal trabeculation of the atrial appendage and a variably prominent ridge at the junction of the left superior pulmonary vein and the LA appendage. Compared with the left superior pulmonary vein, which enters the LA anteriorly with flow directed parallel to the ultrasound beam, the left inferior pulmonary vein enters the atrium with flow perpendicular to the ultrasound beam. The left inferior pulmonary vein

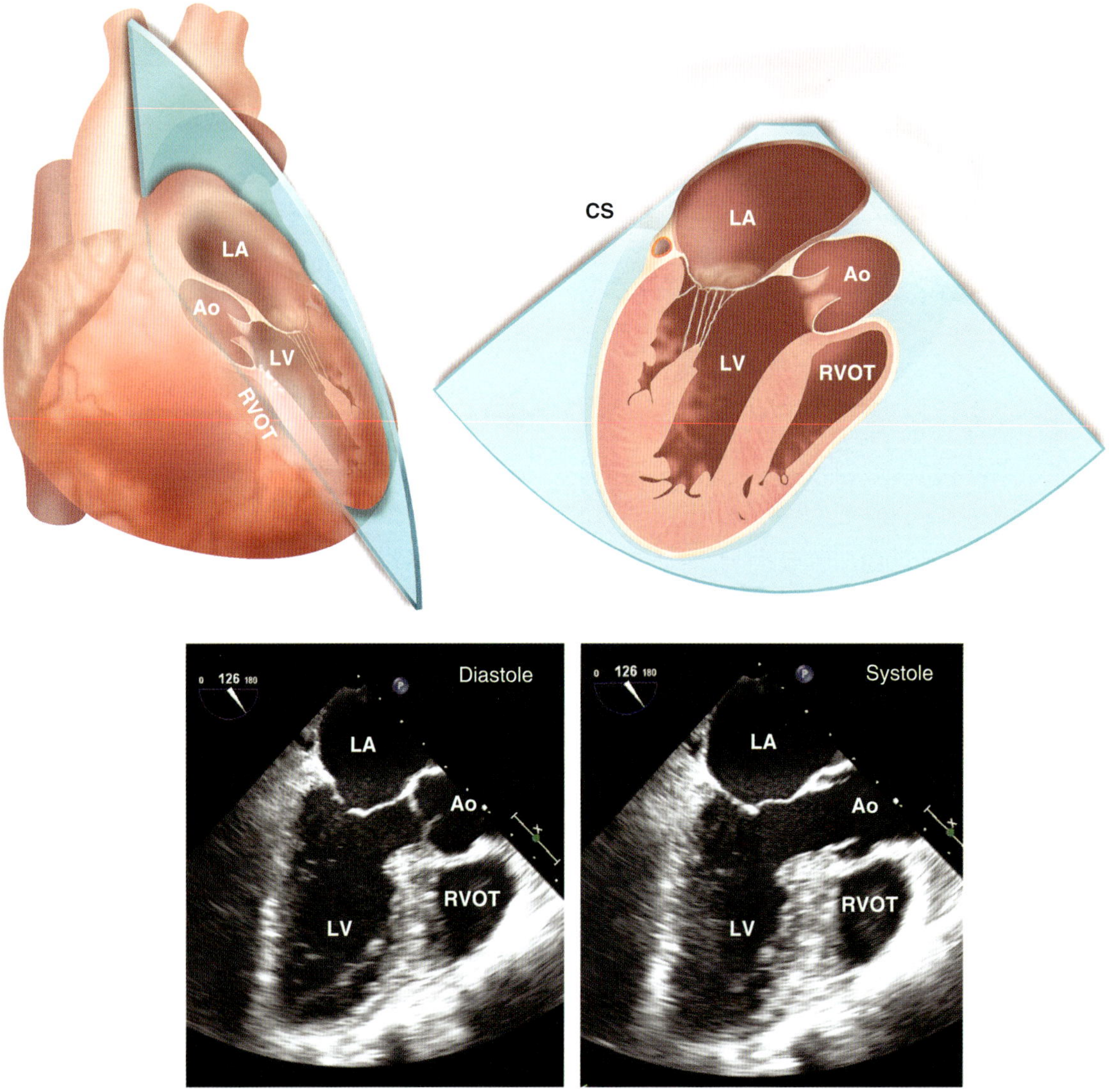

Fig. 3.9 ▶ **Transesophageal echocardiography long-axis view.** The position of the image plane is shown on the 3D heart with the tomographic view rotated to the standard TEE image orientation to correspond to the systolic and diastolic echocardiographic images. This view typically is obtained at approximately 120° rotation, but considerable individual variability exists in the exact image plane needed to show the aorta and LV in a long-axis orientation. The 3D view shows the cross-section of the aortic root *(Ao)*, LV, LA, and RV outflow tract *(RVOT)*. In the long-axis view, the anterior and posterior mitral valve leaflets are seen. *CS*, Coronary sinus.

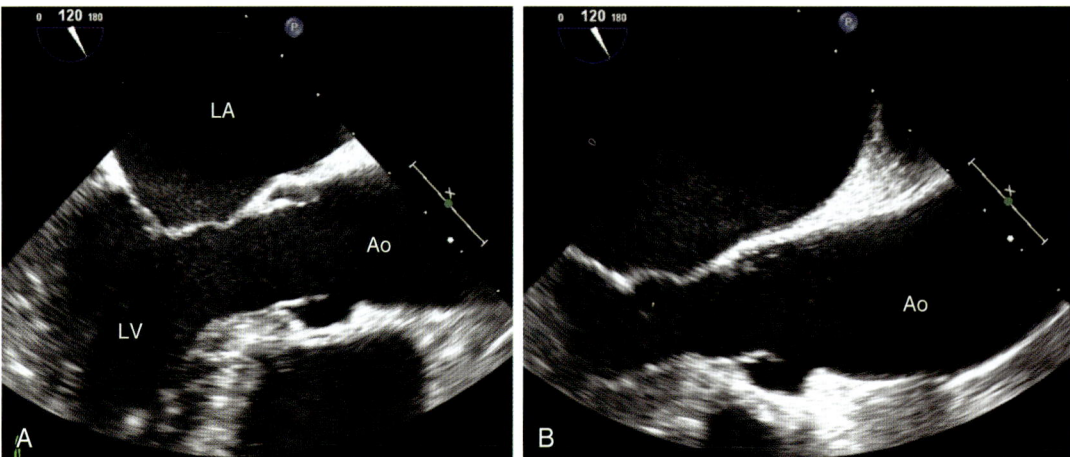

Fig. 3.10 ▶ ▶ **Transesophageal echocardiography view of ascending aorta.** (A) and (B) From the TEE long-axis view, further cephalad segments of the ascending aorta *(Ao)* are seen by slight withdrawal of the transducer in the esophagus.

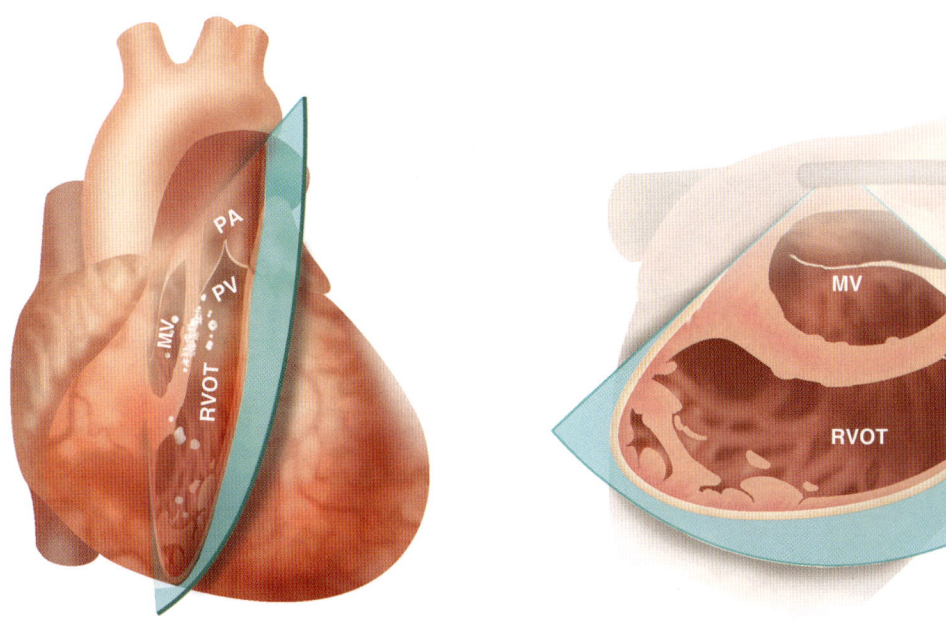
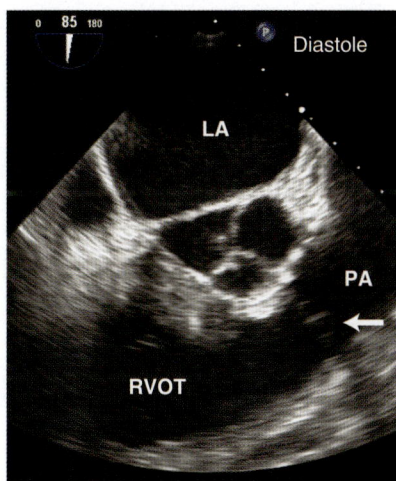
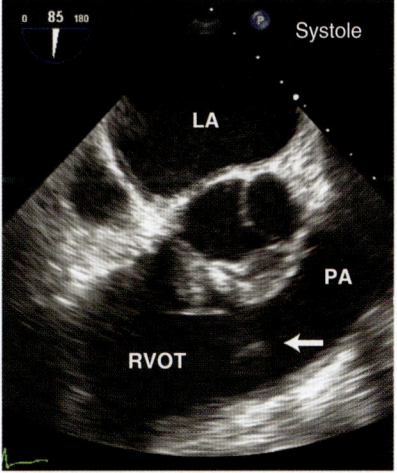

Fig. 3.11 **Transesophageal echocardiography RV outflow tract view.** The position of the image plane is shown on the 3D heart with the tomographic view rotated to the standard TEE image orientation to correspond to the systolic and diastolic echocardiographic images. In the 90° TEE image plane, the RV outflow tract *(RVOT)*, pulmonic valve *(PV, arrow)*, and pulmonary artery *(PA)* are seen. *MV*, Mitral valve.

is seen by advancing the transducer and angulating slightly inferiorly. The right pulmonary veins are imaged by rotating the transducer medially and withdrawing the transducer cephalad (to see the anteriorly directed right superior pulmonary vein) or by angulating the transducer inferiorly (to see the medially directed right inferior pulmonary vein). The pulmonary veins also are identified in the 90° image plane by turning the transducer toward the patient's right to show the right pulmonary veins and to the left for the left pulmonary veins. Again, color flow imaging often facilitates identification of the pulmonary veins based on the characteristic venous inflow patterns.

In many patients, the pulmonary artery can be imaged in the 0° image plane by further withdrawing the probe in the esophagus to obtain a view straight down the main pulmonary artery from the bifurcation to the valve level. In some cases, this view is limited by the position of the air-filled bronchus, and some patients find the probe uncomfortable when it is positioned at this level in the esophagus.

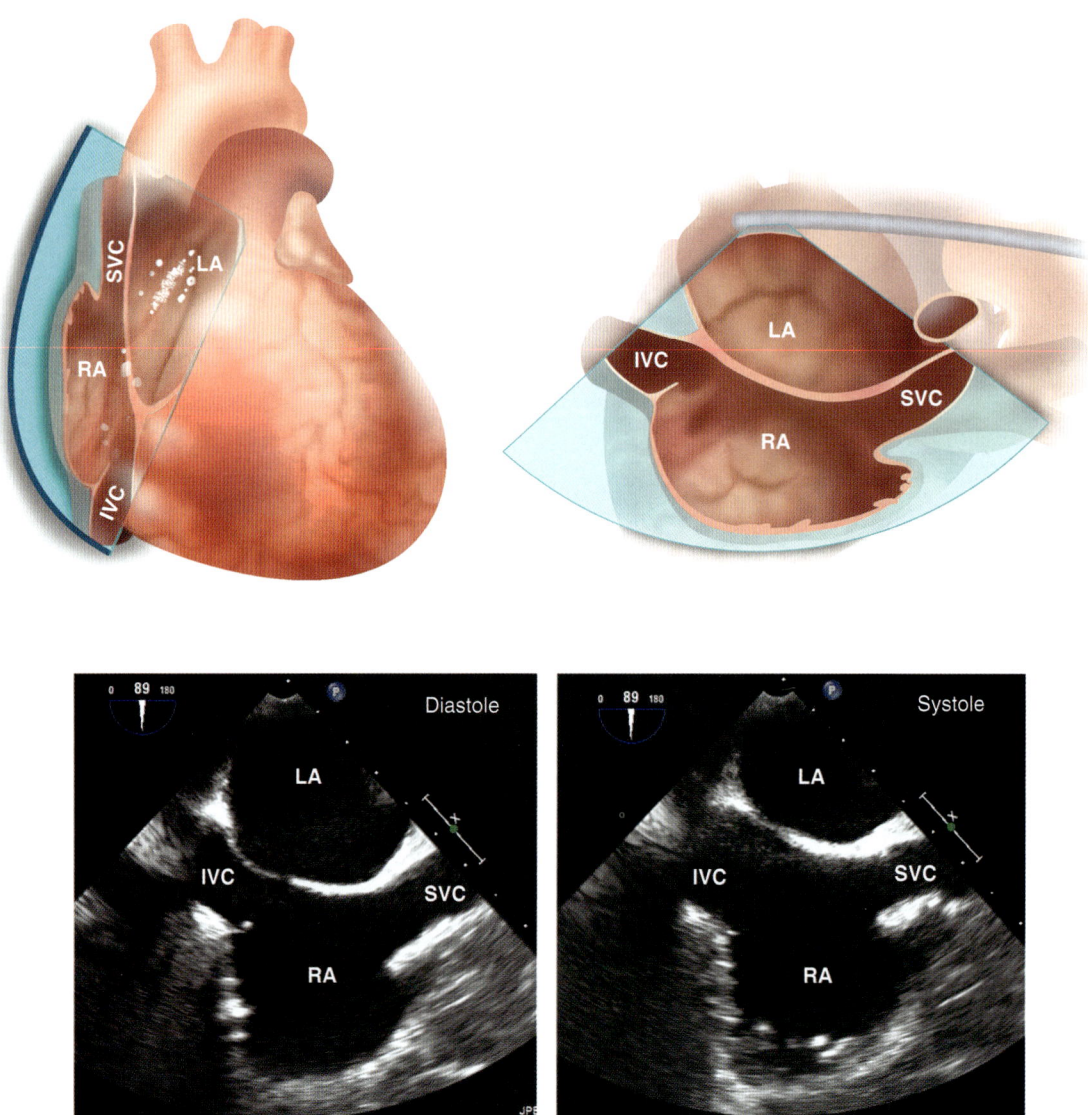

Fig. 3.12 ▶ **Transesophageal echocardiography bicaval view.** The position of the image plane is shown on the 3D heart with the tomographic view rotated to the standard TEE image orientation to correspond to the systolic and diastolic echocardiographic images. With the probe turned toward the patient's right side, the RA, superior vena cava *(SVC)*, and inferior vena cava *(IVC)* are visualized in the 90° TEE image plane. A Eustachian valve often is present at the IVC-RA junction. Part of the trabeculated RA appendage is seen adjacent to the SVC.

Transgastric Position
Short-Axis Plane

As the transducer is passed into the stomach, slight resistance may be encountered at the gastroesophageal junction. With the probe tip in the stomach, superior angulation (flexing the scope) in the 0° image plane results in a short-axis view of the LV at the papillary muscle level (Fig. 3.15). In this view, global LV systolic function, LV dimensions and wall thickness, and regional LV function are evaluated (Fig. 3.16). Depending on the position of the patient's heart with respect to the diaphragm, a short-axis view at the mitral valve level is obtained by slight withdrawal of the transducer toward the esophagus (Fig. 3.17).

Two-Chamber Plane

A two-chamber view of the LV is obtained from the transgastric position by rotating the image plane to the 90° position (Fig. 3.18). From this two-chamber view, turning the entire probe toward the patient's right side results in (1) a view of the LV outflow tract and aortic valve and then, with further turning to the right, (2) a view of the RA, tricuspid valve, and RV similar to a transthoracic RV inflow view. In

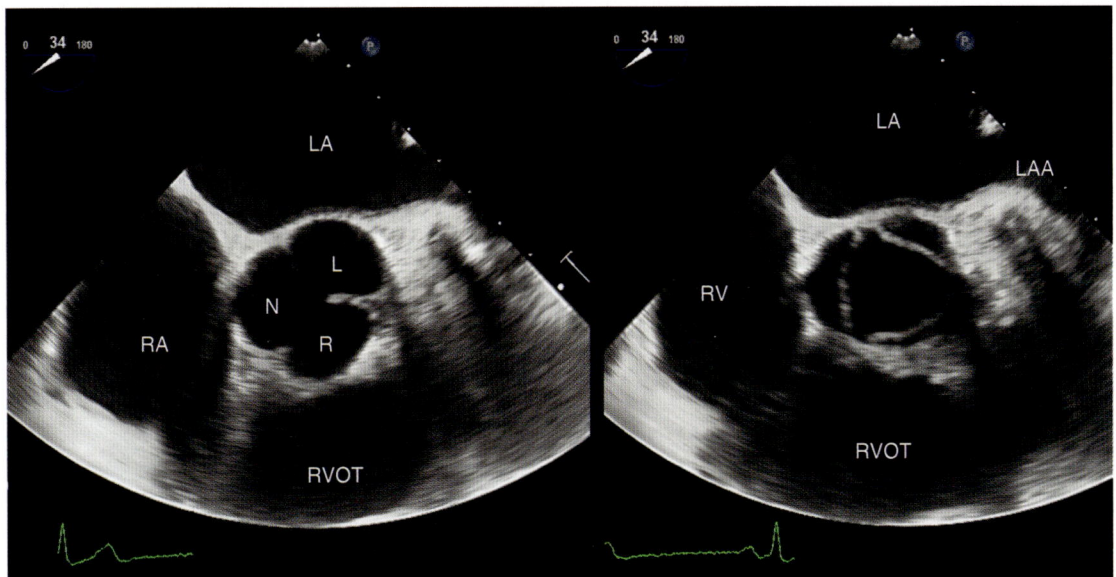

Fig. 3.13 ▶ **Transesophageal echocardiography aortic valve short-axis view.** The aortic valve is seen in diastole *(left)* and systole *(right)* with the degree of rotation needed to obtain this short-axis view varying from approximately 30° to 50°. Oblique image planes may result in artifactual distortion of the valve apparatus. *L,* Left coronary cusp of the aortic valve; *LAA,* LA appendage; *N,* noncoronary cusp of the aortic valve; *R,* right coronary cusp of the aortic valve; *RVOT,* RV outflow tract.

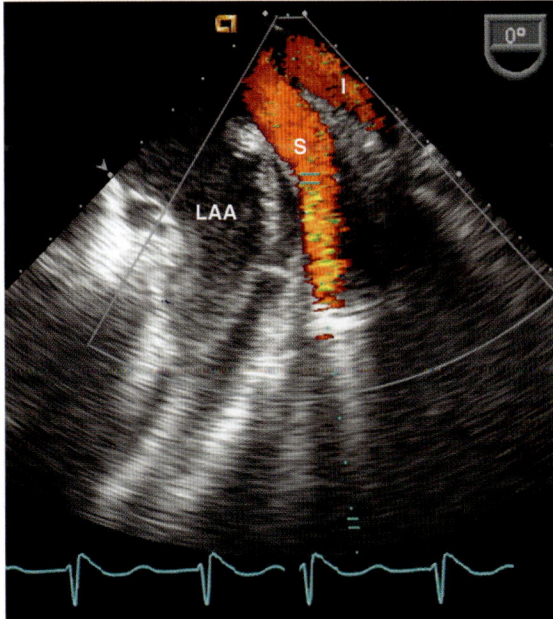

Fig. 3.14 ▶ **Pulmonary veins.** The left superior *(S)* and inferior *(I)* pulmonary veins are seen in the 0° plane with the probe at the level of the LA appendage *(LAA)*. Color flow imaging facilitates identification of the pulmonary views as they enter the LA.

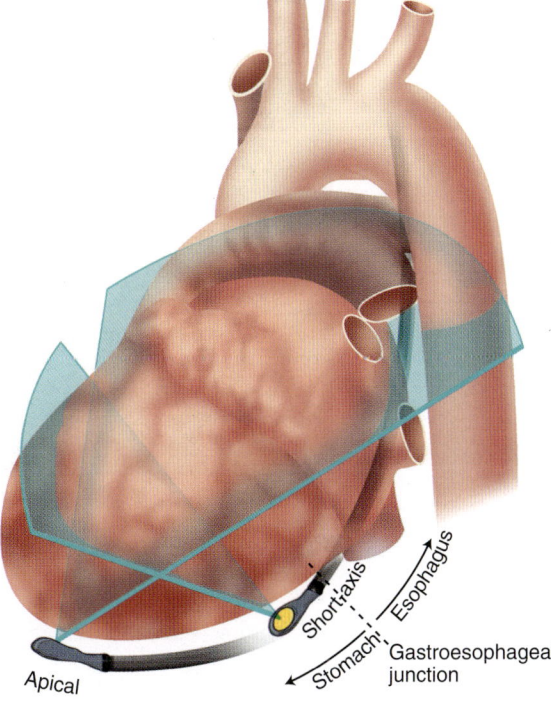

Fig. 3.15 Transgastric image planes. From the transgastric position, the probe is positioned near the gastroesophageal junction to obtain a short-axis view of the LV or is advanced into the stomach to obtain an "apical" view. Transgastric apical images may show a foreshortened LV because the true LV apex often does not lie on the diaphragm.

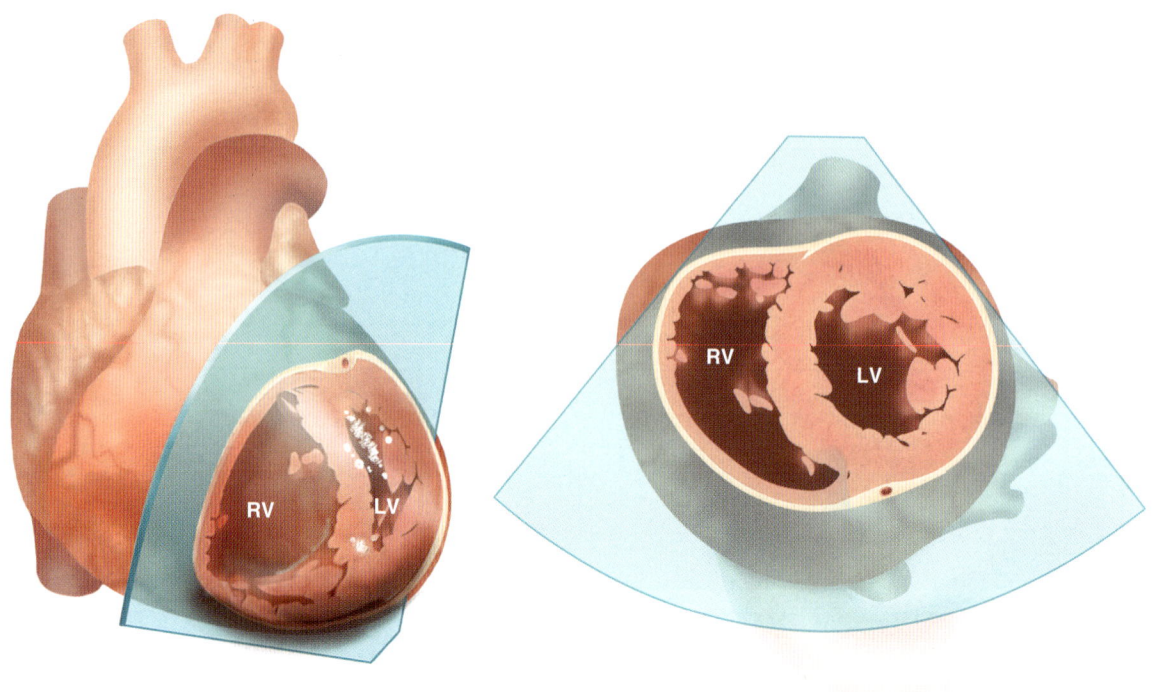

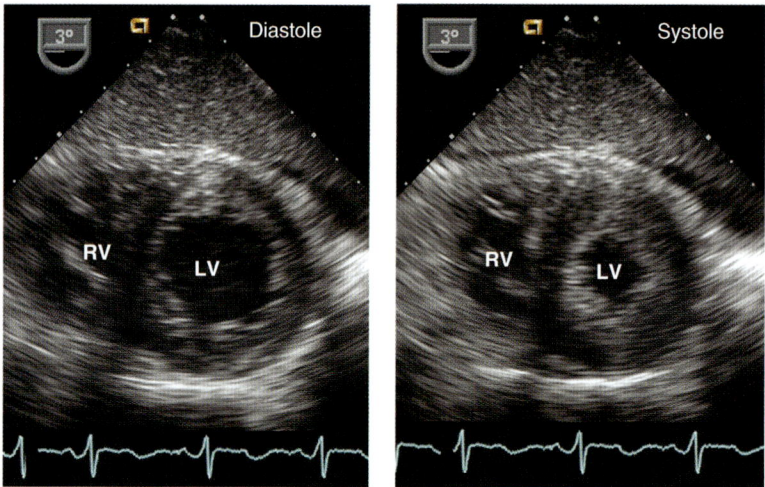

Fig. 3.16 ▶ **Transgastric short-axis views of the left ventricle.** The position of the image plane is shown on the 3D heart with the tomographic view rotated to the standard TEE image orientation to correspond to the systolic and diastolic echocardiographic images. This view is obtained by retroflexion of the transducer from a transgastric position and is particularly valuable for intraoperative monitoring of LV size and global and regional systolic function.

some individuals, the RV outflow tract and pulmonic valve also are visualized.

Four-Chamber Plane

From the transgastric short-axis view, the transducer is advanced farther, into the fundus of the stomach. In most individuals, an "apical" four-chamber view can be obtained using the 0° image plane of the probe if the LV lies on the diaphragm, without intervening lung. Note that the transducer usually is not on the true LV apex, so this view is foreshortened. Anterior angulation shows the aortic valve in a view similar to the transthoracic five-chamber view.

Long-Axis Plane

From the transgastric apical four-chamber plane, rotation of the image plane to 120° results in a long-axis view of the LV outflow tract, thus providing a more parallel intercept angle for Doppler study of outflow tract and aortic velocities. However, this view

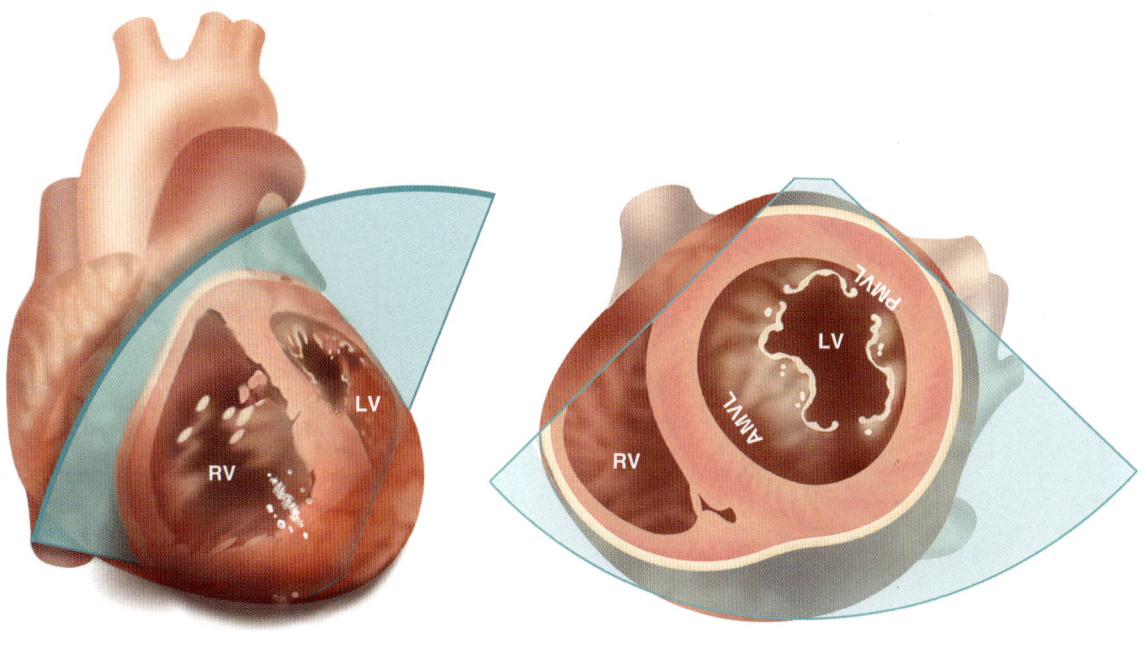

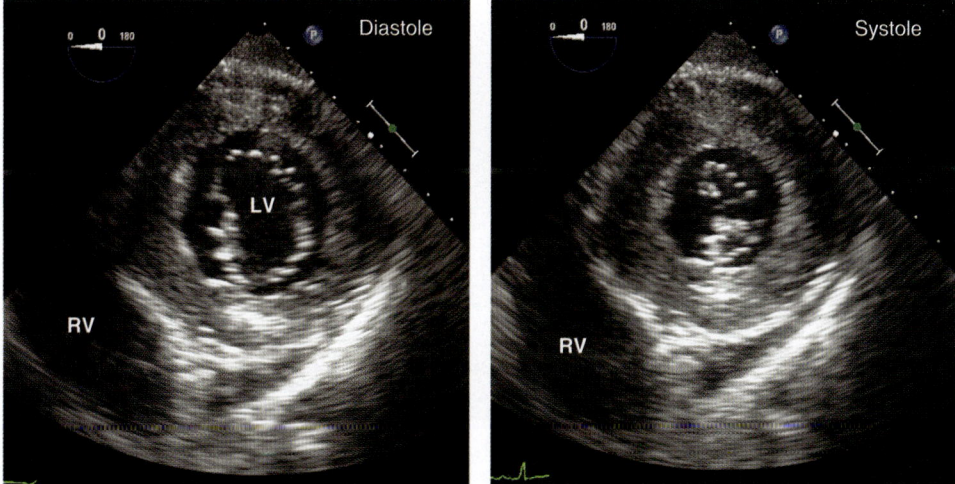

Fig. 3.17 ▶ **Transgastric short-axis at the mitral valve level.** The position of the image plane is shown on the 3D heart with the tomographic view rotated to the standard TEE image orientation to correspond to the systolic and diastolic echocardiographic images. From the transgastric short-axis view of the LV, slight withdrawal of the probe toward the gastroesophageal junction may allow a short-axis view of the mitral valve with definition of the anterior mitral valve leaflets *(AMVL)* and posterior mitral valve leaflets *(PMVL)*.

cannot be obtained in all patients, particularly if the transducer is not on the true LV apex, because lung tissue is interposed between the transducer and cardiac structures as the image plane is rotated.

Descending Thoracic Aorta

From the TEE or transgastric position, the transducer is turned posteriorly until the image plane is directed slightly left of the patient's spine to obtain a short-axis view of the descending thoracic aorta. The aorta appears circular and shows normal systolic pulsations (Fig. 3.19). The descending thoracic aorta is imaged in sequential short-axis views from the transgastric position to the junction with the aortic arch as the probe is slowly withdrawn in the esophagus. When the transducer reaches the level of the arch, turning the transducer medially with inferior angulation allows a long-axis view of the arch itself. Imaging in the short-axis view as the probe is withdrawn along the

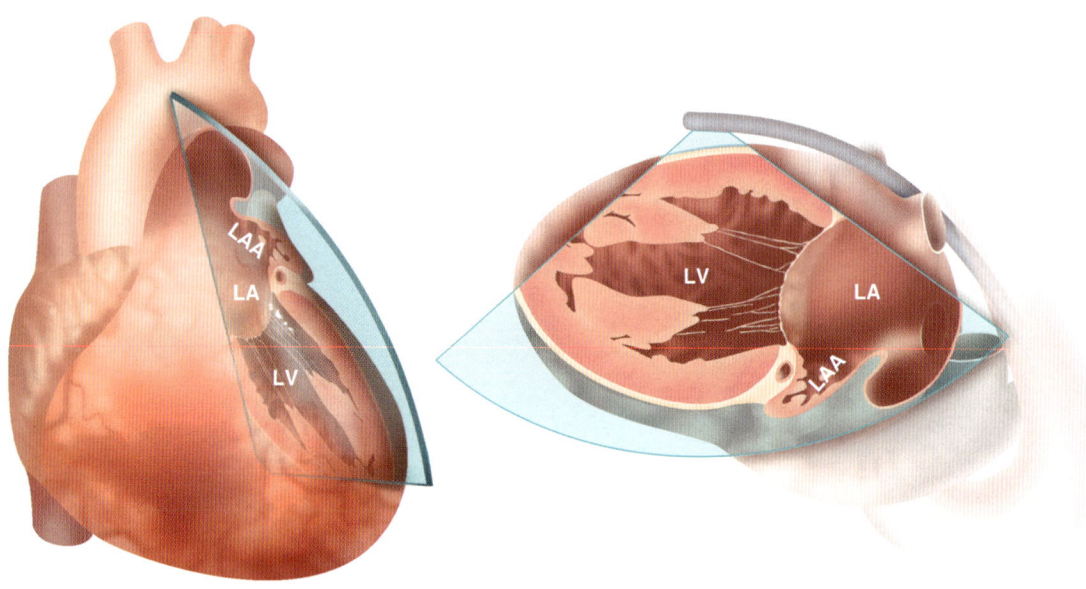

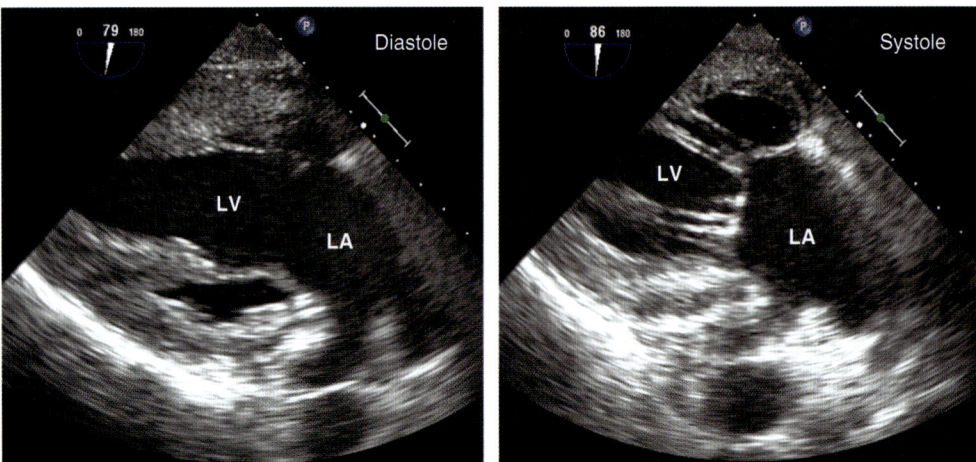

Fig. 3.18 ▶ **Transgastric long-axis views of the left ventricle.** From the transgastric short-axis view, 90° rotation provides a two-chamber view of the LV, LA, and LA appendage *(LAA) (top)*. The tomographic image plane has been rotated with the apex of the sector at the top to correspond to the echocardiographic image *(bottom right)*. Turning the transducer toward the patient's right side from this view provides a two-chamber view of the RA and RV, analogous to a transthoracic RV inflow view.

length of the aorta ensures visualization of the entire aortic endothelium.

A long-axis view of the descending aorta, obtained by centering the aorta in the 2D sector and rotating the image plane to 90°, complements the short-axis view in evaluation of aortic dissections, aneurysms, and atheromas and improves the differentiation of ultrasound artifacts from anatomic abnormalities. The 90° image plane also allows identification of the origin of the left subclavian artery, which is important for describing the proximal extent of dissection and for placement of an intra-aortic balloon pump (see Chapter 16). Biplane imaging allows simultaneous short- and long-axis views of the descending thoracic aorta.

VALVE ANATOMY AND FUNCTION

Optimal evaluation of valve anatomy and function on TEE echocardiography includes the use of at least two standard orthogonal imaging planes (Table 3.3). This approach provides a reasonably complete evaluation of valve anatomy and aids recognition

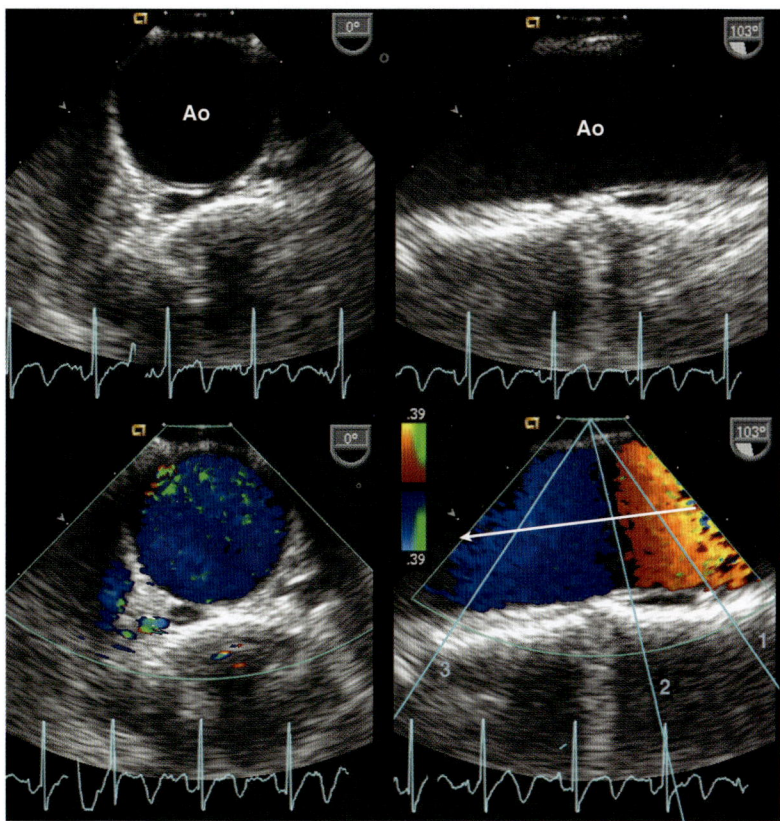

Fig. 3.19 **Transesophageal echocardiography 2D and color flow images of the descending thoracic aorta.** Short-axis ▶ *(left)* (0° rotation) and long-axis ▶ *(right)* (90° rotation) views on 2D echo *(top)* and with color flow imaging *(bottom)* are shown. The short-axis view shows flow filling the aorta *(Ao)* in systole. In the long-axis view, although the direction and velocity of flow are uniform *(arrow)*, the color displayed depends on the angle between the ultrasound beam and the flow direction. Lines for three ultrasound beam angles are shown in cyan *(1, 2, 3)*, illustrating how the color changes from red for flow directed toward the transducer *(1)*, to black where flow is perpendicular to the ultrasound beam *(2)*, and then to blue where flow is directed away from the transducer *(3)*.

of ultrasound artifacts. Continuous-wave (CW) and pulsed Doppler velocities should be recorded with the ultrasound beam aligned parallel to the flowstream. However, a parallel intercept angle is difficult to achieve given the constraints on transducer position from the TEE approach. As with transthoracic imaging, color Doppler is helpful for the evaluation of abnormal flow patterns even at nonparallel intercept angles.

Aortic Valve

The aortic valve and LV outflow tract are imaged in the long-axis view from the high TEE probe position with rotation of the image plane to about 120° (Fig. 3.20). A short-axis view of the aortic valve is obtained by rotating the image plane to about 45° (see Fig. 3.13). In the short-axis view, slight withdrawal of the probe shows the sinuses of Valsalva and left main coronary artery, whereas slight advancement provides a short-axis view of the LV outflow tract. In the 0° four-chamber view, the outflow and aortic valve also are seen by anterior angulation of the image plane (see Fig. 3.5) In both the short- and long-axis views, image quality is optimized by use of a high transducer frequency and adjustment of the depth, or use of zoom mode, to maximize the valve image.

3D images of the aortic valve are helpful in selected patients but can be challenging to acquire in views that are clinically diagnostic. Starting in the 2D short- or long-axis view of the aortic valve, a narrow-angle real-time 3D image is acquired either looking down at the aortic side of the valve or up at the LV side of the valve with the right coronary cusp at the bottom of the image (Fig. 3.21). A full-volume 3D data set also is acquired and then cropped to display the aortic valve in long- or short-axis views.

Color flow imaging in long- and short-axis views of the valve allows evaluation for valvular regurgitation, including vena contracta width and the origin and direction of the regurgitant jet (see Chapter 12). A cross-sectional area of the aortic regurgitant jet can

TABLE 3.3 Transesophageal Imaging and Doppler Assessment of Cardiac Valves

Valve	Probe Position	Imaging View	Rotation Angle	Doppler
Aortic	ME	Long-axis Short-axis 5-chamber	~120°–130° ~30°–50° 0° (anteriorly angulated)	• Color Doppler for regurgitation and level of outflow obstruction
		3D view	3D zoomed image to show aortic valve from LV and aortic side with noncoronary sinus at bottom of the image	—
	TG	Long-axis	90° (from mitral valve view, turn rightward to visualize LVOT)	• Color Doppler for regurgitation and level of outflow obstruction
		Apical	0° (anteriorly angulated)	• CW and pulsed of LVOT is possible, but velocities are likely underestimated due to a nonparallel intercept angle.
Mitral	ME	4-chamber	0° followed by a rotational scan to the long-axis view Record images at 30° to 60° increments depending on valve pathology	• Color Doppler for MR jet direction, vena contracta width, and PISA • Pulsed Doppler LV inflow and pulmonary veins • CW Doppler MR velocity curve
		2-chamber	60° In addition, a 90° view is helpful in some patients.	
		Long-axis	~120°–130°	
	TG	Short-axis	Can be obtained in some patients at 0° with probe flexed	—
	ME	3D	3D zoomed image to show mitral valve from LV or LA side with aortic valve at top of the image	• 3D color Doppler PISA and vena contracta in selected patients
Pulmonic	UE	Long-axis	0° (looking straight down PA from bifurcation)	• Color Doppler for regurgitation • Intercept angle allows pulsed or CW Doppler recording of pulmonary artery antegrade flow if needed.
	ME	Outflow	~90° (turn probe to left)	• Color Doppler for regurgitation
Tricuspid	ME	4-chamber RV inflow (esophageal)	0° ~90° (turn probe to right)	Color Doppler for regurgitation CW Doppler to record TR jet velocity to estimate pulmonary pressures
	TG	RV inflow (transgastric)	~90° (turn probe to right)	

LVOT, LV outflow tract; *ME*, mid-esophageal; *MR*, mitral regurgitation; *PA*, pulmonary artery; *PISA*, proximal isovelocity surface area; *TG*, transgastric; *TR*, tricuspid regurgitation; *UE*, upper esophageal.

be obtained by starting in a short-axis view of the aortic valve and slowly advancing the probe in the esophagus to obtain a short-axis view of the outflow tract.

Measurement of antegrade velocity across the aortic valve is limited by the nonparallel intercept angle between the ultrasound beam and the direction of blood flow from the TEE position. In some patients, a transgastric apical view allows recording of pulsed and CW Doppler flow velocities proximal to and across the aortic valve (Fig. 3.22). However, caution still is needed in interpretation of the Doppler data because the intercept angle may be oblique. If aortic valve pathology is present, transthoracic recording of antegrade velocities is more accurate and should be performed in all cases.

Mitral Valve

The mitral valve is evaluated by slow rotation from the TEE four-chamber view to the long-axis view with image recording at about 30° increments. Transducer depth is decreased to include just the mitral valve, transducer frequency is increased to improve image resolution, and the transducer position is centered relative to the valve annulus. The leaflets

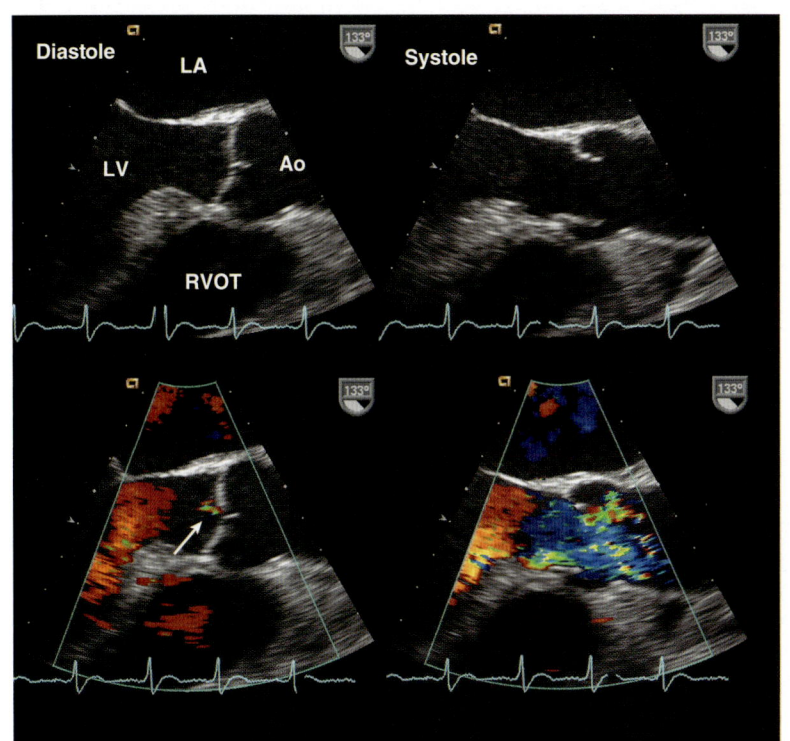

Fig. 3.20 ▶ **Long-axis images of the aortic valve.** Depth is adjusted to optimize evaluation of valve anatomy and motion. The 2D images ▶ *(top)* in diastole *(left)* and systole *(right)* show normal aortic opening and closure. The color flow images ▶ *(bottom)* show trace aortic regurgitation in diastole *(arrow)*, normal antegrade flow in the LV outflow tract, and no mitral regurgitation in systole. *Ao,* Aorta; *RVOT,* RV outflow tract.

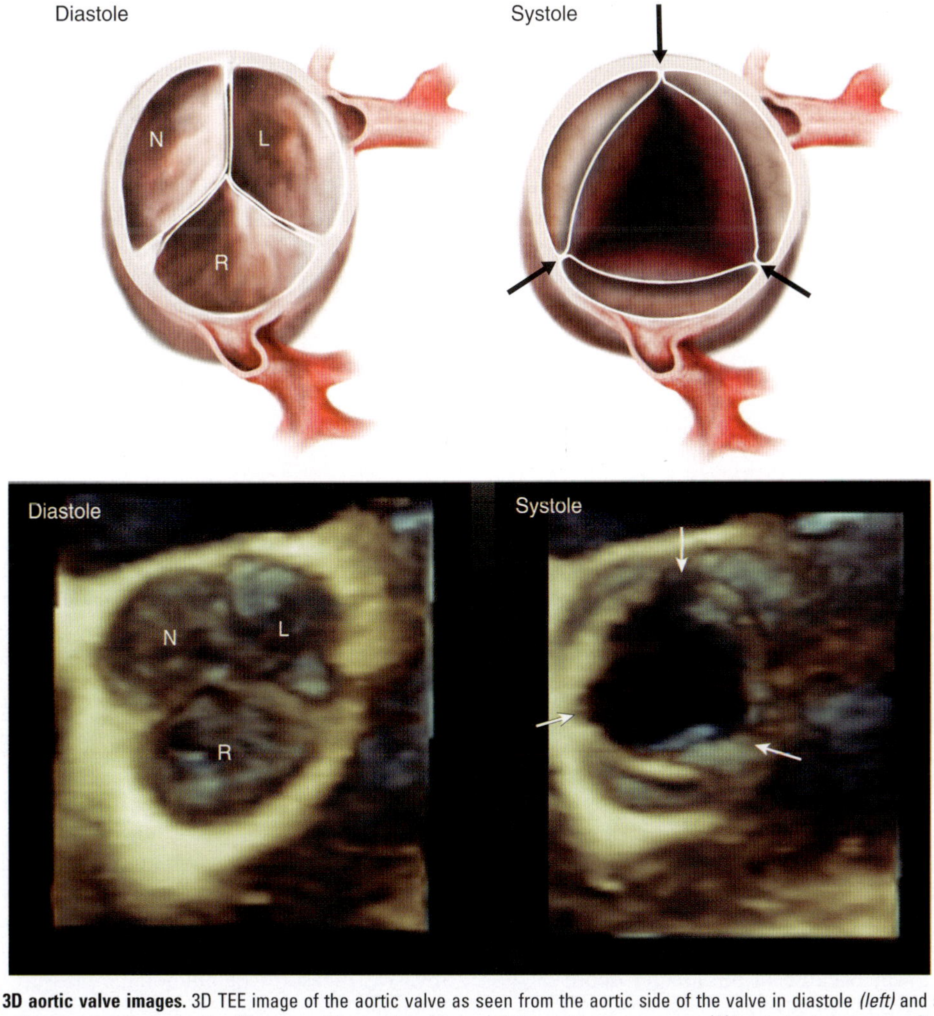

Fig. 3.21 ▶ **3D aortic valve images.** 3D TEE image of the aortic valve as seen from the aortic side of the valve in diastole *(left)* and systole *(right)*. The standard orientation for displaying the 3D image of the aortic valve is with the right coronary cusp *(R)* located inferiorly regardless of whether images are acquired by transthoracic echocardiorgrarphy or TEE. In systole, the three open commissures *(arrows)* of this normal trileaflet valve are seen. *L,* Left coronary cusp; *N,* noncoronary cusp.

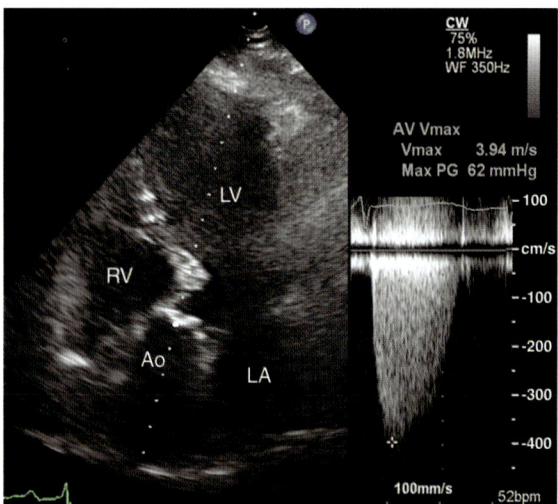

Fig. 3.22 **Transgastric apical view.** The image plane is angulated anteriorly to include aortic valve *(left)* with the line indicating the position of the CW Doppler beam. The aortic valve is calcified and immobile, and the aortic jet velocity recorded with 2D-guided CW Doppler *(right)* is increased to at least 3.9 m/s. When a high-velocity jet is suspected, careful angulation and positioning of the transducer are needed to obtain the highest velocity signal. Because of the constraints on transducer positioning, the possibility of velocity underestimation should be considered. *Ao*, Aorta.

and subvalvular apparatus are usually well seen in these views unless valve calcification with shadowing of distal structures is present. If additional views are needed, transgastric short-axis and two-chamber views of the mitral valve are obtained. The valve also is seen on the transgastric apical view, although image quality often is suboptimal at the depth of the mitral valve.

If the mitral valve is abnormal, 3D imaging is recommended. Real-time 3D imaging showing the LA aspect of the valve provides improved display of spatial relationships, with adequate temporal resolution. A full-volume zoomed 3D acquisition provides the best spatial and temporal resolution. Typically, cropped views show the ventricle and the atrial side of the valve, with the image oriented to show the aortic valve at the top of the image (Fig. 3.23).

The pattern of antegrade flow across the mitral valve (LV diastolic filling) is recorded with pulsed Doppler in the four-chamber or long-axis view at a parallel intercept angle (Fig. 3.24). Because the flow is directly away from the transducer, the velocity curve with the typical early diastolic peak (E) and late diastolic peak (A) velocities is shown below the baseline. Transmitral flow also can be recorded from the transgastric apical approach, although signal strength is lower because of the greater depth of the mitral valve from this position.

Color Doppler is used to evaluate for mitral regurgitation as the image plane is slowly rotated from the four-chamber to two-chamber to long-axis view. The image plane that best shows the proximal jet geometry (proximal isovelocity acceleration and vena contracta) is used for quantitative measures of regurgitant severity, as discussed in Chapter 12. Split screen 2D and color imaging is used if the sector width encompasses the entire mitral annulus, but separate imaging and color Doppler data recordings are needed in some patients. Mitral regurgitation also is evaluated with CW Doppler from the upper esophageal position, using the color flow signal to align the CW Doppler beam with the vena contracta of the regurgitant jet (Fig. 3.25). Color 3D imaging of the proximal jet geometry is an area of active research.

Pulmonic Valve

The pulmonic valve and RV outflow tract are best imaged from an upper esophageal position at 0° rotation with a long-axis view of the pulmonary artery from the valve plane to its bifurcation. Doppler velocities are recorded from this position at a parallel intercept angle as flow is directed straight toward the transducer (Fig. 3.26). The pulmonic valve also is visualized in the 90° long-axis plane with the pulmonic valve seen in its perpendicular relationship with the aortic valve in the far field of the image (see Fig. 3.11). However, velocities cannot be recorded from this approach because of a nonparallel intercept angle. In some patients the pulmonic valve also can be imaged from the transgastric position either in the 90° image plane including the tricuspid valve or in a very anteriorly angulated apical four-chamber view.

Tricuspid Valve

The tricuspid valve is well imaged in the standard four-chamber view, both from the TEE position and from the transgastric apical view. Other useful views include the TEE RV inflow view and the transgastric two-chamber view turned to show the right heart structures. In a transgastric view obtained close to the diaphragm, the entry of the coronary sinus into the RA adjacent to the tricuspid valve is seen. Further advancement of the transducer often allows a short-axis view of the tricuspid valve.

The tricuspid regurgitant jet is recorded from either TEE or transgastric views; however, underestimation of velocity should be considered given the limited ability to vary transducer position to ensure a parallel intercept angle. If high pulmonary pressures are suspected, transthoracic CW Doppler recordings or invasive measures of pulmonary pressure should be obtained.

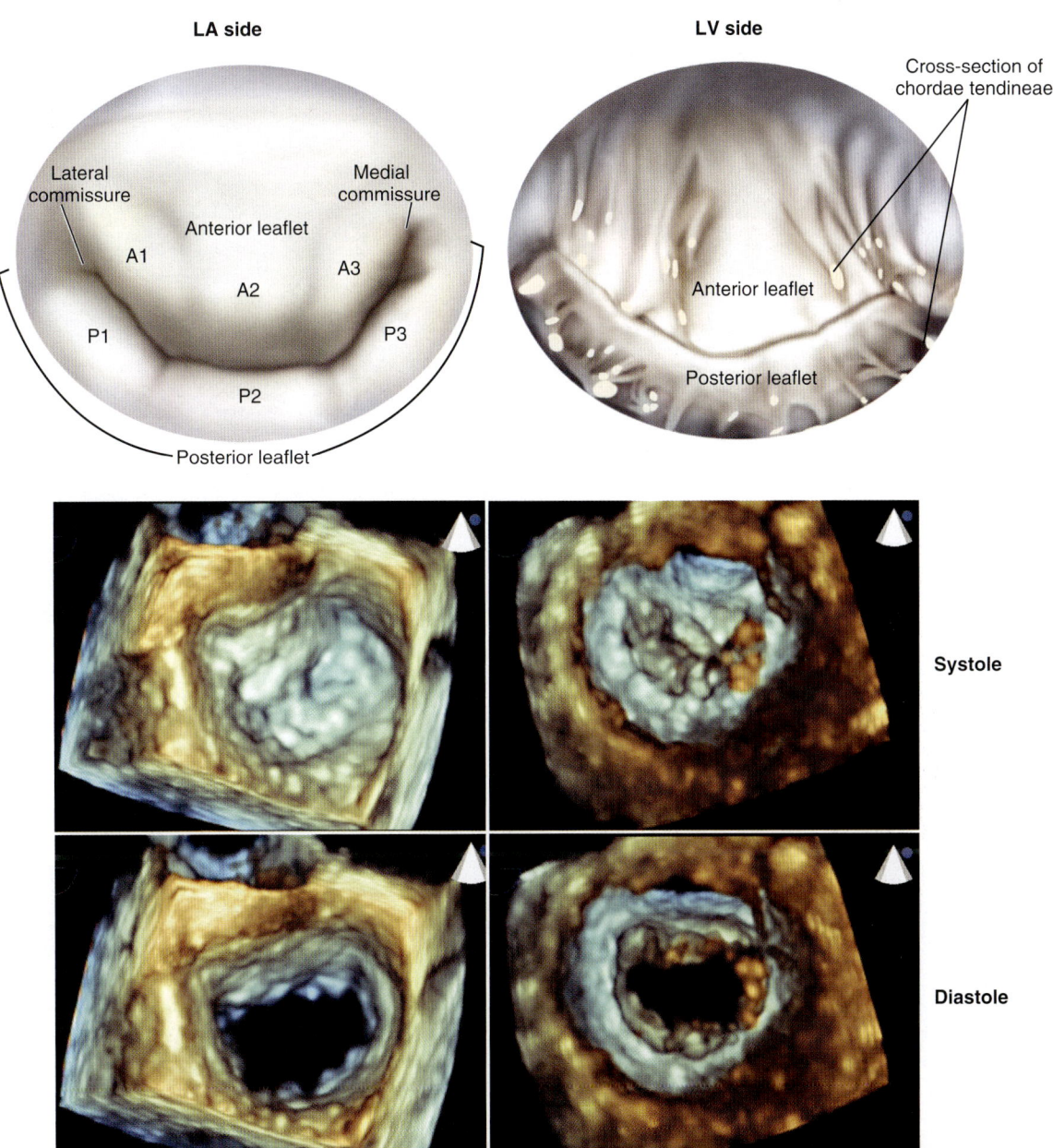

Fig. 3.23 **3D imaging of mitral valve.** Anatomic views of the mitral valve ▶ (top) correspond to 3D volumetric images viewed from the LA side (left) and LV side (right) of the valve in diastole ▶ (middle) and systole (bottom). The recommended orientation of 3D echo images of the mitral valve is with the aortic valve at the top of the image, as shown here. The three scallops of the anterior (A) and posterior (P) mitral leaflets are shown with the medial (P3 and A3) scallops on the right side of the image and the lateral (P1 and A1) scallops on the left side of the image.

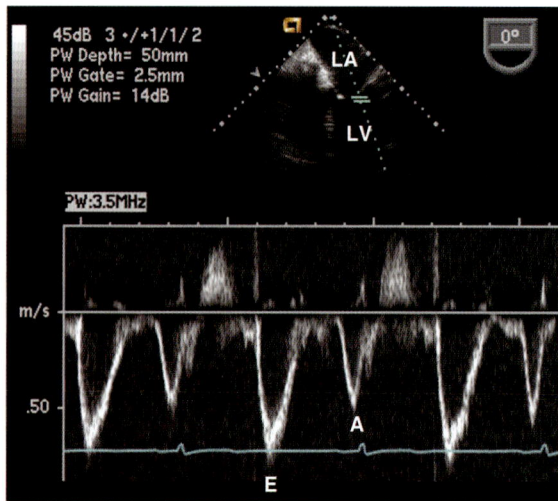

Fig. 3.24 Left ventricular inflow. Pulsed Doppler is recorded with the sample volume positioned at the mitral leaflet tips from an anteriorly angulated TEE four-chamber view. The flow pattern is similar to a transthoracic recording of LV inflow, albeit inverted because the flow is directed away from the transducer.

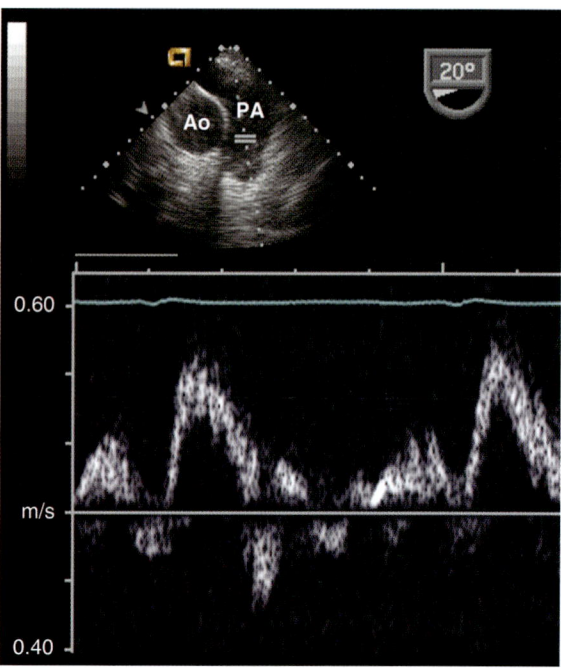

Fig. 3.26 Pulmonary artery flow. A very upper TEE position provides a long-axis view *(top)* of the main pulmonary artery *(PA)* and its bifurcation into right and left pulmonary arteries. The ascending aorta *(Ao)* is seen in the short-axis view. This view allows recording of flow in the pulmonary artery at a parallel intercept angle because flow is directly toward the transducer *(bottom)*.

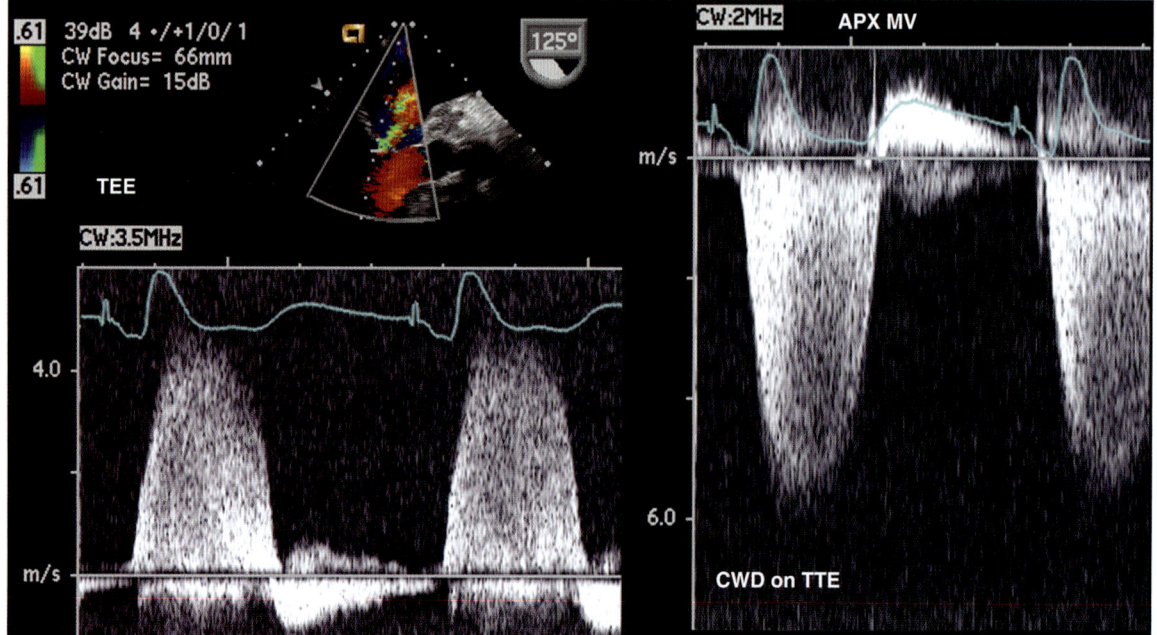

Fig. 3.25 Continuous-wave Doppler recording of mitral regurgitation. From a TEE four-chamber view *(left)*, color flow was used to identify the vena contracta of the regurgitant jet for the initial positioning of the CW Doppler *(CWD)* beam. Transducer position and angulation then were modified as needed to obtain a clear signal with the highest flow velocity. Even so, a higher velocity was obtained with a transthoracic dedicated CW Doppler transducer, immediately after the TEE examination *(right)*. *APX,* Apical; *MV,* mitral valve; *TTE,* transthoracic echocardiography.

CHAMBER ANATOMY AND FILLING PATTERNS

Left Ventricle

Standard views of the LV are obtained from the TEE position in four-chamber, two-chamber, and long-axis views (Table 3.4). A short-axis view is obtained from the transgastric position. These views allow qualitative assessment of LV size and overall systolic function. Regional ventricular function also can be evaluated for each myocardial segment with a high degree of interobserver reproducibility for grading of wall motion in standard segments. In the transgastric short-axis view, the wall segments are the same as in a transthoracic short-axis view, *except* that the entire image has been rotated approximately 180° clockwise. Compared with a transthoracic subcostal short-axis view, the image is rotated 90° clockwise (see Fig. 8.6). Biplane imaging allows faster acquisition of imaging data, but it can be challenging to optimize the image plane and endocardial definition in more than one 2D image at the same time (Fig. 3.27).

LV volumes and ejection fraction can be measured on TEE from 2D four-chamber and two-chamber views. However, 3D calculation of LV volumes and ejection fraction is more accurate because foreshortening of the LV apex is avoided (see Chapter 6 and Fig. 3.27). Measurement of 3D LV volumes and ejection fraction is recommended on all TEE studies

TABLE 3.4   Transesophageal Views for Evaluation of Cardiac Chambers, Great Vessels, and Atrial Septum

Chamber or Structure	Probe Position	Imaging View	Rotation Angle	Doppler or Other
Left ventricle	ME	4-chamber 2-chamber Long-axis	0° 60°–90° 120°	Pulsed Doppler LV inflow for diastolic function Speckle tracking LV strain for global and regional function if needed
		3D	Full-volume 4-beat acquisition for LV volumes and EF Simultaneous multiplane imaging for wall motion	—
	TG	Short-axis 2-chamber Long-axis 4-chamber	0° with probe angulation 90° 90° with probe turned to right 0° at apex with retroflexion	LV outflow velocity with pulsed or CW Doppler, although velocity may be underestimated due to nonparallel intercept angle.
Left atrium	ME	4-chamber 2-chamber Long-axis	0° 60° 120°	—
	ME biplane	LA appendage	0°–90°	Pulsed Doppler atrial appendage flow velocity
Right ventricle	ME	4-chamber Short-axis	0° 60°–90°	TR jet to estimate pulmonary pressures
	TG	RV inflow	90° with probe turned toward patient's right side	TR jet to estimate pulmonary pressures
Right atrium	ME	4-chamber	0° with posterior angulation to visualize coronary sinus	—
		Bicaval	90° with probe turned toward patient's right side	RA appendage visualized in this view
		Low atrial	0° to visualize entry of coronary sinus into RA	Color Doppler to visualize coronary sinus flow
Atrial septum	ME	Rotational	Rotation from 0° to 120°; PFO often best seen at 90°	Color Doppler in each view to detect ASD or PFO Saline contrast to detect interatrial shunt
		3D	Real-time zoon and full-volume acquisition	Measurement of ASD size

Continued

TABLE 3.4 Transesophageal Views for Evaluation of Cardiac Chambers, Great Vessels, and Atrial Septum—cont'd

Chamber or Structure	Probe Position	Imaging View	Rotation Angle	Doppler or Other
Aorta	Long-axis ascending aorta	Long-axis	Long-axis (120°) and short-axis views of aortic sinuses and ascending aorta	Color Doppler of aortic flow
	Thoracic aorta	Descending thoracic aorta	Short-axis view (0°) pullback along length of descending aorta. Supplement with long-axis imaging when pathology present.	Color Doppler of aortic flow Pulsed or CW Doppler for holodiastolic flow reversal when AR present
Pulmonary artery	ME	RV outflow	90°	Color Doppler for pulmonic regurgitation
	UE	Long-axis of PA to bifurcation	0°	Parallel intercept angle allows recording of antegrade pulmonary artery flow with pulsed or CW Doppler
Pulmonary veins	ME	Right and left pulmonary veins	0° with probe turned toward right or left side and angulation to visualize each vein 90° with probe turned toward right or left side to visualize both superior and inferior pulmonary veins	Color Doppler with low aliasing velocity to identify each pulmonary vein Pulsed Doppler for pulmonary venous flow patterns
Systemic venous inflow	ME	Bicaval	90°	Color Doppler of SVC and IVC in bicaval view
	TG	IVC	90°	Color Doppler of IVC at gastroesophageal junction Pulsed Doppler of hepatic veins for RA inflow patterns

AR, Aortic regurgitation; *ASD*, atrial septal defect; *EF*, ejection fraction; *GE*, gastroesophageal; *IVC*, inferior vena cava; *ME*, midesophageal; *PA*, pulmonary artery; *PFO*, patent foramen ovale; *SVC*, superior vena cava; *TG*, transgastric; *TR*, tricuspid regurgitation; *UE*, upper esophageal.

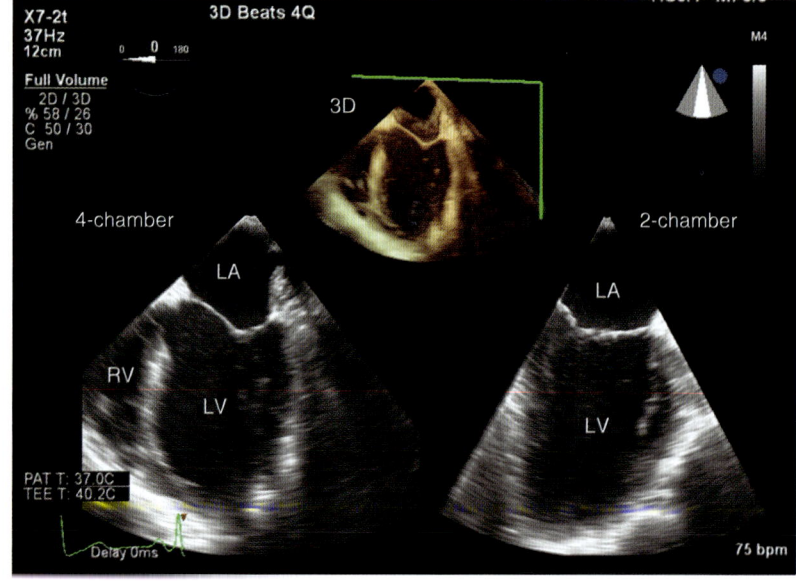

Fig. 3.27 Biplane imaging of the left ventricle. From an upper esophageal probe position, a four-chamber (left) and two-chamber (right) view are seen simultaneously using a three-beat full-volume 3D data acquisition. This view is used for qualitative evaluation of global and regional LV systolic function. This view also is useful to ensure correct positioning and adequate endocardial definition for quantitative measurement of ventricular volumes and ejection fraction, as shown in Fig. 3.28.

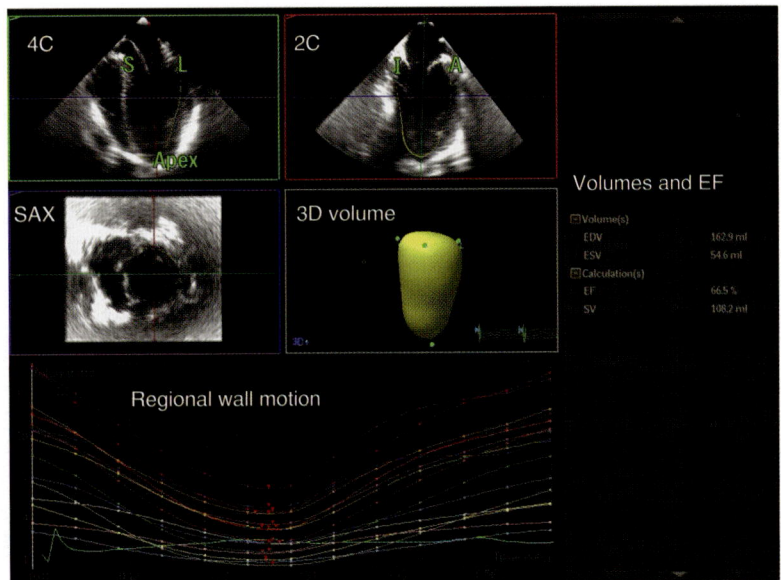

Fig. 3.28 **TEE measurement of left ventricular ejection fraction.** Ejection fraction *(EF)* can be measured on TEE using the apical biplane method by tracing endocardial borders at end-diastole and end-systole in four-chamber *(4C)* and two-chamber *(2C)* 2D views or by using semiautomated border detection with 3D imaging.

unless image quality is inadequate or clinical concerns prevent completion of the exam protocol. Additional modalities for evaluation of ventricular function, such as speckle tracking strain imaging, is helpful in selected cases (see Chapter 4).

Left Atrium

The location and flow patterns of the pulmonary veins are readily assessed by TEE echocardiography (Fig. 3.28). The flow pattern is most easily recorded in the left superior pulmonary vein, where the typical systolic and diastolic antegrade flows and the reversal after atrial contraction can be appreciated (Fig. 3.30). Although flow tends to be more laminar with a narrow band on velocities on the spectral display in the left, compared with the right, superior pulmonary vein, flow patterns generally are similar in all four pulmonary veins. However, exceptions do occur as, for example, when mitral regurgitation is present. In this situation, the regurgitant jet is directed eccentrically, altering flow patterns in some, but not all, pulmonary veins.

If LA thrombus is suspected, the atrial appendage should be examined in at least two orthogonal views or using biplane imaging (see Chapter 15). Recognition of low flow (spontaneous contrast) and appendage thrombi is enhanced by use of a high transducer frequency (7 MHz) and zoom mode. Care is needed to distinguish normal trabeculation from localized thrombus formation. Trabeculae tend to be more linear and are continuous with the atrial wall in more than one view. Thrombi typically protrude into the appendage, often with independent motion.

The flow pattern in the LA appendage is recorded with pulsed Doppler ultrasound with the sample volume positioned in the appendage about 1 cm from the junction with the body of the LA. The normal flow pattern (see Fig. 15.21) is characterized by ejection of blood from the appendage following atrial contraction at a velocity >40 cm/s. Abnormal flow patterns are seen with atrial fibrillation, atrial flutter, and other tachyarrhythmias.

The interatrial septum is well seen in the standard four-chamber view and is evaluated in detail by centering the septum in the image and then slowly rotating the image plane from 0° to 120° while keeping the septum centered in the image plane. The fossa ovalis and primum septum are clearly demarcated, and the "flap valve" of a patent foramen ovale often is identified on 2D imaging, before confirmation with color Doppler or an intravenous contrast injection (see Fig. 15.28). 3D images of the interatrial septum are viewed from the LA side with the right upper pulmonary vein at the 1 o'clock position, or from the RA side with the superior vena cava at the 11 o'clock position. A full-volume multibeat 3D acquisition allows accurate measurement of the size and shape of the atrial septal defect from reconstructed correctly aligned images (see Chapter 17).

Right Ventricle

As with transthoracic imaging quantitation of RV size and systolic function is difficult because of the complex geometry of this chamber. Qualitative assessment of size and function is made from the TEE four-chamber and transgastric short-axis views.

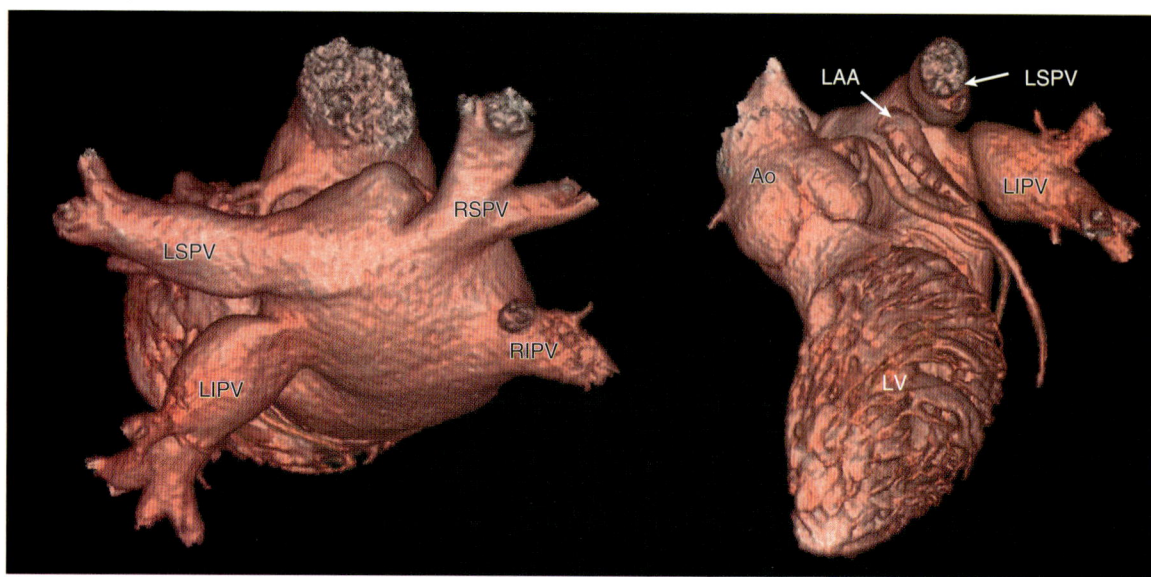

Fig. 3.29 ▶ **Pulmonary vein anatomy.** LA, LA appendage *(LAA)*, and pulmonary vein anatomy obtained from computed tomographic imaging shown looking from a position superior *(left)* and posterior *(right)* to the LA. The left and right superior pulmonary views *(LSPV* and *RSPV)* enter the LA at a superior and anterior angle—on TEE the superior pulmonary venous flow is directed toward the TEE transducer, and the left and right inferior pulmonary veins *(LIPV* and *RIPV)* enter the atrium at a more posterior angle—on TEE the inferior pulmonary venous flow is directed horizontally in the image plane. The LAA is just inferior and anterior to the LSPV. *(Images courtesy James C. Lee.)*

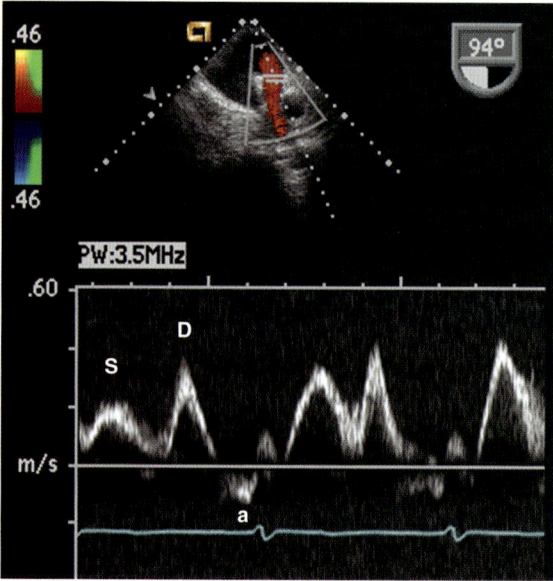

Fig. 3.30 **Pulmonary vein flow.** Pulsed Doppler recording of normal flow in the left superior pulmonary vein shows systolic *(S)* and diastolic *(D)* inflow with a small atrial *(a)* reversal signal.

Right Atrium

The body of the RA is best imaged in the TEE four-chamber view. In addition, the TEE long-axis view of the RA, obtained with the image plane at 90° and the probe rotated toward the patient's right, allows visualization of the atrial appendage (with normal trabeculation) and the entrances of the superior and inferior vena cavae. Movement of the probe up in the esophagus allows evaluation of the cephalad extent of the superior vena cava, whereas movement toward the stomach provides additional views of the inferior vena cava.

The coronary sinus is identified in a posteriorly angled four-chamber view. The entry of the coronary sinus into the RA is best seen in the 0° image plane with the transducer positioned near the gastroesophageal junction and angulated superiorly.

IMAGING SEQUENCE

A standard structured sequence of image acquisition on TEE imaging ensures evaluation with imaging in at least two orthogonal views and Doppler data, as appropriate, of:

- All four cardiac chambers
- All four heart valves
- The interatrial septum and LA appendage
- Both great arteries (aortic and pulmonary artery)
- All major venous inflows (vena cavae and the four pulmonary veins) and
- The descending thoracic aorta

Although this sequence may need to be modified to focus immediately on an acute process in unstable patients or abbreviated in patients who do not tolerate the study, the time needed for a standardized study is relatively short, and these data can be acquired in most patients. A standardized examination ensures that unexpected findings are not missed and provides the data needed for subsequent review of findings in the patient.

The specific sequence used in each laboratory depends on patient populations and physicians' preferences. My preferred sequence starts with an upper TEE view at enough depth to image the LV in four-chamber, two-chamber, and long-axis views. Next, after optimizing the 2D image of the LV, a full-volume multibeat 3D acquisition is performed for calculation of LV volumes and ejection fraction.

Depth is then decreased to focus on 2D imaging of the mitral valve with rotation from the long-axis view back to the four-chamber view, recording images at 30° to 60° increments, with both 2D imaging and color Doppler to detect mitral regurgitation. If mitral regurgitation is present, color Doppler is used to visualize jet direction, measure vena contracta width and the proximal isovelocity surface area (PISA) diameter, along with CW Doppler recording of the mitral regurgitant velocity signal, as detailed in Chapter 12. 3D imaging of the mitral valve is recommended with display of real-time zoom images from the LA and LV sides, as well as a full-volume acquisition for improved 3D image quality and off-line quantitative measurements. Antegrade mitral flow is recorded with pulsed and CW Doppler, if needed, for assessment of LV diastolic function (see Chapter 7) or mitral stenosis (see Chapter 11).

The aortic valve is imaged with 2D and color in the long-axis view. Then the probe is pulled back to show a larger extent of the ascending aorta. The aortic valve short-axis view is obtained with rotation of the image plane to 30° to 50°, again with 3D imaging if appropriate. Pulsed and CW Doppler evaluations of the aortic valve are challenging on TEE. Flow signals may be recorded from transgastric long-axis or apical views, but the possibility that velocities are underestimated must not be forgotten.

Next the pulmonary veins are identified using a combination of 2D and color flow imaging either at a rotation angle of 0° or 90°, by looking at first the left and then the right pulmonary veins. Pulsed Doppler flow should be recorded in at least one pulmonary vein but in more than one if mitral regurgitation or LV diastolic dysfunction is present.

The atrial appendage is visualized either at 90° rotation in the two-chamber view or by angulating superiorly from the 0° (four-chamber) image plane, using a high-frequency transducer and magnified views. Imaging of the atrial appendage is facilitated by biplane imaging, which allow simultaneous recording in two image planes. Atrial appendage flow is recorded with pulsed Doppler if needed.

The atrial septum is examined by centering the septum in the four-chamber view, with identification of the fossa ovalis. Then the image plane is slowly rotated to 90°, while keeping the septum centered in the image. Color flow imaging, either with split screen 2D/color or with separate image acquisition, while rotating back to 0° allows identification of a patent foramen ovale. If an atrial septal defect is present, 3D real-time zoom and full-volume imaging is recommended.

The RV and tricuspid valve are examined in the four-chamber view turned toward the right side and in a low TEE view. Tricuspid regurgitation with color flow imaging is evaluated in these views and in a short-axis view. CW Doppler recording of the tricuspid regurgitant jet velocity allows estimation of pulmonary systolic pressure. The superior and inferior vena cavae are seen in the 90° plane, which also shows the RA appendage.

The pulmonic valve typically is visualized in the 90° image plane and from an upper TEE 0° view with 2D imaging and color Doppler. Recording of antegrade flow in the pulmonary artery is possible from an upper TEE position.

In patients who tolerate transgastric passage of the probe, short-axis and two-chamber views of the LV are obtained. Apical transgastric views are optional, depending on the clinical indication.

After checking with the other medical professionals assisting with the procedure (e.g., the nurse and sonographer) to verify that all the needed data have been recorded, the probe is turned posteriorly to image the descending aorta in the short-axis view with both 2D imaging and color Doppler flow imaging. The probe is slowly withdrawn, keeping the descending aorta centered in the image plane and turning the probe to look down the aortic arch just before probe withdrawal. When aortic pathology is present, long-axis views or biplane images are recommended.

This basic examination is supplemented with additional 3D image acquisitions, additional views, and Doppler flows, depending on the specific clinical question. For example, a study to evaluate for patent foramen ovale also would include a right-sided saline contrast study. The findings on these basic views also may mandate further evaluation. For example, in a patient with endocarditis, findings consistent with a para-aortic abscess would lead to detailed examination for valve dysfunction and any intracardiac shunts or fistula.

THE ECHO EXAM

Basic Transesophageal Echocardiography Exam Sequence

Probe Position	View	Typical Rotation Angle	Modality	Focus on
Mid-esophageal *Set depth to include LV apex*	4-chamber 2-chamber Long-axis	0° 60° 120°	2D and color Doppler 2D and color Doppler 2D and color Doppler	• LV size, global and regional function • In 4-chamber view, angulate anteriorly to see aortic valve. • Aortic and mitral valve anatomy, motion, and flow patterns • RV size and systolic function • LA and RA size • Pericardial effusion
	3D volume	—	Full-volume capture (4 beat)	• 3D LV for calculation of volumes and EF
Mid-esophageal *↓ depth and center mitral valve images*	4-chamber 2-chamber Long-axis	0° 60° 120°	2D and color Doppler 2D and color Doppler 2D and color Doppler	• Mitral valve anatomy and motion • MR • Split screen 2D/color unless wider field of view needed to visualize entire valve • PISA and vena contracta if MR present
	3D volume	—	Real-time zoom mode and full-volume capture (4 beat)	• Mitral valve anatomy and motion from LA and LV views
	Doppler	—	Pulsed and CW Doppler	• Pulsed Doppler LV inflow if needed for diastolic function • CW Doppler of MS or MR jet if more than mild
Mid-upper esophageal *Center aortic valve images*	Long-axis	120°	2D and color Doppler	• Aortic valve • Split screen 2D/color unless wider field of view needed to visualize entire valve
	Long-axis	120°	2D, biplane imaging and color Doppler	• Aorta: start with aortic valve centered and then withdraw transducer slightly to visualize ascending aorta. • Right coronary artery ostium may be visualized.
	Short-axis	30°–50°	2D and color Doppler	• Aortic valve • Split screen 2D/color unless wider field of view needed to visualize entire valve • Withdraw probe slightly to see left main coronary artery ostium. • 3D imaging of aortic valve if number of leaflets not well seen
Mid-esophageal *Move probe to center LAA*	Depth to show LAA	2D scan from 0° to 90°	2D (resolution mode, 7-MHz transducer)	• LAA
	Depth to show LAA	Biplane imaging	2D (resolution mode, 7-MHz transducer)	• LAA
	Doppler	—	Pulsed Doppler	• Flow signal recoded with sample volume about 1 cm into LAA

Basic Transesophageal Echocardiography Exam Sequence—cont'd

Probe Position	View	Typical Rotation Angle	Modality	Focus on
Mid-upper esophageal	Left pulmonary veins	0° or 90°	2D and color Doppler	• At 0° turn probe leftward and angulate to see left superior pulmonary vein. • Advance probe to see inferior vein. • Use of color with low aliasing velocity aids identification of veins. • Also can be seen in 90° view
	Right pulmonary veins	0° or 90°	2D and color Doppler	• At 0° turn probe rightward and angulate to see right superior pulmonary vein. • Advance probe to see inferior vein. • Use of color with low aliasing velocity aids identification of veins. • Also can be seen in 90° view
	Doppler	—	Pulsed Doppler	• Record pulmonary vein flow in one or more pulmonary veins.
Mid-esophageal *Turn rightward to center atrial septum*	Rotational scan	0°→90°	2D and color Doppler	• Atrial septum • Split screen 2D/color unless wider field of view needed to visualize entire atrial septum • Biplane imaging is an alternative option. • 3D imaging if ASD present with real-time zoom and full volume for measurement of ASD size
	SVC/IVC view	90°	2D and color Doppler	• RA and RA appendage • SVC and IVC
Mid-esophageal *Turn rightward to visualize right heart*	4-chamber	0°	2D and color Doppler	• RV • RA • Tricuspid valve
	Short-axis RV	60°	2D and color Doppler	• Tricuspid valve
	RV outflow]	90°	2D and color Doppler	• Pulmonic valve and pulmonary artery
Transgastric	Short-axis	0°	2D or biplane imaging	• LV wall motion, wall thickness, chamber dimensions • RV size and function
	Long-axis	90°	2D or biplane imaging	• LV and mitral valve • Turn medially to image RV and tricuspid valve.
	Right heart	90°	2D	• Turn medially to image RV and tricuspid valve.
Transgastric apical	4-chamber	0°	2D, color and CW Doppler	• Useful for antegrade aortic flow but may still be nonparallel intercept angle
Transgastric to upper esophageal	Descending thoracic aorta	0° 90°	2D or biplane imaging Color, pulsed and CW Doppler	• Image aorta from the diaphragm to aortic arch. • Doppler evaluation of aorta if 2D imaging suggests dissection • CW Doppler for diastolic flow reversal if AR present
	Arch and ascending aorta	0° 90°	2D 2D	• When TEE probe reaches proximal descending thoracic aorta, turn rightward to see arch and ascending aorta.

AR, Aortic regurgitation; *ASD*, atrial septal defect; *EF*, ejection fraction; *IVC*, inferior vena cava; *MR*, mitral regurgitation; *MS*, mitral stenosis; *PISA*, proximal isovelocity surface area; *SVC*, superior vena cava.

SUGGESTED READING

1. Freeman RV: The comprehensive diagnostic transesophageal echocardiogram: integrating 2D and 3D imaging, Doppler quantitation and advanced approaches. In Otto CM, editor: *The Practice of Clinical Echocardiography*, ed 5, Philadelphia, 2017, Elsevier.
   Detailed chapter with numerous tables, figures, and references for performing a complete TEE study. Examples of normal and abnormal findings with linked videos.

2. Otto CM. Transesophageal Echocardiography on Procedures Consult. An online educational module in ClinicalKey, http://www.proceduresconsult.com/medical-procedures/Elsevier. 2016 (this procedure Reviewed 9/19/2013).
   A structured video demonstrates me (C.M.O.) performing a transesophageal echocardiography procedure. The procedure video is divided into steps with narration and is accompanied by a Procedure Checklist that includes indications, contraindications, and postprocedure care. The full details section provides text and illustrations for performing a TEE study, and a self-assessment test is provided. Procedure Consult has 30 other Cardiology Procedures videos, including transthoracic echocardiography (TTE), contrast echocardiography, exercise stress echocardiography, and dobutamine stress echocardiography.

3. Hahn RT, Abraham T, Adams MS, et al: Guidelines for performing a comprehensive transesophageal echocardiographic examination: recommendations from the American Society of Echocardiography and the Society of Cardiovascular Anesthesiologists, *J Am Soc Echocardiogr* 26(9):921–964, 2013.
   This guideline document provides recommendations and practical guidance for performing TEE. The 28 standard views recommended in this document are included in the TEE sequence in The Echo Exam summary in this chapter. Tables and figures demonstrating steps for acquiring and displaying 3D images are especially helpful. 172 references.

4. Hilberath JN, Oakes DA, Shernan SK, et al: Safety of transesophageal echocardiography, *J Am Soc Echocardiogr* 23(11):1115–1127, 2010.
   This detailed review includes summary tables of the incidence of TEE complications stratified by clinical setting (ambulatory, intraoperative, pediatric, intensive care unit). Illustrations show the anatomy of possible malpositions during probe insertion.

5. Statement (dated 10.26.16) on granting privileges to practitioners who are not anesthesia professionals for administration of moderate sedation: American Society of Anesthesiologists Ad Hoc Committee on Credentialing, http://www.asahq.org/quality-and-practice-management/standards-and-guidelines. Accessed September 28, 2017.
   Consensus statement on granting privileges for practitioners; also details the clinical standards for moderate sedation (as is used for TEE procedures). These standards include the knowledge base and training of the practitioner. In addition, this document summarizes standards for patient evaluation, preprocedure preparation, monitoring (level of consciousness, ventilation, oxygenation, and hemodynamics), data recording, and availability of emergency equipment.

6. Wamil M, Newton JD, Rana BS, et al: Transoesophageal echocardiography: what the general cardiologist needs to know, *Heart* 103(8):629–640, 2017.
   A concise review of basic TEE views, indications for TEE studies with illustrative examples of abnormal findings. 77 references.

7. Mahmood F, Shernan SK: Perioperative transoesophageal echocardiography: current status and future directions, *Heart* 102(15):1159–1167, 2016.
   Detailed summary of the qualitative and quantitative information obtained by TEE in the perioperative setting and how this information is used to guide clinical decision making. 59 selected references.

8. Mahmood F, Jeganathan J, Saraf R, et al: A practical approach to an intraoperative three-dimensional transesophageal echocardiography examination, *J Cardiothorac Vasc Anesth* 30(2):470–490, 2016.
   This helpful review article provides guidance on 3D imaging in the perioperative setting. Equipment, key personnel, and technical aspects are summarized with a degree of detail not found in other sources. The different types of 3D imaging and when to use each are illustrated, including multiplane imaging, live zoom and narrow section 3D imaging, single-beat and multibeat full-volume modes, and 3D color Doppler imaging. Different types of image displays are also shown with accompanying drawings.

9. Bertrand PB, Levine RA, Isselbacher EM, et al: Fact or artifact in two-dimensional echocardiography: avoiding misdiagnosis and missed diagnosis, *J Am Soc Echocardiogr* 29(5):381–391, 2016.
   This article addresses the common clinical dilemma of distinguishing an imaging artifact from an abnormal finding on echocardiography. The origin of each type of artifact is explained with figures showing examples from both TTE and TTE imaging.

10. Lee AP, Lam YY, Yip GW, et al: Role of real time three-dimensional transesophageal echocardiography in guidance of interventional procedures in cardiology, *Heart* 96:1485–1493, 2010.
    Nicely illustrated review of the role of TEE in guiding intervention procedures including transcatheter atrial septal defect and patent foramen ovale closure, mitral valve procedures, transcatheter ventricular septal defect closure, placement of LA occluder devices, transseptal catheterization, and catheter ablation of arrhythmias. Brief mention (with references) of transcatheter aortic valve implantation and transcatheter closure of paraprosthetic valve leaks.

11. Stavrakis S, Madden GW, Stoner JA, et al: Transesophageal echocardiography for the diagnosis of pulmonary vein stenosis after catheter ablation of atrial fibrillation: a systematic review, *Echocardiography* 27:1141–1146, 2010.
    Pulmonary vein stenosis can occur after catheter ablation of atrial fibrillation. On TEE, pulmonary vein stenosis can be identified based on an increased pulmonary vein inflow velocity (more than 1.1 m/s) and evidence of flow turbulence. In this systematic review of 344 patients, the sensitivity of TEE for detection of pulmonary vein stenosis ranged from 82% to 100% with a specificity of 98% to 100%. The standards of reference were pulmonary vein angiography, cardiac magnetic resonance, or computed tomographic imaging. Intracardiac echocardiography may be an alternate approach to diagnose pulmonary vein stenosis..

12. Ferrero NA, Bortsov AV, Arora H, et al: Simulator training enhances resident performance in transesophageal echocardiography, *Anesthesiology* 120(1):149–159, 2014.

Anesthesia residents trained with a TEE simulator obtained higher-quality images compared with a control group who did not participate in simulator-based training.

13. Bose RR, Matyal R, Warraich HJ, et al: Utility of a transesophageal echocardiographic simulator as a teaching tool, *J Cardiothorac Vasc Anesth* 25(2):212–215, 2011.

    First year anesthesia residents were randomized to TEE training with a 90-minute simulator session compared with conventional training. The simulator-based training resulted in improved evaluation scores for echo-anatomic correlation, structure identification, and image acquisition..

14. Platts DG, Humphries J, Burstow DJ, et al: The use of computerised simulators for training of transthoracic and transesophageal echocardiography: the future of echocardiographic training?, *Heart Lung Circ* 21(5):267–274, 2012.

    Both sonography students learning TTE imaging and physicians learning TEE found that simulator training was realistic, it improved acquisition of correct image planes, and it helped with understanding spatial anatomic relationships.

4 Specialized Echocardiography Applications

THREE-DIMENSIONAL ECHOCARDIOGRAPHY
  Image Acquisition
  Image Display
  Examination Protocol
  Quantitation From 3D Images
  Clinical Utility
  Limitations

MYOCARDIAL MECHANICS
  Tissue Doppler Strain and Strain Rate
  Speckle Tracking Strain Imaging
  Clinical Utility
  Dyssynchrony, Twist, and Torsion

CONTRAST ECHOCARDIOGRAPHY
  Contrast Agents
  Applications
  Limitations and Safety

INTRACARDIAC ECHOCARDIOGRAPHY
  Instrumentation
  Technique
  Applications
  Limitations and Safety

THE ECHO EXAM

SUGGESTED READING

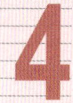

All echocardiographic imaging depends on digital image processing. Ultrasound systems start with raw information (pixels) that are then used for two-dimensional (2D) or three-dimensional (3D) images using intensity, textures, and gradients to highlight edges and structures, thereby creating anatomic-type images of cardiac structures (Fig. 4.1). Automated image analysis is central to display and analysis of 3D images, calculation of 3D LV volumes with semiautomated edge detection, and speckle tracking strain imaging. Currently, image interpretation is primarily based on visual inspection by expert clinicians. In the future, it is likely that imaging systems will offer most complex and accurate computer analysis and interpretation (see Suggested Reading).

THREE-DIMENSIONAL ECHOCARDIOGRAPHY

The term *3D echocardiography* refers broadly to several approaches for the acquisition and display of cardiac ultrasound images. Different 3D approaches are similar in that cardiac structures are shown in relation to one another in all three spatial dimensions and can be rotated or viewed from different orientations, even after image acquisition. One of the challenges of 3D echocardiography is optimizing image resolution in all three dimensions, given the constraints of ultrasound physics and transducer design. Another challenge is ensuring temporal, as well as spatial, resolution.

Image Acquisition

3D imaging uses a complex multiarray transducer that simultaneously acquires ultrasound data from a 3D pyramidal volume. Rapid parallel image processing provides ultrasound images that can be viewed in real time in any orientation on the screen (Fig. 4.2). These matrix array transducers typically include about 3000 piezoelectric elements with a transmission frequency of 2 to 4 MHz for transthoracic echocardiography (TTE) and 5 to 7 MHz for transesophageal echocardiography (TEE). Several approaches exist to the acquisition of echocardiographic data using a 3D matrix array transducer (Table 4.1):

- ■ ***Real-time narrow 3D section:*** A beat-by-beat view with a wider image plane than standard 2D imaging that can be rotated to view from different perspectives. It looks like a "thick" tomographic image.
- ■ ***Real-time 3D-zoom volume-rendered images:*** A full-volume image of an enlarged area of interest that is rotated to show the structure of interest in a "surgical" view. These images are displayed with a perspective-type image similar to a photographic view from inside the heart.

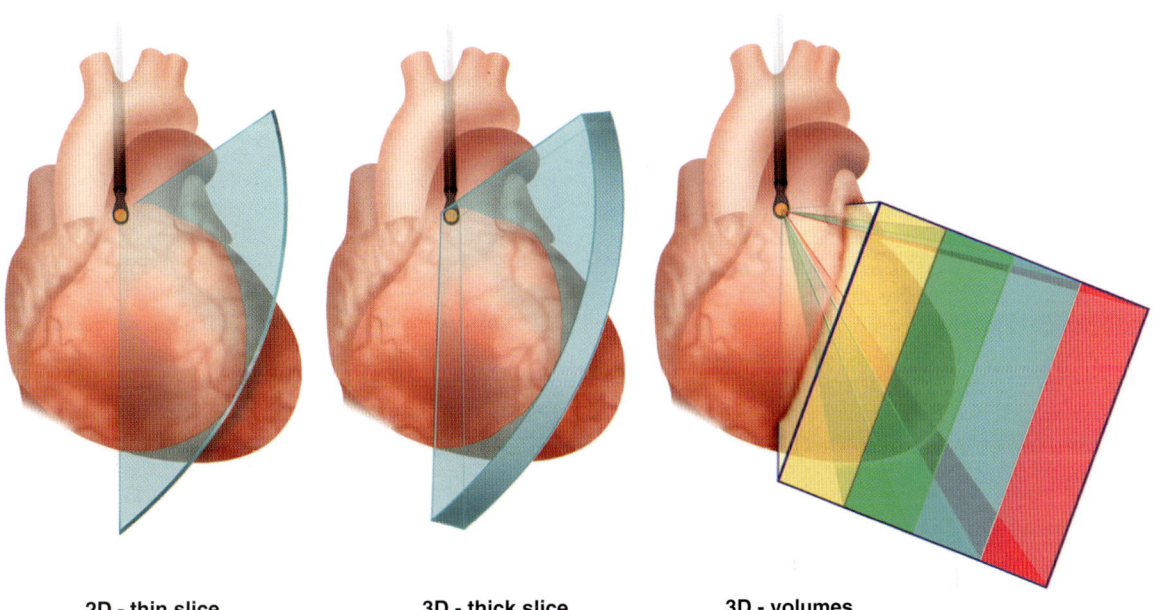

Fig. 4.1 The image interpretation pyramid. Image interpretation depends on a series of steps shown conceptually as a pyramid with a complex overlay of layers starting with the raw pixel values used to generate the image to the final interpretation. *(From Bosch JG. Digital image processing and automated image analysis in echocardiography. In Otto CM, editor:* The Practice of Clinical Echocardiography, *ed 5, Philadelphia, 2017, Elsevier, pp 166–181.)*

Fig. 4.2 3D echocardiography. *(Left)* 3D echocardiographic images are acquired using a fully sampled matrix array transducer. 2D imaging focuses the transducer beam on a single tomographic slice with optimal temporal and spatial resolution. Different 2D image planes are obtained by manually moving, rotating, and tilting the transducer. *(Center)* 3D real-time narrow sector imaging uses a matrix array transducer to display a 300 × 600 pyramidal volume, which maintains high temporal resolution within this narrow volume image. Real-time imaging also can be enlarged to include the entire anatomic structure in "zoom" mode at the expense of decreased spatial and temporal resolution. *(Right)* Full-volume imaging stitches together volumetric image data from more than one cardiac cycle (typically four beats, as shown here) to provide higher temporal and spatial resolution while including the entire cardiac anatomy in the field of view.

TABLE 4.1 3D Imaging Modalities

Modality	Advantages	Limitations
Real-time 3D mode—narrow section, volume-rendered images	• Rapid acquisition, familiar image planes • Image can be rotated; helpful with complex cardiac anatomy	Narrow sector; entire structure does not fit in imaging plane.
Real-time "zoom" volume-rendered cropped images	• Shows anatomy in "surgical" views • Enlarged 3D image of structure of interest	A wider field of view decreases spatial and temporal resolution.
Full-volume gated acquisition for volume-rendered cropped images	• High spatial resolution • High temporal resolution • Quantitation of LV volumes and ejection fraction • Provides 3D LV shape and dyssynchrony	May be difficult to optimize image quality for all structures in the field of view. "Stitch" artifacts occur because of patient and respiratory motion.
Full-volume gated acquisition for multiple 2D tomographic slices	• Accurate measurements of cardiac dimensions • More objective and less operator dependent than standard 2D imaging • Visualization of all myocardial segments simultaneously	Endocardial definition may be suboptimal depending on transducer position.
Simultaneous multiplane 2D imaging	• Simultaneous images in two defined planes • Highest spatial resolution • Highest temporal resolution	Only two planes are visualized.
3D color Doppler	• Visualization of 3D geometry of vena contracta and proximal isovelocity surface area for regurgitant lesions • Location of paravalvular prosthetic leaks and intracardiac shunts	This has a slow frame rate with low temporal resolution.

- ***Full-volume gated acquisition volume-rendered images:*** Multiple-beat volumetric imaging stitches together narrow volumes of data over several cardiac cycles to provide a full volume of data that can be rotated and cropped to show the structures of interest.
- ***Simultaneous multiplane mode:*** This simultaneous display of two 2D image planes has the ability to adjust the rotation angle, tilt, and elevation of the second image plane.
- ***3D color Doppler imaging:*** This uses real-time or full-volume color Doppler data acquisition, but at frame rates lower than for imaging data.

Advantages of real-time narrow sector imaging are rapid image capture, familiar image planes, and evaluation of complex anatomy; however, only a narrow field of view is seen (Fig. 4.3). With focused wide section or real-time "zoom" mode, the entire structure (e.g., the mitral valve) is included in the image, but spatial resolution and temporal resolution are poor, and the image must be rotated and gain carefully adjusted to display the internal cardiac anatomy (Fig. 4.4). Full-volume gated images look similar to real-time zoom-mode images but have better spatial and temporal resolution. Full-volume images also can be analyzed after acquisition to provide additional views. Simultaneous multiplane imaging shows only a few (typically two) tomographic images but provides the highest temporal and spatial resolution within these image planes (Fig. 4.5). The use of 3D color Doppler imaging is helpful for showing the spatial distribution of a flow disturbance, such as prosthetic paravalvular regurgitation or an intracardiac shunt, but it currently has very low temporal resolution.

During the acquisition of 3D images, transducer position is adjusted to optimize visualization of the structure of interest, for example, by imaging the mitral valve from the left atrial (LA) side on TEE imaging with the ultrasound beam perpendicular to the closed mitral leaflets. Next, gain and compression are set in the mid-range (about 50 units), and the time-gain compensation (TGC) curve is adjusted so the image is slightly "overgained" to avoid echo dropout appearing as "holes" in anatomic structures. With real-time imaging, transducer position and gain can be adjusted iteratively to improve image quality and to center the structure of interest in the image. My practice is to optimize position and gain on a zoomed real-time 3D view before the acquisition of a four-beat gated full-volume data set from the same transducer position. Postprocessing, gain, and compression then can be adjusted after image acquisition. With full-volume gated acquisitions, any change in heart position from beat to beat results in a vertical line across the image with misregistration of the image data on both sides of this "stitch" artifact. Causes of a stitch artifact include patient movement, respiratory motion, and an irregular heart rhythm.

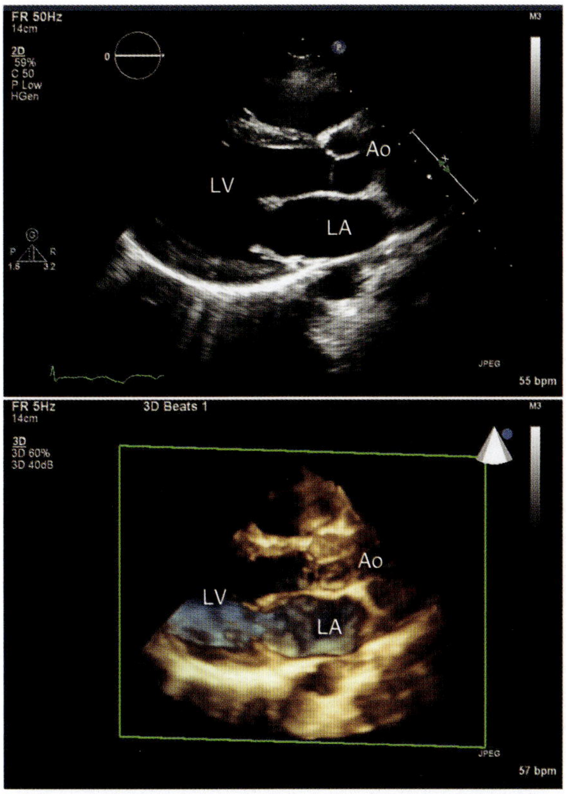

Image Display

There are currently several types of 3D echocardiographic image displays, including:

- Volume-rendered 3D images
- Surface-rendered images
- Wireframe images
- Simultaneous display of multiple 2D images
- Graphic displays of 3D parameters versus time

In both the real-time 3D zoom mode and in full-volume imaging, the display is "cropped" to show different views of the interior structures of the heart. For example, the mitral valve can be viewed from the perspective of the LA; this provides a compelling view of prolapsing segments of the valve in patients with myxomatous mitral valve disease (see Fig. 12.29). The image can then be rotated and recropped to show a long-axis–type image of the mitral valve or to view the valve from the left ventricular (LV) side. Similarly, the aortic valve can be viewed en face from the perspective of the aorta, a view that correlates closely with the surgical view of valve anatomy, from the LV side of the valve or in a long-axis orientation. Real-time 3D images are cropped and rotated as the

Fig. 4.3 **Real-time 3D narrow section volume-rendered imaging.** *(Top)* A standard 2D parasternal long-axis view ▶ has a frame rate of 50 Hz, which drops to 5 Hz in the *(bottom)* 3D mode ▶.

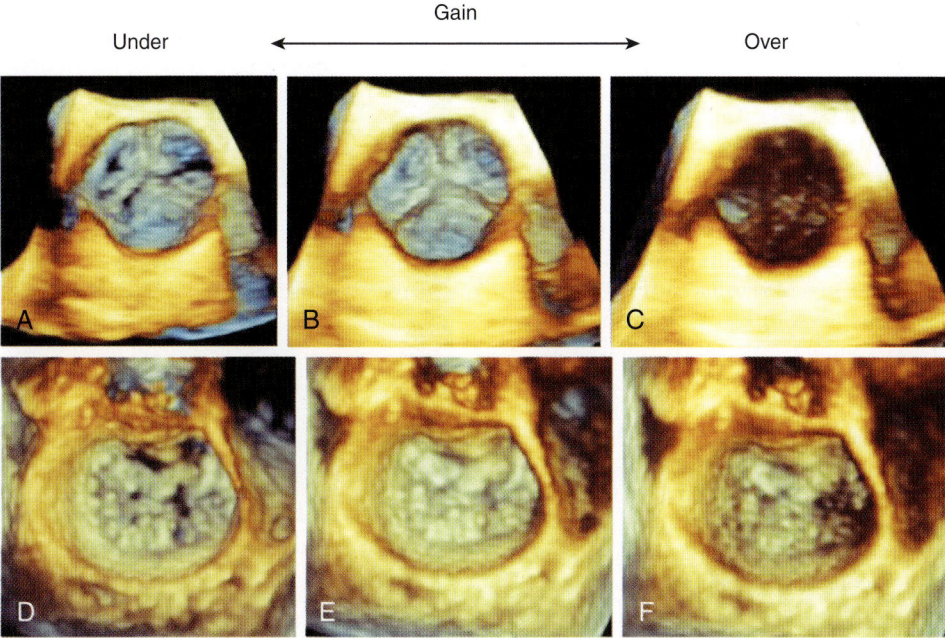

Fig. 4.4 **Effect of gain on 3D imaging.** Real-time zoom 3D images of the (A–C) aortic and (D–F) mitral valves show the effect of gain on the image display. Low gain results in echo dropout, whereas excess gain decreases resolution and obscures the structure of interest. (A) and (D) Dropout of the cusps and leaflets due to low gain. (B) and (E) Normal anatomy without dropout or excess gain. (C) The cusps are obscured by the excess gain. (F) Leaflet visualization is unclear due to excess gain. *(From Tsang W, Lang RO: 3D echocardiography: principles of image acquisition, display and analysis. In Otto CM, editor:* The Practice of Clinical Echocardiography, *ed 5, Philadelphia, 2017, Elsevier, pp 18–36.)*

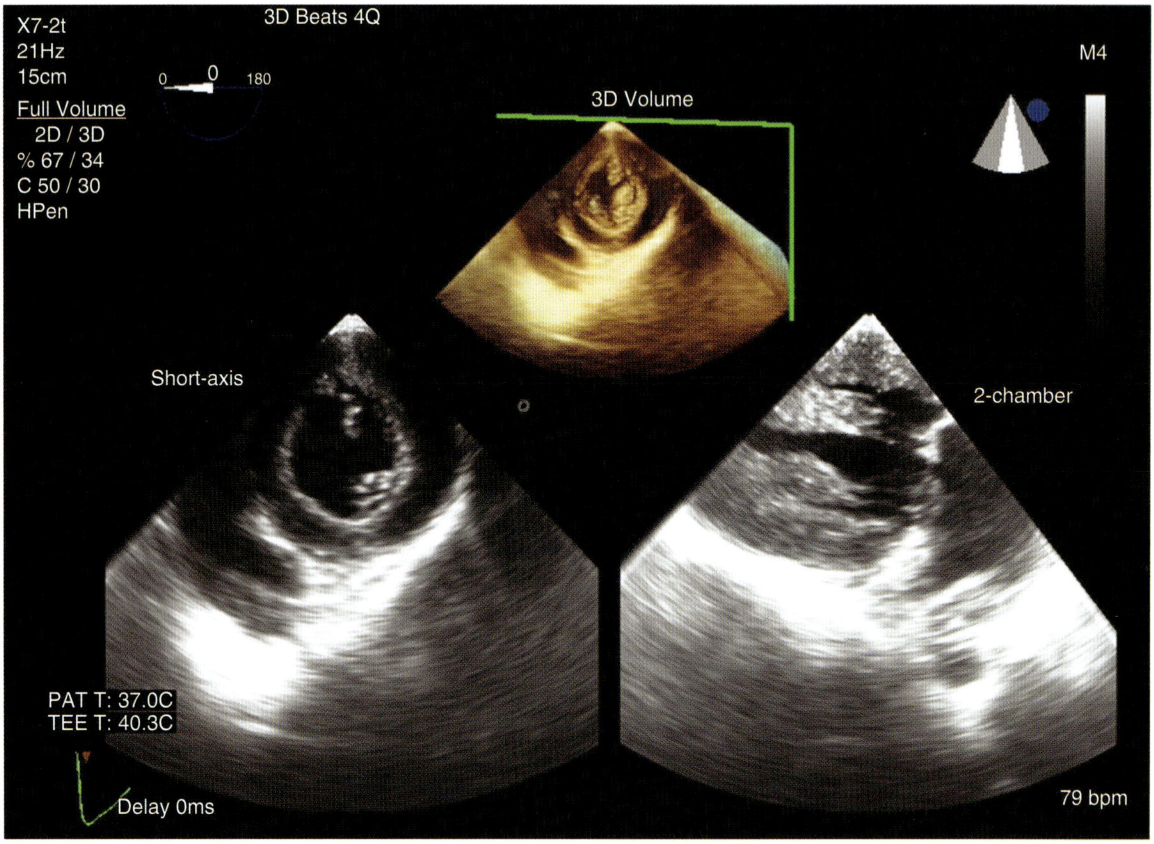

Fig. 4.5 ▶ **Biplane imaging.** On a TEE transgastric view, both the long-axis and short-axis views of the left ventricle can be recorded on the same cardiac cycles.

images are acquired. Full-volume gated acquisitions can be cropped and rotated during the exam but also can be reevaluated later because the full-volume data set is saved digitally.

Surface-rendered images or wireframe displays are based on identifying the boundaries of a cardiac structure, either by using semiautomated methods or by tracing the boundaries on multiple 2D images. For example, the LV endocardial surface is shown as a 3D solid structure with contraction shown by a sequence of 3D volumes over the cardiac cycle, so the rendered volume appears to beat on the display screen (Fig. 4.6). Alternatively, a wireframe-type display can be used. A graphic display also is helpful with time on the horizontal axis and with either LV volume or the position of each myocardial segment shown on the vertical axis.

The 3D echocardiographic data set also can be used for simultaneous display of multiple-image 2D planes (Fig. 4.7). The ability to acquire LV images in multiple planes simultaneously speeds image acquisition during stress echocardiography, thus potentially improving diagnostic accuracy. In addition, the ability to "move through" a 3D data set in any 2D image plane allows better appreciation of cardiac anatomy

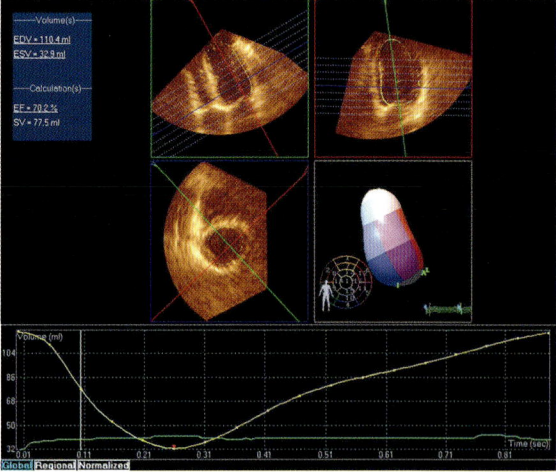

Fig. 4.6 ▶ **Surface-rendered volumetric imaging.** The apical window was used to acquire a full-volume 3D image of the LV. Using three orthogonal planes through the data set for guidance, endocardial borders were traced using semiautomated border detection to provide a surface-rendered image of the ventricular chamber, with color coding for myocardial regions. The graphic curve shows LV volume over a single cardiac cycle.

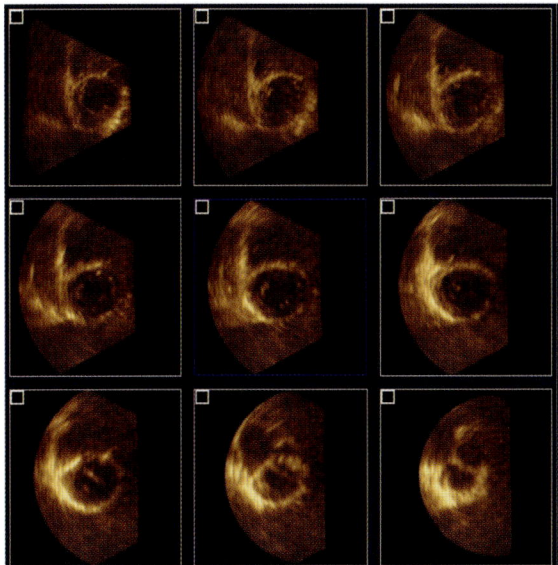

Fig. 4.7 ▶ **Multiple simultaneous 2D image planes.** The 3D full-volume image of the LV recorded from the apical window is displayed as multiple tomographic short-axis views spanning the ventricle from apex *(top left)* to base *(lower right)*.

in patients with complex structural heart disease and allows precise localization of abnormalities.

Examination Protocol

With TTE imaging, only limited 3D imaging is performed to complement a full 2D study, depending on the patient's diagnosis and the reason for the study. Examples of 3D imaging on transthoracic imaging include quantitation of LV volumes and ejection fraction in a patient with heart failure (see Fig. 9.4), 3D measurement of mitral orifice area in a patient with mitral stenosis, or 3D short-axis images of the aortic valve in a patient with calcific aortic valve disease (see Fig. 11.6). With TEE imaging, a systematic approach to 3D image acquisition and display is recommended, with additional views as needed depending on the specific pathology (Table 4.2).

Recommendations for volume-rendered 3D image displays (Fig. 4.8) are:

- *Aortic valve:* The right coronary cusp is located inferiorly (at the 6 o'clock position) for both aortic and LV views of the valve (see Fig. 3.21).
- *Mitral valve:* The aortic valve is located at the top of the image so the anterior mitral leaflet is superior to the posterior leaflet for both LA and LV views of the valve (see Fig. 3.23).
- *LV:* 3D TTE views of the LV are oriented like standard 2D images in either an apical four-chamber view (apex at the top of the image, LV on the right side of the screen) or a short-axis view.
- *Right ventricle (RV):* A four-chamber view or short-axis view is oriented with the LA superior (12 o'clock position).
- *Pulmonic valve:* The anterior valve cusp is located superiorly (12 o'clock position) for both the pulmonary artery and RV sides of valve.
- *Tricuspid valve:* The ventricular septum is placed inferiorly for both the right atrial (RA) and RV views of the valve.
- *Interatrial septum:* From the LA side, the right upper pulmonary view is shown in the 1 o'clock position. From the RA side, the superior vena cava is at the 11 o'clock position.
- *LA appendage:* This display shows the LA appendage en face from the LA perspective with the pulmonary veins shown superiorly or longitudinally.

Quantitation From 3D Images

In addition to volume-rendered images of each chamber and valve, surface-rendered images of the LV are derived from a gated full-volume acquisition with the transducer positioned at the LV apex (for TTE imaging) or in a TEE four-chamber view. A 2D image is used to ensure optimal positioning of the transducer with the entire LV included in the sector scan. Gain and transducer frequency are adjusted to optimize endocardial definition. Acquisition of the gated full-volume data set is guided by a split screen display of orthogonal views, and the patient is asked to suspend respiration to minimize stitch artifacts. Once the full-volume data is acquired, the LV apex and mitral annulus are used as landmarks to initiate the edge detection process. The operator then can adjust the automated tracings as needed to follow the endocardial border accurately. As for 2D measures of LV volumes, trabeculations and the papillary muscles are included in the LV chamber to avoid underestimation of LV volumes. The surface-rendered image data then is used for quantitation of:

- LV end-diastolic and end-systolic volumes
- LV ejection fraction
- LV regional wall motion

Each of these parameters can be displayed on a 3D perspective color-coded LV shape or as a graph over the cardiac cycle (see Fig. 8.7).

Compared with 2D approaches, 3D quantitation of LV function avoids geometric assumptions and is more accurate and reproducible and thus is recommended when technically feasible (see Chapter 6). The 3D measures of LV mass, regional strain, curvature, and wall stress are more complicated and are currently investigational approaches.

TABLE 4.2 American Society of Echocardiography and European Association of Echocardiography Recommendations for a Systematic 3D Study

Structure	TTE Image Acquisition	TEE Image Acquisition	Sequence for TEE Full-Volume Image Orientation (See Fig. 4.7)
Aortic valve	PLAX with and without color, narrow angle and zoomed*	60° mid-esophageal short-axis with and without color, zoomed or full-volume 120° mid-esophageal long-axis with and without color, zoomed or full-volume	2D views at 60° and 120° with aortic valve centered in acquisition boxes Live 3D to optimize gain Full-volume acquisition, and then rotated 90° clockwise around y-axis
Mitral valve	PLAX with and without color, narrow angle and zoomed A4C with and without color, narrow angle and zoomed	0–120° mid-esophageal with and without color, zoomed	2D views at 90° and 120° with mitral valve centered in acquisition boxes Full-volume acquisition, rotated 90° counterclockwise around x-axis and then 90° counterclockwise in plane so aortic valve is superior
Left vetricle	A4C, narrow and wide angle	0–120° mid-esophageal view including entire LV, full-volume	Full-volume acquisition for quantitation of LV volumes, ejection fraction, and regional wall motion Data displayed as a moving 3D surface-rendered image with color coding and as a time graph
Right ventricle	A4C with image tilted to put RV in center of image	0–120° mid-esophageal view, tilted to put RV in center of image, full-volume	
Atrial septum	A4C, narrow angle and zoomed	0° with probe rotated toward atrial septum, zoomed or full-volume	
Pulmonic valve	RV outflow view with and without color, narrow angle and zoomed	90° high-esophageal view with and without color, zoomed 120° mid-esophageal three-chamber view with and without color, zoomed	2D high-esophageal view at 0° with pulmonic valve centered in acquisition box Full-volume acquisition, rotated 90° counterclockwise around x-axis, then rotate in plane 180° counterclockwise so anterior leaflet is superior
Tricuspid valve	A4C with and without color, narrow angle and zoomed RV inflow view with and without color, narrow angle and zoomed	0–30° mid-esophageal four-chamber view with and without color, zoomed 40° transgastric view with anteflexion with or without color, zoomed	TTE[†] 2D views in off-axis A4C view with tricuspid valve centered in acquisition boxes Full-volume acquisition, rotated 90°counterclockwise around x-axis and then rotated 45° in plane so septal leaflet is in 6 o'clock position

*Zoomed, real-time volume-rendered 3D imaging rotated to intracardiac views.
[†]3D images of the tricuspid valve are best obtained from TTE, not TEE, imaging.
A4C, Apical four-chamber view; narrow angle, real-time volume rendered tomographic imaging in standard image planes; PLAX, parasternal long-axis view.
Summarized from Lang RM, Badano LP, Tsang W, et al: EAE/ASE recommendations for image acquisition and display using three-dimensional echocardiography, J Am Soc Echocardiogr 25(1):3–46, 2012.

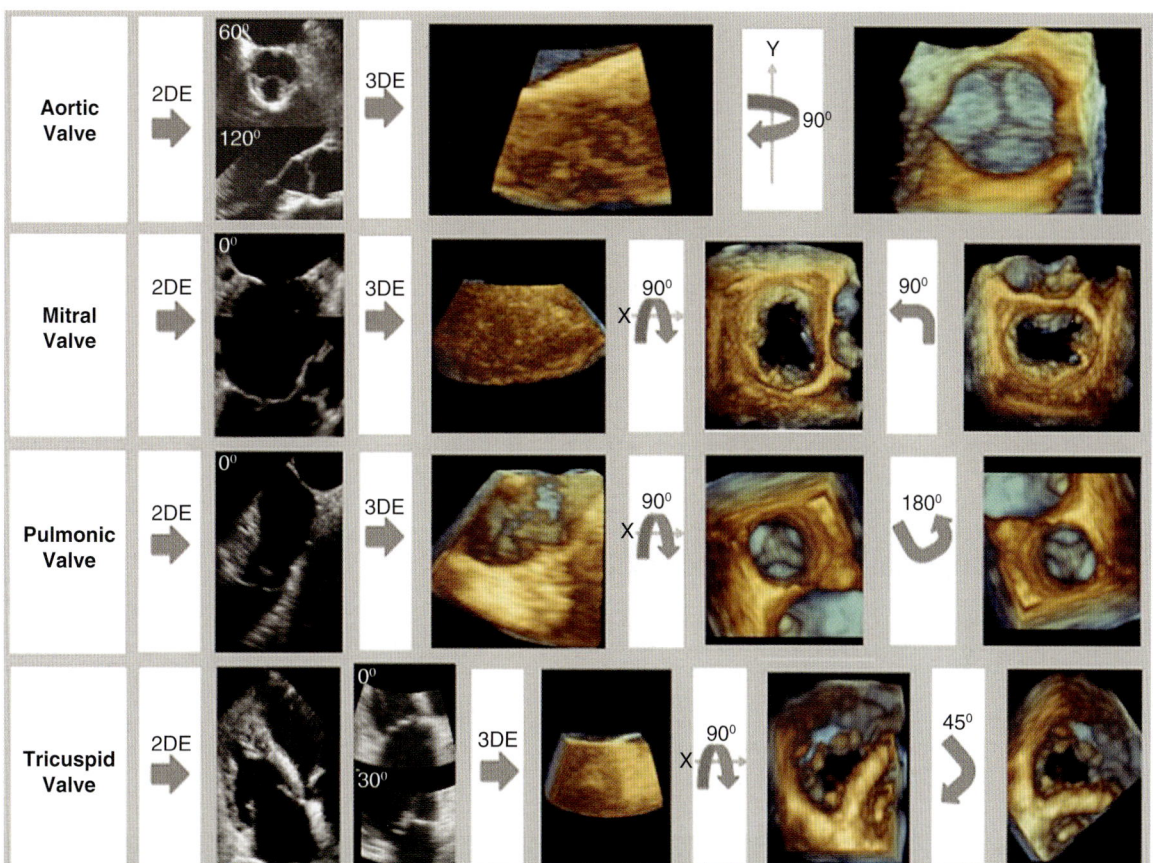

Fig. 4.8 American Society of Echocardiography and European Association of Echocardiography recommendations for image orientation of cardiac valves. The 3D TEE *(3DE)* images of cardiac valves should be recorded in standard orientations as shown in the right column and in Table 4.1. First, the valve is centered in a 2D TEE *(2DE)* view of the valve as shown in the first column. Next, real-time 3D is used to optimize gain settings for visualization of valve anatomy. Then a full-volume image is acquired and is rotated around the x-or y-plane as shown followed by rotation in the image plane (except for the aortic valve) to show the valve in the standard display format. Aortic, mitral, and pulmonic valves are best imaged on TEE as shown. Tricuspid valve 3D TTE imaging is recommended using the TTE views shown. *(From Lang RM, Badano LP, Tsang W, et al: EAE/ASE recommendations for image acquisition and display using 3D echocardiography, J Am Soc Echocardiogr 25[1]:3–46, 2012.)*

Other quantitative measurements from 3D data sets are in evolution. Standard 3D volume-rendered image displays show the cutaway view of the heart as a solid structure using shading and lighting to provide the impression of a 3D perspective on a 2D viewing screen. This display is not conducive to quantitative measurements because only two of the three dimensions are shown. Advances in display and digital processing should alleviate this problem by allowing accurate measurement of distances and areas.

Potentially other 3D measurements have advantages compared with 2D measurements for nonplanar structures, such as a stenotic valve. For example, although experienced operators can accurately measure mitral valve area from 2D images aligned at the minimal orifice area in patients with rheumatic mitral stenosis, inexperienced operators show improved accuracy with 3D imaging, which reliably shows the stenotic orifice and is less dependent on transducer position or image plane positioning. For planimetry of mitral valve area, the 3D volume is acquired, and then a 2D plane is aligned at the minimal orifice with the valve opening traced in mid-diastole (Fig. 4.9). In research applications, more complex structures, such as the mitral leaflets and annulus, can be reconstructed in 3D by tracing the structure in a series of 2D image planes within the 3D volumetric data set (Fig. 4.10).

Clinical Utility

The clinical role of 3D echocardiography will continue to evolve as this technology matures. In addition to providing more detailed anatomic relationships and more accurate quantitation, 3D images are more intuitive than 2D images, thus allowing quicker appreciation of cardiac anatomy by more health care providers (Table 4.3). Potentially, 3D echocardiography could be faster than 2D scanning and could reduce variability in image acquisition. However, because

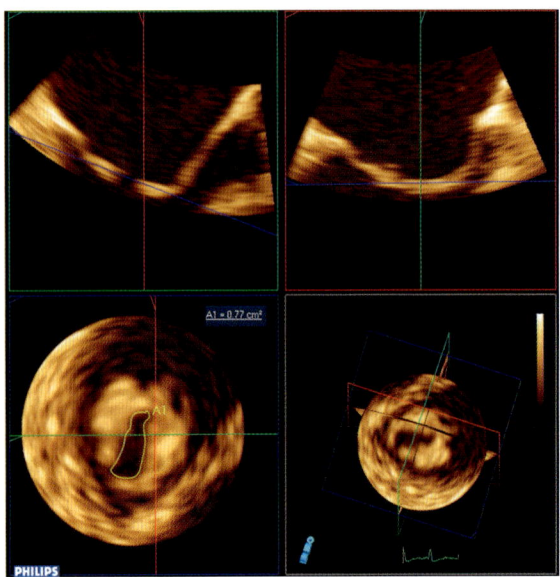

Fig. 4.9 **3D measurement of mitral valve area.** A full-volume image of the mitral valve was acquired (same patient as Fig. 11.10) in a patient with mitral stenosis and asymmetric fusion of the commissures. For measurement of the mitral valve area, off-line analysis of the 3D volume used three orthogonal planes (x, y, z) shown in red, green, and blue to align an image plane at the tips of the stenotic valve. The resulting tomographic image at the minimal orifice area in diastole *(lower left)* was traced to determine mitral valve area.

instrumentation is in development, 3D echocardiography is not yet a routine part of the clinical examination at all centers and typically is used to supplement the 2D study in selected patients, with imaging focused on a specific anatomic structure. The use of 3D imaging is more widespread for intraoperative and intraprocedural imaging because of the improved image quality and the additive value of the 3D perspective in these clinical settings (see Chapter 18).

The American Society of Echocardiography and European Association of Echocardiography guidelines recommend routine use of 3D imaging for:

- Quantitation of LV volumes and ejection fraction
- Evaluation of mitral valve anatomy (valve area in mitral stenosis)
- Guidance of transcatheter procedures

It is likely that other quantitative applications will become available in the near future, including quantitation of RV volumes and ejection fraction and 3D evaluation of aortic valve, outflow tract, and aortic sinus anatomy in adults with valvular aortic stenosis. Further studies are needed for other potential applications including 3D dyssynchrony, strain imaging, and the evaluation of prosthetic valves.

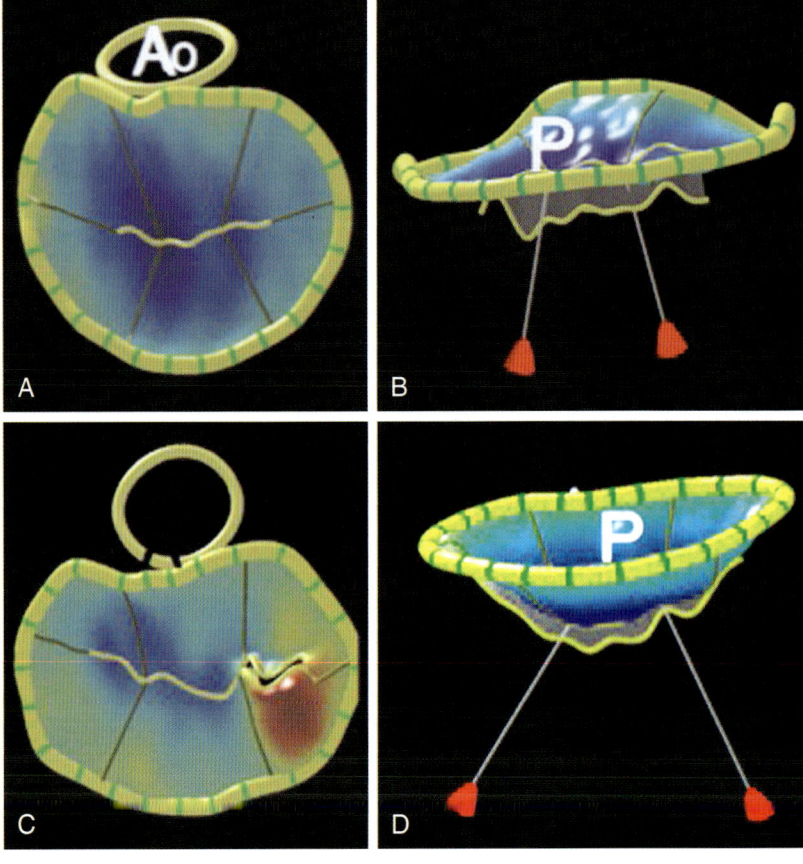

Fig. 4.10 **Mitral valve models.** Mitral valve models with color-encoded parametric maps of leaflet displacement above the mitral annular plane into the left atrium. (A) and (B) When the valve is normal and no leaflet displacement is present, the leaflets remain blue. (C) When prolapse or flail is present, the distance of the leaflet from the mitral annular plane toward the left atrium are indicated by color gradations from yellow (mild) to red (severe). This is an example of a prolapsed P3 scallop. (D) In this model, tenting of the leaflets is appreciated from the profile view. *Ao,* Aorta; *P,* posterior leaflet. *(From Tsang W, Lang RO: 3D echocardiography: principles of image acquisition, display and analysis. In Otto CM, editor:* The Practice of Clinical Echocardiography, *ed 5, Philadelphia, 2017, Elsevier, pp 18–36.)*

TABLE 4.3 Clinical Applications of 3D Echocardiography

Application	3D Approach	Comments
LV function	• Surface-rendered LV volumes, ejection fraction, and regional wall motion derived from gated full-volume 3D acquisition	• 3D echo underestimates LV volumes compared with CMR data. • Trabeculae and papillary muscles are included in the LV chamber.
RV function	• Volume-rendered images allow visualization of entire RV. • Surface-rendered images may allow measurement of volumes and ejection fraction.	• 3D measurement of RV volumes and ejection fraction requires further validation but is a promising approach.
Mitral valve	• Volume-rendered images show mitral valve anatomy en face from the LA or LV side of the valve. • Accurate measurement of valve area in mitral stenosis occurs using 3D-guided 2D image planes. • Annular shape and dimensions are obtained from volumetric images. • 3D color Doppler shows jet origin and direction.	• 3D TEE is recommended for guidance of interventional mitral valve procedures. • 3D TTE or TEE is recommended for clinical evaluation of mitral valve pathology.
Aortic valve and sinuses	• Volume-rendered images obtained from TTE parasternal or TEE high-esophageal views provide optimal spatial resolution. • Planimetry of aortic valve area is possible on 2D images derived from the 3D full-volume data set. • 3D images demonstrate the oval shape of the aortic annulus.	• 3D imaging may be helpful in determining the mechanism of aortic regurgitation and defining the number of valve leaflets. • 3D imaging is recommended for guidance of transcatheter aortic valve implantation.
Pulmonic valve and pulmonary artery	• The pulmonic valve can be imaged using biplane or real-time 3D imaging.	• Routine 3D pulmonic valve imaging is not recommended.
Tricuspid valve	• 3D volume-rendered images of the tricuspid valve are acquired in a fashion similar to those for the mitral valve.	• 3D views of the tricuspid valve may be helpful in determining the mechanism of valve regurgitation.
LA and RA	• 3D volume-rendered images of the atrial septum are helpful for defining the location, size, and shape of atrial septal defects and for guiding transcatheter closure procedures.	• 3D imaging may improve assessment of LA volume but is not a routine measurement.
LA appendage	• 3D volume-rendered images are helpful in guiding transcatheter LA appendage closure.	• Biplane imaging of the LA appendage is useful in evaluating for LA thrombus.
3D stress echocardiography	• 3D imaging provides simultaneous evaluation of wall motion in all myocardial segments, improved visualization of the LV apex, and rapid image acquisition at peak stress.	• Disadvantages of 3D stress imaging include lower frame rates and spatial resolution compared with 2D imaging. • Not all 3D systems allow side-by-side review of rest and stress images.

CMR, Cardiac magnetic resonance.
Summarized from Lang RM, Badano LP, Tsang W, et al: EAE/ASE recommendations for image acquisition and display using three-dimensional echocardiography. *J Am Soc Echocardiogr* 25(1):3–46, 2012.

The use of 3D volume-rendered imaging has proved to be helpful in several clinical settings, both for facilitating communication with other physicians and for providing more detailed anatomic information about shape, size, and 3D anatomic relationships of structures. The benefits of 3D echocardiography for specific clinical settings include:

- Myxomatous mitral valve disease: Evaluation of the number and severity of prolapsed or flail segments and identification of chordal rupture is used for planning surgical repair (see Fig. 12.29).
- Atrial septal defects: Visualization of the location, size, and suitability is used for transcatheter closure (see Figs. 17.19 and 17.20).
- Transcatheter interventions: 3D imaging is used for guidance during procedures, evaluation of procedural results, and detection of complications (see Fig. 18.24).

The 3D color Doppler applications are challenging because of the low frame rates with this modality. Currently, 3D color Doppler is helpful in identifying the location of paravalvular regurgitation. Other potential clinical applications of 3D imaging, such as quantitation of valvular regurgitation based on 3D visualization of proximal jet geometry, require further validation.

Limitations

Although 3D imaging has greatly expanded the capability of echocardiography for the visualization of complex heart disease, this approach does have some limitations. Acquisition of 3D images can be time-consuming, particularly because 3D imaging currently serves as an adjunct, not a replacement, for 2D imaging. However, 3D imaging modalities likely will become more integrated into the standard clinical exam when the instrument interface allows effortless transitions between 2D and 3D imaging and more intuitive approaches to image manipulation. Current display formats attempt to show 3D images on 2D displays; this limitation should be resolved as 3D display systems become more widely available. As with all ultrasound modalities, the direction of the ultrasound beam relative to the structure of interest affects image quality; resolution is optimal in the axial direction for structures perpendicular to the ultrasound beam. In addition, ultrasound artifacts, such as shadowing, reverberations, and poor penetration affect the image, as with any ultrasound modality. Many patients with suboptimal 2D images also have poor 3D images. TEE 3D imaging tends to be much more useful than TTE 3D imaging. Finally, both spatial and temporal resolutions of 3D imaging are inferior to those of 2D imaging, so both modalities are needed for a full imaging study.

MYOCARDIAL MECHANICS

LV function is a complex event that is only partially described by clinical measures of ejection fraction, qualitative changes in regional wall motion, and measures of diastolic filling. Ventricular contraction occurs in the longitudinal direction (the base moves toward the apex), the radial direction (walls thicken), and the circumferential direction (cavity size decreases perpendicular to the long axis of the chamber). In addition, the apex and base rotate in opposite directions during contraction, resulting in a twisting motion called torsion. Several promising approaches to a more complete and quantitative description of myocardial mechanics are used, including:

- **Displacement:** the distance a cardiac structure or myocardial element moves between two consecutive image frames, measured as a distance (cm)
- **Velocity:** the speed (displacement per time unit) of movement of a cardiac structure or myocardial element, reported as velocity (cm/s)
- **Strain:** the fractional change in length of a myocardial segment; a unitless measure of myocardial deformation, reported as a positive or negative percentage
- **Strain rate**: the rate of change in strain with units of 1 per second
- **Rotation:** the circular motion of the LV myocardium around its long axis, measured in degrees
- **Twist:** the absolute difference in rotation between the LV base and apex (degrees)
- **Torsion:** the gradient in rotation angle from base to apex, measured as degrees per cm

Displacement and velocity are vectors with direction in addition to magnitude. Strain and strain rate also are vectors with direction and magnitude and can be measured for regions of the myocardium or averaged over the entire ventricle (global strain) in either the longitudinal or circumferential direction (Table 4.4).

Tissue Doppler Strain and Strain Rate

Doppler blood flow velocity measurements are based on backscatter of low-amplitude, high-velocity signals from moving blood cells (Fig. 4.11). In contrast, Doppler tissue velocity measurements are based on the high-amplitude, low-velocity signals reflected from the myocardium. Thus these signals are easily separated by adjusting the gain, wall filters, and velocity scale of the Doppler spectral or color display.

Tissue Doppler velocity recording at a specific intracardiac site is analogous to pulsed Doppler blood flow velocity recordings. Tissue velocity measurements depend on a parallel alignment between the ultrasound beam and the direction of myocardial motion; in other words, motion is measured only in the direction toward and away from the transducer. For example, a component in evaluation of diastolic function is the tissue Doppler signal recorded in the apical four-chamber view with a 2-mm sample volume positioned about 1 cm apical from the septal side of the mitral annulus (Fig. 4.12). The spectral display is recorded at a velocity range of ±0.2 m/s, using very low gain and wall filter setting. The Doppler velocities show systolic motion of the myocardium toward the apex, corresponding to the apical motion of the annulus in systole seen on 2D imaging. In diastole, an early diastolic motion away from the apex *(E′)* occurs, corresponding to the early phase of diastolic filling, and a late diastolic motion away from the apex *(A′)* occurs, corresponding to the atrial phase of ventricular filling.

TABLE 4.4	Cardiac Mechanics: Approaches and Clinical Applications	
Modality	**Methodology**	**Clinical Applications**
Tissue Doppler imaging	Measurement of the velocity (cm/s) of motion of the myocardium either as a single point with pulsed Doppler or over an image plane with color Doppler	• Tissue Doppler myocardial velocities are standard measures of LV diastolic function.
Tissue Doppler strain rate (SR) and strain imaging	Tissue Doppler velocities at several sites or color Doppler across the image are used to measure SR: $SR = (V_2 - V_1) / D$	• SR is a measure of ventricular contractility. • SR is integrated to determine strain, a measure of regional myocardial function. • The utility of tissue color Doppler is limited by angle dependence and high signal noise for derived SR and strain.
Myocardial speckle tracking strain (STE)	Strain is measured directly from the motion of myocardial speckles across the 2D image or in 3D as: $[L - L_0 / L_0] \times 100\%$	• Myocardial STE is angle independent. • STE analysis can be performed after image acquisition. • STE strain and SR may improve evaluation of LV diastolic function, but further validation is needed. • STE strain and SR can improve accuracy of stress echocardiography by experts.
Myocardial dyssynchrony	Multiple 2D, pulsed Doppler, and tissue Doppler methods	• The degree of dyssynchrony may predict the response to biventricular pacer therapy.
LV rotation, twist, and torsion	**Rotation** is the circular motion of the LV myocardium around its long axis, measured in degrees, using STE. **Twist** is the absolute difference in rotation between the LV base and apex (degrees). **Torsion** is the gradient in rotation angle from base to apex, measured as degrees per centimeter.	• STE-measured abnormalities in LV rotation, twist, and torsion have been described in patients with heart failure and coronary, valve, and pericardial disease. • Limitations of these measurements include lack of standardization of imaging planes and a need to define normal values. • Clinical use of this methodology is not currently recommended.
LV dyssynchrony	Approaches to measuring interventricular dyssynchrony include M-mode, 2D tissue Doppler, STE, and 3D echo.	• Currently there is no clear role for echocardiographic measures of ventricular dyssynchrony in the management of patients with heart failure.

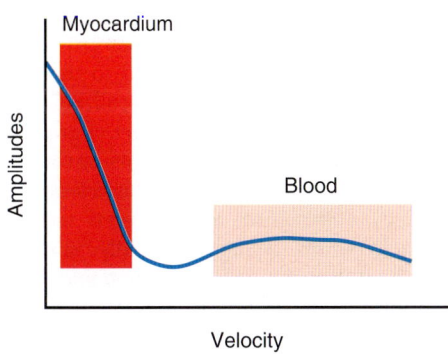 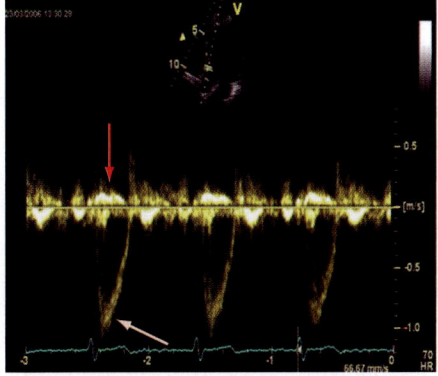

Fig. 4.11 Myocardial velocities and blood flow. Principle for separation of myocardial velocities from blood flow velocities: *(Left)* The difference in velocity and amplitude between myocardial and blood velocities. The myocardium is moving at much lower speed than blood, and therefore Doppler frequencies are lower. Furthermore, the amplitude of myocardial signals is much higher than for blood. *(Right)* A recording in the LV outflow tract that samples both myocardial and blood flow velocities. The *red arrow* points to the high-intensity signals from the myocardium, and the *white arrow* points to the low-intensity, but high-velocity signals from the blood. *(From Smiseth OA, Edvardsen T, Torp H: Myocardial mechanics: velocities, strain, strain rate, cardiac synchrony, and twist. In Otto CM, editor: The Practice of Clinical Echocardiography, ed 5, Philadelphia, 2017, Elsevier, pp 128–146.)*

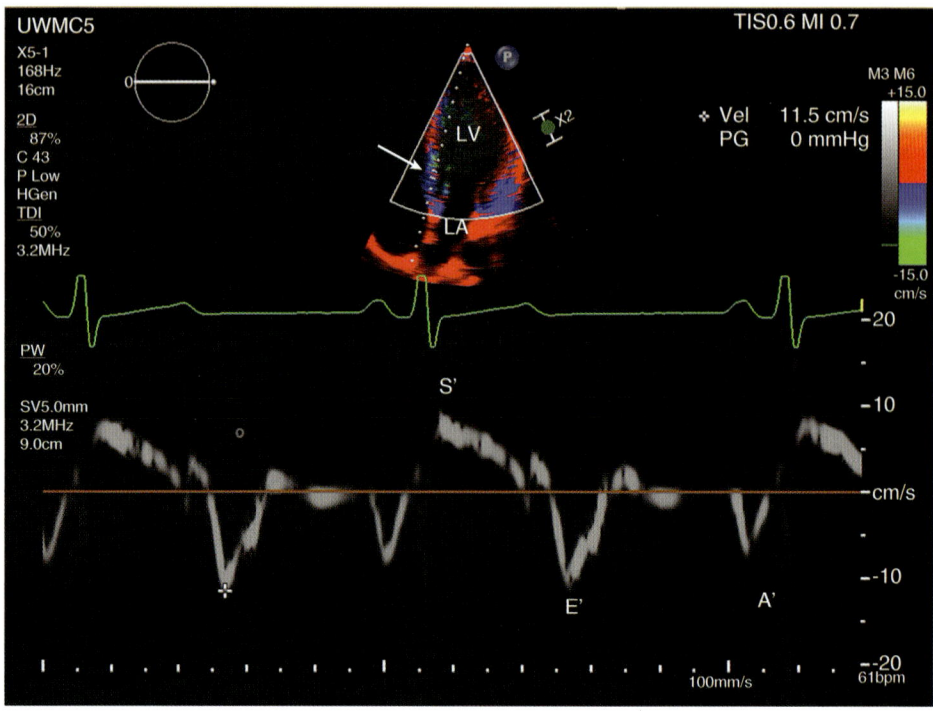

Fig. 4.12 Tissue Doppler velocities. (A) Tissue Doppler imaging *(TDI)* for diastolic function is recorded from the apical window using a 2-mm sample volume positioned in the myocardium about 1 cm from the mitral annulus. (B) A tissue Doppler signal showing that in systole *(S′)*, the myocardium moves toward the apex. In diastole, the myocardial velocity is directed away from the transducer first with early diastolic filling *(E′)* and then with atrial contraction *(A′)*. Myocardial velocities are higher at the base than the apex.

Strain rate imaging is based on the difference in tissue Doppler velocity *(V)* between sample volumes divided by the distance (D) between them (Fig. 4.13). This measures the rate of change in myocardial length, normalized to the original length. Strain rate *(SR)* then is:

$$SR = (V_2 - V_1)/D \qquad \text{(Eq. 4.1)}$$

The units of strain are seconds^{-1} (or /s) because the velocity measured in centimeters per second is divided by the distance in centimeters. Typically, strain rate is measured in the apical-base direction, in the apical four-chamber view with three sample volumes placed in the septal or lateral wall myocardium about 12 mm apart. The tissue Doppler mean velocity curves are examined to ensure a clear signal without excessive noise, lack of aliasing, and avoidance of blood pool signals (see Fig. 4.12). The instrument calculates strain rate from these velocity curves for each time point and displays strain rate in seconds^{-1} as a function of time. The stain rate curve looks like a vertical mirror image of the velocity curve because myocardial shortening is a negative strain and myocardial lengthening is a positive strain. Strain rate provides data on relative timing of myocardial motion and peak systolic and diastolic strain rates. Peak systolic strain rate is a measure of ventricular contractile function that is insensitive to changes in loading conditions.

Strain is a measure of deformation of a material, defined as the difference between the final length *(l)* and the original length *(l₀)*, divided by the original length. Thus strain can be thought of as the percentage change in length:

$$Strain = [(l - l_o)/l_o] \times 100\% \qquad \text{(Eq. 4.2)}$$

Strain can be estimated from the tissue Doppler strain rate by integrating the curve over time.

Thus strain is analogous to ejection fraction (i.e., change in volume normalized to initial volume) with the advantage that spatial localization and temporal localization are possible. In fact, a graph of strain over the cardiac cycle (Fig. 4.14) looks similar to a ventricular volume curve. Because strain is relative to the baseline length, end-diastole is considered zero strain. During systole strain decreases rapidly until end-systole is reached. Isovolumetric relaxation and contraction result in a slight flattening of the curve just before and after systole. In diastole, a rapid increase in strain occurs during the early phase of diastolic filling *(E)*, followed by a plateau during diastasis and then another increase with atrial contraction *(A)* back to the baseline at end-diastole. Peak systolic strain is a measure of regional ventricular function. However, like ejection fraction, strain varies with preload.

Accurate measurements of Doppler strain rate and strain require careful attention to technical aspects of

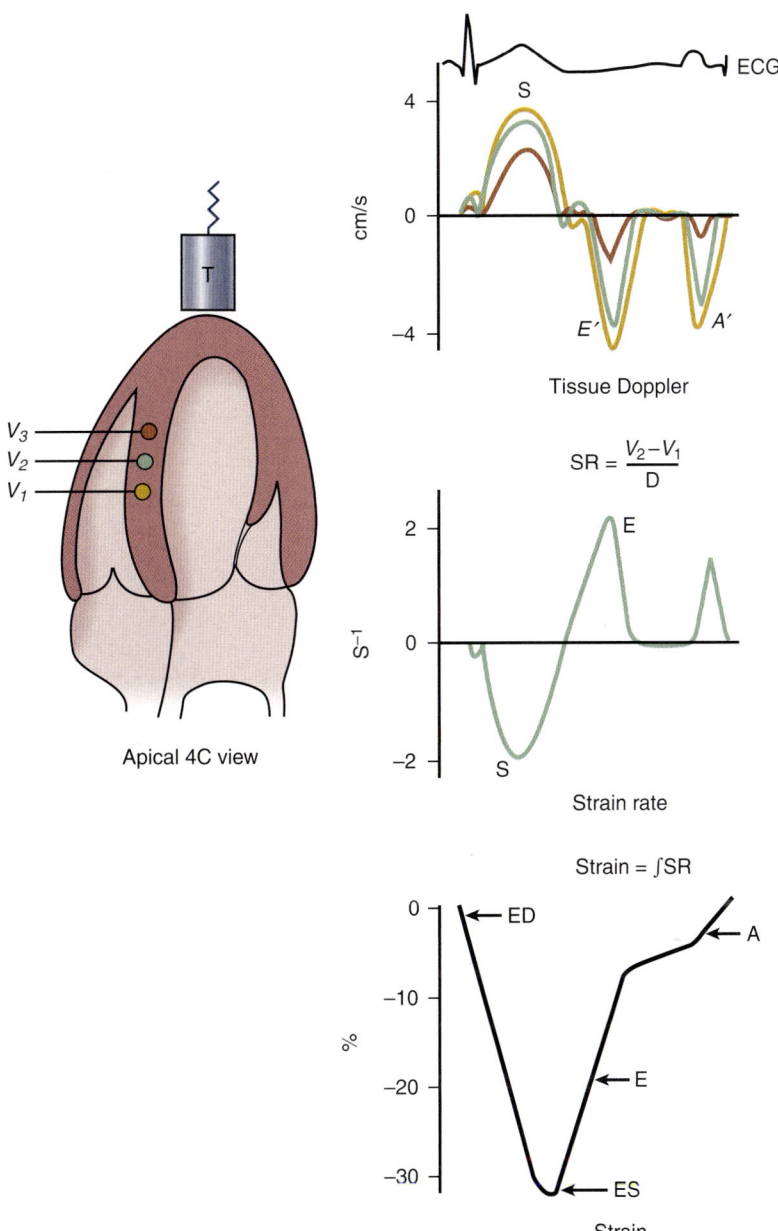

Fig. 4.13 Derivation of strain rate and strain from myocardial tissue velocities. From the apical view, at least three Doppler sample volumes are positioned in the myocardium about 12 mm apart. The three graphs on the right show one cardiac cycle, matched for timing as shown by the electrocardiogram *(ECG)* at the top. The tissue Doppler tracings show mean velocity versus time with the line colors corresponding to each sample volume position. Strain rate *(SR)* is calculated for each time point at the change in velocity *(V)* between each two sample volume positions, divided by the distance *(D)* between them. Strain is determined by integration of the strain rate to generate a curve similar to an LV volume curve with a rapid decrease in strain during ejection (end-diastole *[ED]* to end-systole *[ES]*) and a rapid increase in strain in early diastole *(E)* with another increase in late diastole after atrial contraction *(A)*. *4C*, Four-chamber; *T*, transducer.

data recording. The sample volumes must fit within the myocardium at an adequate distance from each other. In addition, velocity is measured only in the direction toward and away from the transducer. Signal quality is enhanced by the use of harmonic imaging, an adequate pulse repetition frequency, a high frame rate, and by tracking the sample volume to the ventricular wall. The Suggested Reading section provides further details about data acquisition and interpretation.

Speckle Tracking Strain Imaging

Strain imaging also can be based on tracking the motion of small bright spots in the myocardium (speckles) on the gray-scale image as they move during the cardiac cycle. Speckles are natural acoustic markers because of interference patterns caused by backscattered signals from small structures (less than a wavelength) in the myocardium. The advantages

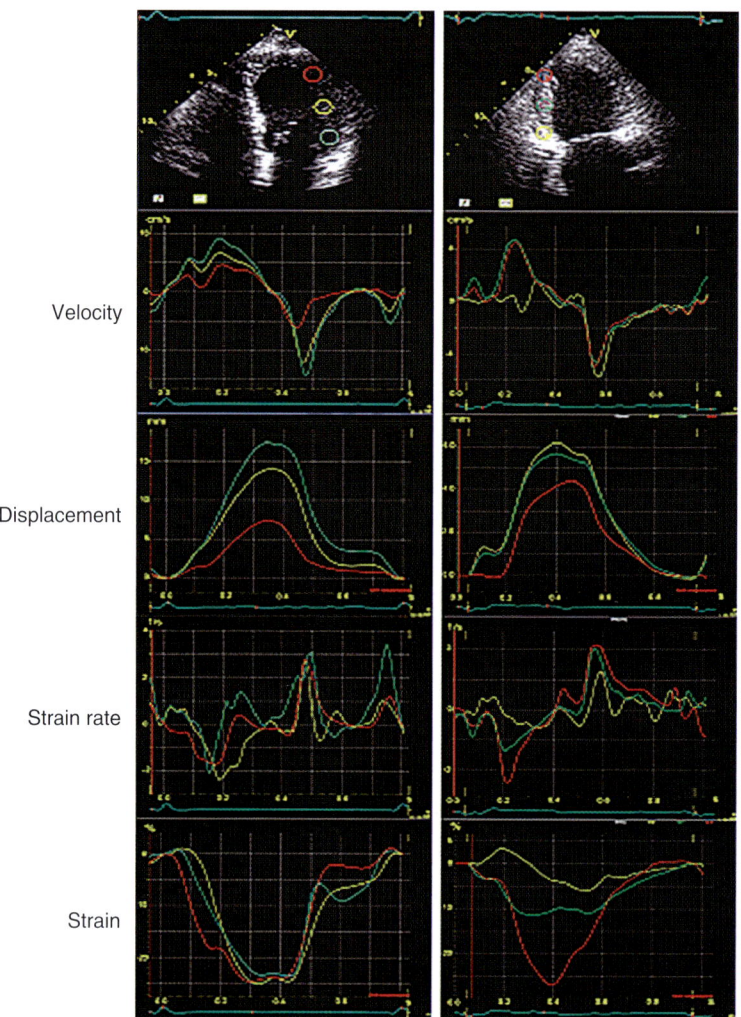

Fig. 4.14 Myocardial mechanics: normal compared with acute myocardial infarction. Recordings from a healthy individual *(left)* and from a patient with posterior myocardial infarction *(right;* be aware of different scales). All tissue Doppler modalities are sampled from three identical levels along the LV lateral wall (healthy individual) and posterior wall (patient with myocardial infarction). In ischemic myocardium, systolic velocities and displacement are typically reduced *(right upper panels)*, and there are reductions in systolic strain rate and strain *(right lower panels)*. *(From Smiseth OA, Edvardsen T, Torp H: Myocardial mechanics: velocities, strain, strain rate, cardiac synchrony and twist. In Otto CM, editor: The Practice of Clinical Echocardiography, ed 5, Philadelphia, 2017, Elsevier, pp 128–146.)*

of speckle tracking compared with Doppler tissue velocities are: (1) simpler data acquisition, (2) lack of angle dependence, (3) direct measurement of strain, (4) multiple simultaneous measurements in the image plane, and (5) the ability to perform the analysis after image acquisition. The ultrasound system tracks speckles and determines the distance between two markers in a defined myocardial region and then plots this distance over the cardiac cycle (Fig. 4.15). Thus speckle tracking provides a direct measure of strain—the change in length of the myocardium relative to the original length. In addition, circumferential strain can be measured from short-axis views, radial strain in multiple segments, and longitudinal strain in long-axis views. Strain rate is the first derivative, or slope, of the graph of strain over the cardiac cycle.

Clinical Utility

Tissue Doppler imaging now is a standard element in the clinical evaluation of diastolic function (see Chapter 7). Other measures of myocardial mechanics have improved our understanding of disease pathophysiology but are not yet routine. For example, Doppler strain rate and strain imaging techniques have been shown to be more sensitive than conventional echocardiographic measurements for the detection of early myocardial involvement in amyloidosis, diabetes, and hypertrophic cardiomyopathy. However, the sensitivity and specificity of these approaches for the detection of subclinical cardiac involvement await further validation. Strain imaging and strain rate imaging have also been proposed as

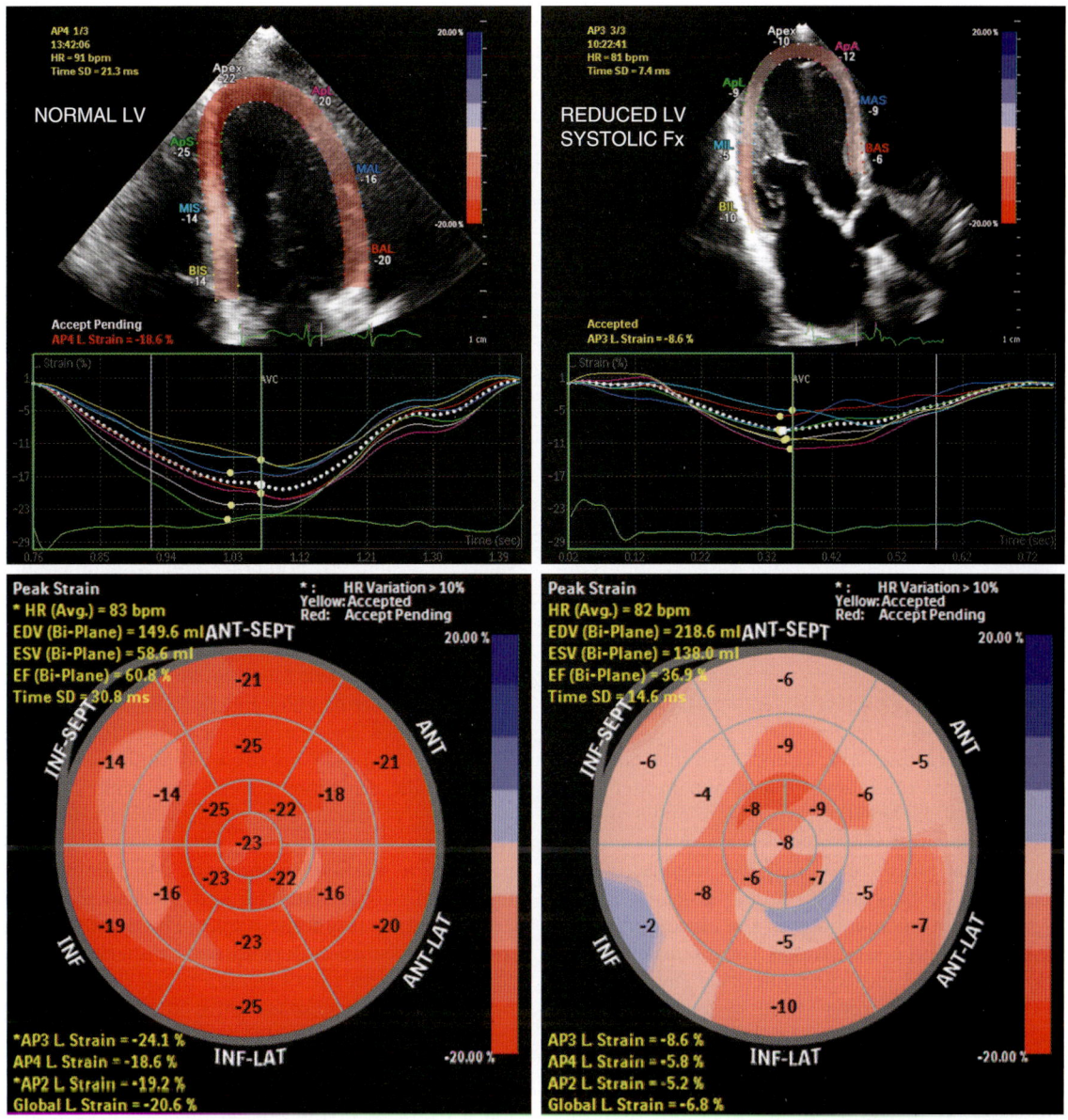

Fig. 4.15 Speckle tracking strain imaging. The figure demonstrates a typical strain pattern from a normal LV. The colors in each strain trace correspond to the colorized LV segments in the in 2D display at the *upper left panel* ▶ ▷. *ANT,* Anterior; *EDV,* end-diastolic volume; *EF,* ejection fraction; *ESV,* end-systolic volume; *Fx,* function; *HR,* heart rate; *INF,* inferior; *LAT,* lateral; *SEPT,* septum. (From Smiseth OA, Edvardsen T: Myocardial mechanics: velocity, strain, strain rate, cardiac synchrony, and twist. In Otto CM, editor: The Practice of Clinical Echocardiography, ed 4, Philadelphia, 2012, Saunders, pp 177–196.)

potentially useful for the detection of myocardial ischemia during stress testing and for the diagnosis of myocardial viability, but they are not currently part of a standard stress echocardiographic study (see Fig. 8.10).

Dyssynchrony, Twist, and Torsion

The term *dyssynchrony* describes a pattern of ventricular contraction in which some areas contract before other areas in an irregular spatial and temporal pattern. Dyssynchrony is primarily seen in patients with a reduced ejection fraction, either from cardiomyopathy or due to ischemic disease, and it may be appreciated on 2D imaging in some cases. Attempts to measure the amount of dyssynchrony have used imaging, conventional Doppler, and tissue Doppler approaches. M-mode echocardiography has been used to measure the time interval from the QRS complex on the electrocardiogram to maximum inward motion of the ventricular wall, by comparing the septum to the posterior wall. This approach is limited by the many other causes of changes in septal motion. Interventricular dyssynchrony has been measured as the difference between LV and RV preejection periods, measured from the QRS complex to the onset of aortic or pulmonic flow, respectively, with abnormal defined as a difference in these measurements >40 ms.

With pulsed tissue Doppler, the variation in time to peak systolic velocity at different locations in the myocardium also provides a measure of dyssynchrony. Tissue Doppler mean velocity data displayed using a color scale superimposed on the 2D image are analogous to color Doppler flow imaging data. With a normal pattern of ventricular contraction, a uniform pattern of red in systole and blue in diastole is present. This can also be displayed using a color M-line display. In contrast, dyssynchrony results in a chaotic pattern of red-blue because different areas of the myocardium contract at different times and rates (see Fig. 9.11).

Abnormalities in LV twist and torsion have been described in patients with heart failure and with coronary, valve, and pericardial disease, but currently these measurements are not recommended for clinical use.

CONTRAST ECHOCARDIOGRAPHY

Contrast echocardiography refers to the injection into the bloodstream of an agent that results in increased echogenicity of the blood or myocardium on ultrasound imaging, thus producing opacification of the cardiac chambers or an increase in echo density of the myocardium. Ultrasound "contrast" is generated by the presence of microbubbles in the ultrasound field. At low ultrasound power outputs, microbubbles scatter ultrasound at the gas-liquid interface and result in the detection of a strong signal by the transducer. Fundamental ultrasound imaging is based on detection of this signal reflected from the gas-liquid interface. In addition, ultrasound causes compression and expansion (i.e., oscillation) of microbubbles, with the resonant frequency of a microbubble inversely related to its diameter. Harmonic imaging detects this nonlinear resonant signal. However, at higher power outputs, ultrasound results in microbubble destruction. Thus careful adjustment of instrument power outputs is needed during contrast imaging.

Contrast Agents

Two types of echo-contrast agents used, those that opacify the:

- Right heart
- Left heart and myocardium

Depending on the size of the microbubbles relative to the lung capillary diameter, the microbubbles are trapped in the pulmonary capillaries so that no contrast material is seen in the left heart in the absence of an intracardiac right-to-left communication (Fig. 4.16). Microbubbles in the 1- to 5-μm size range traverse the pulmonary bed; microbubbles in this size range resonate at a frequency of 1.5 to 7 MHz, corresponding to clinical transducer frequencies.

The most widely used agent for contrast of the right heart is agitated saline. A simple approach is rapidly to push 5 mL of sterile saline, with a small amount (about 0.2 mL) of air, between two syringes connected with a three-way stopcock. This results in the production of large microbubbles that do not pass through the pulmonary vascular bed. When the saline appears opaque, it is injected rapidly into a peripheral vein during echocardiographic imaging, with the total volume and rate of injection adjusted based on image quality. The contrast effect may be enhanced by following the contrast injection with 10 mL of nonagitated saline. Care should be taken to ensure that no visible free air is present in the injection system. In addition, agitated saline should not be used in patients with known significant right-to-left shunts.

Commercially available contrast agents for the left heart consist of air or low-solubility fluorocarbon gas in stabilized microbubbles encapsulated with denatured albumin, monosaccharides, or other formulations. These agents typically are prepared just before injection with specific directions for the preparation and use of each agent. Some require resuspension before each bolus intravenous injection. Others are diluted and given as a continuous infusion. Microbubbles are fragile, so careful handling and infusion techniques are needed for diagnostic results. The optimal volume and rate of infusion depend on the specific contrast agent used, with the objectives being to provide full opacification while minimizing attenuation due to excess microbubble density.

Instrument settings are adjusted to optimize image quality during contrast opacification of the LV, including a decrease in the overall power output (usually to a mechanical index of about 0.5), a focal depth setting at the middle or near field, a lower transducer frequency, and an increase in overall gain and dynamic range.

Applications

Contrast echocardiography has four proposed diagnostic applications (Table 4.5):

- Detection of intracardiac shunts
- Enhancement of Doppler signals
- LV opacification
- Myocardial perfusion

Right heart contrast allows for the detection of right-to-left intracardiac shunts by the appearance of contrast in the left heart within one to two beats

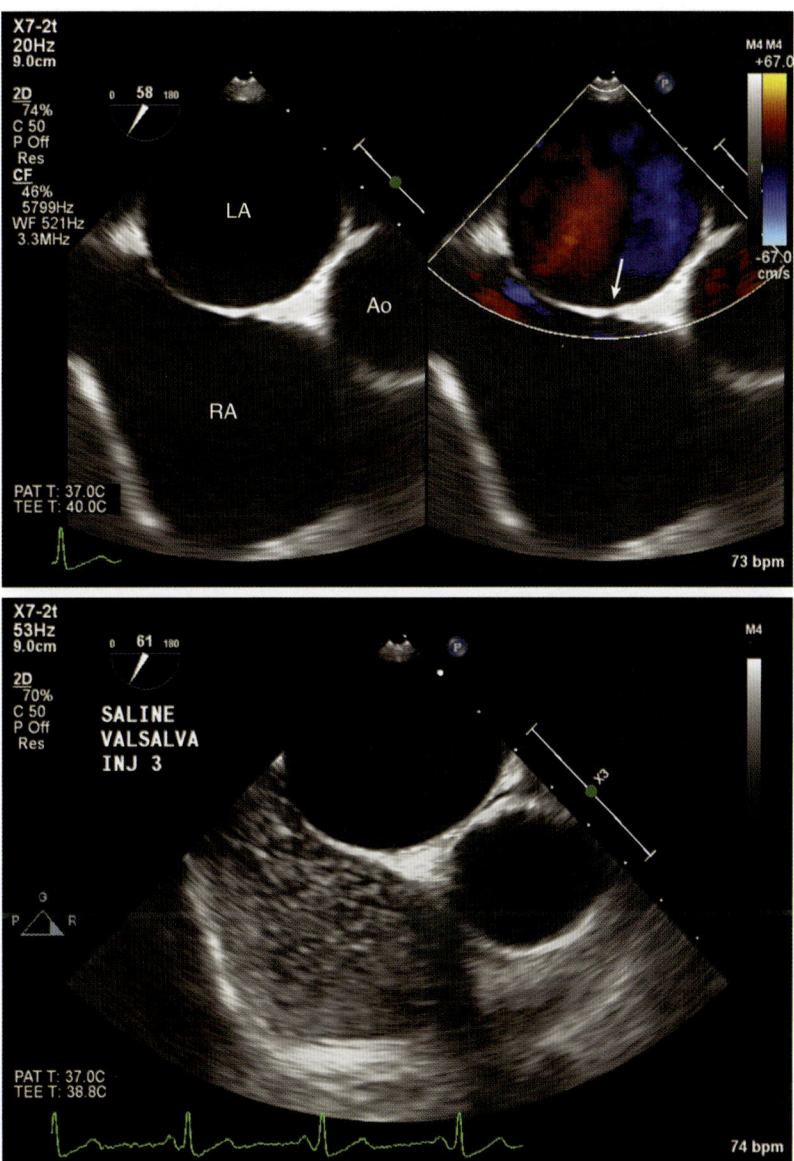

Fig. 4.16 ▶ ▶ **Right heart contrast study.** TEE view showing dense opacification of the RA following a peripheral venous injection *(INJ)* of agitated saline solution, which does not pass through the pulmonary vascular bed. A small amount of contrast *(arrow)* has entered the LA through a patent foramen ovale. *Ao,* Aorta.

of contrast appearance in the right heart. With a patent foramen ovale, right-to-left shunting may be present only after Valsalva maneuver because of the transient increase in RA, compared with LA, pressure (see Figs. 15.26 and 15.28). Even with predominant left-to-right shunts (e.g., with an atrial septal defect), a small amount of right-to-left shunting usually occurs when the pressures on both sides of the defect are similar, thus allowing for the detection of shunting with right heart contrast. Other examples of the utility of right heart contrast include identification of a persistent left superior vena cava or identification of the systemic venous inflow pathway in complex congenital heart disease.

Contrast has been used at some centers to increase Doppler signal strength, for example, the tricuspid regurgitant jet. However, the effect of contrast on the Doppler signal varies with instrument parameters, and this approach has not gained widespread use.

LV opacification in situations that result in poor image quality, either on resting studies or during stress echocardiography, enhances the recognition of segmental wall motion abnormalities and overall LV systolic function (Fig. 4.17). Contrast enhancement improves the accuracy of echocardiographic stress studies when endocardial definition is suboptimal. Recognition of LV thrombus also is improved with opacification of the LV (see Fig. 9.10).

Assessment of myocardial perfusion with contrast echocardiography is technically challenging and rarely used in clinical practice. Only about 6% of the stroke volume perfuses the myocardium, so the relative number of microbubbles in the coronary circulation is small. Mechanical and ultrasound destruction of microbubbles further limits the contrast effect. Thus special imaging modes, such as intermittent imaging, pulse inversion, or power modulation imaging are needed for myocardial contrast imaging. Myocardial contrast perfusion imaging might improve detection of coronary disease on stress studies and allow identification of impaired coronary perfusion at rest. However, other approaches for the evaluation of myocardial viability and perfusion, including nuclear perfusion imaging, cardiac magnetic resonance imaging, and positron emission tomography are superior and are the current clinical standard.

Limitations and Safety

Right heart contrast to detect large intracardiac shunts is needed infrequently given the sensitivity and specificity of color Doppler and TEE imaging. The primary use of right heart contrast is for the detection of a patent foramen ovale. A small ventricular septal defect usually will not be detected with a right heart contrast injection because little right-to-left shunting occurs.

The use of left heart contrast requires considerable experience to judge the infusion rate and volume needed to opacify the LV optimally. When the microbubble density is too high, an excessive contrast effect at the apex results in attenuation of the signal or "shadowing" of the rest of the LV. A swirling appearance is seen with too little contrast or in low-flow states. Bubble destruction due to a high mechanical index also results in a swirling pattern with inadequate ventricular opacification.

The addition of a contrast injection to the echocardiographic examination increases the cost and risk of the procedure. In addition, the added time and personnel needed for placement of an intravenous line during a standard echocardiographic examination or exercise stress study make this approach impractical in many laboratories. Although major adverse reactions

TABLE 4.5	Indications for Contrast Echocardiography

Right heart contrast (e.g., agitated saline)
- Detection of atrial septal defects and patent foramen ovale
- Documentation of persistent left superior vena cava

Left heart contrast (intravenous agents with transpulmonary passage)
- Enhancement of contrast between LV chamber and endocardium (improved border recognition)
- Myocardial perfusion

Intracoronary contrast
- Opacification of myocardium perfused by injected vessel (e.g., during catheter ablation for hypertrophic cardiomyopathy)

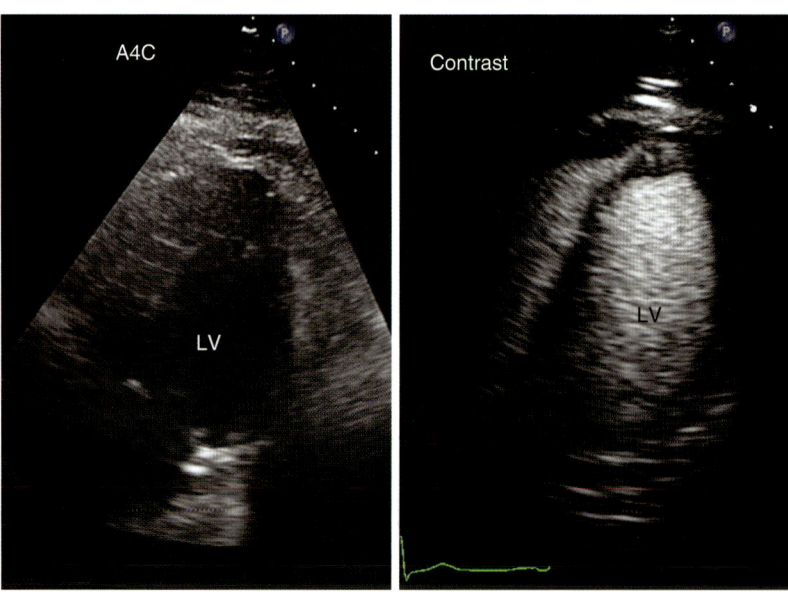

Fig. 4.17 **Left heart echo-contrast.** In this patient with suboptimal image quality on apical views *(left)*, opacification of the LV using left-sided echo contrast enhances endocardial border identification, thus allowing accurate measurement of ejection fraction and evaluation of regional wall motion. *A4C,* Apical four-chamber.

to left-sided contrast agents are rare, patients may experience nausea, vomiting, headache, flushing, or dizziness. Hypersensitivity reactions can occur.

Adverse effects of contrast agents for opacification of the left heart have been reported. Contraindications to the use of left-sided contrast include acute coronary syndromes, acute myocardial infarction, worsening or clinically unstable heart failure, intracardiac shunts, serious ventricular arrhythmias, respiratory failure, pulmonary hypertension, or a history of hypersensitivity to perflutren. Thus use of pharmacologic contrast requires a physician's order, is restricted to studies where improved endocardial definition is necessary, and should be avoided in high-risk patients. Blood pressure and electrocardiographic monitoring for 30 minutes after the contrast injection is recommended in high-risk patients.

INTRACARDIAC ECHOCARDIOGRAPHY

Instrumentation

Intracardiac echocardiography uses a catheter-like ultrasound probe that is passed into the right heart chambers from the femoral vein (Fig. 4.18). The transducer frequency is variable from 5 to 10 MHz to provide adequate penetration to image structures at distances up to 10 cm from the transducer and to provide optimal image resolution. Current devices provide single-plane imaging and pulsed and color Doppler, with a steerable probe connected to a standard ultrasound imaging system.

Technique

Typically, the 10-French 90-cm-long, disposable probe is inserted through a venous sheath as part of an invasive cardiac procedure in the cardiac catheterization or electrophysiology laboratory. The physician performing the interventional or electrophysiologic procedure also acquires the cardiac images because expertise in intracardiac manipulation of catheters is needed for this procedure. Fluoroscopy is used for placement of the probe because it does not accommodate a guidewire. The tip of the probe can be tilted and flexed using dials at the base of the probe, and the image plane also can be adjusted by advancing, withdrawing, or rotating the probe, similar to a single-plane TEE transducer. The transducer can be positioned in the:

- Inferior vena cava
- RA
- RV

The RA location is most useful for monitoring invasive procedures.

From the inferior vena cava the transducer is turned to visualize the abdominal aorta. From the RA position, the following views are obtained:

- Short-axis aortic valve
- Tricuspid valve and RV
- Mitral valve and LV
- Interatrial septum
- LA and left pulmonary veins

The interatrial septum is visualized from an RA position with the catheter retroflexed to show the fossa ovalis, septum primum, and RA and LA. The aortic valve is visualized by straightening and slightly anteflexing the probe and turning it toward the aorta. The tricuspid valve and RV are best visualized by anteflexing the probe after positioning the tip superiorly in the RA. From this position, turning the probe posteriorly allows for visualization of the mitral valve and LV. The left pulmonary veins are visualized by angulation from the atrial septal view inferiorly to image the LA appendage and then the pulmonary views. From this position, the probe is turned clockwise and advanced superiorly in the atrium to visualize the two right pulmonary veins. These views allow diameter measurements and pulsed and color Doppler interrogations of all four pulmonary veins.

From the RV, a view of the outflow tract and pulmonary artery can be achieved. The LV also can

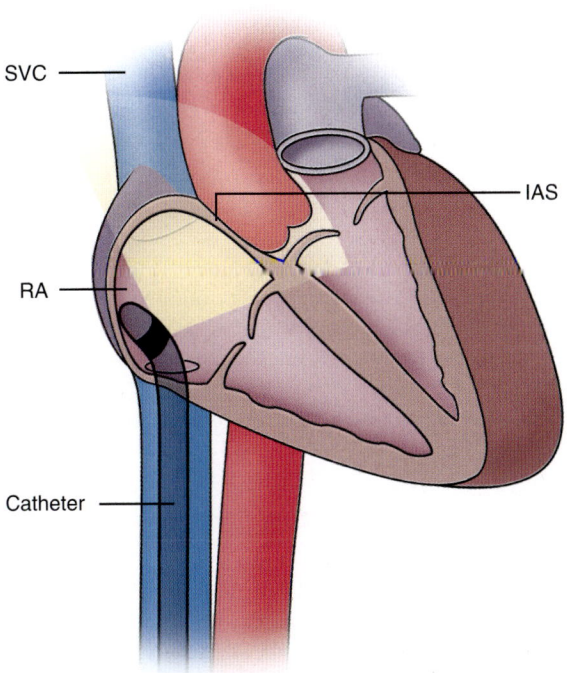

Fig. 4.18 Intracardiac echocardiography. A probe is advanced from the inferior vena cava to the RA. The probe is retroflexed to image the interatrial septum *(IAS)*. *SVC,* Superior vena cava. *(From Bartel T, Muller S, Caspari G, et al: Intracardiac and intraluminal echocardiography: indications and standard approaches,* Ultrasound Med Biol *28[8]:997–1003, 2002.)*

TABLE 4.6 Clinical Applications of Intracardiac Echocardiography

Primary Role in Procedure Guidance	Supplemental or Evolving Role in Procedure Guidance	Investigational Role as Primary Guidance Modality
Closure of interatrial communications (ASD, PFO)	TAVI	Mitral valve clip
Electrophysiology procedures (PVI, CTI, VT ablation)	Less common shunt closure procedures (VSD and PDA)	LAA closure devices
Transseptal catheterization	Transcatheter mitral valve procedures	PVL closure
Percutaneous balloon mitral valvuloplasty	Alcohol septal ablation in hypertrophic cardiomyopathy	LAA thrombus assessment

ASD, Atrial septal defect; *CTI*, cavotricuspid isthmus; *LAA*, left atrial appendage; *PDA*, patent ductus arteriosus; *PFO*, patent foramen ovale; *PVI*, pulmonary vein isolation; *PVL*, paravalvular leak; *TAVI*, transcatheter aortic valve implantation; *VSD*, ventricular septal defect; *VT*, ventricular tachycardia.
From Silvestry FE: Intracardiac echocardiography. In Otto CM, editor: *The Practice of Clinical Echocardiography*, ed 5, Philadelphia, 2017, Elsevier, pp 79–90.

be evaluated, but care in interpretation of wall motion is needed if the catheter is moving in the RV.

Applications

Intracardiac echocardiography is primarily used for monitoring invasive procedures, although the diagnostic potential of this modality has not been fully evaluated (Table 4.6). In a patient undergoing an invasive cardiac procedure, image quality is usually inadequate on TTE imaging, and TEE imaging typically requires general anesthesia, given the length of the procedure. Intracardiac echocardiography is well tolerated, provides accurate information, and provides continuous imaging data to the physician performing the procedure.

The primary applications of intracardiac echocardiography include:

- Guiding device closure of interatrial communications (Fig. 4.19)
- Monitoring percutaneous LA appendage closure
- Guiding radiofrequency pulmonary vein ablation
- Monitoring transcatheter valve implantation
- Peri-interventional imaging of the aorta
- Peri-interventional imaging of the mitral valve

In the cardiac catheterization laboratory, intracardiac echocardiography at baseline before closure of an atrial septal defect allows evaluation of the atrial septal defect size and position and identification of adjacent structures including the pulmonary veins and coronary sinus. During the procedure, intracardiac imaging allows optimal positioning of the device at each stage of the procedure. After the device is deployed, color flow intracardiac imaging allows evaluation for any residual shunt. Advantages of intracardiac echocardiography compared with TEE are that the interventional cardiologist can perform the imaging during the procedure and general anesthesia is not needed.

For electrophysiology procedures, intracardiac echocardiography is used to monitor:

- Transseptal puncture
- Detailed evaluation of LA and pulmonary vein anatomy
- Placement of the radiofrequency ablation probe with optimal probe-tissue contact
- Development of spontaneous contrast during the ablation
- Detection of any complications of the procedure

The transseptal catheter produces "tenting" of the atrial septum when correctly positioned, improving the safety of this procedure. Potential complications that can be detected immediately with intracardiac echocardiography include intracardiac thrombus formation, pericardial effusion, and pulmonary vein obstruction.

Limitations and Safety

The major limitations of intracardiac echocardiography are cost and the risks of an invasive procedure. However, because most patients undergo intracardiac echocardiography as part of an invasive therapeutic procedure, little additional risk is incurred. The current cost of the disposable catheter is substantial, which limits use of this technology for diagnostic purposes. The single-plane probe design is adequate, but a biplane or multiplane probe would improve image acquisition.

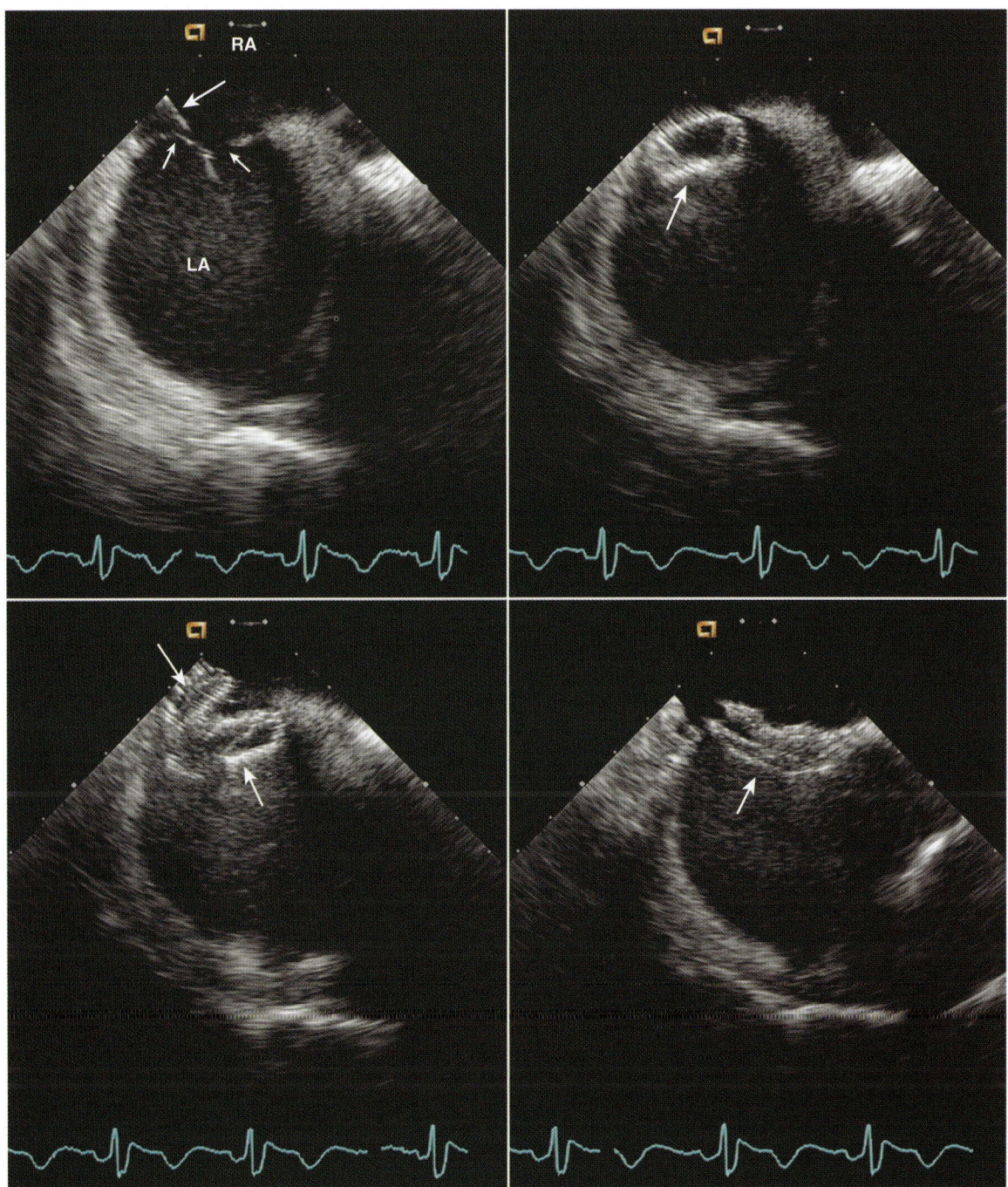

Fig. 4.19 Intracardiac echocardiographic guidance during placement of an atrial septal closure device. The catheter is guided across the atrial septal defect *(top left)*, ▶ and the LA side of the device is deployed first *(top right)*, followed by deployment of the RA side of the device *(bottom left)*. ▶ When the device is correctly positioned, the guiding catheter is detached and the two sides of the device are flattened to close the atrial septal defect *(bottom right)*. *(Images courtesy Steve Goldberg, MD.)*

THE ECHO EXAM

Specialized Echo Applications

Modality	Instrumentation	Clinical Utility	Special Training
3D echo	Volume-rendered images Surface-rendered LV volumes Simultaneous 2D images	• LV volumes, EF, and regional wall motion • Mitral valve anatomy • Procedural guidance	• Image acquisition and analysis
Tissue Doppler strain rate and strain	Tissue Doppler and 2D imaging are used to measure strain rate: $SR = (V_2 - V_1) / D$	• Strain rate is a measure of ventricular contractility. • Strain rate is integrated to determine strain, a measure of regional myocardial function.	• Data acquisition and analysis • Clinical interpretation of data
Myocardial speckle tracking	Strain is measured directly from the motion of myocardial speckles as: $[(L - L_0) / L_0] \times 100\%$	• Myocardial speckle tracking is angle independent. • Analysis can be performed after image acquisition.	• Data acquisition and analysis • Clinical interpretation of data
Myocardial dyssynchrony	Multiple 2D pulsed Doppler and tissue Doppler methods	• The degree of dyssynchrony is altered in various disease states.	• Data acquisition and analysis • Clinical interpretation of data
Contrast echo	Microbubbles for right or left heart contrast	• Detection of patent foramen ovale • LV endocardial definition	• Intravenous administration of contrast agents • Knowledge of potential risks
Intracardiac echo (ICE)	5–10-MHz catheter-like intracardiac probe	• Interventional procedures (ASD closure) • EP procedures	• Invasive cardiology training and experience
Point-of-care ultrasound study (POCUS)	Small, inexpensive ultrasound instruments	• Bedside evaluation by physician for pericardial effusion, LV global function, and LV regional function	• At least level 1 echo training
Procedural guidance	Complete TEE and/or TTE ultrasound system	• Intraoperative evaluation of structural heart disease immediately before and after the procedure • Procedural guidance of transcatheter procedures for structural heart disease	• Echocardiography training (often performed by cardiac anesthesiologists)

ASD, Atrial septal defect; *EF,* ejection fraction; *EP,* electrophysiology.

SUGGESTED READING

General

1. Bosch JG: Digital image processing and automated image analysis in echocardiography. In Otto CM, editor: *The Practice of Clinical Echocardiography,* ed 5, Philadelphia, 2017, Elsevier, pp 166–181.
   Advanced level discussion of digital image processing with specific details of relevance to 3D, strain and speckle tracking imaging.
2. Gillam LD, Otto CM, editors: *Advanced Approaches in Echocardiography,* Philadelphia, 2012, Saunders.
   This concise book is part of the Otto Practical Echocardiography Series, which provides a step-by-step approach to the implementation of advanced imaging techniques in clinical practice. The text is presented as bulleted lists with frequent illustrations and summary tables. Online cases and videos supplement the printed text. The 12 chapters include 3D echocardiography, intracardiac interventions, strain and strain rate imaging, contrast echocardiography, and stress echocardiography for structural heart disease.

3D Echocardiography

3. Tsang W, Lang RO: 3D Echocardiography: Principles of Image Acquisition, Display and Analysis. In Otto CM, editor: *The Practice of Clinical Echocardiography,* ed 5, Philadelphia, 2017, Elsevier, pp 18–36.
   Comprehensive, nicely illustrated, chapter on approaches to 3D echocardiographic imaging including a discussion of image resolution, data acquisition, image optimization, image display, and 3D analysis. Protocols for 3D acquisition and analysis for evaluation of each cardiac chamber and each valve are provided.
4. Lang RM, Badano LP, Tsang W, et al: EAE/ASE recommendations for

image acquisition and display using three-dimensional echocardiography, *J Am Soc Echocardiogr* 25(1):3–46, 2012.
Guidelines for the clinical use of 3D echocardiography are presented with excellent descriptions of the details of image acquisition, presentation of display formats, and clear illustrations and tables. The published data validating 3D echocardiography are summarized. 153 references.

Myocardial Mechanics

5. Smiseth OA, Edvardsen T, Torp H: Myocardial mechanics: Velocities, Strain, Strain Rate, Cardiac Synchrony and Twist. In Otto CM, editor: *The Practice of Clinical Echocardiography*, ed 5, Philadelphia, 2017, Elsevier, pp 128–146.
Advanced-level discussion of the principles of tissue Doppler echocardiography and the physiology of ventricular contraction. The clinical applications of strain rate and strain imaging in myocardial ischemia and diastolic dysfunction are reviewed. Approaches to measurement of ventricular dyssynchrony and LV twist and torsion are summarized and illustrated.

6. Mor-Avi V, Lang RM, Badano LP, et al: Current and evolving echocardiographic techniques for the quantitative evaluation of cardiac mechanics: ASE/EAE consensus statement on methodology and indications endorsed by the Japanese Society of Echocardiography, *Eur J Echocardiogr* 12(3):167–205, 2011.
Consensus document with clear definitions of cardiac mechanics terms, detailed descriptions of the methodology for accurate data recording, and a concise and well-referenced summary of the literature. Includes evaluation of LA and right-sided function using strain and strain rate imaging.

7. Kalam K, Otahal P, Marwick TH: Prognostic implications of global LV dysfunction: a systematic review and meta-analysis of global longitudinal strain and ejection fraction, *Heart* 100(21):1673–1680, 2014.
A systematic review of 16 studies (total of 5721 adults) showed that left ventricular global longitudinal strain was more predictive of mortality than ejection fraction. Each standard deviation of change in global longitudinal strain was associated with a 1.62 (95% CI: 1.13 to 2.33;

$P = 0.009$) *times reduction in mortality times compared with a similar change in ejection fraction.*

8. Geyer H, Caracciolo G, Abe H, et al: Assessment of myocardial mechanics using speckle tracking echocardiography: fundamentals and clinical applications, *J Am Soc Echocardiogr* 23(4):351–369, 2010.
This review of the basic principles and clinical applications of speckle tracking echocardiography includes excellent summary tables of studies evaluating strain and twist in coronary artery disease, myocardial strain in valvular disease, speckle tracking in patients with physiologic hypertrophy, myocardial strain in hypertensive heart disease, and cardiac strain in cardiomyopathies.

9. Tops LF, Delgado V, Marsan NA, et al: Myocardial strain to detect subtle left ventricular systolic dysfunction, *Eur J Heart Fail* 19(3):307–313, 2017.
A discussion of the utility of myocardial strain for detection of subclinical left ventricular systolic dysfunction.

Contrast Echocardiography

10. Porter TR, Abdelmoneim S, Belcik JT, et al: Guidelines for the cardiac sonographer in the performance of contrast echocardiography: a focused update from the American Society of Echocardiography, *J Am Soc Echocardiogr* 27(8):797–810, 2014.
Detailed information on optimal (low mechanical index) instrument settings for contrast echocardiography, common problems and artifacts encountered with contrast imaging, interpretation of imaging findings, and clinical applications. Includes 18 online videos and detailed protocols for contrast preparation and administration. 41 references.

11. Porter TR, Xie F: Contrast echocardiography: latest developments and clinical utility, *Curr Cardiol Rep* 17:11, 2015.
Review of recent developments in ultrasound enhancing agents and their effectiveness for 3D quantitation of left ventricular function and myocardial perfusion imaging. 33 references.

12. Seol SH, Lindner JR: A primer on the methods and applications for contrast echocardiography in clinical imaging, *J Cardiovasc Ultrasound* 22(3):101–110, 2014.
Illustrated review of contrast echocardiography in current clinical practice. An excellent introduction to this topic with 48 references.

13. Davidson BP, Lindner JR: Future applications of contrast echocardiography, *Heart* 98(3):246–253, 2012.
Newer applications of contrast echocardiography in development include visualization of neovascularization in atherosclerotic plaques, detection of microvascular dysfunction, stress/rest limb perfusion imaging for peripheral vascular disease, molecular imaging, and delivery of pharmaceutical agents to specific anatomic sites and improved thrombolysis.

Intracardiac Echocardiography

14. Silvestry FE: Intracardiac Echocardiography. In Otto CM, editor: *The Practice of Clinical Echocardiography*, ed 5, Philadelphia, 2017, Elsevier, pp 79–90.
This chapter reviews the instrument and imaging approach to intracardiac ultrasound. The use of intracardiac echocardiography in monitoring procedures, including atrial septal defect and patent foramen ovale closure, LA appendage closure, radiofrequency pulmonary vein ablation, myocardial septal ablation, percutaneous mitral valve procedures, and perioperative imaging of the aortic valve and aorta, is described and illustrated.

15. Bartel T, Müller S, Biviano A, et al: Why is intracardiac echocardiography helpful? Benefits, costs, and how to learn, *Eur Heart J* 35(2):69–76, 2014.
Beautifully illustrated review of the use of intracardiac echocardiography (ICE) for guidance of interventional and electrophysiological procedures. 12 figures, 43 references.

16. Ruisi CP, Brysiewicz N, Asnes JD, et al: Use of intracardiac echocardiography during atrial fibrillation ablation, *Pacing Clin Electrophysiol* 36(6):781–788, 2013.
Detailed and well-illustrated review of atrial anatomy as appreciate on ICE followed by a discussion of ICE-guided transseptal puncture, guidance of catheters during atrial fibrillation ablation, and identification of complications.

5 Clinical Indications and Quality Assurance

TYPES OF ECHOCARDIOGRAPHIC STUDIES
BASIC PRINCIPLES OF DIAGNOSTIC TESTING
    Reliability of a Diagnostic Test
        Accuracy
        Precision
        Expertise
    Integration of Clinical Data and Test Results
        Predictive Value
        Likelihood Ratio
        Pre-test and Post-test Probability
    Cost-Effectiveness
    Clinical Outcomes
INDICATIONS AND APPROPRIATENESS CRITERIA
INDICATIONS FOR DIAGNOSTIC ECHOCARDIOGRAPHY
    Transthoracic Echocardiography
    Transesophageal Echocardiography
    Stress Echocardiography

POINT OF CARE CARDIAC ULTRASOUND STUDIES
    Instrumentation
    Applications
    Providers
    Safety and Limitations
QUALITY ASSURANCE IN ECHOCARDIOGRAPHY
    Sonographer Education and Training
    Physician Education and Training
    Echocardiography Reporting
    Echocardiography Laboratory Structure
THE ECHO EXAM
SUGGESTED READING

TYPES OF ECHOCARDIOGRAPHIC STUDIES

Cardiac ultrasound examinations now are performed in various practice settings by health care providers with differing types of clinical and imaging expertise. *Diagnostic echocardiography* is defined as an echocardiographic examination performed under the supervision of a cardiologist with expertise in echocardiography (Level 2 or 3 training) for the purposes of diagnosis, measurement of disease severity, evaluation of disease progression, or assessment of response to therapy. A diagnostic echocardiogram includes a formal interpretation in the medical record that meets American Society of Echocardiography quality standards and archiving of a complete set of diagnostic images. Diagnostic echocardiography typically is performed in the context of a medical center–based echocardiography service or outpatient cardiology practice with established technical standards, imaging protocols, and quality control measures (Table 5.1). Diagnostic studies also may include contrast enhancement, 3D echocardiography, and strain imaging. In addition to transthoracic echocardiography (TTE) and transesophageal echocardiography (TTE), additional diagnostic echocardiographic modalities used by cardiologists include exercise and pharmacologic stress echocardiography.

Cardiac ultrasound imaging also is used in other clinical settings by physicians with special expertise in areas other than echocardiography. For example, TEE to provide *procedural guidance* in the operating room and interventional suite usually is performed and simultaneously interpreted by cardiac anesthesiologists or cardiologists participating in the procedure (see Chapter 18). Intracardiac echocardiography may be used in conjunction with (or instead of) TEE imaging for procedural guidance in some situations (see Chapter 4). The results of monitoring studies are included in the procedure report, and selected images should be archived.

Focused cardiac ultrasound imaging often is performed in other clinical settings in which a rapid evaluation of basic cardiac function is needed for acute patient management. These *point of care cardiac ultrasound* (POCUS) studies typically are performed

TABLE 5.1 Cardiac Ultrasound Examination Types Defined by Purpose of Study, Clinical Setting, and Health Care Provider

	Diagnostic Echocardiogram	PROCEDURAL GUIDANCE			Point of Care Echocardiography
		Cardiac Surgery	Interventional Procedures	Electrophysiology Procedures	
Purpose of imaging	Diagnose and measure disease severity, evaluate progression or response to therapy, integrate with clinical information and other imaging approaches.	Comprehensive perioperative exam and/or procedure guidance (baseline data, measure results, detect complications)	Direct catheter and device positioning, evaluate procedural results, detect complications.	Direct catheter and device positioning, detect complications.	Immediate patient triage and management or monitoring cardiac parameters
Clinical setting	Any inpatient or outpatient location under the auspices of a structured echocardiography laboratory*	Operating room	Interventional suite or hybrid operating room	Electrophysiology laboratory	Inpatient bedside, emergency department or outpatient clinic
Heath care provider	Images recorded by cardiac sonographer and interpreted by cardiologist with expertise in echocardiography	Interventional echocardiographer or cardiac anesthesiologist with expertise in echocardiography	Interventional echocardiographer, interventional cardiologist or anesthesiologist†	Clinical cardiac electrophysiologist or anesthesiologist†	Physician with limited training in echocardiography who provides direct care to the patient
Ultrasound modalities	All echocardiographic modalities as appropriate	TEE Epicardial	TEE ICE TTE	TEE ICE TTE	TTE, primarily 2D imaging and color Doppler
Documentation	Formal written report in medical record	Results integrated into anesthesiology procedure note	Results integrated into interventional procedure report	Results integrated into EP procedure report	Results reported in clinical progress note
Quality improvement	Long-term PACS storage of digital images documenting entire study	Long-term PACS storage of representative digital images	Optional long-term PACS storage of representative images	Optional long-term PACS storage of representative images	Images typically not recorded, although key images may be saved for CQI

*Ideally, the echocardiography laboratory is accredited by the Intersocietal Commission for the Accreditation of Echocardiology Laboratories.
†Imaging may be performed by an anesthesiologist with expertise in echocardiography, a cardiologist, or the interventional cardiologist.
CQI, Continuous quality improvement; EP, electrophysiology; ICE, intracardiac echocardiography; PACS, picture archiving and communication system. TEE, transesophageal echocardiography; TTE, transthoracic echocardiography.
From Otto CM: Echocardiography: the transition from master of the craft to admiral of the fleet, Heart 102(12):899–901, 2016.

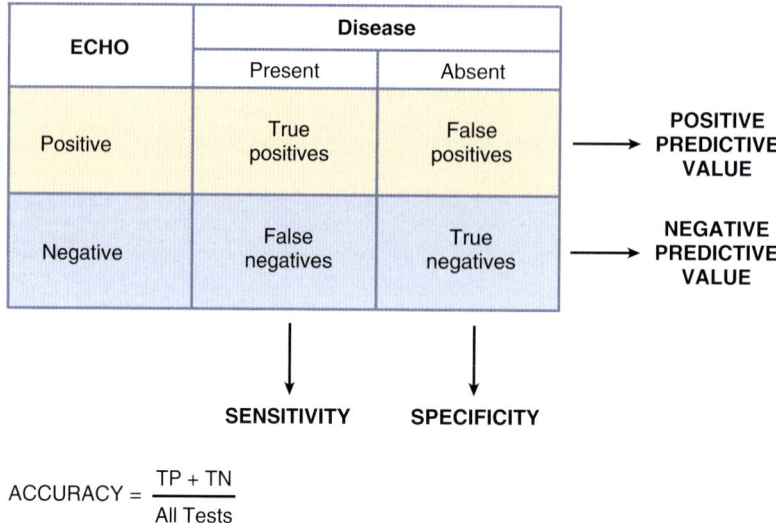

Fig. 5.1 Sensitivity and specificity in comparison with positive and negative predictive value. Note that predictive values are dependent on the prevalence of the disease in the study population and thus cannot be extrapolated to other patient groups. *TN,* True negatives; *TP,* true positives.

by providers in the emergency department or intensive care unit as an integral component of clinical care. POCUS studies also are used for screening at risk populations, for example, in evaluation for structural heart disease in athletes or detection of rheumatic valve disease in endemic areas.

Appropriate education and training in cardiac ultrasound are needed by all providers performing cardiac ultrasound examinations. Each medical center also has procedures to ensure monitoring and quality improvement for all imaging studies.

BASIC PRINCIPLES OF DIAGNOSTIC TESTING

Reliability of a Diagnostic Test

The reliability of a diagnostic test includes two components: accuracy and precision. Accuracy is the ability of the test to make a correct numeric measurement (e.g., left ventricular [LV] volume) or to diagnose the presence or absence of a condition correctly (e.g., coronary artery disease). Precision reflects the agreement of repeated evaluations, including the acquisition, measurement, and interpretation of data. The combination of accuracy and precision determines the value of echocardiography in different clinical situations.

Accuracy

The accuracy of a numeric measurement, such as wall thickness, aortic jet velocity, or aortic diameter, is expressed as the agreement between the echocardiographic measurement and a reference standard. These measurements reflect continuous variables; a continuous range of values is recognized from the smallest to largest seen in clinical practice. For example, aortic jet velocity ranges from <1 m/s to as high as 6 m/s. The numeric reference standard may be an anatomic measurement at surgery or autopsy, direct measurements in an experimental model, or comparison of echocardiography with other imaging techniques or hemodynamic recordings. Published data on the accuracy of echocardiography are shown in tables in each chapter of this book. More recent studies use an approach called Bland-Altman analysis, which compares the deviation of each measurement (echocardiography and the reference standard) with the mean of both measurements. Older validation studies typically report correlation coefficients and regression equations with standard errors for each measurement.

For echocardiographic diagnoses that are either present or absent (called categorical variables), accuracy reflects the certainty with which a specific diagnosis can be confirmed or excluded based on the test results (Fig. 5.1). An example is echocardiography for the diagnosis of endocarditis: the patient either has or does not have endocarditis; no range of values exists. Accuracy for this type of test is described in terms of sensitivity and specificity. The sensitivity of a test is the degree to which it identifies all patients with the disease; specificity is the degree to which a test identifies all patients without the disease.

- Sensitivity = "True-positive" test results / All patients with the disease = TP / (TP + FN)
- Specificity = "True-negative" test results / All patients without the disease = TN / (TN + FP)

where TP is true positive, FN is false negative, TN is true negative, and FP is false positive.

Accuracy indicates the percentage of patients in whom the test results are correct in identifying the presence or absence of disease.

- Accuracy = True positives + True negatives / Total number of tests = (TP + TN) / All tests

Using a diagnostic test to determine whether a disease is present or absent depends on the cutoff value or breakpoint used to define the test as abnormal. Sensitivity and specificity are related inversely to each other; in general, the higher the sensitivity, the lower is the specificity and vice versa. Whether a higher sensitivity is preferable to a higher specificity depends on the clinical question. If the goal of the test is identification of all patients with the disease, a high sensitivity is preferable. If the goal is confirmation of the diagnosis in an individual patient, a high specificity is preferable.

The relationship between sensitivity and specificity can be evaluated quantitatively for any given diagnostic test by graphing the sensitivity (y-axis) versus $1 -$ specificity (x-axis), with each point on the curve representing a different breakpoint defining the test as abnormal. The area under the curve reflects the clinical value of the test, with a larger area indicating a more reliable diagnostic test. The point on the receiver-operator curve where sensitivity and specificity are maximized indicates an appropriate breakpoint (Fig. 5.2).

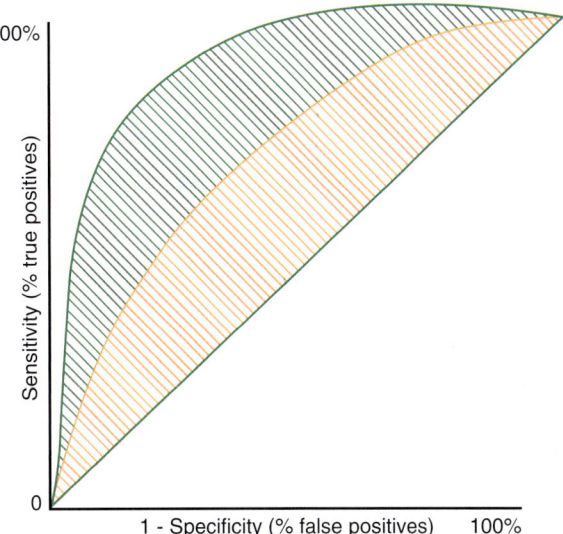

Fig. 5.2 Receiver-operator curve for a diagnostic test. A receiver-operator curve is a graph of sensitivity (the percentage of positive test results that are true positives) versus 1 minus specificity (the percentage of positive test results that are false positives). Each point on the curve defined by a threshold value for the test result. If the test has no value in making a correct diagnosis, points would fall on the line of identity *(diagonal green line)*. For a useful test, a curve can be drawn to the left of the line of identity; hypothetic curves for two different tests are shown by the *green* and *orange lines*. The area between each curve and the line of identity indicates the overall value of the test, with a larger area indicating a more useful test.

Precision

The reproducibility of echocardiographic imaging and Doppler data is affected by variability in:

- Recording
- Measurement
- Interpretation

In addition, variability can occur both when the same person repeats the data acquisition or measurement at a different time (intraobserver variability) and when data acquisition or measurement is performed by different people (interobserver variability). These sources of imprecision are major limitations of echocardiography in clinical practice. Several approaches to improving the precision, and thus reliability, of echocardiographic data are used. Appropriate training and experience help ensure correct acquisition of data, including correctly aligned image planes and Doppler recordings, optimization of instrument parameters, and standardized study protocols. Measurement precision is improved with adherence to published standards, quality control in each laboratory, and comparison with reference standards when possible. Interpretation variability is minimized by using standard terminology and diagnostic criteria, developing a consensus approach to reporting in each laboratory, and comparing images and Doppler data with previous recordings in that patient whenever possible; that is, the report should specify whether a change from previous studies has occurred based on direct comparison of the recorded data, with side-by-side measurements as needed. Measurement variability is reported in each chapter when this information is available.

Expertise

The quality of an echocardiographic examination is highly dependent on the expertise of the sonographer performing the study, the physician interpreting the data, and the expertise of the laboratory. Optimal acquisition of image and Doppler data requires experience, in addition to education and training. A physician's interpretation is affected both by the data acquired (e.g., if images of a ventricular thrombus are not recorded, the physician will not see it) and by the education, training, and experience of that physician. Laboratory expertise affects data quality in terms of study protocols, time allocation and efficiency, instrumentation, and the group expertise of the sonographers and physicians. Thus, echocardiographic studies performed in different laboratories are not always comparable, and published studies on the accuracy of echocardiographic diagnosis may not apply to all diagnostic examinations.

Integration of Clinical Data and Test Results

Predictive Value

A major limitation of applying sensitivity and specificity data to an individual patient is the problem of whether a particular patient has a "true" or a "false" test result. Predictive values indicate the percentage of patients with a positive test result who have the suspected disease and the percentage with a negative test result who do not have the suspected disease:

- Positive predictive value = true positives divided by all positives
- Negative predictive value = true negatives divided by all negatives

However, predictive values are determined by the prevalence of disease in the population studied and also by the sensitivity and specificity of the test. Intuitively, this is obvious, comparing the use of echocardiography to "screen" healthy young subjects for endocarditis (many false-positive results because of ultrasound imaging artifacts) versus the same test in patients who have a new murmur, fever, and positive blood culture results, with a high prevalence of disease. The finding of a valvular vegetation on echocardiography in the latter group has a much higher predictive value for a diagnosis of endocarditis than in the healthy subjects, even though the sensitivity and specificity of echocardiography for diagnosing endocarditis are the same in both groups. Thus, the positive or negative predictive value of a test reflects disease prevalence as well as test accuracy.

Likelihood Ratio

The likelihood ratio indicates the relative likelihood of disease in an individual patient, based on a positive or negative test result. The likelihood ratio for a positive test result is calculated as:

$$+\text{Likelihood ratio} = \text{sensitivity}/(1-\text{specificity})$$

or

$$+\text{Likelihood ratio} = \frac{\text{True} - \text{positive rate}}{\text{False} - \text{positive rate}}$$

A positive likelihood ratio >10 indicates an excellent test, and a ratio of 5 to 10 indicates a good test.

The likelihood ratio for a negative test result is calculated as:

$$-\text{Likelihood ratio} = (1-\text{sensitivity})/\text{specificity}$$

or

$$+\text{Likelihood ratio} = \frac{\text{False} - \text{negative rate}}{\text{True} - \text{negative rate}}$$

A negative likelihood ratio <0.1 indicates an excellent test, and a ratio of 0.1 to 0.2 indicates a reasonably good test.

For example, diagnosis of left ventricular (LV) thrombus by echocardiography, assuming a sensitivity of 95% and a specificity of 88%, has a positive likelihood of 7.9 (a good diagnostic test) and a negative likelihood ratio of 0.06 (an excellent diagnostic test). The positive likelihood is not excellent because ultrasound artifacts may be mistaken for a ventricular thrombus. The excellent negative likelihood depends on a high-quality echocardiographic study and the expertise of the sonographer to ensure that an apical thrombus is not missed by echocardiographic imaging.

Pre-test and Post-test Probability

Another approach to the use of sensitivity and specificity data in patient management is to consider relevant clinical data along with the test result (Fig. 5.3). The value of a diagnostic test increases when the pre-test likelihood of disease is integrated with the test results to derive a post-test likelihood of disease. This approach is known as Bayesian analysis. For example, the pre-test likelihood of severe aortic stenosis in an asymptomatic 30-year-old woman without a systolic murmur is very low. An echocardiogram purporting to show severe aortic stenosis most likely is an erroneous interpretation (a false-positive test result). In this setting, the result does not increase the post-test likelihood of disease very much. In contrast, in an elderly man with a 4/6 aortic stenosis murmur and symptoms of angina, syncope, and heart failure, the diagnosis of severe valvular aortic stenosis can be made with a high level of certainty even before any test is performed. The echocardiogram serves only to confirm the diagnosis and define the severity of obstruction. In general, diagnostic tests are most helpful when the pre-test likelihood of disease is intermediate so that the test result will substantially change the post-test likelihood of disease.

The most comprehensive approach to the evaluation of a diagnostic test is clinical decision analysis. Clinical decision analysis incorporates several rigorous approaches to the problem of clinical prediction, with the method most applicable to a diagnostic test (e.g., echocardiography) being the threshold approach. The basic tenet of clinical decision analysis as applied to a diagnostic test is that the test results should have an impact on patient care by either:

- Prompting a change in therapy or
- Leading to a change in the subsequent diagnostic strategy in that patient

This basic assumption is formalized in the threshold model of decision analysis. In this approach, two

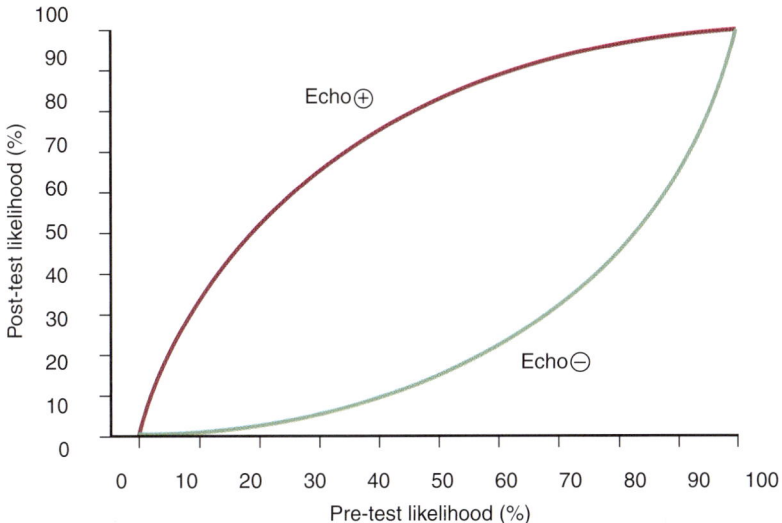

Fig. 5.3 Bayesian analysis. The pre-test and post-test likelihoods of coronary artery disease in patients undergoing exercise echocardiography are shown for inducible ischemia (+echo) or a normal result (−echo). These curves were generated based on a sensitivity of 85% and a specificity of 82% of exercise echocardiography for diagnosis of significant (>70% luminal narrowing) coronary artery disease. In clinical practice, the pre-test likelihood is based on the patient's clinical history, age, and sex. The post-test likelihood then depends on the result of the exercise echocardiogram. For example, if the pre-test likelihood is 50%, an exercise echocardiogram showing inducible ischemia indicates an 83% likelihood of coronary disease, whereas a negative test indicates only a 15% likelihood of coronary disease.

disease probability thresholds are defined for the diagnostic test:

- A lower threshold below which the risk of the test is greater than the risk of not treating the patient and
- An upper threshold above which treating the patient is a lower risk than performing the test

The intermediate range—in which the risk of treating or not treating the patient is greater than the risk of the diagnostic test—is known as the testing zone (Fig. 5.4). For any specific indication, the testing zone for echocardiography generally is wide because of the low risk and high accuracy of this technique. However, both an upper threshold and a lower threshold still are definable for echocardiography. The upper threshold is reached in situations in which the diagnosis is clear, and echocardiographic examination would only delay appropriate treatment. For example, a patient with a classic presentation of an ascending aortic dissection (chest pain, wide mediastinum, peripheral pulse loss) requires prompt surgery. Any delay caused by unnecessary diagnostic testing could result in additional morbidity or mortality.

It is tempting to assume that no lower end to the test zone for echocardiography exists, given the absence of known adverse biologic effects of this procedure. However, the risk of the test also includes the risks of additional diagnostic tests or even erroneous treatment choices resulting from a false-positive or false-negative echocardiographic findings. For example, an

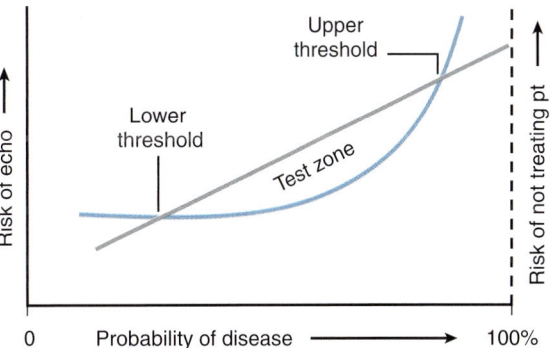

Fig. 5.4 Threshold approach to clinical decision making. The risk of the diagnostic test—in this case, echocardiography—is shown by the *curved blue line* (*left* y-axis), with the risk of not treating the patient *(pt)* for the suspected disease shown by the *straight gray line* (*right* y-axis). The probability of disease based on the clinical presentation is shown from 0% to 100% on the x-axis. The lower threshold is the point at which the risk of not treating the patient is greater than the risk of echocardiography. The upper threshold is the point at which the risk of echocardiography (including false-negative results, delay in treatment) is greater than the risk of not treating the patient. The test zone is the pre-test likelihood of disease between these two thresholds.

echocardiogram is not indicated to evaluate for aortic dissection in a young patient with atypical chest pain and a normal physical examination, electrocardiogram, and chest radiograph. If a false-positive echocardiographic diagnosis leads to further evaluation with cardiac catheterization, any complications from the invasive procedure ultimately can be considered a consequence of the echocardiographic results. Thus, a lower limit to the test zone does exist for echocardiography and can be defined for each specific diagnostic indication by applying decision analysis techniques. Other clinical decision analysis approaches have been applied to specific clinical problems that use echocardiographic data as a branch point in the decision analysis tree.

Cost-Effectiveness

An additional consideration in medical practice is the cost-effectiveness of a diagnostic procedure. Note that this term includes not only the cost of the test (echocardiography compares favorably with other cardiac diagnostic tests) but also the effectiveness of the test—that is, test accuracy and its impact on patient management. This type of analysis has been applied to some echocardiographic diagnostic issues, but more widespread use of this approach is needed.

Clinical Outcomes

The most important measure of the value of a diagnostic test is its impact on subsequent clinical outcome (Fig. 5.5). Although the first step in evaluation of the clinical utility of a test includes various measures of diagnostic accuracy in comparison with some accepted standard, the more important assessment is whether the diagnostic test changes the subsequent diagnostic or therapeutic plan in each patient. The definitive value of echocardiography depends on its ability to predict prognosis, for example, survival in patients with dilated cardiomyopathy, timing of valve surgery in patients with chronic regurgitation, or the rate of hemodynamic progression in patients with valvular stenosis. Echocardiographic data are increasingly used in clinical outcome studies, as referenced in the suggested readings throughout this textbook.

INDICATIONS AND APPROPRIATENESS CRITERIA

The indications for echocardiography are based on the reliability of this approach for diagnosis in a wide range of cardiovascular diseases and are summarized in consensus guidelines developed by the American Heart Association and the American College of Cardiology. In addition, specific recommendations on the use of echocardiography often are included in disease-specific guidelines, for example, guidelines for the management of valvular heart disease and for heart failure.

Appropriateness criteria go beyond indications to consider the clinical setting in which a diagnostic test is appropriate. For example, exercise echocardiography is sensitive and specific for the diagnosis of coronary artery disease, but it should not be used as a routine screening test in all patients. Appropriateness criteria have been developed by the American College of Cardiology in collaboration with other organizations that provide helpful guidance, although not all possible clinical situations are included. These criteria can be used to improve appropriateness of referrals for diagnostic imaging (Fig. 5.6).

Ideally, the echocardiogram request should indicate an appropriate clinical question (not "evaluate heart") based on the patient's symptoms or exam findings and, when possible, an estimate of the probability of the diagnosis in that patient. Next, the reliability of

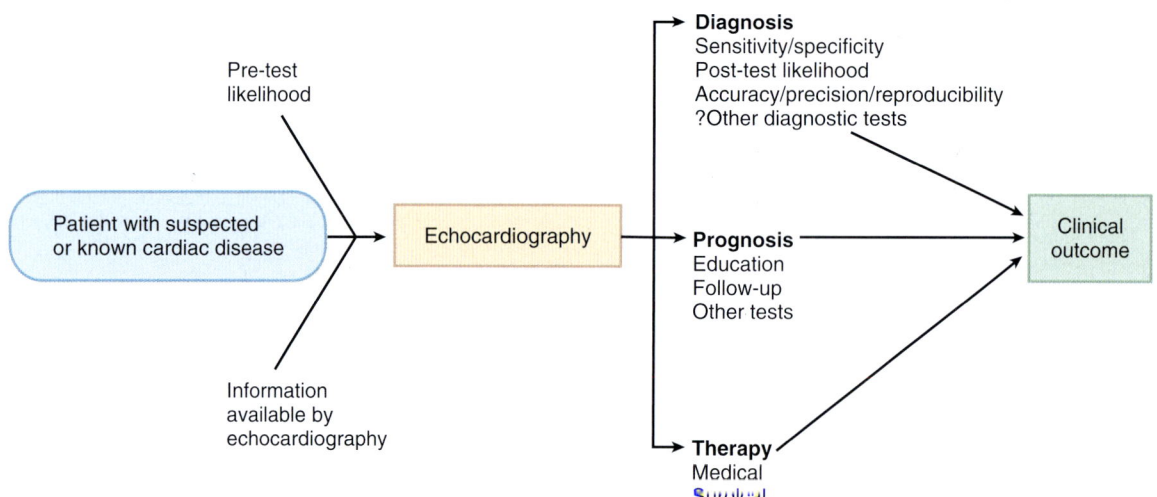

Fig. 5.5 Flow chart illustrating the importance of the impact of the echocardiographic results on diagnosis, prognosis, and therapy. Ultimately, the effect of the echocardiographic examination on clinical outcome is the best measure of the usefulness of the test result.

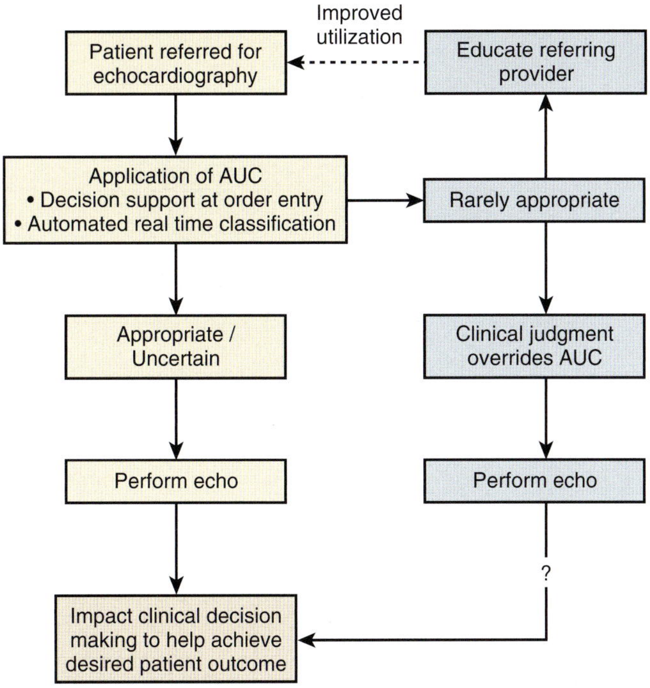

Fig. 5.6 Appropriate selection of patients for echocardiography. A potential approach for application of Appropriate Use Criteria (AUC) in real time to help improve patient selection and minimize rarely appropriate echocardiograms. Adherence to AUC and the subsequent impact on clinical outcomes warrant further study.

echocardiography for that diagnosis and the likelihood that the echocardiographic results will alter patient management are considered before performing the study. Often it is helpful to consider the specific branch point in the diagnostic and therapeutic plans that the echocardiographic results will be applied to in the clinical decision process.

With these considerations in mind, in certain situations the use of echocardiography clearly changes patient management. These situations include:

- Making the correct anatomic diagnosis. For example, differentiating a primary valvular problem from systolic LV dysfunction in a patient with heart failure symptoms.
- Providing important prognostic data in a patient with a known anatomic diagnosis. For example, LV ejection fraction in cardiomyopathy or severity of asymptomatic mitral regurgitation.
- Identifying complications of a known diagnosis. For example, paravalvular abscess in endocarditis or LV thrombus in cardiomyopathy.
- Assessing the effect of therapy. For example, reevaluation of LV systolic function after optimization of heart failure therapy.

Throughout this text, the accuracy (sensitivity and specificity) of echocardiography for each specific diagnosis will be indicated, if known. The clinician then should integrate these data with the pre-test likelihood of disease in each patient. Critical evaluations of the diagnostic utility of echocardiography in specific patient populations and clinical settings will be highlighted, including evaluation of chest pain in the emergency room (see Chapter 8), decision making in adults with aortic stenosis (see Chapter 11) and aortic regurgitation (see Chapter 12), the diagnosis and prognosis of endocarditis (see Chapter 14), and intraoperative assessment of mitral valve repair (see Chapter 18).

INDICATIONS FOR DIAGNOSTIC ECHOCARDIOGRAPHY

Transthoracic Echocardiography

Common clinical signs and symptoms in patients referred for echocardiography include an enlarged heart (Fig. 5.7), a murmur on auscultation (Fig. 5.8), chest pain (Fig. 5.9), heart failure (Fig. 5.10), and fever or bacteremia (Fig. 5.11). When the echocardiographer evaluates a patient with one of these indications, it is important that the differential diagnosis be considered and each possibility excluded or confirmed during the course of the examination.

Echocardiography is appropriate in the acute setting when the likelihood of a cardiac cause is high and the imaging results would affect patient management, as shown in Table 5.2.

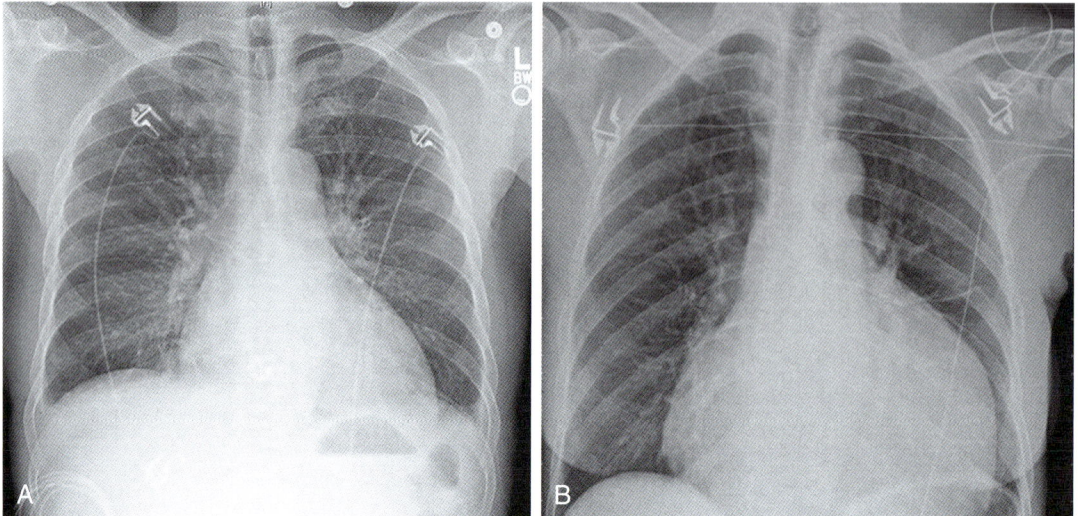

Fig. 5.7 Enlarged heart. Chest radiographs demonstrating cardiomegaly caused by dilated cardiomyopathy with four-chamber enlargement (A) or caused by a large pericardial effusion (B). Echocardiography reliably identifies the cause of an enlarged cardiac silhouette.

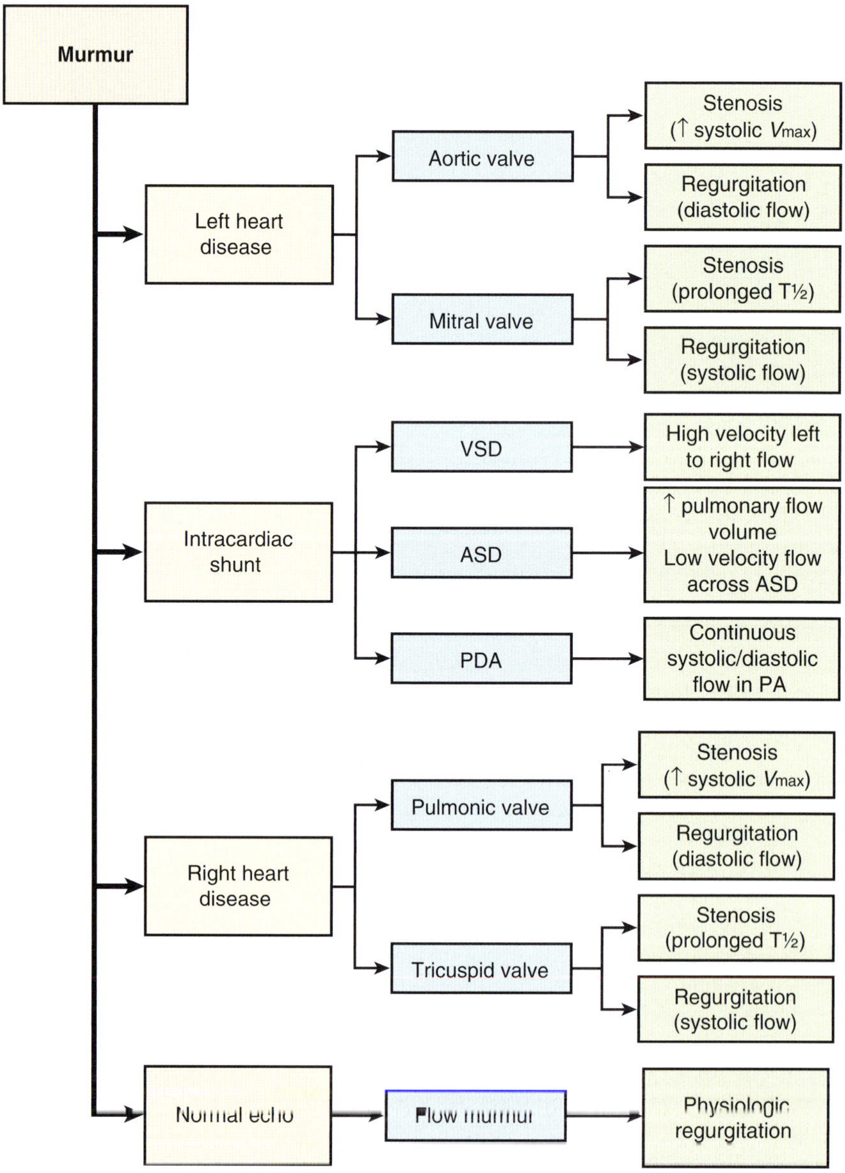

Fig. 5.8 Flow chart for the echocardiographic differential diagnosis of a murmur. The flow chart is arranged by anatomy because the echocardiographer often is not provided information about the type of murmur or other clinical findings. The basic echocardiographic examination includes measurement of antegrade flows and evaluation for regurgitation of all four valves. Additional evaluation for murmur includes careful interrogation of flow in the pulmonary artery *(PA)* to detect a patent ductus arteriosus or increased flow because of an atrial septal defect *(ASD)*. Flow in the septal region is examined with color and CW Doppler to exclude a ventricular septal defect *(VSD)*. Normal physiologic amounts of mitral and tricuspid regurgitation are not audible and do not explain the presence of a murmur. *PDA,* Patent ductus arteriosus; $T\frac{1}{2}$, pressure half-time; V_{max}, maximum antegrade velocity.

Clinical Indications and Quality Assurance | Chapter 5

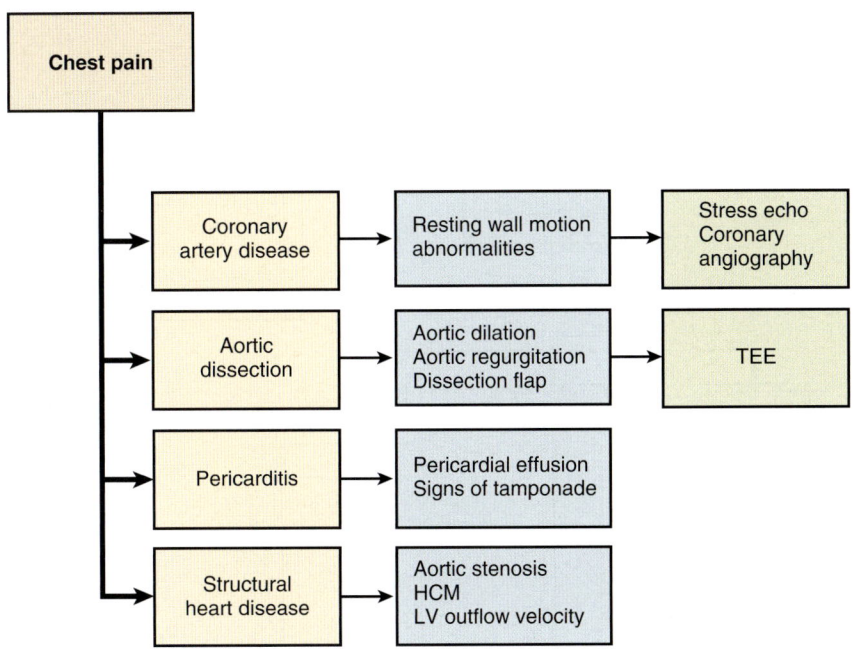

Fig. 5.9 Echocardiographic approach to evaluation of chest pain. The primary goal in the acute setting is to exclude life-threatening conditions, such as an acute coronary syndrome or acute aortic dissection. With both acute and chronic chest pain, further diagnostic evaluation often is needed. *HCM*, Hypertrophic cardiomyopathy.

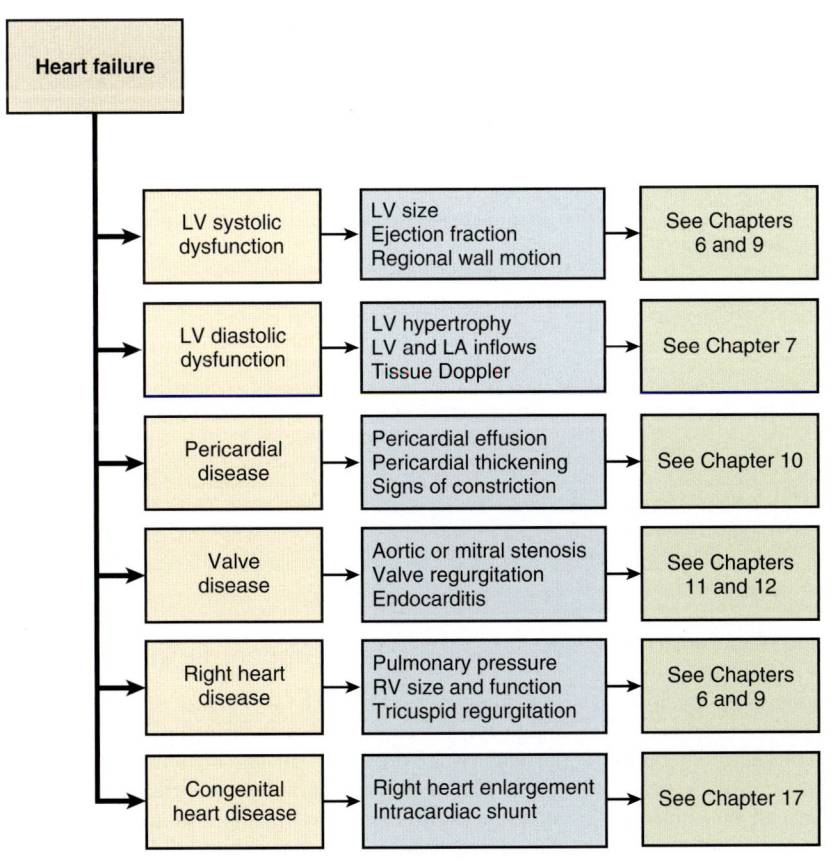

Fig. 5.10 Echocardiographic approach to the patient referred for heart failure. A systemic echocardiographic study will include the 2D views and Doppler flows to identify each of these possible diagnoses. In addition, the sonographer should mentally "check off" each of these conditions as the exam progresses to ensure that the entire differential diagnosis is considered. If the echocardiographic study result is normal, a noncardiac cause of symptoms is likely.

Fig. 5.11 Flow chart for a suggested approach to evaluation of patients with fever and/or bacteremia who are referred for echocardiography. *AV,* Atrioventricular.

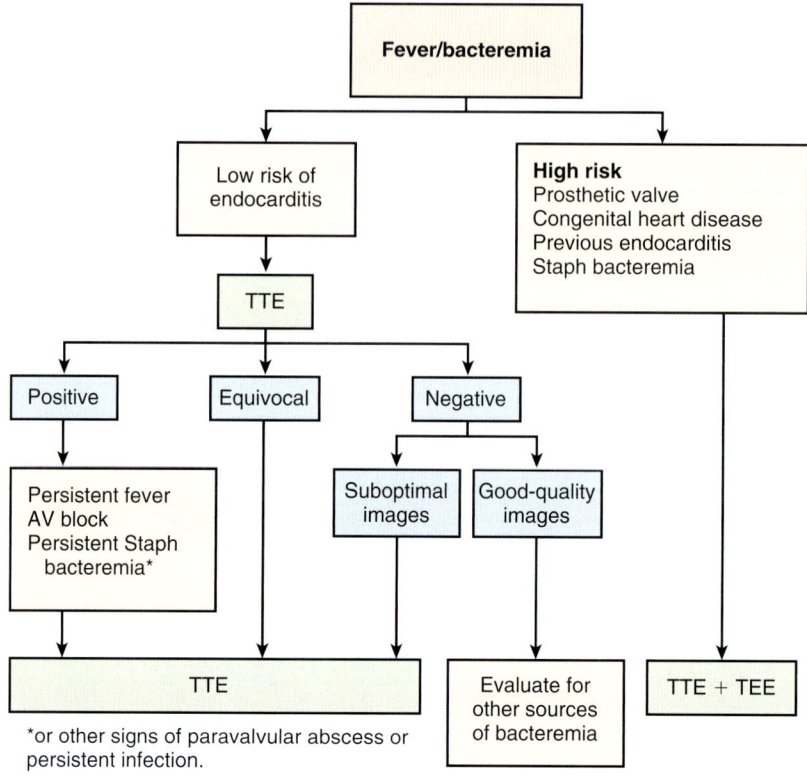

TABLE 5.2 Indications for Transthoracic Echocardiography in the Acute Setting and in Patients With Cardiac Signs or Symptoms

Cardiac Signs and Symptoms	Acute Setting
• Cardiac symptoms including chest pain, shortness of breath, palpitations, syncope/presyncope, TIA, stroke, or peripheral embolic event • Abnormal cardiac murmur (any diastolic murmur or systolic murmur grade 3 or louder) • Prior testing suggesting structural heart disease • Atrial fibrillation, SVT, VT, frequent or exercise-induced VPCs • Evaluation of pulmonary hypertension • Suspected infective endocarditis (native or prosthetic valve) with positive blood culture results or a new murmur	• Hypotension or hemodynamic instability of suspected cardiac etiology • Acute chest pain with suspected MI but nondiagnostic ECG • Elevated cardiac biomarkers without other features of ACS • Suspected complications of acute MI • Evaluation of ventricular function following ACS • Respiratory failure of uncertain etiology • Guidance of therapy with acute pulmonary embolism • Chest trauma or severe deceleration injury with possible cardiac consequences

ACS, Acute coronary syndrome; *ECG,* electrocardiogram; *MI,* myocardial infarction; *SVT,* supraventricular tachycardia; *TIA,* transient ischemic attack; *VPCs,* ventricular premature contractions; *VT,* ventricular tachycardia.
Adapted from Douglas PS, Garcia MJ, Haines DE, et al: ACCF/ASE/AHA/ASNC/HFSA/HRS/SCAI/SCCM/SCCT/SCMR 2011 appropriate use criteria for echocardiography, *J Am Coll Cardiol* 57:1126–1166, 2011 (see Suggested Reading).

In patients with a known cardiac diagnosis, such as valvular heart disease (Table 5.3), heart failure (Table 5.4), or aortic disease (Table 5.5), periodic echocardiographic monitoring often is needed for decisions about medical therapy and timing of interventions. In these patients, the echocardiographer needs to be aware of the information that can be obtained by echocardiography, the limitations of echocardiography, and alternative diagnostic approaches.

Transesophageal Echocardiography

The indications for TEE are based on its superior image quality compared with transthoracic imaging, particularly of posterior cardiac structures. In many cases, TEE echocardiography is performed after a complete transthoracic examination. However, in some clinical situations it is appropriate to begin with a TEE examination (Table 5.6). Some echocardiographers

TABLE 5.3 Appropriate Indications for Transthoracic Echocardiography in Patients With Valvular Heart Disease

Valve Regurgitation
- Initial evaluation
- Routine reevaluation of moderate or severe valve regurgitation (6-month to 1-year intervals)
- Reevaluation for a change in clinical status

Valve Stenosis
- Initial evaluation
- Routine reevaluation of mild valve stenosis (typically 3-year intervals)
- Routine reevaluation of moderate or severe valve stenosis (typically 1-year intervals)
- Reevaluation for a change in clinical status

Prosthetic Valves
- Initial postoperative study
- Routine reevaluation, depending on valve type
- Reevaluation for suspected dysfunction, thrombosis or a change in clinical status

Endocarditis
- Initial evaluation of suspected infective endocarditis (native or prosthetic valve) with positive blood cultures or a new murmur
- Reevaluation of infective endocarditis in high-risk patients—virulent organism, severe hemodynamic lesion, aortic involvement, persistent bacteremia, a change in clinical status, or symptomatic deterioration

ASE/AHA/ASNC/HFSA/HRS/SCAI/SCCM/SCCT/SCMR 2011 appropriate use criteria for echocardiography, *J Am Coll Cardiol* 57:1126–1166, 2011 (see Suggested Reading) and from American College of Cardiology/American Heart Association and European Society of Cardiology valve guidelines.

TABLE 5.4 Appropriate Indications for Transthoracic Echocardiography in Patients With Hypertension, Heart Failure, and Cardiomyopathies

Hypertension
- Initial evaluation of suspected hypertensive heart disease

Heart Failure
- Initial evaluation of known or suspected HF (systolic or diastolic)
- Reevaluation of known HF with a change in clinical status or exam, without a clear precipitating factor, or to guide therapy
- Pacer, ICD, and CRT devices—determine candidacy and device type, evaluate symptoms possibly caused by device complication or suboptimal device settings
- Ventricular assist devices—determine candidacy, optimize settings, evaluate for complications
- Monitor for rejection after heart transplantation
- Evaluation of potential heart donor

Cardiomyopathies
- Initial evaluation of known or suspected cardiomyopathy
- Reevaluation of known cardiomyopathy with a change in clinical status to guide therapy
- Screening evaluation in first-degree relatives of a patient with an inherited cardiomyopathy
- Baseline and serial reevaluation in patients receiving cardiotoxic agents

CRT, Cardiac resynchronization therapy; *HF*, heart failure; *ICD*, implantable cardioverter-defibrillator.
Adapted from Douglas PS, Garcia MJ, Haines DE, et al: ACCF/ASE/AHA/ASNC/HFSA/HRS/SCAI/SCCM/SCCT/SCMR 2011 appropriate use criteria for echocardiography, *J Am Coll Cardiol* 57:1126–1166, 2011 (see Suggested Reading).

advocate the use of TEE imaging whenever transthoracic images are nondiagnostic. However, given that the threshold approach to clinical testing predicts a narrower test window as the risk of the test increases, it is appropriate to consider TEE studies somewhat more critically. The indications for a TEE study should be discussed with the referring physician on a case-by-case basis to determine whether the information potentially obtained justifies the slight but definite risk of the TEE approach.

Several definite indications for TEE are apparent when the limitations of transthoracic imaging are considered. The improved sensitivity of TEE versus transthoracic imaging for detection of paravalvular abscess in patients with endocarditis has been demonstrated convincingly (see Chapter 14). TEE clearly is indicated for the evaluation of prosthetic mitral valve dysfunction because the shadows and reverberations from the prosthetic valve no longer obscure the left atrium (LA) from this approach as they do on transthoracic imaging (Fig. 5.12) (see also Chapter

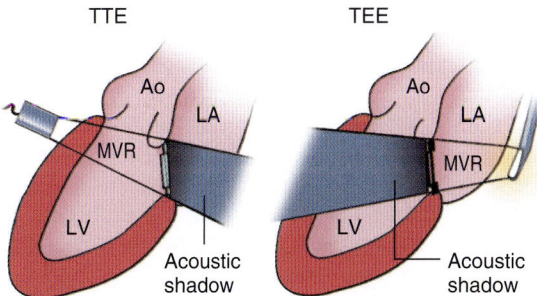

Fig. 5.12 Acoustic shadowing from a prosthetic mitral valve. *(Left)* With TTE, the acoustic shadow obscures the LA, thus limiting assessment of valvular incompetence by Doppler techniques. *(Right)* With TEE, the LA now can be evaluated for valvular incompetence. However, the acoustic shadow now obscures the LV outflow tract. *Ao*, Aorta; *MVR*, mitral valve replacement.

13). Abnormalities of the posterior aspect of a prosthetic aortic valve also are seen well with the TEE approach, although the anterior portion of the paravalvular region is shadowed by the posterior aspect of the prosthetic valve.

TABLE 5.5 Additional Indications for Transthoracic Echocardiography

Cardiac Masses
- Suspected cardiac mass
- Suspected cardiovascular source of embolus

Pericardial Disease
- Suspected pericardial disease
- Reevaluation of known pericardial effusion to guide management
- Guidance of percutaneous noncoronary cardiac procedures (e.g., pericardiocentesis, septal ablation, or RV biopsy)

Aortic Disease
- Known or suspected connective tissue disorder or genetic condition associated with aortic dilation
- Reevaluation of known ascending aortic dilation or history of aortic dissection to establish rate of expansion, when rate of change is excessive, or with a change in clinical status when findings may alter management or therapy

Adult Congenital Heart Disease
- Initial evaluation of known or suspected adult congenital heart disease
- Reevaluation to guide therapy or for a change in clinical symptoms or signs
- Routine surveillance (≥1 year) following incomplete or palliative repair

Adapted from Douglas PS, Garcia MJ, Haines DE, et al: ACCF/ASE/AHA/ASNC/HFSA/HRS/SCAI/SCCM/SCCT/SCMR 2011 appropriate use criteria for echocardiography, *J Am Coll Cardiol* 57:1126–1166, 2011 (see Suggested Reading).

TABLE 5.6 Indications for Use of TEE as the Initial or Supplemental Test

- Patients with a high likelihood of a nondiagnostic TTE because of patient-related characteristics or ability to visualize the structures of interest
- Suspected acute aortic pathology including dissection or transection
- Suspected endocarditis with a moderate or high pre-test probability (e.g., staphylococcal bacteremia, fungemia, prosthetic heart valve, or intracardiac device)
- Evaluation of valve structure and function to evaluate suitability for surgical or transcatheter valve interventions
- Guidance of percutaneous noncoronary cardiac interventions including but not limited to septal ablation, mitral valvuloplasty, PFO/ASD closure, radiofrequency ablation
- Evaluation of patients with atrial fibrillation or flutter to facilitate clinical decision making with regard to anticoagulation and/or cardioversion and/or radiofrequency ablation
- Evaluation for cardiac source of embolus with no identified source on TTE
- Reevaluation for interval changes compared with prior TEE when a change in therapy is anticipated.
- Suspected complications of endocarditis (e.g., abscess, fistula)*
- Suspected prosthetic mitral valve dysfunction*
- Evaluation of posterior structure (e.g., atrial baffles) in patients with congenital heart disease*

*Not considered in the appropriateness guidelines document but generally accepted as appropriate indications for TEE as the initial approach.
PFO/ASD, Patent foramen ovale/atrial septal defect.
Adapted from Douglas PS, Garcia MJ, Haines DE, et al: ACCF/ASE/AHA/ASNC/HFSA/HRS/SCAI/SCCM/SCCT/SCMR 2011 appropriate use criteria for echocardiography, *J Am Coll Cardiol* 57:1126–1166, 2011 (see Suggested Reading).

Improved evaluation of mitral valve anatomy and the degree of mitral regurgitation is especially useful in the perioperative evaluation of patients undergoing surgical mitral valve repair (see Chapter 18). In patients with congenital heart disease, TEE imaging improves diagnostic certainty, particularly in evaluation of posterior structures such as an interatrial baffle surgical repair or a sinus venosus atrial septal defect. The sensitivity of TEE echocardiography for detection of LA thrombus far exceeds that of transthoracic imaging. Finally, excellent images of the thoracic aorta, arch, and ascending aorta allow accurate diagnosis of aortic dissection by TEE. Other indications for TEE imaging include the evaluation for a patent foramen ovale in patients with a systemic embolic event and the exclusion of endocarditis when this diagnosis is a possibility.

Stress Echocardiography

In many cardiac conditions, abnormalities of cardiac function are manifested only when increased oxygen consumption results in increased cardiac demands that cannot be met by the usual compensatory changes (Table 5.7). This basic concept has led to the widespread use of stress testing in patients with cardiovascular disease. Increased cardiac demand can be induced by exercise or with appropriate pharmacologic interventions. The risk of this approach is related to the risk of stress testing with no significant additive effect of echocardiographic imaging.

Exercise echocardiography is performed by recording images of the LV immediately before and immediately after treadmill exercise or by recording images during supine or upright bicycle exercise. The most common indication for exercise echocardiography is suspected or known coronary artery disease. At rest, LV endocardial motion and wall thickening are normal, even if significant coronary disease is present, unless prior myocardial infarction has occurred. Increased myocardial oxygen demands (e.g., with exercise) result in ischemia when significant stenosis of an epicardial coronary artery is present. This results sequentially in myocardial metabolic changes, decreased wall thickening and endocardial motion, electrocardiographic changes, and angina. Echocardiographic

TABLE 5.7 Appropriate Indications for Exercise or Pharmacologic Stress Echocardiography*

Low Pre-test Probability of CAD (10-Year Risk <10%) With:
- Angina or equivalent and an uninterruptable ECG or inability to exercise
- New-onset heart failure or LV dysfunction and no plans for coronary angiography
- Stress test–induced arrhythmias including sustained and nonsustained VT or frequent PVCs

Intermediate (10-Year Risk 10%-20%) to High (10-Year Risk >20%) Probability of CAD With:
- Angina or equivalent
- Acute chest pain without diagnostic ECG changes or elevated cardiac enzymes
- New-onset atrial fibrillation

Prior Abnormal Test Results
- Abnormal catheterization or stress study with worsening symptoms on medical therapy
- Coronary calcium score (Agatston) ≥400
- Coronary stenosis of unclear significance by invasive or CT angiography

Risk Assessment
- Before noncardiac surgery with at least one cardiac risk factor and poor exercise tolerance (<4 METs)
- Following acute coronary syndrome when early catheterization not planned
- Recurrent chest pain late after coronary revascularization
- Incomplete revascularization after coronary intervention

Other
- Assessment of myocardial viability with known CAD eligible for revascularization
- Evaluation of low output aortic stenosis (dobutamine stress only)
- Symptomatic patients with moderate mitral stenosis at rest
- Asymptomatic moderate to severe mitral regurgitation with LV size not meeting surgical criteria
- Contrast is appropriate when one or more contiguous segments are not seen on noncontrast images.

*The stress modality is exercise, unless the patient is unable to exercise.
CAD, Coronary artery disease; *CT,* computed tomography; *ECG,* electrocardiogram; *MET,* metabolic equivalent; *PVCs,* premature ventricular contractions; *VT,* ventricular tachycardia.
Adapted from Douglas PS, Garcia MJ, Haines DE, et al: ACCF/ASE/AHA/ASNC/HFSA/HRS/SCAI/SCCM/SCCT/SCMR 2011 appropriate use criteria for echocardiography, *J Am Coll Cardiol* 57:1126–1166, 2011 (see Suggested Reading).

---

echocardiography, as discussed in detail in Chapter 8, has been found to be more sensitive than exercise electrocardiography (and as sensitive as nuclear perfusion imaging) for detection of significant coronary artery disease. Exercise echocardiography is particularly helpful in patients with an abnormal resting electrocardiogram (e.g., bundle branch block or LV hypertrophy). It also has been used to assess the extent of disease, to document functional improvement after revascularization, and to detect restenosis after angioplasty.

In addition to changes in segmental wall motion with exercise stress testing, parameters of global ventricular function, including ventricular volumes, ejection fraction, and the Doppler LV ejection velocity curve, can be evaluated. Other Doppler parameters are helpful in specific settings. For example, a patient with mitral stenosis will show an excessive rise in pulmonary artery systolic pressure (estimated from the tricuspid regurgitant jet) with exercise. In a patient with aortic coarctation, the increase in gradient across the coarctation with exercise can be demonstrated with Doppler recordings.

Pharmacologic stress echocardiography replaces exercise testing when the patient is unable to exercise (e.g., peripheral vascular disease, musculoskeletal limitation). In addition, pharmacologic stress testing allows monitoring by echocardiography as the dose is increased and permits evaluation at sequential stress levels. Pharmacologic stress testing most often is performed using a beta-agonist, such as dobutamine, which increases myocardial contractility, myocardial oxygen demands, and the degree of peripheral vasodilation. An alternate pharmacologic agent is adenosine, which vasodilates coronary vessels, thus resulting in relative inequalities in blood flow between myocardium supplied by normal coronary arteries and myocardium supplied by stenosed coronary arteries.

POINT OF CARE CARDIAC ULTRASOUND STUDIES

Instrumentation

The term *point of care cardiac ultrasound* (POCUS) refers to the bedside use of small, lightweight ultrasound systems. Some of these systems are very small ("pocket-size") and have only limited capabilities, whereas others have nearly all the features of a standard ultrasound system and are still easily carried in one hand (Table 5.8).

Applications

Small, relatively inexpensive, portable or handheld echocardiography instruments are of great clinical utility in the emergency department, intensive care

---

images recorded during ischemia show abnormalities of wall motion, thus allowing for the detection of significant coronary artery disease. The specific coronary arteries involved can be identified by the anatomic pattern of induced wall motion abnormalities. Exercise

TABLE 5.8 Comparison of Features of State-of-the-Art, Intermediate, and Handheld Ultrasound Platforms

Variable	State-of-the-Art	Laptop or Intermediate	Handheld or Pocket Size
Power source	Electricity	Electricity or battery	Rechargeable battery; requires recharging after approximately 1–2 hours of use
Storage	Storage of multiple full length studies	Storage of multiple full length studies	Limited storage of images
Connectivity	DICOM connectivity for connection and storage to PACS or other review and storage systems	DICOM connectivity for connection and storage to PACS or other review and storage systems	Not DICOM compatible, but can be transferred to a computer or interfaced with a cloud-based system
Components	3D, 2D, pulsed wave, and CW Doppler, color flow, biplane, stress echo quad screen, and strain	2D, pulsed wave, and CW Doppler, and color flow, with stress echo available on most and strain available on some platforms	2D with or without rudimentary color flow
Image acquisition modifications	Zoom option, adjustment of focus, gray-scale, transducer frequency, dynamic range, and sector width, harmonic imaging, multiple varied settings for contrast and difficult to image patients	Many features similar to state-of-the-art systems	Most modifications are absent; frame rates are lower.
Image viewing	Large, high-resolution screen	Intermediate screen	Small, low-resolution screen
Quantification	3D, 2D, Doppler, color flow, and strain measurements, with varying degrees of automaticity	2D, Doppler, and color flow measurements, with strain measurements available on some systems	2D linear measurements

DICOM, Digital Imaging and Communications in Medicine; *PACS*, picture archiving and communication system.
From Pellikka PA, Cullen MW, Sekiguchi H: Point of care cardiac ultrasound: scope of practice, quality assurance and impact on patient outcomes. In Otto CM, editor: *The Practice of Clinical Echocardiography*, ed 5, Philadelphia, 2017, Elsevier, pp 91–104.

unit, and other clinical settings for triage of acutely ill patients. POCUS allows for rapid diagnosis of:

- Pericardial effusion
- Overall LV and RV systolic function
- Segmental wall motion abnormalities

For example, a point of care study showing a dilated, hypokinetic LV in a patient with shortness of breath supports a diagnosis of heart failure, not pulmonary disease. POCUS also is useful in patients with chest pain and a nondiagnostic electrocardiogram; for this situation, an akinetic anterior wall indicates coronary disease, whereas a pericardial effusion suggests pericarditis. Another example is the hypotensive patient; severe global LV hypokinesis indicates heart failure, whereas a small hyperdynamic LV suggests an alternate diagnosis, such as septic shock (Fig. 5.13).

POCUS also may identify the *presence* of valve disease based on visualization of aortic valve calcification on 2D imaging or mitral regurgitation on color flow imaging. However, in general, evaluation of valve disease, diastolic function, suspected aortic dissection, and congenital heart disease requires a full echocardiographic examination with a standard ultrasound system.

In addition, POCUS is a useful tool for patient triage, for screening populations at risk of heart disease, and in medical education (Table 5.9). As these devices become more widely available, with better image quality and lower cost, we can expect that POCUS will become a routine part of bedside diagnosis.

Providers

Point of care cardiac imaging typically is performed by health care providers with limited ultrasound training who perform a quick study to answer a specific clinical question. Diagnostic accuracy is highest for major findings such as the presence or absence of a pericardial effusion or the presence or absence of LV systolic dysfunction. Accuracy is lower for more

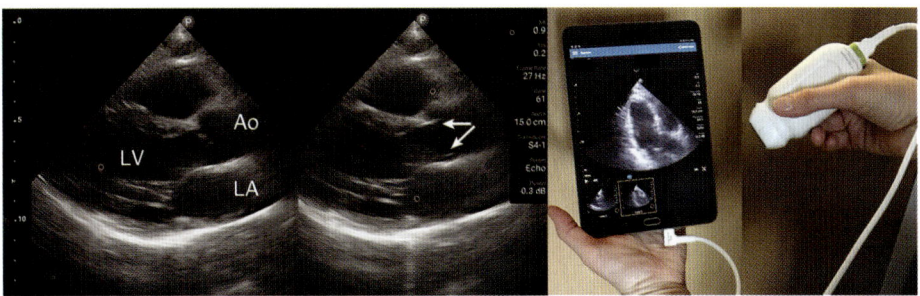

Fig. 5.13 ▶ **Point of care ultrasound.** Example of images obtained with a small handheld ultrasound system showing the parasternal long-axis view in diastole *(left)* and in systole *(center)*. Image resolution allows identification of the thin, open aortic valve leaflets in systole *(arrows)*. This system (Lumify, Philips North America, Andover, MA) uses software on a smart device with a portable, relatively inexpensive transducer *(right)*. *Ao,* Aorta.

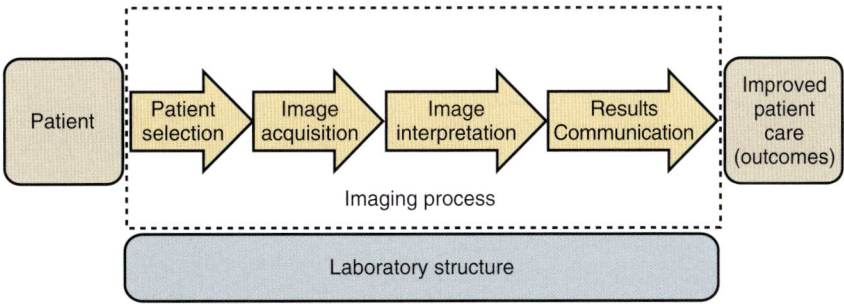

Fig. 5.14 Dimensions of care framework for evaluating quality of cardiovascular imaging. The quality of an imaging study depends on multiple processes, as well as appropriately educated and trained sonographers and physicians and high-quality imaging systems. The value of clinical imaging depends on appropriate patient selection, optimal image acquisition, correct interpretation, and clear communication of results.

TABLE 5.9	Point of Care Cardiac Ultrasound: Typical Indications
Urgent clinical evaluation (emergency department or intensive care unit) • LV size (volume status) and systolic function • RV size and systolic function • Pericardial effusion or tamponade	
Screening at risk populations (e.g., athletes, rheumatic heart disease)	
Frequent serial exams for known abnormality (e.g., response to heart failure therapy)	

complex diagnoses such as regional wall motion or valvular heart disease. Recommendations for training have been published by the American Society of Echocardiography and other groups. However, as the use of ultrasound imaging is disseminated further and instrumentation improves, each medical center or practice group will need to establish standards for training and competency, study documentation, scope of practice, and continuous quality improvement.

Safety and Limitations

The greatest limitation of these instruments is a missed diagnosis due to an inexperienced operator or suboptimal image quality. When handheld images suggest a new cardiac diagnosis or when diagnostic images cannot be obtained, it may be prudent to obtain a complete echocardiographic examination. Most handheld systems provide only limited recording capacity, so accurate reporting in the clinical notes, similar to reporting of physical examination findings, is essential. Quality assurance and improvement are important for POCUS as for any type of ultrasound imaging.

QUALITY ASSURANCE IN ECHOCARDIOGRAPHY

Several steps should be taken to ensuring that high-quality echocardiographic studies are provided to our patients (Fig. 5.14). These include documentation of sonographer and physician competency, appropriate laboratory standards and procedures, and continuous quality improvement measures. Documentation of competency typically is based on:

- Accreditation—endorsement of a training program or laboratory by a recognized national accreditation agency
- Certification—documentation of appropriate training and successful completion of an examination in the area of expertise by each physician and sonographer

- Credentialing—standards set by each health care organization for health care professionals providing patient care at that institution

In addition, innovative approaches to quality assurance based on statistical analysis of physician or laboratory performance have been proposed. Statistical database approaches will be increasingly useful as medical record systems are computerized.

Sonographer Education and Training

The sonographer must be familiar with patterns of disease in clinical cardiology and also with the technical aspects of performing the examination. A sonographer's education and training include a knowledge base of cardiac anatomy and physiology, cardiac pathology, and clinical cardiology, in addition to ultrasound physics and the echocardiographic examination. Training also includes patient interaction skills, basic medical procedures (e.g., sterile technique), patient privacy, and so forth.

Guidelines for the education and training of cardiac sonographers have been published by the American Society of Echocardiography and are periodically updated. Education and training in an accredited program are recommended with accreditation for cardiac sonographer programs provided by two Joint Review Commissions (JRCs) under the auspices of the Commission on Accreditation of Allied Health Educational Programs (CAAHEP), the JRC-Diagnostic Medical Sonography (JRC-DMS), and the JRC-Cardiovascular Technology (JRC-CVT). Education and training include the acquisition of both cognitive and technical skills with demonstration of competency in each area. After completion of training, sonographers can be credentialed by the American Registry of Diagnostic Medical Sonographers (ARDMS), with separate examinations for adult and pediatric echocardiography, or they can be accredited by Cardiovascular Credentialing International (CCI). Cardiac sonographers must attend formal continuing medical education meetings to maintain these credentials.

Physician Education and Training

The physician must have expertise in the technical aspects of the examination, in addition to the expected findings in each disease state, to guide the sonographer in optimizing data quality and to interpret the recorded data correctly. Details such as transducer frequency, gain controls, processing curves, and depth settings significantly affect image quality. The appropriate choice of Doppler modality for the flow of interest—pulsed, color flow, or continuous-wave (CW) Doppler—affects the data obtained. Factors such as wall filters, gain, sample volume size, and color sector width also significantly affect data collection. Knowledge of how these factors affect data quality and knowledge of which views and approaches yield optimal data allow the physician to assess the reliability of recorded data, to suspect abnormalities that may not have been noted explicitly during the examination, to recognize imaging and flow artifacts, and to direct the sonographer in optimal data acquisition.

Physician education and training in echocardiography most often take place during Cardiology Fellowship Training in a program accredited by the American Council of Graduate Medical Education (ACGME). In addition, specific recommendations for training in echocardiography have been published, and are periodically updated, by the American College of Cardiology (ACC) and the American Heart Association (AHA). These recommendations divide training into three levels of expertise:

Level 1: Basic introduction to echocardiography needed by all cardiologists
Level 2: Qualified to independently interpret echocardiographic studies
Level 3: Additional qualifications to supervise an echocardiography laboratory

It is recommended that Level 2 training in TTE be achieved before training is undertaken in advanced procedures, including TEE and stress echocardiography. Recommended numbers of procedures during training are indicated in Table 5.10.

Most physicians completing a 3- or 4-year program in cardiology will have achieved Level 2 training. Successful completion of the American Board of Internal Medicine (ABIM) examination in Cardiovascular Disease, in conjunction with at least Level 2 training as documented by the program director, provides verification of competence in TTE.

Other physicians achieve competency in echocardiography based on the same training guidelines recommended for cardiology trainees. Physicians who receive echocardiography training outside of Cardiology Fellowship programs have the option of taking the examination provided by the National Board of Echocardiography (NBE) to document competency. In addition, specific guidelines for training of cardiovascular anesthesiologists in echocardiography have been published by the American Society of Echocardiography with a focus on expertise in TEE and intraoperative echocardiography. The NBE offers a special examination for cardiovascular anesthesiology.

To maintain competency in echocardiography, physicians should document continuing medical education and should interpret a minimum of 300 studies per year for Level 2 and 500 studies per year for Level 3, with performance of some studies recommended. For maintaining competency in TEE echocardiography, 25 to 50 studies should be performed and interpreted annually, with 100 studies per year recommended for stress echocardiography.

TABLE 5.10 Summary of American College of Cardiology/American Heart Association and European Association of Echocardiography Recommendations for Physician Training in Echocardiography

Level of Expertise	Cumulative Duration (Months)	TRAINING			MAINTENANCE OF COMPETENCY	
		ACC/AHA[1]		EAE[2]	ACC/AHA	EAE
		Studies Performed	Studies Interpreted	Studies Performed and Interpreted	Studies Performed	Studies Performed and Interpreted
1	3	75	150			
2 (Basic)	6	150	300	350	300	*
3 (Advanced)	9	300	750	750	500	100
Stress echo		100		100	100	100
TEE		50		75	25–50	50

*Reasonable case volume and mix are recommended without a specific number.
ACC/AHA, American College of Cardiology/American Heart Association; EAE, European Association of Echocardiography.
Summarized from American Heart Association/American College of Cardiology, European Society of Cardiology/European Association of Echocardiography training guideline documents:
1. Ryan T, Berlacher K, Lindner JR, et al: COCATS 4 Task Force 5: training in echocardiography, *J Am Coll Cardiol* 65(17):1786–1799, 2015.
2. Popescu BA, Andrade MJ, Badano LP, et al: European Association of Echocardiography recommendations for training, competence, and quality improvement in echocardiography, *Eur J Echocardiogr* 10(8):893-905, 2009.

Echocardiography Reporting

It is essential that sonographers relay technical concerns to the physician and direct attention to abnormalities noted during the examination. Conversely, the physician should give feedback to the sonographer about the completeness and quality of data recorded and offer suggestions for future patient studies. The physician review also should indicate whether additional echocardiographic recordings are needed, either before the patient leaves the laboratory or at a later examination.

The echocardiographic report serves at least two purposes: (1) it conveys the results of the test to the referring physician, and (2) it serves as a narrative summary of the echocardiographic examination for comparison with future studies. Given the wide variety of views and flows that can be recorded, it is helpful for the report to document the structures imaged (even if normal), the flow signals recorded, the different Doppler modalities used, and the overall quality of the study. Any areas of limitation in the study are noted.

In each patient, the various echocardiographic findings then are integrated with each other in the final interpretation. For example, a report describing mitral regurgitation also would include a clear description of valve anatomy with an indication of the most likely cause of regurgitation or the differential diagnosis if the cause were unclear. Mitral regurgitant severity is estimated, and the methods used to generate this estimate are indicated. In addition, the degrees of LA and LV dilation are described, with attention to serial changes if previous studies are available. LV systolic function is quantitated, and the degree of pulmonary hypertension is estimated. All these findings fit together physiologically and thus can be reported in a logical integration of the data. For example, significant mitral regurgitation results in LV and LA enlargement because of volume overload, whereas the chronically elevated LA pressure leads to pulmonary hypertension.

Finally, these findings are reviewed in the context of the patient's clinical presentation, potential implications of the findings are discussed with the referring physician, and additional diagnostic tests or follow-up studies are recommended as clinically indicated. If principles of clinical decision analysis are being used in patient management, the pre-test and post-test likelihood of disease can be estimated. Ideally, the overall impact of the echocardiographic findings on the patient's therapy or subsequent diagnostic evaluation is reviewed with the referring physician both before and after the examination. Specific comments about timing of periodic echocardiography or consideration of referral to a cardiologist also may be appropriate. Of course, any unexpected or serious findings should promptly be relayed to the referring physician. In some cases, the echocardiography attending physician may need to assume immediate care of the patient, for example, if results indicate persistent abnormalities after stress testing or with the unexpected finding of an aortic dissection.

Echocardiography Laboratory Structure

The essential components of the echocardiography laboratory structure are shown in Table 5.11. Accreditation of echocardiography laboratories is available

TABLE 5.11 Components of Echocardiography Laboratory Structure

Component	Requirements
Physical laboratory	• IAC accreditation (and reaccreditation every 3 years) • Sufficient support staff (assist with scheduling and disseminating reports to ordering clinicians) • Sanitizing equipment (high-level disinfection of TEE probes; cleansing products for TTE transducers, ultrasound machines, and beds; readily available sinks and approved hand cleaners)
Equipment	• Machines capable of performing 2D, M-mode, and color and spectral (both flow and tissue) Doppler • Machine display must identify the institution, patient's name, and date and time of study. • Electrocardiogram and depth or flow velocity calibrations must be present on all displays; capability to display other physiologic signals (i.e., respiration) • Stress echocardiogram machines with software for split screen and quad-screen display • TTE transducers that can provide high- and low-frequency imaging, and dedicated nonimaging CW Doppler • Machines with harmonic imaging capabilities and settings to optimize standard and contrast-enhanced exams • Capability for 3D and strain imaging • Multiplane TEE probes • Machines with a digital image storage method • Availability of contrast agents and intravenous supplies • Patient beds that include a drop-down portion of the mattress to facilitate apical imaging • Equipment required to treat medical emergencies (e.g., oxygen suction, "code carts") • Adherence to manufacturers' recommendations for preventive maintenance and accuracy testing; service records maintained in the laboratory
Sonographer	• Achieve and maintain minimum standards in education and credentialing within 2 years of employment for all sonographers. • Credentialing can be as a registered diagnostic cardiac sonographer through ARDMS or a registered cardiac sonographer through CCI. • Fulfillment of any local or state requirements, including licensure
Physician	• Minimum of level II training in TTE imaging for all physicians independently interpreting echocardiograms and meeting annual criteria to maintain that competence • Physicians who trained before this level of training in fellowship programs must achieve adequate training through an experience-based pathway. • Special competency and board certification by passing NBE exam is desired. • Physician director who has completed level III training • Adequate supervision of studies as determined by the Centers for Medicare and Medicaid Services: general supervision (general oversight, not on site), direct supervision (physician in the office suite and immediately available), or personal supervision (physician in the room)

ARDMS, American Registry of Diagnostic Medical Sonographers; *CCI*, Cardiovascular Credentialing International; *IAC*, Intersocietal Accreditation Commission; *NBE*, National Board of Echocardiography.
From Weiner RB, Douglas PS. The diagnostic echocardiography laboratory: structure, standards, and quality improvement. In Otto CM, editor: *The Practice of Clinical Echocardiography*, ed 5, Philadelphia, 2017, Elsevier, pp 3–15. Based on Picard MH, Adams D, Bierig SM, et al: American Society of Echocardiography recommendations for quality echocardiography laboratory operations, *J Am Soc Echocardiogr* 24:1–10, 2011.

through the Intersocietal Commission for the Accreditation of Echocardiography Laboratories (ICAEL, http://www.intersocietal.org/echo/). This accreditation process reviews all aspects of the echocardiographic examination, including:

- Physician training and experience
- Sonographer training and experience
- Continuing medical education of physicians and sonographers
- Physical facilities (e.g., instruments, exam area)
- Echocardiography performance
- Laboratory procedures and protocols
- Echocardiographic reporting and data storage
- Quality assurance measures

The detailed recommendations of the ICAEL provide a useful starting point for laboratory policies and procedures that then can be modified as needed for each institution. The recommendations also include the essential components of TTE, TEE, and stress echocardiography examinations.

THE ECHO EXAM

Indications for Transthoracic Echocardiography

Clinical Diagnosis	Key Echo Findings	Limitations of Echo	Alternate Approaches
Valvular Heart Disease			
Valve stenosis	Cause of stenosis, valve anatomy Transvalvular ΔP, valve area Chamber enlargement and hypertrophy LV and RV systolic function Associated valvular regurgitation	Possible underestimation of stenosis severity Possible coexisting CAD	Cardiac cath CMR
Valve regurgitation	Mechanism and cause of regurgitation Severity of regurgitation Chamber enlargement LV and RV systolic function PA pressure estimate	TEE indicated for evaluation of MR severity and valve anatomy (especially before MV repair)	Cardiac cath CMR
Prosthetic valve function	Evidence for stenosis Detection of regurgitation Chamber enlargement Ventricular function PA pressure estimate	TTE is limited by shadowing and reverberations. TEE is needed for suspected prosthetic MR due to "masking" of the LA on TTE.	Cardiac cath Fluoroscopy
Endocarditis	Detection of vegetations (TTE sensitivity 70%–85%) Presence and degree of valve dysfunction Chamber enlargement and function Detection of abscess Possible prognostic implications	TEE more sensitive for detection of vegetations (>90%) A definite diagnosis of endocarditis also depends on bacteriologic criteria. TEE more sensitive for abscess detection	Blood cultures and clinical findings also are diagnostic criteria for endocarditis.
Coronary Artery Disease			
Acute myocardial infarction	Segmental wall motion abnormality reflects "myocardium at risk." Global LV function (EF) Complications: Acute MR vs. VSD Pericarditis LV thrombus, aneurysm, or rupture RV infarct	Coronary artery anatomy itself not directly visualized	Coronary angio (cath or CT) Radionuclide or PET imaging
Angina	Global and segmental LV systolic function Exclude other causes of angina (e.g., AS, HCM).	Resting wall motion may be normal despite significant CAD. Stress echo needed to induce ischemia and wall motion abnormality.	Coronary angio (cath or CT) Radionuclide or PET imaging ETT
Pre-revascularization/ post-revascularization status	Assess wall thickening and endocardial motion at baseline. Improvement in segmental function postprocedure	Dobutamine stress and/or contrast echo needed to detect viable but nonfunctioning myocardium	CMR Coronary angio (cath or CT) Radionuclide or PET imaging Contrast echocardiography

Continued

Indications for Transthoracic Echocardiography—cont'd

Clinical Diagnosis	Key Echo Findings	Limitations of Echo	Alternate Approaches
End-stage ischemic disease	Overall LV systolic function (EF) PA pressures Associated MR LV thrombus RV systolic function		Coronary angio (cath or CT) Radionuclide or PET imaging CMR for myocardial viability
Cardiomyopathy			
Dilated	Chamber dilation (all four) LV and RV systolic function (qualitative and EF) Coexisting atrioventricular valve regurgitation PA systolic pressure LV thrombus	Indirect measures of LVEDP Accurate EF may be difficult if image quality is poor.	CMR for LV size, function, and myocardial fibrosis LV angiography with left and right heart hemodynamics
Restrictive	LV wall thickness LV systolic function LV diastolic function PA systolic pressure	Must be distinguished from constrictive pericarditis	Cardiac cath with direct, simultaneous RV and LV pressure measurement after volume loading CMR
Hypertrophic	Pattern and extent of LV hypertrophy Dynamic LVOT obstruction (imaging and Doppler) Coexisting MR Diastolic LV dysfunction	Exercise echo needed to detect inducible LVOT obstruction	CMR Strain and strain rate imaging
Hypertension			
	LV hypertrophy LV diastolic dysfunction LV systolic function Aortic valve sclerosis, MAC	Diastolic dysfunction precedes systolic dysfunction, but detection is challenging because of impact of age and other factors.	Speckle tracking strain and strain rate imaging LV twist and torsion
Pericardial Disease			
	Pericardial thickening Detection, size, and location of PE 2D signs of tamponade physiology Doppler signs of tamponade physiology	Diagnosis of tamponade is a hemodynamic and clinical diagnosis. Constrictive pericarditis is a difficult diagnosis. Not all patients with pericarditis have an effusion.	Intracardiac pressure measurements for tamponade or constriction CMR or CT to detect pericardial thickening
Aortic Disease			
Aortic dilation	Cause of aortic dilation Accurate aortic diameter measurements Anatomy of sinuses of Valsalva (especially Marfan syndrome) Associated aortic regurgitation	The ascending aorta is only partially visualized on TTE in most patients.	CT, CMR, TEE
Aortic dissection	2D images of ascending aorta, aortic arch, descending thoracic, and proximal abdominal aorta Imaging of dissection "flap" Associated aortic regurgitation Ventricular function	TEE more sensitive (97%) and specific (100%) Cannot assess distal vascular beds	Aortography CT CMR TEE

Indications for Transthoracic Echocardiography—cont'd

Clinical Diagnosis	Key Echo Findings	Limitations of Echo	Alternate Approaches
Cardiac Masses			
LV thrombus	High sensitivity and specificity for diagnosis of LV thrombus. Suspect with apical wall motion abnormality or diffuse LV systolic dysfunction.	Technical artifacts can be misleading. 5-MHz or higher frequency transducer and angulated apical views needed	LV thrombus may not be recognized on radionuclide or contrast angiography.
LA thrombus	Low sensitivity for detection of LA thrombus, although specificity is high. Suspect with LA enlargement, or MV disease.	TEE is needed to detect LA thrombus reliability.	TEE
Cardiac tumors	Size, location, and physiologic consequences of tumor mass	Extracardiac involvement not well seen. Cannot distinguish benign from malignant or tumor from thrombus	TEE CT CMR Intracardiac echo
Pulmonary Hypertension			
	PA pressure estimate. Evidence of left-sided heart disease to account for increased PA pressures. RV size and systolic function (cor pulmonale). Associated TR	Indirect PA pressure measurement. Difficult to determine pulmonary vascular resistance accurately	Cardiac cath
Congenital Heart Disease			
	Detection and assessment of anatomic abnormalities. Quantitation of physiologic abnormalities. Chamber enlargement. Ventricular function	No direct intracardiac pressure measurements. Complicated anatomy may be difficult to evaluate if image quality is poor (TEE helpful).	CMR with 3D reconstruction. Cardiac cath. TEE. 3D Echo

angio, Angiography; *AS,* aortic stenosis; *CAD,* coronary artery disease; *cath,* catheterization; *CMR,* cardiac magnetic resonance; *CT,* computed tomography; *EF,* ejection fraction; *ETT,* exercise treadmill test; *HCM,* hypertrophic cardiomyopathy; *LVEDP,* LV end-diastolic pressure; *LVOT,* LV outflow tract; *MAC,* mitral annular calcification; *MR,* mitral regurgitation; *MV,* mitral valve; *ΔP,* pressure gradient; *PA,* pulmonary artery; *PET,* positron emission tomography; *TR,* tricuspid regurgitation; *VSD,* ventricular septal defect.

SUGGESTED READING

Types of Echocardiography

1. Otto CM: Echocardiography: the transition from master of the craft to admiral of the fleet, *Heart* 102(12):899–901, 2016.
   An editorial discussing the types of echocardiography currently performed across the medical spectrum and the need for quality control at all levels.
2. Weiner RB, Douglas PS: The diagnostic echocardiography laboratory: structure, standards, and quality improvement. In Otto CM, editor: *The Practice of Clinical Echocardiography,* 5th ed, Philadelphia, 2017, Elsevier, pp 3–15.
   Textbook chapter with sections on laboratory structure and standards, recommended imaging protocols, and quality improvement.
3. Porter TR, Shillcutt SK, Adams MS, et al: Guidelines for the use of echocardiography as a monitor for therapeutic intervention in adults: a report from the American Society of Echocardiography, *J Am Soc Echocardiogr* 28(1):40–56, 2015.
   This guideline document from the American Society of Echocardiography discusses the use of echocardiographic monitoring for patients with acute heart failure, pericardial tamponade, pulmonary embolism, prosthetic valve thrombosis, and chest trauma. Use of echocardiography monitoring in the intensive care unit and for patients undergoing noncardiac surgical procedures also is reviewed.

Diagnostic Testing Principles

4. Lee TH: Using data for clinical decisions. In Goldman, Schafer AI, editor: *Goldman's Cecil Medicine,* 25th ed, Philadelphia, 2016, Saunders, pp 37–41.
   A readable, concise textbook chapter summarizing the entire spectrum of medical decision making from sensitivity and specificity to cost-benefit analysis.
5. Mahutte NG, Duleba AJ: Evaluating diagnostic tests, Up-to-Date www.uptodate.com This topic last updated March 23, 2017. (Accessed October 2, 2017).
   Concise primer on evaluation of diagnostic tests including sensitivity and specificity, accuracy and precision, likelihood ratios, the appropriate choice of a reference standard,

and the impact of disease prevalence. Essential information for the evaluation of echocardiographic diagnostic measures.
6. Roberts MS, Tsevat J: Decision analysis, Up-to-Date. www.uptodate.com: This topic last updated Jan 29, 2016 (Accessed October 2, 2017).
This article defines the types of clinical problems amenable to decision analysis and provides a step-by-step approach to performing decision analysis for a specific problem.

Indications for Echocardiography

7. Douglas PS, Garcia MJ, Haines DE, et al: ACCF/ASE/AHA/ASNC/HFSA/HRS/SCAI/SCCM/SCCT/SCMR 2011 appropriate use criteria for echocardiography, *J Am Coll Cardiol* 57:1126–1166, 2011.
The appropriateness of echocardiography as a diagnostic test was ascertained for 200 clinical situations by a panel of experts grading each clinical situation on a 1 (inappropriate) to 9 (definitely appropriate) scale. Echocardiography was considered appropriate for scores 7 to 9, inappropriate for scores 1 to 3, and of uncertain appropriateness for scores 4 to 6. Tables in this chapter summarize the appropriate indications from this document. Echocardiography laboratories should refer to the complete document for quality assurance programs.

Point of Care Echocardiography

8. Pellikka PA, Cullen MW, Sekiguchi H: Point of care cardiac ultrasound: scope of practice, quality assurance and impact on patient outcomes. In Otto CM, editor: *The Practice of Clinical Echocardiography*, ed 5, Philadelphia, 2017, Elsevier, pp 91–104.
This chapter covers the clinical utility of POCUS, the scope of practice in different clinical settings, the impact on outcomes, and approaches to quality assurance with integration into clinical practice. 102 references.
9. Spencer KT, Kimura BJ, Korcarz CE, et al: Focused cardiac ultrasound: recommendations from the American Society of Echocardiography, *J Am Soc Echocardiogr* 26(6):567–581, 2013.
This article discusses the approach, equipment, and personnel needed for point of care echocardiography. Sections on scope of practice, potential limitations, and appropriate uses of this approach are provided.
10. Sicari R, Galderisi M, Voigt JU, et al: The use of pocket-size imaging devices: a position statement of the European Association of Echocardiography, *Eur J Echocardiogr* 12(2):85–87, 2011.
This position statement emphasizes that point of care echocardiography with small handheld devices is a powerful clinical tool but can address only a limited number of clinical diagnoses. To ensure quality patient care, the European Association of Echocardiography recommends that point of care echocardiography users remember that: (1) point of care echocardiography devices do not provide a complete diagnostic study; (2) imaging results should be reported as part of the physical examination; (3) appropriate training and certification are recommended for all users, relevant to their scope of practice; and (4) patients should be informed that a point of care study is not a complete echocardiogram.

Sonographer Education and Training

11. Ehler D, Carney DK, Dempsey AL, et al: Guidelines for cardiac sonographer education: recommendations of the American Society of Echocardiography Sonographer Training and Education Committee, *J Am Soc Echocardiogr* 14:77–84, 2001.
Detailed summary of the educational requirements for education in cardiac sonography. A useful outline for training programs for curriculum development. Physicians should review these guidelines to ensure appropriate education of sonographers performing studies under their supervision.
12. Commission on Accreditation of Allied Health Education Programs (CAAHEP): http://www.caahep.org.
Includes essentials and guidelines for accreditation of programs in cardiac sonography by the Joint Review Commission for Diagnostic Medical Sonography (JRC-DMS) and the Joint Review Commission for Cardiovascular Technology (JRC-CVT). Also includes lists of accredited programs. Currently, the JRC-DMS provides accreditation to a total of 216 programs, with 76 echocardiography programs. The JRC-CVT provides accreditation to a total of 53 programs, with 38 adult echocardiography programs. One program is accredited for Advanced Cardiovascular Sonography.
13. Cardiovascular Credentialing International (CCI): http://www.cci-online.org.
CCI offers nine examinations including credentialing as a Registered Cardiac Sonographer (RCS), Registered Congenital Cardiac Sonographer (RCCS), and Advanced Cardiac Sonographer ACS).
14. American Registry of Diagnostic Medical Sonography (ARDMS): http://www.ardms.org.
The ARDMS offers four credentials, one of which is Registered Diagnostic Cardiac Sonographer (RDCS), with examination options in adult and pediatric echocardiography.

Physician Education and Training

15. Ryan T, Berlacher K, Lindner JR, et al: COCATS 4 Task Force 5: training in echocardiography: endorsed by the American Society of Echocardiography, *J Am Soc Echocardiogr* 28(6):615–627, 2015.
Detailed guidelines for training in echocardiography as part of an accredited fellowship training program in cardiovascular disease. Detailed tables list core competencies for medical knowledge, patient care/procedural skills, systems-based practice, practice-based learning and improvement, professionalism, and communication skills. This guideline establishes standards for physician Level I, II and III training in echocardiography.
16. National Board of Echocardiography (NBE): http://www.echoboards.org.
The National Board of Echocardiography offers five examinations including the Examination of Special Competency in Adult Echocardiography (ASCeXAM) and the Examination of Special Competency in Basic or Advanced Perioperative Transesophageal Echocardiography (PTEeXAM), along with recertification examinations in both areas. Certification is based on documentation of training and experience and passing the examination.
17. Cahalan MK, Abel M, Goldman M, et al: American Society of Echocardiography and Society of Cardiovascular Anesthesiologists task force guidelines for training in perioperative echocardiography, *Anesth Analg* 94(6):1384–1388, 2002.
This guideline document sets standards for training of anesthesiologists in echocardiography with detailed lists of learning objectives for basic and advanced training.
18. Pustavoitau A, Blaivas M, Brown SM, et al; Ultrasound Certification Task Force on behalf of the Society of Critical Care Medicine. Recommendations for achieving and maintaining competence and credentialing in critical care ultrasound with focused cardiac

ultrasound and advanced critical care echocardiography. Society of Critical Care Medicine. http://journals.lww.com/ccmjournal/Documents/Critical%20Care%20Ultrasound.pdf. (Accessed 21 March 2016).
Detailed guidelines for achieving and maintaining competency in POCUS by critical care physicians.

19. Labovitz AJ, Noble VE, Bierig M, et al: Focused cardiac ultrasound in the emergent setting: a consensus statement of the American Society of Echocardiography and American College of Emergency Physicians, *J Am Soc Echocardiogr* 23(12):1225–1230, 2010.
Consensus statement on use of POCUS in the emergency department including a statement on training of emergency department physicians for performance of cardiac ultrasound studies.

Laboratory Quality Assurance

20. Popescu BA, Stefanidis A, Nihoyannopoulos P, et al: Updated standards and processes for accreditation of echocardiographic laboratories from the European Association of Cardiovascular Imaging: an executive summary, *Eur Heart J Cardiovasc Imaging* 15(11):1188–1193, 2014.
Standards for echocardiography laboratories including quality control and accreditation standards.

21. Picard MH, Adams D, Bierig SM, et al: American Society of Echocardiography recommendations for quality echocardiography laboratory operations, *J Am Soc Echocardiogr* 24:1–10, 2011.
Concise document with recommendations to improve the quality of echocardiography. Sections include laboratory structure (space, equipment, sonographers, physicians) and the imaging process (patient selection, image acquisition, image interpretation, results communication). Tables detail recommended image acquisition protocols and recommended elements of the report. Reference list includes all of the American Society of Echocardiography guidelines.

22. Intersocietal Accreditation Commission for Echocardiography http://www.intersocietal.org/echo/. (Accessed October 2, 2017).
Standards for accreditation of echocardiography laboratories in the United States. Detailed standards and guidelines provide a reference point for optimal echocardiograph laboratory operations and quality assurance.

23. European Association of Cardiovascular Imaging (EACVI). https://www.escardio.org/Sub-specialty-communities/European-Association-of-Cardiovascular-Imaging-(EACVI)/Certification-Accreditation. (Accessed October 2, 2017).
The EACVI offers individual accreditation for Europeans in adult TTE and TEE, as well as congenital heart disease echocardiography. EACVI Laboratory Accreditation also is offered to European programs.

6 Left and Right Ventricular Systolic Function

BASIC PRINCIPLES
 Cardiac Cycle
 Physiology of Systolic Function
 Ventricular Volumes and Geometry
 Cardiac Output
 Response to Exercise
IMAGING THE LEFT VENTRICLE
 Qualitative Evaluation of Systolic Function
 Quantitative Evaluation of Systolic Function
  Linear Dimensions
  2D and 3D Ventricular Volumes
  Left Ventricular Wall Stress, Strain, and Strain Rate Imaging
  Left Ventricular Speckle Tracking Strain Imaging
 Left Ventricular Geometry and Mass
 Limitations and Alternate Approaches
  Endocardial Definition
  Geometric Assumptions
  Accuracy and Reproducibility
  Alternate Approaches
DOPPLER EVALUATION OF LEFT VENTRICULAR SYSTOLIC FUNCTION
 Stroke Volume Calculation
 Sites for Stroke Volume Measurement
  Left Ventricular Outflow
  Mitral Valve
  Right Heart
 Differences in Transvalvular Volume Flow Rates
 Other Doppler Measures of Systolic Function
  Ejection Acceleration Times
  Rate of Ventricular Pressure Rise (dP/dt)
 Limitations and Alternate Approaches
ECHO APPROACH TO RIGHT VENTRICULAR SYSTOLIC FUNCTION
 Right Ventricle Size
 Right Ventricular Systolic Function
 Patterns of Ventricular Septal Motion
 Limitations and Alternate Approaches
PULMONARY VASCULATURE
 Pulmonary Systolic Pressure Estimates
  Tricuspid Regurgitant Velocity
  Pulmonic Regurgitant Velocity
 Estimation of Right Atrial Pressure
 Pulmonary Vascular Resistance
  Pulmonary Artery Velocity Curve
  Pulmonary Vascular Resistance Calculations
 Limitations and Alternate Approaches
THE ECHO EXAM
SUGGESTED READING

The degree of ventricular systolic dysfunction is a potent predictor of clinical outcome for a wide range of cardiovascular disease, including ischemic cardiac disease, cardiomyopathies, valvular heart disease, and congenital heart disease. Echocardiographic estimates of global and regional function, quantitative ventricular volumes and ejection fractions, and Doppler echocardiographic ejection phase indices all are valuable clinical tools. Even when evaluation of ventricular systolic function is not the primary focus of the echocardiographic examination, evaluation of ventricular systolic function is a key component of every clinical study. For research applications, echocardiographic measures of left ventricular (LV) systolic function provide important baseline data on disease severity and clinical endpoints for intervention trials in patients with ventricular dysfunction.

BASIC PRINCIPLES

Cardiac Cycle

Systole is defined as the segment of the cardiac cycle from mitral valve closure to aortic valve closure (Fig. 6.1). The onset of systole is identified on the electrocardiogram as ventricular depolarization (onset of the QRS complex), with the end of systole occurring after repolarization (end of T wave). In terms of ventricular pressure curves over time, systole begins when LV pressure exceeds left atrial (LA) pressure, resulting in closure of the mitral valve. Mitral valve closure is followed by isovolumic contraction, during which the cardiac muscle depolarizes, calcium influx and myosin-actin shortening occur, and ventricular pressure rises rapidly at a constant ventricular volume

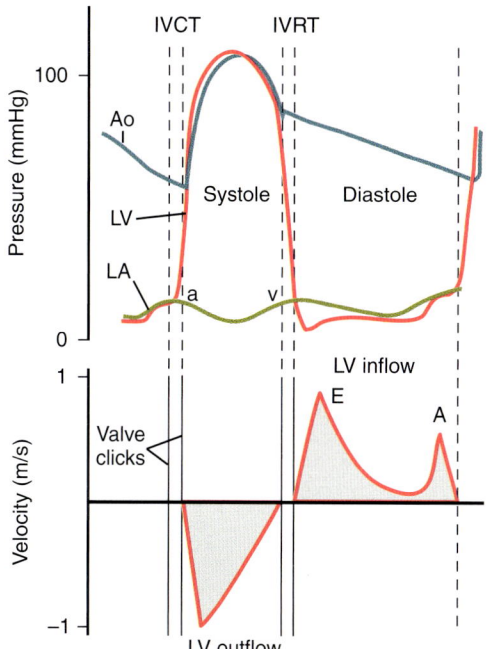

Fig. 6.1 The cardiac cycle. LV, aortic *(Ao)*, and LA pressures are shown with the corresponding Doppler LV outflow and inflow-velocity curves. The isovolumic contraction time *(IVCT)* represents the time between mitral valve closure and aortic valve opening, whereas the isovolumic relaxation time *(IVRT)* represents the time between aortic valve closure and mitral valve opening.

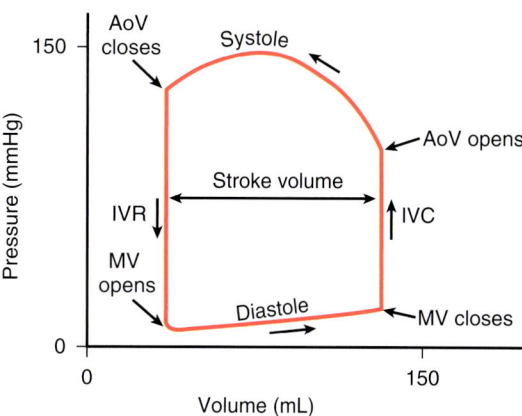

Fig. 6.2 Pressure-volume loop. LV volume is graphed on the horizontal axis, with pressure on the vertical axis. The temporal direction of pressure-volume changes is shown by the *arrows*. During diastole, volume increases with little rise in pressure. After mitral valve *(MV)* closure, isovolumic contraction *(IVC)* results in a rapid rise in pressure with no change in volume. At the onset of ejection, the aortic valve *(AoV)* opens with a rapid decrease in LV volume during systole. Aortic valve closure is followed by isovolumic relaxation *(IVR)*.

(although shape changes do occur). When ventricular pressure exceeds aortic pressure, the aortic valve opens. During ejection (aortic valve opening to closing), LV volume falls rapidly as blood flows from the LV to the aorta. LV pressure exceeds aortic pressure for approximately the first half of systole, corresponding to a rapid acceleration of blood flow and a small pressure difference from the ventricle to the aorta. In the normal heart, pressure crossover occurs in mid-systole, so during the second half of systole, aortic pressure exceeds LV pressure, thus resulting in continued forward blood flow but at progressively slower velocities (deceleration). Aortic valve closure occurs at the dicrotic notch of the aortic pressure tracing, immediately following end-ejection. In sum, systole includes isovolumic contraction and ventricular ejection (acceleration and deceleration phases). Ventricular volume ranges from a maximum at end-diastole (or onset of systole) to a minimum at end-systole.

Physiology of Systolic Function

During systole, ventricular myocardial fibers contract circumferentially and longitudinally, resulting in myocardial wall thickening and inward motion of the endocardium. The simultaneous decrease in ventricular size and increase in pressure result in ejection of a volume of blood (stroke volume) from the ventricle.

Stroke volume reflects the *pump performance* of the heart. The decrease in chamber volume relative to end-diastolic volume, or ejection fraction, reflects overall *ventricular function*. Ventricular function and pump performance depend on:

- Contractility (the basic ability of the myocardium to contract)
- Preload (initial ventricular volume or pressure)
- Afterload (aortic resistance or end-systolic wall stress)
- Ventricular geometry

Contractility is the intrinsic ability of the myocardium to contract, independent of loading conditions or geometry. Evaluation of contractility itself thus requires measurement of ventricular ejection performance under different loading conditions. Experimentally, contractility often is described by the slope of the end-systolic pressure-volume relationship (E_{max}). To derive this value, LV pressure is graphed on the vertical axis, with volume (not time) on the horizontal axis (Fig. 6.2). This pressure-volume "loop" then represents a single cardiac cycle, with different pressure-volume loops for the same ventricle representing different loading conditions (e.g., increasing or decreasing ventricular end-diastolic volume or changing afterload). E_{max} is the slope of the line that intersects the end-systolic pressure-volume point for each curve. A decrease in contractility results in a decrease in stroke volume and larger LV volumes (Fig. 6.3). Contractility itself can be affected by several physiologic parameters including heart rate, coupling interval, and metabolic factors, in addition to disease processes and pharmacologic agents.

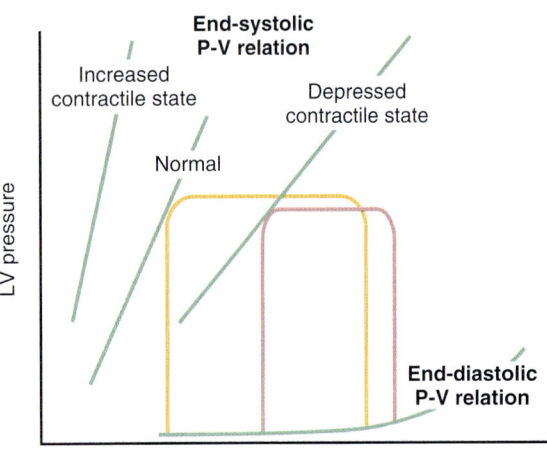
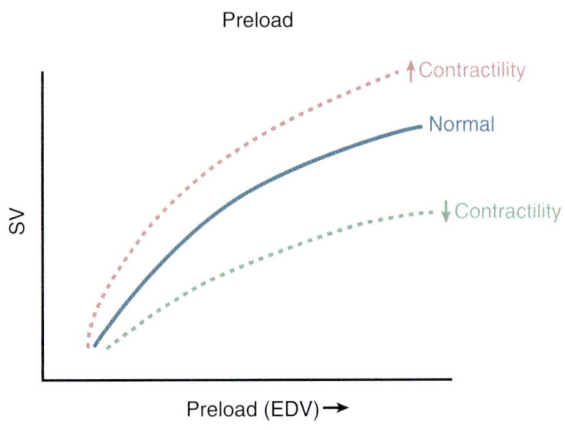
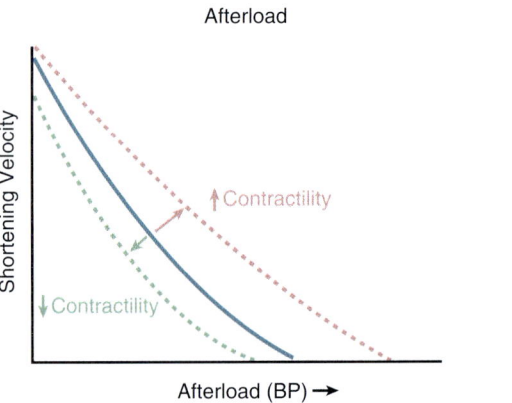

Fig. 6.3 Effect of changes in contractility on left ventricular pressure-volume loops. A normal ventricle is shown in yellow and an acute decrease in contractile state in pink. The slope of the line intersecting the end-systolic pressure-volume (P-V) points at different loading conditions, shown as a green line for each P-V loop, is a measure of contractility known as elastance (E_{max}), which is insensitive to changes in loading conditions. With decreased contractility, the P-V loop is displaced to the right, and the end-systolic P-V line shifts downward and to the right. The effect of an acute increase in contractile state is illustrated by the line on the left; the slope of the end-systolic P-V line is increased (the corresponding loop is not shown). *(From Aurigemma GP, Gaasch WH, Villegas B, et al: Noninvasive assessment of left ventricular mass, chamber volume, and contractile function. Curr Probl Cardiol 20:418, 1995.)*

Fig. 6.4 Preload and afterload. *(Top)* The relationship between preload, often defined by end-diastolic volume *(EDV)*, and stroke volume *(SV)* is shown for a normal *(blue line)* LV. With increased contractility, one sees a greater increase in SV for an increase in EDV *(red line)*; with decreased contractility, one sees a smaller increase in SV for an increase in EDV *(green dashed line)*. *(Bottom)* The inverse relationship between afterload, approximated by blood pressure *(BP)* or systemic vascular resistance, and LV myocardial shortening velocity is shown for a normal ventricle *(blue line)*. With increased contractility, shortening velocity (and stroke volume) can be maintained at higher afterloads *(red line)*; with decreased contractility, shortening velocity is lower for any given afterload *(green dashed line)*.

The effect of *preload* on ventricular ejection performance is summarized by the Frank-Starling curve showing ventricular end-diastolic volume (or pressure) on the horizontal axis and stroke volume on the vertical axis (Fig. 6.4). For a given degree of contractility, a curvilinear relationship exists between these variables such that increasing end-diastolic volume results in a greater stroke volume. An increase in contractility results in a greater increase in stroke volume for a given increase in preload; a decrease in contractility has the opposite effect.

Afterload, defined by resistance or impedance, has an inverse relationship with myocardial fiber shortening such that increasing vascular resistance results in a decreased stroke volume (see Fig. 6.4). An increase in contractility allows maintenance of a normal stroke volume with a higher afterload. With a decrease in contractility, even slight increases in afterload further decrease myocardial fiber shortening and stroke volume.

Measurement of LV systolic function independent of loading conditions is difficult using echocardiographic or other clinical approaches. It rarely is possible to construct pressure-volume loops under different loading conditions because of the problem of measuring instantaneous LV volumes and the potential risk of altering loading conditions in ill patients. Thus clinical evaluation of ventricular function has focused on measurements of cardiac output, ejection fraction, and end-systolic dimension or volume, even though the load dependence of these measures is a clearly acknowledged limitation. Strain and strain rate measurements offer another approach to evaluation of ventricular function and are becoming more widely used.

Ventricular Volumes and Geometry

The normal shape of the LV is symmetric, with two relatively equal short axes and with the long axis running from the base (mitral annulus) to the apex. In long-axis views, the apex is slightly rounded, so the apical half of the ventricle resembles a hemiellipse. The basal half of the ventricle is more cylindrical, so the ventricle appears circular in short-axis views. Various assumptions about LV shape have been used to derive formulas for calculating ventricular volumes from linear dimensions (M-mode) and cross-sectional areas (two-dimensional [2D] echo). Formulas using linear or cross-sectional measurements are simplifications to greater or lesser degrees, and variability exists among patients in the shape of the ventricle. Calculation of LV size from three-dimensional (3D) images avoids inaccuracy related to geometric assumptions.

ECHO MATH: Stroke Volume and Ejection Fraction

> Although instantaneous ventricular volumes throughout the cardiac cycle are of interest, usually only end-diastolic volume (EDV) and end-systolic volume (ESV) are measured in the clinical setting.
>
> Stroke volume (SV) is calculated as:
>
> $$SV = EDV - ESV \quad \text{(Eq. 6.1)}$$
>
> with cardiac output obtained by multiplying stroke volume by heart rate.
>
> Ejection fraction (EF) is:
>
> $$EF(\%) = (SV/EDV) \times 100\% \quad \text{(Eq. 6.2)}$$
>
> For example, if EDV is 106 mL and ESV is 62 mL, stroke volume and ejection fraction are:
>
> $$SV = EDV - ESV = 44 \text{ mL}$$
> $$EF = [(EDV - ESV)/EDV] \times 100\%$$
> $$= (106 - 62)/106 \times 100\% = 42\%$$

Cardiac Output

The basic function of the heart is as a pump, so measurements of cardiac output are useful in routine day-to-day patient management. Cardiac output is the volume of blood pumped by the heart per minute, with stroke volume being the amount pumped on a single beat. Although cardiac output can be derived from ventricular volumes, as described earlier, various other approaches to measurement are available, including right heart catheterization with indicator dilation methods (Fick, thermodilution); inert gas rebreathing approaches; angiographic, radionuclide, or cardiac magnetic resonance) ventricular volumes; and cardiac magnetic resonance or Doppler flow-velocity methods.

Response to Exercise

Ventricular systolic function and cardiac output are dynamic, responding rapidly to the metabolic demands of the individual. Cardiac output increases from a mean of 6 L/min at rest to 18 L/min with exercise in young, healthy adults. Most of this increase in cardiac output is mediated by an increase in heart rate. With supine exercise, only a minimal increase in stroke volume (about 10%) occurs, whereas with upright exercise, the increase in stroke volume is approximately 20% to 35%. With exercise, end-diastolic volume is unchanged or slightly decreased, but ejection fraction increases and end-systolic volume decreases. With imaging techniques, endocardial motion and myocardial wall thickening are augmented, with an appearance of "hypercontractility" during and immediately following exercise.

IMAGING THE LEFT VENTRICLE

Qualitative Evaluation of Systolic Function

Both global and regional ventricular function can be evaluated with 2D echocardiography on a semiquantitative scale by an experienced observer. On transthoracic (TTE) imaging, overall LV systolic function is evaluated best from multiple tomographic planes, typically:

- Parasternal long-axis view
- Parasternal short-axis view
- Apical four-chamber view
- Apical two-chamber view
- Apical long-axis view

On transesophageal (TEE) imaging, equivalent views from a high TEE and transgastric position are used. Attention to image acquisition is needed to obtain adequate endocardial definition. 3D image acquisition from the TTE or TEE approach allows simultaneous display of two or more tomographic planes and likely will be more widely used as 3D image quality and endocardial definition are improved.

The echocardiographer then integrates the degree of endocardial motion and wall thickening from these views to classify overall systolic function as normal, mildly reduced, moderately reduced, or severely reduced. Some experienced observers can estimate ejection fraction visually from 2D images with a reasonable correlation with ejection fractions measured quantitatively by echocardiography or other techniques. Typically, ejection fraction is estimated in intervals of 5% to 10% (i.e., 20%, 30%, 40%, and so on), or an estimated ejection fraction range is reported (e.g., 20% to 30%).

Several other imaging parameters provide a qualitative measure of LV systolic function. M-mode signs include:

- The separation between the maximum anterior motion of the anterior mitral leaflet and

maximum posterior motion of the ventricular septum (E-point septal separation)
- The degree of anteroposterior motion of the aortic root

With normal systolic function, the anterior mitral leaflet opens to nearly fill the ventricular chamber, thus resulting in little (0 to 5 mm) E-point septal separation. With systolic dysfunction, this distance is increased because of a combination of LV dilation and reduced motion of the mitral valve as a result of low transmitral volume flow. Similarly, LV systolic dysfunction results in reduced LA filling and emptying (low cardiac output), seen on M-mode as reduced anteroposterior motion of the aortic root (see Fig. 9.5).

On 2D echocardiography, the mitral annulus moves toward the ventricular apex in systole, with the magnitude of this motion proportional to the extent of shortening in ventricular length—a useful measure of overall LV systolic function. Normal subjects have motion of the mitral annulus toward the apex ≥8 mm, with a mean value of 12 ± 2 mm in both four- and two-chamber views. The sensitivity of mitral annulus motion <8 mm is 98%, with a specificity of 82% for identification of an ejection fraction <50%.

Qualitative evaluation of overall systolic function is a simple and highly predictive index that is of great clinical utility. Conversely, several factors can limit the usefulness of this evaluation. First, the accuracy of the estimated ejection fraction is dependent on the experience of each observer. Second, inadequate endocardial definition can result in incorrect estimates of systolic function. Third, integration of data from multiple tomographic images can be difficult when the pattern of contraction is asynchronous (with conduction defects, pacers, postoperative septal motion) or when the pattern of contraction is asymmetric (with prior myocardial infarction or with ischemia), especially when dyskinesis is present. To some extent, these limitations are minimized by an experienced observer, optimal endocardial definition, use of contrast to enhance border recognition, and integration of data from multiple views. However, when possible, it is preferable to avoid the limitations of estimates of systolic function by performing quantitative measurements.

Regional ventricular function also can be evaluated by imaging in multiple tomographic planes on TTE or TEE imaging. Regional function is evaluated qualitatively by dividing the ventricle into segments corresponding to the coronary artery anatomy and then grading wall motion on a 1 to 4+ scale as normal (score = 1), hypokinetic (score = 2), akinetic (score = 3), or dyskinetic (score = 4). In some cases, hyperkinesis (i.e., a compensatory increase in wall motion in regions remote from an acute myocardial infarction or the normal increase seen with exercise) also is scored. Evaluation of segmental wall motion is discussed in detail in Chapter 8.

Quantitative Evaluation of Systolic Function

Linear Dimensions

LV internal dimensions and wall thickness are routinely measured using 2D echocardiography. Measurements of LV size are most accurate when the ultrasound beam is perpendicular to the blood-endocardium interface because of the precision of axial, compared with lateral, resolution. In some specific situations, such as serial evaluation of the patient with chronic aortic or mitral regurgitation, 2D guided M-mode measurements are recommended, particularly when identification of the endocardium is suboptimal on the 2D images (Table 6.1).

On a standard examination, ventricular size is measured in the parasternal long-axis view, at the level of the mitral leaflet tips (mitral chordal level), perpendicular to the long axis of the ventricle (Fig. 6.5). Biplane imaging or scanning between the long- and short-axis views is also helpful to ensure that the measurements are centered in the short-axis plane. TEE measurements of LV internal dimensions are made in a transgastric two-chamber view at the junction between the basal third and apical portion of the ventricle. Wall thickness is measured in the transgastric short-axis view. On 2D images, LV internal dimensions are measured at end-diastole and end-systole from the tissue-blood interface (white-black transition). End-diastole is defined as the onset of the QRS complex, the first frame after mitral valve closure or maximum ventricular volume. End-systole is defined as the smallest ventricular volume or the frame just after aortic valve closure.

When 2D guided M-mode measurements are used, the transducer often needs to be moved cephalad to obtain a perpendicular angle between the M-line and the long axis of the ventricle. If only an oblique orientation is possible, correctly aligned measurements should be made from the 2D image instead. The major advantage of M-mode echocardiography is high time resolution, which facilitates recognition of endocardial motion and thus a more accurate measurement of ventricular internal dimensions. On M-mode, the LV posterior wall endocardium is the most continuous line with the steepest systolic motion (Fig. 6.6). The posterior wall epicardium is identified as the echo reflection immediately anterior to the pericardium. The septal endocardium also shows the steepest slope in systole with a continuous reflection through the cycle. On the right ventricular (RV) side of the septum, it is important to exclude any reflections that are caused by RV trabeculations. Conversely, a dark "mid-septal" stripe often is noted and should not be confused with the endocardial borders. LV wall thickness and dimensions are measured from the leading edge to leading edge of each interface of interest for optimal measurement accuracy. For example,

TABLE 6.1 Left Ventricular Dimension Measurements

	TTE-2D	TTE-2D Guided M-Mode	TEE
Transducer position	Parasternal	Parasternal	Transgastric
Image plane	Long-axis	Long-axis	Two-chamber view (rotation angle 60°–90°)
Measurement position in LV chamber	Perpendicular to LV long axis in the center of the LV Biplane imaging or rotation between long- and short-axis views helps ensure a centered measurement.	Perpendicular to LV long axis in the center of the LV Correct M-line orientation often requires moving the transducer up an interspace.	Perpendicular to LV long axis in the center of the LV Ensuring a centered measurement is more difficult on TEE.
Measurement site along LV length	Just apical to the mitral leaflet tips (chordal level)	Just apical to the mitral leaflet tips (chordal level)	At the junction of the basal third and apical two thirds of the LV
Measurement technique	White-black interface	Leading edge-to-leading edge	White-black interface
Timing in cardiac cycle End-diastole End-systole	Onset of QRS frame just before MV closure, or maximum LV volume Minimum LV volume or frame just before aortic valve closure	Onset of QRS frame just before MV closure, or maximum LV volume Minimum LV volume or frame just before aortic valve closure	Onset of QRS frame just before MV closure, or maximum LV volume Minimum LV volume or frame just before aortic valve closure
Advantages	It is feasible in most patients. Measurements can be made perpendicular to LV long axis.	High sampling rate facilitates identification of endocardium. Reproducible	It allows intraoperative monitoring preload. Ultrasound beam is perpendicular to endocardium from TG view, improving border recognition.
Disadvantages	Endocardial and epicardial borders may be difficult to identify accurately. It has a slow frame rate compared with M-mode.	M-line measurements should be made only if a perpendicular LV measurement is possible. This requires more attention to transducer and M-line position.	Image plane may be oblique. Wall thickness is measured in a transgastric short-axis view.

MV, Mitral valve; *TG*, transgastric.

ventricular internal dimensions are measured from the leading edge of the septal endocardium to the leading edge of the posterior wall endocardium. Normal values for linear ventricular dimensions depend on age and sex (Fig. 6.7).

In addition to LV wall thickness and internal dimensions (LVID) at end-diastole (d) and end-systole (s), endocardial fractional shortening (FS) can be calculated as:

$$FS (\%) = (LVID_d - LVID_s)/LVID_d \times 100\% \quad \text{(Eq. 6.3)}$$

Fractional shortening is a rough measurement of LV systolic function, with the normal range being about 25% to 45% (95% confidence limits). Instead of endocardial fractional shortening, as shown in Eq. 6.3, mid-wall fractional shortening is a better reflector of contractility because it reflects both the inward motion of the endocardium and the degree of wall thickening. However, mid-wall shortening calculations are rarely used in clinical practice because 2D measures of ventricular systolic function are more robust.

2D and 3D Ventricular Volumes

The 2D echocardiographic calculation of ventricular volumes is based on endocardial border tracing at

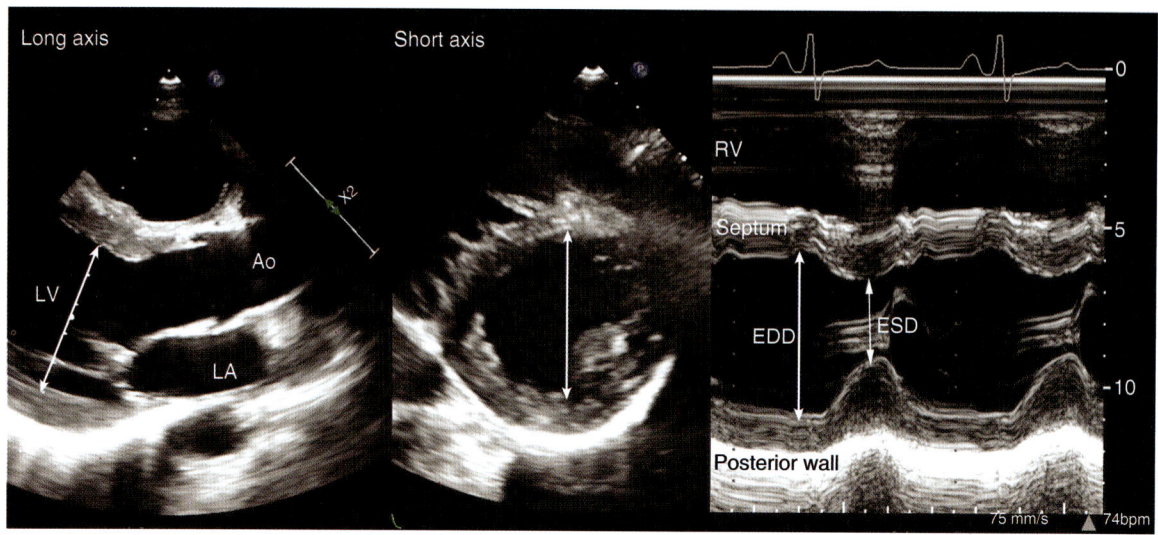

Fig. 6.5 Left ventricular M-mode measurements. LV end-diastolic dimension *(EDD)* and end-systolic dimension *(ESD)* are measured from the parasternal window. 2D measurements are made for the white-black interface of the septum to the posterior wall, while taking care to measure perpendicular to the long axis of the ventricle and centered in the short axis. Similarly, 2D-guided M-mode measurements are made after verifying that the M-line is centered in the LV in the short-axis view and perpendicular to the long axis of the LV in the long-axis view. The transducer should be in a high intercostal space to ensure that the M-line is not oblique. The high sampling rate of the M-mode recording allows more precise identification of the endocardium. *Ao,* Aorta.

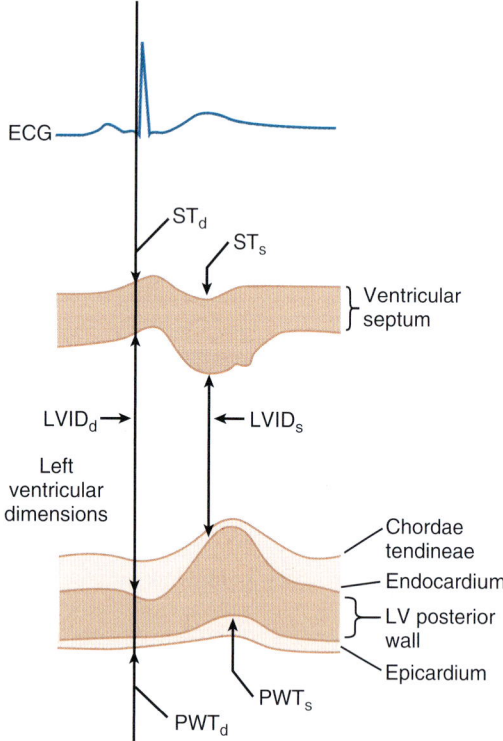

Fig. 6.6 Left ventricular M-mode schematic diagram. From a 2D-guided M-mode recording, diastolic measurements are made coincident with the Q-wave of the simultaneous electrocardiogram *(ECG)*. Systolic measurements are made at the maximum posterior motion of the septum, when septal motion is normal. *d,* Diastolic; *LVID,* LV internal dimensions; *PWT,* posterior wall thickness; *s,* systolic; *ST,* ventricular septal thickness in diastole. *(From Aurigemma GP, Gaasch WH, Villegas B, et al: Noninvasive assessment of left ventricular mass, chamber volume, and contractile function,* Curr Probl Cardiol *20:381, 1995.)*

end-diastole and end-systole in one or more tomographic planes on TTE or TEE images (Table 6.2 and Appendix A, Table A.1). Prerequisites for quantitative evaluation by 2D echocardiography are:

- Nonoblique standard image planes or image planes of known orientation relative to the long and short axis of the LV
- Inclusion of the apex of the ventricle
- Adequate endocardial definition
- Accurate identification of the endocardial borders

When image quality is suboptimal, use of left-sided echo contrast improves endocardial definition. Currently, 2D or contrast-enhanced endocardial borders must be traced manually by an experienced physician or sonographer for accurate quantitation of LV systolic function. Because 2D echocardiography is a tomographic technique, LV volume calculations are based on geometric assumptions about the shape of the LV. By convention, the papillary muscles are included in the ventricular chamber, with endocardial borders extrapolated along the base of the papillary muscle, following the expected curvature of the ventricular wall. Obviously, accuracy in individual patients will be highest with methods that have the fewest geometric assumptions and that use data from multiple tomographic images (see Appendix B, Table B.1).

Several approaches for the calculation of LV volumes from tomographic data, based on different geometric assumptions, have been proposed, ranging from a simple ellipsoid shape to complex

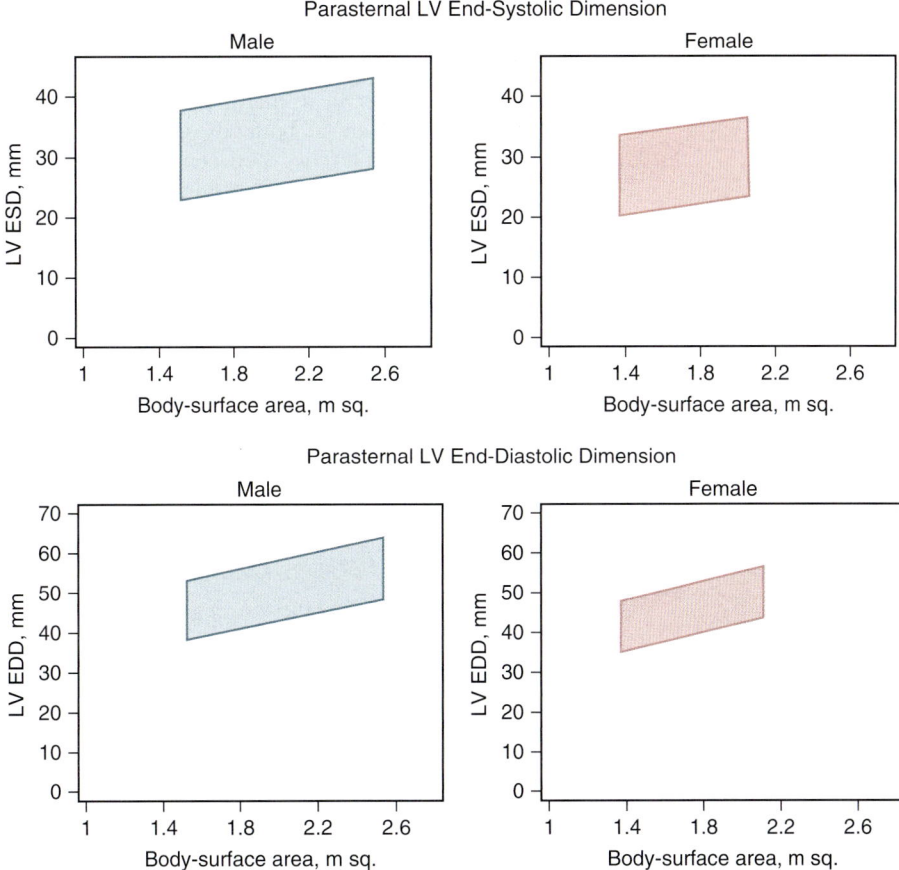

Fig. 6.7 Normal left ventricular dimensions in males and females by body surface area. LV end-diastolic dimension *(EDD)* and end-systolic dimension *(ESD)* measured from a parasternal long-axis for men *(left)* and women *(right)*. The 95% confidence intervals are shown by the *shaded box*. *(From Lang RM, Badano LP, Mor-Avi V, et al. Recommendations for cardiac chamber quantification by echocardiography in adults: an update from the American Society of Echocardiography and the European Association of Cardiovascular Imaging, J Am Soc Echocardiogr 28(1):1–39.e14, 2015.)*

TABLE 6.2 2D and 3D Echocardiographic Measurement of LV Volumes and Ejection Fraction

	2D	3D
Window	Apical • Patient in steep left lateral position • Apical cutout in exam stretcher • Avoid apical foreshortening.	Apical • Patient in steep left lateral position • Apical cutout in exam stretcher • Adjust transducer position to ensure inclusion of entire LV.
Image acquisition	Four-chamber and two-chamber views • Adjust depth to mitral annulus level. • Adjust gain, time-gain compensation, harmonic imaging, and other instrument parameters to optimize endocardial definition. • Left-sided contrast enhances endocardial border identification when image quality is suboptimal.	Apical volumetric acquisition • Full-volume gated acquisition • Use 2D images for initial positioning and adjusting gain. • Use split screen display of orthogonal views to optimize acquisition. • Breath hold during acquisition to minimize stitch artifacts. • Left-sided contrast enhances endocardial border identification when image quality is suboptimal.
Endocardial borders	Manual tracing at ED and ES • ED defined as onset of QRS • ES defined as minimal LV volume Trace borders at time of image acquisition and adjust, if needed, on final review.	Semiautomated endocardial border detection • Exclude papillary muscles and trabeculations from LV chamber. • Review and adjust borders after acquisition.
Volume calculations	• Apical biplane formula	• Surface-rendered LV volumes

ED, End-diastole; *ES,* end-systole.

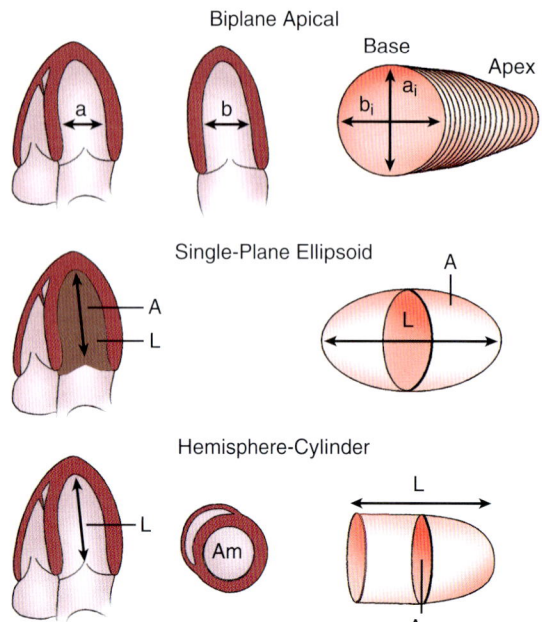

Fig. 6.8 2D left ventricular volume calculations. Examples of three formulas for LV volume calculations showing the 2D echocardiographic views and measurements on the *left* and the geometric model on the *right*. For the biplane apical method, endocardial borders are traced in apical four-chamber and two-chamber views, which are used to define a series of orthogonal diameters *(a and b)*. A "Simpson's rule" assumption based on stacked disks is used to calculate volume. The single-plane ellipsoid method uses the 2D area *(A)* and length *(L)* in a single (usually apical four-chamber) view. The hemisphere-cylinder method uses a short-axis endocardial area at the midventricular level *(Am)* and a long-axis length *(L)*. For each method, both end-diastolic and end-systolic measurements are needed for calculation of end-diastolic and end-systolic volumes, respectively, and for ejection fraction determination.

hemicylindrical or hemiellipsoid shapes (Fig. 6.8). The most robust and practical method for clinical use is Simpson's rule or *method of disks*, which calculates ventricular volume as the sum of a series of parallel "slices" from apex to base.

$$\text{LV volume} = \sum_{i=1}^{n} A_i T \qquad \text{(Eq. 6.4)}$$

Where A is the area and T is the thickness of each of n slices. For example, if 20 disks are summated, LV volume is:

$$\text{LV volume} = \sum_{n=20} [A_i \times L/20] \qquad \text{(Eq. 6.5)}$$

This approach is recommended in consensus guidelines because it is accurate even when ventricular geometry is distorted (Table 6.3). The apical biplane approach requires tracing of endocardial borders at end-diastole and end-systole in both four-chamber and two-chamber views, from either TTE or TEE images (Fig. 6.9). These borders are then used to calculate cross-sectional areas of a series of elliptical disks. End-diastolic volume is calculated from end-diastolic images, and end-systolic volume is calculated from end-systolic images. Normal LV volumes are smaller in women compared with men and decrease with age in both sexes (Fig. 6.10). Stroke volume is the difference between end-diastolic volume (EDV) and end-systolic volume (ESV) (Eq. 6.2), whereas ejection fraction (EF) is calculated with Eq. 6.1.

When only a four-chamber view is available, a single-plane ejection fraction can be calculated that summates a series of disks with a circular cross-sectional area. Another alternative is the area-length method, which assumes that the base of the ventricle is approximated by a cylinder and the apex by an ellipsoid, sometimes called the "bullet" formula; this formula uses a long-axis length L and the cross-sectional area A_m of an orthogonal short-axis view at the mid-papillary level:

$$\text{LV volume} = 5/6 \times A_m L \qquad \text{(Eq. 6.6)}$$

In the presence of a distorted ventricular shape or regional wall motion abnormalities, these alternate methods are less accurate because, if the region of abnormal wall motion is included in the dimension or area measurements, volumes will be overestimated and vice versa.

3D echocardiography provides more accurate measurements of LV volumes and ejection fraction that are independent of geometric assumptions (Appendix B, Table B.2). Current instrumentation allows semiautomated border detection from the 3D volumetric data set with calculation of end-diastolic and end-systolic volumes and ejection fraction. From an apical window, the key steps in 3D data acquisition for evaluation of the LV are as follows:

- Start with 2D apical views to optimize gain settings, typically higher than for 2D imaging.
- Guide the 3D acquisition by use of a split screen display of orthogonal views of the LV.
- Acquire the 3D volume data set during a breath hold to minimize stitch artifacts.
- Consider use of contrast to opacify the LV to improve endocardial border identification.

Data are displayed as a cine loop 3D-rendered LV volume, a graph of LV volume over the cardiac cycle, and images showing regional wall motion or regional ejection fraction, depending on the specific ultrasound system (Fig. 6.11). In clinical practice, limitations of 3D evaluation of the LV include lower temporal and spatial resolution compared with 2D imaging and difficulty including the entire LV chamber within the 3D volume data set. However, 3D volumes and ejection fraction are more accurate than 2D measurements, so quantitative evaluation of LV systolic function 3D echocardiography is recommended, whenever possible.

TABLE 6.3 American Society of Echocardiography and European Association of Cardiovascular Imaging Recommendations for Left Ventricular Chamber Quantification

Parameter	Recommended Measurements	Comments	
LV size	2D LV volumes (biplane method, indexed to BSA)	Should be routinely assessed on all diagnostic echo studies.	Upper limits of normal EDV • Men 74 mL/m² • Women 61 mL/m² LV ESV • Men 31 mL/m² • Women 24 mL/m²
	3D LV volumes (indexed to BSA)	Recommended when feasible depending on image quality.	
	LV linear dimensions	Useful when accurate volumes are not available.	
LV global systolic function	2D ejection fraction (biplane method of disks)	Should be routinely assessed on all diagnostic echo studies.	Lower limit of normal • Men <52% • Women <54%
	3D ejection fraction	Recommended when feasible depending on image quality.	
	GLS (2D speckle tracking)	GLS is most often calculated using midwall deformation. Serial GLS measurements in patients should use same equipment and software for each study.	Normal About negative 20% but depends on equipment and software.
LV regional function	16-segment model with visual grading of wall motion as normal, hypokinetic, akinetic, or dyskinetic	See Chapter 8 for details. For perfusion studies, a 17-segment model is recommended.	
	Regional longitudinal strain (speckle tracking)	Not routine due to lack of standardization.	
LV mass	M-mode or 2D calculated mass indexed to BSA	Important research tool but not routine on clinical studies. 3D methods are promising, but reference values are not yet established.	Upper limits of normal LV mass by linear measurement • Men 115 g/m² • Women 95 g/m² LV mass from 2D imaging • Men 102 g/m² • Women 88 g/m²

BSA, Body surface area; *EDV*, end-diastolic volume; *ESV*, end-systolic volume; *GLS*, global longitudinal strain.
Summarized from the American Society of Echocardiography and European Association of Cardiovascular Imaging Recommendations published in 2015 in Lang RM, Badano LP, Mor-Avi V, et al: Recommendations for cardiac chamber quantification by echocardiography in adults: an update from the American Society of Echocardiography and the European Association of Cardiovascular Imaging, *J Am Soc Echocardiogr* 28(1):1–39.e14, 2015.

Left Ventricular Wall Stress, Strain, and Strain Rate Imaging

Wall stress is the force per unit area exerted on the myocardium. Wall stress is dependent on:

- Cavity radius (R)
- Pressure (P), and
- Wall thickness (Th)

The basic equation for wall stress (σ) is:

$$\sigma = PR/2\,Th \quad \text{(Eq. 6.7)}$$

Wall stress can be described in three dimensions as circumferential, meridional (longitudinal), or radial. End-systolic calculations of circumferential and meridional wall stress reflect ventricular afterload, whereas end-diastolic wall stress reflects preload. Both meridional and circumferential wall stress can be calculated from 2D echocardiographic measures of chamber size and wall thickness. Although the concept of wall stress is important in understanding ventricular function, especially in ventricular pressure or volume overall states (e.g., hypertension, aortic stenosis, aortic or

Fig. 6.9 Apical biplane left ventricular volumes. Examples of apical four-chamber *(A4C; top)* ▶ and two-chamber *(A2C; bottom)* ▶ views at end-diastole *(left)* and end-systole *(right)*, showing the traced endocardial borders for calculation of biplane LV systolic (76 mL) and diastolic (205 mL) volumes and ejection fraction *(EF; 63%)*. *EDV,* End-diastolic volume; *ESV,* end-systolic volume.

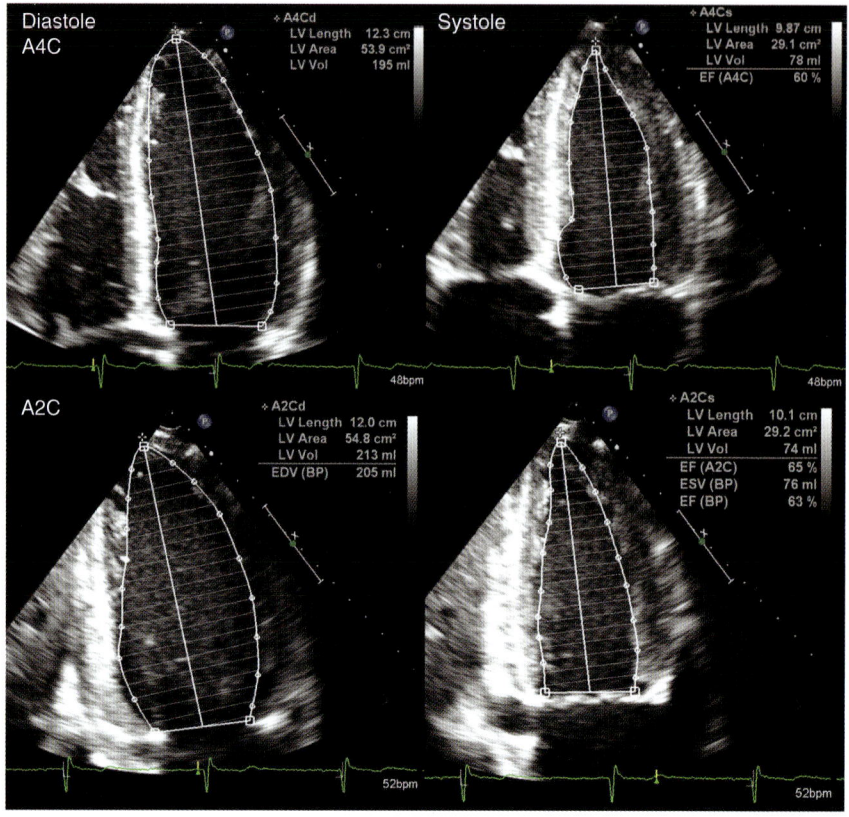

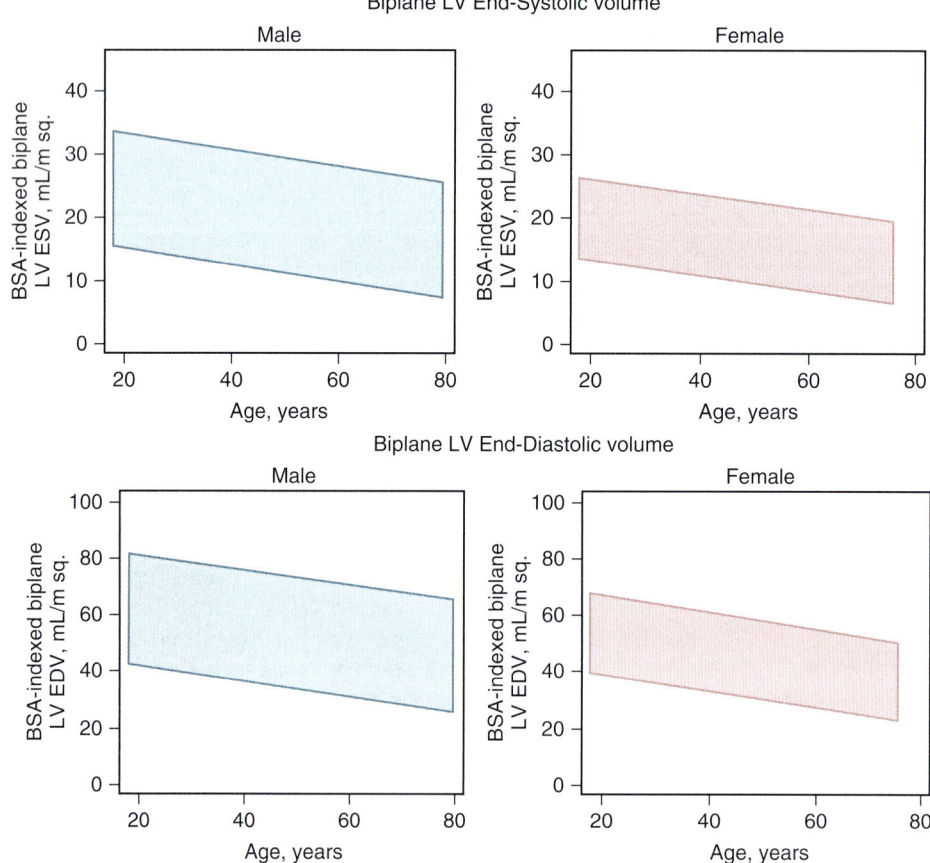

Fig. 6.10 Normal left ventricular volumes in males and females by age. LV end-diastolic and end-systolic dimensions measured from a parasternal long-axis for men *(left)* and women *(right)*. The 95% confidence intervals are shown by the *shaded boxes*. *BSA,* Body surface area; *EDV,* end-diastolic volume; *ESV,* end-sysyolic volume. *(From Lang RM, Badano LP, Mor-Avi V, et al: Recommendations for cardiac chamber quantification by echocardiography in adults: an update from the American Society of Echocardiography and the European Association of Cardiovascular Imaging. J Am Soc Echocardiogr 28(1):1–39.e14, 2015.)*

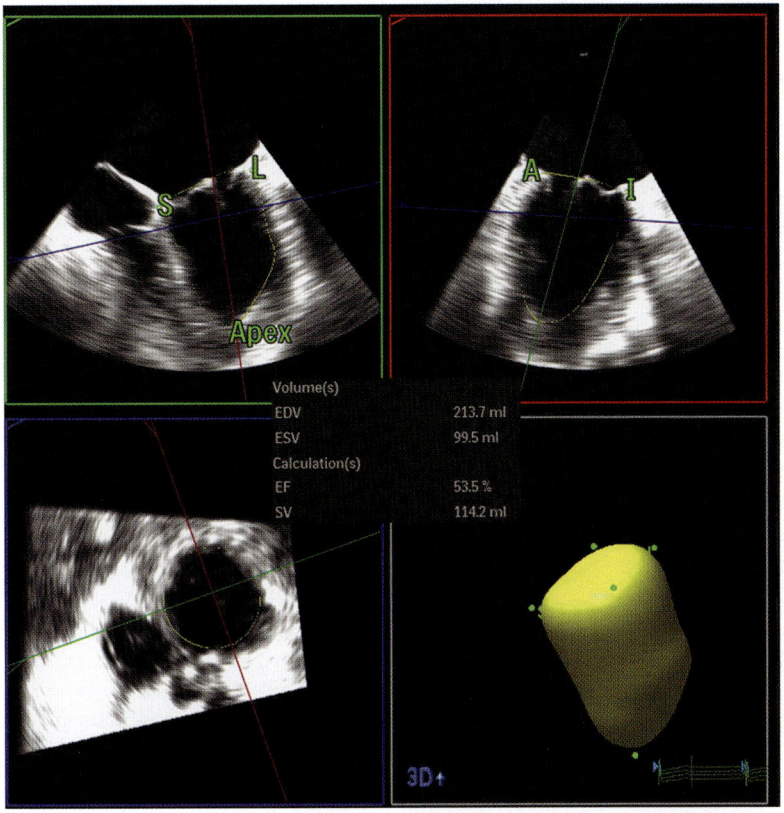

Fig. 6.11 ▶ **3D left ventricular volumes.** LV volumes are derived from a 3D volume acquisition with three orthogonal planes corresponding to four-chamber *(green box)*, two-chamber *(red box)*, and short-axis *(blue box)* views shown along with the 3D volume *(lower right)* rendered from semiautomated border tracing. The 3D calculations for end-diastolic volume *(EDV)*, end-systolic volume *(ESV)*, ejection fraction *(EF)*, and stroke volume *(SV)* are shown.

mitral regurgitation), wall stress calculations are not yet widely utilized in clinical practice.

Left Ventricular Speckle Tracking Strain Imaging

Speckle tracking strain is less load dependent compared with other echocardiographic parameters and allows detection of early LV systolic dysfunction before overt evidence of a fall in ejection fraction, as detailed in Chapter 4 (Fig. 6.12). Most often global longitudinal strain (GLS) is measured with images acquired in apical four-chamber, two-chamber, and long-axis views. Longitudinal strain is a negative number with the normal value varying among different ultrasound systems, but typically it is about 20%. Global longitudinal strain includes data from all three apical views, with results presented in a target-type color-coded chart, a graph of strain over the cardiac cycle for each myocardial wall, and a single number representing global longitudinal systolic LV function.

Left Ventricular Geometry and Mass

LV mass is the total weight of the myocardium, derived by multiplying the volume of myocardium by the specific density of cardiac muscle. LV mass can be estimated from M-mode dimensions of septal thickness (ST), posterior wall thickness (PWT), and LV internal dimensions (LVID) at end-diastole as:

$$\text{LV mass} = 0.80 \times [1.04\,(ST_d + PWT_d + LVID_d)^3 - LVID_d^3] + 0.6\,g$$

(Eq. 6.8)

On 2D or 3D echocardiography, LV mass theoretically can be determined by tracing epicardial borders to calculate the total ventricular volume (walls plus chamber), subtracting the volumes determined from endocardial border tracing, and then multiplying by the specific density of myocardium:

$$\text{LV mass} = 1.05\,(\text{total volume} - \text{chamber volume})$$

(Eq. 6.9)

However, epicardial definition rarely is adequate for this approach. Instead, mean wall thickness is calculated from epicardial (A_1) and endocardial (A_2) cross-sectional areas in a short-axis view at the papillary muscle level. LV mass measurements often are indexed for body size (either as body surface area or height)

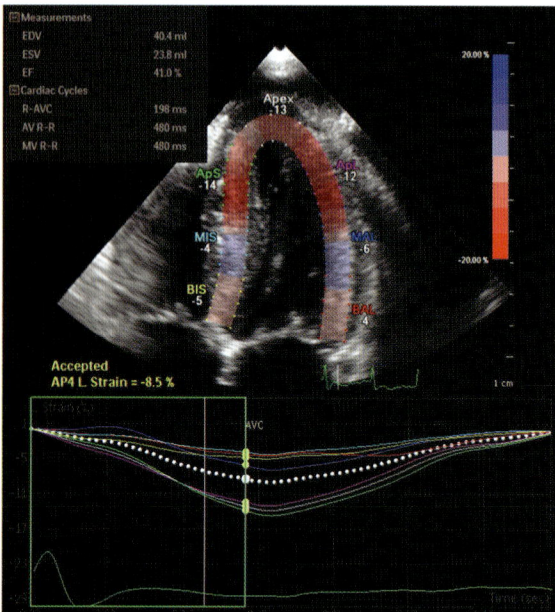
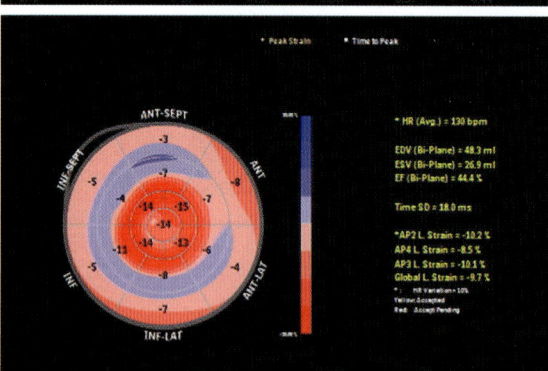

Fig. 6.12 **3D speckle tracking echocardiography.** *(Top)* Example of strain imaging with speckle tracking echocardiography in an apical four-chamber view. The strain measurement for each segment is displayed as a color overlay on the 2D image with the *dashed line* indicating automated endocardial and epicardial borders. *(Middle)* The graph shows instantaneous strain for each color-coded (to match labels on 2D image) myocardial segment as a function of time over one cardiac cycle, with the electrocardiogram in green. The maximum strain is used to determine the valve displayed of −8.5%. *(Bottom)* The target diagram integrates strain data from multiple image planes with the apex in the center and the base around the edges of the circle. In this example, apical strain has a large absolute value indicating better systolic function than basal segments. Global longitudinal strain is reduced (−9.7%), as is ejection fraction (*EF*; 44.4%) calculated from strain imaging. *AP2*, Apical two-chamber; *AP3*, apical long-axis; *AP4*, apical four-chamber; *ApL*, apical lateral wall; *ApS*, apical septum; *AVC*, aortic valve closure; *BAL*, basal anterior-lateral wall; *BIS*, basal inferior septum; *EDV*, end-diastole volume; *ESV*, end-systolic volume; *HR*, heart rate; *L*, longitudinal; *MIS*, mid-inferior septum; *MAL*, mid-anterior lateral wall.

using sex-specific normal values (see Appendix A, Table A.2).

Relative wall thickness is a simpler measure of ventricular geometry in patients with hypertrophy that reflects the relative thickness of the walls compared with chamber size. Relative wall thickness (RWT) is calculated from posterior wall thickness (PWT) and LV internal dimension (LVID), both at end-diastole, as:

$$\text{RWT} = 2\text{PWT}_d/\text{LVID}_d \quad \text{(Eq. 6.10)}$$

Ventricular geometry can be classified based on relative wall thickness (normal <0.42) and LV mass as:

- Normal geometry—Normal LV mass and normal relative wall thickness
- Concentric hypertrophy—Increased LV mass and increased relative wall thickness
- Eccentric hypertrophy—Increased LV mass with normal relative wall thickness
- Concentric remodeling—Normal LV mass with increased relative wall thickness

Concentric hypertrophy is typical of ventricular pressure overload caused by aortic stenosis with a small chamber and thick walls, whereas eccentric hypertrophy is typical of chronic volume overload caused by aortic regurgitation with a dilated chamber with normal wall thickness but an increased total weight of the ventricle. Hypertensive heart disease most often results in concentric remodeling with a normal total ventricular weight but walls that are relatively thick compared with the chamber size.

Limitations and Alternate Approaches
Endocardial Definition

Accurate identification of the ventricular endocardium is key in the echocardiographic evaluation of LV systolic function regardless of whether M-mode, 2D, or 3D approaches are used. Speckle tracking stain also is most accurate with high-quality images of the myocardium. Endocardial definition is affected by the physics of ultrasound instrumentation, by anatomic factors, and by technical factors, including the skill of the sonographer. The endocardial-ventricular cavity interface is curved from any imaging window, so the endocardium appears as a thin, bright line where it is perpendicular to the ultrasound beam (axial resolution), but as a broad, "blurred" line where the beam is parallel to the endocardial-ventricular cavity interface (lateral resolution). As for other ultrasound targets, lateral resolution is depth dependent. In addition, "dropout" of signals may result from attenuation, a parallel intercept angle, acoustic shadowing, or reverberations.

Anatomically, the endocardium is not a smooth surface but has numerous trabeculations that are most prominent at the LV apex. The ultrasound beam is reflected from the inner edge of these trabeculations, so that the "endocardium" identified by echocardiography differs from the "endocardium" identified by contrast ventriculography or cardiac magnetic resonance imaging, in which contrast fills these trabeculations and outlines their outer edges.

Several technical factors affect endocardial definition during image acquisition, and meticulous examination technique is needed for optimal image quality. First, acoustic access can be optimizing by:

- Patient positioning
- Use of an echo-stretcher with an apical cutout
- Having the patient suspend respiration
- Careful adjustment of transducer position

Instrument settings can dramatically affect image quality, including:

- Transducer frequency
- Gain
- Gray-scale settings
- Focal depth
- Tissue harmonic imaging

2D endocardial borders are traced from digitally acquired images using the real-time motion of the images to aid in identification of the endocardial border during the tracing process. End-diastolic and end-systolic images are traced on the same cardiac cycle, with end-diastole defined as onset of the QRS complex and end-systole defined as minimal ventricular volume. The trained human observer remains the most accurate means for endocardial border tracing, thus limiting the wide application of quantitative methods because manual tracing of endocardial borders at end-diastole and end-systole in at least two views remains a tedious and time-consuming task. 3D imaging uses semiautomated border detection but continues to rely on manual identification of key anatomic landmarks and usually requires adjustment of the automated borders for accurate volumes measurements. Similarly, the speckle tracking strain images are visually inspected and adjusted to ensure that the myocardium is tracked correctly.

For 3D, 2D, and speckle tracking apical imaging, the patient is positioned in a steep left lateral position on a stretcher with an apical cutout to avoid fore-shortening the LV length. A higher-frequency transducer is used for optimal image quality, and the focal depth of the transducer is adjusted to the depth of interest. The sector depth and width are adjusted to maximize the size of the LV on the screen and to optimize frame rate. Tissue harmonic imaging improves 2D endocardial definition in most patients. In addition, the patient is asked to suspend respiration, while avoiding a Valsalva maneuver, at the phase of respiration where image quality is optimal. When endocardial definition remains poor despite these measures, the use of an intravenous contrast agent to opacify the LV is appropriate.

Geometric Assumptions

Quantitation of LV volumes depends on accurate visualization of the endocardium along the entire length of the chamber. 3D data sets or 2D views that foreshorten the LV will result in underestimation of LV length, which affects both TTE and TEE approaches. With TTE imaging, adequate apical views require a steep left lateral decubitus position with an apical cutout in the echo-stretcher mattress to visualize the true long axis of the chamber. On TEE imaging, even with adjustment of transducer position and angulation of the image plane, it is not always possible to include the apex on 3D data sets or in the 2D four-chamber and two-chamber views.

Respiratory motion and cardiac motion within the chest during the cardiac cycle further confound the geometric assumptions of LV volume calculations. The effect of respiratory motion of the heart relative to the transducer can be avoided by measuring beats at the same phase of respiration or by having the patient briefly suspend respiration during data acquisition. In some cases, optimal images are obtained when the patient suspends respiration after taking in a small breath, rather than at end-expiration. It is more difficult to correct for the motion of the heart itself when using a tomographic imaging procedure. Cardiac translation (movement of the heart in the chest), rotation (movement around the long axis of the heart), and torsion (unequal rotational motion of the heart) can result in images of different segments of the LV during systole and diastole, even with a fixed image plane. Although cardiac motion has only a limited effect on the accuracy of LV volume calculations, it can have a pronounced effect on quantitative evaluation of regional ventricular function, as discussed in Chapter 8.

Accuracy and Reproducibility

Qualitative comparison of LV systolic function from different studies on the same patient is facilitated by the standard digital cine loop side by side format. Of course, the influence of loading conditions on LV systolic function still must be considered when comparing studies performed at different time points in a patient's clinical course.

In most reported series, intraobserver variability for 2D LV volumes ranges from 5% to 10%. Interobserver variability is greater, ranging from 7% to 25% for 2D ventricular volumes. Because ejection fraction is a calculated percentage, reproducibility is better, with variability of about 10%. These values are similar to reported variability for ventricular volumes and ejection fraction determined by contrast or radionuclide ventriculography. Note that variability between studies in an individual patient includes:

- Physiologic variability (loading condition, heart rate, volume states)
- Image acquisition or test-retest variability (endocardial definition, image orientation)

- Measurement variability in tracing the endothelial borders

With optimal data, a significant change between studies is a difference in ejection fraction >2%, end-diastolic volume >2%, and end-systolic volume >5%.

Although LV volumes are underestimated by 3D echocardiography compared with cardiac magnetic resonance imaging, measurements are more accurate and reproducible than 2D-derived data. For example, the mean difference between observers for 3D echocardiographic LV end-diastolic volume is −3 ± 10 mL compared with 13 ± 17 mL for 2D LV volumes. Similarly, the interobserver mean difference of LV ejection fraction is 0 ± 3% for 3D versus 2 ± 8% for 2D imaging.

Alternate Approaches

Cardiac magnetic resonance imaging provides precise and accurate measures of LV volumes, mass, ejection fraction, and cardiac output. Other approaches include contrast angiography in the cardiac catheterization laboratory and radionuclide ventriculography. The choice of imaging technique in an individual patient depends on what other clinical questions are present in addition to availability and cost.

DOPPLER EVALUATION OF LEFT VENTRICULAR SYSTOLIC FUNCTION

Stroke Volume Calculation

Doppler echocardiographic evaluation of LV systolic function usually is based on calculation of stroke volume and cardiac output (see Appendix B, Table B.3).

Cardiac output (CO) is calculated using the LVOT diameter to calculate the circular cross-sectional areas of flow:

$$CSA_{LVOT} = \pi(LVOT_D/2)^2 = 3.14(2.3/2)^2 = 4.2 \text{ cm}^2$$

Stroke volume across the aortic valve (cm^3 = mL), then, is:

$$SV_{LVOT} = (CSA_{LVOT} \times VTI_{LVOT})$$
$$= 4.2 \text{ cm}^2 \times 11 \text{ cm} = 46 \text{ cm}^3$$

Cardiac output is:

$$CO = SV \times HR = 46 \text{ mL} \times 88 \text{ beats/min}$$
$$= 4048 \text{ mL/min or } 4.05 \text{ L/min}$$

Cardiac index (CI) normalizes flow to body surface area (BSA):

$$CI = CO/BSA = 4.05 \text{ L/min}/1.8 \text{ m}^2 = 2.25 \text{ L/min/m}^2$$

This indicates a low cardiac output and index (normal >2.5 $L/min/m^2$)

Conceptually, the LV ejects a volume of blood into the cylindrical aorta on each beat (Fig. 6.13). The base of this cylinder is the systolic cross-sectional area of the outflow tract, whereas its height is the distance the average blood cell traveled during ejection for that beat. This distance is expressed as the integral of the Doppler systolic velocity-time curve because velocity is the first derivative of distance. Alternatively, this distance also can be thought of as mean velocity (cm/s) multiplied by ejection duration (seconds). Again, because the volume of a cylinder is base times height, stroke volume is cross-sectional area multiplied by the velocity-time integral.

ECHO MATH: Doppler Stroke Volume and Cardiac Output

Using Doppler and 2D echo data, stroke volume (SV in cm^3 or mL) is calculated as cross-sectional area (CSA in cm^2) of flow times the velocity-time integral (VTI in cm) of flow through that region:

$$SV = CSA \times VTI \quad \text{(Eq. 6.11)}$$

and

$$CO = SV \times HR \quad \text{(Eq. 6.12)}$$

Where CO is cardiac output and HR is heart rate.

For example, if LV outflow tract diameter is 2.3 cm, LV outflow-velocity time integral is 11 cm, and heart rate is 88 bpm:

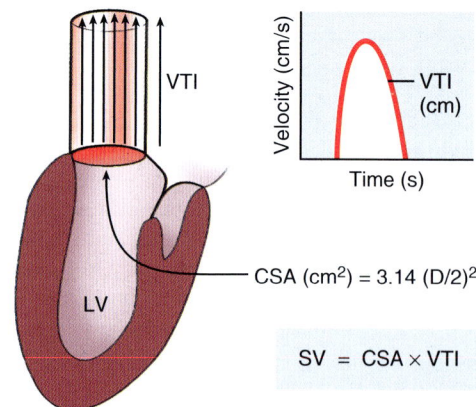

Fig. 6.13 Doppler stroke volume concept. The cross-sectional area *(CSA)* of flow is calculated as a circle based on a 2D echo diameter *(D)* measurement. The length of the cylinder of blood ejected through this cross-sectional area on a single beat is the velocity-time integral *(VTI)* of the Doppler curve. Stroke volume *(SV)* then is calculated as CSA × VTI.

This approach to stroke volume calculation depends on several basic assumptions:

- Accurate cross-sectional flow area measurement
- Laminar flow with spatially "flat" flow-velocity profile
- Parallel intercept angle between Doppler beam and direction of blood flow
- Velocity and diameter measurements are made at the same anatomic site

First, the cross-sectional area must be measured accurately. Typically, diameter is measured and 2D area calculated as $\pi(D/2)^2$ based on the assumption of a circular geometry. Deviations from a circular geometry or changes in cross-sectional area during the flow period will result in inaccuracies unless appropriate corrections are included in the calculations. Small errors in 2D diameter measurements become large errors in cross-sectional area calculations because radius (half the diameter) is squared in the calculations. Using a transducer orientation and instrument settings that maximize image quality, performing measurements based on axial (rather than lateral) resolution, performing diameter measurements in two orthogonal planes (when possible), and averaging several beats can help minimize this source of error.

Second, the pattern of flow is assumed to be laminar, and the spatial flow profile across the flowstream is assumed to be relatively flat. These assumptions ensure that the velocity curve represents the spatial (and temporal) average flow in that region. The validity of the assumption of laminar flow in the great vessels and across normal cardiac valves is demonstrated by the narrow band of velocities and smooth spectral signal seen on pulsed Doppler echo recordings. A flat flow profile also is a reasonable assumption at the inlet to the great vessels and across the valve planes because of the effects of geometric convergence and acceleration. A flat flow-velocity profile can be confirmed by moving the sample volume across the flowstream in two orthogonal views to demonstrate uniform velocities at the center and the edges of the flowstream.

Third, the Doppler signal is assumed to have been recorded at a parallel intercept angle to flow, resulting in an accurate velocity measurement (based on a cos θ = 1 in the Doppler equation). In practical terms, the sonographer aligns the Doppler beam in the presumed direction of flow and then carefully moves the ultrasound beam across the image plane and in the elevational plane to obtain the highest-velocity signal, thus indicating the most parallel alignment with flow. Note that the optimal window for Doppler interrogation is when the ultrasound beam and flowstream are parallel, whereas the optimal window for diameter measurement is when the ultrasound beam and tissue-blood interfaces are perpendicular.

Fourth, it is crucial that the diameter and velocity measurements be made at the same anatomic site because the cross-sectional area and flow-velocity curves must be temporally and spatially congruent for accurate volume flow rate calculations. As the cross-sectional area of flow narrows or expands, flow velocity will increase or decrease correspondingly, so that conjoining information from two different anatomic sites will result in erroneous stroke volume data. Similarly, dynamic changes in stroke volume occur with changes in heart rate, loading conditions, exercise, and so on, so that measurements made at disparate times cannot be combined. In clinical practice, diameter and velocity recordings are made in close sequence and are repeated if any question of an interval physiologic change exists.

Sites for Stroke Volume Measurement

Stroke volume can be measured by this approach at any intracardiac site where both cross-sectional area and the flow-velocity integral can be recorded, given the assumptions of laminar flow and a flat flow profile.

Left Ventricular Outflow

The standard site for stroke volume measurement is the LV outflow tract at the level of the aortic annulus just proximal to the valve leaflets. The LV outflow tract offers several advantages: (1) the spatial flow profile is relatively flat because of tapering geometry and flow acceleration, (2) the needed data can be recorded in nearly all patients, and (3) flow remains laminar proximal to a stenosis (allowing transaortic stroke volume calculations in patients with aortic valve disease). LV outflow tract diameter is measured in a parasternal long-axis view parallel and immediately adjacent to the aortic valve, in mid-systole, from the white-black edge of the septal endocardium to the black-white edge of the anterior mitral leaflet (Fig. 6.14). Pulsed Doppler is used from an apical approach to record the velocity curve, by using the closing click of the aortic valve to ensure that the sample volume is located at the annulus (the same site as the diameter measurement). The small region of flow convergence proximal to the narrowed aortic valve is avoided by moving the sample volume slightly apically until a narrow spectral width is seen at the velocity peak.

On TEE imaging, outflow tract diameter is measured in a long-axis view with improved accuracy because of the higher-resolution images on TEE. LV outflow velocity sometimes may be recorded from a transgastric apical view or, starting from a transgastric short-axis view, rotating the image plane 90° to the two-chamber view and then turning the transducer slightly medially to visualize the LV outflow tract. However, it is difficult to ensure a parallel intercept angle between the ultrasound beam and LV outflow, so underestimation of stroke volume is likely.

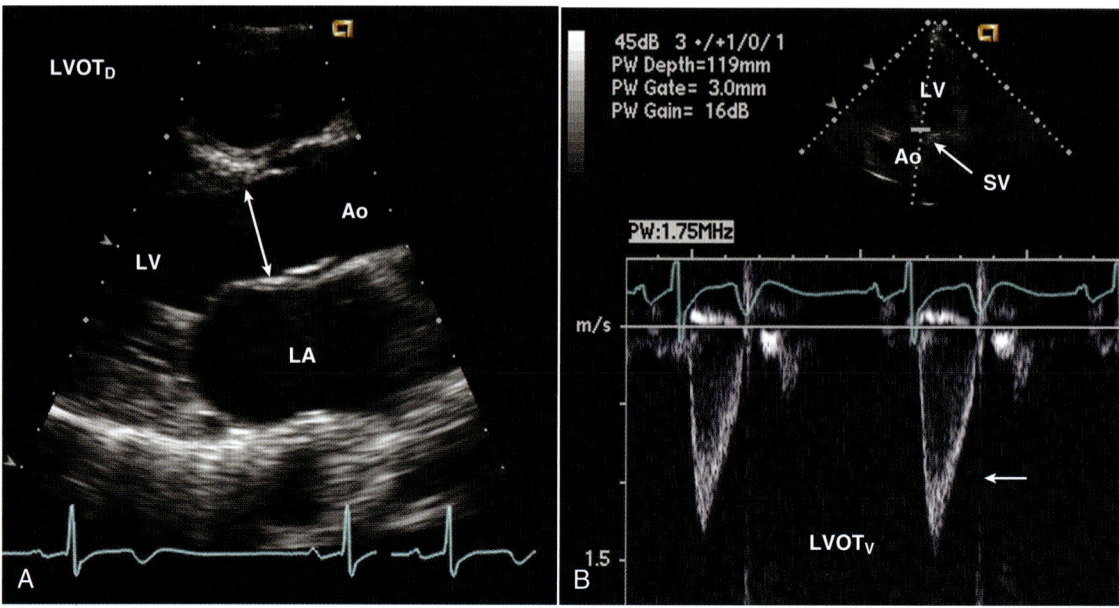

Fig. 6.14 **Doppler left ventricular outflow stroke volume calculation.** (A) LV outflow tract diameter *(LVOT$_D$)* measurement from a parasternal long-axis view and (B) the pulsed Doppler recording of LV outflow just proximal to the aortic valve *(Ao)* from an apical approach for stroke volume calculation. The aortic valve closing click *(arrow)* on the outflow tract velocity *(LVOT$_V$)* recording ensures that the sample volume *(SV)* location is immediately adjacent to the valve, corresponding with the site of outflow tract diameter measurement.

LV stroke volume also can be measured in the ascending aorta with diameter measured from a parasternal long-axis view and the flow-velocity curve recorded from either an apical or a suprasternal notch window. If continuous-wave (CW) Doppler ultrasound is used, the highest velocities along the path of the beam will be recorded, so the narrowest segment of the aorta (the sinotubular junction) is used for diameter measurements. If pulsed Doppler is used, the aortic diameter measurement should correspond to the Doppler sample volume location. Note that if aortic valve disease is present, stroke volume measurement in the ascending aorta will be inaccurate because of nonlaminar flow distal to the valve.

Mitral Valve

Transmitral stroke volume calculations assume that the mitral annulus is the limiting cross-sectional flow area, with the leaflets moving passively in response to the flowstream. Transmitral stroke volume is calculated as the product of the cross-sectional annulus area and the velocity-time integral of flow recorded at the mitral annulus level. On TEE imaging, transmitral flow rate is measured in the four-chamber view with the pulsed Doppler sample volume placed at the annulus level and the diameter measured from the 2D image (Fig. 6.15). Although the mitral annulus is most accurately described as a curved ellipse with the major (more apical) axis seen in the four-chamber view and the minor (more basal) axis seen in the long-axis view, for most clinical applications, the mitral annulus is assumed to be circular. Mitral annulus diameter can be measured in a parasternal long-axis view, which has the advantage of using axial resolution (which improves accuracy) but the disadvantage of ambiguity in the correct measurement location because the site of Doppler recording must be estimated. Alternatively, diameter can be measured in the apical four-chamber view, which has as the advantage that diameter can be measured on the same image that displays the sample volume (ensuring a correct measurement site) but the disadvantage of lateral resolution, which limits the accuracy of the measurement.

Right Heart

Stroke volume can be calculated by analogous methods in the pulmonary artery or across the tricuspid valve (Fig. 6.16). In adult patients, use of the pulmonary artery site on TTE imaging often is limited by poor image quality, which results in unobtainable or inaccurate pulmonary artery diameter measurements. However, from a TEE approach, pulmonary artery flow and diameter often can be measured using a very high transducer position looking from the pulmonary artery bifurcation toward the pulmonic valve.

Differences in Transvalvular Volume Flow Rates

In a normal heart, stroke volume across each of the four valves is equal, and measurement at more than

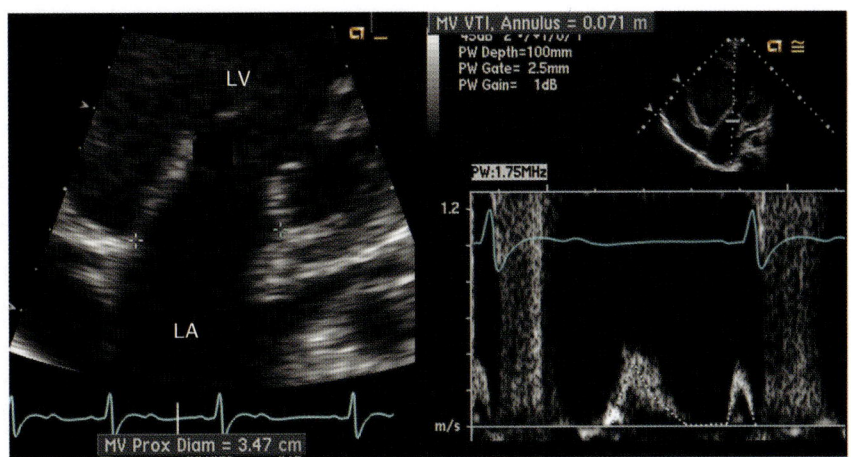

Fig. 6.15 Doppler transmitral stroke volume calculation. The mitral valve *(MV)* annulus area in diastole is multiplied by the velocity-time integral *(VTI)* of flow at the annulus. In this example, annulus diameter *(left)* is 3.5 cm, so the circular cross-sectional area is 9.6 cm². The velocity-time integral of transmitral flow is 7.7 cm for a stroke volume of 74 mL or a cardiac output of 4.4 L/min at a heart rate of 60 bpm.

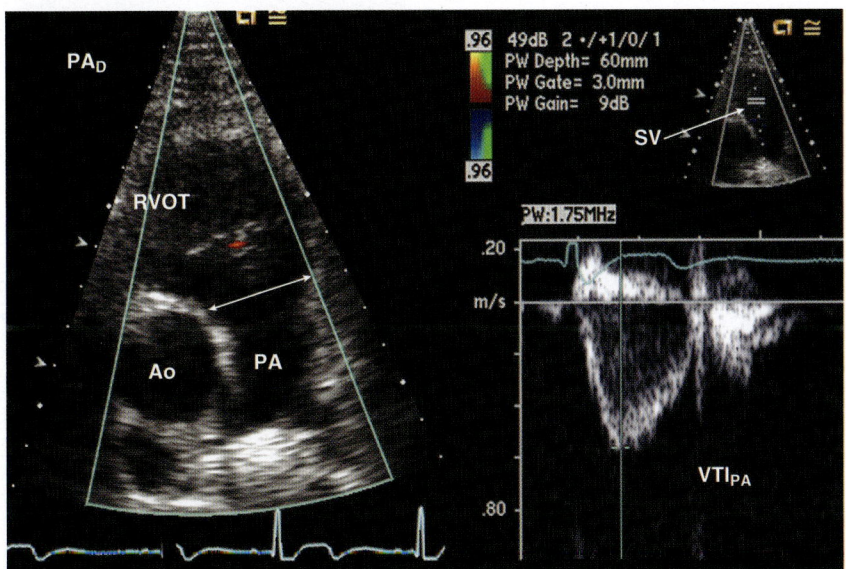

Fig. 6.16 Doppler stroke volume in the pulmonary artery. Diameter is measured in a parasternal RV outflow view *(RVOT; left)* and pulsed Doppler pulmonary artery *(PA)* flow recorded from a parasternal approach *(right)* for transpulmonic stroke volume *(SV)* calculation. PA_D, pulmonary artery diameter; VTI_{PA}, pulmonary artery velocity-time integral.

one site only serves as an internal accuracy check. However, in the presence of valvular regurgitation or an intracardiac shunt, calculation of stroke volume at two intracardiac sites allows quantitation of the degree of regurgitation or pulmonic-to-systemic shunt ratio, as detailed in Chapters 12 and 17.

Other Doppler Measures of Systolic Function

Ejection Acceleration Times

In addition to stroke volume calculations, the shape of the Doppler ejection curve provides information about ventricular function. When systolic function is normal, the isovolumic contraction period is short, and the rate of pressure rise in early systole is rapid. These features are reflected in the Doppler velocity curve, which shows a short isovolumic contraction time, a rapid acceleration of blood in early systole, and a short time interval from the onset of flow to maximum velocity. With impaired LV systolic function, the isovolumic contraction time (also known as the pre-ejection period) becomes progressively longer, the rate of acceleration diminishes, and the time to maximum velocity increases, with all these changes mirrored in the Doppler velocity curve. In addition to measuring these variables at rest, some centers have found evaluation of aortic ejection curves with exercise useful in detection of LV systolic dysfunction.

Rate of Ventricular Pressure Rise (dP/dt)

When mitral regurgitation is present, the CW Doppler velocity curve indicates the instantaneous pressure difference between the LV and the LA in systole, assuming a constant intercept angle between the mitral regurgitant jet and the ultrasound beam. Given the rapid rate of rise of LV pressure with normal systolic function (and the low LA pressure), mitral regurgitation typically shows a rapid rise to maximum velocity as per the Bernoulli equation. If the rate of rise in ventricular pressure is reduced because of LV systolic dysfunction, the rate of increase in velocity of the mitral regurgitant jet also is reduced. For example, in patients with premature ventricular beats, the altered contractility of the premature beat is evidenced by a marked difference in the rate of velocity increase of the mitral regurgitant jet.

ECHO MATH: Left Ventricular dP/dt

The slope of the mitral regurgitant jet can be quantitated as the rate of change in pressure over time *(dP/dt)* by measuring the time interval between the mitral regurgitant jet velocity at 1 and at 3 m/s (Fig. 6.17). At each velocity, the corresponding pressure gradient is $4v^2$ per the Bernoulli equation. Then,

$$dP/dt = [4(3)^2 - 4(1)^2]/\text{time interval} \quad \text{(Eq. 6.13)}$$
$$= 32 \text{ mmHg/time interval}$$

Thus a longer time interval indicates a depressed *dP/dt*, and vice versa. Of course, the calculation of *dP/dt* can be performed only when a recordable mitral regurgitant jet is present and assumes a constant (and parallel) intercept angle between the mitral regurgitant jet and the ultrasound beam during the measurement period.

For example, if the time interval is 36 ms (0.036 seconds) between the points on the mitral regurgitant velocity curve at 1 and 3 m/s,

$$dP/dt = [4(3)^2 - 4(1)^2]/0.036 \text{ s} = 32 \text{ mmHg}/0.036 \text{ s}$$
$$= 889 \text{ mmHg/s}$$

which is mildly reduced (normal >1000 mmHg/s).

Limitations and Alternate Approaches

The major limitation of Doppler evaluation of LV systolic function in adults is accurate diameter measurement for cross-sectional area calculations. Although

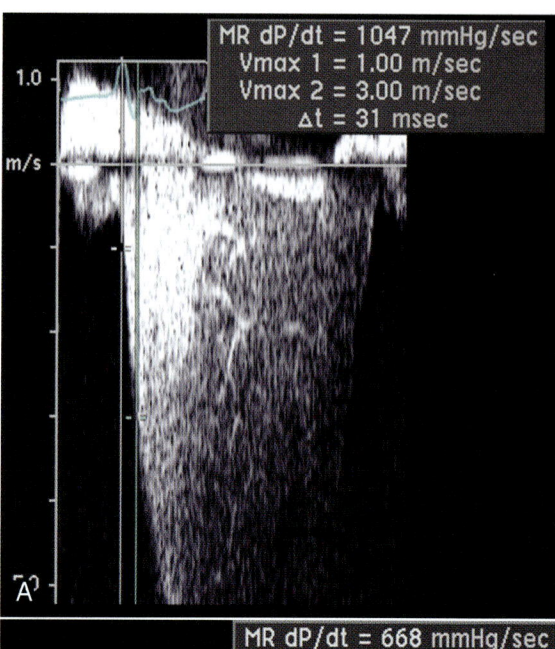
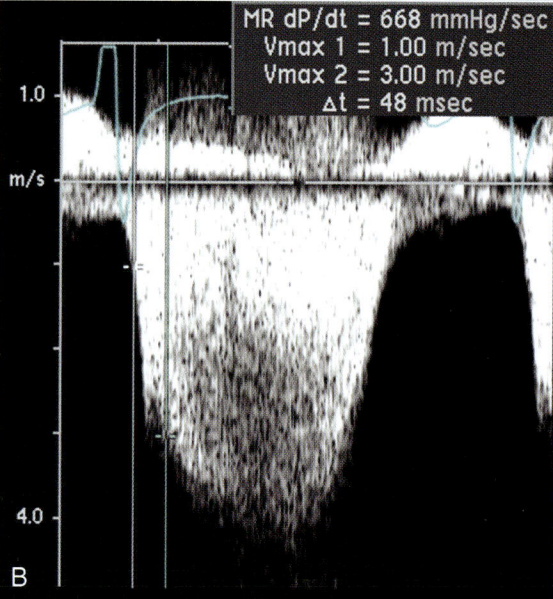

Fig. 6.17 Left ventricular *dP/dt*. The time interval between 1 and 3 m/s on the mitral regurgitant *(MR)* velocity curve is measured with the scale expanded to optimize accuracy. Examples of (A) normal ventricular systolic function (*dP/dt* >1000 mmHg/s) and (B) the slow rate of rise in mitral regurgitant velocity in a patient with dilated cardiomyopathy, corresponding to a *dP/dt* of 668 mmHg/s, are shown by the parallel vertical lines.

Doppler velocity curves can be recorded consistently with little interobserver measurement variability (2% to 5%), the variability of 2D diameter measurements is significantly greater (8% to 12%). For Doppler velocity data, the major source of measurement variability is data recording, given the critical importance of obtaining a parallel intercept angle between the ultrasound beam and the flow of interest. For 2D diameters, the major source of variability is measuring the 2D images, particularly when image quality is suboptimal or when lateral resolution limits accurate border recognition. Despite these potential limitations, Doppler measurement of stroke volume has been well validated in a variety of clinical and research settings.

Measurement of *dP/dt* is limited by the need for enough mitral regurgitation to generate a Doppler signal with a well-defined velocity curve. Changes during ejection in the intercept angle between the ultrasound beam and the regurgitant jet will result in an erroneous measurement because the assumption that $\cos\theta = 1$ in the Doppler equation will not be valid.

When more precise or repeated measures of flow are needed, cardiac output can be measured by the thermodilution or Fick techniques through a right-sided heart catheter both in the catheterization laboratory and in the coronary care unit.

ECHO APPROACH TO RIGHT VENTRICULAR SYSTOLIC FUNCTION

The normal shape of the RV is complex in 3D, with the inflow segment located medial to the LV, the body and apex located anterior to the LV, and the RV outflow tract located superior to the LV and aortic valve (Fig. 6.18). No simple geometric shape approximates the RV chamber; rather, it is "wrapped around" the LV in a U-shaped fashion. Because echocardiographic long- and short-axis views are oriented with respect to the LV, the RV appears abnormal in some individuals because of an oblique image plane compared with the position of the RV, particularly from the parasternal window. Both subcostal and apical four-chamber windows tend to offer more consistent views of the RV, with the RV appearing somewhat triangular, with a broad base and narrow apex. The RV apex is slightly closer to the base than the LV apex (by about one third of the LV length) in normal individuals.

On TTE 2D imaging, the RV is evaluated from several different windows:

- Parasternal long- and short-axis
- RV inflow
- Apical four-chamber
- Subcostal four-chamber

On TEE imaging, similar views are obtained including the high TEE four-chamber view, a TEE short-axis view obtained by rotating the image plane to about 90°, and the transgastric RV inflow view. In each view on either TTE or TEE imaging, evaluation of the RV includes:

- Area of the chamber (relative to the LV chamber)
- Shape of the RV cavity
- Wall thickness
- Motion of the RV free wall
- Ventricular septal curvature and motion

Right Ventricle Size

With RV dilation, the RV outflow tract may be enlarged in the parasternal and TEE long-axis view. On apical and subcostal views and TEE transgastric views, the RV chamber is larger, and the RV apex is either closer to or encompasses the LV apex. The degree of RV dilation is best evaluated in the apical or subcostal four-chamber view in relation to the size of the LV, while taking into consideration any abnormalities in LV size. Qualitatively, RV size is described as:

- Normal (smaller than LV with RV apex more basal than LV apex)
- Mildly dilated (enlarged but RV < LV area)
- Moderately dilated (RV = LV area)
- Severely dilated (RV > LV area)

Quantitative end-diastolic 2D echocardiographic measurements for quantitation of RV size (Fig. 6.19 and Table 6.4) include:

- Basal and mid-RV dimensions measured in the four-chamber view
- RV wall thickness measured on the subcostal view
- RV outflow tract proximal and distal diameters measured in parasternal views

RV dilation is the normal response of the ventricle to volume overload, and its presence mandates a careful search for etiology, such as an atrial septal defect, tricuspid regurgitation, or pulmonic regurgitation.

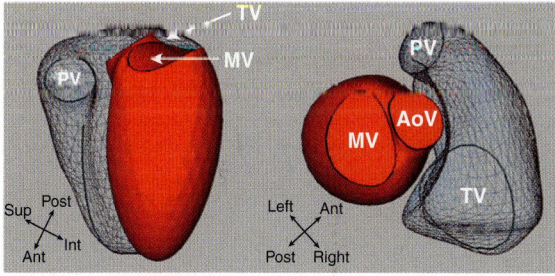

Fig. 6.18 Anatomy of the normal right ventricle. *Left,* Left lateral view. *Right,* Basal view. Endocardial surfaces were generated by reconstruction using 3D echo and knowledge-based reconstruction. The hollow mesh is the RV endocardial surface; the solid red is that of the LV. The RV is crescentic in short-axis section, with tricuspid and pulmonic valve orifices widely separated by the crista supraventricularis. *Ant,* Anterior; *AoV,* aortic valve; *Inf,* inferior; *MV,* mitral valve; *Post,* posterior; *PV,* pulmonic valve; *Sup,* superior; *TV,* tricuspid valve. (Images courtesy Dr. Florence H. Sheehan, University of Washington Cardiovascular Research and Training Center. From Kurtz C: Right ventricular anatomy, function, and echocardiographic evaluation. In Otto CM, editor: The Practice of Clinical Echocardiography, ed 5, Philadelphia, 2017, Elsevier, p 620.)

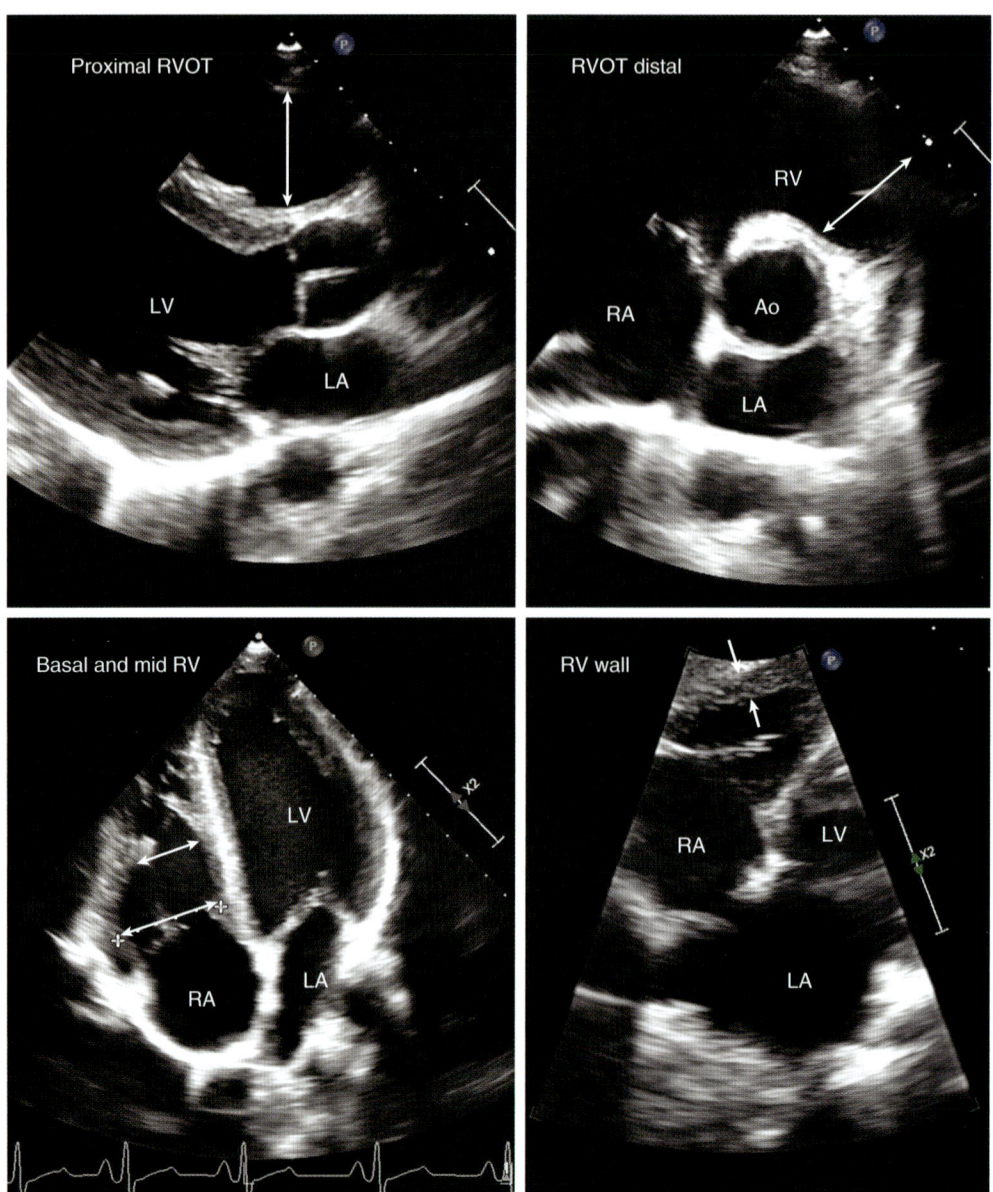

Fig. 6.19 Standard 2D right ventricle views and measurements. Evaluation of RV size and systolic function is based on multiple views including the parasternal long-axis *(upper left)* ▶ and short-axis *(upper right)* ▶ apical four-chamber *(lower left)* ▶ views angulated to focus on the RV and the subcostal four-chamber view *(lower right)* ▶. Standard measurements (*arrows* in each view) include the proximal and distal RV outflow tract *(RVOT)*, the basal and mid-RV diameters at end-diastole, and the RV free wall thickness, as shown. *Ao,* Aorta.

Pressure overload of the RV also leads to dilation, so evaluation of pulmonary pressures is mandatory when the RV is abnormal.

RV hypertrophy is manifested as an RV free wall thickness >0.5 cm. RV wall thickness is best measured by 2D or 2D-guided M-mode in a subcostal four-chamber view at the tricuspid chordal level at the peak of the R wave on the electrocardiogram. Epicardial fat and myocardial trabeculations are excluded from this measurement. The presence of RV hypertrophy suggests RV pressure overload and prompts a search for evidence of elevated pulmonary pressures or pulmonic valve stenosis. Increased thickness of the RV free wall also is seen in some infiltrative cardiomyopathies or in hypertrophic cardiomyopathy.

Right Ventricular Systolic Function

RV systolic function is evaluated qualitatively as:

- Normal
- Mildly reduced
- Moderately reduced
- Severely reduced

TABLE 6.4 American Society of Echocardiography and European Association of Cardiovascular Imaging Recommendations for Right Ventricular Chamber Quantification

Parameter	Recommended Measurements	Comments	Reference Values
RV size	• RV linear ED internal dimensions at base and mid-RV (apical views) • RV outflow tract ED diameter proximally and at pulmonic annulus (parasternal views) • 2D imaging from multiple acoustic window • 3D RV volumes	• Both qualitative and quantitative measures should be routinely assessed on all diagnostic echo studies. • End-diastolic diameter, inner edge to inner edge (white-black interface) Recommended when feasible depending on image quality. Not routine in most laboratories.	*Upper limits of normal RV size* Basal RV <42 mm Mid-RV <36 mm Proximal RVOT <36 mm Distal RVOT <28 mm
RV wall thickness	Linear measurement of RV free wall on subcostal view	Zoomed image at ED	*Normal RV wall thickness* 1–5 mm
RV systolic function	RIMP	Measure IVCT, IVRT, and ET from same heartbeat using pulsed Doppler or DTI of tricuspid annulus.	*Normal RIMP* PW Doppler <0.42 DTI <0.53
	TAPSE	Reflects longitudinal RV systolic function. Measured by M-mode of tricuspid annulus.	*Normal TAPSE* 15 mm or higher
	RV 2D FAC	2D area of RV at ED and ES in apical view Include trabeculations, papillary muscles and moderator band in cavity area.	*Normal FAC* 35% or higher
	DTI annular systolic velocity	S' velocity is easy to measure, reliable, and reproducible	*Normal S'* 10 cm/s or greater
	RV speckle tracking longitudinal strain	Promising approach, but additional normative data are needed.	
	3D RV ejection fraction	Helpful in experienced laboratories.	*Normal RV 3D EF* 45% or higher

DTI, Doppler tissue imaging; *ED*, end-diastole; *EF*, ejection fraction; *ES*, end-systole; *ET*, ejection time; *FAC*, fractional area change; *IVCT*, isovolumic contraction time; *IVRT*, isovolumic relaxation time; *PW*, pulsed wave; *RIMP*, RV index of myocardial performance; *RVOT*, RV outflow tract; *TAPSE*, tricuspid annular plane systolic excursion.
Summarized from American Society of Echocardiography and European Association of Cardiovascular Imaging Recommendations published in 2015 in Lang RM, Badano LP, Mor-Avi V, et al: Recommendations for cardiac chamber quantification by echocardiography in adults: an update from the American Society of Echocardiography and the European Association of Cardiovascular Imaging, *J Am Soc Echocardiogr* 28(1):1–39.e14, 2015.

When ventricular systolic function is normal, the relative function of the two ventricles can be compared. When LV systolic function is depressed, the severity of LV dysfunction is used as an index of RV function (e.g., a normal RV compared with a reduced LV ejection fraction appears hyperdynamic). If both ventricles have a similar qualitative pattern of contraction, the degree of RV dysfunction will be similar to the degree of LV dysfunction.

Quantitative evaluation of RV systolic function is challenging. Standard geometric formulas for volume calculations have only limited applicability given the shape of the RV and 3D methods require further evaluation. Instead, clinical evaluation is based on simpler measures including:

- Tricuspid annular plane systolic excursion (TAPSE)
- RV fractional area change
- Tissue Doppler peak systolic velocity at the tricuspid annulus
- Pulsed or tissue Doppler myocardial performance index

TAPSE measures RV longitudinal shortening based on the distance the tricuspid annulus moves toward the RV apex from end-diastole to end-systole. TAPSE

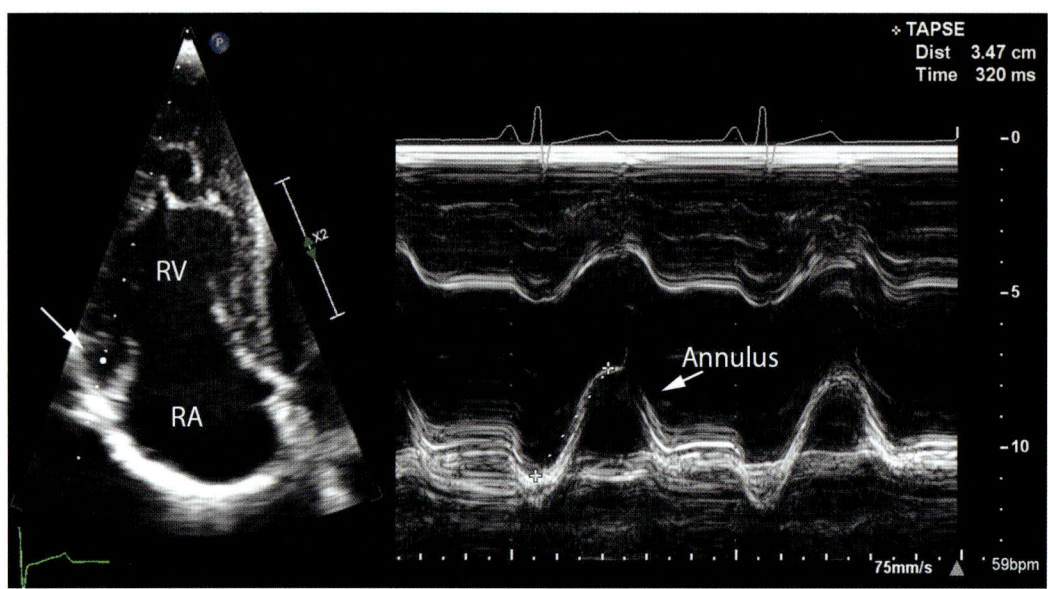

Fig. 6.20 Tricuspid annular systolic plane excursion. From an apical view focused on the RV *(left)*, an M-line cursor is placed through the lateral tricuspid annulus *(arrow)*. The M-mode tracing *(right)* allows measurement of the vertical distance between the end-diastolic and end-systolic position of the annulus *(white and green lines)*. *TAPSE,* Tricuspid annular systolic plane excursion.

is measured from an RV-optimized apical four-chamber view, with an M-mode intersecting the lateral tricuspid annulus (Fig. 6.20). RV fractional area change is measured by tracing the RV endocardial borders at end-diastole and end-systole in the apical four-chamber view, while taking care to include the RV apex and lateral wall in the image plane (Fig. 6.21). The tissue Doppler annular velocity signal (Fig. 6.22) allows measurement of the peak systolic velocity (with a measurement over 10 cm/s indicating normal RV systolic function).

ECHO MATH: RV Index of Myocardial Performance

The RV index of myocardial performance (RIMP) is the ratio of isovolumic contraction time (IVCT) plus isovolumic relaxation time (IVRT) divided by ejection time (ET):

$$RIMP = (IVCT_{RV} + IVRT_{RV})/ET \quad \text{(Eq. 6.14)}$$

RIMP can be measured using intervals measured from conventional pulsed Doppler or from the Doppler tissue imaging signal with time intervals measured on the same heartbeat. Ejection time is measured as the pulmonic systolic flow duration or as the tissue Doppler systolic velocity duration. Tricuspid valve closure time (TCO) is measured as the total duration of tricuspid regurgitation or as the interval between the end of the tissue Doppler A' velocity and the onset of the next E' velocity. Tricuspid valve closure time includes RV ejection time (ET_{RV}) plus isovolumic relaxation (IVR_{RV}) and isovolumic contraction (IVC_{RV}):

$$TCO = IVC_{RV} + IVR_{RV} + ET_{RV} \quad \text{(Eq. 6.15)}$$

so that

$$TCO - ET_{RV} = IVC_{RV} + IVR_{RV} \quad \text{(Eq. 6.16)}$$

Thus,

$$RIMP = (TCO - ET)/ET \quad \text{(Eq. 6.17)}$$

For example, if the ejection time is 300 ms and the tricuspid closure time is 430 ms,

$$RIMP = (430 - 300)/430 = 0.30$$

which indicates normal RV systolic function. Abnormal RV function is indicated by an RIMP >0.43 by pulsed and > 0.54 by tissue Doppler.

Patterns of Ventricular Septal Motion

The interventricular septum functions as part of the LV in the normal heart. During diastole, the LV is circular in a short-axis view, with the normal septal curvature convex toward the RV and concave toward the LV. With the onset of systole, the septal myocardium thickens, and the septal endocardium moves toward the center of the LV such that at end-systole the short-axis image shows a circular LV chamber.

Several cardiac disorders alter the pattern of ventricular septal motion, the most prominent being RV pressure and volume overload. The basic principle

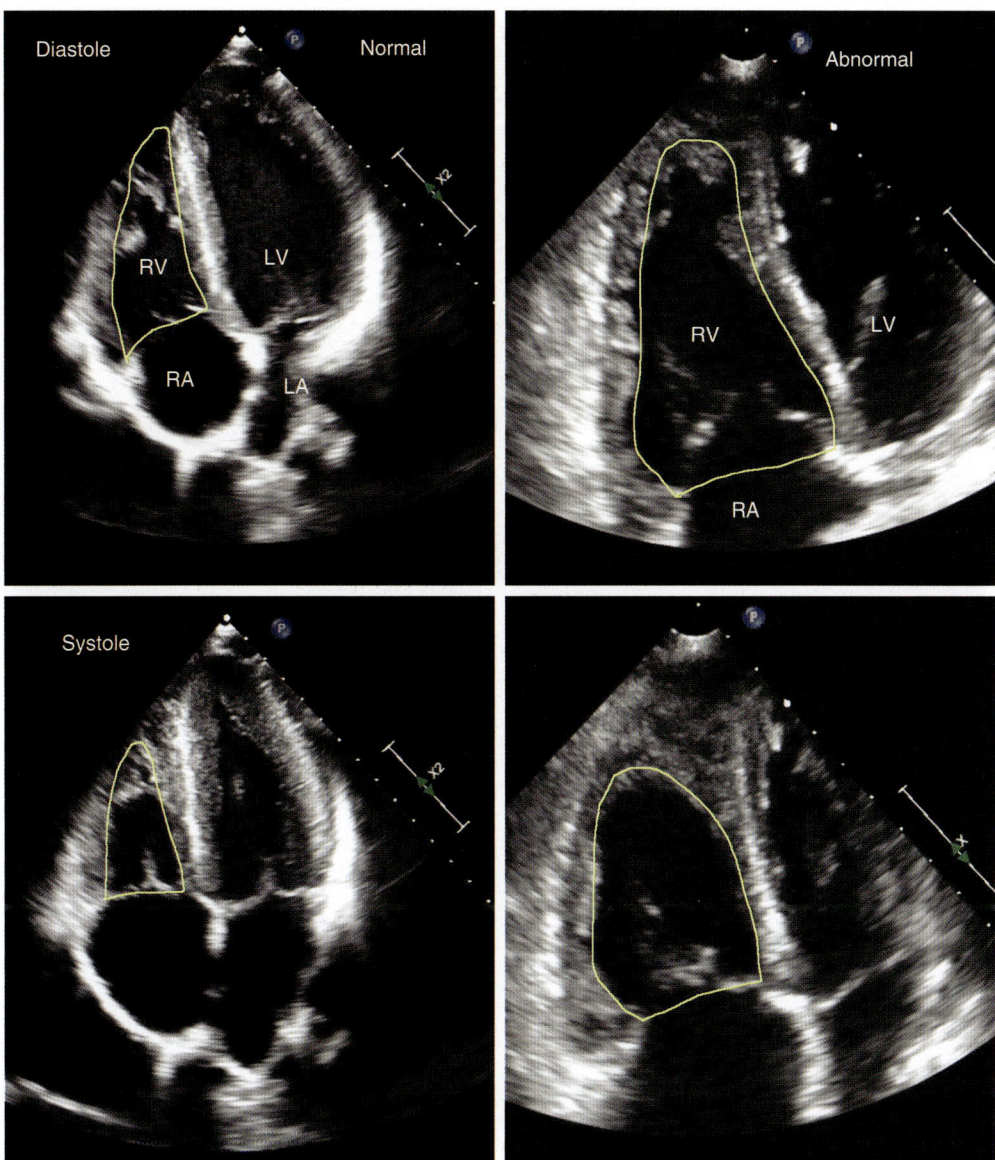

Fig. 6.21 Right ventricular fractional area change. In the apical four-chamber view, the end-diastolic *(top)* and end-systolic *(bottom)* RV areas are traced to calculate fractional area change in a patient with normal RV size and systolic function *(left)* ▶ and a patient with a dilated, hypertrophied, and hypocontractile RV *(right)*. ▶

underlying the pattern of septal motion with RV dilation or hypertrophy is that the septum moves toward the center of mass of the entire heart. Normally, the center of cardiac mass coincides with the center of the LV. When RV and LV masses are equal, septal motion is "flat" (on M-mode) or minimal (on 2D echo). When RV mass exceeds LV mass, the septum moves "paradoxically" anterior in systole (on M-mode) and flattens or reverses its curvature in diastole (on 2D echo) (Fig. 6.23).

On 2D echocardiography, pressure overload of the RV (increased mass as a result of increased wall thickness with a nondilated chamber) results in a leftward shift of septal motion throughout the cardiac cycle with the maximum reversed curvature at end-systole. With predominant RV volume overload, the maximum reversed curvature is seen in mid-diastole with normalization of curvature in systole. With increased RV mass resulting from volume overload, the additional factor of increased RV filling and emptying accentuates the diastolic reverse motion of the septum (because of rapid RV diastolic filling), resulting in a D shape of the LV chamber in early diastole, with the reversed curvature of the septum persisting throughout diastole. Anterior motion with systole appears less prominent than with isolated pressure overload as the septum moves from its abnormal diastolic position back toward the center

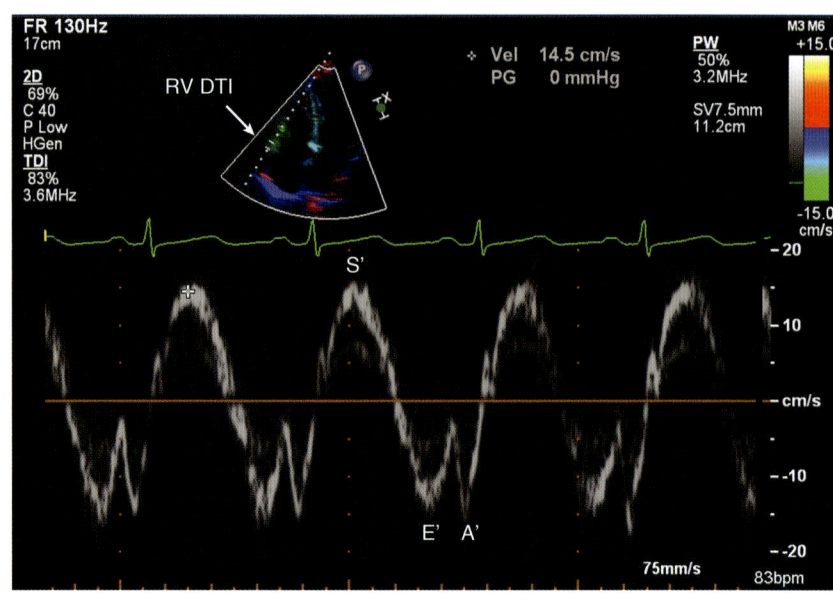

Fig. 6.22 Right ventricular annular tissue Doppler imaging. In an apical four-chamber view angled toward the right heart, a Doppler sample volume is placed about 1 cm apical to the tricuspid annulus (arrow). Tissue Doppler imaging (TDI) shows apical motion toward the transducer in systole (S′) with a normal velocity over 10 cm/s, as in this example. In diastole, E′ and A′ tissue Doppler velocities are seen, analogous to those seen on mitral TDI recordings.

of the heart, thereby resulting in a more convex curve relative to the RV chamber. Often, the observation of abnormal septal motion during the examination is the first clue of RV pressure, volume overload, or both.

Other abnormalities that affect the pattern of ventricular septal motion are summarized in Fig. 6.24. Conduction defects affect the pattern of motion by altering the sequence of RV and LV contraction. Valvular disease can affect the timing of RV versus LV diastolic filling, particularly in early diastole. Pericardial tamponade or constriction results in a fixed total cardiac volume so that respiratory changes in RV filling result in respiratory shifts in the pattern of septal motion.

An abnormal pattern of septal motion may be appreciated on 2D imaging; however, M-mode echo offers more detailed time resolution for studying the pattern of motion. Abnormal septal motion rarely is diagnostic in and of itself, but it may raise a diagnostic possibility that had not been considered previously or support a suspected diagnosis. For example, a pattern of paradoxical septal motion in association with RV and right atrial (RA) enlargement suggests the possibility of an atrial septal defect. This possibility then can be specifically excluded (or confirmed) during the echocardiographic examination. Another example is the patient with a pericardial effusion; in this situation a changing pattern of septal motion with respiration supports a diagnosis of tamponade physiology.

Limitations and Alternate Approaches

Echocardiographic measures of RV size and systolic function generally are adequate in most clinical situations, despite the challenges related to RV geometry and image quality. However, when precise measurements are needed, alternate approaches are appropriate. Cardiac magnetic resonance imaging provides accurate measurement of RV volumes and ejection fraction and is increasingly used when these measurements are needed for clinical decision making, particularly in adults with congenital heart disease. RV contrast angiography can be performed at catheterization, but wide variability in the appearance of the normal RV has been observed. Radionuclide ventriculography can be used to derive an RV ejection fraction.

PULMONARY VASCULATURE

Pulmonary Systolic Pressure Estimates

Clinically, one of the most important quantitative parameters affecting RV systolic function is pulmonary artery pressure or resistance. Pulmonary hypertension often occurs in response to chronic left-sided heart diseases, such as mitral stenosis, mitral regurgitation, cardiomyopathy, and ischemic cardiac disease, but it also occurs in patients with pulmonary disease or primary pulmonary hypertension. Knowledge of the degree of pulmonary pressure elevation is critical in patient management and is a key component of the echocardiographic examination (Table 6.5).

Tricuspid Regurgitant Velocity

The most reliable method for estimating pulmonary artery pressures noninvasively is based on measurement of the velocity in the tricuspid regurgitant jet.

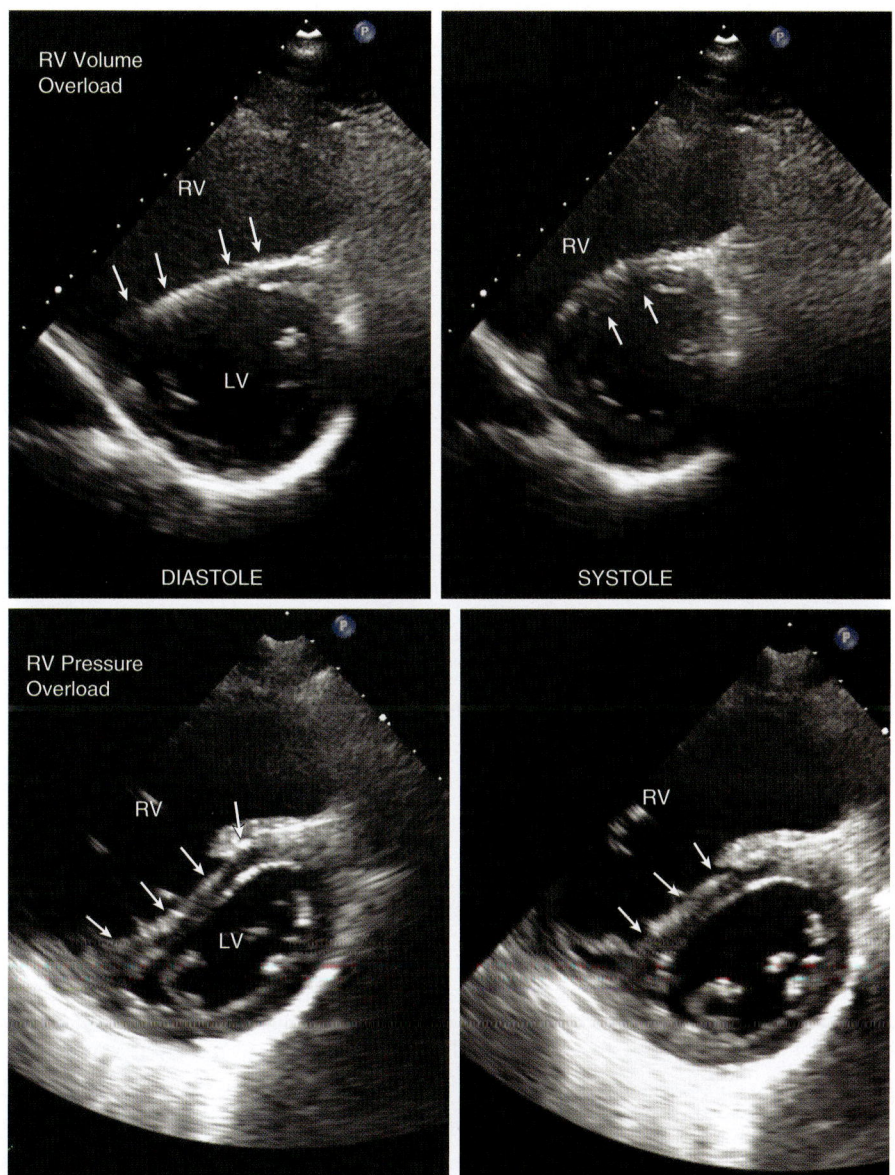

Fig. 6.23 Paradoxical septal motion. *(Top)* In a patient with RV volume overload ▶ due to severe tricuspid regurgitation, the parasternal short-axis view shows a dilated RV with a flat contour of the septum in diastole *(arrows)* but with a normal sepal contour and round appearance of the LV chamber in systole. *(Bottom)* In contrast, with RV pressure overload caused by primary pulmonary hypertension, ▶ although the diastolic image is similar to the volume-overloaded RV, with a markedly dilated RV with reverse curvature of the normal septal contour *(arrows)*, the systolic image shows persistent flattening of the septal contour, with a D-shaped LV in both systole and diastole.

TABLE 6.5 Doppler Echo Methods for Estimation of Right Heart Pressures

	Method	Advantages	Potential Limitations
Systolic PA pressure	Tricuspid regurgitant jet: $PAP_{systolic} = 4(V_{TR})^2 + RAP$	• Accurate • Measurable in a high percentage of patients overall (90%)	• Underestimation because of nonparallel intercept angle or inadequate signal strength • Overestimation because of measurement outside well-defined spectral envelope or misidentification of jet signal • Presence of pulmonic stenosis where RV pressure is greater than PA pressure • RA pressure estimate needed
Diastolic PA pressure	PR end-diastolic velocity (V): $PAP_{diastolic} = 4(V_{PR})^2 + RAP$	• Reflects pulmonary diastolic pressure • Adequate signal in 85% of patients	• Nonparallel intercept angle between jet and ultrasound beam • RA pressure estimate needed
Mean PA pressure	TR jet tracing for mean RV to RA pressure gradient plus RA pressure estimate PA acceleration time	• Mean PA pressure is more accurate for identification of pulmonary hypertension. • Readily measured in nearly all patients, including patients with chronic lung disease • Estimates *mean* PA pressure	• Nonparallel intercept angle between jet and ultrasound beam • Inadequate signal in some patients • Skewed flow profile in PA • Measurement variability
RA pressure	IVC diameter and change with respiration or sniff	• Obtainable from subcostal window in most patients • Reliably identifies normal versus severely elevated RA pressure	• IVC collapse not accurate for RA pressure estimates in patients on mechanical ventilation • Less reliable for intermediate values of RA pressure

IVC, Inferior vena cava; *PA*, pulmonary artery; *RA*, right artrial; *TR*, tricuspid regurgitation.

ECHO MATH: Estimated Pulmonary Systolic Pressure

The tricuspid regurgitant velocity V_{TR} reflects the RV to RA pressure difference ΔP, as stated in the Bernoulli equation (Fig. 6.25):

$$\Delta P_{RV-RA} = 4(V_{TR})^2 \quad \text{(Eq. 6.18)}$$

When added to an estimate of RA pressure, RV systolic pressure (RVP) is obtained:

$$RVP = \Delta P_{RV-RA} + RAP \quad \text{(Eq. 6.19)}$$

In the absence of pulmonic stenosis (which is rare in adults), RV systolic pressure equals pulmonary artery systolic pressure, so that:

$$RVP = PAP_{systolic} = 4(V_{TR})^2 + RAP \quad \text{(Eq. 6.20)}$$

as diagrammed in Fig. 6.25.

For example, with a tricuspid regurgitant velocity of 2.7 m/s and an estimated right atrial pressure of 10 mmHg,

$$\text{Estimated PA systolic pressure} = 4(2.7)^2 + 10 \text{ mmHg} = 39 \text{ mmHg}$$

When pulmonic stenosis (PS) is present, the peak gradient (ΔP_{PS}) is subtracted from the estimated RV systolic pressure:

$$PAP_{systolic} = [4(V_{TR})^2 + RAP] - \Delta P_{PS} \quad \text{(Eq. 6.21)}$$

Mean pulmonary systolic pressure can be estimated by tracing the tricuspid regurgitant jet velocity to obtain the mean RV to RA pressure difference in systole, which is then added to the estimated RA pressure:

$$PAP_{mean} = \text{Mean } \Delta P_{RV-RA} + RAP \quad \text{(Eq. 6.22)}$$

This method has been shown to be highly accurate compared with invasive measurements of pulmonary artery pressure over a wide range of values (Appendix B, Table B.4). Of course, the reliability of this approach is dependent on obtaining a parallel intercept angle between the tricuspid regurgitant jet and the ultrasound beam. Most often the apical or RV inflow view yields the highest-velocity signal given careful angulation of the ultrasound beam in 3D (Fig. 6.26). Occasionally, the highest-velocity tricuspid regurgitant jet is recorded

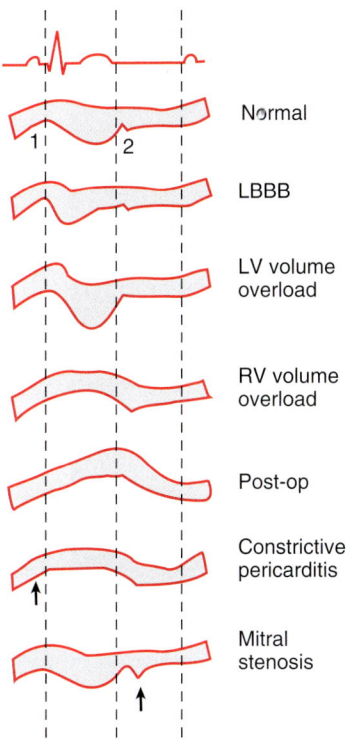

Fig. 6.24 Patterns of septal motion on M-mode echocardiography. The normal pattern is characterized by systolic brief anterior motion *(1)* followed by posterior motion and myocardial thickening. In diastole, a small diastolic dip *(2)* following mitral valve opening may be seen. Left bundle branch block *(LBBB)* is characterized by systolic rapid downward septal motion. LV volume overload results in exaggerated septal (and posterior wall) motion. RV volume overload results in paradoxical anterior motion of the septum in systole. A similar pattern is seen in patients after cardiac surgery *(Post-op)*. Constrictive pericarditis is characterized by anterior motion of the septum with atrial filling (before the QRS), whereas mitral stenosis typically shows a prominent early diastolic dip.

from a subcostal approach. Although this method requires the presence of tricuspid regurgitation, this rarely is a limitation because about 90% of normal individuals and patients have some degree of tricuspid regurgitation.

Pulmonic Regurgitant Velocity

The same concept can be applied to the pulmonic regurgitant velocity curve. The end-diastolic pulmonic regurgitant velocity (V_{PR}) reflects the pulmonary artery to RV end-diastolic pressure gradient per the Bernoulli equation. When added to an estimate of RA pressure, this provides a noninvasive estimate of diastolic pulmonary artery pressure (Fig. 6.27).

$$PAP_{diastolic} = 4(V_{PR})^2 + RAP \quad \text{(Eq. 6.23)}$$

Estimation of Right Atrial Pressure

RA pressure is best estimated from evaluation of the inferior vena cava during respiration (Fig. 6.28). From a subcostal window, this segment of the inferior vena cava is imaged during quiet respiration. If the inferior vena cava diameter is normal (≤2 cm diameter) and the segment adjacent to the RA collapses by at least 50% with respiration, then RA pressure is equal to normal intrathoracic pressures (i.e., 5 to 10 mmHg). Failure to collapse with respiration, dilation of the inferior vena cava and hepatic veins, or both is associated with higher RA pressures (Table 6.6). When no response is noted with normal respiration, the patient is asked to sniff. This generates a sudden decrease in intrathoracic pressure, normally resulting in a decrease in inferior vena cava diameter. Echocardiographic estimates of RA pressure are most accurate for normal and severely elevated pressures, so it is prudent to indicate a range of possible pressures for intermediate values.

Pulmonary Vascular Resistance

Pulmonary pressure is not an ideal measure of the vascular properties of the pulmonary bed because pressure is affected by volume flow rate (increased pressures with higher flow rates and vice versa) and by the LA pressure.

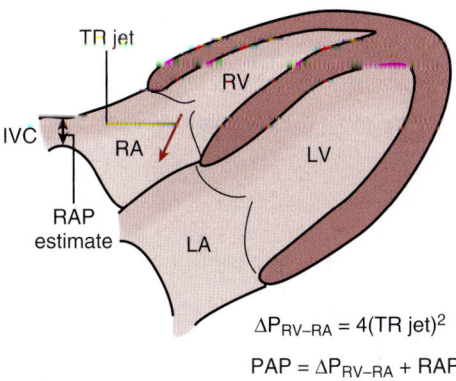

Fig. 6.25 Pulmonary artery pressure calculation. The velocity in the tricuspid regurgitant *(TR)* jet provides the RV-to-RA systolic pressure difference. Respiratory variation in inferior vena cava *(IVC)* size is used to estimate RA pressure *(RAP)*. PAP, Pulmonary artery pressure.

Pulmonary Artery Velocity Curve

LV ejection curves show very rapid acceleration with a short time from flow onset to maximum velocity, whereas RV ejection curves show slower acceleration, a longer time from onset of flow to peak flow, and a more "rounded" velocity curve. As pulmonary vascular resistance increases, the shape of the RV ejection curve more closely approximates an LV

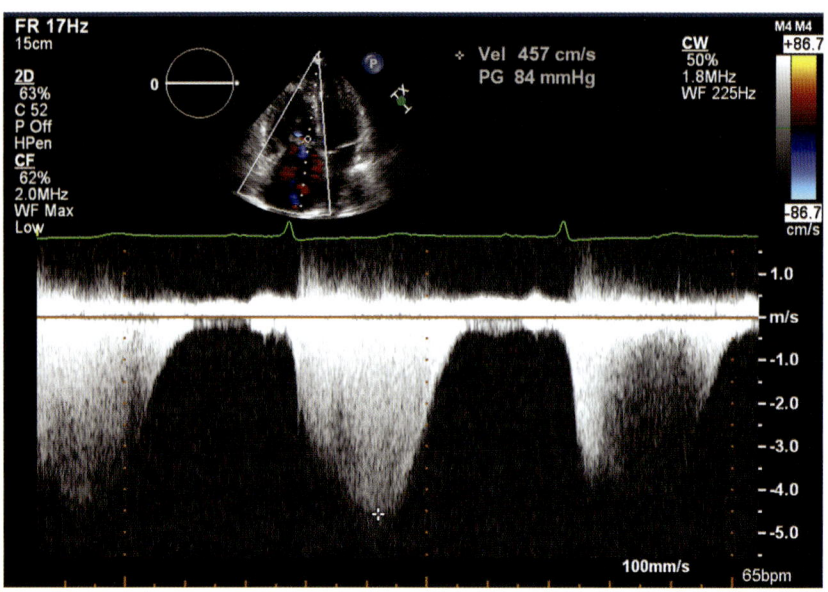

Fig. 6.26 Tricuspid regurgitant velocity for pulmonary artery pressure calculations. The tricuspid regurgitant jet is recorded with CW Doppler from the window yielding the highest velocity signal, the apical four-chamber view in this example, to calculate the peak RV-to-RA systolic pressure difference. The velocity curve also can be traced for calculation of the mean pressure difference for determination of mean pulmonary artery pressure.

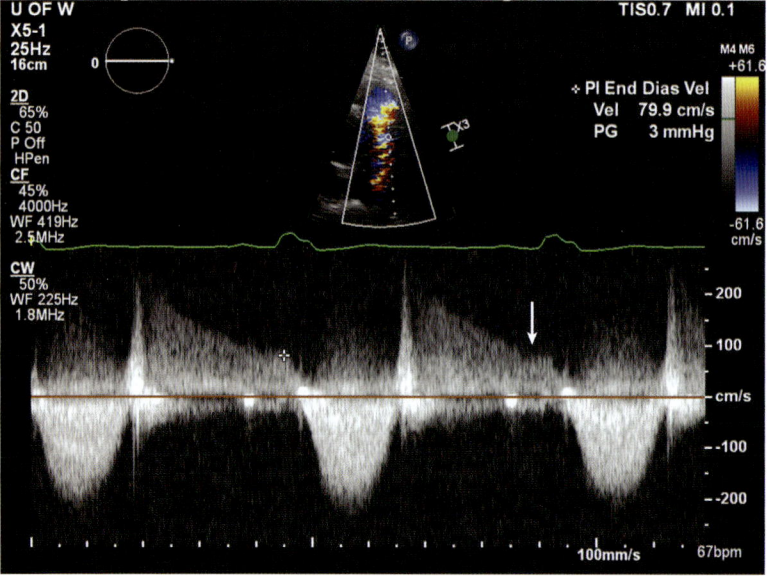

Fig. 6.27 Pulmonic regurgitation for diastolic pulmonary artery pressure estimate. Pulmonic regurgitation recorded from a parasternal approach with CW Doppler shows an end-diastolic velocity *(PI End Dias Vel)* of about 1 m/s, indicating low diastolic pulmonary pressures.

ejection curve, with a shorter time to peak velocity, findings suggesting that the shapes of these velocity curves are related to the downstream resistance or impedance. However, estimates of pulmonary pressures based on the pulmonary artery velocity curve are not as reliable as those based on the tricuspid regurgitant velocity, because an apparent short time to peak velocity can be due to measurement variability or to a nonuniform spatial flow-velocity distribution in the pulmonary artery.

Pulmonary Vascular Resistance Calculations

Pulmonary vascular resistance (PVR) is calculated as the pressure drop across the pulmonary bed (mean systolic pulmonary pressure minus mean LA pressure) divided by stroke volume (SV):

$$\text{PVR} = (\text{PA}_{mean} - \text{LA}_{mean})/\text{SV} \quad \text{(Eq. 6.24)}$$

Pulmonary vascular resistance is expressed in dimensionless Wood units where normal is <1.5 Wood

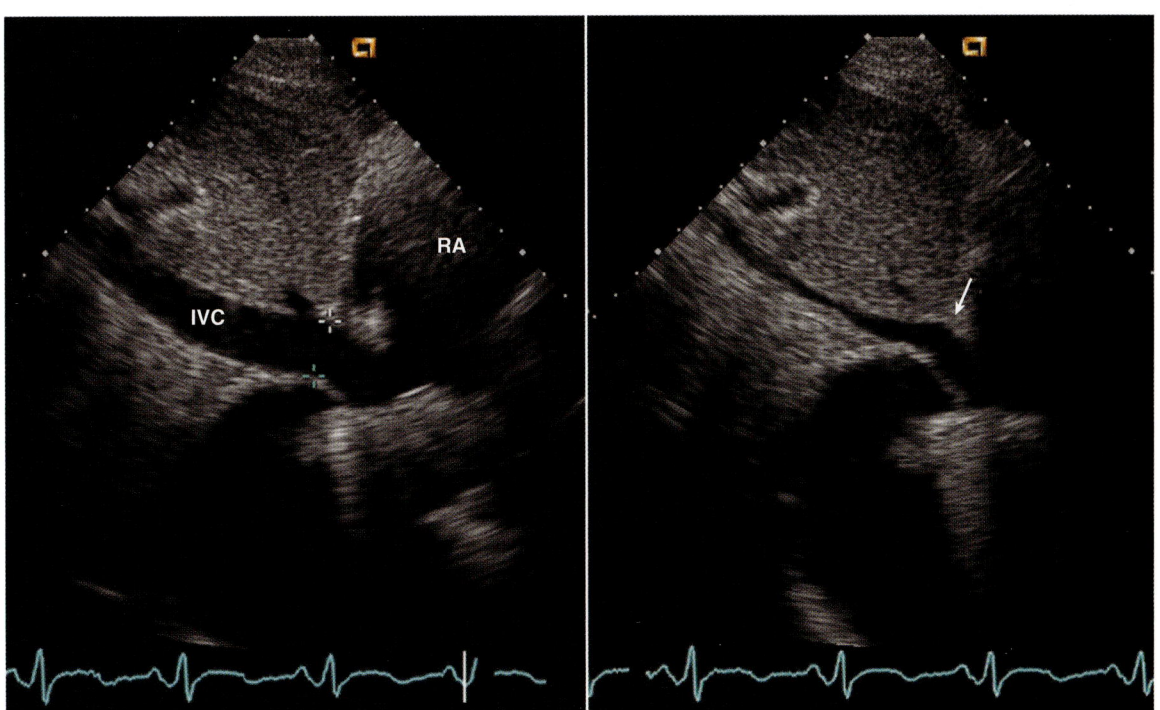

Fig. 6.28 ▶ **Right atrial pressure estimate.** Subcostal view of the junction between the inferior vena cava *(IVC)* and the RA during normal expiration *(left)* and inspiration *(right)*.

TABLE 6.6 Estimation of Right Atrial Pressure

		RA PRESSURE ESTIMATE	
IVC Diameter*	**Change With Sniff**	**Range Estimate**[†]	**ASE Guidelines**[‡]
Normal (≤2.1 cm)	Decrease >50%	0–5 mmHg	3 mmHg
Normal (≤2.1 cm)	Decrease ≤50%	5–10 mmHg	8 mmHg[§]
Dilated (>2.1 cm)	Decrease >50%	10–15 mmHg	
Dilated (>2.1 cm)	Decrease ≤50%	15–20 mmHg	15 mmHg

*Inferior vena cava diameter (IVC) is measured just proximal to entrance of hepatic veins in a subcostal view. Changes in IVC diameter during the respiratory cycle are not reliable indicators of RA pressure in patients on mechanical ventilation.
[†]Data integrated from multiple sources, including: Brennan JM, Blair JE, Goonewardena S, et al: Reappraisal of the use of interior vena cava for estimating right atrial pressure, *J Am Soc Echocardiogr* 20:857–861, 2007; Kircher BH, Himelmann RB, Schiller NG: Noninvasive estimation of right atrial pressure from the inspiratory collapse of the inferior vena cava, *Am J Cardiol* 66:493, 1990; Lang RM, Bierig M, Devereux RB, et al: Recommendations for chamber quantification, *J Am Soc Echocardiogr* 18:1440, 2005.
[‡]Data from Rudksi LG, Lai WW, Afilalo J, et al: Guidelines for the echocardiographic assessment of the right heart in adults, *J Am Soc Echocardiogr* 23:685–713, 2010.
[§]For intermediate values, the RA pressure estimate should be lowered or increased depending on the absence or presence of other signs of elevated RA pressures including restrictive right-sided diastolic filling pattern, tricuspid E/E' >6, diastolic flow predominance in the hepatic veins (systolic filling fraction <55%), and dilated RA with bulging of the septum toward the LA.

units, or a conversion factor is used for units of dynes/s/cm^{-5}, where normal is <120 dynes/s/cm^{-5}.

Noninvasive calculation of pulmonary resistance is problematic because of difficulty in measuring mean LA pressure and because of the measurement variability in noninvasive pulmonary artery pressure and right heart cardiac output calculations. One approach is to estimate the pressure drop across the pulmonary bed using the peak tricuspid regurgitant jet velocity (V_{TR} in m/s) (ignoring LA pressure) and to estimate stroke volume using the velocity-time integral of flow in the RV outflow tract (VTI_{RVOT} in cm). This ratio is multiplied by 10 to approximate pulmonary vascular resistance (PVR) in Wood units:

$$PVR \cong 10(V_{TR})/VTI_{RVOT} \quad \text{(Eq. 6.25)}$$

This approach is not recommended for routine use, but it may be helpful in identification of patients with normal resistance despite a high pulmonary systolic pressure and, conversely, patients with high resistance but low pressures resulting from a low cardiac output. However, this method may not be accurate in patients with primary pulmonary hypertension, elevated pulmonary diastolic pressures, pulmonary artery or outflow tract dilation, severe elevation of RA pressure, or severe pulmonic regurgitation.

Limitations and Alternate Approaches

Determination of pulmonary artery systolic pressure derived from the CW Doppler tricuspid regurgitant jet velocity is only as accurate as the primary data. Underestimation of tricuspid regurgitant jet velocity because of a nonparallel intercept angle between the jet and the ultrasound beam results in underestimation of pulmonary artery pressures. Overestimation of pulmonary artery pressures can occur if the mitral regurgitant jet is mistaken for tricuspid regurgitation. Although both signals occur in systole and are directed away from the LV apex, the duration of tricuspid regurgitation is slightly longer than that of mitral regurgitation (when RV and LV systolic function are normal) because of a slightly longer RV systolic ejection period. The shapes of the velocity curves tend to differ as well, with tricuspid regurgitation having a slower upstroke and a peak later in systole, although the shapes of both velocity curves are affected by changes in ventricular function or atrial pressure. Note that the velocity of mitral regurgitation always is high because it reflects the systolic LV (approximately 100 mmHg) to LA (approximately 10 mmHg) pressure difference. With normal pulmonary artery pressures, tricuspid regurgitant jet velocity is 2 to 2.5 m/s. With severe pulmonary hypertension, pulmonary pressure approaches systemic pressures, with a corresponding tricuspid regurgitant jet velocity in the range of 5 m/s.

It is important to keep separate the concepts of regurgitant *volume flow rate*—which relates to regurgitant severity—and regurgitant jet *velocity*—which reflects the instantaneous pressure gradient across the valve.

The estimate of RA pressure from the appearance of the inferior vena cava also can affect the accuracy of Doppler pulmonary artery pressure estimates. The importance of this source of error is greatest at intermediate tricuspid regurgitant jet velocities: a tricuspid regurgitant jet velocity of 2.5 m/s with an RA pressure of 5 mmHg indicates a pulmonary artery pressure of only 30 mmHg (normal to mildly elevated), but if RA pressure is 20 mmHg, then pulmonary artery pressure is 45 mmHg (moderate pulmonary hypertension). At the extreme (e.g., a tricuspid regurgitant jet of 5 m/s), pulmonary hypertension clearly is severe regardless of the RA pressure estimate.

If images of the inferior vena cava are suboptimal, or if the degree of change with respiration is equivocal, it is appropriate to report the range of possible pulmonary artery pressures or to indicate that the RV-to-RA pressure gradient is added to a clinical estimate of RA pressure. Evaluation of respiratory variation in inferior vena cava diameter can be confounded by respiratory motion in the position of the inferior vena cava such that the center of the vessel moves in and out of the image plane. Of course, evaluation of inferior vena cava size and respiratory variation is not helpful in patients supported by positive-pressure ventilation because intrathoracic pressures are abnormal.

When clinical and echocardiographic data are discrepant, invasive measurement of pulmonary artery pressure is appropriate. In many types of heart disease, accurate measures of pulmonary vascular resistance are needed, requiring direct measurement of pulmonary pressures with simultaneous cardiac output measurements.

Left and Right Ventricular Systolic Function | Chapter 6

THE ECHO EXAM

Ventricular Systolic Function

	TTE	TEE
LV size and wall thickness	• Linear LV internal dimensions and wall thickness • LV volumes calculated from apical biplane method • 3D volumes when possible	• Linear dimensions can be measured on transgastric short-axis views. • LV volumes can be calculated by the 2D biplane method or by 3D volumes.
LV ejection fraction	• 3D EF when possible • 2D biplane method using 4-chamber and 2-chamber views, taking care to image from tip of LV apex	• 3D volumes and EF recommended on all TEE studies.
LV regional wall motion	• Apical 4-chamber, 2-chamber, and long-axis views plus parasternal long- and short-axis views	• TEE 4-chamber, 2-chamber, and long-axis views plus TG short-axis view • Apical wall motion may be difficult to assess.
Doppler cardiac output	• LVOT and transmitral flows from apical approach • PA flow from parasternal views	• Transmitral flow in 4-chamber view • PA flow from high TEE view • LVOT flow sometimes obtained from TG long-axis view, but intercept angle may be nonparallel.
Speckle tracking strain imaging	• Global longitudinal strain measured from apical views	• Global longitudinal strain measurements may supplement 2D and 3D imaging.
LV dP/dt	• CW Doppler mitral regurgitant jet	• CW Doppler mitral regurgitant jet
RV size and systolic function	• Apical and subcostal 4-chamber views plus parasternal long- and short-axis views • TAPSE	• TEE 4-chamber view plus transgastric short-axis and RV-inflow views
PA pressure estimates	• TR jet recorded from parasternal and apical views with dedicated CW Doppler transducer	• TR jet may be recorded on TEE 4-chamber or short-axis views, but underestimation is possible due to a nonparallel intercept angle.

EF, Ejection fraction; *LVOT*, left ventricular outflow tract; *PA*, pulmonary artery; *TAPSE*, tricuspid annular plane systolic excursion; *TG*, transgastric; *TR*, tricuspid regurgitation.

Technical Details in Evaluation of Left Ventricular Systolic Function

Parameter	Modality	View	Recording	Measurements
Ejection fraction	3D or 2D	Apical 4-chamber and 2-chamber	Adjust depth, optimize endocardial definition, harmonic imaging, contrast if needed	Careful tracing of endocardial borders at end-diastole and end-systole in both views
Global longitudinal strain	Speckle tracking strain	Apical 4- chamber, 2 chamber, and long-axis views	Adjust depth, optimize myocardial tracking, record each view and composite data	Global longitudinal strain measurement if myocardial tracking is accurate, regional ventricular function and synchrony
dP/dt	CW Doppler	MR jet, usually from apex	Patient positioning and transducer angulation to obtain highest velocity MR jet, decrease velocity scale, increase sweep speed	Time interval between 1 m/s and 3 m/s on Doppler MR velocity curve
PA pressures	CW Doppler	Parasternal and apical	Patient positioning and transducer angulation to obtain highest-velocity TR jet	Estimate of RA pressure from size and appearance of IVC
Cardiac output	2D and pulsed Doppler	Parasternal LVOT diameter	Ultrasound beam perpendicular to LVOT with depth decreased and gain adjusted to see mid-systolic diameter	LVOT diameter from inner edge to inner edge in mid-systole, adjacent and parallel to aortic valve
		Apical LVOT velocity-time integral	LVOT velocity from anteriorly angulated apical four-chamber view with sample volume just on LV side of aortic valve	Trace modal velocity of LVOT spectral Doppler envelope

IVC, Inferior vena cava; *LVOT*, left ventricular outflow tract; *MR*, mitral regurgitation; *PA*, pulmonary artery; *TR*, tricuspid regurgitation.

SUGGESTED READING

Left Ventricular Anatomy and Physiology

1. Gaasch WH, Zile MR: Left ventricular structural remodeling in health and disease: with special emphasis on volume, mass, and geometry, *J Am Coll Cardiol* 58(17):1733–1740, 2011.

   Changes in LV structure and geometry that occur with myocardial injury or overload result in chamber dilation or hypertrophy that is best classified based on measures of LV volume, mass, and the relative wall thickness (ratio of wall to chamber). The type of LV remodeling is predictive of long-term outcomes.

2. Thomas JD, Popović ZB: Assessment of left ventricular function by cardiac ultrasound, *J Am Coll Cardiol* 48:2012–2025, 2006.

   Review of basic principles of ventricular function including cardiac hemodynamics (conservation of mass, energy, and momentum), cardiac mechanics (global and regional function), and measures of diastolic function (relaxation, compliance, pressure differences, and shear strain and torsion).

Echocardiographic Measures of Left Ventricular Function

3. Lang RM, Badano LP, Mor-Avi V, et al: Recommendations for cardiac chamber quantification by echocardiography in adults: an update from the American Society of Echocardiography and the European Association of Cardiovascular Imaging, *J Am Soc Echocardiogr* 28(1):1–39.e14, 2015.

   Detailed discussion of methods for quantitation of LV and RV systolic function by 2D echocardiography and measurement of atrial size and aortic root dimensions. Technical details of image acquisition, diagrams illustrating quantitative methods, and tables of normal values are included.

4. Aurigemma GP: Quantitative evaluation of left ventricular structure, wall stress and systolic function. In Otto CM, editor: *The Practice of Clinical Echocardiography*, ed 5, Philadelphia, 2017, Elsevier, pp 107–127.

   Advanced-level discussion of ventricular geometry, wall stress, and systolic function. This chapter provides a detailed and critical discussion of these approaches, which include LV ejection fraction, mass, and circumferential and meridional stress. Pressure-volume analysis and stress-shortening relationships are emphasized.

5. Lang RM, Badano LP, Tsang W, et al: American Society of Echocardiography; European Association of Echocardiography. EAE/ASE recommendations for image acquisition and display using three-dimensional echocardiography, *J Am Soc Echocardiogr* 25(1):3–46, 2012.

   Specific recommendations for routine quantitation of LV volumes and ejection fraction by 3D echocardiography with semiautomated border detection and surface-rendered volumes are provided. Technical aspects of data acquisition are provided along with illustrations demonstrating this approach.

6. Chandra S, Skali H, Blankstein R: Novel techniques for assessment of left ventricular systolic function, *Heart Fail Rev* 16(4):327–337, 2011.

   Contemporary review of multimodality imaging for evaluation of LV systolic function including newer echocardiographic approaches such as strain and strain rate imaging and 3D echocardiography. Context is provided by inclusion of newer nuclear and cardiac magnetic resonance images approaches. 95 references.

7. Mor-Avi V, Lang RM, Badano LP, et al: Current and evolving echocardiographic techniques for the quantitative evaluation of cardiac mechanics: ASE/EAE consensus statement on methodology and indications endorsed by the Japanese Society of Echocardiography, *J Am Soc Echocardiogr* 24(3):277–313, 2011.

   This comprehensive consensus document reviews the basic parameters of myocardial function, Doppler tissue imaging, speckle tracing echocardiography (both 2D and 3D), and use of strain in clinical practice. Both LV and RV systolic function and diastolic function are reviewed. 30 figures and 185 references.

Right Ventricular Size and Systolic Function

8. Rudski LG, Lai WW, Afilalo J, et al: Guidelines for the echocardiographic assessment of the right heart in adults: a report from the American Society of Echocardiography endorsed by the European Association of Echocardiography, a registered branch of the European Society of Cardiology, and the Canadian Society of Echocardiography, *J Am Soc Echocardiogr* 23:685–713, 2010.

   Summary recommendations for evaluation of RV size and systolic and diastolic function. Numerous figures illustrate each of the recommended measurements. Tables summarize normal values for chamber dimensions, measures of systolic function, longitudinal strain and strain rate, and diastolic function.

9. Vaidya A, Kirkpatrick JN: Right ventricular anatomy, function, and echocardiographic evaluation. In Otto CM, editor: *The Practice of Clinical Echocardiography*, ed 5, Philadelphia, 2017, Elsevier, pp 619–632.

   This chapter provides a detailed review of RV anatomy and physiology followed by a detailed discussion of the approach to echocardiographic imaging and Doppler assessment. Algorithms for routine evaluation of RV size and function are provided.

10. Horton KD, Meece RW, Hill JC: Assessment of the right ventricle by echocardiography: a primer for cardiac sonographers, *J Am Soc Echocardiogr* 22(7):776–792, quiz 861–862, 2009.

    Concise, well-written review of RV anatomy, imaging, and Doppler measurements. Methodology and technical hints for RV pulsed and color tissue Doppler imaging and for speckle tracking strain and strain rate are provided, along with 3D imaging. Video loops are available online.

11. Mertens LL, Friedberg MK: Imaging the right ventricle—current state of the art, *Nat Rev Cardiol* 7(10):551–563, 2010.

    Review of RV anatomy and function. Clinical imaging of the RV by echocardiography, cardiac magnetic resonance imaging, and the use of newer Doppler techniques is reviewed. 102 references.

12. Ahmad H, Mor-Avi V, Lang RM, et al: Assessment of right ventricular function using echocardiographic speckle tracking of the tricuspid annular motion: comparison with cardiac magnetic resonance, *Echocardiography* 29(1):19–24, 2012.

    In a series of 63 patients with echo and CMR imaging on the same day, TAPSE measured by speckle tracking echocardiography was quick and easy to do, was feasible in all patients, and correlated better with CMR RV ejection fraction than standard M-mode TAPSE.

Noninvasive Pulmonary Pressures

13. Celermajer DS, Playford D: Pulmonary hypertension: role of echocardiography in diagnosis and patient management. In Otto CM, editor: *The Practice of Clinical*

Echocardiography, ed 5, Philadelphia, 2017, Elsevier, pp 633–650.

This chapter provides a detailed review of RV anatomy and physiology followed by a detailed discussion of the approach to echocardiographic imaging and Doppler assessment. Algorithms for routine evaluation of RV size and function are provided.

14. Milan A, Magnino C, Veglio F: Echocardiographic indexes for the non-invasive evaluation of pulmonary hemodynamics, *J Am Soc Echocardiogr* 23:225–239, 2010.

    Summary article with detailed tables and clear illustrations of Doppler recordings and calculations for echocardiographic measurement of right heart pressures. 142 references.

15. Freed BH, Tsang W, Bhave NM, et al: Right ventricular strain in pulmonary arterial hypertension: a 2D echocardiography and cardiac magnetic resonance study, *Echocardiography* 32(2):257–263, 2015.

    In 30 patients with pulmonary arterial hypertension (PAH), RV speckle tracking strain correlated well with CMR-derived RV ejection fraction and had lower interobserver variability than 2D echocardiographic measures of RV systolic function.

16. Schiller NB, Ristow B: Doppler under pressure: it's time to cease the folly of chasing the peak right ventricular systolic pressure, *J Am Soc Echocardiogr* 26(5):479–482, 2013.

    This editorial comments on three papers that evaluated the accuracy of echocardiography for estimation of pulmonary pressures. Instead of defining pulmonary pressures by a single number, such as the peak RV systolic pressure calculated from the tricuspid regurgitant jet velocity, the authors suggest we use multiple parameters for evaluation of the pulmonary vasculature. Specifically, they recommend measuring the pulmonary artery velocity time integral (stroke distance) as a measure of the pulmonary volume flow rate. Other useful parameters include calculations of pulmonary mean pressure and pulmonary vascular resistance.

17. Lafitte S, Pillois X, Reant P, et al: Estimation of pulmonary pressures and diagnosis of pulmonary hypertension by Doppler echocardiography: a retrospective comparison of routine echocardiography and invasive hemodynamics, *J Am Soc Echocardiogr* 26(5):457–463, 2013.

    In a database of 301 patients, a good correlation was observed between Doppler-echo and direct measurement of pulmonary systolic pressure. A Doppler-derived systolic pulmonary pressure >38 mmHg had a high sensitivity (88%) and specificity (83%) for diagnosis of pulmonary hypertension, defined as a pulmonary systolic mean pressure >25 mmHg at catheterization.

18. Steckelberg RC, Tseng AS, Nishimura R, et al: Derivation of mean pulmonary artery pressure from noninvasive parameters, *J Am Soc Echocardiogr* 26(5):464–468, 2013.

    In series of 307 patients undergoing right heart catheterization, a regression equation for calculation of mean pulmonary artery pressure (MPAP) from pulmonary artery systolic pressure (PASP).

    $\text{MPAP} = 0.61\,\text{PASP} + 1.95\ \text{mmHg}.$

    Mean pressures calculated with this equation from the echo PASP correlated well with direct measurement at catheterization.

7. Ventricular Diastolic Filling and Function

BASIC PRINCIPLES
   Phases of Diastole
   Parameters of Diastolic Function
      Ventricular Relaxation
      Ventricular Compliance
      Ventricular Diastolic Pressures
      Ventricular Diastolic Filling (Volume) Curves
      Atrial Pressures and Filling Curves
   Normal Respiratory Changes
   Causes of Diastolic Dysfunction

ANATOMIC PARAMETERS
   Left Ventricular Changes
   Left Atrial Volume and Function
   Other Imaging Parameters

DOPPLER EVALUATION OF LV FILLING
   Nomenclature and Measurements
   Volumetric Flow Rates
   Doppler Data Recording

TISSUE DOPPLER MYOCARDIAL IMAGING

LEFT ATRIAL FILLING
   Nomenclature and Measurements
   Doppler Data Recording

OTHER APPROACHES
   Isovolumic Relaxation Time
   Propagation Velocity
   Rate of Left Ventricular Relaxation (−dP/dt)
   LV and LA Myocardial Mechanics

CONFOUNDING FACTORS
   Physiologic Factors
      Respiration, Heart Rate, and PR Interval
      Age
      Preload
   Pathophysiology
      LV Systolic Function
      Mitral Valve Disease
      Cardiac Rhythm and Atrial Contractile Function

CLINICAL CLASSIFICATION OF DIASTOLIC DYSFUNCTION
   Estimates of Diastolic Filling Pressures
   Mild Diastolic Dysfunction
   Moderate Diastolic Dysfunction
   Severe Diastolic Dysfunction

RIGHT VENTRICULAR DIASTOLIC FUNCTION
   Right Ventricular Filling
   Doppler Data Recording
   Physiologic Factors That Affect RV Filling
   Right Atrial Filling

ALTERNATE APPROACHES

DIASTOLIC FUNCTION REPORTING

THE ECHO EXAM

SUGGESTED READING

Ventricular emptying and filling are complex interdependent processes, with the cardiac cycle conceptually divided into systole and diastole to allow clinical measurements of disease severity. *Diastolic* ventricular dysfunction plays a key role in the clinical manifestations of disease in patients with a wide range of cardiac disorders. In patients with clinical heart failure who have a preserved ejection fraction (HFpEF), diastolic dysfunction is the predominant cause of symptoms. Diastolic dysfunction often is an early sign of cardiac diseases (as in hypertension) and frequently antedates clinical or echocardiographic evidence of systolic dysfunction. In addition, in patients with heart failure with reduced ejection fraction, the degree of diastolic dysfunction may explain differences in clinical symptoms among patients with similar ejection fractions.

Echocardiographic techniques allow evaluation of right ventricular (RV) and left ventricular (LV) diastolic filling patterns, the velocity of myocardial motion, and right atrial (RA) and left atrial (LA) filling patterns. Newer approaches to the evaluation of diastolic function include strain imaging of the LV and LA. The relationship between these noninvasive measures and ventricular diastolic function and the utility of these measures in patient evaluation are discussed in this chapter. Specific patterns of diastolic dysfunction are discussed in chapters relevant to each disease process.

Ventricular Diastolic Filling and Function | Chapter 7

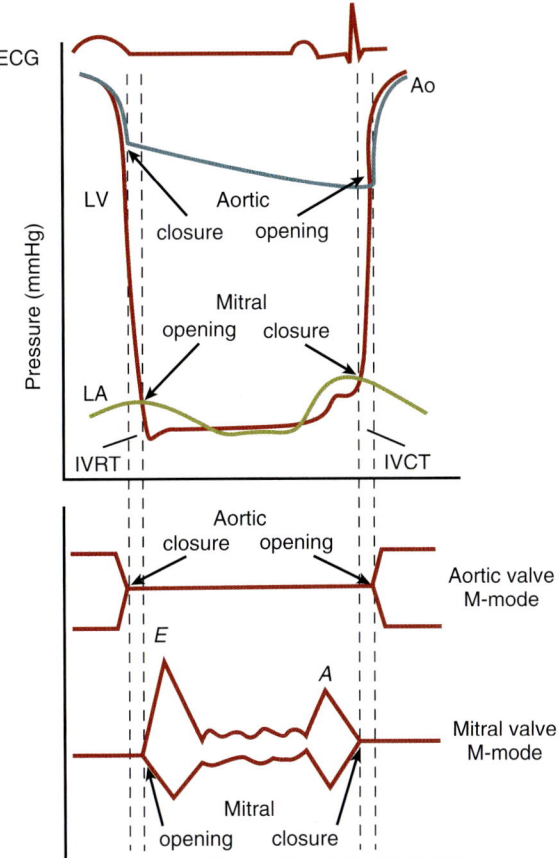

Fig. 7.1 Diastolic pressure curves. The relationships among LV, LA, and aortic (Ao) pressures and M-mode tracings of the aortic and mitral valve are shown. The isovolumic relaxation time *(IVRT)* is the interval from aortic valve closure to mitral valve opening. During this interval, LV pressure declines rapidly. A rapid rise in LV pressure occurs during the isovolumic contraction time *(IVCT)*, the interval between mitral valve closure and aortic valve opening.

BASIC PRINCIPLES

Phases of Diastole

Diastole is the interval from aortic valve closure (end-systole) to mitral valve closure (end-diastole) (Fig. 7.1). The isovolumic contraction period, from mitral valve closure to aortic valve opening, is part of systole.

Diastole can be divided into four phases:

- Isovolumic relaxation
- Early rapid diastolic filling
- Diastasis
- Late diastolic filling caused by atrial contraction

Isovolumic relaxation starts with aortic valve closure, followed by a rapid decline in LV pressure. When LV pressure falls below LA pressure, the mitral valve opens, ending the isovolumic relaxation period. Maximal opening of the mitral leaflets occurs rapidly, within 100 ± 10 ms of valve opening, in normal individuals. Mitral valve opening is followed by *rapid*

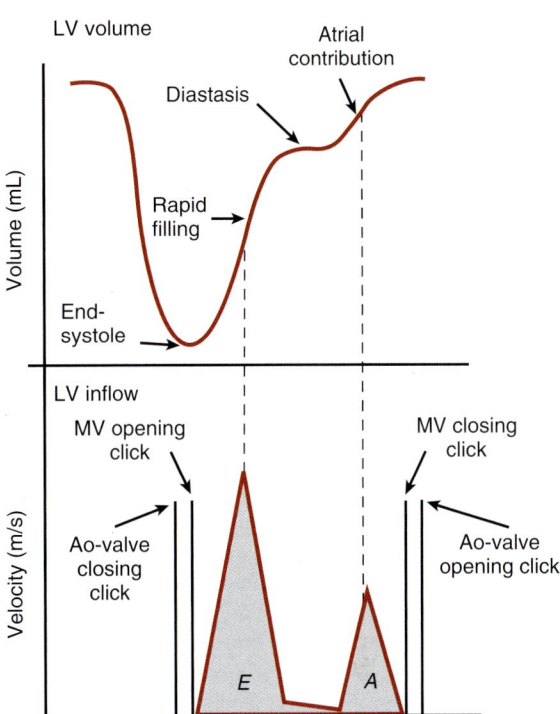

Fig. 7.2 Diastolic filling curves. The relationship between LV volume and the diastolic LV Doppler filling pattern is shown. Early rapid filling coincides with the *E* velocity, followed by diastasis (with little or no flow from the LA to the LV), and atrial contraction (which coincides with the late diastolic *A* velocity). The Doppler velocity curve, in effect, is the first derivative of the LV volume curve. *Ao*, Aortic; *MV*, mitral valve.

early diastolic filling, with the rate and time course of LA to LV flow determined by several factors, including the pressure difference along the flow stream, ventricular relaxation, and the relative compliances of the two chambers.

As the ventricle fills, pressures in the atrium and ventricle equalize, resulting in a period of *diastasis*, during which little movement of blood between the chambers occurs, and the mitral leaflets remain in a semiopen position. The duration of diastasis depends on heart rate; it is longer at slow heart rates and entirely absent at faster heart rates. With *atrial contraction*, LA pressure again exceeds LV pressure, thus resulting in further mitral leaflet opening and a second pulse of LV filling. In normal individuals this atrial contribution accounts for only about 20% of total ventricular filling (Fig. 7.2).

The phases of diastole for the RV are analogous to those described for the LV, with the difference that the total duration of diastole is slightly shorter in normal individuals because of a slightly longer RV systolic ejection period.

Parameters of Diastolic Function

Several physiologic parameters can be used to describe different aspects of diastolic function, but no single measure of overall diastolic function exists. The most clinically relevant parameters of diastolic function are:

- Ventricular relaxation
- Myocardial or chamber compliance
- Filling pressures

Additional parameters of interest include elastic recoil of the ventricle and the effect of pericardial constraint, but the importance of these factors in normal diastolic ventricular function remains controversial.

Ventricular Relaxation

LV relaxation, occurring during isovolumic relaxation and the early diastolic filling period, is an active process involving the use of energy by the myocardium. Factors affecting isovolumic relaxation include internal loading forces (cardiac fiber length), external loading conditions (wall stress, arterial impedance), inactivation of myocardial contraction (metabolic, neurohumoral, and pharmacologic), and nonuniformity in the spatial and temporal patterns of these factors. Abnormal relaxation results in prolongation of the isovolumic relaxation time, a slower rate of decline in ventricular pressure, and a consequent reduction in the early peak filling rate (due to a smaller pressure difference between the atrium and the ventricle when the atrioventricular valve opens). Measures of LV relaxation include the isovolumic relaxation time (IVRT), the maximum rate of pressure decline $(-dP/dt)$, and the time constant of relaxation (tau or τ). Several different mathematical approaches to the calculation of τ are available, but basically it reflects the rate of pressure decline from the point of maximum $-dP/dt$ to mitral valve opening. Although peak rapid filling rate is affected by ventricular relaxation, it is only an indirect measure of this physiologic parameter because several other factors also affect peak filling (Fig. 7.3).

Ventricular Compliance

Compliance is the ratio of change in volume to change in pressure (dV/dP). Stiffness is the inverse of compliance: the ratio of change in pressure to change in volume (dP/dV). Conceptually, compliance can be divided into myocardial (the characteristics of the isolated myocardium) and chamber (the characteristics of the entire ventricle) components. Chamber compliance is influenced by ventricular size and shape, in addition to the characteristics of the myocardium. Extrinsic factors also affect measurement of compliance, including the pericardium, RV volume, and pleural pressure. Evaluation of ventricular compliance is based on diastolic passive pressure-volume curves showing the degree to which pressure and volume change in relation to each other over the physiologic range (Fig. 7.4).

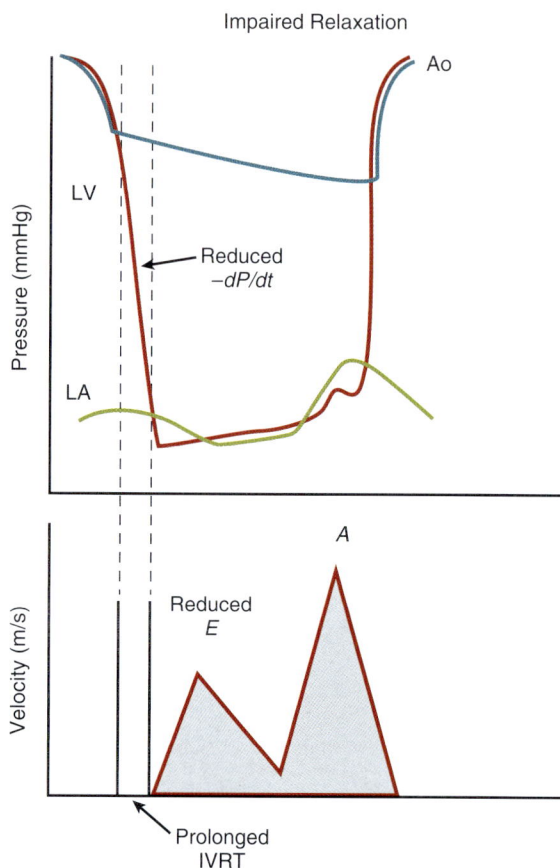

Fig. 7.3 Impaired left ventricular relaxation. A reduced $-dP/dt$ and a prolonged time constant of relaxation are noted. The Doppler velocity curve shows a prolonged isovolumic relaxation time *(IVRT)*, reduced *E* velocity (corresponding to a low LA-LV gradient at mitral valve opening), and an increased *A* velocity. *Ao,* Aortic.

Ventricular Diastolic Pressures

Clinically, evaluation of diastolic pressures alone often is used in patient management. Diastolic "filling" pressures include LV end-diastolic pressure and mean LA pressure. LV end-diastolic pressure reflects ventricular pressure after filling is complete, and LA pressure reflects the average pressure in the LA during diastole. Clinically, LA pressure is estimated by the pulmonary wedge pressure either at a single time point in the cardiac catheterization laboratory or at many time points with an indwelling right heart (Swan-Ganz) catheter in the intensive care unit.

Ventricular Diastolic Filling (Volume) Curves

Another clinically available measure related to diastolic function is the time course of ventricular filling. In theory, an LV volume curve can be generated by multiplying mitral annulus area by the integral of the Doppler velocity curve for each time point in diastole. LV filling curves also can be generated from

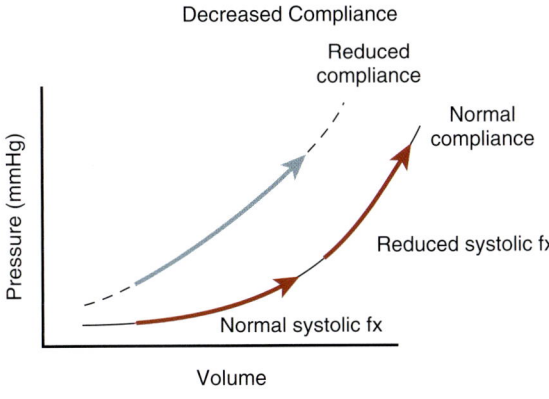

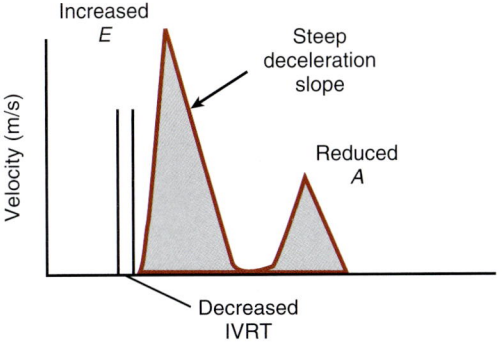

Fig. 7.4 Reduced diastolic compliance. The passive pressure-volume relationship of the LV is steeper than normal. As LV volume increases in diastole, pressure rises rapidly, resulting in an initial high LA-LV pressure gradient with a rapid decrease in the filling gradient during diastole. The Doppler velocity curve shows a decreased isovolumic relaxation time *(IVRT)*, a steep deceleration slope, and a reduced *A* velocity. Note that even with normal compliance, reduced systolic function *(fx)* results in a rightward shift along the normal pressure-volume relationship, resulting in a pattern of diastolic filling similar to decreased compliance.

frame-by-frame measurements of ventricular volumes using three-dimensional (3D) echocardiography. The accuracy, reproducibility, and diagnostic value of LV filling curve data require further study before widespread clinical application.

Ventricular *diastolic function* is one of the major factors affecting the pattern of *diastolic filling*, but these two concepts are not identical. Several physiologic parameters other than diastolic function affect diastolic filling. Given no change in diastolic function (e.g., relaxation, compliance), the peak **early diastolic filling rate** will be affected by:

- Changes in preload that affect the initial pressure difference between the ventricle and the atrium (e.g., increased with volume loading, decreased with volume depletion)
- A change in transmitral volume flow rate (e.g., increased with coexisting mitral regurgitation)
- A change in atrial pressure (e.g., elevated LV end-diastolic pressure or a *v*-wave caused by mitral regurgitation)

Late diastolic filling is affected by:

- Cardiac rhythm
- Atrial contractile function
- Ventricular end-diastolic pressure
- Heart rate
- The timing of atrial contraction (PR interval)
- Ventricular diastolic function

The importance of considering how these factors affect the Doppler pattern of diastolic filling is discussed in more detail in the following sections. In addition, it is obvious that the utility of ventricular diastolic filling patterns for assessing diastolic function is valid only in the absence of mitral valve disease because, with mitral stenosis, LV filling velocity and timing are predominantly affected by the severity of valve obstruction, whereas with mitral regurgitation, the transmitral volume flow rate is increased, altering the LV inflow velocity curve. In patients with rhythms other than normal sinus rhythm (e.g., atrial fibrillation), evaluation of diastolic function with Doppler is more challenging because of the absence of atrial contraction and the varying length of the diastolic filling period.

Atrial Pressures and Filling Curves

Another component in the evaluation of ventricular diastolic function is the measurement of atrial filling patterns and pressures. The atrium serves as a "conduit" for flow from the venous circulation to the ventricle, especially in early diastole, when the atrium is not contracting. In addition, elevations in ventricular diastolic pressures are reflected in elevated pressures in the atrium (Fig. 7.5).

RA pressures normally are quite low (0 to 5 mmHg), with only small increases in pressure following atrial (*a*-wave) and ventricular (*v*-wave) contraction.

Right atrial filling is characterized by:

- A small reversal of flow following atrial contraction (*a*-wave)
- A systolic phase (which is effectively "diastole" for the atrium) when blood flows from the superior and inferior vena cavae into the atrium
- A small reversal of flow at end-systole (*v*-wave)
- A diastolic filling phase when the atrium serves as a conduit for flow from the systemic venous return to the RV

These filling phases are reflected in the patterns of jugular venous pulsation familiar to the clinician: the *a*-wave following atrial contraction, the *x*-descent corresponding to atrial filling during ventricular systole, the *v*-wave at end-systole, and the *y*-descent corresponding to atrial filling during ventricular diastole. Disease processes affect the jugular venous pulsations and the Doppler pattern of RA filling in similar ways.

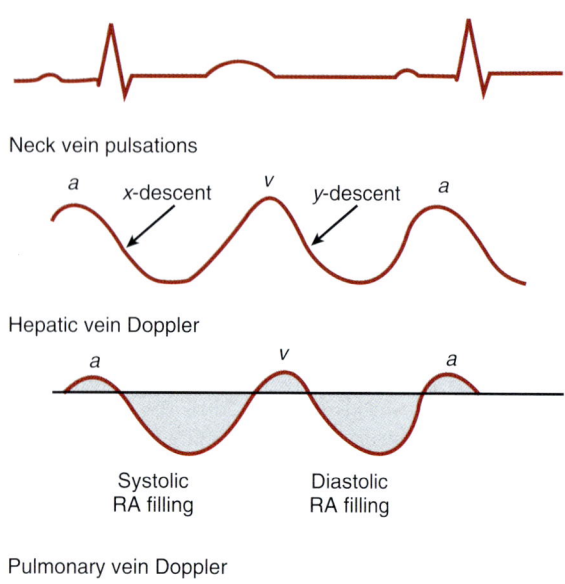

Fig. 7.5 Right atrial (hepatic vein) and left atrial (pulmonary vein) filling patterns. Atrial filling patterns are similar to the pattern of jugular venous pulsations seen on physical examination with atrial *(a)* and ventricular *(v)* "waves." Pulmonary and hepatic vein patterns appear "opposite" in direction because the direction of flow in the hepatic vein using a transthoracic subcostal view is away from the transducer (into the RA), whereas the direction of flow from a transthoracic apical view of the pulmonary vein is toward the transducer (into the LA).

LA filling from the pulmonary veins also is characterized by:

- A small reversal of flow following atrial contraction (*a*-wave)
- A systolic filling phase
- A blunting of flow or brief reversal at end-systole (*v*-wave)
- A diastolic filling phase

In normal individuals, the systolic and diastolic filling phases are approximately equal in volume. Normal LA pressure is low (5 to 10 mmHg), corresponding to the normal LV end-diastolic pressure, with slight increases in pressure following atrial (*a*-wave) and ventricular (*v*-wave) contraction.

Normal Respiratory Changes

Normal LV and RV diastolic filling shows respiratory variation. With inspiration, negative intrapleural pressure results in an increase in systemic venous return into the thorax and thus into the RA. This increase in RA volume and pressure results in a transient increase in RV diastolic filling volumes and velocities, with a normal magnitude of increase of up to 20% compared with end-expiratory values.

TABLE 7.1	Causes of Diastolic Dysfunction (Examples)
Cause	**Examples**
Primary myocardial disease	Dilated cardiomyopathy Restrictive cardiomyopathy Hypertrophic cardiomyopathy
Secondary hypertrophy	Hypertension Aortic stenosis Congenital heart disease
Coronary artery disease	Ischemia Infarction
Extrinsic constraint	Pericardial tamponade Pericardial constriction

LA filling does *not* increase with inspiration because pulmonary venous return is entirely intrathoracic and thus not affected significantly by respiratory changes in intrathoracic pressure. In fact, LA and, consequently, LV diastolic filling is slightly higher at end-expiration than during inspiration. The mechanism of this observation remains controversial. Some investigators postulate a delay in transit of the increased RV filling to the left side of the heart. Others suggest a decrease in LA filling during inspiration because of an increased volume (or "pooling") in the pulmonary venous bed. Less likely in normal individuals is impaired LV diastolic filling due to an increase in RV diastolic volume within a fixed-volume pericardium. This last mechanism becomes important in patients with pericardial disease (e.g., constriction, tamponade) and partly accounts for the exaggerated respiratory changes in RV and LV diastolic filling seen in these conditions.

Causes of Diastolic Dysfunction

Although diastolic dysfunction can be seen with a wide range of cardiac disorders, the four basic mechanisms of disease (Table 7.1) that lead to diastolic dysfunction are:

- Primary myocardial disease
- Secondary LV hypertrophy
- Coronary artery disease
- Extrinsic constraint

ANATOMIC PARAMETERS

Left Ventricular Changes

Evaluation of ventricular chamber dimensions and wall thickness is an integral part of the echocardiographic evaluation of diastolic function. The relative degree of systolic and diastolic dysfunction in patients with heart failure ranges from severe diastolic dysfunction with a normal ejection fraction to severe systolic dysfunction with normal filling pressures. However, most patients with systolic dysfunction have some degree of diastolic dysfunction, and most patients with diastolic dysfunction have anatomic cardiac changes evident on echocardiographic imaging. Typically, diastolic heart failure (HFpEF) occurs in patients with a thick-walled, small ventricle due to either restrictive cardiomyopathy or hypertensive heart disease. The presence and severity of LA enlargement reflect chronically elevated filling pressures, so that measurement of LA size or volume is integral to evaluation of diastolic function (see Fig. 2.16).

In patients with heart failure due primarily to systolic ventricular dysfunction (heart failure with reduced ejection fraction), typical imaging findings include a dilated LV with global or regional dysfunction and a reduced ejection fraction. Diastolic dysfunction usually accompanies systolic dysfunction, and measures of diastolic function and LV filling pressures are important for patient management and prognosis.

Left Atrial Volumes

LA volume is a key element in the evaluation of diastolic dysfunction. Measurement of LA volumes by two-dimensional (2D) or 3D imaging is feasible and accurate and is a strong predictor of clinical outcome. However, LA volume is nonspecific because, in addition to diastolic dysfunction, LA volume increases with age, athletic conditioning, cardiac arrhythmias, high-output states (e.g., anemia), and mitral valve disease.

Other Imaging Parameters

Other imaging findings that raise the question of diastolic dysfunction include pericardial thickening (as in constrictive pericarditis), the pattern of ventricular septal motion with respiration (especially with tamponade physiology), and dilation of the inferior vena cava and hepatic veins (consistent with elevated RA pressures). Elevated pulmonary artery systolic pressures, in the absence of another cause such as mitral valve disease or primary pulmonary disease, also raise the concern for LV diastolic dysfunction.

DOPPLER EVALUATION OF LV FILLING

Nomenclature and Measurements

Doppler recordings of LV diastolic filling velocities correspond closely with ventricular filling parameters measured by other techniques. The normal Doppler ventricular inflow pattern is characterized by a brief time interval between aortic valve closure and the onset of ventricular filling (the isovolumic relaxation time). Immediately following mitral valve opening rapid acceleration of blood flow from the LA to the ventricle occurs with an early peak filling velocity of 0.6 to 0.8 m/s 90 to 110 ms after the onset of flow in young, healthy individuals (Table 7.2). This early maximum filling velocity (E velocity) occurs simultaneously with the maximum pressure gradient between the atrium and the ventricle. After this maximum velocity, flow decelerates rapidly (i.e., with a steep slope) in normal individuals with a normal deceleration slope of 4.3 to 6.7 m/s^2 (Table 7.3). Deceleration time, defined as the time interval from the E peak to where a line following the deceleration slope intersects with the zero baseline, ranges from 140 to 200 ms. Early diastolic filling is followed by a variable period of minimal flow (diastasis), depending on the total duration of diastole. With atrial contraction, LA pressure again exceeds ventricular pressure, with a resulting second velocity peak (late diastolic or atrial velocity), which typically ranges from 0.19 to 0.35 m/s in young, normal individuals (Fig. 7.6).

Quantitative measurements that can be made from the Doppler velocity curve include (Fig. 7.7):

- *Maximum velocities:* The E velocity, the A velocity, and their ratio (E/A ratio)
- *Velocity-time integrals:* Total, early diastolic, atrial contribution, first third or half of diastole, and their ratios
- *Time intervals:* The isovolumic relaxation time, the total duration of diastole, the deceleration time, and the atrial filling period
- *Measures of acceleration and deceleration:* The time from onset of flow to the E velocity, the maximum rate of rise in velocity, and the slope of early diastolic deceleration

Volumetric Flow Rates

To convert the Doppler ventricular inflow *velocity* curve to a *volume* curve, the cross-sectional area of flow must be taken into account. Volumetric flow rates can be calculated as the product of velocity and cross-sectional area in regions where flow is laminar with a spatially symmetric flow pattern (Fig. 7.8). Thus the instantaneous volume flow rate across the mitral valve can be calculated as instantaneous velocity times the flow cross-sectional area (CSA). Similarly, transmitral stroke volume (SV) can be determined from the integral of the flow velocity curve (VTI) over the diastolic filling period:

$$SV_{transmitral} = VTI \times CSA \quad (Eq. 7.1)$$

The standard approach to determining the cross-sectional area of flow across the mitral valve is to calculate the cross-sectional area of flow at the mitral annulus level. Motion of the mitral leaflets is a passive

TABLE 7.2 Quantitation of Diastolic Function

Parameter	Modality	TTE View	TEE View	Recording	Measurements
LV inflow at leaflet tips	Pulsed Doppler	A4C with 2–3-mm sample volume positioned at mitral leaflet tips	High TEE 4-chamber view with sample volume at leaflet tips	Parallel to flow, normal expiration, low wall filters	E = early diastolic filling velocity (m/s) A = filling velocity after atrial contraction (m/s) E/A ratio DT = deceleration time (ms)
LV inflow at annulus	Pulsed Doppler	A4C with 2-mm sample volume at mitral annulus	High TEE 4-chamber view with sample volume at mitral annulus	Parallel to flow, normal expiration, low wall filters	A_{dur} = duration of atrial filling velocity in ms
Myocardial tissue Doppler	Pulsed Doppler	A4C with 2–4-mm sample volume placed within basal segment of septal wall	High TEE 4-chamber view with 2–3-mm sample volume placed within basal segment of septal wall	Very low gain settings, low wall filters	E' = early diastolic filling velocity (m/s) A' = filling velocity after atrial contraction (m/s) E/E' = ratio of LV inflow E velocity to tissue Doppler E' velocity
Isovolumic relaxation time (IVRT)	Pulsed Doppler	Anteriorly angulated A4C with 3–5-mm sample volume midway between aortic and mitral valves	High TEE 4-chamber view angulated toward aortic valve with a 3–5-mm sample volume midway between aortic and mitral valves	Clear aortic closing click and clear onset of transmitral flow, low wall filters	IVRT (ms)
Pulmonary vein (PV)	Pulsed Doppler (color to guide location)	Right superior PV in A4C view using color flow to visualize flow	Left superior PV from high TEE view (all four veins can be used)	1–3-mm sample volume, 1–2 cm into pulmonary vein	PV_S = peak systolic velocity PV_D = peak diastolic velocity PV_a = peak atrial reversal velocity a_{dur} = PV atrial reversal duration

A4C, Apical four-chamber.

process, with the degree of motion reflecting flow across the valve (in the absence of mitral stenosis). Although flow area tapers from the annulus to the leaflet tips, the more rigid mitral annulus is a preferable site for flow measurement rather than the flexible, mobile leaflets. Even though the shape of the mitral annulus is complex in 3D, in clinical practice assuming either a circular or elliptical geometry is a reasonable approximation, based on a diameter measurement in the apical four-chamber or parasternal long-axis view or both (see Fig. 6.15).

Combining Doppler LV inflow velocity data with the cross-sectional area of the mitral annulus, additional filling parameters that can be calculated include:

- *Peak filling rates:* Peak rapid filling rate, atrial peak filling rate, and their ratio
- *Stroke volume*
- *Fractional filling rates:* For example, first third filling fraction or the ratio of early to late filling

For each of these parameters, the filling rate is calculated by multiplying the appropriate velocity or

TABLE 7.3 Selected Normal Parameters of Diastolic Function

Parameters	Normal Value
Velocities	
E/A ratio	1.32 ± 0.42
Deceleration slope	5.0 ± 1.4 m/s²
Intervals	
IVRT	63 ± 11 ms
Deceleration time	150–200 ms
$A_{dur} - a_{dur}$	<20 ms
Derived Measures	
τ	33 ± 6 ms
−dP/dt	2048 ± 335 mmHg/s
Filling Rates	
Peak filling rate	288 ± 66 mL/s
Peak filling rate normalized to LVEDV	2.9 ± 1.0 s⁻¹
Atrial filling rate	229 ± 83 mL/s
Myocardial Doppler Velocities	
E′	10.3 ± 2.0 cm/s
A′	5.8 ± 1.6 cm/s
Ratio of E′/A′	2.1 ± 0.9
Ratio of E/E′	≤10

A_{dur}, Transmitral A-velocity duration; a_{dur}, pulmonary venous a-velocity duration; *IVRT*, isovolumic relaxation time; *LVEDV*, left ventricular end-diastolic volume.
Data from Tebbe U, Hoffmeister N, Sauer G, et al: *Clin Cardiol* 3:19, 1980; Shapiro LM, McKenna WJ: *Br Heart J* 51:637, 1984; Pearson AC, Labovitz AJ, Mrosek D: *Am Heart J* 113:1417, 1987; Snider AR, Gidding SS, Rocchini AP: *Am J Cardiol* 56:921, 1985; García-Fernández MA, Azevedo J, Moreno M: *Eur Heart J* 20:496, 1999.

velocity-time integral by cross-sectional area. For example, peak rapid filling rate (PRFR) is:

$$\text{PRFR (mL/s)} = E \text{ velocity (cm/s)} \times \text{CSA (cm}^2\text{)} \quad \text{(Eq. 7.2)}$$

Of course, volume flow measurements are accurate only when velocities and diameters are measured at the same anatomic location, for example, at the annulus level.

Doppler Data Recording

LV inflow can be recorded in nearly all patients from an apical approach in either a four-chamber or long-axis view on transthoracic (TTE) imaging. This window allows parallel alignment between the ultrasound beam and the direction of LV filling. On transesophageal (TEE) echocardiography, LV inflow can be recorded from a high esophageal position, while taking care to align the Doppler beam parallel to the inflow stream (Fig. 7.9). In some patients, a transgastric apical view also allows recording of LV inflow, although caution is needed to avoid a nonparallel intercept angle (with resultant underestimation of velocities) and a foreshortening of the ventricle from this window.

Inflow velocities should be recorded using pulsed Doppler with a 2- to 3-mm sample volume positioned either at the mitral leaflet tips (for evaluation of diastolic function) or at the mitral annulus level (for measurement of volume flow rates and the duration of atrial filling) (see Fig. 7.6). For diastolic function evaluation, with the beam aligned parallel to the flow stream, the sample volume is moved slowly along the length of the ultrasound beam to identify the site of maximal velocity, usually at the mitral leaflet tip level. The velocity range is adjusted to maximize the display of the velocity of interest and avoid signal aliasing. The sweep speed of the spectral display is maximized (100 cm/s), and wall filters are reduced (as allowed by signal quality) so that the velocities approach the baseline, thus allowing accurate time interval measurements. Flows are recorded at end-expiration during normal breathing.

Standard clinical measurements of LV inflow include:

- Early diastolic filling velocity *(E)*
- Atrial filling velocity *(A)*
- Deceleration time (DT) all at the leaflet tips
- Atrial filling duration (A_{dur}) is measured at the mitral annulus.

TISSUE DOPPLER MYOCARDIAL IMAGING

As the LV fills in diastole, the chamber lengthens from base to apex and expands in both radial and circumferential directions. The velocity of longitudinal myocardial lengthening in diastole (and shortening in systole) can be measured using pulsed tissue Doppler with the velocity scale, gain, and wall filters adjusted to display the velocity of the movement of the myocardium, rather than the intracavity blood flow velocities. Tissue Doppler myocardial velocities are less dependent on preload than are transmitral flow velocities and thus are useful measures in evaluation of diastolic function.

Compared with transmitral blood flow velocity, the myocardial velocity curve is similar but inverted and lower in velocity (Fig. 7.10). When myocardial tissue velocities are recorded near the mitral annulus from an apical approach, there is a brief early systolic velocity peak away from the transducer, corresponding

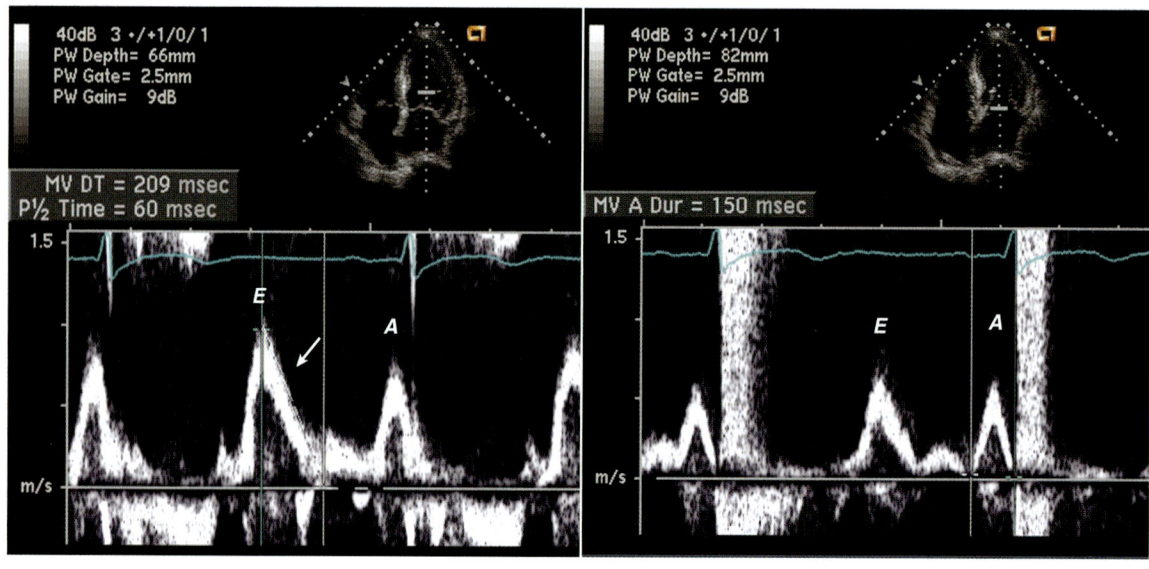

Fig. 7.6 Normal pattern of left ventricular diastolic filling. Pulsed Doppler recording in an apical four-chamber view with the sample volume positioned at the mitral leaflet tips *(left)* is used to measure E velocity, A velocity, and the deceleration time *(arrow)*. The flow signal recorded with the sample volume positioned at the level of the mitral annulus level *(right)* is used for measurement of atrial flow duration. If transmitral stroke volume is calculated, the annular flow signal is used for the velocity-time integral.

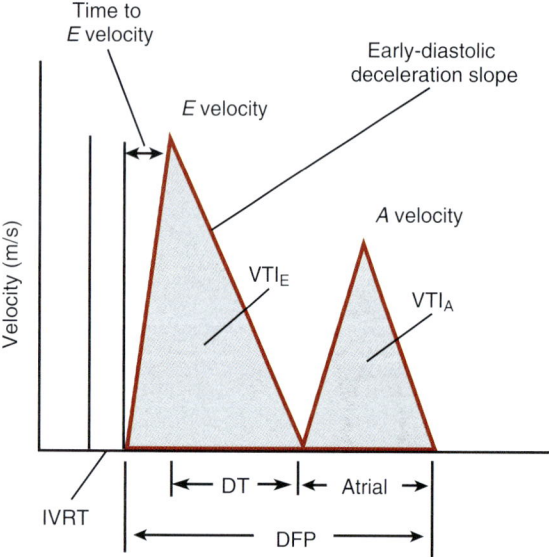

Fig. 7.7 Schematic diagram of quantitative measurements that can be made from the Doppler left ventricular filling curve. *DFP,* Diastolic filling period; *DT,* deceleration time; *IVRT,* isovolumic relaxation time; *VTI,* velocity-time integral.

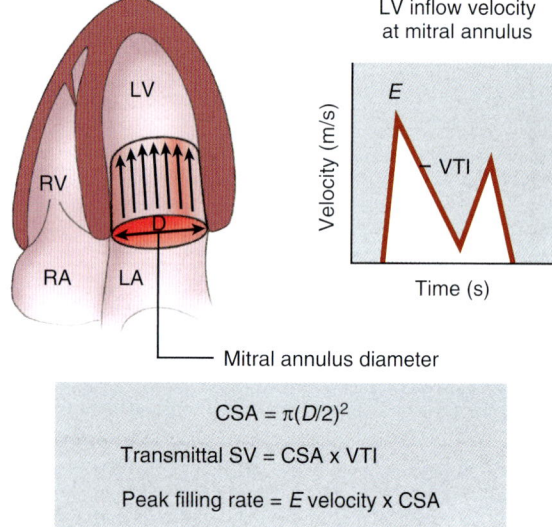

Fig. 7.8 Transmitral volume flow rate. Volumetric flow rates across the mitral annulus can be calculated as shown. Mitral annular diameter can be measured from both apical four-chamber and parasternal long-axis views to calculate an elliptical cross-sectional area *(CSA)*. Alternatively, a circular cross-sectional area is used as an approximation using a single annular diameter measurement. *SV,* Stroke volume; *VTI,* flow velocity curve.

to early diastolic relaxation, with a normal velocity between 0.10 and 0.14 cm/s. This early diastolic velocity is abbreviated as E' (E-prime) in this book, but other common abbreviations include e' (small e' instead of capital E') E_m (for mitral annular), and E_a (for annular). Following atrial contraction, a second velocity peak away from the apex is seen (A') with a normal ratio of E'/A' greater than 1.0. A reduced E'/A' ratio indicates impaired relaxation. The pattern of E'/A' also helps distinguish normal LV filling from the pseudo-normalized pattern seen in patients with moderate to severe diastolic dysfunction.

Myocardial tissue Doppler signals are recorded using pulsed Doppler in an apical four-chamber view with a small sample volume (1 to 3 mm in length) positioned within the basal ventricular wall, within

1 cm of the mitral annulus. For evaluation of diastolic function, recordings from the basal septum (medial annulus) typically are used. Tissue Doppler velocities recorded from the lateral annulus usually are slightly higher in velocity but are not as reproducible as medial annulus measurements. Some experts recommend averaging medial and lateral annular tissue velocities. For Doppler tissue recordings, the velocity scale is decreased to show a range of only about 0.2 m/s, gain is turned to very low levels, and wall filters are reduced to obtain a well-defined signal with clear E' and A' peaks. Some instruments have a tissue Doppler setting that automatically makes these adjustments to the pulsed Doppler modality. Recordings are made at end-expiration during normal quiet respiration. Standard clinical measurements from the myocardial tissue Doppler include:

- Early diastolic filling velocity (E')
- Filling velocity after atrial contraction (A')
- Ratio of early to atrial diastolic myocardial velocity (E'/A')
- Ratio of transmitral blood flow velocity to tissue Doppler velocity (E/E')

The rationale for the ratio of blood flow to tissue velocity is that the transmitral E velocity reflects both the LA to LV opening pressure gradient and the amount of blood entering the ventricle in diastole. In contrast, the tissue Doppler velocity reflects only the amount of blood entering the ventricle (the volume increase in ventricular size), so this ratio normalizes the E velocity for volume flow rate, thus providing a measure of filling pressure. A very high E/E' ratio (>15) is specific for an elevated filling pressure, but this ratio is not very sensitive, so many patients with elevated filling pressures have a ratio between 8 and 15.

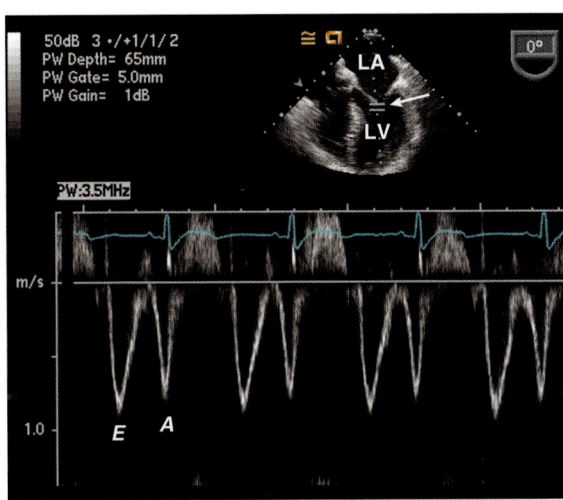

Fig. 7.9 Transesophageal echocardiography transmitral flow velocities. The typical pattern of LV diastolic filling is seen with a parallel alignment between the ultrasound beam and flow direction from a TEE four-chamber view. The only difference from a TTE flow recording is that flow is directed away from the transducer on TEE.

LEFT ATRIAL FILLING

Nomenclature and Measurements

LA filling is evaluated by Doppler recordings of pulmonary vein flow either from a TEE or a TTE approach. Again, the Doppler pattern of velocities parallels the normal filling curves, with inflow into the LA occurring in two phases, systolic and diastolic. In addition, flow deceleration following ventricular contraction and a small reversal of flow after atrial contraction occur (Fig. 7.11). On TEE recordings, the systolic inflow pattern is biphasic in some patients, with an early systolic peak related to atrial relaxation and a second late systolic peak related to displacement of the mitral annulus toward the LV apex. Respiratory variation in flow is seen in left heart filling patterns

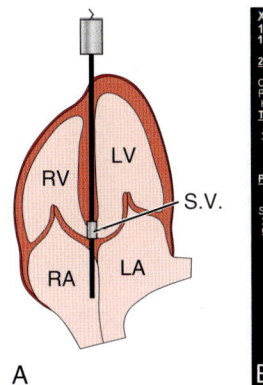
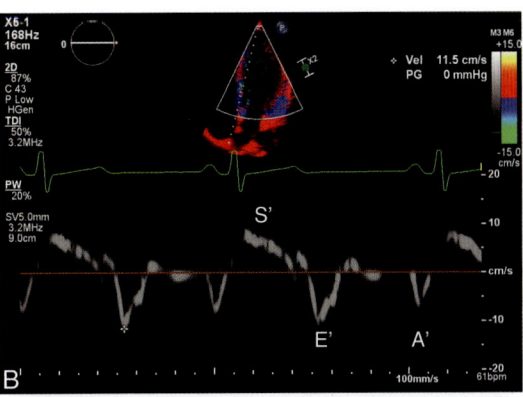

Fig. 7.10 Tissue Doppler imaging at the mitral annulus. (A) The Doppler sample volume (S.V.) is located in the basal septum, adjacent to the mitral annulus, in the apical four-chamber view. (B) The tissue Doppler imaging *(TDI)* recording in a young normal patient shows an early myocardial velocity (E') greater than the atrial velocity (A'). The systolic velocity toward the transducer is termed S'. Note that the velocity scale has a maximum of only 0.15 m/s, compared with 1.5 m/s for LV inflow in Fig. 7.6 in the same patient.

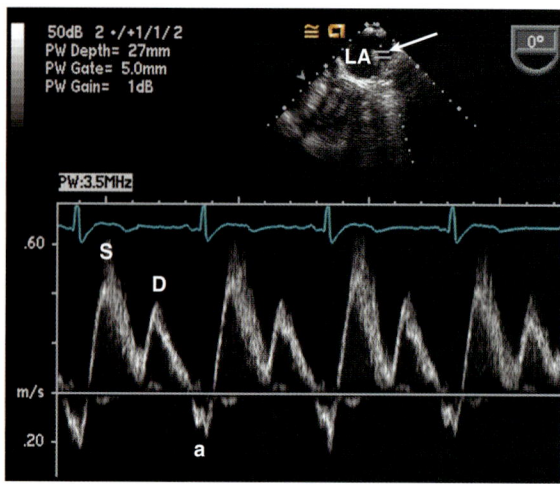

Fig. 7.11 Left atrial inflow on transesophageal echocardiography. Normal pattern of LA inflow recorded in the left superior pulmonary vein from a TEE approach. *a*, Atrial contraction; *D*, diastolic; *S*, systolic.

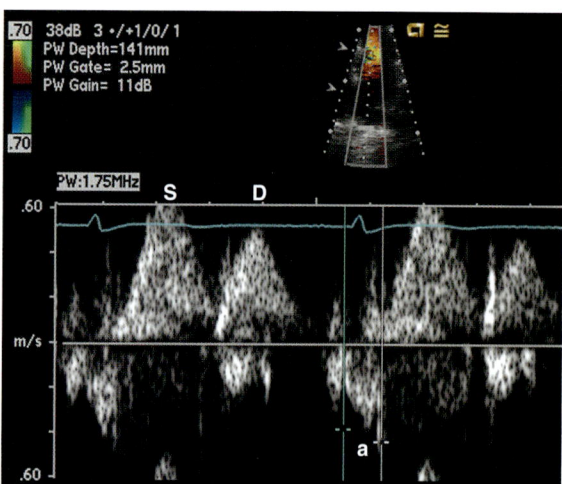

Fig. 7.12 Left atrial inflow on transesophageal echocardiography. Normal pattern of LA inflow recorded in the right superior pulmonary vein from a transthoracic apical four-chamber view using color flow imaging to aid in positioning the sample volume approximately 1 to 2 cm into the vein. Filling shows systolic *(S)* and diastolic *(D)* filling phases with a slight flow reversal following atrial contraction *(a)*.

(atrial and ventricular) but is less prominent than the variation seen in right heart filling patterns, *and* it is directionally opposite: left heart filling diminishes slightly with inspiration. Both the pulmonary veins and the LA are intrathoracic in their entirety, so negative intrathoracic pressure does not result in a pressure gradient between them. Instead, atrial filling diminishes during inspiration as blood "pools" briefly in the expanded pulmonary veins, which then empty during expiration.

Doppler Data Recording

From a TEE approach, LA inflow patterns can be easily recorded in each of the four pulmonary veins in the transverse plane. Careful positioning and angulation are needed to ensure that the pulsed Doppler sample volume is located in the pulmonary vein itself rather than in the adjacent LA. A sample volume size of 2 to 3 mm typically is used, with wall filters lowered to show the low-velocity components associated with atrial and ventricular contraction. The flow pattern varies somewhat with distance from the pulmonary vein orifice. A distance about 1 cm from the orifice provides optimal signal strength with the most consistent inflow pattern.

The left superior pulmonary vein is most easily visualized adjacent to the LA appendage, directed somewhat anteriorly. The left inferior pulmonary vein can be visualized by advancing the transducer a short distance to see the inflow pattern from this horizontally directed vein. The right pulmonary veins can be imaged by turning the transducer medially to identify the superior right pulmonary vein (again anteriorly directed) and advancing the probe slightly to image the horizontally positioned right inferior pulmonary vein.

From a TTE approach, recording pulmonary venous flow patterns is more challenging. Most echocardiographers use the apical four-chamber view, which allows a parallel alignment between the right superior pulmonary vein flow stream and the ultrasound beam. Signal strength is a limiting factor at this depth of interrogation (typically about 14 cm), so careful attention to sample volume position, wall filters, and gain settings is needed to optimize the velocity data. Sample volume positioning is facilitated by the use of color flow imaging to identify the flow stream from the pulmonary vein into the LA. Again, the sample volume should be positioned in the pulmonary vein, 1 to 2 cm from the orifice. Of note, atrial reversal and the biphasic pattern of systolic inflow are more difficult to demonstrate on TTE compared with TEE imaging because of a lower signal-to-noise ratio (Fig. 7.12). In addition, the flow pattern in the left upper pulmonary vein on TEE echocardiography shows a more laminar flow pattern than the right upper pulmonary vein. Alternate transthoracic windows for recording of pulmonary vein flow in some individuals include subcostal and parasternal short-axis views at the aortic valve level or suprasternal notch views of the LA and pulmonary veins. However, the intercept angle tends to be suboptimal from these windows.

Standard clinical measures of **pulmonary venous inflow** include:

- Peak systolic velocity (PV_S)
- Peak diastolic velocity (PV_D)
- Peak atrial reversal velocity (PV_a)
- Duration of pulmonary vein atrial reversal (a_{dur})

OTHER APPROACHES

Isovolumic Relaxation Time

The isovolumic relaxation time (IVRT) is simply the time interval between aortic valve closure and mitral valve opening. A normal isovolumic relaxation time is approximately 50 to 100 ms, but the normal range varies with age and heart rate. Impaired relaxation is associated with a prolonged isovolumic relaxation time, whereas decreased compliance and elevated filling pressures are associated with a shortened isovolumic relaxation time. Thus this measurement is useful in determining the severity of diastolic dysfunction, particularly in serial studies of patients receiving medical therapy or with disease progression.

The isovolumic relaxation time is measured from an apical four-chamber view angulated anteriorly to show the outflow tract and aortic valve. Using pulsed Doppler, a 3- to 5-mm sample volume is positioned midway between the aortic and mitral valves to obtain a clear signal showing both aortic outflow and mitral inflow, optimally with a defined aortic valve closing click. After adjusting gain and decreasing the wall filters, the isovolumic relaxation time is measured as the time interval in milliseconds from the middle of the aortic closure click to the onset of mitral flow (Fig. 7.13).

Propagation Velocity

Color Doppler M-mode recordings of LV inflow from an apical approach can be used to measure the propagation velocity as blood moves from the annulus to the apex. The flow propagation velocity is decreased with restrictive ventricular filling and increased with constrictive pericarditis.

Color M-mode propagation velocity is recorded from an apical four-chamber view using color flow imaging to place a color M-mode cursor parallel to mitral inflow in the center of the flow stream (Fig. 7.14). Using a narrow sector, minimum depth needed to include the annulus and apex, and an aliasing velocity of 0.5 to 0.7 m/s, the color M-mode signal is recorded at a fast sweep speed (100 to 200 mm/s). With normal diastolic function, the blood flows quickly from the annulus toward the apex, resulting in a nearly vertical M-mode color pattern. The slope of the line along the edge of the color Doppler M-mode in early diastole is termed the propagation velocity, with a normal value greater than 50 cm/s. With decreased relaxation, the movement of blood from the annulus to the apex is slower, so the slope of color M-mode is prolonged. Accurate recording and measurement of the propagation velocity require considerable expertise and are not used in all laboratories.

Rate of Left Ventricular Relaxation (−dP/dt)

The rate of decline in velocity of the mitral regurgitant jet at end-systole reflects the rate of decrease in LV pressure in early diastole (Fig. 7.15). This allows measurement of negative dP/dt from the end-systolic segment of the mitral regurgitant jet, analogous to measurement of positive dP/dt from the initial segment of the jet (see Fig. 6.17). Unfortunately, the mitral regurgitant jet velocity is also affected by LA pressure, which often is elevated with mitral regurgitation independent of abnormalities in diastolic function. In addition, reproducibility of this

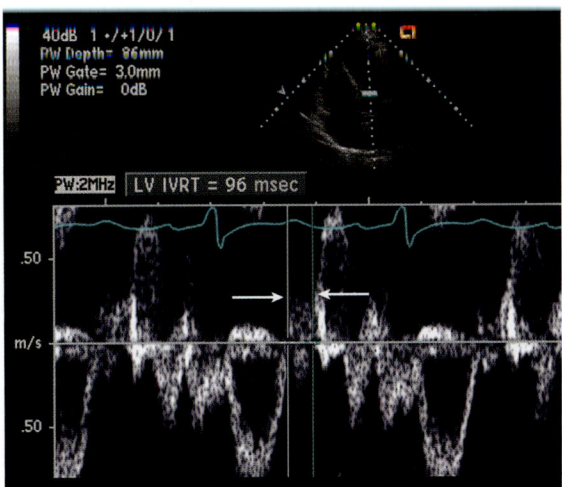

Fig. 7.13 Isovolumic relaxation time. The isovolumic relaxation time *(IVRT)* is measured from aortic valve closure and the onset of mitral flow *(arrows)* and measures 96 ms in this example.

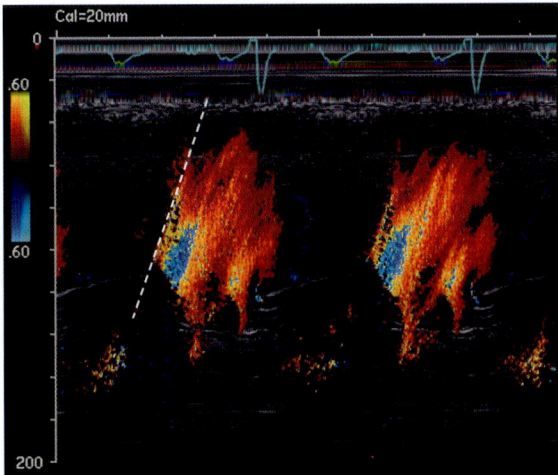

Fig. 7.14 Color Doppler M-mode propagation velocity. Propagation velocity *(dashed line)* recorded with the color Doppler M-mode cursor positioned in the center of the mitral annulus in an apical four-chamber view. The slope of the Doppler flow as it moves from the annulus *(bottom of scale)* to the apex *(top of the scale)* reflects the rate of LV relaxation.

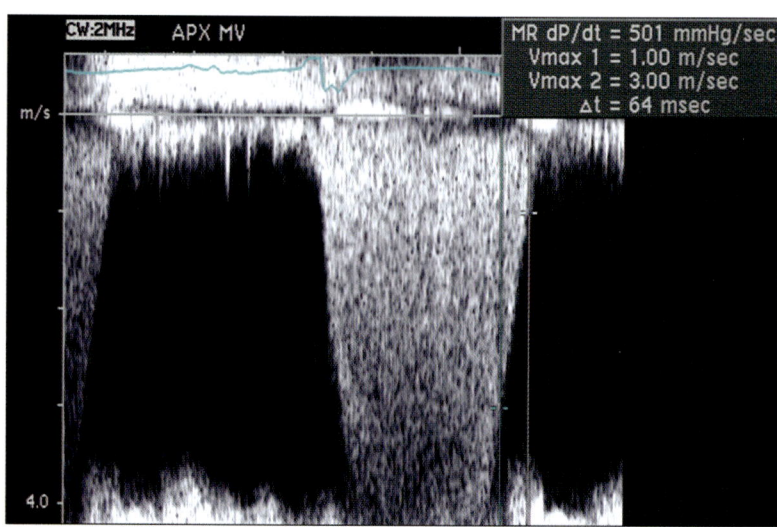

Fig. 7.15 Early diastolic −dP/dt. The time interval between 1 and 3 m/s on the mitral regurgitant velocity deceleration curve is used to calculate −dP/dt as Δt/32 mmHg.

measurement is suboptimal because of poor signal strength in some patients and measurement of a short time interval, so it has not been widely accepted as a standard method for evaluation of diastolic dysfunction.

LV and LA Myocardial Mechanics

Measures of LV strain and strain rate derived from tissue Doppler imaging or speckle tracking echocardiography (see Fig. 4.14) can be used to evaluate regional diastolic dysfunction. This approach may be helpful for the diagnosis of coronary disease, assessment of myocardial viability, and detection of interstitial fibrosis. Other potential measures of diastolic function that can be derived from tissue Doppler imaging include the time interval from E' to E velocity, which reflects end-diastolic pressure and global myocardial deformation measures such as strain rate during isovolumetric relaxation (which is not affected by loading conditions). Tissue Doppler imaging and speckle tracking echocardiography also allow evaluation of rotation and twist of the LV in systole and of untwisting in diastole, although the clinical utility of this approach has not been established.

LA function can be assessed using tissue Doppler imaging or speckle tracking echocardiography. Indices that can be derived from these approaches include:

- Maximal strain during LV systole (LA reservoir function)
- Early diastolic strain (LA conduit function)
- Strain during LA systole (LA contractile function)

LA strain measures may be useful in the evaluation of patients with diastolic heart failure and in predicting persistence of sinus rhythm after cardioversion for atrial fibrillation. However, further study of these measures is needed before they can be recommended for routine clinical use.

CONFOUNDING FACTORS

Physiologic Factors

Evaluation of LV diastolic function is confounded by the normal variation in ventricular filling related to:

- Respiration
- Heart rate
- PR interval
- Age
- Preload

Pulmonary venous flow patterns also are affected by physiologic factors other than diastolic function, with the *systolic filling phase* most affected by:

- LA size
- LA pressure
- LA compliance
- Atrial contractile function

The velocity and duration of the *atrial reversal* is affected by:

- LA contraction
- LA compliance
- Cardiac rhythm

Despite the potential influence of all these factors on the pattern of LV diastolic filling, the Doppler velocity data still can provide useful information on diastolic dysfunction if they are carefully interpreted.

Respiration, Heart Rate, and PR Interval

A normal slight variation (<20%) in LV inflow velocities occurs with respiration. At higher heart rates, diastole is shorter—particularly the period of diastasis—so that the *A* velocity more closely succeeds the *E* velocity. When overlap of these two velocity curves occurs, the *A* velocity, in effect, is "added" to the *E*-velocity curve, resulting in a higher *A* velocity and a lower *E/A* ratio (Fig. 7.16). Similarly, a longer PR interval results in an *A* velocity earlier in diastole that becomes superimposed on the *E*-velocity curve. At very high heart rates (short diastolic filling periods), the *E*- and *A*-velocity curves become merged into a single *E/A* velocity. Evaluation of a patient with heart block or an atrial arrhythmia often demonstrates this nicely, with the location of the *A* velocity relative to the *E* velocity affecting its magnitude accordingly (Fig. 7.17).

LA filling is affected by many of the same variables that affect LV diastolic filling. Higher heart rates result in merging of the systolic and diastolic phases of LA filling, whereas lower heart rates result in clearer separation between them.

Age

In children and young adults, the majority of ventricular filling occurs in early diastole, with a prominent *E* velocity and only a small contribution to ventricular filling due to atrial contraction (20% of total LV volume). With age, the *E* velocity diminishes, and the atrial contribution becomes more prominent, with equalization of *E* and *A* velocities at approximately age 50 years and reversal of the *E/A* ratio after that age in normal individuals (Appendix A, Table A.5). Early diastolic deceleration time also is progressively prolonged, and a slight increase in isovolumic relaxation time occurs with age (Fig. 7.18). Presumably the mechanism of the changes in LV filling patterns with age is a gradual reduction in the rate of early diastolic relaxation. Keeping in mind that *E* velocity and *E/A* ratio usually decrease with age, the finding of a "normal" LV filling pattern in an older patient should raise the question of abnormal ventricular compliance.

Changes in LA inflow with aging have been described, including a reduction in the diastolic filling phase, a compensatory increase in the systolic filling phase, and a more prominent atrial reversal in subjects older than age 50 years.

Preload

LA pressure and volume *preload* dramatically affect the pattern of LV filling (Fig. 7.19). Increased LA pressure results in an increase in the *E* velocity, a shortened isovolumic relaxation time, and steeper deceleration slope of early diastolic filling. As the LV fills rapidly in early diastole LV diastolic pressure rises, so atrial contraction results in only a small pressure gradient between the LA and the LV and a small *A* velocity. Examples of elevated preload include volume infusion or an elevated LA pressure due to elevation of LV end-diastolic pressure.

Situations with a reduced preload also affect diastolic filling parameters. Reduced LA pressures have

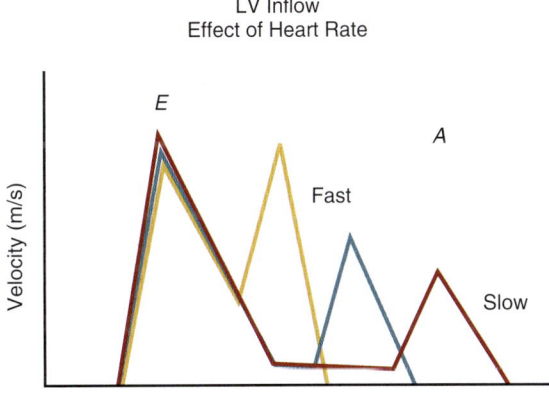

Fig. 7.16 Effect of heart rate on E/A ratio. Schematic diagram showing the overlap or "summation" of *A* velocity with *E* velocity that occurs with higher heart rates.

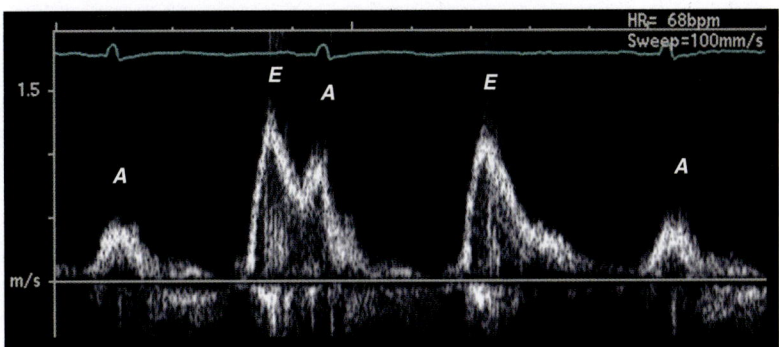

Fig. 7.17 Effect of diastolic filling interval on E/A ratio. LV filling in a patient with an atrial arrhythmia showing the effect of a shorter diastolic interval on the *E/A* pattern.

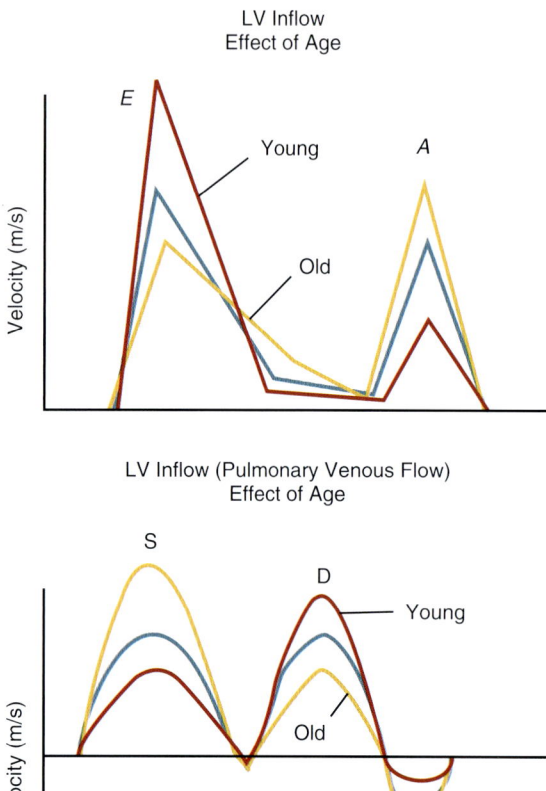

Fig. 7.18 Aging changes in left ventricular and left atrial inflow patterns. Schematic diagram showing the changes in LV *(top)* and LA inflow and pulmonary venous flow *(bottom)* patterns that occur with age. The typical pattern seen in younger (age 50 years) subjects *(pink)* is compared with middle-aged *(blue)* and older (age 70 years) subjects *(yellow)*. A, atrial; D, diastolic; S, systolic.

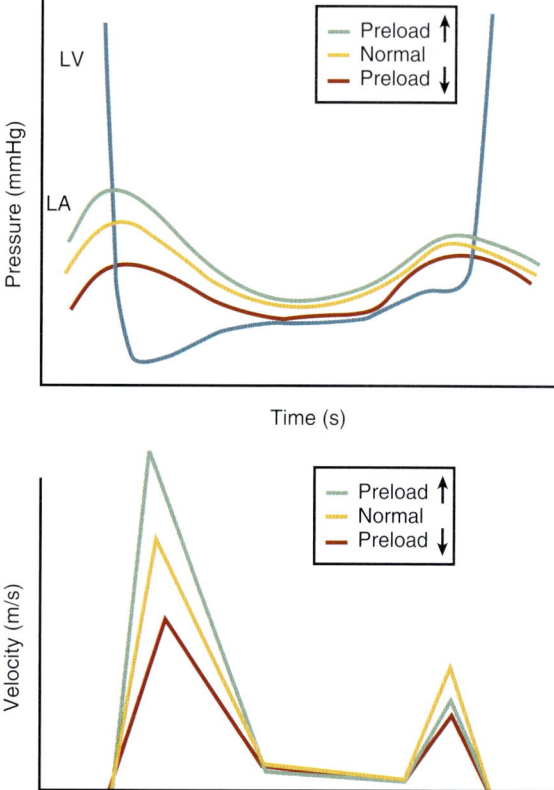

Fig. 7.19 Effect of preload on left ventricular filling patterns. With increased preload, an increased pressure gradient from the LA to the LV at the time of mitral valve opening results in a higher *E* velocity. The *A* velocity remains the same or is reduced if a high end-diastolic pressure results in a smaller LA to LV pressure gradient following atrial contraction. The opposite changes occur with decreased preload.

- LV systolic function
- Mitral valve disease
- Cardiac rhythm and atrial contractile function

a reduced *E* velocity because of a smaller gradient between the LA and LV at mitral valve opening. Thus hypovolemia or use of a venodilator (e.g., nitroglycerin) results in a decrease in the *E* velocity, with a much smaller effect on *A* velocity. Preload is transiently decreased during the strain phase of the Valsalva maneuver. Thus if the *E/A* ratio appears normal but preload is elevated, with the Valsalva maneuver the decrease in *E* velocity results in normalization or reversal of the *E/A* ratio. This response to the Valsalva maneuver may be used to separate a normal from a pseudo-normal pattern of diastolic filling and to distinguish reversible from irreversible severe diastolic dysfunction.

Pathophysiology

Several pathophysiologic variables, other than LV diastolic function, that also affect the pattern of LV diastolic filling include:

LV Systolic Function

LV systolic function affects the pattern of diastolic filling in that, for a given diastolic pressure-volume curve, an increased end-systolic volume results in a shift to a steeper portion of the pressure-volume curve. Diastolic filling then occurs with a greater increase in pressure for a given increase in volume. This results in an increased *E* velocity and reduced *A* velocity, similar to the pattern seen with decreased compliance due to a shift to a different diastolic pressure-volume curve (see Fig. 7.4).

Mitral Valve Disease

The use of transmitral and pulmonary vein flow curve in assessment of LV diastolic function depends on the assumption that the mitral valve itself does not affect filling patterns. Obviously this assumption is invalid when mitral valve disease is present. Mitral valve area is the rate-limiting step for LV filling when mitral stenosis is present; Doppler echo cannot be used for evaluation of LV diastolic function if significant mitral stenosis is present. When more than mild mitral regurgitation is present, an increased initial pressure gradient is present when the valve opens and an increased volume flow rate across the mitral valve occurs in early diastole. Thus diastolic function cannot be accurately evaluated when significant mitral regurgitation is present (Fig. 7.20).

Cardiac Rhythm and Atrial Contractile Function

Evaluation of diastolic function is challenging except with normal sinus rhythm (Fig. 7.21) because the E/A ratio is a key diagnostic measure. In addition, some patients with sinus rhythm on the electrocardiogram may have ineffective atrial contraction, resulting in a small or absence A velocity. In atrial fibrillation, diastolic filling time varies from beat to beat, and the LV inflow A velocity and pulmonary venous inflow atrial reversal are absent. In addition, because forward pulmonary vein flow in systole reflects atrial filling after atrial contraction, systolic pulmonary vein flow typically is blunted when atrial fibrillation is present, even in the absence of mitral regurgitation or LV diastolic dysfunction. Measures of LV diastolic function that indicate elevated filling pressures in the presence of atrial fibrillation, when averaged from several beats, include:

- Mitral deceleration time (DT) ≤160 ms
- Isovolumic relaxation time (IVRT) ≤ 65 ms
- $E/E' \geq 11$

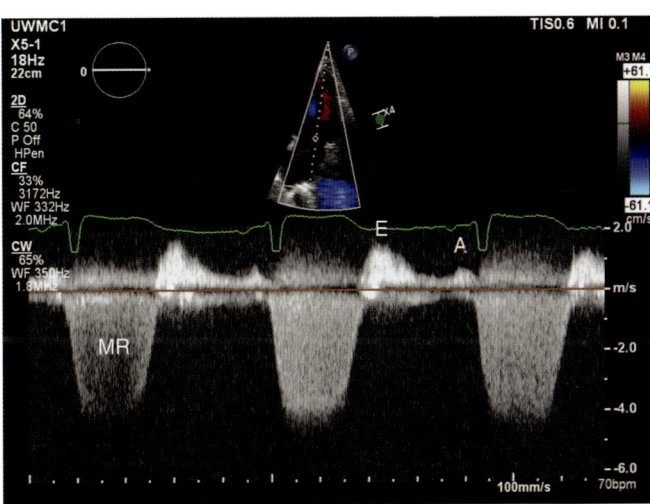

Fig. 7.20 Effect of volume flow rate on left ventricular filling. LV inflow in a patient with severe mitral regurgitation *(MR)* showing a high E velocity because of increased volume flow across the mitral valve and an increased LA pressure.

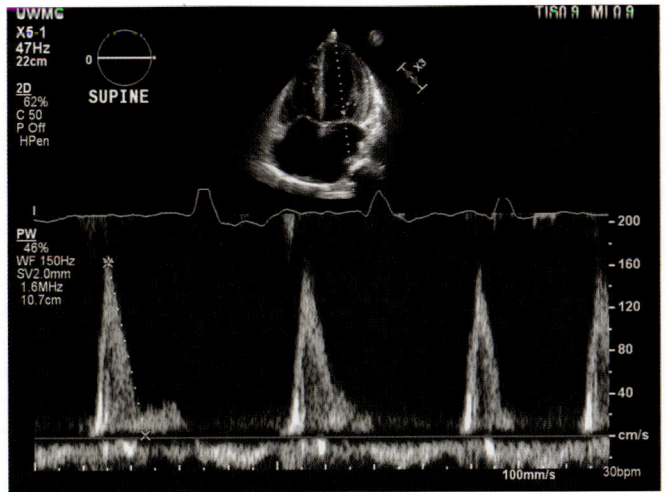

Fig. 7.21 Atrial fibrillation. LV inflow in a patient with atrial fibrillation shows a single velocity peak and no A velocity with an irregular rhythm.

TABLE 7.4 Classification of Diastolic Dysfunction (Key Measures Highlighted)

	Normal	Mild (Grade I)	Moderate (Grade II)	Severe* (Grade III)
Pathophysiology		↓ Relaxation and normal LVEDP	↓ Relaxation and ↑ LVEDP	↓ Compliance and ↑↑ LVEDP
E/A ratio[†]	≥0.8	<0.8	>0.8 to <2.0[‡]	≥2.0
Valsalva ΔE/A		<0.5	≥0.5	≥0.5
DT (ms)	150–200	>200	150–200	<150
E' velocity (cm/s)	≥10	<8	<8	<5
E/E' ratio	≤10	≤10	10–14	>14
IVRT (ms)	50–100	≥100	60–100	≤60
PV S/D	≅1	S > D	S < D	S ≪ D
PV_a (m/s)	<0.35	<0.35[§]	≥0.35	≥0.35
$a_{dur}-A_{dur}$ (ms)	<20	<20[§]	≥30	≥30
LA volume index	<34 mL/m²	Mildly enlarged	Moderately enlarged	Severely enlarged

*An additional grade of irreversible severe dysfunction is characterized by the absence of a decrease in E velocity with the strain phase of the Valsalva maneuver.
[†]Only the yellow rows are included in the American Society of Echocardiography guidelines plus consideration of tricuspid regurgitant jet velocity. In the absence of other causes for elevated pulmonary pressures, a tricuspid regurgitant velocity greater than 2.8 m/s is consistent with moderate to severe LV diastolic dysfunction.
[‡]E/A with the Valsalva maneuver is <1.
[§]Pulmonary vein a duration and velocity may be increased if filling pressures are elevated.
A, Late diastolic ventricular filling velocity with atrial contraction; DT, deceleration time; E, early diastolic peak velocity; E', early diastolic tissue Doppler velocity; $IVRT$, isovolumic relaxation time; $LVEDP$, LV end-diastolic pressure; PV, pulmonary vein.
Data from Nagueh SF, Smiseth OA, Appleton CP, et al: [ASE guidelines.] *J Am Soc Echocardiogr* 29:277–314, 2015; Rakowski H, Appleton C, Chan KL, et al: [Canadian consensus guidelines.] *J Am Soc Echocadiogr* 9:736–760, 1996; Yamada H, Goh PP, Sun JP, et al: *J Am Soc Echocardiogr* 15:1238–1244, 2002; Redfield MM, Jacobsen SJ, Burnett JC Jr, et al: *JAMA* 289:194–202, 2003; Lester SJ, Tajik AJ, Nishimura RA, et al: *J Am Coll Cardiol* 51:679–689, 2008.

CLINICAL CLASSIFICATION OF DIASTOLIC DYSFUNCTION

In the clinical setting, evaluation of diastolic ventricular function is complicated by the coexistence of more than one of the factors that affect diastolic filling. For example, patients with reduced compliance often have an elevated preload. Thus an older adult patient with reduced compliance has a pattern of LV filling similar to a younger patient with normal diastolic function (a pattern referred to as *pseudo-normalization*). Conversely, a patient with impaired relaxation has coexisting mitral regurgitation, resulting in an increased E/A ratio due to the increased transmitral volume flow rate instead of the expected decrease in E/A ratio due to impaired relaxation. As these examples illustrate, sorting out the relative contribution of diastolic dysfunction from other physiologic parameters can be difficult in an individual patient. Furthermore, the factors that affect diastolic filling are not independent. A change in one physiologic parameter (e.g., LA pressure) affects other parameters (e.g., atrial compliance and LV contractility). However, from a practical point of view, the combination of transmitral flow, myocardial tissue velocity, and pulmonary venous inflow patterns allows a clinically useful classification of the type and severity of diastolic dysfunction (Table 7.4).

The clinical indications and optimal examination for diastolic dysfunction continue to evolve, so each laboratory needs to develop a protocol for when and how to evaluate diastolic function. My recommendation is that detailed evaluation of diastolic dysfunction be performed in patients referred for evaluation of heart failure symptoms, including dyspnea, particularly if LV systolic function is normal, and in patients with evidence of any of the conditions listed in Table 7.1 based on clinical or echocardiographic criteria (Fig. 7.22).

Estimates of Diastolic Filling Pressures

In clinical practice, it can be difficult to separate the effects of changes in ventricular relaxation and compliance from changes due to elevated filling pressures. Nevertheless, these parameters are conceptually different. Although Doppler data are not accurate or precise enough to replace invasive pressure measurements in critically ill patients when treatment is being titrated based on hemodynamic parameters, several Doppler parameters are useful for identification of patients with elevated filling pressure, even when an

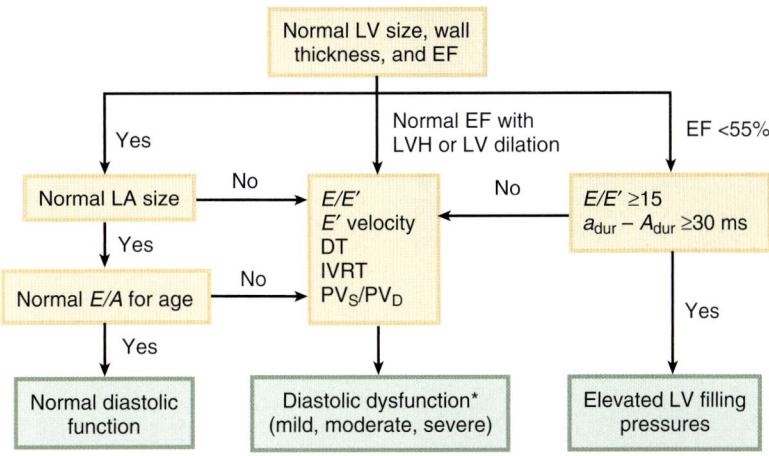

*See Table 7.4 for classification of diastolic dysfunction.

Fig. 7.22 Practical approach to clinical evaluation of diastolic dysfunction. When LV size, wall thickness, and ejection fraction *(EF)* are normal, further evaluation of diastolic function is needed only in the presence of LA enlargement or an abnormal *E/A* ratio for age. In patients with ventricular hypertrophy or dilation with a normal ejection fraction, diastolic function should be fully evaluated, particularly if clinical concern exists that diastolic dysfunction is the cause of symptoms. When ejection fraction is reduced, the first step is to evaluate for elevated filling pressures. If simple criteria for elevated filling pressures are not present, a more complete evaluation of diastolic function is appropriate. *DT*, Deceleration time; *IVRT*, isovolumic relaxation time; *LVH*, LV hypertrophy; PV_D, peak diastolic velocity; PV_S, peak systolic velocity.

exact numeric value cannot be provided (see Appendix B, Table B.5).

Doppler parameters that indicate an elevated LV filling pressure include a:

- Ratio of transmitral *E* velocity to the myocardial tissue *E′* velocity *(E/E′)* >15
- Pulmonary vein atrial reversal velocity (PV_a) >0.35 m/s
- Pulmonary atrial reversal duration (a_{dur}) at least 20 ms > transmitral atrial flow duration (A_{dur})
- Pulmonary venous systolic flow less than diastolic flow (S < D)
- Ratio of the early to atrial transmitral velocity *(E/A* ratio) >2
- Deceleration time <140 ms

In clinical practice, several of these variables are considered in the examination of patients with suspected diastolic dysfunction, with the confounding factors of diastolic relaxation and compliance affecting the data in each patient. In patients with a low LV ejection fraction, an *E/E′* ratio greater than 15 is a reasonably accurate indicator of elevated filing pressures. When LV systolic function is normal, a very low (≤8) or very high (>15) *E/E′* ratio is diagnostic, but the additional parameters listed earlier should be considered when the *E/E′* ratio is between 8 and 15. The diagnosis of elevated filling pressures is most secure when multiple parameters are congruent. Additional findings, such as LA enlargement and pulmonary hypertension, improve diagnostic reliability.

Mild Diastolic Dysfunction

Mild diastolic dysfunction is characterized by impaired ventricular relaxation with a classic pattern of impaired early diastolic filling and an increased atrial contribution to total LV filling (Fig. 7.23). *Impaired relaxation* is associated with a:

- Reduced *E* velocity
- Longer early diastolic deceleration time (DT) (>200 ms)
- Tissue Doppler *E′* velocity <10 cm/s
- Prolonged isovolumic relaxation time (≥100 ms)

If filling pressures are normal despite impaired relaxation, the *E/E′* ratio is less than 8, and the pulmonary venous pattern is normal with a:

- Systolic phase greater than a diastolic phase
- Normal atrial reversal duration and velocity

If impaired relaxation is accompanied by elevated filling pressures, the LV inflow pattern will continue to show an *E/A* ratio less than 0.8 with a prolonged deceleration time. However, the ratio of early diastolic blood flow to tissue velocity *(E/E′)* now is elevated, the isovolumic relaxation time is in the normal range, and the pulmonary venous atrial reversal is prolonged in duration and increased in velocity. This pattern is consistent with mild to moderate diastolic dysfunction.

Moderate Diastolic Dysfunction

Moderate diastolic dysfunction is characterized by abnormal compliance, often in addition to impaired

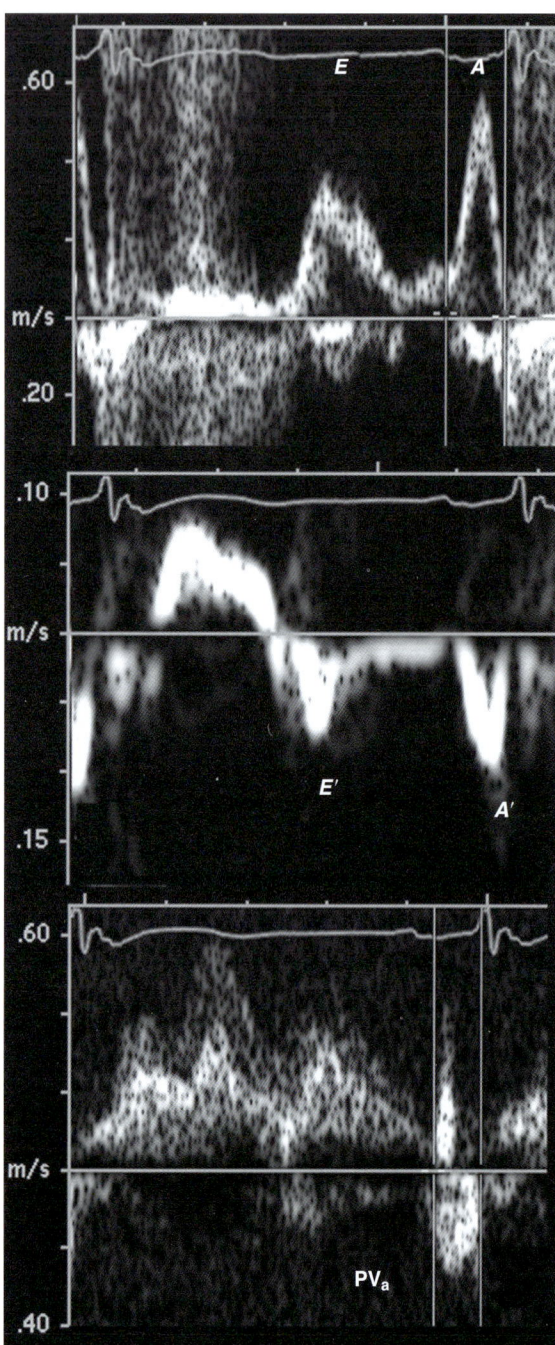

Fig. 7.23 Mild diastolic dysfunction. In this patient with LV hypertrophy and decreased relaxation, the mitral inflow at the leaflet tips (*top*) shows an E/A <1 and a prolonged deceleration time. The myocardial tissue Doppler (*center*) confirms impaired relaxation with an E'A' <1, indicating the mitral flow pattern is not related to loading conditions. The pulmonary venous inflow (*bottom*) shows relatively slightly greater systolic flow compared with diastolic flow and a normal atrial reversal velocity and duration (PV_a), consistent with normal LV filling pressures. In addition, the E/E' ratio is only 4.

relaxation. Abnormal ventricular compliance results in rapid early diastolic filling following mitral valve opening with a short isovolumic relaxation time and acceleration time. As the ventricle fills, LV diastolic pressure rises rapidly because of a stiff ventricle with decreased compliance, so a high E velocity is followed by a steep deceleration slope (Fig. 7.24). The atrial contribution to filling is relatively small because filling is now occurring on the steep portion of the pressure-volume relationship. In addition, LV end-diastolic pressure typically is elevated, so only a small LA to LV pressure gradient is present following atrial contraction. This pattern of ventricular filling often is referred to as "pseudo-normal" because the *E/A* ratio looks similar to normal even though diastolic dysfunction is present.

Moderate diastolic dysfunction, with a normal *E/A* ratio (pseudo-normal), is distinguished from normal ventricular filling by a:

- Low *E'* velocity (<8 cm/s)
- Short, early diastolic deceleration time (150 to 200 ms)
- Tissue Doppler *E'/A'* <1
- Ratio of *E* to *E'* between 10 and 14
- Short isovolumic relaxation time (60 to 100 ms)
- Pulmonary venous diastolic velocity greater than systolic velocity

In addition, the pulmonary venous flow pattern shows a prominent diastolic phase with an increased velocity and duration of atrial flow reversal, thus confirming the diagnosis of moderate diastolic dysfunction. Although the *E/A* ratio is typically 0.8 to 2 at rest, with the strain phase of the Valsalva maneuver (decreased preload), the *E* velocity decreases more than the *A* velocity, resulting in an *E/A* ratio less than 1.

Severe Diastolic Dysfunction

With severe diastolic dysfunction, the progressive reduction in compliance and elevation of filling pressures results in a further increase in the *E* velocity and a decrease in the deceleration time. The myocardial tissue velocities decrease to less than 5 cm/s, and the ratio of *E/E'* increases to 15 or greater. The isovolumic relaxation time becomes very short, and the pulmonary venous inflow pattern is dominated by diastolic flow. Atrial reversal is prominent as well, with an increased velocity and duration of atrial flow caused by a high LV diastolic pressure that reduces late diastolic LV filling so that atrial contraction results in reversal of flow in the pulmonary veins (Fig. 7.25).

In summary, severe diastolic dysfunction with *reduced compliance* is associated with:

- Increased *E* velocity and *E/A* ratio
- Decreased deceleration time
- Low *E'* velocity with an *E/E'* ratio ≥15

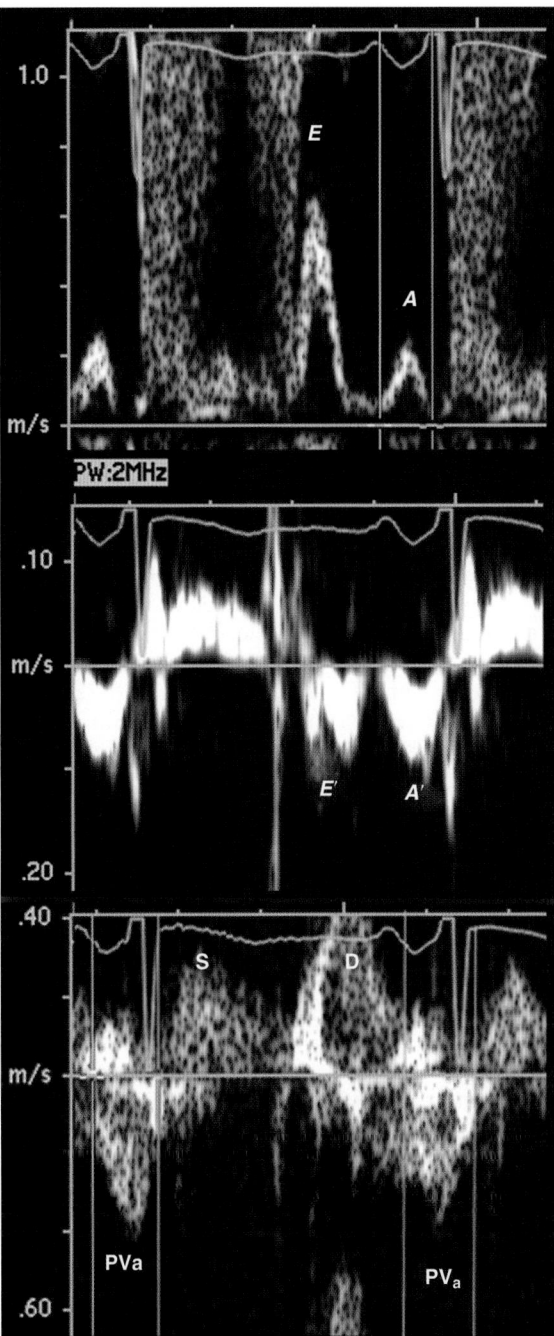

Fig. 7.24 Moderate diastolic dysfunction. In a patient with impaired compliance and an elevated LV end-diastolic pressure, the mitral inflow at the leaflet tips (*top*) shows an E/A >1 and a short deceleration time. The myocardial tissue Doppler (*center*) shows about equal E' and A' velocities, with an E' <0.8 m/s, consistent with decreased compliance. The E/E' ratio is slightly higher than 8. The pulmonary venous inflow (*bottom*) shows a relatively larger diastolic component than systolic component and an increased atrial reversal velocity (PV$_a$) (approximately 0.40 m/s) and duration, consistent with elevated LV filling pressures.

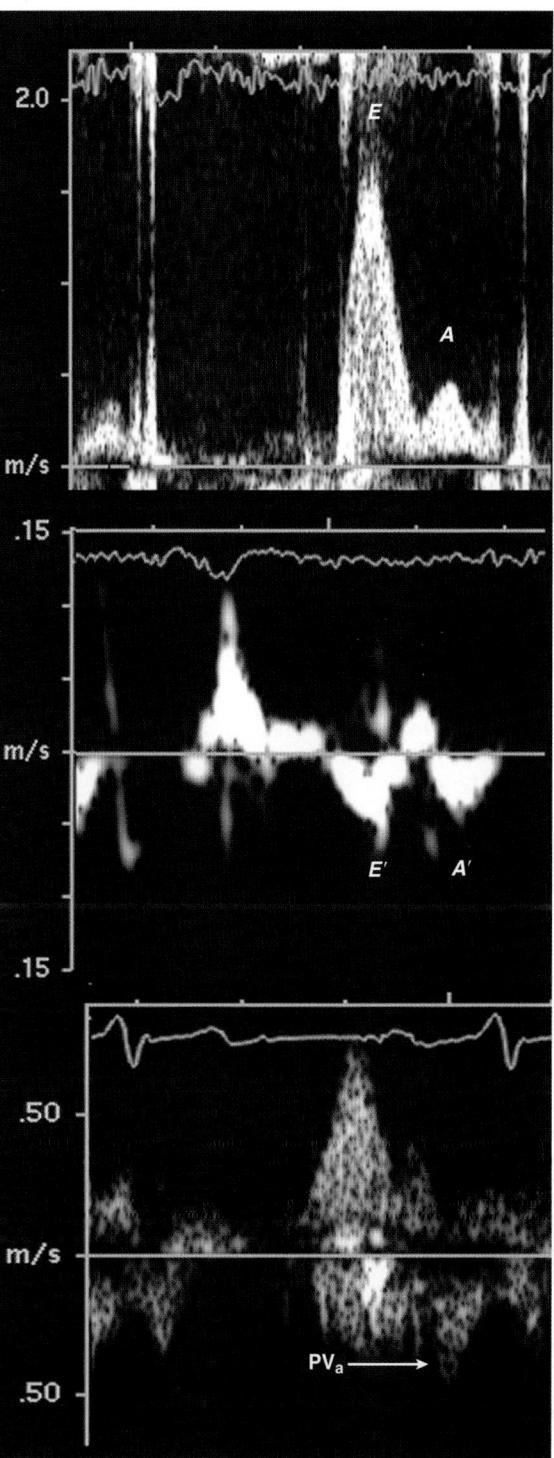

Fig. 7.25 Severe diastolic dysfunction. In this patient with heart failure and a low ejection fraction, the transmitral inflow shows a very high E/A ratio of 4 and a steep deceleration time (*top*). The myocardial tissue Doppler (*center*) shows a very low E' velocity of 0.5 m/s and a very high E/E' ratio of 32. The pulmonary venous inflow pattern (*bottom*) is suboptimal, but diastolic flow is seen with no systolic component and the atrial reversal velocity (PV$_a$) is at the upper limits of normal (approximately 0.35 m/s) (*arrow*), with a duration slightly longer than the mitral A duration, also supporting the diagnosis of elevated LV filling pressures.

- Short isovolumic relaxation time
- Pulmonary venous diastolic flow greater than systolic flow
- Increased velocity and prolonged duration of pulmonary vein atrial reversal

Some classifications of diastolic dysfunction include another category of severe irreversible diastolic dysfunction characterized by the lack of a decrease in E velocity with the Valsalva maneuver, along with even more severe abnormalities in the other parameters of diastolic function. Examples of clinical patterns of diastolic dysfunction are shown in Table 7.5.

RIGHT VENTRICULAR DIASTOLIC FUNCTION

Right Ventricular Filling

The pattern of RV diastolic filling is similar to LV diastolic filling, except that maximal velocities are lower (because the tricuspid annulus is larger), the diastolic filling period is slightly shorter, and greater normal respiratory variation in RV filling occurs (Fig. 7.26). Although few studies have addressed RV diastolic filling, the same measurements described for LV diastolic filling are applicable.

Doppler Data Recording

On TTE, RV inflow can be recorded from the parasternal RV inflow view or from the apical four-chamber view. Pulsed Doppler is used with the same technical considerations that apply to recording LV inflow velocities. Evaluation of respiratory variation of inflow velocities is complicated by the respiratory motion of the heart, so care is needed to ensure a parallel intercept angle between the ultrasound beam and inflow stream throughout the respiratory cycle. This can be accomplished in most patients by using a window where 2D echo shows little respiratory variation in the image plane itself or in the Doppler beam orientation relative to the 2D image.

Physiologic Factors That Affect Right Ventricular Filling

RV filling appears to be affected by all the same physiologic parameters that affect LV filling. Again, the major differences between RV and LV filling are (1) timing, (2) reciprocal respiratory variation (as described earlier), and (3) absolute velocities, which are lower for RV inflow because the tricuspid annulus is larger than the mitral annulus.

Right Atrial Filling

Doppler velocity curves of RA filling can be recorded in the superior vena cava (from a suprasternal notch approach) or the central hepatic vein (from a subcostal approach) because these central veins empty directly into the RA without intervening venous valves. The pattern of RA filling recorded by Doppler parallels the jugular venous pressure curves seen clinically (Fig. 7.27). However, the Doppler data represent a more reliable approach given that evaluation of jugular venous patterns is difficult in some patients because of body habitus and the fact that interpretation is subjective (with no recorded data).

Again, RA filling patterns show respiratory variation in normal individuals with augmentation of RA inflow during inspiration, as is seen in the RV inflow pattern. A plausible explanation for these observations is that the negative intrathoracic pressure with voluntary inspiration (but not with mechanical ventilation) results in an extrathoracic to intrathoracic pressure gradient from the great veins into the RA, thus leading to increased blood flow into the right side of the heart. RA pressure can be estimated by echocardiographic evaluation (from the subcostal window) of the inferior vena cava as blood flow enters the RA, as discussed in Chapter 6.

RA filling is most often evaluated from the subcostal window. After the long-axis view of the inferior vena cava is obtained, the transducer is rotated and angulated to visualize the central hepatic vein, which tends to be directed toward the transducer in this view, to allow a parallel intercept angle between the pulsed Doppler beam and hepatic vein flow. Hepatic vein flow is assumed to be representative of inferior vena caval flow because both enter into the RA without intervening venous valves. Direct study of inferior vena caval flow is limited by a nearly perpendicular intercept angle.

RA inflow also can be recorded in the superior vena cava from the suprasternal notch window. From the standard aortic arch view, the transducer is angulated toward the patient's right to visualize the superior vena cava adjacent and slightly anterior to the ascending aorta. The pulsed Doppler sample volume is positioned in the superior vena cava, with adjustment of transducer angle and sample volume depth to obtain a well-defined velocity curve. As for other inflow patterns, wall filters are minimized (as allowed by signal-to-noise ratio) to demonstrate the low-velocity flows associated with atrial filling.

From both the superior vena cava and hepatic vein recordings, it is important to distinguish respiratory variation in the Doppler curves due to (1) respiratory variation in the angle between the ultrasound beam and blood flow direction from (2) true variations in atrial filling volumes. The hepatic vein is small, so several positions often need to be tried

TABLE 7.5 Examples of Diastolic Dysfunction in Clinical Practice

Condition	Typical Findings	Clinical Implications	Limitations
Heart failure with preserved ejection fraction (HFpEF)	• Normal ejection fraction (>50%) • Normal to mildly dilated LV (EDVI <97 mL/m^2) • Diastolic dysfunction, grades I–III • Elevated filling pressures (LVEDP >16 mmHg; PWP >12 mmHg)	• Clinical symptoms and signs of heart failure are related to diastolic dysfunction. • Clinical decompensation is associated with elevated filling pressures.	• Normal aging changes in LV filling patterns are similar to grade I diastolic dysfunction. • Other noncardiac causes of symptoms should be excluded.
Dilated cardiomyopathy	• Reduced ejection fraction • Dilated LV • Diastolic dysfunction with reduced compliance • Elevated filling pressures	• Clinical signs and symptoms are due to combined systolic and diastolic dysfunction. • Lower filling pressures are seen with effective medical therapy.	• Noninvasive measures of LV filling, PA, and RA pressures often are not adequate for medical management in decompensated patients (see Chapter 9).
Amyloidosis	• LV hypertrophy (with no history of hypertension) • Impaired relaxation with early disease (grade I) • Decreased compliance with advanced disease (grades II–III)	• Severity of diastolic dysfunction predicts clinical outcomes.	• Concurrent changes in LV systolic function, MR, and LA filling pressures also occur, which confounds evaluation of diastolic function.
Hypertrophic cardiomyopathy (HCM)	• Asymmetric LV hypertrophy • Impaired relaxation is typical. • Filling pressures may be elevated. • Subclinical disease can be detected with strain or strain rate imaging.	• Effective medical therapy results in normalization of LV diastolic filling. • Changes in estimated filling pressures can guide therapy. • Detection of early disease has prognostic value.	• Changes in MR severity affect LV filling velocities. • HCM manifests clinically over a wide age range in genetically affected individuals.
Hypertensive heart disease	• Concentric LV hypertrophy • Impaired relaxation with E/A <1	• Diastolic dysfunction is a marker of hypertensive heart disease. • Diastolic dysfunction is seen before overt LV hypertrophy.	• With advanced disease, elevated LVEDP results in a pseudo-normal pattern (grade II). • Coexisting MR related to MAC results in an increased E velocity.
Ischemic heart disease	• Segmental wall motion abnormalities if prior MI • Acute MI associated with impaired relaxation (grade I) • With transmural infarction, more severe diastolic dysfunction is seen long term. • With ischemia, diastolic dysfunction precedes systolic dysfunction.	• Diastolic dysfunction contributes to clinical symptoms with acute MI. • With successful reperfusion, diastolic dysfunction may resolve. • With stress testing for chronic coronary disease, diastolic dysfunction may be seen.	• Diastolic dysfunction may be present only during ischemic episodes and thus missed on a resting echocardiogram. • A complete evaluation of diastolic function is needed to distinguish pseudo-normal filling from normal filling in patients with coronary artery disease (see Chapter 8).
Pericardial constriction	• Normal early-diastolic filling with marked impairment of late diastolic filling • Elevated (and equal) filling pressures in all four cardiac chambers	• Doppler evaluation of diastolic dysfunction helps distinguish restrictive cardiomyopathy from constrictive pericarditis (see Table 10.4).	• Diagnosis of pericardial constriction is challenging and requires correlation with other clinical and imaging data (see Chapter 10).

Grades refer to grades of diastolic dysfunction shown in Table 7.4.
EDVI, End-diastolic volume index; *LVEDP*, LV end-diastolic pressure; *MAC*, mitral annular calcification; *MI*, myocardial infarction; *MR*, mitral regurgitation; *PA*, pulmonary artery; *PWP*, pulmonary wedge pressure.

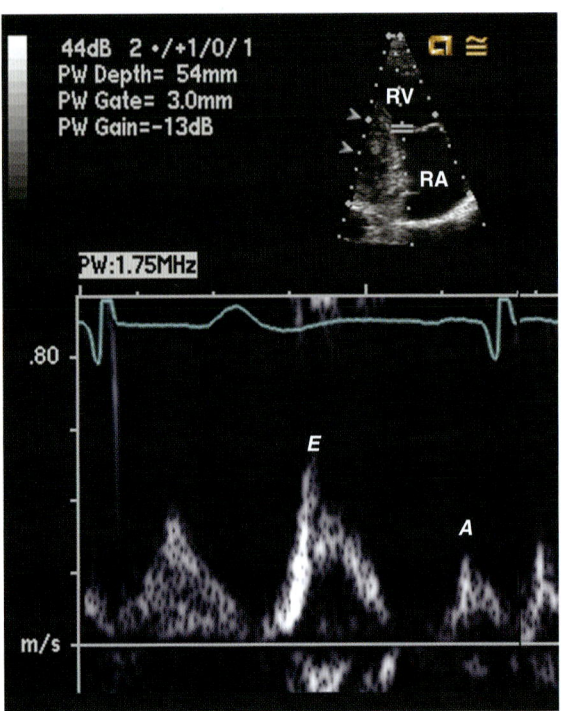

Fig. 7.26 Doppler right ventricular inflow. The RV inflow pattern is similar to LV inflow with an *E* velocity and *A* velocity.

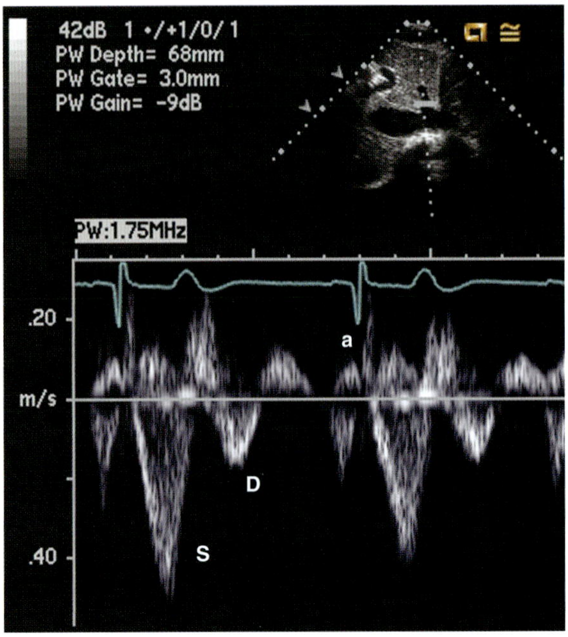

Fig. 7.27 Normal pattern of right atrial inflow. From a subcostal view, flow is recorded in the central hepatic vein showing systolic *(S)* and diastolic *(D)* antegrade filling, with slight flow reversal following atrial *(a)* contraction.

to find one that maintains the sample volume in the hepatic vein throughout the respiratory cycle.

The physiologic factors that affect LA filling also affect RA filling, although less attention has been focused on physiologic parameters affecting the right side of the heart. Respiratory variation in RA filling typically is much more prominent than the respiratory variation seen in LA filling. When a nonsinus cardiac rhythm is present, the lack of atrial contraction results in an absent atrial reversal; systolic forward flow (the filling phase following atrial emptying) may be blunted or reversed.

ALTERNATE APPROACHES

Despite the numerous potential shortcomings of Doppler echocardiographic evaluation of diastolic filling, it has proven to be a repeatable, noninvasive, widely available method for the evaluation of diastolic function (Fig. 7.28). Techniques used in the research laboratory (e.g., time constant of relaxation, pressure-volume curves) rarely are applicable to clinical patient management. The other available clinical modalities for the evaluation of diastolic function include:

- Direct intracardiac pressure measurements
- Radionuclide high-resolution time-activity curves
- Cardiac magnetic resonance tissue tracking methods

The roles of tissue Doppler or speckle tracking strain rate and strain measurements and other newer approaches for clinical evaluation of diastolic dysfunction are in evolution.

DIASTOLIC FUNCTION REPORTING

Essential data on diastolic dysfunction in the echocardiographic report includes key numeric measures as established by each laboratory protocol along with a plain language interpretation of the findings. Key information includes the presence or absence of evidence for diastolic dysfunction, the presence or absence of evidence for elevated filling pressures, the severity of diastolic dysfunction (mild, moderate, or severe), and concurrent factors that affect this diagnosis (e.g., age, heart rate, rhythm, mitral valve disease). Evaluation of diastolic dysfunction is complex, requiring integration with other echocardiographic and clinical data in each patient. Specific measures of diastolic function are most useful in an individual patient when comparing changes over time or in response to medical or interventional therapy.

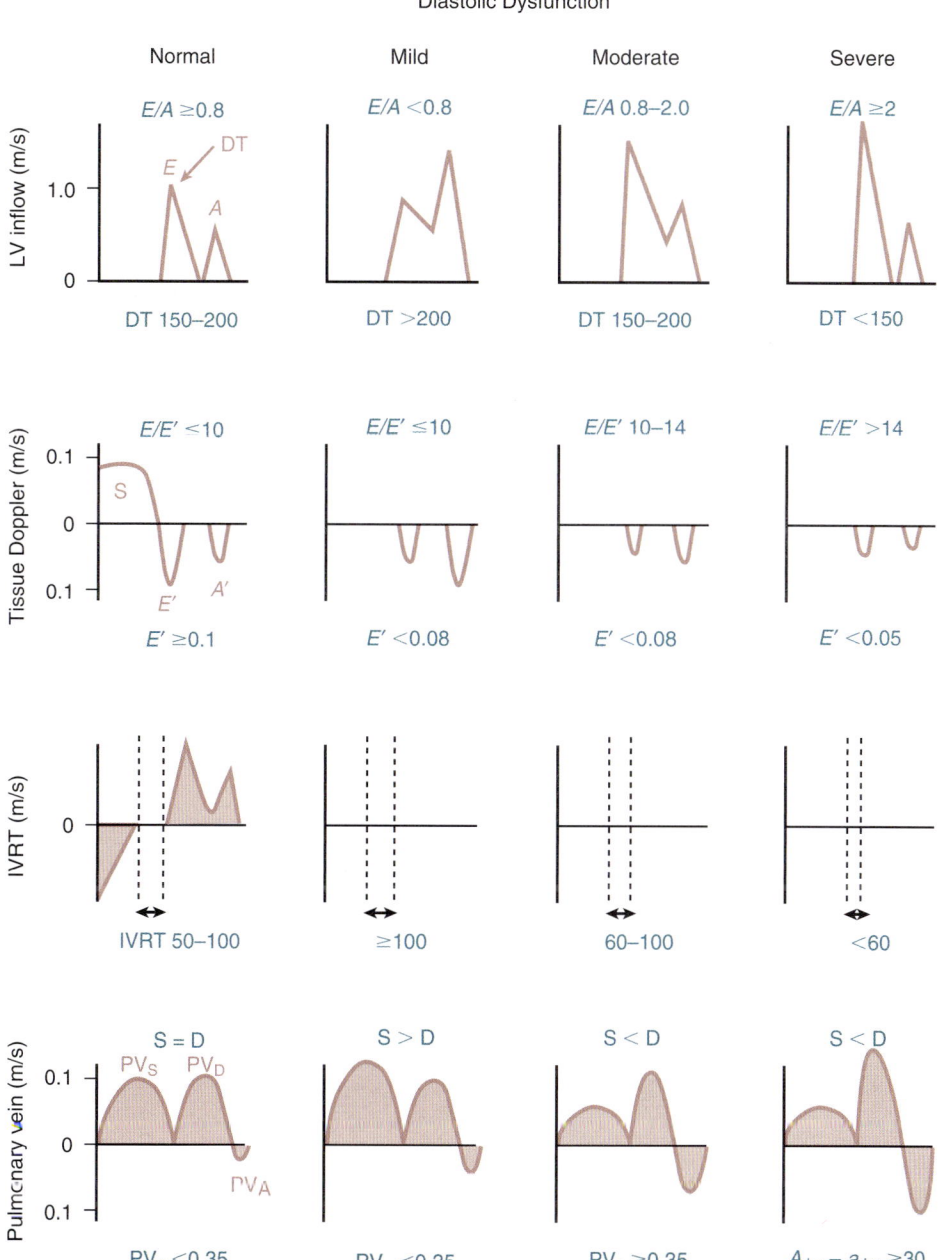

Fig. 7.28 Doppler findings in patients with normal diastolic function and with mild, moderate, and severe diastolic dysfunction. The *top row* shows LV inflow with early *(E)* and atrial *(A)* phases of diastolic filling, the *second row from the top* shows tissue Doppler imaging recorded at the septal side of the mitral annulus with the myocardial early *(E′)* and atrial *(A′)* velocities and the expected ratio of *(E/E′)*, the *third row from the top* shows the isovolumic relaxation time *(IVRT)*, and the *bottom row* shows the pulmonary venous inflow pattern with systolic *(S)* and diastolic *(D)* antegrade flow and the pulmonary vein atrial *(PV$_a$)* reversal of flow.

THE ECHO EXAM

Echocardiographic Techniques in Assessment of Diastolic Function

	Clinical Utility	Technical Points	Limitations
Mitral inflow	• Assess LV compliance, relaxation, filling pressures. • Short DT associated with poor prognosis • Best used with combined systolic and diastolic heart failure	• Sample volume 1–3 mm, filter at 200 Hz, sweep speed 50–100 mm/s • Measure E- and A-waves, DT, IVRT. • A_{dur} measured at mitral annulus	• Preload dependent • E/A ratio can be pseudo-normalized.
Pulmonary vein flow	• Assess LV compliance, relaxation, filling pressures. • Blunted S and D velocities associated with poor prognosis • Best used with combined systolic and diastolic heart failure • PV_a used to assess pseudo-normalization	• Sample volume 2–3 mm, placed 1–2 cm into the PV, filter at 200 Hz, sweep speed 50–100 mm/s • Measure S, D, and PV_a waves.	• Relatively preload independent • Technically difficult to obtain in all patients • Blunted S/D from other conditions including atrial fibrillation and mitral regurgitation
Tissue Doppler imaging	• Assess LV compliance, relaxation, filling pressures. • E/E′ ≥15 associated with elevated filling pressures • Best used with primary diastolic heart failure	• Sample volume 2–4 mm at mitral annulus, filter at 200 Hz, sweep speed 50–100 mm/s • Measure S′, E′, and A′ waves.	• Relatively preload independent • Angle and translation dependent • Different velocities at annuli (lateral > medial)
Color M-mode	• Assess LV compliance, relaxation, filling pressures. • E/V_p >1.5 associated with elevated filling pressures • Best used with primary diastolic heart failure	• Slope of flow propagation (first aliasing velocity) for 4 cm into LV • 2D depth reduced to 16 cm • Move baseline to set color aliasing velocity about 40 cm/s. • M-mode sweep recorded at 100 mm/s • Measure V_p slope.	• Relatively preload independent • Technically difficult to obtain in all patients • Influenced by LV geometry
Strain imaging	• High time resolution of deformation (sampling rates >200/min) • Allows assessment of regional diastolic deformation	• Global measures include peak early and late diastolic strain rates and time to early peak strain rate.	• Circumferential strain should be measured in addition to radial and longitudinal strain. • Diastolic strain rate measurements are complex and not yet clinically validated

A, Filling wave due to atrial contraction; D, diastolic flow; DT, deceleration time; IVRT, isovolumic relaxation time; PV, pulmonary vein; PV_a, pulmonary vein atrial reversal; S, systolic flow; V_p, velocity of propagation.
Modified from Plana JC, Desai MY, Klein AL: Assessment of diastolic function by echocardiography. In Otto CM, editor: *The Practice of Clinical Echocardiography*, ed 4, Philadelphia, 2012, Elsevier.

SUGGESTED READING

1. Abraham TP, Mayer SA: Left ventricular diastolic function. In Otto CM, editor: *The Practice of Clinical Echocardiography*, ed 5, Philadelphia, 2017, Elsevier, pp 147–165 *Advanced discussion of Doppler echocardiographic measures for evaluation of diastolic dysfunction with emphasis on clinical applications. Numerous figures and tables supplement the concise text. 95 references.*

2. Flachskampf FA, Biering-Sørensen T, Solomon SD, et al: Cardiac imaging to evaluate left ventricular diastolic function, *JACC Cardiovasc Imaging* 8(9):1071–1093, 2015. *Review of the physiology of diastole with diagrams showing the relationship between pressure and Doppler measures of diastolic function. Simple diagrams illustrate concepts including early diastolic lengthening velocity,*

compliance, and strain imaging. 115 references.

3. Nagueh SF, Smiseth OA, Appleton CP, et al: Recommendations for the evaluation of left ventricular diastolic function by echocardiography: an update from the American Society of Echocardiography and the European Association of Cardiovascular Imaging, *J Am Soc Echocardiogr* 29(4):277–314, 2016.
This consensus statement from the American Society of Echocardiography and the European Society of Echocardiography reviews the physiology of diastole, provides a detailed discussion of parameters of diastolic function (including validation), includes tables of normal values, proposes algorithms for clinical diagnosis of diastolic function, and classifies diastolic dysfunction (grades I, II, and III) based on LV filling and tissue Doppler parameters.

4. Gillebert TC, De Pauw M, Timmermans F: Echo-Doppler assessment of diastole: flow, function and haemodynamics, *Heart* 99(1):55–64, 2013.
Review of the physiology of diastole, Doppler echo measures of diastolic function, and grading of diastolic dysfunction.

5. Oh JK, Park SJ, Nagueh SF: Established and novel clinical applications of diastolic function assessment by echocardiography, *Circ Cardiovasc Imaging* 4(4):444–455, 2011.
Review of the physiology of normal diastolic function and the echocardiographic approach to recognition and classification of diastolic dysfunction. In addition to standard clinical parameters, newer approaches including strain imaging for evaluation of regional diastolic dysfunction, torsion for detection of mild diastolic dysfunction, and LA strain to assess LA function and LV diastolic pressure. 63 references.

6. Shah SJ, Kitzman DW, Borlaug BA, et al: Phenotype-specific treatment of heart failure with preserved ejection fraction: a multiorgan roadmap, *Circulation* 134(1):73–90, 2016.
Review article on the differing mechanisms of HFpEF and how understanding the specific phenotype might inform therapy. Clinical presentation phenotypes are divided into lung congestion, chronotropic incompetence, pulmonary hypertension, skeletal muscle weakness, and atrial fibrillation. Common predisposing phenotypes include obesity/metabolic syndrome, arterial hypertension, renal dysfunction, and coronary artery disease. The echocardiographer should consider the diagnosis of HFpEF and record appropriate imaging and Doppler data in patients undergoing imaging for these indications.

7. Erdei T, Smiseth OA, Marino P, et al: A systematic review of diastolic stress tests in heart failure with preserved ejection fraction, with proposals from the EU-FP7 MEDIA study group, *Eur J Heart Fail* 16(12):1345–1361, 2014.
The use of stress testing to evaluate changes in diastolic function in patients with HFpEF is emerging as a potential clinical approach to diagnosis. In this meta-analysis, the various types of stress testing used and the echocardiographic parameters measured are summarized. The authors recommend a ramped exercise protocol on a semisupine bicycle, starting at 15 W, with increments of 5 W/min to a submaximal target (heart rate 100–110 bpm, or symptoms) in older adult subjects with HRpEF. Changes from rest to exercise in LV long-axis function and indirect e indices of LV diastolic pressure, such as E/E′, should be measured.

8. Erdei T, Aakhus S, Marino P, et al: Pathophysiological rationale and diagnostic targets for diastolic stress testing, *Heart* 101(17):1355–1360, 2015.
Diastolic stress testing is based on the concept that impaired diastolic function during exercise may account for symptoms in patients with HFpEF. Older adults have a greater and more rapid rise in left atrial pressure with exercise, compared with younger patients, but diastolic relaxation and compliance also may be abnormal. Mechanisms and diagnostic targets for diastolic stress testing are summarized in a table.

9. Nakatani S: Left ventricular rotation and twist: why should we learn?, *J Cardiovasc Ultrasound* 19:1–6, 2011.
Concise review of the basic principles of LV rotation and twist in addition to echocardiographic approaches to measurement. 3D speckle tracking is recommended for measurement of twist to avoid effects of cardiac motion through any given tomographic plane. Measurement of twist and untwist offer promise for improved diagnosis, but further evaluation of the clinical utility of these approaches is needed.

10. Singh A, Addetia K, Maffessanti F, et al: LA strain categorization of LV diastolic dysfunction, *JACC Cardiovasc Imaging* 10(7):735–743, 2017.
Left atrial strain measurements were feasible and allowed categorization of LV diastolic function in a series of 229 patients with heart failure with preserved ejection fraction.

11. Morris DA, Gailani M, Vaz Pérez A, et al: Right ventricular myocardial systolic and diastolic dysfunction in heart failure with normal left ventricular ejection fraction, *J Am Soc Echocardiogr* 24(8):886–897, 2011.
In patients with HFpEF, the presence of abnormal LV global longitudinal strain was associated with RV diastolic dysfunction, and both the LV and RV showed similar degrees of impairment of subendocardial function. These findings suggest that RV diastolic dysfunction may contribute to symptoms in patients with HFpEF.

12. Pagourelias ED, Efthimiadis GK, Parcharidou DG, et al: Prognostic value of right ventricular diastolic function indices in hypertrophic cardiomyopathy, *Eur J Echocardiogr* 12(11):809–817, 2011.
In 386 patients with hypertrophic cardiomyopathy, the presence of an increased RV E/E′ ratio was associated with a 1.8 times greater risk of heart failure mortality (95% confidence intervals 1.1 to 2.4). This study demonstrates that evaluation of RV diastolic dysfunction may be useful in predicting prognosis in patients with hypertrophic cardiomyopathy.

8 Coronary Artery Disease

BASIC PRINCIPLES
  Coronary Artery Anatomy
  Evaluation of Left Ventricular Wall Motion
    Transthoracic Imaging
    Transesophageal Imaging
  Sequence of Events in Ischemia
  Evaluation of Global and Regional Ventricular Function

MYOCARDIAL ISCHEMIA
  Basic Principles of Stress Echocardiography
  Exercise Echocardiography
  Dobutamine Stress Echocardiography
    Evaluation for Ischemia
    Evaluation for Myocardial Viability
  Other Stress Modalities
  Limitations and Technical Aspects
  Alternate Approaches
  Clinical Utility
    Diagnosis of Coronary Artery Disease
    Extent and Location of Ischemic Areas
    Prognostic Implications

MYOCARDIAL INFARCTION
  Basic Principles
  Echocardiographic Imaging
  Limitations and Alternate Approaches
  Clinical Utility
    Diagnosis in the Emergency Department
    Evaluation of Interventional Therapy
    Myocardial Viability
    Mechanical Complications of Myocardial Infarction

END-STAGE ISCHEMIC CARDIAC DISEASE
  Differentiation From Other Causes of Left Ventricular Systolic Dysfunction
  Echocardiographic Approach
  Limitations and Alternate Approaches

THE ECHO EXAM

SUGGESTED READING

Evaluation of patients with suspected or documented coronary artery disease is one of the most common indications for echocardiography. Evaluation typically focuses on functional changes due to coronary artery narrowing or occlusion—specifically systolic wall thickening and endocardial motion—rather than on direct imaging of the coronary arteries. Although the proximal left main and right coronary arteries often can be identified, even on transthoracic images, ultrasound imaging currently does not provide the detailed knowledge of distal vessel anatomy or the location and severity of coronary artery narrowing that is needed for patient management. Invasive coronary angiography remains the procedure of choice for direct assessment of coronary artery anatomy because diagnosis often is combined with interventional treatment. Computed tomographic (CT) coronary angiography provides an alternative approach in some clinical situations.

However, echocardiography offers detailed functional assessment of segmental and global left ventricular (LV) systolic function both at rest and with stressors to induce ischemia. Functional assessment provides critical data for patient management. For example, stress echocardiography is a reliable approach for the initial diagnosis of coronary artery disease, especially in patients with a nondiagnostic stress electrocardiogram (ECG). Another example is the use of echocardiography in the emergency department for early diagnosis of acute myocardial infarction in patients with equivocal ECG changes. In addition, the central role of echocardiography in evaluation for complications of acute myocardial infarction has long been recognized. Finally, echocardiography often provides important prognostic data in patients with coronary artery disease.

BASIC PRINCIPLES

Coronary Artery Anatomy

Coronary anatomy varies to some degree from patient to patient, but the overall pattern of coronary artery branching is relatively uniform (Fig. 8.1). The left main coronary artery arises from the superior aspect of the left coronary sinus of Valsalva and divides into (1) the left anterior descending (LAD) artery, which extends by the interventricular groove down the anterior wall to (and sometimes around) the LV apex; and (2) the circumflex (Cx) artery, which continues laterally in the atrioventricular groove. The right coronary artery (RCA) arises from the superior aspect

Coronary Artery Disease | Chapter 8

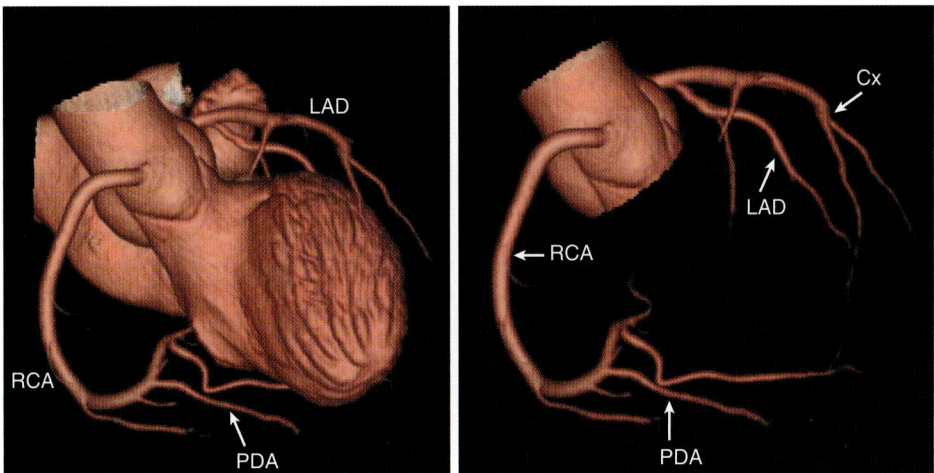

Fig. 8.1 ▶ ▶ **Normal coronary anatomy.** A computed tomographic reconstruction of the coronary arteries shows *(left)* the origin of the right and left coronary arteries from the aorta with the left ventricular chamber shown for orientation. The right coronary artery *(RCA)* gives rise to the posterior descending artery *(PDA)* in most people, although a few have the PDA arising from the distal circumflex coronary artery *(Cx)*. With the heart chambers removed and the image rotated *(right)*, the left main coronary artery bifurcates into the left anterior descending coronary artery *(LAD)* (with a septal branch) and the circumflex coronary artery, which branches into obtuse marginal branches. *(Images courtesy Dr. Kelley Branch.)*

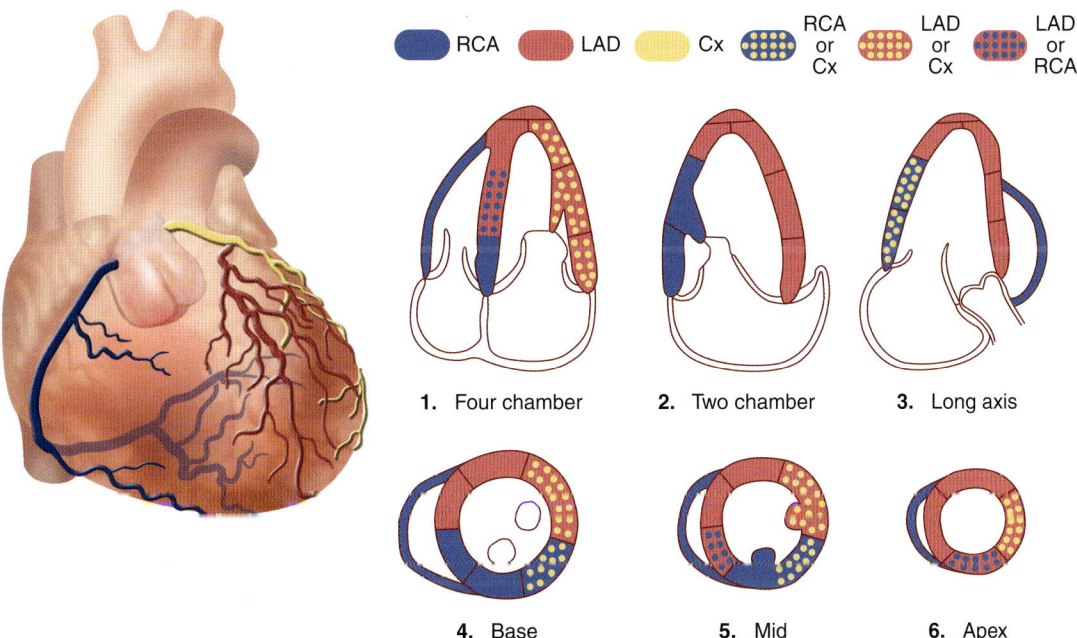

Fig. 8.2 **Typical myocardial segments supplied by the right coronary artery, left anterior descending artery, and circumflex coronary arteries.** The coronary anatomy is shown on the *left*, with the corresponding wall segments in standard echocardiographic views on the *right*. The arterial distribution varies among patients. Some segments have variable coronary perfusion, as indicated by the *hatched regions*. *Cx*, Circumflex coronary artery; *LAD*, left anterior descending coronary artery; *RCA*, right coronary artery. *(From Lang RM, Bierig M, Devereux RB, et al: Recommendations for chamber quantification: a report from the American Society of Echocardiography's Guidelines and Standards Committee and the Chamber Quantification Writing Group, developed in conjunction with the European Association of Echocardiography, a branch of the European Society of Cardiology. J Am Soc Echocardiogr 18:1440–1463, 2005.)*

of the right coronary sinus of Valsalva and extends inferomedially following the atrioventricular groove. Approximately 80% of patients have a *right-dominant* coronary circulation; the right coronary artery gives rise to the posterior descending artery (PDA), which lies in the inferior interventricular groove. In about 20% of patients the coronary circulation is *left dominant;* the circumflex artery gives rise to the posterior descending artery.

Segmental wall motion abnormalities seen by echocardiography correspond closely to the coronary artery blood supply to the myocardium (Fig. 8.2). The left anterior descending artery supplies the anterior portion of the interventricular septum through septal

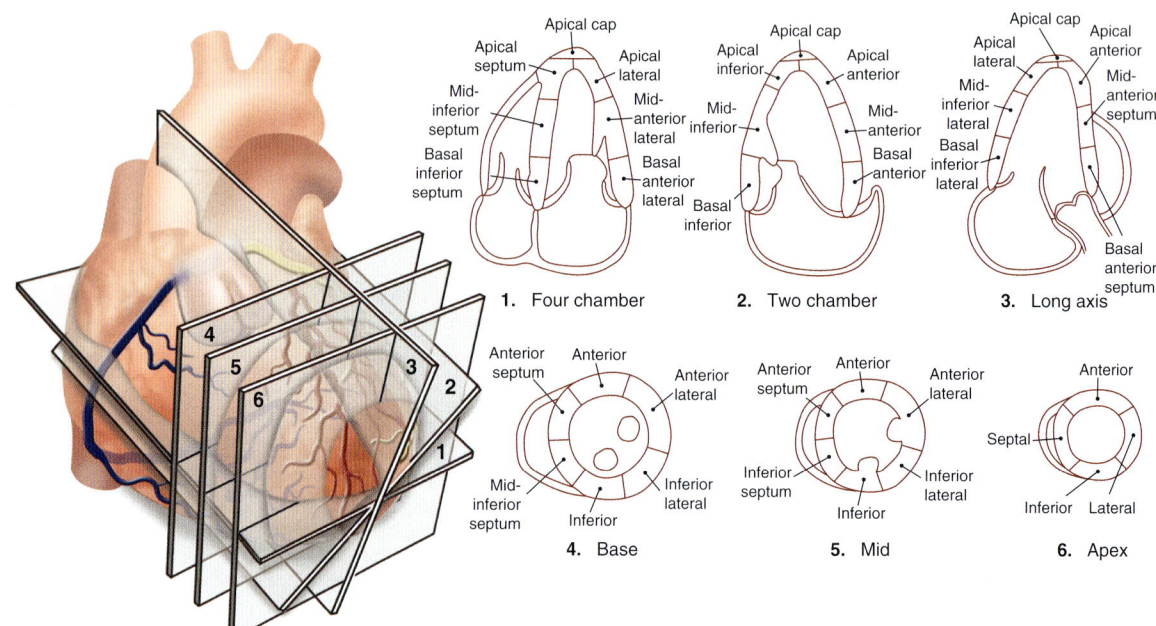

Fig. 8.3 Segmental analysis of left ventricular endocardial motion and wall thickening. The LV is divided into three levels from base to apex, with wall segment nomenclature as shown. The apex segments are usually visualized from apical four-chamber, apical two-chamber, and apical three-chamber views. The apical cap can be appreciated only on contrast studies in some patients. *(From Lang RM, Bierig M, Devereux RB, et al: Recommendations for chamber quantification: a report from the American Society of Echocardiography's Guidelines and Standards Committee and the Chamber Quantification Writing Group, developed in conjunction with the European Association of Echocardiography, a branch of the European Society of Cardiology. J Am Soc Echocardiogr 18:1440–1463, 2005.)*

perforating branches and the anterior wall through diagonal branches. The posterior descending artery supplies the inferior aspect of the ventricular septum and the inferior free wall. The lateral wall is supplied by obtuse marginal branches of the circumflex artery. The inferolateral (or posterior) LV wall may be supplied by extension branches from the right coronary artery or by obtuse marginal branches of the circumflex arteries. Marked individual variability is noted in the blood supply to the LV apex. In some cases, the left anterior descending artery extends around the apex to supply the apical segment of the inferior wall. In other cases, the posterior descending artery extends around the apex to supply the apical segment of the anterior wall. More commonly, the blood supply to the apex arises from both the left anterior descending and the posterior descending coronary arteries.

Standardized nomenclature for tomographic imaging of the heart allows consistency of terms, correlations among different imaging techniques, and a known relationship of each segment with coronary anatomy. Standard tomographic planes on echocardiography are short axis, long axis, four chamber, and two chamber. In each image plane, the LV is divided into three segments from base to apex—basal, mid-cavity, and apical—which correspond to proximal, middle, and apical lesions of the coronary arteries (Fig. 8.3). In a short-axis view, both at the basal (mitral valve) and mid-cavity (or papillary muscle) levels, the ventricle is divided clockwise, beginning with the interventricular groove, into six segments: the anterior wall, the anterolateral wall, the inferolateral (or posterior) wall, the inferior wall, the inferior septal wall, and the anterior septal wall. The apical region is divided into four segments because of the normal tapering of the ventricle toward the apex: anterior, lateral, inferior, and septal, with an additional segment for the tip of the apex. This results in a total of 17 myocardial segments. On standard echocardiographic imaging, the apical cap is difficult to visualize, so a 16-segment model typically is used in clinical practice. The location of wall motion abnormalities can be reported in two-dimensional (2D) or three-dimensional (3D) formats, descriptively, using colors to signify wall motion abnormalities or using more quantitative display formats.

The segmental wall motion abnormalities seen with ischemia or infarction correspond to the coronary anatomy as follows:

1. Left anterior coronary artery disease
   - Anterior septum
   - Anterior free wall, at the base and mid-cavity level
   - Apical segments of the septum and anterior wall, plus the apical cap

Depending on the degree to which diagonal branches supply the lateral wall, the anterolateral wall also may be affected. If the left anterior descending artery extends around the apex, the affected area includes apical segments of the inferior and inferolateral walls. The location of the lesion along the length of the coronary artery affects the pattern of wall motion. A lesion in the distal third of the vessel affects only the apex, and a lesion in the mid-segment of the vessel affects the mid-cavity and apical segments, whereas a proximal lesion affects the entire wall including the basal segments.

2. Circumflex coronary artery disease
   - Anterolateral wall
   - Inferolateral (posterior) wall

Again the extent of segmental wall motion is related to the exact coronary anatomy in an individual patient. Echocardiography is particularly helpful in patients with circumflex artery disease because this myocardial region often is "silent" electrocardiographically and is not well seen on a single-plane right anterior oblique LV angiogram.

3. Posterior descending coronary artery disease
   - Inferior septum
   - Inferior free wall

If the posterior descending artery is a short vessel, the apex will not be affected, whereas extensive wall motion abnormalities of the apex may be seen if the posterior descending artery extends to supply the ventricular apex.

Other patterns of abnormal wall motion are seen with lesions of the branches of the three major coronary arteries. For example, isolated disease in a diagonal branch of the left anterior descending artery results in a discrete wall motion abnormality in the portion of the anterolateral wall supplied by that vessel. Proximal right coronary artery disease can result in ischemia or infarction of the right ventricular (RV) free wall.

Collateral vessels and previous coronary stenting or bypass surgery also affect the pattern of wall motion. If a myocardial segment has a balanced oxygen demand-to-supply ratio, wall motion will be normal whether blood flow is supplied antegrade by the native vessel, by collateral vessels, or by a bypass graft.

Evaluation of Left Ventricular Wall Motion

Transthoracic Imaging

Regional systolic function for each segment of the LV can be assessed on transthoracic imaging by combining data from multiple image planes or using 3D echocardiography.

With 2D imaging, standard views for evaluation of wall motion are (Fig. 8.4):

- Short-axis (base, mid-LV, and apex) view
- Four-chamber view
- Two-chamber view
- Long-axis view

In the parasternal long-axis view, the basal and midventricular segments of the anterior septum and posterior LV walls are seen. In the parasternal short-axis view, circumferential images of the LV at the base and midventricular levels are obtained. Note that if the transducer is angulated toward the apex from a fixed parasternal position, progressively more

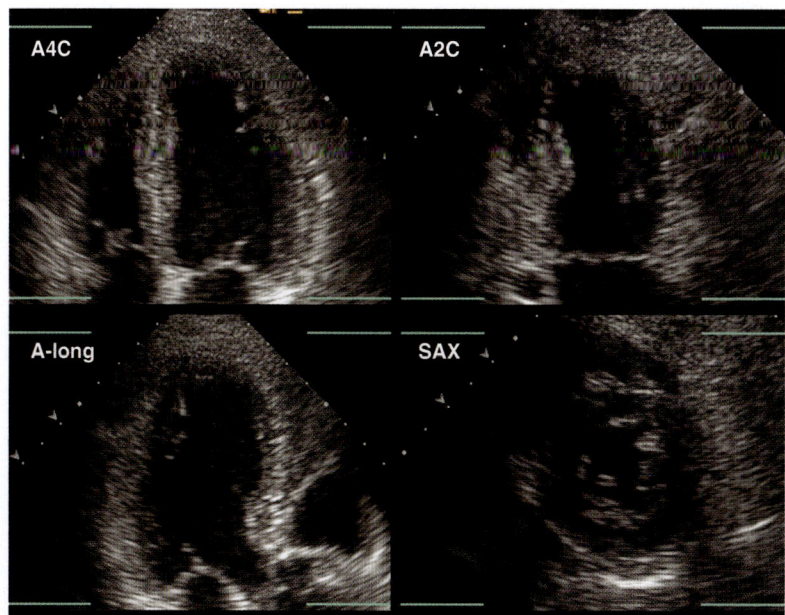

Fig. 8.4 **Example of the standard image planes used for stress echocardiography.** These planes are apical four-chamber *(A4C)*, apical two-chamber *(A2C)*, apical long-axis *(A-long)*, and parasternal short-axis *(SAX)*. Images are acquired in a digital cine-loop format at each stress stage and are then re-sorted to show the baseline and peak stress images side by side for each view. Images are gated to show only systole, so that endocardial motion and wall thickening appear to occur in the same time frame, even though a substantial difference is present in heart rate between baseline and peak stress. Image depth is adjusted to show only the LV.

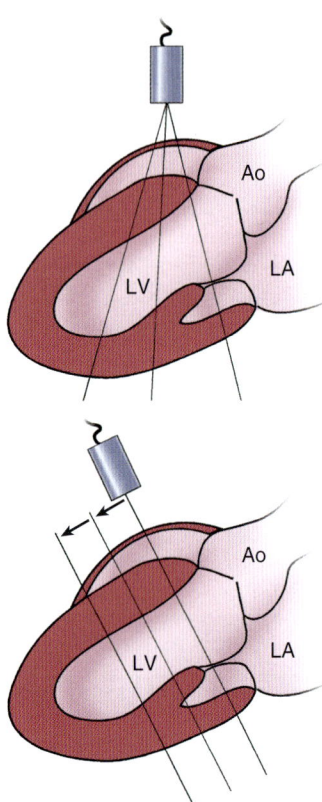

Fig. 8.5 Effect of transducer angulation on left ventricle imaging. Angulation of the transducer from a fixed parasternal position results in short-axis views that intersect similar segments of the septum but progressively more apical segments of the posterior wall. By moving the transducer apically, more parallel image planes can be obtained. *Ao,* Aorta.

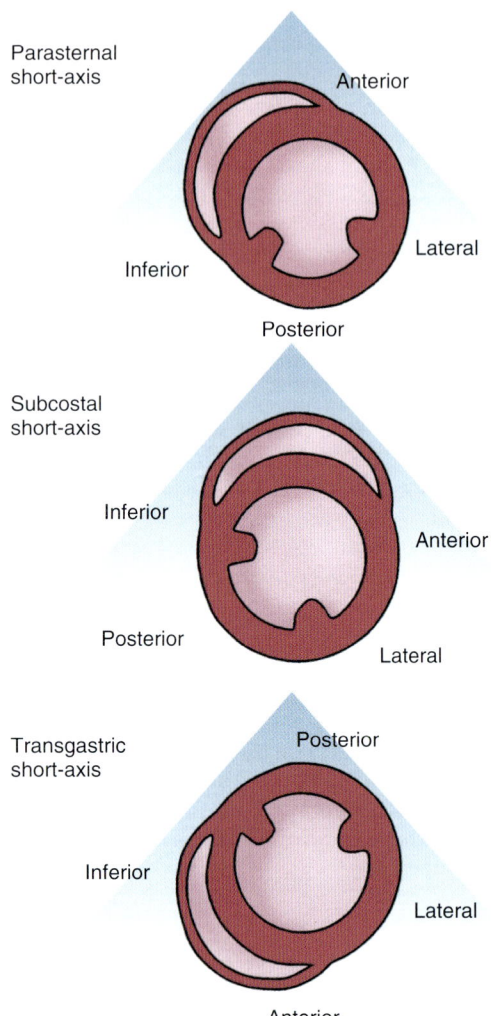

Fig. 8.6 Comparison of parasternal, subcostal, and transesophageal echocardiography transgastric short-axis views of the left ventricle. Correct identification of wall segments is facilitated by noting the position of the septum and the papillary muscles.

apical segments of the posterior wall are imaged while the *same* segment of the septum is included in the ultrasound image plane. A more parallel alignment between image planes is obtained by moving the transducer apically to obtain short-axis mid-cavity and (sometimes) apical views of the LV (Fig. 8.5) or by using 3D imaging. The apical segments rarely are adequately visualized from the parasternal window or on transesophageal (TEE) images.

From the apical window, evaluation of LV wall motion is performed in four-chamber, two-chamber, and long-axis views. Detailed evaluation of the extent of abnormal myocardium is possible on 2D imaging by slow rotation of the image plane between the standard views. In the four-chamber view, the inferior septum and anterolateral wall are seen. Anterior angulation to include the aortic valve allows visualization of portions of the anterior septum. In the two-chamber view, the anterior and inferior free walls are seen. Endocardial and epicardial definition of the anterior wall often is difficult due to attenuation by adjacent overlying lung tissue. This problem can be alleviated by careful patient positioning and imaging during held respiration. In the apical long-axis view, the anterior septum and inferolateral (posterior) wall are seen (analogous to the parasternal long-axis view). Care is needed in positioning the transducer at the apex to avoid foreshortening of the ventricle from this approach. Integration of data from parasternal and apical approaches, while taking into account image quality in each view, allows assessment of each myocardial segment in at least two views. Evaluation from a subcostal approach also is helpful. In the subcostal four-chamber view, the inferior septum and anterolateral wall are imaged. In the subcostal short-axis view, the inferior and inferolateral (posterior) walls are nearest the transducer and the anterior and anterolateral walls are most distal (Fig. 8.6).

Real-time 3D multiplane or volumetric imaging from an apical approach has the potential to provide more rapid and complete assessment of wall motion.

With 3D echocardiography, wall motion is assessed using:

- Multiple simultaneous 2D views or
- 3D volumetric LV image

Simultaneous apical views at set angles of rotation or multiple parallel short-axis views can be generated from the 3D volume set, thus allowing rapid evaluation of wall motion in multiple myocardial segments on the same cardiac cycles. A limitation of apical volumetric scans is that the endocardium is imaged using the lateral, rather than axial, resolution of the ultrasound beam, and this limits identification of endocardial borders for quantitative analysis. The 3D volumetric image can be displayed in motion in a cine-loop format, with rotation of the image to show different wall segments. In addition to qualitative measures of wall motion, semiquantitative measures of timing and magnitude of wall motion can be displayed in a "target diagram" with the apex in the center and the base around the edges of the circular display (Fig. 8.7).

When endocardial definition is suboptimal with either 2D or 3D imaging, opacification of the LV with left-sided contrast is recommended for evaluation or regional function (Fig. 8.8). Contrast to enhance endocardial border definition is recommended when two or more segments are poorly visualized with standard imaging and is particularly important for stress echocardiography to ensure detection of ischemic segments. Most laboratories find that contrast enhancement is needed for 30% to 50% of stress echocardiographic studies, depending on the patient population.

Transesophageal Imaging

When transthoracic images are inadequate, or in certain monitoring situations (e.g., intraoperative monitoring of LV function), regional LV function can be evaluated from a TEE approach. From the high left atrial (LA) position a four-chamber view of the LV is obtained (in the 0° plane of the TEE probe), showing the inferior septum and lateral wall. Rotating the image plane to approximately 60° provides a two-chamber view with visualization of the anterior and inferior walls, whereas further rotation to about 120° results in a long-axis view with imaging of the anterior septum and inferolateral (posterior) wall, although the exact

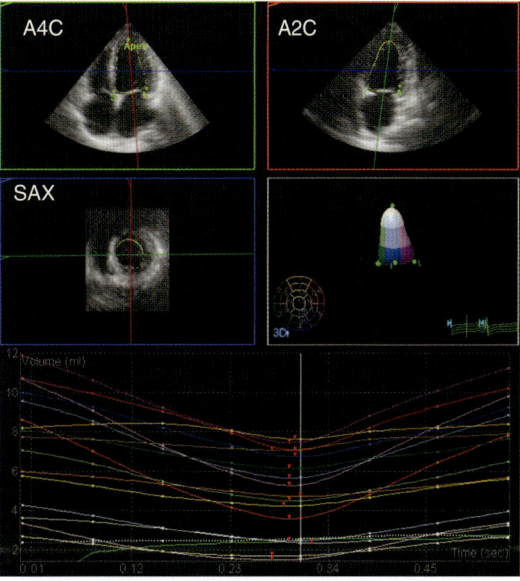

Fig. 8.7 3D echocardiographic wall motion assessment. Wall motion can be assessed based on 3D volume acquisition image planes corresponding to four-chamber (A4C), two-chamber (A2C), and short-axis (SAX) images. Wall motion is then displayed graphically on a cine or still image coded by color on the 3D LV reconstruction *(middle right)*, as a graph of motion versus time with each segment shown in a different color *(bottom)*.

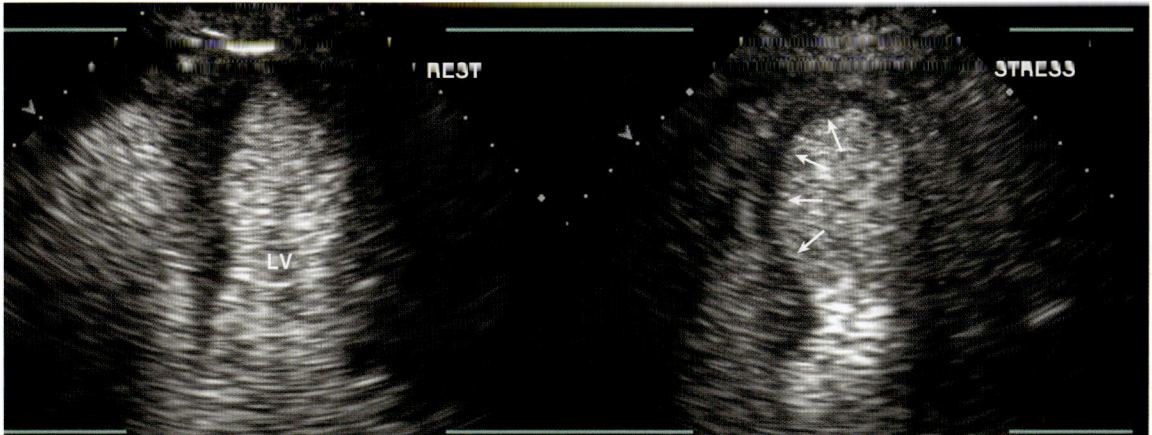

Fig. 8.8 ▶ **Contrast enhancement of left ventricular endocardial borders.** This patient had suboptimal endocardial definition even with harmonic imaging and careful patient positioning. After intravenous injection of a left heart contrast agent, opacification of the LV chamber is seen with clear definition of the endocardial border, at rest *(left)* and with stress *(right)* in the apical four-chamber view, demonstrating inducible ischemia in the middle and apical inferior septum *(arrows)*.

degree of rotation to obtain these views varies slightly from patient to patient. Transducer position and angulation require adjustment as the image plane is rotated using anatomic landmarks to ensure proper alignment. Even with optimal technique these views are usually foreshortened; that is, the apparent apex represents an oblique plane through the anterolateral wall, whereas the true LV apex is not seen.

From the transgastric position, the transverse image plane provides short-axis views of the LV at the base (mitral valve) and mid-cavity (papillary muscle) levels. Rotation of the image plane at this position provides a two-chamber view, though the apex often is foreshortened. Further advancement of the probe allows acquisition of an "apical" four-chamber view (in the 0° plane) by flexing the probe tip. Often, the true apex is missed in this view because the LV apex does not lie on the diaphragm without intervening lung tissue in a position accessible from the transgastric approach.

With all TEE studies, a 3D volumetric image acquisition is recommended for measurement of LV volumes and ejection fraction, as well as assessment of regional wall motion.

TEE imaging of LV wall motion is indicated:

- For intraoperative assessment of global and segmental LV function
- In critically ill patients when transthoracic views are inadequate

TEE imaging also may be used with stress protocols, although this is not a routine approach.

Sequence of Events in Ischemia

Irreversible myocardial damage (e.g., infarction) results in wall motion abnormalities that are present at rest. With an acute infarction, wall thickness is normal, but systolic wall thickening and endocardial motion are reduced or absent. An old myocardial infarction is characterized by thinning and increased echogenicity of the affected segments due to scarring and fibrosis, in addition to abnormal motion and absent wall thickening.

In contrast, ischemia is a reversible imbalance in the myocardial oxygen demand-to-supply ratio. Even with substantial coronary artery narrowing, blood flow is adequate for myocardial oxygen demands at rest. However, when the narrowing exceeds approximately 70% of the luminal cross-sectional area, blood flow becomes inadequate to meet increased myocardial oxygen demands with exercise, pharmacologic interventions, or mental stress, with resulting ischemia. When oxygen demand returns to baseline, blood flow again is adequate, ischemia resolves, and wall motion returns to normal. Thus wall motion *at rest* is normal in patients with coronary artery disease if no prior myocardial infarction occurred.

The sequence of changes as a region of myocardium becomes ischemic is as follows (Fig. 8.9). The first detectable changes associated with heterogeneity of flow to the LV are biochemical, followed by a significant perfusion defect (detectable by radionuclide and magnetic resonance techniques). Next, regional myocardial dysfunction, characterized by both abnormal diastolic function and impaired systolic wall thickening, occurs in rapid succession (within a few cardiac cycles). Ischemic ST-segment depression on ECG and clinical angina are relatively late manifestations of ischemia and are not seen consistently. Echocardiography, by detecting abnormal regional wall motion, provides a useful noninvasive method for evaluating ischemia that is more sensitive than ECG given this sequence of events. Echocardiography differs from radionuclide techniques in that the functional consequences of ischemia, rather than the pattern of myocardial perfusion, are assessed.

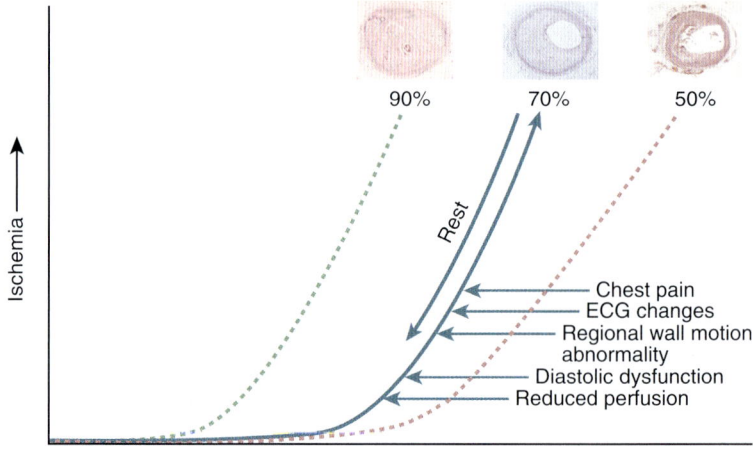

Fig. 8.9 Schematic diagram of the sequence of events in myocardial ischemia. The level of stress is shown on the horizontal axis, often estimated by the heart rate *(HR)* × blood pressure *(BP)* product, with the degree of ischemia shown on the vertical axis. With a 70% coronary artery narrowing *(blue)*, ischemia begins when the stress level results in inadequate coronary blood flow to that region of myocardium. As ischemia increases, the sequence of events is shown. With rest *(downward blue arrow)*, these events reverse unless the duration of ischemia is long enough to cause infarction. The onset and slope of the ischemic response are earlier and steeper with more severe coronary stenosis (as shown for a 90% lesion), and they are later and less steep with milder coronary disease (as shown for a 50% stenosis).

Evaluation of Global and Regional Ventricular Function

Global LV systolic function can be evaluated either qualitatively or quantitatively in patients with coronary artery disease by using the approaches described in Chapter 6. Because the pattern of LV dysfunction typically is *not* uniform, it is important that qualitative and quantitative evaluation be based on multiple tomographic views or 3D imaging. In patients with coronary artery disease, LV ejection fraction measurement provides essential clinical data because it is an essential variable in clinical decision making.

Segmental (or regional) LV systolic function most often is evaluated using a semiquantitative scoring system based on 2D or 3D imaging. The endocardial motion for each defined myocardial segment is graded as normal, hypokinetic, akinetic, dyskinetic, or aneurysmal (Table 8.1). Some clinicians prefer to subclassify the degree of hypokinesis as mild, moderate, or severe, but such a subclassification often has significant interobserver and intraobserver variability. Ischemia results both in a decrease in the total amplitude and velocity of endocardial motion and wall thickening and in a delay in the onset of contraction and relaxation. Some centers use a numeric scoring system for wall motion from 1 (normal) to 4 (dyskinetic) for each segment. An overall wall motion score index can be derived by dividing the sum of scores for each segment by the number of segments evaluated:

$$\text{Wall motion score} = \frac{\text{Sum of individual segment scores}}{\text{Number of segments visualized}}$$

(Eq. 8.1)

Several more sophisticated approaches to quantitation of wall motion have been proposed based on the total amplitude of endocardial motion, the extent of wall thickening, the velocity of myocardial motion, or the timing of the onset of contraction. Quantitative evaluation of regional function based on imaging the myocardium requires:

- Identification of the endocardial border at end-diastole and end-systole
- Evaluation of wall motion for all segments of the myocardium
- Knowledge of the degree of variability of normal wall motion
- Correction for the effects of LV translation, rotation, and torsion
- High temporal resolution for analysis of the onset and velocity of myocardial thickening

Approaches that incorporate 3D reconstruction of the LV improve data acquisition times and diminish the effects of cardiac motion that potentially result in imaging different regions of myocardium in systole versus diastole for a given tomographic plane. Although wall thickening or the timing and velocity of motion may be more sensitive methods for evaluation of regional ventricular function, most current approaches continue to rely on endocardial motion.

Contrast now is routinely used to enhance endocardial definition with improved reliability for detection of abnormal wall motion; typically contrast is needed in about one half of stress echo studies. Other promising techniques include (1) contrast echocardiography for evaluation of myocardial perfusion and (2) tissue Doppler or speckle tracking strain and strain rate imaging (Fig. 8.10). However, these newer approaches are not commonly used in clinical practice because evidence to show improved diagnostic accuracy or better prediction of clinical outcomes is inadequate (see Suggested Reading and Chapter 4).

MYOCARDIAL ISCHEMIA

Because echocardiographic wall motion at rest is normal in a patient with significant coronary artery disease and no prior myocardial infarction, imaging *during ischemia* is needed for diagnosis. Inducing ischemia during echocardiographic imaging is referred to as *stress echocardiography*. Ischemia can be induced by increasing myocardial oxygen demand either with exercise or by pharmacologic interventions (Table 8.2).

Basic Principles of Stress Echocardiography

Stress echocardiography is based on the concept that an increased cardiac workload is needed to elicit signs of physiologic dysfunction in many types of cardiac

TABLE 8.1   Qualitative Scale for Assessment of Segmental Wall Motion

Wall Motion Grade	Definition
Normal	Normal endocardial inward motion and wall thickening in systole
Hypokinesis	Reduced amplitude (<5 mm) and velocity of endocardial motion and wall thickening in systole; delay in the onset of contraction and relaxation
Akinesis	Absence of inward endocardial motion (<2 mm) or wall thickening in systole
Dyskinesis	Outward motion or "bulging" of the segment in systole, usually associated with thin, scarred myocardium.
Aneurysmal	Diastolic contour abnormality with dyskinesis

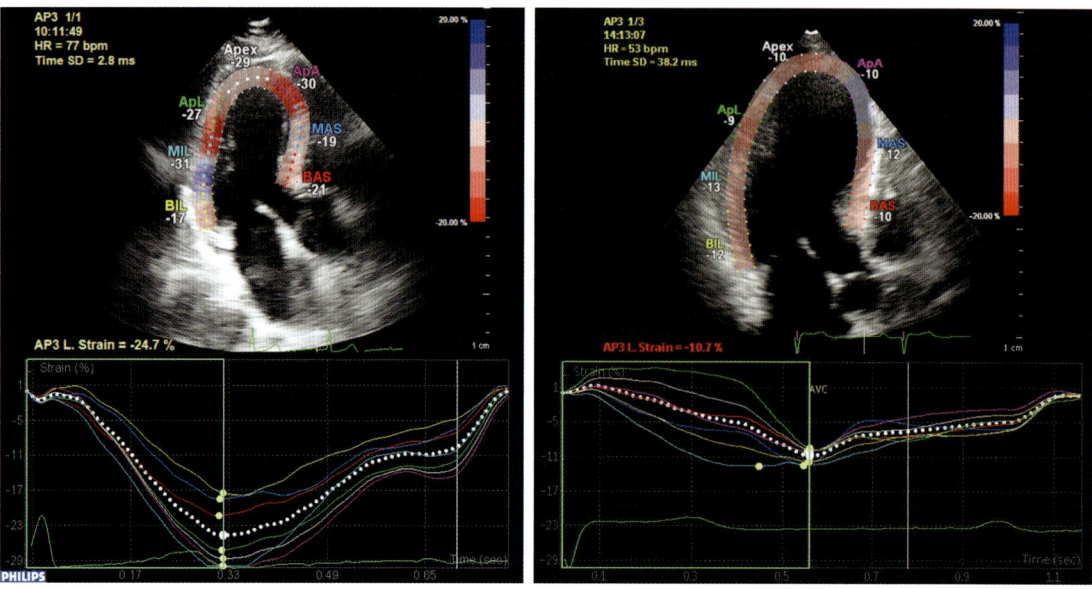

Fig. 8.10 🔵 🔵 **3D strain for regional wall motion.** Apical long-axis view with speckle tracking strain in a patient with normal wall motion and normal longitudinal strain *(L. strain)* of −24.7% *(left)* and in a patient an anterior-apical myocardial infarction resulting in differing degrees and rates of strain during systolic with a reduced overall long-axis strain of −10.7% *(right)*.

TABLE 8.2	Stress Echocardiography	
Type of Stress	**Advantages**	**Disadvantages**
Treadmill exercise	Widely available High workload Validated data on exercise duration and heart rate recovery	Imaging post–exercise tread mill only
Bicycle ergometry	Imaging during exercise	Imaging may be technically difficult. Lower workload Less validated data on exercise duration and prognosis
Dobutamine + atropine	Continuous imaging. Does not require physically active patient	Potential adverse effects of dobutamine Level of stress achieved
Vasodilator	Continuous imaging Does not require physically active patient	Potential adverse effects of vasodilator agent Induction of relative flow inequality rather than ischemia per se
Atrial pacing	Continuous imaging Does not require physically active patient	Requires permanent pacer Does not simulate exercise

disease. For example, in patients with coronary artery disease, resting myocardial blood flow is adequate, so myocardial function, seen on echocardiography as wall thickening and endocardial motion, is normal at rest. However, when cardiac workload is increased, the increased oxygen demands of the myocardium cannot be balanced by an increase in flow in the coronary artery, with resulting ischemia with impairment of myocardial thickening and endocardial motion (Fig. 8.11). An increase in cardiac workload typically is achieved by having the patient exercise, either on a supine bicycle or an upright treadmill, or by infusion of a pharmacologic agent, such as dobutamine, that increases heart rate and blood pressure. In addition to echocardiographic imaging, key elements in interpretation of stress test results include the:

- Duration of exercise
- Maximum workload—approximated by multiplying heart rate by systolic blood pressure
- Symptoms
- Blood pressure response
- Arrhythmias
- ST-segment changes on ECG

The basic principles of image acquisition for stress echocardiography are to use standard image planes, ensure that all myocardial segments are visualized in at least one (and preferably two) views, use comparable views at rest and stress, and record images in a digital cine-loop format with side-by-side display of rest and stress images. The cine-loop format is essential because otherwise the change in heart rate between rest and stress makes interpretation of wall motion difficult.

For evaluation of regional ventricular function, optimal endocardial definition is essential. When endocardial definition remains suboptimal despite careful patient positioning, use of harmonic imaging and other imaging adjustments, contrast echocardiography, or a nonechocardiographic imaging approach should be considered.

The sensitivity of stress echocardiography for detection of coronary disease depends on acquiring stress images at the maximal cardiac workload. With pharmacologic stress testing, this is rarely an issue because the stress level can be maintained until image acquisition is complete. However, with exercise stress, the workload declines rapidly on cessation of exercise, so that images must be acquired as quickly as possible after exercise. Both the time from stopping exercise and the heart rate at the time of image acquisition compared with maximum heart rate are recorded as indicators of workload. 3D echocardiographic acquisition systems that allow simultaneous real-time imaging in multiple image planes offer the promise of faster acquisition times at peak stress, with the potential for improved diagnostic sensitivity (Fig. 8.12).

Exercise Echocardiography

Exercise echocardiography typically is performed using standard exercise test protocols. Supine or upright bicycle exercise protocols have the advantage that echocardiographic imaging can be performed during exercise at each progressive level of exertion, including maximal exercise. Treadmill exercise protocols have the advantage that a higher total workload can be achieved but the disadvantage that imaging can be performed only after exercise. Wall motion abnormalities that resolve very rapidly after exercise may be missed.

Resting images are acquired in digital cine-loop format for standard views of the LV. Standard exercise protocols are used with monitoring of the 12-lead ECG, blood pressure, and symptoms by a qualified medical professional during and following the exercise protocol. The risks of exercise echocardiography are the risks of the exercise test itself. Either during

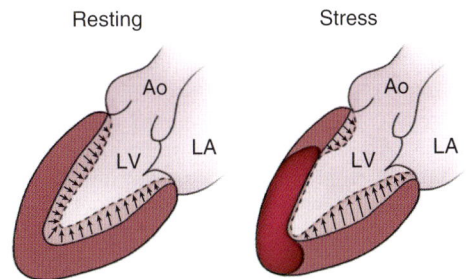

Fig. 8.11 Concept of stress echocardiography. This schematic illustrates a patient with a 70% stenosis in the proximal third of the left anterior descending coronary artery (LAD). At rest (*left*), endocardial motion and wall thickening are normal. After stress (*right*), either exercise or pharmacologic, the middle and apical segments of the anterior wall become ischemic, showing reduced endocardial wall motion and wall thickening. If the LAD extends around the apex, the apical segment of the posterior wall also will be affected, as shown here. The normal segment of the posterior wall shows compensatory hyperkinesis. *Ao,* Aorta.

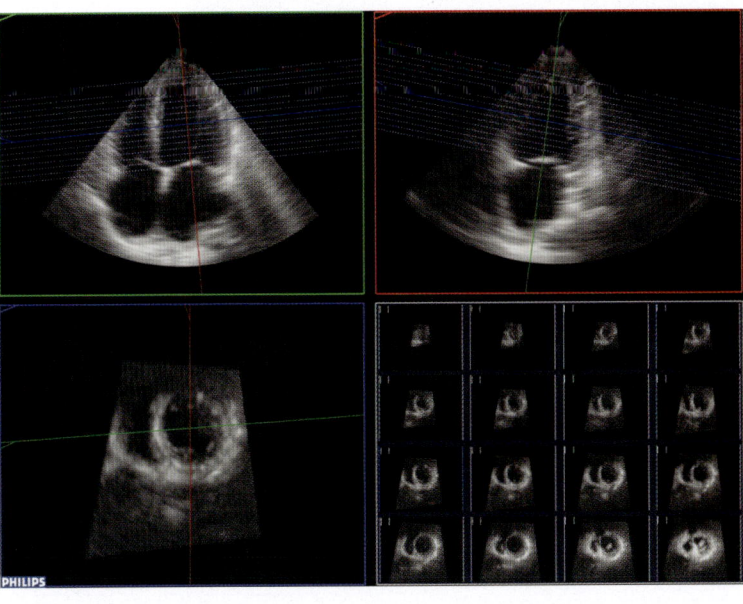

Fig. 8.12 Multiplane imaging for evaluation of regional function. Example of a multiplane display derived from a full volume 3D stress echocardiogram. The *lower right* panel displays simultaneous short-axis views from apex *(upper left)* to base *(lower right)* of the left ventricle. The distance between each adjacently displayed short-axis image is equal, and positions of these transverse cropping planes are shown as *white lines* on the coronal and sagittal crops.

maximal exercise (supine or sitting bicycle) or immediately after exercise (treadmill), digital cine-loop image acquisition is repeated. The patient exercises to maximum capacity rather than a target heart rate because accuracy is highest with a high workload. Heart rate starts to decline immediately on stopping exercise; thus all four standard poststress images should be acquired as quickly as possible (within 90 seconds) after exercise, and heart rate at the time of image acquisition should be displayed on the screen. Typically, four or more sequential cycles are recorded digitally, and the examiner subsequently chooses the best image for comparison with the baseline views (Fig. 8.13). This allows elimination of poor-quality images due to respiratory motion. Next, the rest and exercise cine-loop digital images are displayed side by side so that endocardial motion and wall thickening for each myocardial region can be compared.

Interpretation of an exercise stress echocardiogram includes incorporation of data on the maximum workload achieved (exercise duration), the heart rate and blood pressure response to exercise, the presence of arrhythmias, and clinical symptoms, as well as evaluation of the echocardiographic images. A systematic approach, comparing each segment in turn, is needed for detection of subtle abnormalities (Fig. 8.14).

Dobutamine Stress Echocardiography
Evaluation for Ischemia

Pharmacologic stress testing with intravenous dobutamine is based on the increased heart rate and contractility induced by this potent beta-agonist. Dobutamine is started at a low dose (5 µg/kg/min) and increased incrementally every 3 minutes with a calibrated intravenous infusion pump to (10, 20, 30, and 40 µg/kg/min) until the maximum dose or an endpoint has been reached. Atropine is used as needed, in divided doses of 0.25 to 0.5 mg (maximum total 2.0 mg), to achieve the target goal of 85% of the patient's maximum predicted heart rate. To minimize the likelihood of significant adverse effects and to

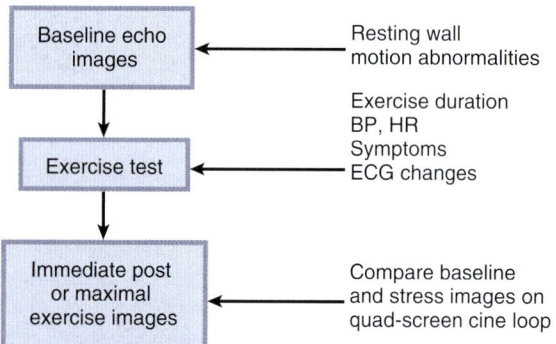

Fig. 8.13 Flow chart of an exercise echocardiography protocol. *BP*, Blood pressure; *ECG*, electrocardiogram; *HR*, heart rate.

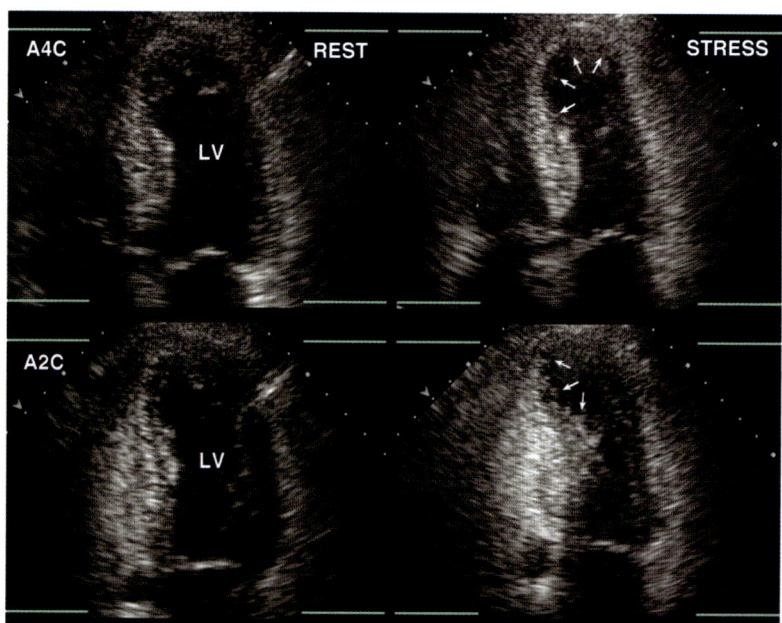

Fig. 8.14 Abnormal exercise echocardiogram. Compared with rest images, this study shows development of apical akinesis *(arrows)* with exercise. End-systolic images are shown at rest on the *left* and immediately after exercise on the *right* in the apical four-chamber *(A4C)* view *(top)* and the apical two-chamber *(A2C)* view *(bottom)*. Regional function was normal at rest, with normal endocardial motion and wall thickening in all segments. With stress, the apical inferior septum and inferior wall become akinetic, consistent with inducible ischemia in the distal left anterior descending coronary artery territory.

optimize the quality of the data obtained, a dobutamine stress echocardiography examination requires a well-defined study protocol performed in the appropriate clinical setting.

Patient monitoring during dobutamine stress echocardiography includes:

- Periodic blood pressures (usually every 2 to 3 minutes)
- Continuous ECG monitoring
- Careful observation for clinical symptoms or signs

Appropriate equipment, medications, and trained personnel should be immediately available in the event of an adverse effect, including a cardiac defibrillator, emergency cardiac medications, intravenous esmolol (a beta-blocker that counteracts the effects of dobutamine), and a qualified physician.

After an intravenous line for administration of the dobutamine has been placed, the patient is positioned in a left lateral decubitus position on an echo-stretcher with an apical cutout to allow optimal image acquisition throughout the study protocol. Initially the intravenous line is filled only with saline solution while resting data are obtained. Data collection at baseline, at each dosage level, and during recovery includes heart rate, blood pressure, symptoms, a 12-lead ECG, and echocardiographic images (Fig. 8.15). Standard views include parasternal short-axis images at the base and mid-cavity levels and apical four-chamber, two-chamber, and long-axis images with digital image acquisition in each view or with 3D image acquisition at each stage. Some centers also record Doppler LV filling and ejection velocities at each stage of the stress protocol.

Endpoints for stopping the test are:

- Reaching the maximum protocol dose
- Patient's discomfort
- A definite wall motion abnormality involving two or more adjacent segments
- ST-segment elevation on ECG
- Reaching 85% of maximum predicted heart rate for age
- A systolic blood pressure >200 or <100 mmHg or a diastolic blood pressure >120 mmHg, or
- Significant ventricular arrhythmias

Although serious complications are uncommon when appropriate precautions are observed, reported adverse effects include anxiety, tremulousness, palpitations, arrhythmias, paresthesias, and chest pain. About 10% of patients have premature atrial or ventricular beats, and up to 4% of patients experience nonsustained supraventricular or ventricular tachycardia. Because the purpose of the test is to induce ischemia, some patients have either echocardiographic changes or ECG evidence of ischemia and may experience angina. However, the frequency of angina may be less than with standard ECG stress testing because the protocol can be stopped as soon as wall motion abnormalities are seen (which often is before angina occurs). Hypotension occurs in up to 10% of patients because of peripheral β_2-receptor–mediated vasodilation, but unlike hypotension with exercise testing, it is *not* a predictor of severe coronary disease or a worse prognosis. Overall, the risk of myocardial infarction or ventricular fibrillation is about 1 in 2000 studies. Contraindications to dobutamine stress echocardiography include unstable angina, uncontrolled hypertension, or sensitivity to dobutamine.

The echocardiographic images are interpreted after reformatting the digital images, with each quadrant of the screen showing a different stress stage (Fig. 8.16). For each myocardial segment, wall motion is compared on matched images in a systematic fashion. Because wall thickening and endocardial motion normally increase with dobutamine, an abnormal test result is defined as the observation of hypokinesis or akinesis in a region that had normal wall motion at rest (Fig. 8.17).

Evaluation for Myocardial Viability

In addition to detection of ischemic myocardium, dobutamine stress echocardiography has been proposed as a method to evaluate for myocardial viability in regions that are "stunned" or "hibernating." For example, after treatment of myocardial infarction with thrombolytic therapy, the extent of residual viable myocardium in the area at risk may be unclear early after the event because of myocardial "stunning." Alternatively, a patient with chronic coronary artery disease may have hypokinesis or akinesis at baseline due to "hibernating" myocardium, which may recover

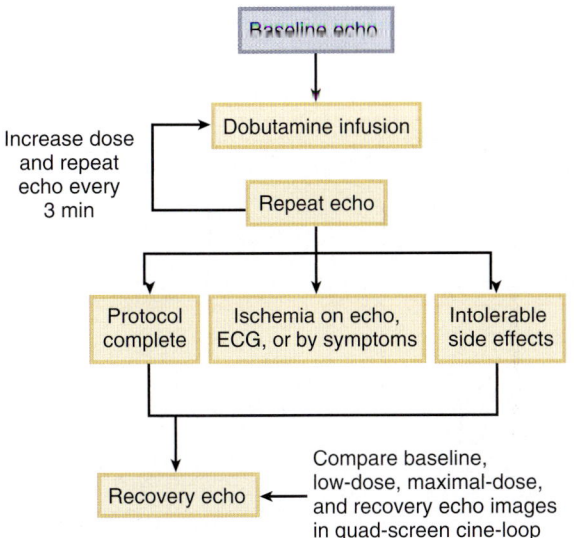

Fig. 8.15 Flow chart of dobutamine stress echo protocol.

Fig. 8.16 ▶ ▶ **Normal dobutamine stress echocardiography.** The standard display format shows the apical four-chamber view at end-systole at baseline, low-dose (5 µg/kg/min) dobutamine, high-dose (40 µg/kg/min) dobutamine, and recovery images. This example shows the end-systolic images in the apical four-chamber *(A4C)* view *(top)* and the apical two-chamber *(A2C)* view *(bottom)* at baseline and at peak dose dobutamine.

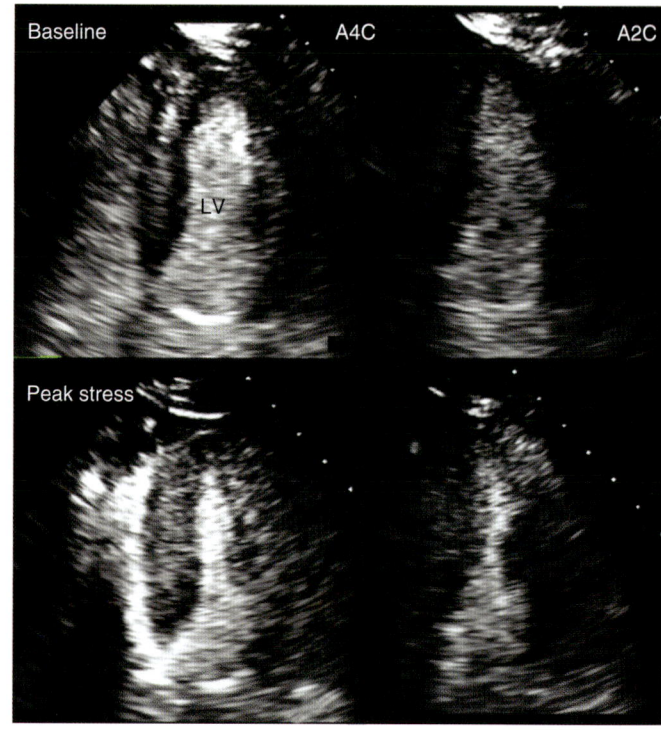

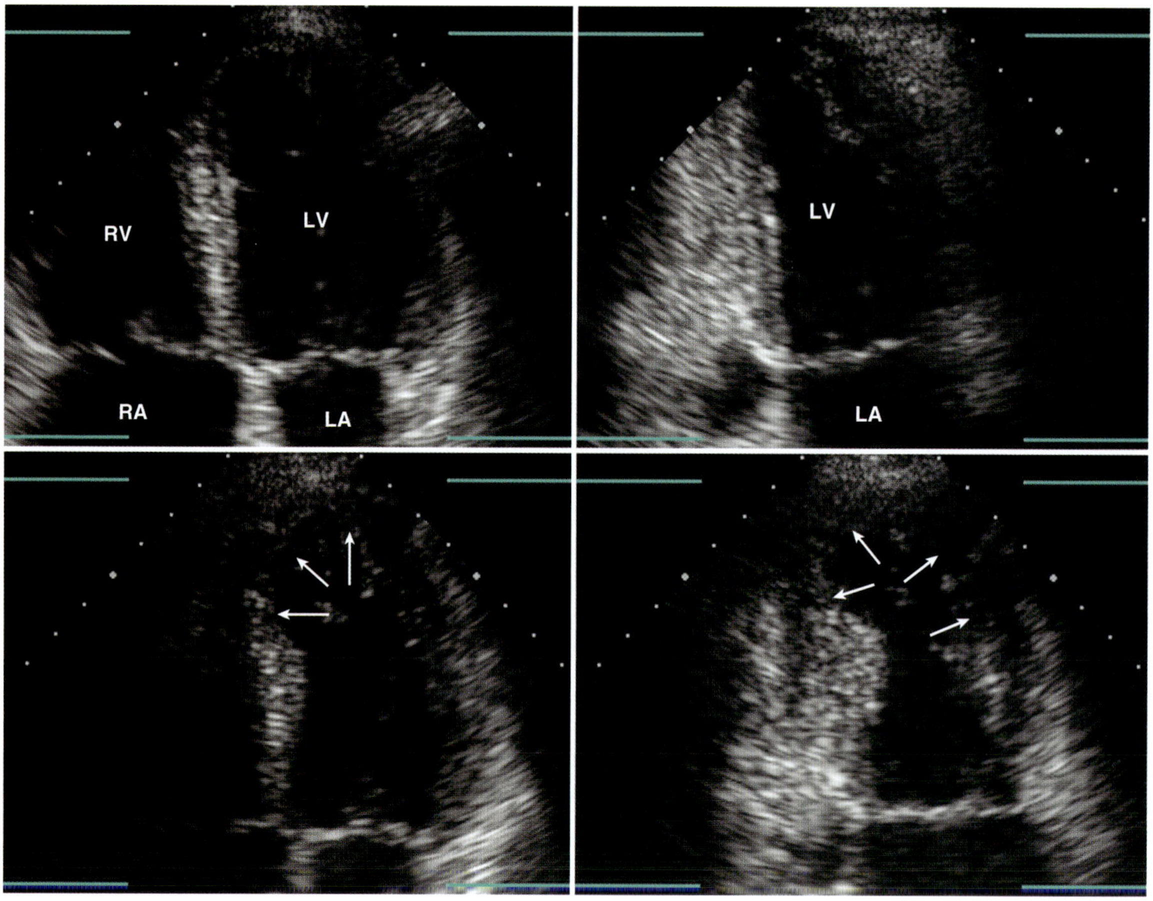

Fig. 8.17 Abnormal dobutamine stress echocardiographic study. Baseline images *(top)* at end-systole in an apical four-chamber view *(left)* and apical two-chamber view *(right)* are compared with peak dose (40 µg/kg/min dobutamine plus 0.5 mg atropine) end-systole images on the *bottom*. The apical segments of the septum, anterior, and inferior walls became akinetic at peak dobutamine dose *(arrows)*, indicating significant coronary artery disease in the left anterior descending coronary artery distribution.

with revascularization. In both these settings, echocardiographic imaging during low-dose (5 to 10 μg/kg/min) dobutamine infusion has been reported to show improved wall thickening and endocardial motion in viable segments of the myocardium. Of course, at higher dobutamine doses, worsening of regional function may occur due to induction of ischemia. This pattern of initial improvement at low dose, with subsequent worsening of myocardial function at higher dobutamine doses, is referred to as a *biphasic response*.

Other Stress Modalities

Vasodilators (dipyridamole or adenosine) have been proposed for echocardiographic stress testing by some investigators based on the differential pattern of coronary blood flow induced by these agents: increased blood flow in normal coronary arteries with a *relative* decrease in blood flow in diseased vessels. Overall success with this approach has been higher with nuclear perfusion imaging because the difference in blood flow between regions supplied by normal versus abnormal coronary arteries can be seen on the radionuclide images. Results with echocardiographic imaging have been less consistent because actual ischemia (not just a relative difference in blood flow) is needed to discern a wall motion abnormality. In patients with a permanent pacemaker, atrial pacing to achieve the target heart rate is another option.

Limitations and Technical Aspects

Stress echocardiography has high sensitivity and specificity for diagnosis of significant coronary artery disease. In addition, it allows reliable definition of the anatomic location and extent of ischemic myocardium. However, stress echocardiography does have potential technical and physiologic limitations:

- Endocardial definition
- Cardiac and respiratory motion
- Inadequate stress or workload
- Abnormal resting LV function

Assessment of endocardial wall motion and wall thickening requires adequate delineation of the endocardium for each myocardial segment. Careful attention to patient positioning, transducer orientation, and image-processing parameters can improve image quality, but definition of certain segments, particularly the anterior wall, is difficult in some individuals due to adjacent lung tissue. Contrast agents that opacify the LV after intravenous administration should be used to enhance detection of regional wall motion abnormalities when endocardial definition is suboptimal.

Exercise and postexercise imaging can be limited by respiratory interference due to a rapid respiratory rate. Digital acquisition in cine-loop format of several cycles, followed by selection of the best images, is necessary for correct interpretation. The possible effects of cardiac translation and rotation, both between systole and diastole and between baseline and stress, should be considered in comparisons of wall motion. The interpretation of a stress echocardiographic study includes a description of image quality as an indicator of the reliability of these results. Suboptimal images should be interpreted with caution.

Potential physiologic limitations are related to the fact that abnormal wall motion occurs only *during* ischemia. First, if the "stress" used does *not* induce ischemia, no wall motion abnormality will be seen even if significant coronary disease is present. For example, a patient with limited exercise duration due to hip pain will not achieve a level of exertion that results in ischemia. Similarly, a pharmacologic "stress" that does not induce ischemia will not induce a wall motion abnormality. Second, the duration of ischemia is important. If ischemia has resolved by the time imaging is performed, the wall motion abnormality will not be detected. This is of particular concern with treadmill exercise because echocardiographic imaging is performed after exertion, although this possible limitation is offset by the higher maximum workload achieved before the recovery period compared with bicycle exercise protocols.

Stress echocardiography in patients with abnormal global or regional function at rest is more difficult to interpret than in subjects with normal resting LV systolic function. The presence of a segmental motion abnormality at rest implies that coronary artery disease, with prior myocardial infarction, is present. With stress imaging, new wall motion abnormalities in regions remote from the site of resting abnormal wall motion indicate additional areas of ischemia. Evaluation of areas adjacent to the resting wall motion abnormality is problematic due to a potential tethering effect by the abnormal region. In patients with global systolic dysfunction at rest—which may be due to end-stage ischemic disease, cardiomyopathy, or chronic valvular disease—stress echocardiography is less specific for the diagnosis of coronary disease.

Alternate Approaches

In patients with suspected or known coronary artery disease, the choice of stress and imaging modality depends on patient-related factors and on the specific clinical question. Optimally, the method of stress is chosen to allow an adequate workload in that patient—with pharmacologic testing used in patients who cannot exercise to a maximal workload due to orthopedic, neurologic, pulmonary, or other conditions. The choice of imaging modality is based on image quality in each patient and the type of information needed (Table 8.3).

The origins of the right and left coronary arteries often can be identified on transthoracic imaging (Fig. 8.18). On TEE imaging the proximal left coronary can be followed to its bifurcation into left anterior descending and circumflex arteries (Figs. 8.19 and 8.20),

TABLE 8.3 Approaches for Evaluation of Myocardial Ischemia

Diagnostic Approach	Methodology	Advantages	Disadvantages
Stress ECG	Exercise testing on a treadmill or bicycle with continuous 12-lead ECG recording	• Low cost; widely available; appropriate for initial diagnosis in many patients • Exercise testing provides data on exercise capacity, blood pressure and heart rate response, and possible provoked symptoms.	• Low sensitivity and specificity, particularly in women; requires ability to exercise to adequate workload
Stress echo	Exercise or pharmacologic stress with echo imaging of wall motion	• Higher sensitivity and specificity compared with stress ECG; identifies affected coronary distribution and area of myocardial at risk; noninvasive, no ionizing radiation	• Image quality may be suboptimal in larger patients but can be improved with contrast.
Stress SPECT nuclear perfusion imaging	Exercise or pharmacologic stress testing with radiotracer visualization of myocardial perfusion	• Noninvasive, more sensitive and specific than stress ECG testing; identifies affected coronary distribution and area of myocardial at risk. It is highly prognostic of outcomes. • Late reperfusion imaging allows evaluation of myocardial viability.	• Ionizing radiation • Poor image quality in very obese patients. Attenuation correction with SPECT improves this.
Stress PET imaging	Exercise or pharmacologic stress testing with radiotracer visualization of myocardial perfusion	• Noninvasive, sensitive and specific for diagnosis of coronary disease. Improved image quality in larger patients provides prognosis. • Quantification of absolute myocardial blood flow and coronary flow reserve	• Small amount of ionizing radiation; not widely available; cost • Pharmacologic stress only (no exercise)
Coronary angiography	Injection of contrast dye in coronary arteries at cardiac catheterization.	• Direct and detailed visualization of coronary anatomy • Can be combined with intravascular ultrasound and fractional flow reserve measurements • Allows prompt therapeutic intervention following diagnosis	• Invasive, use of contrast dye, ionizing radiation exposure, cost Poor correlation between stenosis severity and physiology
CT coronary angiography	High-resolution ECG-gated CT imaging with IV contrast administration	• Noninvasive detailed images of coronary anatomy and ability to characterize intracoronary plaque	• Use of contrast dye, ionizing radiation exposure, cost
CMR imaging	Resting images for evaluation of coronary artery anatomy and for evaluation of myocardial infarction and fibrosis; stress perfusion imaging possible	• Allows identification of coronary anomalies • Viable myocardium can reliably be distinguished from infarcted tissue. • Wall motion at rest and stress and myocardial perfusion can be evaluated using CMR cine images with a pharmacologic stress test.	• Cost, complexity; not widely available

CMR, Cardiac magnetic resonance; *CT*, computed tomographic; *ECG*, electrocardiography; *IV*, intravenous; *PET*, positron emission tomography; *SPECT*, single photon emission computed tomography.

Coronary Artery Disease | Chapter 8

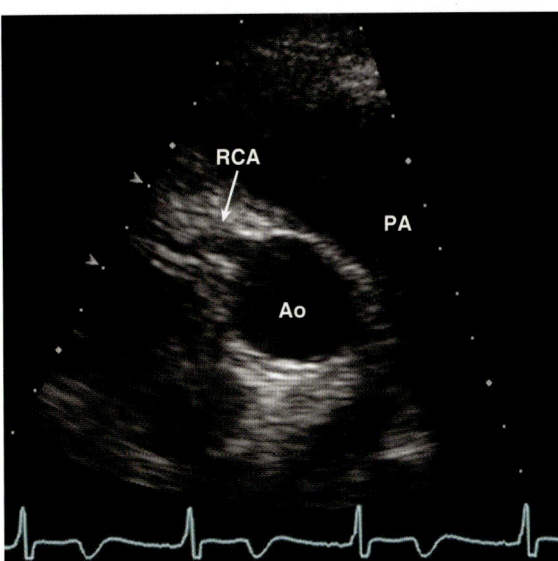

Fig. 8.18 Right coronary artery seen on a transthoracic echocardiography parasternal short-axis view. *Ao*, Aorta; *PA*, pulmonary artery.

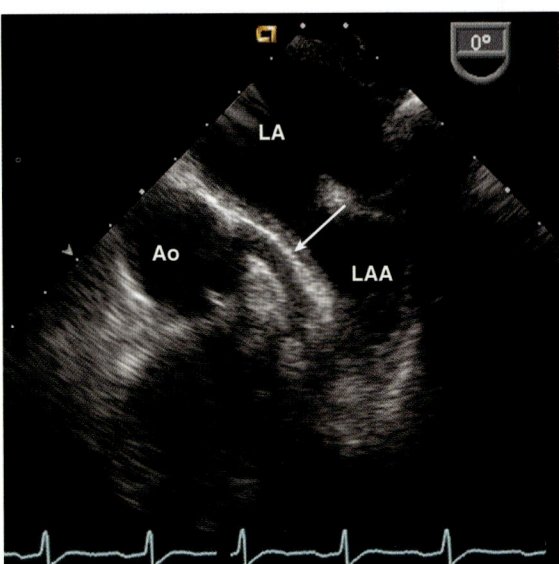

Fig. 8.20 Left anterior descending coronary artery on transesophageal echocardiography. In the same patient as Fig. 8.18, slight withdrawal of the probe with angulation toward the apex shows the left main coronary artery continuing into the left anterior descending coronary artery *(arrow)*. The circumflex coronary artery extends out of the image plane. *Ao*, Aorta; *LAA*, left atrial appendage.

- Detection of coronary artery disease
- Assessment of the area of myocardium at risk
- Risk stratification after myocardial infarction
- Evaluation after revascularization
- Detection of myocardial viability

Stress echocardiography is particularly useful for detection of coronary artery disease in specific patient groups, including:

- Women with chest pain symptoms or cardiac risk factors, or both
- Patients after heart transplantation
- Patients being considered for renal transplantation
- Patients undergoing vascular surgery

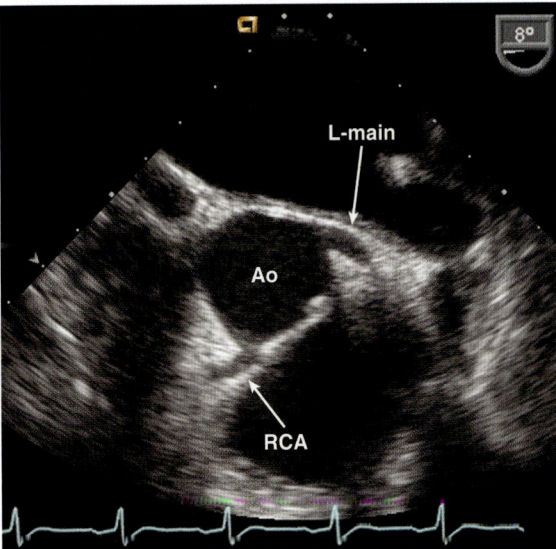

Fig. 8.19 ▶ Transesophageal echocardiography short-axis view showing the origins of the left main and right coronary arteries. *Ao*, Aorta; *L-main*, left main coronary artery; *RCA*, right coronary artery.

Stress echocardiography also can be used to evaluate changes in cardiac hemodynamics including valve gradients and areas, regurgitant severity, and pulmonary pressures. As discussed in Chapters 11 and 17, echocardiography is used in patients with valvular or congenital heart disease for evaluation of changes with stress in:

and often these branches can be imaged for a portion of their length, as can the right coronary artery. However, clinical decision making usually requires detailed knowledge of the entire extent of the coronary anatomy. Ultrasound imaging is a suboptimal method for evaluation of the relatively small coronary vessels that move with the epicardial surface of the heart.

Clinical Utility

The utility of stress echocardiography in patients with known or suspected coronary artery disease includes (Table 8.4):

- Aortic valve gradient and area in calcific aortic stenosis
- Mitral regurgitant severity in myxomatous mitral valve disease
- Pulmonary pressures in mitral stenosis or regurgitation
- Aortic coarctation pressure gradients
- Dynamic outflow obstruction in hypertrophic cardiomyopathy

TABLE 8.4 Coronary Artery Disease: Clinical-Echocardiographic Correlates

	Coronary Anatomy	Clinical Presentation	Echocardiographic Findings
Asymptomatic coronary disease	Coronary artery narrowing <70% typically does not cause symptoms or myocardial ischemia.	Stress echo may be requested in asymptomatic patients at high risk of coronary disease (e.g. to assess risk before noncardiac surgery).	A normal stress echo does not exclude atherosclerotic coronary disease but indicates a low likelihood of significant ischemia.
Chronic stable angina	Coronary stenosis ≥70% narrowing usually is asymptomatic at rest but causes symptoms with exertion.	Typical angina on exertion	Normal resting LV regional and global systolic function. Stress echo shows inducible wall motion abnormalities in the distribution of the affected coronary artery.
Acute coronary syndrome	Coronary occlusion or severe stenosis with rupture of an atherosclerotic plaque and luminal thrombus	Acute chest pain. Differential diagnosis includes aortic dissection, pericarditis, AS, HCM.	Akinesis or hypokinesis of the myocardium supplied by the occluded vessel with normal wall thickness. With unstable angina, wall motion may be normal between pain episodes.
Old myocardial infarction	Occluded coronary artery with attenuated distal vessel. Collateral vessels often are present.	Asymptomatic if other coronary vessels are not stenosed. Heart failure if significant LV dysfunction is present	Thinning increased echogenicity and akinesis in the distribution of the affected coronary artery. Ischemic MR may be present.
End-stage ischemic disease	Multiple old coronary occlusions, small distal vessels	Heart failure	Dilated LV with severely reduced ejection fraction. Areas of akinesis and areas of normal LV function are present. LV diastolic dysfunction. RV systolic function is normal, unless RV infarction is present. Ischemic MR may be present.

AS, Aortic stenosis; *HCM*, hypertrophic cardiomyopathy; *MR*, mitral regurgitation.

Diagnosis of Coronary Artery Disease

The accuracy of stress echocardiography for diagnosis of significant coronary artery disease is highly dependent on image quality, specifically endocardial definition, with most investigators reporting success rates for obtaining diagnostic images after treadmill exercise of 85% to 100% in their patients. The success rate for image acquisition and the quality of the images obtained tend to be greater with supine exercise (in which the patient can be positioned optimally) and with pharmacologic stress (which has the added advantage of little increase in respiratory interference).

Compared with coronary angiography, with significant disease defined as 50% narrowing of an epicardial coronary artery, exercise echocardiography has an overall sensitivity of 74% to 97% and a specificity of 64% to 100% for diagnosing the presence of coronary artery disease (see Appendix B, Tables B.6 and B.7). Sensitivity is highest for multivessel disease (>90%) and lowest for single-vessel disease (60% to 80%) in these studies. In comparison, exercise ECG had a much lower sensitivity at 51% to 63% and specificity at 62% to 74%, whereas exercise thallium-201 perfusion imaging tends to have an accuracy similar to that of echocardiography, with a sensitivity of 61% to 94% and a specificity of 81%.

Extent and Location of Ischemic Areas

When image quality is adequate, stress echocardiography also allows accurate evaluation of the location and extent of the area of ischemic myocardium. By integrating data from multiple views or using 3D imaging, a reasonable estimate of the location of significant coronary lesions can be made. Echocardiographic estimates of which and how many coronary arteries are affected correlate well with angiographic findings.

Prognostic Implications

The relationship between stress echocardiographic results and clinical outcome has been evaluated in several studies and in a meta-analysis (Appendix B, Tables B.8 and B.9). In patients with known or suspected coronary artery disease, a normal stress echocardiogram has a 98% negative predictive value for myocardial infarction or cardiovascular death over the next 3 years. Interpretation of a stress test depends on the pretest likelihood of disease, including clinical risk factors such as age, sex, diabetes, smoking, hypertension, and hypercholesterolemia. In addition, indicators of a higher likelihood of an adverse outcome with exercise echocardiography, as with all exercise stress tests, include exercise capacity, exercise-induced angina, and the blood pressure response to exercise. However, echocardiographic images provide additional prognostic information, with the key predictors of clinical outcome including resting wall motion abnormalities, ejection fraction, and the extent of ischemia. Similarly, with dobutamine stress, echocardiography provides incremental value with resting wall motion and evidence of inducible ischemia predicting cardiovascular events.

MYOCARDIAL INFARCTION

Basic Principles

Acute coronary syndrome includes patients presenting with acute chest pain due to transient rest ischemia (unstable angina), those with non–ST-elevation myocardial infarction, and those with ST-elevation (or transmural) myocardial infarction. Pathologically, myocardial infarction is defined as irreversible injury to the myocardium due to prolonged ischemia, usually secondary to acute thrombotic occlusion of an epicardial coronary artery at the site of an atherosclerotic plaque. Initially the affected myocardium becomes akinetic, with normal wall thickness. Over time (4 to 6 weeks), an un-reperfused ST-elevation myocardial infraction results in a definite area of akinesis and wall thinning. A non–ST-elevation myocardial infarction results in a lesser degree of wall thinning and in hypokinesis rather than akinesis. However, in the current era, the extent of myocardial damage in patients presenting with an acute coronary syndrome depends on the speed and success of reperfusion therapy. A corresponding range of findings is seen on echocardiography, with the extent of wall motion abnormalities ranging from a large transmural infarction to a nearly normal LV.

Echocardiographic Imaging

The myocardial segments affected and the echocardiographic views for assessment of myocardial infarction are the same as described for myocardial ischemia. An occlusion of the left anterior descending artery results in akinesis of the anterior septum, anterior free wall, and apex (Fig. 8.21). Imaging in parasternal long-and short-axis views and in apical views demonstrates these segmental wall motion abnormalities. In the acute setting (Fig. 8.22), the unaffected walls are hyperkinetic. Overall LV systolic function typically is moderately depressed with an average ejection fraction of 41 ± 11% after an un-reperfused anterior myocardial infarction due to a proximal left anterior descending artery occlusion.

Occlusion of the posterior descending artery results in an inferior myocardial infarction with akinesis of the inferior septum, the inferior free wall, and (to a variable extent) the inferolateral (posterior) wall. Parasternal and apical views again are used. The subcostal approach is particularly helpful in patients with poor image quality from parasternal and apical windows. Typically, overall LV systolic function is only mildly depressed, with an average postinfarction ejection fraction of 53 ± 10% after an un-reperfused inferior infarction. With inferior infarction the echocardiographer also should evaluate for possible concurrent RV infarction.

Occlusion of the circumflex artery, resulting in a lateral myocardial infarction, is less common and often is electrocardiographically "silent." Akinesis of the anterolateral and posterolateral walls is seen, with a mild to moderately depressed ejection fraction depending on the extent of myocardium supplied by the circumflex artery in that individual.

Note that these "classic" patterns of wall motion abnormalities vary with individual variation in coronary anatomy and the location of the occlusion along the length of the coronary artery. Also, these patterns are altered by the use of reperfusion therapy.

In acute myocardial infarction, diastolic function, as well as systolic function, is abnormal. Acutely, diastolic relaxation is impaired with normalization over the subsequent 1 to 2 weeks when reperfusion is successful. With late or ineffective reperfusion resulting in a large infarction, an initial pattern of impaired relaxation is followed by pseudo-normalization of diastolic filling with a high E velocity reflecting an increased LV end-diastolic pressure. In patients with moderate to severely reduced systolic function, the E/A ratio correlates positively with LV end-diastolic and LA pressures (i.e., a higher E/A ratio indicates a higher LV end-diastolic pressure) due to the overriding effect of LA pressure on the early diastolic filling velocity. It is most helpful to interpret patterns of LV diastolic filling in a patients with coronary artery disease over time with side-by-side comparisons of the echocardiographic findings and integration with other clinical data (see Chapter 7).

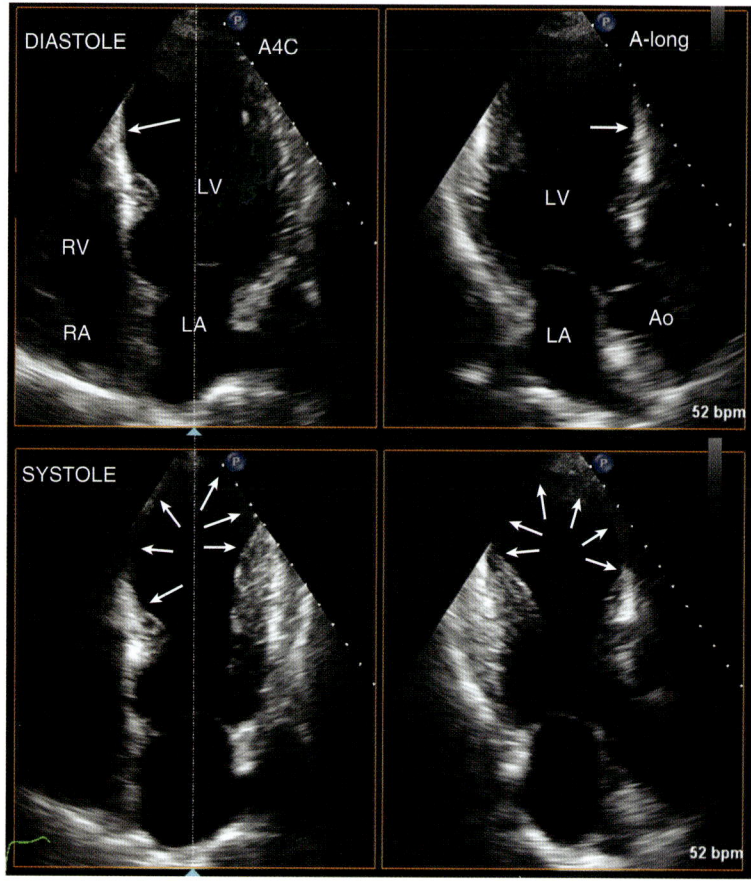

Fig. 8.21 ▶ **Old anterior myocardial infarction.** Biplane imaging in an apical four chamber *(A4C)* and apical long-axis *(A-long)* view at end-diastole *(top)* shows thinning and increased echogenicity of the apical inferior and anterior septum *(arrows)*. In systole *(bottom)*, akinesis of the apical one half of the anterior and inferior septum, as well as the entire apical cap and apical segments of the lateral and posterior walls, is noted, as indicated by *the arrows*. These findings are consistent with prior infarction in the territory of the left anterior descending coronary artery. *Ao,* Aorta.

Limitations and Alternate Approaches

As for other applications of echocardiography, image quality can be a limiting factor in patients with poor ultrasound tissue penetration. However, with optimal patient positioning, an experienced sonographer, and a state-of-the-art instrument, diagnostic images can be obtained in nearly all patients.

The standard approach to the diagnosis of acute myocardial infarction includes two of the following three findings:

- A typical clinical presentation
- Diagnostic ECG changes
- A consistent pattern of elevation in serum cardiac enzyme levels

When typical findings of acute myocardial infarction are present, the diagnosis rarely is in doubt. Unfortunately, many patients have an atypical clinical presentation, and ECG changes often are nondiagnostic.

Radionuclide imaging for acute myocardial infarction is based on the principle of detection of areas of hypoperfusion. The finding of a normal radionuclide perfusion pattern in patients presenting with chest pain has a high specificity for the absence of acute myocardial infarction. Sensitivity for acute infarction is lower because an old infarction cannot be distinguished from an acute infarction with this approach.

Noninvasive computed tomographic imaging of the coronary arteries is useful for screening for coronary disease in patients undergoing other cardiac surgery or with a low pretest likelihood of disease.

Invasive coronary angiography remains the standard of reference for identification of an occluded coronary artery. Concurrent left ventriculography can identify wall motion abnormalities. The current standard of care for acute myocardial infarction includes percutaneous coronary revascularization, so most patients go directly to the catheterization laboratory at the time of presentation.

Clinical Utility

Diagnosis in the Emergency Department

In a patient presenting to the emergency department with chest pain and a nondiagnostic ECG, echocardiographic assessment of global and segmental wall motion can be helpful in clinical decision making. The presence of a segmental wall motion abnormality indicates that coronary artery disease is present—which may be acute infarction, unstable angina, or an old infarction. Associated hyperkinesis of uninvolved

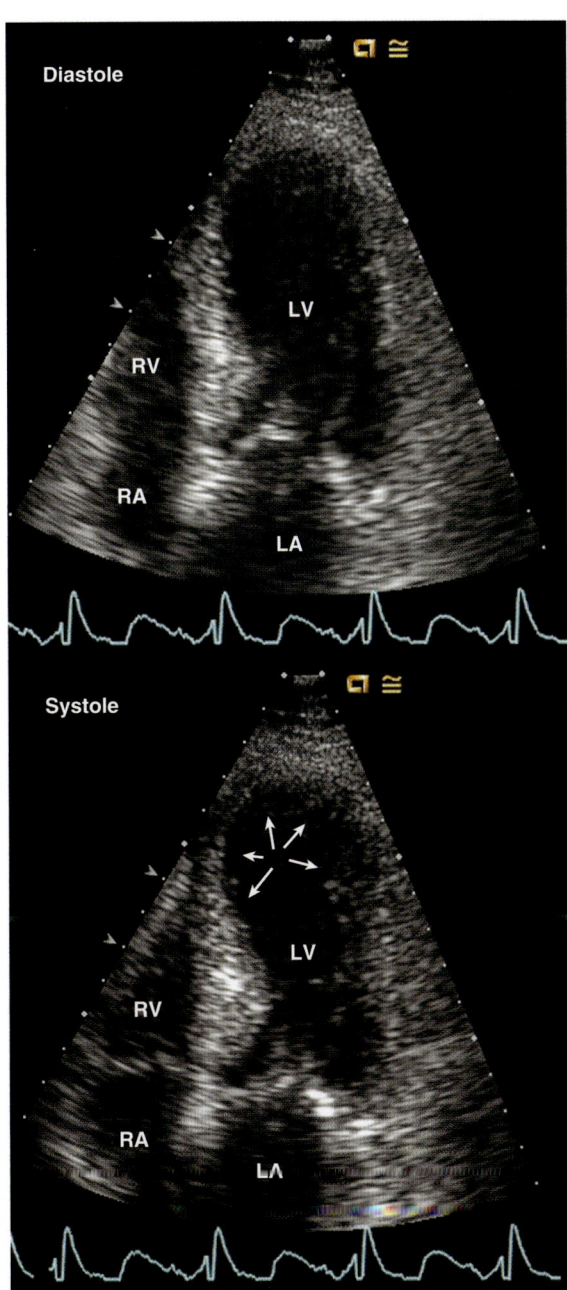

Fig. 8.22 ▶ ▶ ▶ **Acute anterior myocardial infarction.** Comparing the apical four-chamber view in diastole *(top)* and systole *(bottom)* demonstrates the akinetic septum *(arrows)*, although the myocardium is not yet thinned and scarred, as in the old infarction shown in Fig. 8.21.

not exclude a diagnosis of unstable angina. In patients presenting with chest pain, a nondiagnostic ECG, and normal cardiac enzymes, some clinical centers now use exercise echocardiography to allow triage to further inpatient versus outpatient evaluation.

Evaluation of Interventional Therapy

In a patient with a definite myocardial infarction by clinical and ECG criteria, echocardiography allows assessment of the location and extent of "myocardium at risk." Once reperfusion therapy has been initiated, echocardiography can be used to assess its effects. However, a several-day time lag often occurs between successful reperfusion and normalization of wall motion ("stunned" myocardium), so evaluation is most meaningful just before hospital discharge or at outpatient follow-up. Prolonged persistence of wall motion abnormalities that can be reversed by reperfusion also can occur—termed *hibernating myocardium*. Echocardiographic imaging at rest cannot distinguish between these conditions because it shows the regional myocardial function at the time imaging is performed. In patients with postinfarction chest pain, echocardiography helps separate those with recurrent ischemia, and new wall motion abnormalities, from those with postinfarction pericarditis or noncardiac chest pain. At long-term follow-up after myocardial infarction, echocardiography allows assessment of global ventricular function and long-term ventricular dilation due to infarct expansion.

Myocardial Viability

Distinguishing irreversibly infarcted myocardial from viable myocardium that might benefit from reperfusion therapy is important in clinical decision making. Akinesis or hypokinesis at rest may be due to myocardial stunning or hibernation rather than to irreversible myocardial damage. Viable myocardium shows an increase in wall thickening and endocardial motion in response to low-dose (5 to 10 µg/kg/min) dobutamine. At higher dobutamine doses, myocardium supplied by a patent coronary artery shows further enhancement of myocardial thickening, whereas ischemia with hypokinesis or akinesis is seen when significant coronary stenosis is present. This biphasic response—wall motion improvement at low-dose and worsening at high-dose dobutamine—identifies areas of myocardium likely to benefit from percutaneous or surgical reperfusion, even late after myocardial infarction, with a sensitivity of 80% and specificity of 78%. Factors that affect the response to dobutamine include:

- Extent of viable tissue
- Degree of residual coronary stenosis
- Extent of collateral coronary blood flow
- Tethering from adjacent segments
- Medical therapy

segments suggests an acute event. Many emergency departments now use point of care ultrasound devices for this indication.

Because ischemic myocardium also is akinetic in a patient with chest pain, echocardiography cannot distinguish acute infarction from ongoing ischemia. Normal wall motion implies that no ischemia was present *at the time* the images were acquired. Thus normal wall motion *between* episodes of chest pain does

A uniphasic response (improvement at low dose with no change or further improvement at higher dobutamine doses) is less specific for myocardial viability. Alternate approaches for evaluation of myocardial viability include nuclear perfusion, positron emission tomography (PET) and cardiac magnetic resonance (CMR) imaging.

Mechanical Complications of Myocardial Infarction

Echocardiography is the procedure of choice for initial evaluation of the post–myocardial infarction patient with a new systolic murmur (Table 8.5) with a differential diagnosis of:

- Mitral regurgitation
- Ventricular septal defect
- Ventricular rupture with pseudoaneurysm formation

Most commonly, the etiology of the murmur is *mitral regurgitation* due to papillary muscle dysfunction, abnormal wall motion of the segment underlying a papillary muscle, or papillary muscle rupture. The presence and severity of mitral regurgitation are evaluated using Doppler techniques (see Chapter 12), and the etiology is inferred from 2D or 3D imaging. Ischemic mitral regurgitation typically results from failure of adequate coaptation of the anterior leaflet against a tethered posterior leaflet resulting in a posteriorly directed regurgitant jet. Partial or complete rupture of the papillary muscle is a catastrophic complication that can be recognized as a flail leaflet with an attached mass (the papillary muscle head) that prolapses into the LA in systole (Fig. 8.23). TEE imaging is indicated when this diagnosis is suspected unless the diagnosis is clear on transthoracic images.

Another cause of a new systolic murmur after myocardial infarction is a *ventricular septal defect* due

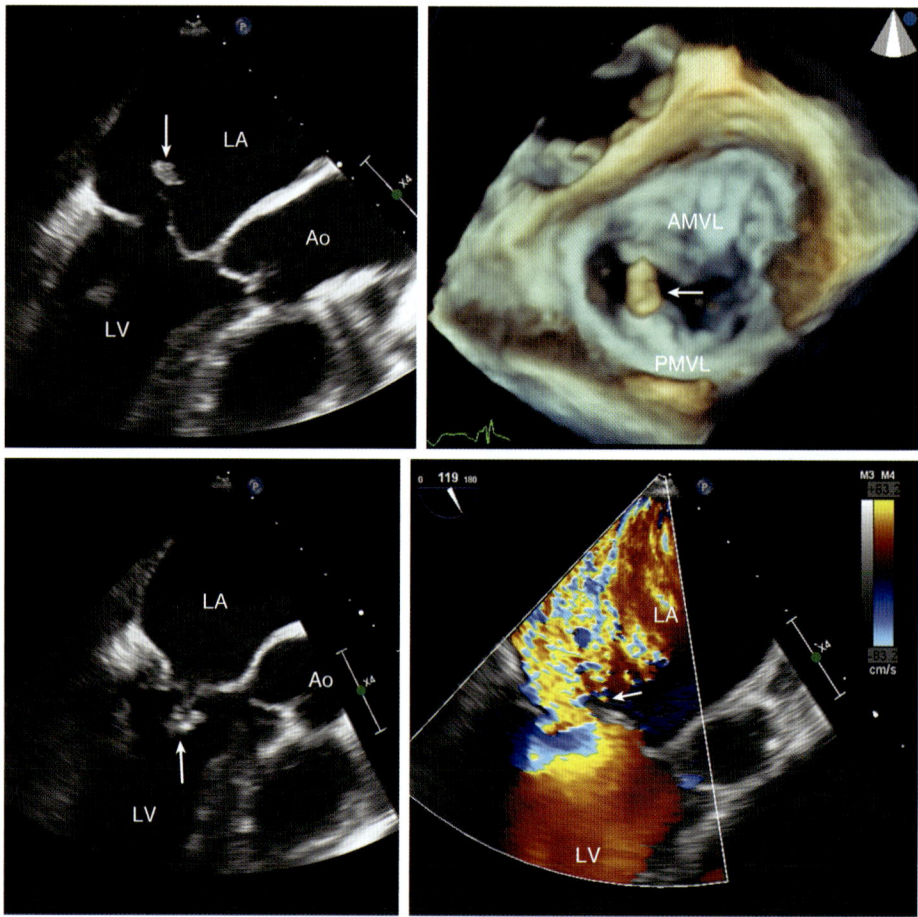

Fig. 8.23 ▶ **Papillary muscle rupture.** On a TEE image in the four-chamber view *(top left)*, papillary muscle rupture is seen with prolapse of the papillary muscle head *(arrow)* into the LA in systole *(top left)* and back into the LV chamber in diastole *(bottom left)*. 3D imaging from the LA perspective *(upper right)* ▶ shows the detached papillary muscle head, and color Doppler imaging shows an eccentric posteriorly directed jet of severe mitral regurgitation *(bottom right)* ▶ with a wide vena contracta *(arrow)*. The patient underwent emergency mitral valve repair. *AMVL*, Anterior mitral valve leaflet; *Ao*, aorta; *PMVL*, posterior mitral valve leaflet.

TABLE 8.5 Complications of Acute Myocardial Infarction: Clinical-Echocardiographic Correlates

	Incidence	Pathophysiology	Echocardiographic Findings
Pericarditis and pericardial effusion	5%	• Occurs in first 4 days after reperfused acute MI	• Small circumferential pericardial effusion • Larger effusion raises concern for LV rupture.
RV infarction	30%–50% of patients with inferior MI	• Occlusion of the acute marginal branch of the RCA; often associated with inferior LV myocardial infarction	• Dilated hypokinetic or akinetic RV • Infarction of adjacent inferior LV wall
Ischemic MR	25%	• Infarction or ischemia of the papillary muscle results in MR. • No audible murmur in 50% • More common with inferior-posterior MI • Papillary muscle rupture is uncommon, but ischemic MR is seen in about $\frac{1}{4}$ of patients with MI.	• Moderate to severe mitral regurgitation • TEE often needed to identify cause of MR
Ventricular septal defect	< 0.5%	• Transmural infarction with hemorrhage in necrotic zone • Occurs most often 24 h after reperfusion in older women with single vessel disease	• Discrete septal defect in area of akinesis with left to right flow seen on color and CW Doppler
Free wall rupture and tamponade	0.8%	• Transmural infarction with hemorrhage in necrotic zone • Most likely involves inferolateral wall with circumflex or LAD occlusion	• Large pericardial effusion with tamponade • Acute fatal event unless temporarily sealed by fibrinous pericardial adhesions
LV pseudoaneurysm	Rare	• Free wall rupture contained by organized thrombus and pericardium • Occurs most often with circumflex and RCA occlusion in the basal inferior-posterior walls	• Discrete akinetic dilated area with a narrow neck between the LV and pseudoaneurysm cavity • Lined with thrombus, which may be mistaken for a thick wall.
LV aneurysm	8%–15%	• Myocardial thinning and dilation due to infarct expansion 24 to 72 h after acute MI • The thin aneurysm walls are composed of fibrotic myocardium. • Occurs most often at the LV apex with LAD occlusion	• Thin, bright, dyskinetic LV segment with a diastolic contour abnormality • Often with associated thrombus
LV thrombus	5%–10%	• Peak incidence is 3 days post MI but may occur within hours in areas of infarction and akinesis, most commonly at the apex.	• Echogenic mass, distinct from myocardium, often protruding into the chamber, with underlying akinesis, typically at the apex
LV systolic dysfunction	Variable	• Extent of LV regional and global systolic dysfunction depends on infarct size, timing and success of reperfusion, and medical therapy.	• Location and size of the regional wall motion abnormalities correspond to infarct size. • Overall ejection fraction also reflects adverse LV remodeling.

LAD, Left anterior descending coronary artery; *MI*, myocardial infarction; *MR*, mitral regurgitation; *RCA*, right coronary artery.

Fig. 8.24 Post–myocardial infarction ventricular septal defect (VSD). (A) On transthoracic imaging, short-axis views do not show an obvious defect, but color Doppler demonstrates flow from the LV to the RV (arrow). (B) CW Doppler confirms high-velocity flow, although velocity likely is underestimated due to a nonparallel intercept angle. TEE images in an oblique long-axis view more clearly show the septal defect (arrow) with color flow across the septum.

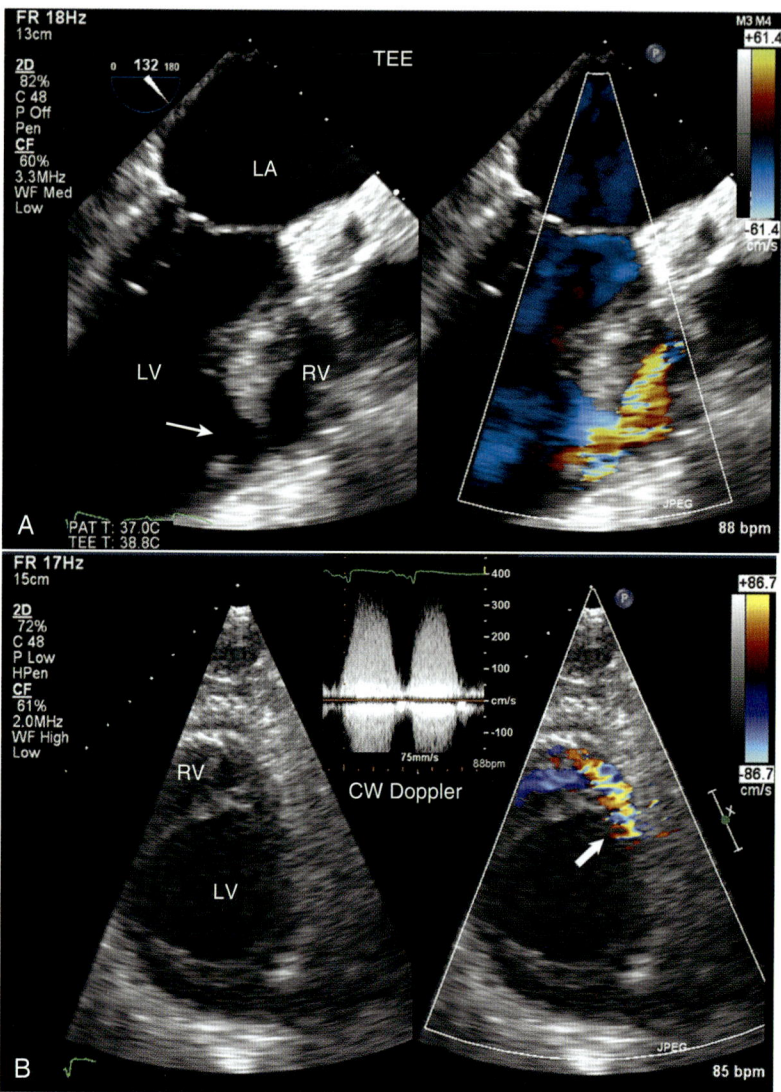

to necrosis and rupture of a focal area of the interventricular septum (Fig. 8.24). Identification of the rupture site is difficult with 2D imaging, especially because this complication tends to occur with *small* infarcts, so the wall motion abnormality may be subtle. Evaluation with Doppler ultrasound establishes the diagnosis, with a high-velocity left-to-right systolic jet recorded with continuous-wave Doppler ultrasound and systolic turbulence on the RV side of the septum recorded with conventional pulsed Doppler or color flow imaging.

When *ventricular rupture* occurs in the free wall of the LV (instead of in the septum), the mortality rate is extremely high due to extravasation of blood into the pericardial space and acute pericardial tamponade. However, some patients have a temporary respite due to containment of the rupture by pericardial adhesions or by thrombosis at the rupture site. In these patients, echocardiography may establish the diagnosis, thus prompting emergency surgery (Fig. 8.25). Echocardiographic clues of ventricular rupture (in the appropriate clinical setting) include a diffuse or localized pericardial effusion and a discrete segmental wall motion abnormality. Occasionally, the site of rupture can be visualized on 2D imaging, and rarely, flow from the ventricle into the pericardial space can be demonstrated with Doppler techniques.

A chronic, contained ventricular rupture is called a *pseudoaneurysm* (Fig. 8.26). An LV pseudoaneurysm has a wall composed of pericardium (no myocardial fibers). Characteristic features are:

- An abrupt transition from normal myocardium to the aneurysm
- An acute angle between the normal myocardium and aneurysm
- A narrow "neck" at the site of rupture

Coronary Artery Disease | Chapter 8

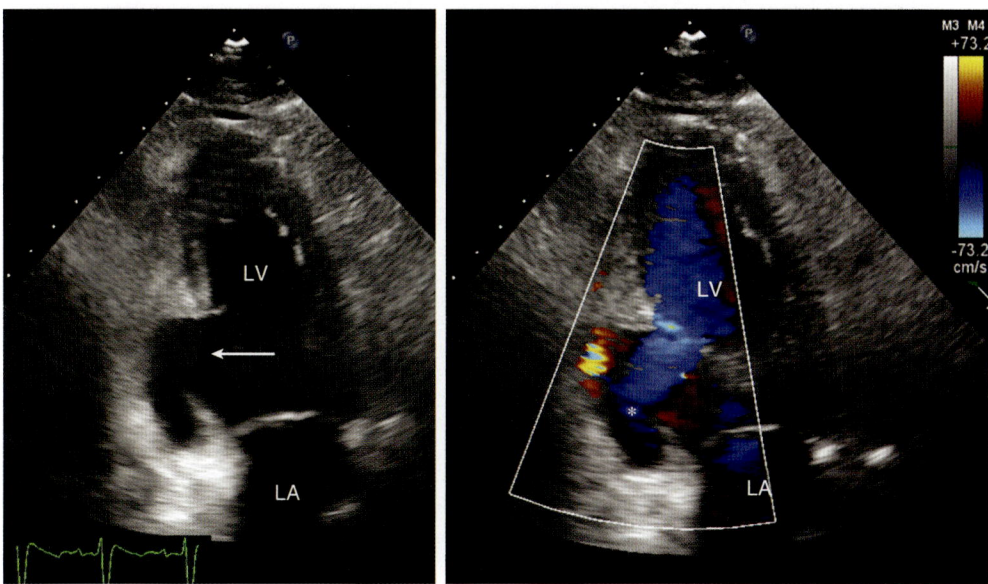

Fig. 8.25 ▶ **Left ventricular pseudoaneurysm.** The apical two-chamber view shows acute rupture of the basal inferior LV wall after myocardial infarction. An abrupt discontinuity in the LV wall *(arrow)* is noted, with flow in and out of a thrombus-lined section of the pericardium. Rapid diagnosis allowed surgical intervention in this patient.

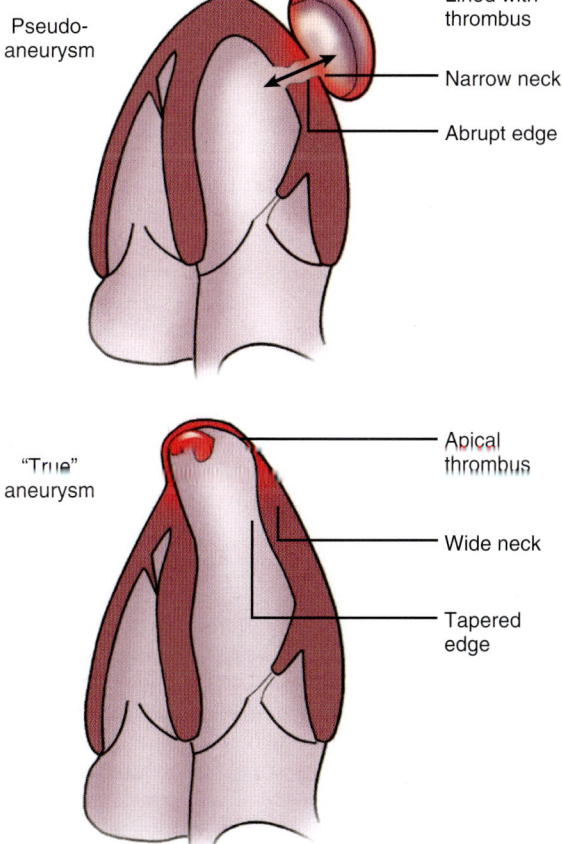

Fig. 8.26 Schematic diagram of a pseudoaneurysm versus a true aneurysm.

- A ratio of the "neck" diameter to the maximum diameter <0.5
- Partial filling of the aneurysm with thrombus

Often, flow into and out of the pseudoaneurysm is seen, and clinically, a corresponding apical murmur may be appreciated on auscultation. Although long-term survival has been described occasionally in patients with a pseudoaneurysm, correct echocardiographic diagnosis is essential. Surgical repair usually is recommended given a high likelihood of spontaneous rupture.

Other complications of acute myocardial infarction include:

- Pericardial effusion
- RV infarction
- LV aneurysm
- LV thrombus

A *pericardial effusion* also can be seen after myocardial infarction as a nonspecific response to transmural infarction. This effusion may be asymptomatic or associated with clinical symptoms (chest pain) and signs (ECG changes) of acute pericarditis. Although usually benign, an effusion may be complicated by tamponade physiology.

RV infarction may accompany an inferior infarction of the LV. Echocardiographic findings include RV hypokinesis or akinesis with variable degrees of RV dilation. With ECG leads placed on the right chest (in a mirror image pattern to the normal positions), ST-segment elevation may be seen, but this finding is not as sensitive or specific as echocardiographic features.

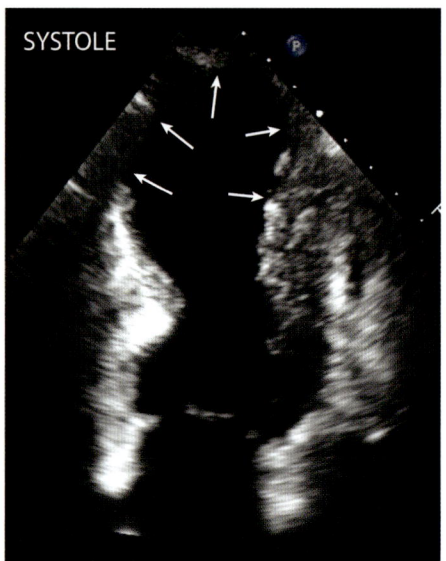

Fig. 8.27 ▶ **Apical aneurysm.** The end-diastolic image *(left)* shows increased echogenicity and thinning of the basal two thirds of the septum with dilation (e.g., a diastolic contour abnormality; *arrows*) of the apex. The end-systolic image *(right)* shows persistent apical dyskinesis (*arrows*). No obvious thrombus is noted, but evaluation with a higher-frequency transducer and oblique views is needed.

Longer-term complications of acute myocardial infarction include aneurysm formation, LV thrombi, and the sequelae of the irreversible decrease in LV systolic function. An *LV aneurysm* is defined echocardiographically as a dyskinetic region with a diastolic contour abnormality (Fig. 8.27). Apical aneurysms are most common, but inferior-basal aneurysms also are seen. Note that a "true" LV aneurysm, unlike a "false" aneurysm or pseudoaneurysm, is lined by (thinned) myocardium. A smooth transition is seen from normal myocardium to the thinned area, with an obtuse angle between the aneurysm and body of the LV. The ratio of the diameter of the junction between the aneurysm and the remainder of the LV to the maximum aneurysm diameter is >0.5.

LV thrombi form in regions of stasis of blood flow, such as in an apical aneurysm or overlying an area of akinesis in other regions of the LV. Evidence of severely reduced overall ventricular function, an aneurysm, an akinetic area, and the appearance of a spontaneous contrast effect in the LV all increase the likelihood of LV thrombus formation. Only rarely (as in hypereosinophilic syndrome) do ventricular thrombi occur in the absence of an underlying wall motion abnormality.

A thrombus is identified as an area of increased echogenicity within the ventricular chamber, distinct from the endocardium (see Fig. 15.18). Often, the thrombus protrudes into the chamber with a convex contour, but laminated thrombus with a concave contour following the endocardial curve also can be seen. Care is needed to distinguish a thrombus from prominent apical trabeculation with a false tendon or "web" traversing the apex of the LV chamber (see Fig. 15.1).

Diagnosis of apical thrombi is enhanced by using a 5-MHz transducer (improved near-field resolution), sliding the transducer laterally from the apical window, and then angulating it medially and superiorly to obtain a short-axis view of the apex. These procedures allow clear definition of the apical endocardium in most individuals. However, if images are suboptimal, appropriate interpretation should indicate that a thrombus "cannot be excluded," especially if the patient is at high risk of LV thrombus formation. Note that TEE imaging is less helpful for this diagnosis because the apex often is not fully visualized and is in the far field of the image plane.

END-STAGE ISCHEMIC CARDIAC DISEASE

Differentiation From Other Causes of Left Ventricular Systolic Dysfunction

The diagnosis of coronary artery disease is clear in patients with definite segmental wall motion abnormalities that correspond to the distribution of coronary blood flow. In end-stage ischemic disease, repeated transmural and subendocardial infarctions result in a diffuse pattern of abnormal wall thickening and endocardial motion. Thus when global systolic dysfunction is present, it is difficult to differentiate between end-stage ischemic disease and systolic dysfunction due to long-standing valvular disease or dilated cardiomyopathy (Fig. 8.28).

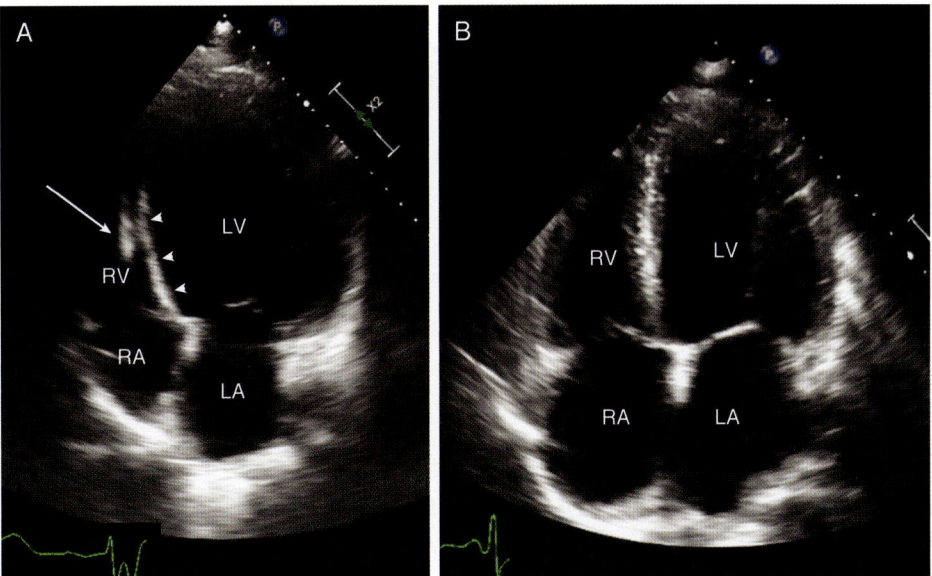

Fig. 8.28 ▶ ▶ **End-stage ischemic heart disease versus dilated cardiomyopathy.** Although the 2D images are superficially similar, the patient with ischemic disease (A) has apical dilation and dyskinesis, thinning and brightness of the septum due to prior infarction *(arrowheads)*, and a cardiac implanted electronic device lead in a relatively normal right heart. (B) The patient with dilated cardiomyopathy has more diffuse and severe four-chamber enlargement and biventricular dysfunction.

Echocardiographic Approach

Several features of the echocardiographic examination help in this differentiation. The segmental pattern of LV wall motion is examined carefully in each tomographic plane. Although patients with dilated cardiomyopathy often have a somewhat asymmetric pattern of wall motion with relative preservation at the ventricular base, definite areas of akinesis or wall thinning suggest ischemic disease. The degree of reduction in overall ventricular function (ejection fraction) is important in patient management but does not assist in determining the etiology of disease.

RV size and systolic function are normal in patients with ischemic disease unless they have had a previous RV infarction. Dilated cardiomyopathy occasionally affects the two ventricles in differing degrees but most often results in a symmetric pattern of RV and LV dilation and reduced systolic function.

Mitral valve regurgitation typically accompanies both dilated cardiomyopathy and end-stage ischemic disease due to one of several mechanisms, including mitral annular dilation, reduced papillary muscle systolic function, or malalignment of the papillary muscles. LV dilation and systolic dysfunction *due to* chronic mitral regurgitation, in contrast to mitral regurgitation due to ventricular dilation and dysfunction, usually are associated with anatomic abnormalities of the mitral leaflets themselves (e.g., myxomatous or rheumatic disease).

Pulmonary artery pressures are elevated to variable degrees in patients with LV dysfunction of any etiology, due to chronic elevation in LV end-diastolic pressure. Pulmonary pressures can be estimated from the tricuspid regurgitant jet velocity or from the pulmonary artery systolic velocity curve, as described in Chapter 6. Mild degrees of tricuspid valve regurgitation are common in ischemic disease, but moderate or severe regurgitation usually is a response to chronic pulmonary hypertension or chronic RV dilation and systolic dysfunction.

Note that aortic regurgitation is *not* a consequence of LV dilation or systolic dysfunction. LV dilation typically does not result in an increase in the diameter of the aortic annulus or adjacent outflow tract. The finding of moderate or severe aortic regurgitation implies primary valvular disease or aortic root dilation.

LV thrombi are possible with severe LV dysfunction of any etiology. The observation of reduced systolic function should prompt a search for apical thrombi, but this finding does not help in the differential diagnosis.

Limitations and Alternate Approaches

If a diagnosis of end-stage ischemic disease versus a primary cardiomyopathy would alter patient management, coronary angiography will be needed for a definitive diagnosis, to document the exact site and severity of coronary lesions, and to assess the distal vessel anatomy. Other useful approaches include computed tomographic coronary angiography or cardiac magnetic resonance imaging for visualization of coronary anatomy and identification of myocardial scar.

THE ECHO EXAM

Echocardiographic Diagnosis of Coronary Disease

Modality	Clinical Utility	Echocardiographic Findings	Recording	Interpretation
Resting regional wall motion	• Acute coronary syndrome • Chronic CAD	• Akinesis or hypokinesis of infarcted or acutely ischemic regions	• 2D or 3D imaging of the LV • Optimize endocardial definition. • Use contrast if images are suboptimal.	• Use standard wall segment nomenclature for location. • Categorize wall motion as normal, hypokinetic or akinetic. • Use 3D display when possible.
Exercise stress echocardiography	• Diagnosis of CAD • Evaluation for ischemia with known CAD	• Normal wall motion at rest • Hypokinesis or akinesis with stress in ischemic segments • Return of normal wall motion with rest	• Depth that includes only LV; optimize endocardial definition, use contrast if needed. • Same depth for baseline and stress images. • Select optimal images from series of digital cine loops.	• Include exercise duration, blood pressure and heart rate response, symptoms, and ECG changes in report. • Compare baseline and stress images in same views. • Maximal workload affects accuracy of echo results for detection of ischemia.
Dobutamine stress echocardiography	• Diagnosis and evaluation of CAD in patients unable to exercise	• Normal wall motion at rest • Hypokinesis or akinesis with stress in ischemic segments • Return of normal wall motion with rest	• Depth that includes only LV; optimize endocardial definition, use contrast if needed. • Same depth for baseline and stress images. • Select optimal images from series of digital cine loops.	• Include symptoms and peak heart rate as percent of maximum predicted in report. • Blood pressure response and ECG changes are not diagnostic for CAD. • Compare baseline and stress images in same views. • Maximal workload affects accuracy of echo results for detection of ischemia.
Myocardial viability	• Diagnosis of hibernating or stunned myocardium	• Biphasic response on DSE	• Standard DSE protocol with additional low-dose stages	• Improvement in wall thickening at low dose followed by ischemia at high-dose DSE is consistent with viable myocardium supplied by a stenosed vessel.
Overall LV systolic function	• All patients with CAD	• Ejection fraction by 2D and 3D imaging • dP/dt	• 3D Biplane apical ejection fraction • CW Doppler mitral regurgitant jet	• The degree of reduction in EF after acute MI depends on infarct size and success of reperfusion.
LV diastolic function	• All patients with CAD	• Diastolic dysfunction and elevated filling pressures depend on type and severity of CAD.	• Standard approaches to evaluation of LV diastolic function and filling pressures (see Chapter 7)	• Transient diastolic dysfunction with ischemia • End-stage CAD is associated with severe diastolic dysfunction.

CAD, Coronary artery disease; *DSE*, dobutamine stress echocardiography; *EF*, ejection fraction; *MI*, myocardial infarction.

Coronary Anatomy and Echo Wall Segments

Coronary Artery	Echo Wall Segments	Variations
Left anterior descending (LAD)	Anterior septum Anterior wall Apex	Diagonal branches of the LAD may supply some segments of the lateral wall. Extension of the LAD around the LV apex is variable.
Circumflex (Cx)	Anterior-lateral wall Posterior-lateral wall	The number and distribution of obtuse marginal branches supplying the lateral wall are variable.
Posterior descending artery (PDA)	Inferior wall Inferior septum	The PDA arises from the right coronary artery in about 80% of patients. Length of the PDA is variable, extending to the apex in some patients. An LV extension branch from the PDA may supply parts of the lateral wall.

Complications of Acute Myocardial Infarction

Complication	Echocardiographic Findings	Imaging Approach
Pericardial effusion	• Small circumferential pericardial effusion	• Standard views for evaluation of effusion • Larger effusion raises concern for LV rupture.
RV infarction	• Dilated hypokinetic or akinetic RV • Infarction of adjacent inferior LV wall	• Apical and subcostal views to evaluate RV free wall motion • Measure TAPSE, DTI S-velocity, and fractional area change.
Ischemic MR	• Tethering of posterior leaflet with posteriorly directed MR • Papillary muscle rupture (rare) with mass attached to flail leaflet • Moderate to severe mitral regurgitation (may be intermittent, present only during ischemic episodes)	• Evaluate mitral valve anatomy in standard views. • Evaluate and quantitate mitral regurgitant severity (see Chapter 12). • TEE and 3D imaging is often needed to identify the cause of MR.
Ventricular septal defect	• Discrete septal defect in area of akinesis with left-to-right flow seen on color and CW Doppler	• Use color Doppler to detect VSD in focal region of akinesis or when imaging suggests discontinuity in septum. • CW Doppler confirms velocity and direction of blood flow.
Free wall rupture and tamponade	• Large pericardial effusion with tamponade • Acute fatal event unless temporarily sealed by fibrinous pericardial adhesions	• Pericardial hematoma or localized effusion after MI should be promptly reported to referring MD. • Use color Doppler to search for communication from LV to pericardial space; subcostal views are helpful.
LV pseudoaneurysm	• Abrupt transition from normal myocardium to aneurysm • Acute angle between myocardium and aneurysm • Narrow neck • Ratio of neck diameter to aneurysm diameter <0.5 • Often lined with thrombus	• Most often located at inferior base of LV • Parasternal views and apical 2-chamber views are helpful. • TEE imaging is often needed for diagnosis.
LV aneurysm	• Thin, bright, dyskinetic LV segment with a diastolic contour abnormality, often with associated thrombus	• Most often located at LV apex • Best seen in apical views or with 3D imaging from apex

Continued

Complications of Acute Myocardial Infarction—cont'd

Complication	Echocardiographic Findings	Imaging Approach
LV thrombus	• Echogenic mass, distinct from myocardium, often protruding into the chamber, with underlying akinesis, typically at the apex	• Use high-frequency transducer, zoom mode, adjust gain and instrument settings; off-axis lateral apical views are helpful. • Contrast to opacify the LV better demonstrates the thrombus. • Apical thrombi may be missed on TEE.
LV systolic dysfunction	• Location and size of the regional wall motion abnormalities correspond to infarct size. Overall ejection fraction also reflects adverse LV remodeling.	• 3D or 2D biplane ejection fraction calculations

DTI, Doppler tissue imaging; *MI*, myocardial infarction; *MR*, mitral regurgitation; *TAPSE*, tricuspid annular plane systolic excursion; *VSD*, ventricular septal defect.

Differentiation of Left Ventricular Systolic Dysfunction Due to End-Stage Ischemic Disease From Dilated Cardiomyopathy or Chronic Valvular Disease

Findings	End-Stage Ischemic Disease	Dilated Cardiomyopathy	Chronic Valvular Disease
LV ejection fraction	Moderately-severely depressed	Moderately-severely depressed	Moderately-severely depressed
Segmental wall motion abnormalities	May be present	Absent	Absent
RV systolic function	Normal	Decreased	Variable
Pulmonary artery pressures	Elevated	Elevated	Elevated
• Mitral regurgitation	Moderate	Moderate	Moderate-severe
• Aortic regurgitation	Not significant	Not significant	Moderate-severe

SUGGESTED READING

General

1. Lang RM, Badano LP, Mor-Avi V, et al: Recommendations for cardiac chamber quantification by echocardiography in adults: an update from the American Society of Echocardiography and the European Association of Cardiovascular Imaging, *J Am Soc Echocardiogr* 28(1):1–39.e14, 2015.
   This comprehensive standards document includes a section on nomenclature for describing regional wall motion. These definitions are unchanged from prior documents. The standard reference for cardiac displays is defined as the long axis of the LV. The names used for image planes are short axis (90° to long axis), vertical long axis (apical two-chamber plane), and horizontal long axis (four-chamber plane). Myocardial segments are defined at the basal and midventricular level as (clockwise from the anterior septal insertion) as anterior, anterolateral, inferolateral, inferior, inferoseptal, and anteroseptal. There are four apical segments (anterior, septal, inferior, and lateral).

2. Porter TR, Abdelmoneim S, Belcik JT, et al: Guidelines for the cardiac sonographer in the performance of contrast echocardiography: a focused update from the American Society of Echocardiography, *J Am Soc Echocardiogr* 27(8):797–810, 2014.
   This guideline document provides details on when and how to use contrast echocardiography. Technical details of contrast preparation and injection and instrument settings can be used in laboratory imaging protocols. Practical advice is provided for dealing with common artifacts seen with contrast including swirling, shadowing, and inadequate chamber opacification.

Exercise Echocardiography

3. Siegel R, Rader F: Stress echocardiography for diagnosis of coronary disease. In Otto CM, editor: *The Practice of Clinical Echocardiography*, 5th ed, Philadelphia, 2017, Elsevier.
   The clinical application of exercise echocardiography is discussed in detail, including necessary equipment and personnel, interpretation of stress images, a comparison of treadmill versus bicycle exercise testing, and the relative advantages and disadvantages of exercise echocardiography compared with other diagnostic approaches. 68 references.

4. Fihn SD, Gardin JM, Abrams J, et al: American College of Cardiology Foundation: 2012 ACCF/AHA/ACP/AATS/PCNA/SCAI/STS guideline for the diagnosis and management of patients with stable ischemic heart disease: executive summary: a report of the American College of Cardiology Foundation/American Heart Association task force on practice guidelines, and the American College of Physicians,

American Association for Thoracic Surgery, Preventive Cardiovascular Nurses Association, Society for Cardiovascular Angiography and Interventions, and Society of Thoracic Surgeons, Circulation 126:3097–3137, 2012.
This guideline document provides a detailed discussion and summary of the evidence for selecting the most appropriate diagnostic test for evaluation of patients with possible coronary artery disease. Exercise stress echocardiography is recommended when ECG changes would be uninterpretable due to an abnormal resting ECG, with pharmacologic stress testing in patients unable to exercise.

5. Banerjee A, Newman DR, Van den Bruel A, et al: Diagnostic accuracy of exercise stress testing for coronary artery disease: a systematic review and meta-analysis of prospective studies, Int J Clin Pract 66:477–492, 2012.
This systematic review identified 34 studies with 3352 participants in studies published between 1996 and 2009 that evaluated the diagnostic accuracy of exercise stress echocardiography for diagnosis of coronary disease at angiography. As expected, diagnostic accuracy depended on age, sex, clinical characteristics, and the prevalence of coronary disease in the study group. Exercise echocardiography was more useful for excluding coronary disease than for confirming the diagnosis. This finding is consistent with those of other studies showing a high sensitivity of stress echo and the low likelihood of adverse cardiac outcomes in patients with a normal stress echocardiogram.

6. Danad I, Szymonifka J, Twisk JW, et al: Diagnostic performance of cardiac imaging methods to diagnose ischaemia-causing coronary artery disease when directly compared with fractional flow reserve as a reference standard: a meta-analysis, Eur Heart J 38(13):991–998, 2017.
Using fractional flow reserve measured at cardiac catheterization as the reference standard for diagnosis of coronary disease, this meta-analysis showed that stress echocardiography had a sensitivity of 77% (95% confidence interval: 61 to 88) and specificity of 75% (95% confidence interval: 63 to 85). However, the number of patients with both stress echocardiography was low (n = 115), and this group of subjects undergoing invasive fractional flow reserve measurements may not be representative of most patients referred for stress studies.

Dobutamine Stress Echocardiography

7. Delgado V, Bax JJ: Non-exercise stress echocardiography for diagnosis of coronary disease. In Otto CM, editor: *The Practice of Clinical Echocardiograph*, 5th ed, Philadelphia, 2017, Elsevier.
Concise summary of the principles, technical aspects, and clinical utility of pharmacologic stress echocardiography. Comprehensive tables summarize clinical studies evaluating the sensitivity and specificity of dobutamine stress echocardiography as well as discussion of the use of contrast, 3D imaging, tissue Doppler, and speckle trading strain imaging. 72 references.

8. Geleijnse ML, Krenning BJ, Nemes A, et al: Incidence, pathophysiology, and treatment of complications during dobutamine-atropine stress echocardiography, Circulation 121:1756–1767, 2010.
Meta-analysis of complications with pharmacologic stress echocardiography based on 26 studies with more than 400 patients each for a total of 55,071 patients. Total major complications occurred in 1 out of 475 patients. Rare complications (< 0.01%) included death, cardiac rupture, asystole, and cerebrovascular events. The risk of myocardial infarction was 0.02% and the risk of ventricular fibrillation was approximately 0.04%. This meta-analysis has a comprehensive list of references.

9. Uusitalo V, Luotolahti M, Pietilä M, et al: Two-dimensional speckle-tracking during dobutamine stress echocardiography in the detection of myocardial ischemia in patients with suspected coronary artery disease, J Am Soc Echocardiogr 29(5):470–479.e3, 2016.
In a series of 50 patients with an intermediate pretest likelihood of coronary artery disease, the combination of an increased postsystolic strain index and reduced strain during early recovery was better than qualitative analysis of regional wall motion for diagnosis of significant coronary stenosis on angiography.

10. Joyce E, Delgado V, Bax JJ, et al: Advanced techniques in dobutamine stress echocardiography: focus on myocardial deformation analysis, Heart 101:72–81, 2015.
The use of tissue Doppler imaging and speckle tracking echocardiography, specific types of myocardial deformation analysis, may improve the accuracy of dobutamine stress echocardiography for diagnosis of coronary artery disease. Tissue Doppler imaging provides high temporal resolution and evaluation of all myocardial segments but is angle dependent, mostly used for longitudinal shortening. Speckle tracking strain is angle independent, which allows measurement of twist and torsion, as well as strain for each myocardial segment.

11. Joyce E, Debonnaire P, Leong DP, et al: Differential response of LV sublayer twist during dobutamine stress echocardiography as a novel marker of contractile reserve after acute myocardial infarction: relationship with follow-up LVEF improvement, Eur Heart J Cardiovasc Imaging 17(6):652–659, 2016.
In 61 patients with a first ST-elevation myocardial infarction, the response of subepicardial twist on dobutamine stress echocardiography performed 3 months later was predictive of subsequent improvement in LV systolic function. This new approach is promising but requires further validation.

Chest Pain in the Emergency Department

12. Fleischmann KE, Weeks SG: Echocardiography in the emergency department: role in patients with acute chest pain. In Otto CM, editor: *The Practice of Clinical Echocardiography*, 5th ed, Philadelphia, 2017, Elsevier.
Review of the potential utility of echocardiography for triage, risk stratification, and detection of other causes of chest pain in patients with suspected myocardial infarction. The concept of a chest pain center and the cost-effectiveness of various approaches are discussed.

13. Wei K, Peters D, Belcik T, et al: A predictive instrument using contrast echocardiography in patients presenting to the emergency department with chest pain and without ST-segment elevation, J Am Soc Echocardiogr 23:636–642, 2010.
A risk model was developed in 1166 patients presenting with chest pain and a nondiagnostic ECG and then validated in a subsequent group of 720 patients. A simple risk score from 0 to 4 can be calculated by adding one point for each of the following:

- *Nonspecific ST-T changes on ECG*
- *Any abnormality on ECG*
- *Abnormal regional function on echocardiography*
- *Abnormal myocardial perfusion on contrast echocardiography*

The risk of cardiac events during the next 48 hours increases with this score: 0.4% with a score of 0 to as high as 55.3% with a score of 4.

14. Rybicki FJ, Udelson JE, Peacock WF, et al: 2015 ACR/ACC/AHA/AATS/ACEP/ASNC/NASCI/SAEM/SCCT/SCMR/SCPC/SNMMI/STR/STS appropriate utilization of cardiovascular imaging in emergency department patients with chest pain: a joint document of the American

College of Radiology Appropriateness Criteria Committee and the American College of Cardiology Appropriate Use Criteria Task Force, *J Am Coll Cardiol* 67(7):853–879, 2016.

This appropriate use consensus document suggests resting echocardiography may be appropriate in patients presenting with chest pain and a suspected non–ST-elevation myocardial infarction when serial troponin levels and ECG findings are borderline or positive for infarction. Exercise echocardiography is appropriate when serial troponin levels and ECG results are negative for an acute coronary syndrome. Other imaging approaches also are discussed including nuclear perfusion imaging, computed tomographic coronary angiography and cardiac magnetic resonance imaging.

Complications of Acute Myocardial Infarction

15. Gerber IL, Foster E: Echocardiography in the coronary care unit: management of acute myocardial infarction, detection of complications, and prognostic implications. In Otto CM, editor: *The Practice of Clinical Echocardiography*, 5th ed, Philadelphia, 2017, Elsevier.

    This chapter summarizes the pathophysiologic correlates of the echocardiographic findings in acute myocardial infarction, the role of echocardiography in patient management, and the utility of echocardiography for detecting complications of acute myocardial infarction. Post–myocardial infarction complications and risk stratification are reviewed. 100 references.

16. Moreyra A, Huang M, Wilson A, et al: Trends in incidence and mortality rates of ventricular septal rupture during acute myocardial infarction, *Am J Cardiol* 106:1095–1100, 2010.

    In this database of 148,881 patients with first acute myocardial infarction, the 408 patients with a post–myocardial infarction ventricular septal defect (0.3%) were more likely to be older, women, and have increased rates of chronic renal disease, heart failure, and cardiogenic shock. The hospital mortality rate with a post–myocardial infarction ventricular septal defect was 41%, with a 1 year mortality rate 60%, with no significant change in mortality rates between 1990 and 2007

17. Solheim S, Seljeflot I, Lunde K, et al: Frequency of left ventricular thrombus in patients with anterior wall acute myocardial infarction treated with percutaneous coronary intervention and dual antiplatelet therapy, *Am J Cardiol* 106:1197–1200, 2010.

    In 100 patients with an ST-elevation anterior myocardial infarction who underwent revascularization with acute percutaneous coronary intervention and antiplatelet therapy, LV thrombi were detected in 15 patients by echocardiography, two thirds within the first week after infarction. Patients with an LV thrombus had higher cardiac enzyme levels, larger infarct sizes, and lower ejection fractions compared with patients with no LV thrombus.

9. Cardiomyopathies, Hypertensive and Pulmonary Heart Disease

DILATED CARDIOMYOPATHY
  Basic Principles
  Echocardiographic Approach
  Limitations and Technical Considerations
  Clinical Utility
  Alternate Approaches

HYPERTROPHIC CARDIOMYOPATHY
  Basic Principles
  Echocardiographic Approach
    Asymmetric Left Ventricular Hypertrophy
    Left Ventricular Diastolic Function
    Dynamic Subaortic LV Outflow Tract Obstruction
    Mitral Valve Abnormalities
  Limitations and Technical Considerations
  Clinical Utility
    Diagnosis and Screening
    Evaluation of Medical Therapy
    Selection of Patients for Implantable Cardiac Defibrillators
    Monitoring of Alcohol Septal Ablation
    Surgical Therapy
  Alternate Approaches

RESTRICTIVE CARDIOMYOPATHY
  Basic Principles
  Echocardiographic Approach
    Anatomic Features
    Diastolic Function
  Limitations and Technical Considerations
  Clinical Utility
  Alternate Approaches

OTHER CARDIOMYOPATHIES
  Arrhythmogenic Right Ventricular Dysplasia
  Left Ventricular Noncompaction

ADVANCED HEART FAILURE THERAPIES
  Cardiac Resynchronization Therapy
  Left Ventricular Assist Devices
  Total Artificial Heart
  Cardiac Transplantation
    Cardiac Allograft Structure and Function
    Acute Transplant Rejection
    Post-Transplant Monitoring
  Limitations, Technical Considerations, and Alternate Approaches

HYPERTENSIVE HEART DISEASE
  Basic Principles
  Echocardiographic Approach
    Ventricular Hypertrophy
    Diastolic Function
    Systolic Function
    Other Echocardiographic Findings
  Limitations and Technical Considerations
  Clinical Utility
    Diagnosis and Prognosis
    Evaluation of Heart Failure Symptoms in a Patient With Hypertension
  Alternate Approaches

PULMONARY HEART DISEASE
  Chronic Versus Acute Pulmonary Disease
  Echocardiographic Approach
    Pulmonary Pressures
    Right Ventricular Pressure Overload
    Secondary Tricuspid Regurgitation
  Limitations and Technical Considerations
  Clinical Utility
  Alternate Approaches

THE ECHO EXAM

SUGGESTED READING

Cardiomyopathy is defined as a primary disease of the myocardium, excluding myocardial dysfunction due to ischemia or chronic valvular disease. Several approaches to the classification of cardiomyopathies are possible, such as etiology or anatomy, but a physiologic classification is most useful clinically. The three basic physiologic categories of cardiomyopathy are:

- Dilated
- Hypertrophic
- Restrictive

The disease process in an individual patient tends to correspond closely with one of these physiologic categories; however, overlap among these categories (particularly between dilated and restrictive) can occur. Echocardiographic evaluation focuses on confirming the diagnosis and type of cardiomyopathy present and on defining the physiologic consequences of the disease process in that individual.

Although hypertensive and pulmonary heart diseases are not primary diseases of the heart muscle, they are included in this chapter because their clinical and echocardiographic presentations often mimic those of cardiomyopathy. In addition, evaluation of patients receiving advanced heart failure therapies is outlined. End-stage coronary disease resulting in left ventricular (LV) systolic dysfunction, sometimes referred to as ischemic cardiomyopathy, is discussed in Chapter 8.

DILATED CARDIOMYOPATHY

Basic Principles

Dilated cardiomyopathy manifests clinically as heart failure with reduced ejection fraction (HFrEF). Typically, all four chambers are enlarged, and impaired systolic function of both the LV and right ventricle (RV) occurs, due to a wide range of underlying causes (Table 9.1). The physiology of dilated cardiomyopathy (Fig. 9.1) is characterized predominantly by:

- Impaired LV contractility
- Reduced cardiac output
- Elevated LV end-diastolic pressure

Clinically, patients most often have heart failure, with initial complaints ranging from symptoms of pulmonary or systemic venous congestion to symptoms of low forward cardiac output. Secondary mitral regurgitation frequently is present secondary to LV and mitral annular dilation. In addition, pulmonary hypertension develops in many patients in response to the chronic elevation in left atrial (LA) pressure.

Typically, LV diastolic dysfunction coexists with systolic dysfunction, although separating the hemodynamic effects of diastolic dysfunction from concurrent systolic dysfunction is challenging.

Echocardiographic Approach

The echocardiographic approach to the patient with heart failure symptoms should start with an evaluation of LV size, wall thickness, and systolic function (Figs. 9.2 and 9.3). Echocardiographic imaging from standard windows allows evaluation of the size and function

TABLE 9.1	Examples of Causes of Cardiomyopathies: Functional Classification

Dilated Cardiomyopathy

Genetic
Infectious
- Postviral (myocarditis)
- Chagas disease

Toxins and drugs
- Alcohol
- Anthracycline medications

Metabolic
- Hypothyroidism or hyperthyroidism
- Pheochromocytoma

Nutritional
- Beriberi (thiamine)

Peripartum
Systemic inflammatory disease
Neuromuscular diseases
- Duchenne-Becker muscular dystrophy

Stress induced
- Tako-tsubo

Hypertrophic Cardiomyopathy

Nonobstructive
Obstructive
Latent obstructive

Restrictive Cardiomyopathy

Infiltrative systemic diseases
- Amyloidosis
- Gaucher disease

Inflammatory (granulomatous)
- Sarcoidosis

Storage diseases
- Hemochromatosis
- Fabry disease

Endomyocardial
- Hypereosinophilic syndrome
- Radiation induced

Noninfiltrative
- Scleroderma

Other Cardiomyopathies

Arrhythmogenic RV dysplasia
Isolated LV noncompaction

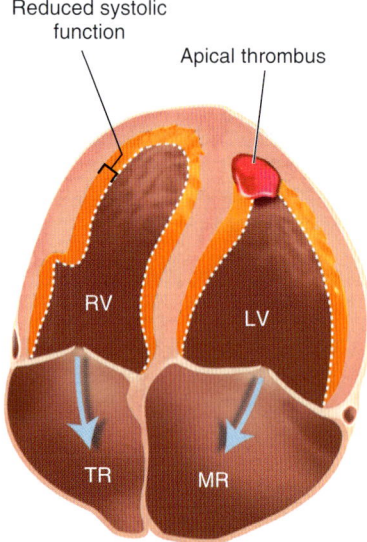

Four-chamber dilation

Fig. 9.1 Dilated cardiomyopathy. Four-chamber enlargement is present with reduced LV and RV systolic function. *Dashed lines* indicate the limited extent of endocardial motion between end-diastole and end-systole. An apical thrombus is present. Secondary mitral regurgitation *(MR)* and tricuspid regurgitation *(TR)* are indicated by the *arrows*.

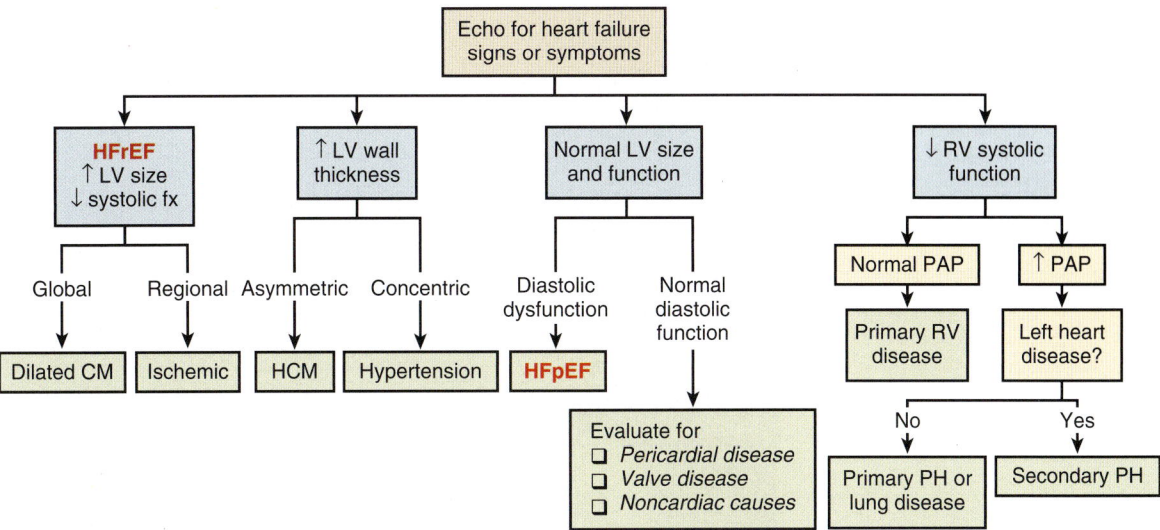

Fig. 9.2 Echocardiographic approach to the patient with heart failure. Key features that help distinguish the cause of heart failure symptoms include LV chamber size, wall thickness, and systolic function in addition to RV systolic function. Heart failure with reduced ejection fraction *(HFrEF)* is characterized by global myocardial dysfunction versus regional dysfunction with ischemic disease. Asymmetric hypertrophy suggests hypertrophic cardiomyopathy *(HCM)*, whereas concentric hypertrophy is more typical of hypertensive heart disease. When LV size and function are normal, diastolic dysfunction or heart failure with preserved ejection fraction *(HFpEF)* is likely in the absence of pericardial or valve disease. RV dysfunction may be due to primary myocardial disease, such as RV infarction or arrhythmogenic RV cardiomyopathy, or to elevated pulmonary artery pressure *(PAP)* with primary or secondary pulmonary hypertension *(PH)*. *CM,* Cardiomyopathy; *fx,* function.

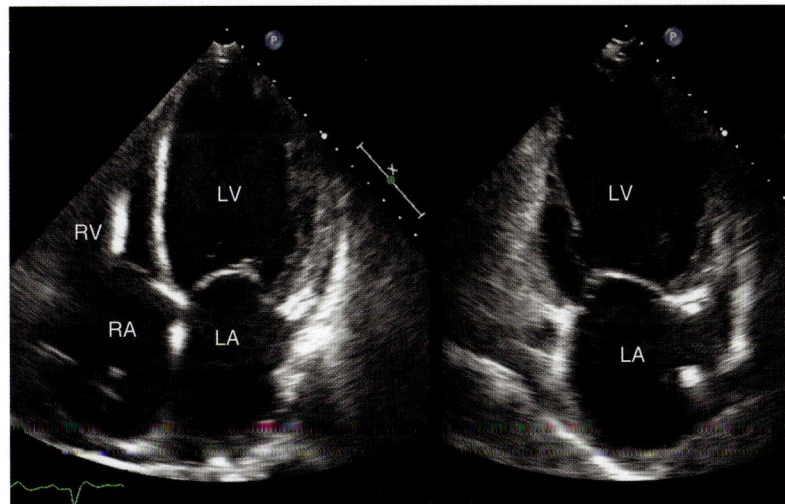

Fig. 9.3 Echocardiographic images in a patient with dilated cardiomyopathy. In the apical four-chamber view *(left),* ▶ dilation of all four cardiac chambers is seen. In the apical two-chamber view *(right),* ▶ the LV and atrium are seen. In real time, RV and LV systolic functions are severely reduced.

of all four cardiac chambers using two-dimensional (2D) or three-dimensional (3D) imaging (Fig. 9.4):

❐ LV systolic function
  ■ Qualitative global and regional systolic function
  ■ Quantitative end-diastolic and end-systolic dimensions or volumes
  ■ Ejection fraction
❐ RV systolic function
  ■ Qualitative size and systolic function
  ■ Pulmonary artery systolic pressure and estimated resistance

❐ LA size
  ■ Qualitative size and linear dimensions
  ■ Quantitation of LA volumes

In addition to 2D and 3D imaging, other signs of poor LV systolic function include:

❐ M-mode
  ■ Increased mitral E-point to septal separation (EPSS)
  ■ Reduced anteroposterior aortic root motion
  ■ Delayed mitral valve closure

Fig. 9.4 **3D ventricular volumes in dilated cardiomyopathy.** A 3D volume is acquired from the apical window with semiautomated borders in x, y, and z planes, corresponding to four-chamber, two-chamber, and short-axis (not shown) views. The volumetric reconstruction allows calculation of end-diastolic volume *(EDV)* and end-systolic volume *(ESV)*, stroke volume *(SV)*, and ejection fraction *(EF)*.

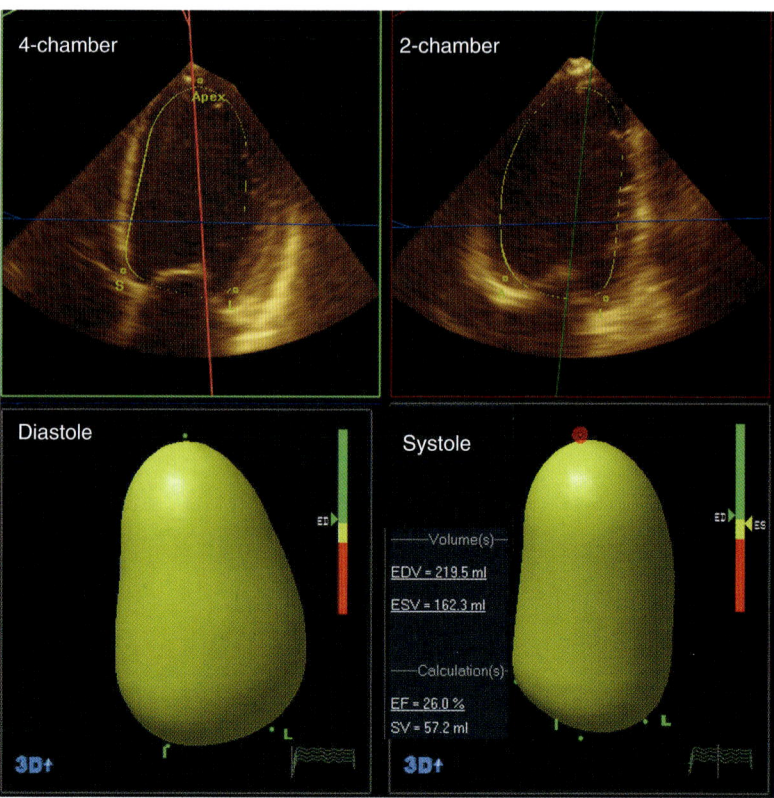

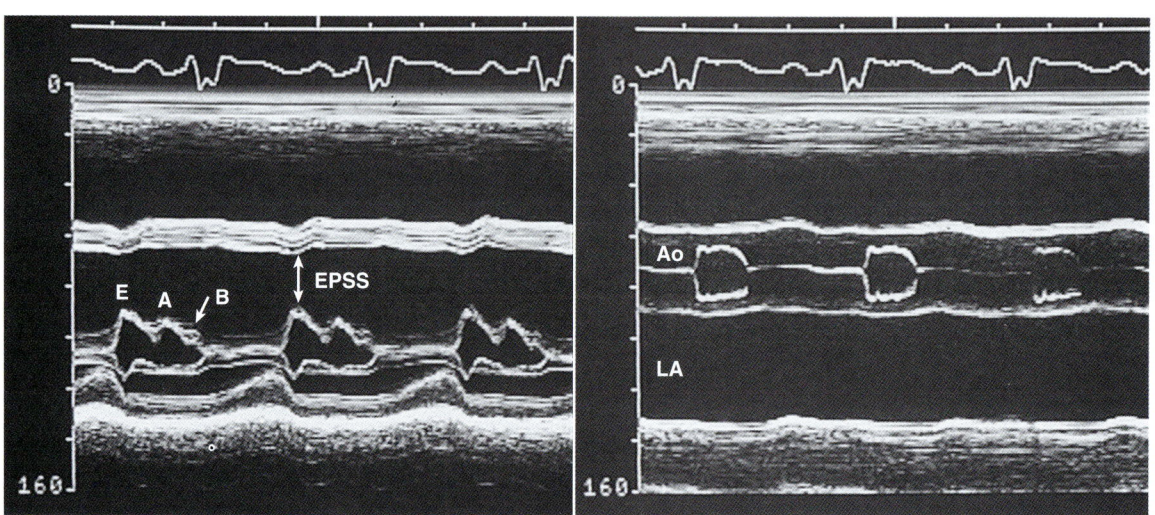

Fig. 9.5 M-mode findings in dilated cardiomyopathy. The mitral M-mode shows increased mitral E-point septal separation *(EPSS)* and a "B-bump" *(left)*. The aortic M-mode shows decreased aortic root motion with early closure of the aortic valve *(right)*.

- Doppler
    - Reduced aortic ejection velocity
    - Reduced rate of rise in ventricular pressure (dP/dt)
    - Secondary mitral regurgitation
    - Diastolic dysfunction

The increase in E-point to septal separation is due to a combination of LV dilation and reduced mitral leaflet motion caused by low transmitral flow rates. Reduced anteroposterior aortic root motion reflects reduced LA filling and emptying (Fig. 9.5). A reduced aortic ejection velocity indicates a reduced stroke

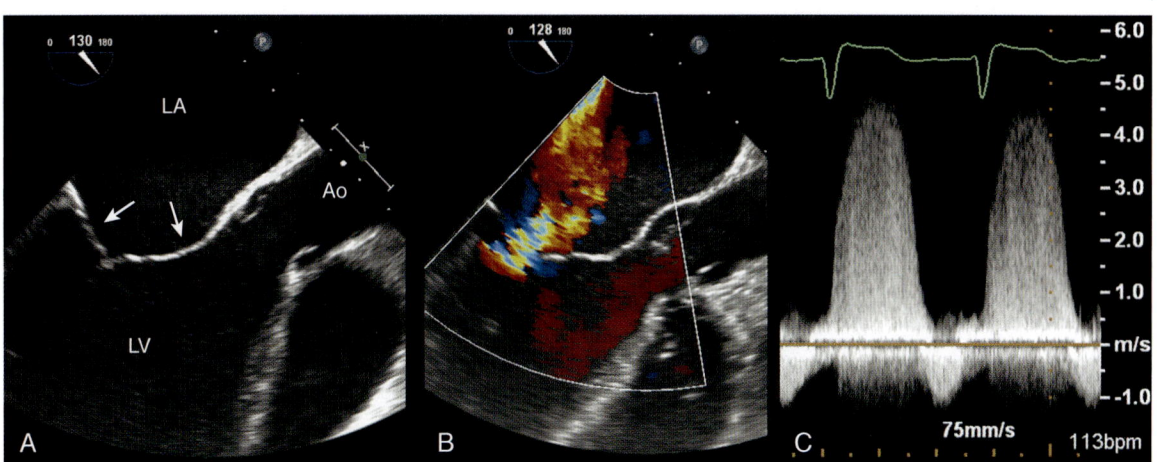

Fig. 9.6 Secondary mitral regurgitation. TEE imaging in this 62-year-old man with severe LV dilation and an ejection fraction of 21% shows (A) ▶ normal leaflet anatomy with tethering *(arrows)* preventing complete coaptation, (B) ▶ a central jet of mitral regurgitation with a vena contracta width of 5 mm, and (C) a CW Doppler signal consistent with moderate to severe mitral regurgitation. *Ao*, Aorta.

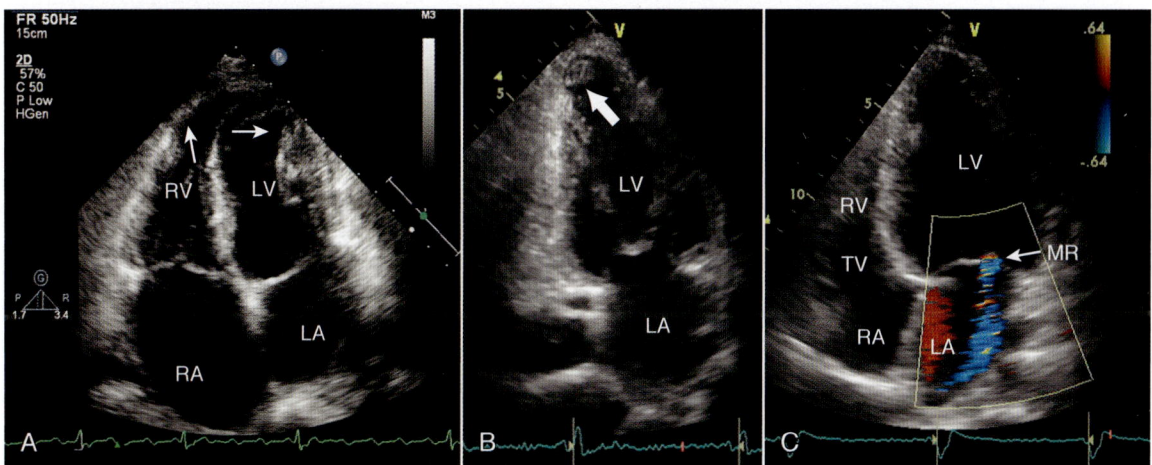

Fig. 9.7 Chagas disease. (A) The four-chamber view shows typical localized biventricular apical aneurysms *(arrows)*. ▶ (B) In the two-chamber view an apical thrombus is seen *(arrow)*. ▶ Inferior akinesis was present, which is a typical finding in Chagas cardiomyopathy. (C) Color Doppler demonstrates mild to moderate secondary mitral regurgitation *(MR)*. *TV*, Tricuspid valve. *(Courtesy Dr. Marcia Barbosa and Dr. Maria P. Nunes, Belo Horizonte, Brazil.)*

volume, although compensatory mechanisms (including LV dilation) often result in a normal stroke volume at rest. A slow rate of rise in velocity of the mitral regurgitant jet indicates a reduced rate of rise in LV pressure in early systole *(dP/dt)*.

The cause of secondary mitral valve regurgitation (with an anatomically normal valve) is related to misalignment of the papillary muscles, ventricular systolic dysfunction, and annular dilation. Regurgitant severity ranges from mild to severe, as assessed with Doppler techniques (Fig. 9.6; see Table 12.8). Pulmonary pressures usually are elevated and can be estimated from the velocity of the tricuspid regurgitant jet, as described in Chapter 6.

The echocardiographic appearance of dilated cardiomyopathy is fairly uniform despite a wide range of disease processes. Exceptions include fulminant myocarditis, in which little ventricular dilation is present, despite severe systolic dysfunction. In Chagas heart disease, an LV apical aneurysm is seen in about half of patients; thrombus formation is often seen, although global hypokinesis is typical with advanced disease (Fig. 9.7). Tako-tsubo cardiomyopathy is an acute, transient, stress-induced cardiomyopathy characterized by "apical ballooning" with apical dilation and dyskinesis but preserved dimensions and function of the cardiac base (Fig. 9.8).

Diastolic dysfunction typically accompanies systolic heart failure in patients with dilated cardiomyopathy, and noninvasive estimates of filling pressures are helpful in clinical management. When systolic dysfunction is present, the elevated end-systolic volume results in a

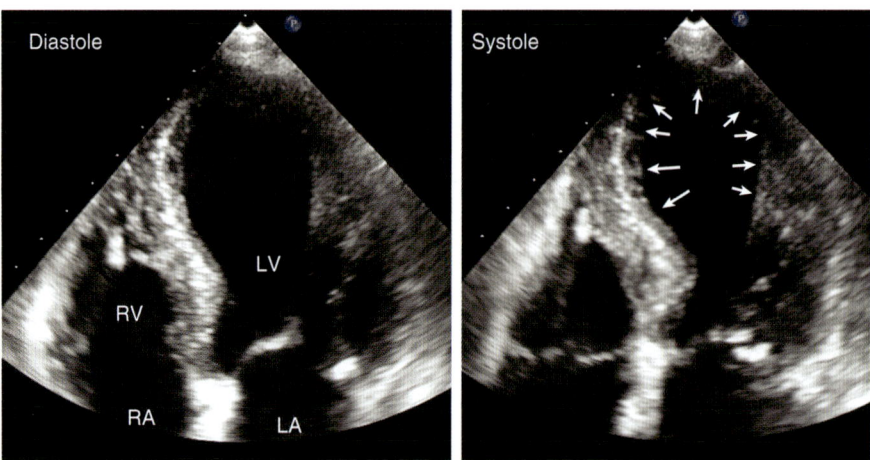

Fig. 9.8 ▶ **Tako-tsubo cardiomyopathy.** This older woman developed acute heart failure after emergency noncardiac surgery. In the apical four-chamber view, the LV apex is dilated with systolic dyskinesis *(arrows)* with relatively preserved contraction at the myocardial base. Coronary angiography was normal, and ventricular systolic function returned to normal within 2 weeks.

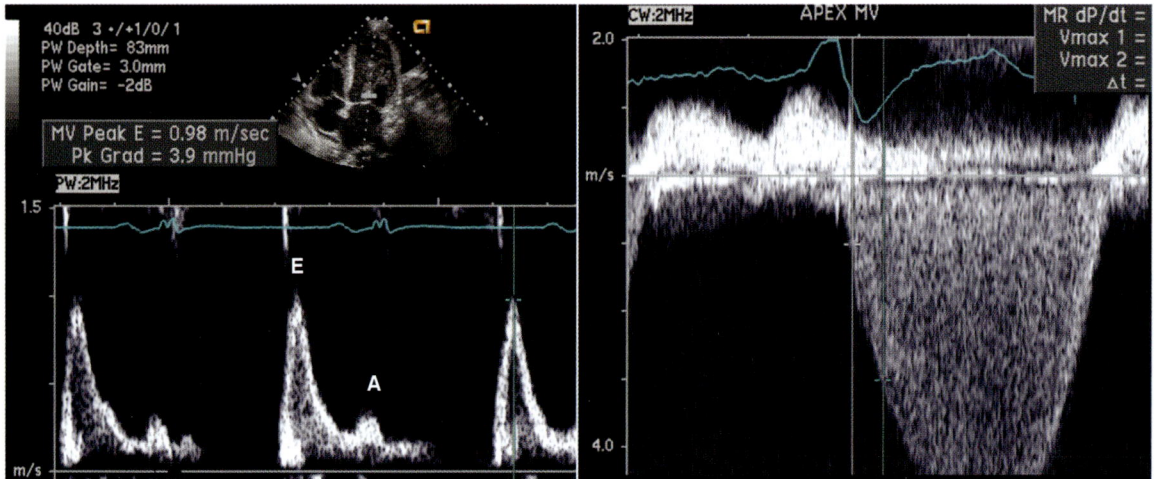

Fig. 9.9 **Doppler findings in dilated cardiomyopathy.** LV diastolic inflow shows a high *E* velocity and low *A* velocity suggestive of "pseudonormalization" due to an elevated end-diastolic pressure *(left)*. The mitral regurgitant *(MR)* jet shows a slow rate of rise in velocity consistent with a reduced *dP/dt* *(right)*.

shift along the pressure-volume curve to a steeper segment. This means that, for a given diastolic pressure-volume relationship, compliance is reduced at higher LV volumes. Thus the expected pattern of diastolic filling in dilated cardiomyopathy is that of reduced compliance: a high E velocity, rapid deceleration slope, low A velocity, and an E/A ratio >1 (Fig. 9.9). When filling pressures are elevated, the E/E' ratio is increased to 15 or higher, and the pulmonary vein *a*-wave velocity and duration are increased. The M-mode finding of a delayed rate of mitral valve closure, termed a "B-bump" or "AC-shoulder" also correlates with an elevated end-diastolic pressure (see Fig. 9.5). However, patterns of diastolic dysfunction can be complex in patients with a dilated cardiomyopathy and vary with volume status, medical therapy, and phase of the disease course.

When significant LV systolic dysfunction is present (ejection fraction <35%), a careful search for apical LV thrombus is indicated, although prevalence is low with current medical therapy (Fig. 9.10). Details on the technical aspects of identifying an LV thrombus are given in Chapter 8.

Limitations and Technical Considerations

Echocardiography rarely can establish the etiology of dilated cardiomyopathy, even though it is instrumental both in confirming the presence of ventricular dysfunction and in providing prognostic data. The accuracy of measures of ventricular volumes and ejection fraction depend on attention to data acquisition and analysis, as discussed in Chapter 6. In addition to the technical aspects in the evaluation of diastolic dysfunction, as

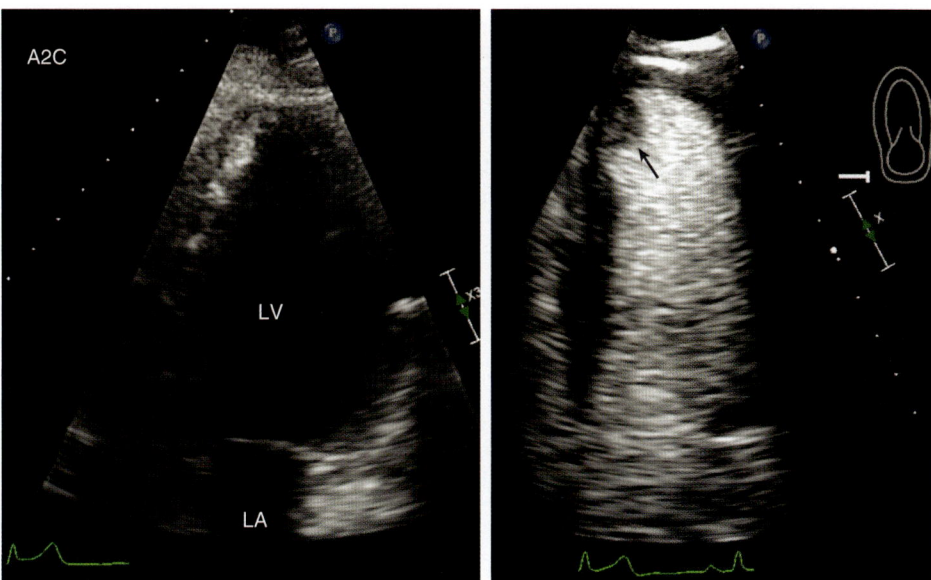

Fig. 9.10 Left ventricular apical thrombus. In the apical two-chamber *(A2C)* view *(left)* ▶ in a patient with dilated cardiomyopathy, endocardial definition is poor, but no obvious LV mass is noted. With left-sided contrast to opacify the LV, a nonopacified apical mass consistent with thrombus *(arrow)* is seen. The use of left-sided echo contrast *(right)* ▶ improves sensitivity for detection of thrombus by enhancing the blood-thrombus border.

discussed in Chapter 7, diastolic function and systolic function are inseparable parts of cardiac performance. Isolating the effects of diastolic dysfunction from the altered loading conditions related to systolic dysfunction can be problematic. Most patients have combined systolic and diastolic dysfunction, with both contributing to clinical symptoms and outcomes.

Clinical Utility

Echocardiography plays a key role in the evaluation and management of patients with heart failure. The correlation between echocardiographic findings and specific causes of heart failure is shown in Table 9.2. If echocardiography shows no significant impairment of LV systolic dysfunction, other possible diagnoses includes

- Coronary artery disease
- Valve disease
- Hypertensive heart disease
- Pericardial disease
- Pulmonary heart disease

Whenever the clinical presentation suggests heart failure, a comprehensive examination of systolic and diastolic function is needed, even when the core echocardiographic examination does not show obvious evidence of dysfunction. If the echocardiogram is consistent with the clinical diagnosis of dilated cardiomyopathy, detailed information on ventricular function, chamber sizes, associated valvular disease, and pulmonary artery pressures should be obtained.

Periodic echocardiography is essential for optimal care of patients with dilated cardiomyopathy. The detailed assessment available by echocardiography aids in the appropriate tailoring of medical therapy. In addition, repeat echocardiography is helpful when a change in clinical status suggests an interval change in ventricular function. Myocardial dyssynchrony can be evaluated by tissue Doppler and speckle tracking techniques (Fig. 9.11) although the role of this information in clinical practice not well established.

In patients with dilated cardiomyopathy in the intensive care unit, echocardiographic evaluation can be helpful in to assess LV function, pulmonary artery pressures, and the degree of coexisting mitral regurgitation and to estimate LV filling pressure. Evaluation of an individual patient's response to afterload reduction therapy can be performed by repeat ejection fraction measurements or by sequential noninvasive measurements of pulmonary pressures and cardiac output (Fig. 9.12).

Alternate Approaches

Evaluation of a patient with new-onset heart failure typically includes a careful clinical evaluation and laboratory data. In many patients with dilated cardiomyopathy, an exact etiology cannot be identified, even when all diagnostic modalities are used. Cardiac magnetic resonance imaging provides evaluation of myocardial fibrosis and inflammation. The possibility of an ischemic cause of LV systolic dysfunction relies on visualization of coronary anatomy by computed tomography or at cardiac catheterization. If exact

TABLE 9.2 Cardiomyopathies: Clinical Echocardiographic Correlation

Cardiomyopathy	Pathophysiology	Clinical Presentation	Echocardiographic Findings
Dilated			
Idiopathic	Primary myocardial dysfunction of unknown cause	• Heart failure signs and symptoms	• Dilation of all four chambers with RV and LV systolic dysfunction • Secondary mitral regurgitation occurs in some patients, but valve leaflets are normal. • LV thrombus can occur with severe LV dysfunction. • Elevated LV filling pressures with variable elevation in PA pressures
Familial	Inherited primary myocardial dysfunction	• Heart failure signs and symptoms	• Dilation of all four chambers with RV and LV systolic dysfunction • Secondary mitral regurgitation may be present, but valve leaflets are normal. • LV thrombus can occur with severe LV dysfunction. • Elevated LV filling pressures with variable elevation in PA pressures
Chagas	Protozoan infection, due to *Trypanosoma cruzi*, that affects the heart, esophagus, and colon	• Acute phase is characterized by fever, myalgias, hepatosplenomegaly, and myocarditis. • Chronic Chagas heart disease has a high mortality rate (44% at 4 years) due to sudden death (55%–65%), heart failure (25%–30%), and stroke (10%–15%).	• LV dilation and systolic dysfunction, ranging from mild to severe • Wall motion may be regional but not in a pattern consistent with coronary artery disease. • Apical abnormalities are common with apical aneurysm in about 5% of asymptomatic patients and about 55% of those with heart failure.
Duchenne MD	Inherited myopathic disorder that affects both skeletal and cardiac muscle	• Patients often have asymptomatic LV dysfunction, likely due to limited physical activity. • Late in disease, heart failure and arrhythmias are seen.	• Echocardiography is consistent with dilated cardiomyopathy.
Hypertrophic			
Hypertrophic	Inherited autosomal-dominant myocardial disease	• Wide age range of clinical presentation • Often diagnosed in asymptomatic patients on screening echo • Manifests with symptoms of heart failure and angina or as sudden death with no previous diagnosis	• Asymmetric LV hypertrophy with normal systolic function but abnormal diastolic function • About one third have resting dynamic outflow obstruction, and one third have a provoked gradient with exercise.
Fabry	Inherited X-linked glycolipid storage disease, now recognized in women as well as men	• Manifests in boys younger age 10 years with skin and neurologic findings • Manifests in women later in life with unexplained LV hypertrophy • Diagnosis based on plasma alpha-galactosidase A activity • Conduction system abnormalities and arrhythmias are common.	• LV hypertrophy may be asymmetric but in an atypical pattern for HCM. • An endocardial hyperechoic layer is typical of Fabry heart disease. • About 50% have aortic and mitral valve thickening and mild regurgitation.

TABLE 9.2 Cardiomyopathies: Clinical Echocardiographic Correlation—cont'd

Cardiomyopathy	Pathophysiology	Clinical Presentation	Echocardiographic Findings
Restrictive			
Amyloid	Extracellular tissue deposition of serum protein subunit fibrils—cardiac involvement in 50% of primary AL amyloidosis (monoclonal light chains) cases but only 5% with secondary AA amyloidosis	• Conduction system disease • Myocardial involvement	• Increased LV and RV wall thickness with increased myocardial echogenicity, but "sparkling" appearance is not specific or sensitive for diagnosis • Progressive diastolic dysfunction • Valve thickening • Intracardiac thrombus
Sarcoidosis	Systemic disease with pulmonary involvement in most patients Subclinical cardiac involvement in up to 20% of patients	• Cardiac involvement most often results in conduction system abnormalities, ventricular arrhythmias, or heart failure.	• Nonspecific • Regional wall motion abnormalities in a non–coronary disease pattern • LV systolic and diastolic dysfunction
Other			
Isolated LV noncompaction	Rare, primary genetic cardiomyopathy	• Clinical presentation with heart failure, angina, arrhythmias, and thromboembolic events	• Deep ventricular trabeculations, particularly in the inferior and lateral walls • Color Doppler shows communication between the intertrabecular recesses and LV chamber. • Ejection fraction may be reduced. • Ratio of noncompacted to compacted myocardium >2:1 at end-systole in short-axis view
Tako-tsubo (Stress-induced cardiomyopathy)	Catecholamine-induced acute myocardial dysfunction	• Sudden onset of chest pain, dyspnea, electrocardiogram changes, and elevated cardiac enzymes with normal coronary arteries • Occurs in the setting of intense emotional or physical stress or with an acute medical illness • More than 80% of patient are women, typically age 50–75 years.	• Apical dilation and systolic dysfunction resulting in a significant reduction in LV ejection fraction • A pattern of regional myocardial dysfunction is atypical for coronary disease. • LV systolic function typically returns to normal in 1 to 4 weeks, although recurrences have been reported.
Arrhythmogenic RV cardiomyopathy	Familial inheritance occurs in at least 30%, most often in an autosomal dominant pattern. Autosomal recessive inheritance also has been described.	• Manifests with sudden cardiac death or ventricular arrhythmias	• RV dilation and systolic dysfunction • Echo findings are nonspecific; diagnosis depends on magnetic resonance imaging and electrophysiologic evaluation.

HCM, Hypertrophic cardiomyopathy; *MD*, muscular dystrophy; *PA*, pulmonary artery.

Fig. 9.11 Dyssynchrony on speckle tracing strain. (A) In the apical four-chamber view, speckle tracking strain shows marked dyssynchrony with wide separation in the strain curves for each myocardial segment on the graph of strain versus time. (B) A bulls-eye view of the strain pattern shows normal apical strain with basal and mid-ventricular reductions in strain. This pattern is typical of amyloid heart disease. *ANT*, Anterior; *EDV*, end-diastolic volume; *EF*, ejection fraction; *ESV*, end-systolic volume; *HR*, heart rate; *INF*, inferior; *L. strain*, longitudinal strain; *LAT*, lateral; *SEPT*, septum.

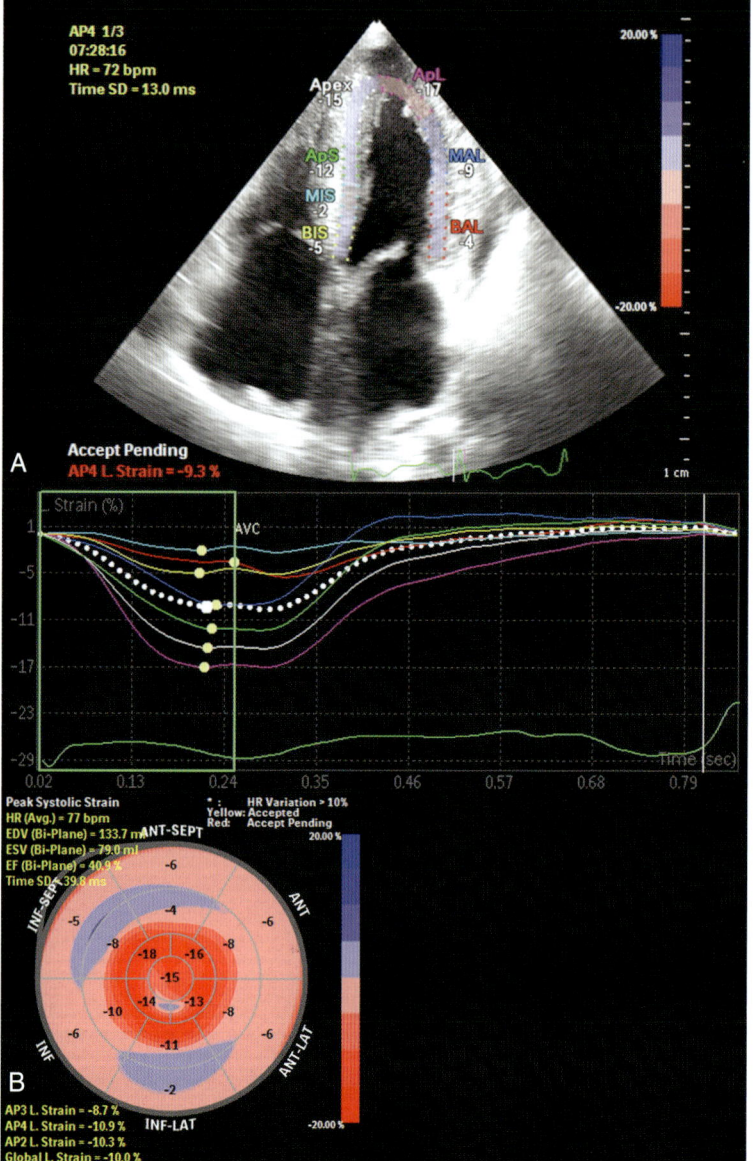

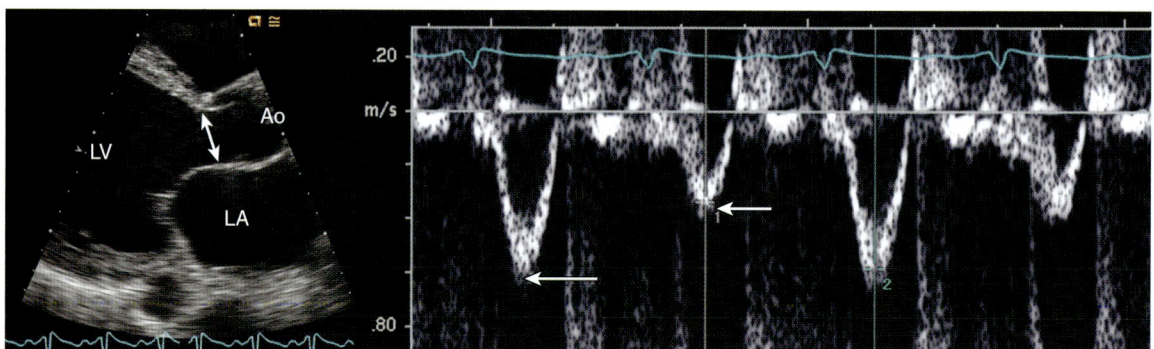

Fig. 9.12 Stroke volume calculation in a patient with dilated cardiomyopathy. LV outflow tract diameter is measured from a parasternal long-axis view *(left)* for calculation of a circular cross-sectional area (CSA), and the LV outflow tract velocity-time integral (VTI) is recorded just proximal to the aortic valve from an apical approach using a pulsed Doppler sample volume length of 5 to 10 mm *(right)*. Stroke volume is calculated as VTI ×CSA. Cardiac output is stroke volume multiplied by heart rate. Calculation of stroke volume in this patient is complicated by mechanical alternans related to severe systolic dysfunction with marked variation in the outflow velocity *(arrows)* on alternating beats despite normal sinus rhythm. *Ao*, Aorta.

measurement of pulmonary vascular resistance is needed (e.g., in a heart transplant candidate), cardiac catheterization is indicated because noninvasive approaches provide only an estimate of pulmonary vascular resistance.

HYPERTROPHIC CARDIOMYOPATHY
Basic Principles

Hypertrophic cardiomyopathy is an autosomal dominant inherited disease of the myocardium (with variable penetrance) related to abnormalities in genes coding for contractile proteins. Characteristic anatomic features of this disease (Fig. 9.13) include:

- Asymmetric hypertrophy of the LV
- Normal LV systolic function
- Impaired diastolic LV function
- Dynamic subaortic LV outflow obstruction

Other important clinical features of this disease are a high risk of sudden death (especially during exertion); symptoms of angina, exercise intolerance, and syncope; a high prevalence of atrial fibrillation; and a systolic murmur on cardiac auscultation.

The pattern and degree of LV hypertrophy in patients with hypertrophic cardiomyopathy can be quite variable (Fig. 9.14). The septum often is primarily hypertrophied at the base with a sigmoid shape of the septum, or severe septal hypertrophy can occur, with bulging into the LV chamber. With apical hypertrophic cardiomyopathy severe hypertrophy is confined to the LV apex, sometimes with near obliteration of the LV cavity in systole. The common feature of all these hypertrophy patterns is normal thickness (or "sparing") of the basal posterior LV wall.

Hypertrophic cardiomyopathy is classified as:

- Nonobstructive (about one third of patients) if the outflow gradient at rest and with provocation is <30 mmHg
- Obstructive if the gradient at rest is ≥30 mmHg (>2.7 m/s)
- Provocable or latent if the resting gradient is <30 mmHg but obstruction occurs with exercise (or other maneuvers)

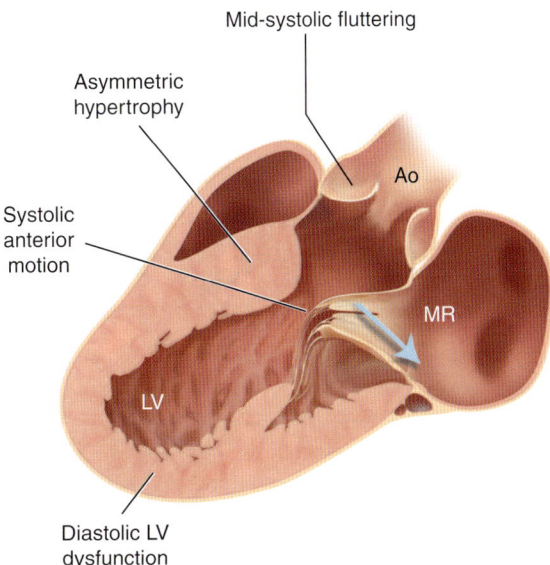

Fig. 9.13 Hypertrophic cardiomyopathy. Typical findings include asymmetric septal hypertrophy with sparing of the basal posterior wall and normal LV systolic function with impaired diastolic function. When dynamic outflow tract obstruction is present, systolic anterior motion of the mitral valve leaflets, mid-systolic closure and coarse fluttering of the aortic valve leaflets, and mitral regurgitation (MR; *blue arrow*) are noted. *Ao,* Aorta.

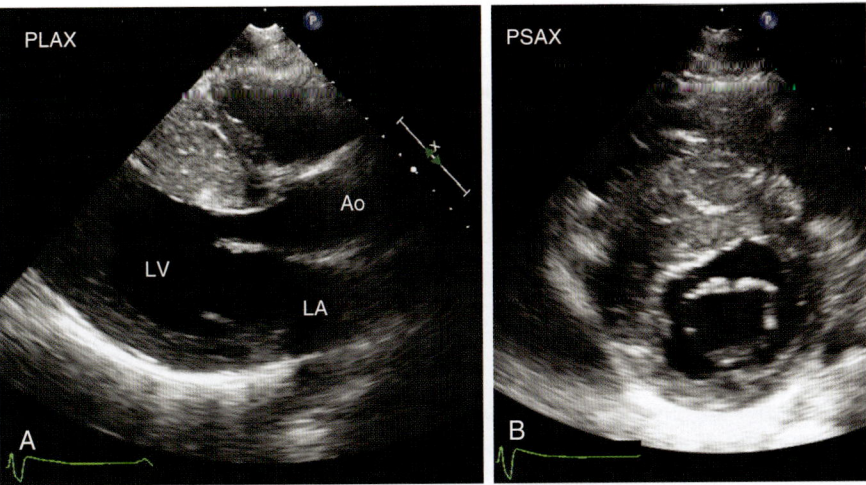

Fig. 9.14 Septal hypertrophy. 2D images of hypertrophic cardiomyopathy in (A) a parasternal long-axis *(PLAX)* view at end-diastole for measurement of septal and posterior wall thickness. The septum is markedly thickened with a normal thickness of the basal inferior-lateral (posterior) wall. (B) The parasternal short-axis *(PSAX)* view shows hypertrophy involving the anterior and inferior septum. *Ao,* Aorta.

Fig. 9.15 Dynamic subaortic outflow obstruction. In patients with hypertrophic cardiomyopathy, hemodynamics are characterized by a small gradient in late systole between the LV and aorta *(Ao)* at rest. The CW Doppler curve shows a late-peaking velocity of 2.5 m/s, with the origin of this velocity being the subaortic region. With alterations in loading conditions (decreased preload), the degree of obstruction increases dramatically. A late-peaking, high-velocity (3.5 m/s) Doppler curve now is obtained.

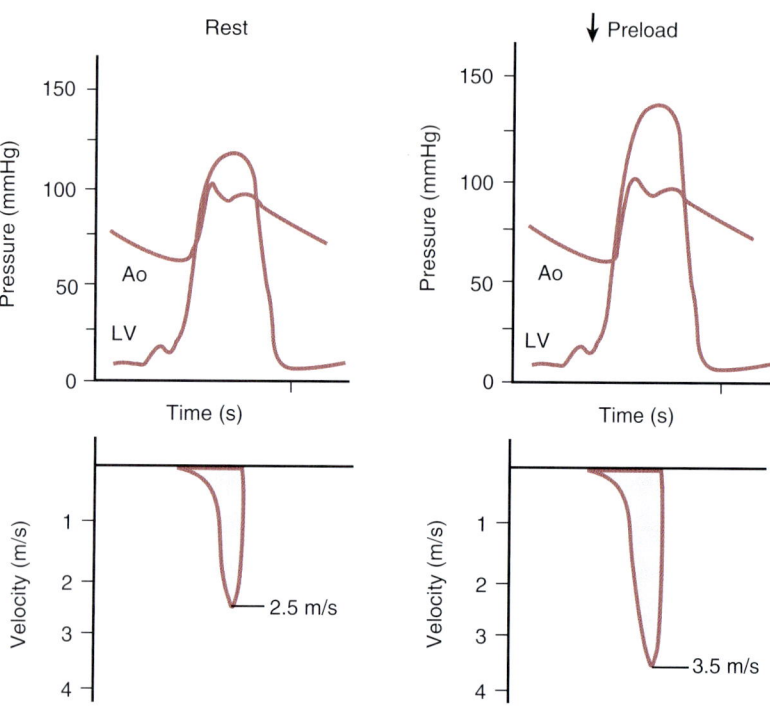

With dynamic obstruction, one sees an increase in flow velocity, and corresponding pressure gradient, proximal to the aortic valve, in association with systolic anterior motion of the mitral valve toward the hypertrophied ventricular septum (Fig. 9.15). Obstruction is dynamic rather than fixed, both in the sense that it occurs only in mid to late systole and in the sense that the presence and severity of obstruction can be altered by loading conditions. These features contrast with the relatively fixed obstruction of aortic valve stenosis, which persists from the onset to the end of ejection and in which the severity of the stenosis is relatively insensitive to changes in loading conditions. Dynamic outflow obstruction in hypertrophic cardiomyopathy typically has a pattern of onset in mid-systole, with the maximum LV to aortic pressure gradient occurring in late systole.

Obstruction can be diminished by maneuvers that increase ventricular volume (e.g., an increase in preload or a decrease in contractility) or by maneuvers that increase afterload. Conversely, the degree of obstruction is increased by:

- Reduced preload
- Increased contractility
- Decreased afterload

Each of these physiologic changes results in a decrease in LV volume and an increase in the degree of dynamic obstruction, with a louder murmur and an increased Doppler velocity.

Dynamic outflow obstruction usually is associated with mitral regurgitation because the systolic anterior motion of the leaflets disrupts normal coaptation. A posteriorly directed mitral regurgitant jet of mild to moderate severity originates at the malcoapted segment of the leaflets (Fig. 9.16).

LV systolic function typically is normal in patients with hypertrophic cardiomyopathy. However, LV diastolic function is abnormal, with impaired relaxation and decreased compliance, thus accounting for many of the heart failure symptoms in patients with hypertrophic cardiomyopathy.

Echocardiographic Approach

Asymmetric Left Ventricular Hypertrophy

Evaluation of the pattern and extent of LV hypertrophy is made from multiple tomographic 2D image planes. In the parasternal long-axis view, particular attention is focused on the posterior basal wall between the papillary muscle and the mitral annulus. Although the wall in this region is not thickened in most patients with hypertrophic cardiomyopathy, it is thickened in patients with concentric hypertrophy due to other etiologies (e.g., hypertension, infiltrative cardiomyopathy). 2D guided M-mode tracings are used for the measurement of septal and posterior wall thickness, by using both long- and short-axis views to ensure that the measurements are perpendicular to the LV wall and to avoid inclusion of RV trabeculation in the septal wall thickness. Careful measurements of diastolic septal thickness provide prognostic information (e.g., risk of sudden death) and are essential for decision making about septal reduction procedures.

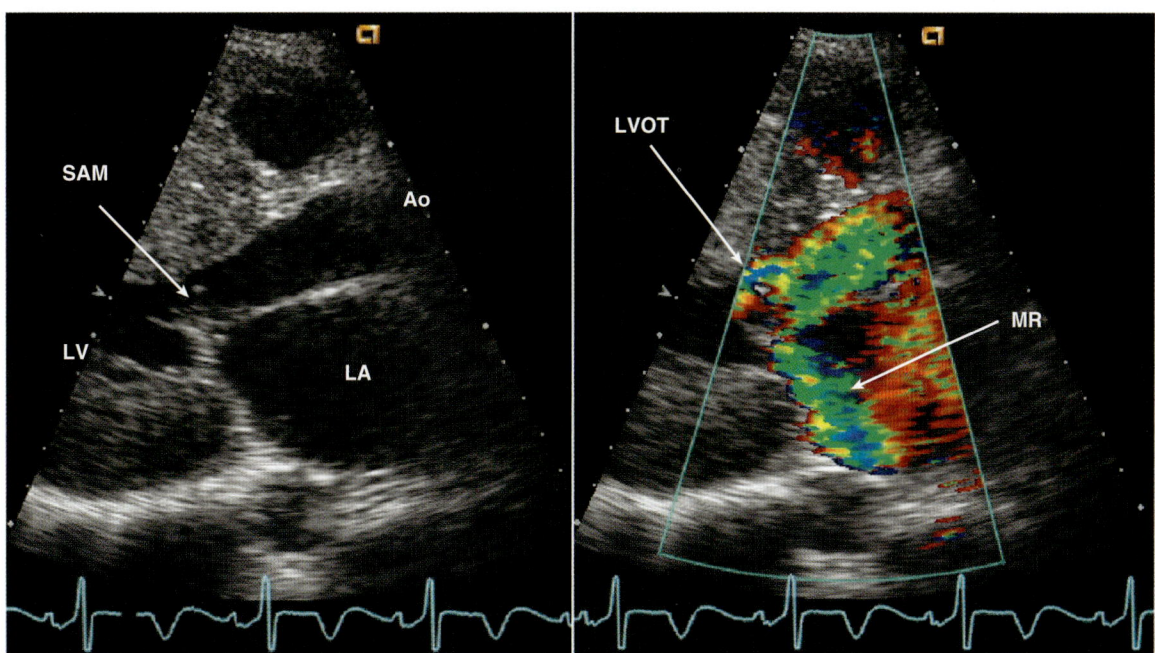

Fig. 9.16 **Mitral systolic anterior motion and mitral regurgitation in hypertrophic cardiomyopathy.** In this parasternal long-axis 2D image *(left)* and color flow image *(right)*, systolic anterior motion *(SAM)* and mitral regurgitation *(MR)* are seen. The posteriorly directed MR jet originates from malcoaptation of a mitral leaflet segment in association with systolic anterior motion. Turbulence in the LV outflow tract *(LVOT)* is seen because of subaortic dynamic obstruction. *Ao,* Aorta.

The parasternal long-axis view also offers the best opportunity to define the exact relationship between the pattern of septal hypertrophy and the outflow tract. This is important when a surgical approach, such as septal myectomy, is being considered because surgical visualization usually is retrograde across the aortic valve, thereby allowing only limited direct inspection of the septal endocardium and little information on the extent of septal thickening or the degree of septal curvature. The extent and pattern of hypertrophy also are relevant if alcohol septal ablation is being considered. Parasternal short-axis views from base to apex allow assessment of the medial to lateral extent of the hypertrophic process.

It is important to recognize that some degree of bulging of the septum into the LV outflow tract, often called a septal "knuckle," is seen in normal older individuals. This apparent septal prominence most likely is due to increased tortuosity of the aorta that results in a more acute angle between the basal septum and aortic root. Most patients with this anatomy do not have convincing clinical features of hypertrophic cardiomyopathy.

Apical views are essential for complete visualization of the pattern and extent of hypertrophy. Diagnosis of apical hypertrophy can be difficult because endocardial definition may be poor, and the endocardial surface (which is located up to one third the distance from the apical epicardium to the base) is missed if image quality is suboptimal (Fig. 9.17). In some cases, the

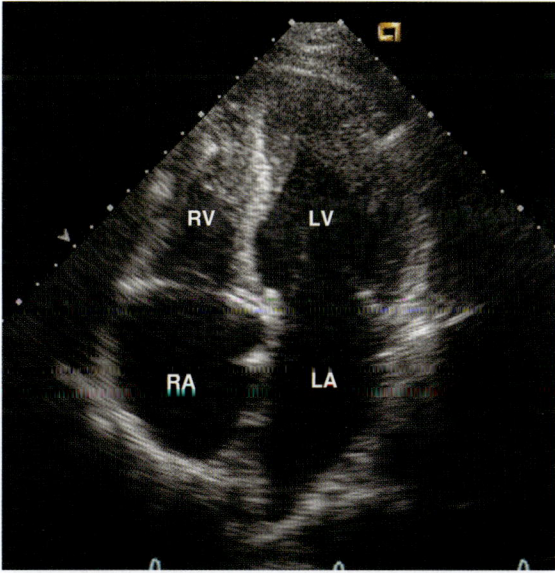

Fig. 9.17 **Apical hypertrophic cardiomyopathy.** Marked thickening of the apical segments is noted in the apical four-chamber view.

epicardium is mistaken for the apical endocardium. A careful examination, when the referring physician has alerted the echocardiographer to this possible diagnosis, avoids this potential pitfall. Color or pulsed Doppler examination is helpful in demonstrating the absence of blood flow in the "apical" region, which is occupied by the hypertrophied myocardium. If needed, echo contrast can be used to define the endocardial border more clearly. Qualitative and quantitative evaluations of LV systolic function are performed using standard approaches (see Chapter 6).

Left Ventricular Diastolic Function

Patients with hypertrophic cardiomyopathy often have a pattern of LV diastolic filling consistent with impaired relaxation. Typical changes include a reduced E velocity, enhanced A velocity, and increased duration and velocity of the pulmonary vein a-reversal. These findings are consistent with impaired diastolic relaxation and an elevated LV end-diastolic pressure. However, the evaluation of diastolic dysfunction in patients with hypertrophic cardiomyopathy is problematic because of the numerous confounding factors in these patients. Many of the parameters validated in other patient groups are not accurate in patients with hypertrophic cardiomyopathy, including only a modest correlation between E/E' and LV filling pressures.

Dynamic Subaortic LV Outflow Tract Obstruction

In about 70% of patients with hypertrophic cardiomyopathy, subaortic obstruction is present, at rest or with exercise, and characterized by:

❐ Systolic anterior motion of the mitral leaflet
❐ Mid-systolic closure of the aortic valve
❐ Late-peaking, high-velocity flow in the outflow tract
❐ Variability in the severity of obstruction with maneuvers:
  ■ Post-premature ventricular contraction beats
  ■ Valsalva maneuver
  ■ Exercise

IMAGING. In a patient with dynamic LV outflow tract obstruction, long-axis images show the classic finding of systolic anterior motion of the mitral valve with apposition of the mitral leaflet and septum in mid to late systole. M-mode recordings are helpful in that, with pathologic systolic anterior motion, the rate of anterior leaflet motion is more rapid than the anterior motion of the posterior wall in systole (Fig. 9.18). A "contact lesion" on the ventricular septum at the site of mitral leaflet impingement is seen in some patients.

Short-axis views also show the systolic anterior motion of the mitral valve leaflets. Frame-by-frame analysis shows the cross-sectional area of the outflow tract throughout systole.

Apical 2D views are helpful for demonstrating the abnormal mitral leaflet motion, especially the apical long-axis and the anteriorly angulated four-chamber views. Note that the degree of systolic anterior motion is not always uniform from medial to lateral across the mitral leaflets, so imaging in multiple planes with slight adjustments in transducer angulation are needed to demonstrate the presence and extent of dynamic outflow obstruction.

The aortic valve shows normal leaflet opening in early systole, followed by mid-systolic abrupt partial closure with coarse fluttering of the aortic valve leaflets in late systole due to late systolic dynamic outflow obstruction. Again, these rapid leaflet movements are

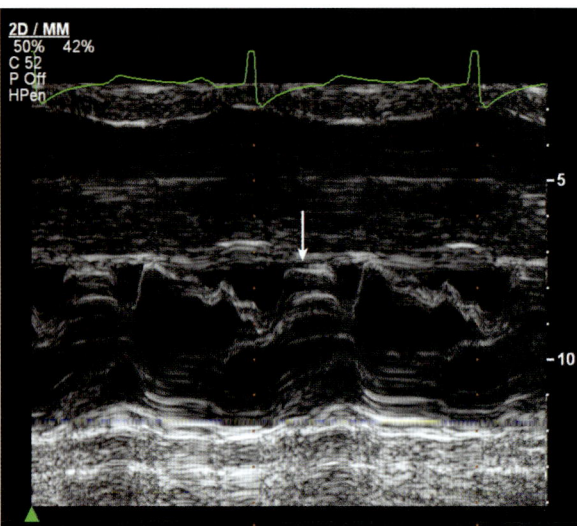
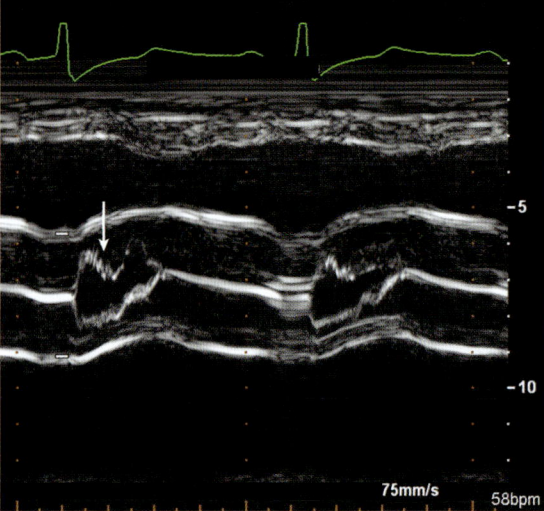

Fig. 9.18 M-mode findings in hypertrophic cardiomyopathy. M-mode at the mitral valve level *(left)* in a patient with dynamic outflow obstruction shows classic septal hypertrophy and systolic anterior motion of the mitral leaflets *(arrows)*. An M-mode view at the aortic valve level *(right)* shows mid-systolic closure of the aortic valve *(arrow)* followed by coarse fluttering of the leaflets.

best documented on M-mode recordings. Often the aortic leaflets themselves are sclerotic because of the long-term effect of a turbulent jet as a result of subaortic obstruction, with some degree of coexisting aortic regurgitation.

DOPPLER EVALUATION. Doppler studies provide a more direct evaluation of the presence, location, and degree of dynamic subaortic obstruction than do imaging techniques. With conventional pulsed or color flow imaging, the site of obstruction is identified based on the location of the poststenotic turbulence. Both parasternal and apical long-axis views are useful for this examination.

Using pulsed Doppler from an apical approach, the sample volume is slowly moved from the apex progressively toward the base, recording the velocity curve at each step. Proximal to the outflow obstruction, velocities are normal. At the site of obstruction, the velocity increases abruptly to a velocity reflecting the degree of obstruction (as stated in the Bernoulli equation). This approach, using stepwise evaluation with pulsed Doppler ultrasound, is advantageous in that intracavity gradients due to apical hypertrophy or apposition of the papillary muscle with the septum will be recognized and not mistaken for subaortic dynamic obstruction.

Continuous-wave (CW) Doppler from an apical approach typically shows a late-peaking, high-velocity systolic jet in patients with a dynamic LV outflow tract obstruction (Fig. 9.19). The shape of this curve is distinctive, corresponding to the temporal course of the LV to aortic pressure gradient (see Fig. 9.15).

LATENT OUTFLOW OBSTRUCTION. Some patients with hypertrophic cardiomyopathy have dynamic outflow obstruction with exercise but not at rest. Traditionally, maneuvers to "provoke" outflow obstruction at rest were performed during the echocardiography examination. A spontaneous premature ventricular contraction (PVC) results in an increased degree of obstruction on the post-PVC beat due to increased LV contractility. The strain phase of the Valsalva maneuver increases obstruction by decreasing preload (smaller LV cavity size), but it is difficult to perform simultaneously with echocardiography because of changes in cardiac position and lung interference as the patient performs the maneuver. In the past, amyl nitrate inhalation was used to induce a brief decrease in preload (venodilation) and decrease in afterload (arterial dilation), both of which increase the degree of obstruction. However, these maneuvers are no longer recommended because of low reproducibly and limited clinical value.

The optimal approach to evaluate for provocable obstruction is a supine bicycle or upright treadmill exercise stress test. CW Doppler outflow velocity recordings are made at rest and immediately after exercise to assess for inducible outflow obstruction, defined as an exercise outflow tract gradient ≥30 mmHg (velocity ≥2.7 m/s) (Fig. 9.20). Pharmacologic stress testing with dobutamine is not recommended because it is nonspecific (mid-cavity obstruction is seen even in normal individuals) and does not provide information on exercise capacity or the relationship of symptoms to exertion.

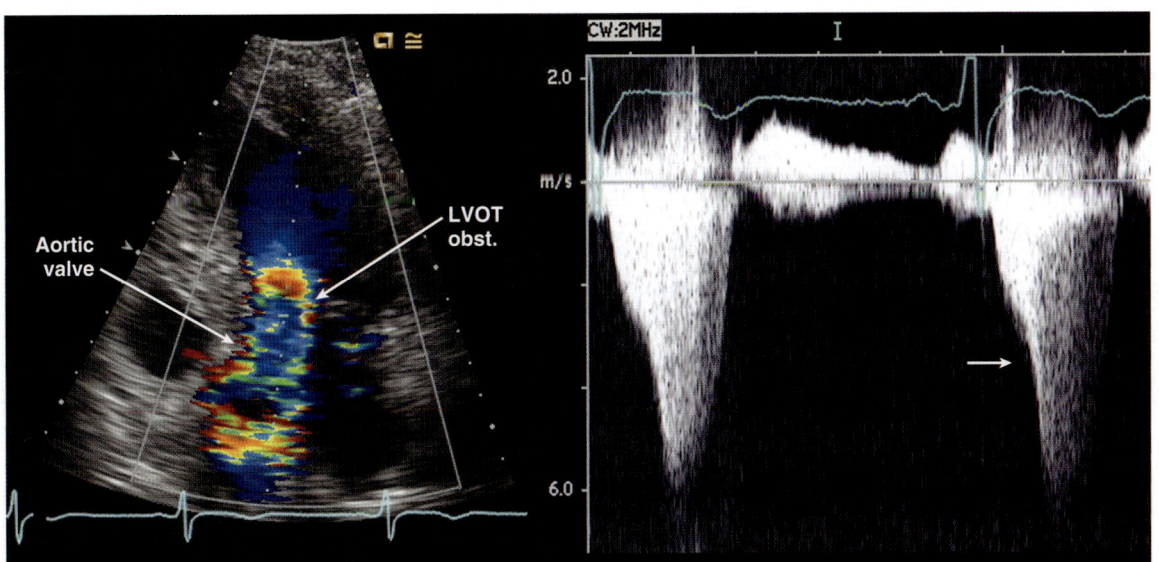

Fig. 9.19 **Dynamic outflow obstruction in hypertrophic cardiomyopathy.** Resting outflow obstruction in this patient with hypertrophic cardiomyopathy was evaluated from the apical view *(left)* with color and pulsed Doppler to localize the level of obstruction. The pulsed Doppler sample volume was moved sequentially from the ventricular cavity toward the aortic valve to identify the site of increased velocity. CW Doppler *(right)* shows the high-velocity, late-peaking *(arrow)* jet typical of dynamic outflow obstruction. *LVOT obstr.,* LV outflow tract obstruction.

Mitral Valve Abnormalities

The mitral valve is anatomically and functionally abnormal in the majority of patients with hypertrophic cardiomyopathy. Anatomically, the leaflets are larger than in normal individuals. Functionally, mitral regurgitation results from systolic anterior motion of the leaflets into the outflow tract that leads to late systolic failure of coaptation and a consequent posteriorly directed regurgitant jet. Mitral regurgitant severity typically is moderate but ranges from mild to severe and varies dynamically with the severity of outflow obstruction. Evaluation of mitral valve anatomy and severity of regurgitation is detailed in Chapter 12.

Limitations and Technical Considerations

When a high-velocity outflow signal is detected with CW Doppler, other techniques are needed to determine the depth of origin of the signal because velocities are measured along the entire length of the ultrasound beam. In some patients with hypertensive heart disease or hypovolemia, the combination of LV hypertrophy and hyperdynamic systolic function results in a late-peaking, high-velocity systolic waveform (Fig. 9.21) similar to that seen in hypertrophic cardiomyopathy. However, in these patients the site of obstruction is not subaortic; it is closer to the apex, at the mid-ventricular level.

The distinction between hypertrophic cardiomyopathy and a hyperdynamic concentrically hypertrophied ventricle can be made by careful attention to the 2D images (sparing of the basal posterior wall in hypertrophic cardiomyopathy) and by evaluating the depth of origin of the high-velocity jet using conventional pulsed, high pulse repetition frequency (HPRF), and color Doppler techniques. The patient's clinical and family histories also are important for making this distinction. Genetic testing is increasingly a routine part of the diagnostic evaluation.

Distinguishing between the signal due to dynamic subaortic obstruction and mitral regurgitation can be challenging because both are common with hypertrophic cardiomyopathy, and both are high-velocity systolic signals directed away from the apex. The two features that are helpful in this distinction are: (1)

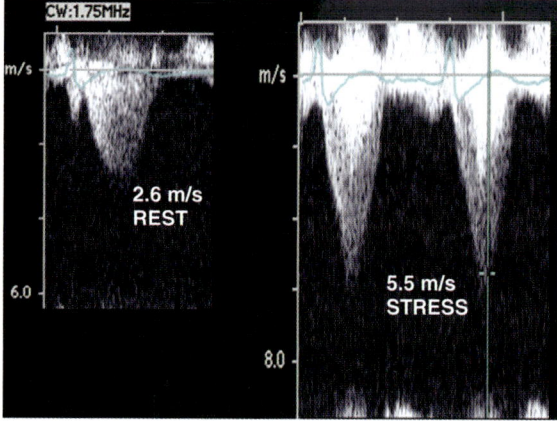

Fig. 9.20 Provoked dynamic outflow obstruction. Supine bicycle stress testing in a 45-year-old man with hypertrophic cardiomyopathy showed an LV outflow tract velocity that peaked in mid-systole at 2.6 m/s during rest *(left)* consistent with no significant obstruction. Peak stress Doppler data *(right)* documented provoked obstruction with a late-peaking LV outflow signal with a maximum velocity of 5.5 m/s. The velocity scale on the baseline and peak Doppler recordings have matched in this example. *(From Owens DS, Otto CM: Exercise testing for structural heart disease. In Gillam L, Otto CM, editors:* Advanced Approaches in Echocardiography: Practical Echocardiography Series, *Philadelphia, 2012, Saunders, Fig. 11-14.)*

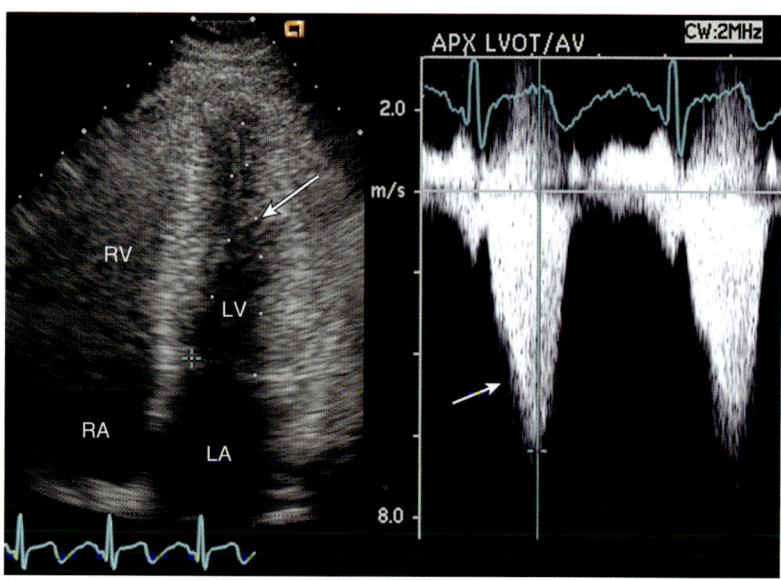

Fig. 9.21 Mid-cavity left ventricular outflow obstruction in hypertensive heart disease. In an apical four-chamber view, mid-cavity obliteration at end-systole *(left)* results in a late-peaking, high-velocity, outflow tract Doppler curve *(right)*. This patient was anemic and febrile at the time of this examination. Hypertensive hyperdynamic mid-cavity obstruction must be distinguished from the dynamic subaortic obstruction seen in hypertrophic cardiomyopathy.

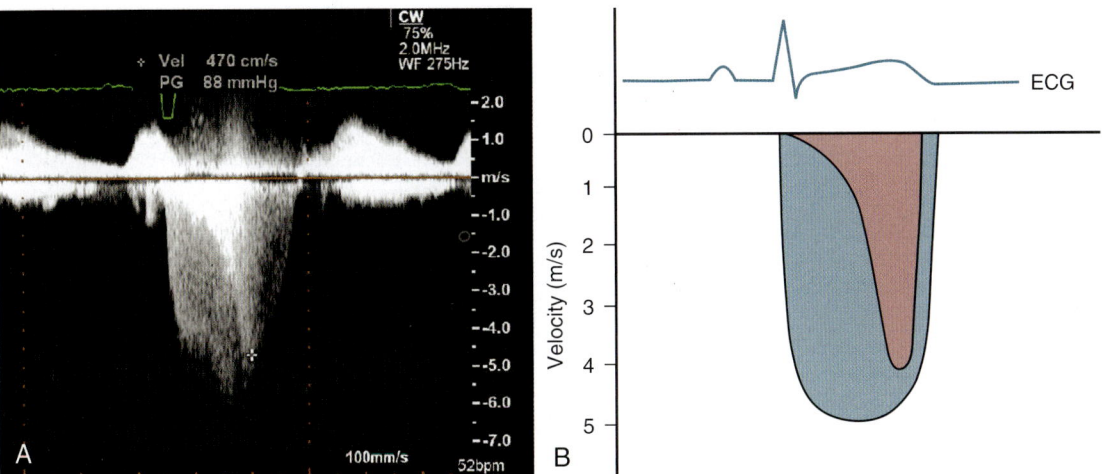

Fig. 9.22 Comparison of continuous-wave Doppler velocity signal for subaortic dynamic outflow obstruction and mitral regurgitation. (A) These signals often are both present and overlap each other and often are difficult to separate. (B) The mitral regurgitation signal *(blue)* starts earlier and ends later in systole, has a high velocity throughout the ejection period, and is higher in velocity than LV outflow. Dynamic subaortic obstruction *(red)* starts later in systole, typically is low in early systole with a peak near end-ejection. *ECG,* Electrocardiogram. *(From Owens DS, Otto CM: Exercise testing for structural heart disease. In Gillam L, Otto CM, editors: Advanced Approaches in Echocardiography: Practical Echocardiography Series, Philadelphia, 2012, Saunders, Fig. 11-15.)*

the shape of the velocity curve (late peaking with subaortic obstruction versus a rapid early systolic rise in velocity with mitral regurgitation) and (2) the timing of flow (mitral regurgitation is longer in duration, starting earlier and ending later in the cardiac cycle) (Fig. 9.22).

Clinical Utility

Diagnosis and Screening

Echocardiography is the procedure of choice for the accurate diagnosis of hypertrophic cardiomyopathy. Because this is an inherited disorder, screening with echocardiography is indicated for all first-degree relatives of the affected individual. This diagnosis significantly affects clinical management even in asymptomatic individuals, given the high risk of sudden death with exertion, and it has important implications for genetic counseling. Doppler diastolic tissue velocities are reduced even in the absence LV hypertrophy and help identify genetically affected family members early in the disease course.

Evaluation of Medical Therapy

In patients with a definite diagnosis of hypertrophic cardiomyopathy, Doppler findings can be used to assess the impact of medical therapy. Specifically, the pattern of LV diastolic filling after the institution of therapy to improve diastolic function (e.g., beta blockers or calcium channel blockers) shows an improvement in early diastolic filling. The degree of dynamic outflow obstruction also may be reduced with medical therapy.

Selection of Patients for Implantable Cardiac Defibrillators

Primary prevention of sudden cardiac death in patients with hypertrophic cardiomyopathy is based on implantable cardiac defibrillator (ICD) placement in patients with a combination of risk factors for sudden death. Definite risk factors are sustained or frequent nonsustained ventricular tachycardia, recurrent unexplained syncope, a family history of sudden death, an abnormal blood pressure response to exercise, and extreme LV hypertrophy (septal diastolic wall thickness >30 mm). Other risk factors include high-risk genetic defects. Outflow obstruction is considered only a minor risk factor for sudden cardiac death.

Monitoring of Alcohol Septal Ablation

Echocardiography plays a key role in patient selection for catheter septal ablation procedures and for monitoring the procedure in the catheterization laboratory. In the patient being considered for alcohol septal ablation or surgical treatment for hypertrophic cardiomyopathy, knowledge of the extent, distribution, and curvature of septal hypertrophy determines the location and size of the muscle segment to be removed or ablated. In the catheterization laboratory, contrast is injected during echocardiographic imaging, with the catheter positioned in a septal coronary branch to show the specific location and extent of the area perfused by that vessel before the delivery of the ablation agent (Fig. 9.23). Baseline and postprocedure Doppler data are used in conjunction with invasive hemodynamics to assess the reduction in outflow

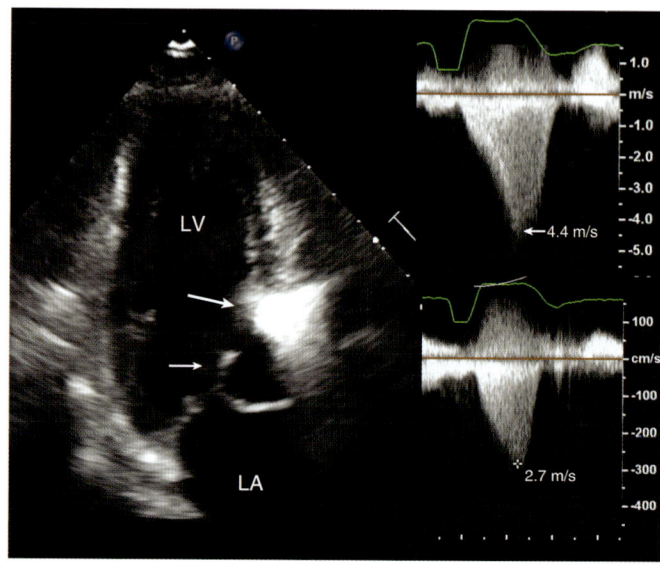

Fig. 9.23 **Catheter septal ablation for hypertrophic cardiomyopathy.** An apical four-chamber view shows contrast in the septum *(arrows)* defining the area perfused by the septal branch that will be injected with the ablation agent. At baseline, Doppler demonstrated severe obstruction with a late-peaking outflow tract velocity of 5 m/s *(top)*. After the septal ablation, the maximum velocity was 1.4 m/s *(bottom)*.

obstruction. After the procedure, sequential echocardiographic studies may show continued improvement in the extent of outflow obstruction due to healing and fibrosis of the infarcted septal myocardium.

Surgical Therapy

Intraoperative monitoring of septal myectomy allows evaluation of the adequacy of the procedure in relieving outflow tract obstruction. Transesophageal echocardiographic (TEE) imaging often provides adequate images of the myectomy site; however, epicardial imaging can be helpful because the septum is located anteriorly relative to the esophagus. Doppler evaluation for residual obstruction following cardiopulmonary bypass should be performed under hemodynamic conditions as similar as possible to the baseline state because the degree of obstruction is influenced by loading conditions. Color flow imaging is helpful in excluding residual obstruction, but when the subaortic flow pattern remains abnormal, quantitative Doppler velocity data are needed. Careful examination for a postoperative ventricular septal defect also should be performed.

It often is difficult to obtain an accurate CW Doppler recording of the degree of outflow obstruction in the operating room because the TEE approach rarely provides a transgastric apical view from which the beam can be aligned parallel to the jet. An epicardial apical position may not be obtainable with a median sternotomy because the transducer often is too large to fit under the ribs at the apex. Placement of a sterile transducer on the ascending aorta with inferior angulation toward the outflow tract allows a parallel intercept angle in some patients (see Chapter 18).

Alternate Approaches

Cardiac magnetic resonance imaging provides an accurate and detailed assessment of the pattern and degree of hypertrophy. Cine images demonstrate systolic anterior motion of the mitral valve and outflow obstruction. Patchy areas of late gadolinium enhancement in the myocardium are supportive of a diagnosis of hypertrophic cardiomyopathy.

In some patients, cardiac catheterization is helpful. First, evaluation of coronary anatomy may be indicated because coexisting epicardial coronary artery disease explains symptoms in some patients with hypertrophic cardiomyopathy. Second, recordings of LV and aortic pressures at rest and after provocative maneuvers to increase or decrease dynamic outflow obstruction and with slow "pullback" across the outflow tract and aortic valve allow more detailed hemodynamic evaluation. This is particularly helpful in the patient with sequential stenoses in the subaortic region and at the aortic valve level. In the operating room, direct LV and aortic pressure measurements after myectomy are helpful if residual obstruction is suspected.

RESTRICTIVE CARDIOMYOPATHY

Basic Principles

Restrictive cardiomyopathy is characterized by heart failure with preserved ejection fraction (HFpEF) and predominant diastolic dysfunction due to a stiff and thickened myocardium (Fig. 9.24). Heart failure is due to the inability to maintain a normal cardiac output or maintenance of a normal cardiac output only with an elevated LV end-diastolic pressure. Thus the initial clinical presentation tends to include signs and symptoms of low cardiac output, including fatigue and decreased exercise tolerance; right heart failure may also be prominent, with peripheral edema and ascites.

As the disease progresses, an individual patient progresses from an anatomic or hemodynamic pattern consistent with restrictive cardiomyopathy to a pattern showing some features of dilated cardiomyopathy, ending with a picture indistinguishable from dilated cardiomyopathy. Compared with dilated cardiomyopathy, restrictive cardiomyopathy is an uncommon diagnosis. Causes of restrictive cardiomyopathy include systemic diseases with accumulation of cells or protein in the myocardial interstitium, storage diseases with accumulation of material within myocardial cells, and processes that affect the endocardium (see Table 9.1).

Echocardiographic Approach

Anatomic Features

Typical echocardiographic features (Fig. 9.25) in the untreated patient with restrictive cardiomyopathy include:

- Nondilated, thick-walled LV
- Normal LV systolic function
- Abnormal LV diastolic function
- RV free wall thickening
- Biatrial enlargement
- Moderate pulmonary hypertension
- Elevated right atrial (RA) pressure (dilated inferior vena cava)

Fig. 9.24 Restrictive cardiomyopathy. Typical features include a thick-walled, small LV with impaired diastolic function, LA and RA enlargement, and signs of secondary pulmonary hypertension, including paradoxical septal motion and a high-velocity tricuspid regurgitant *(TR)* jet.

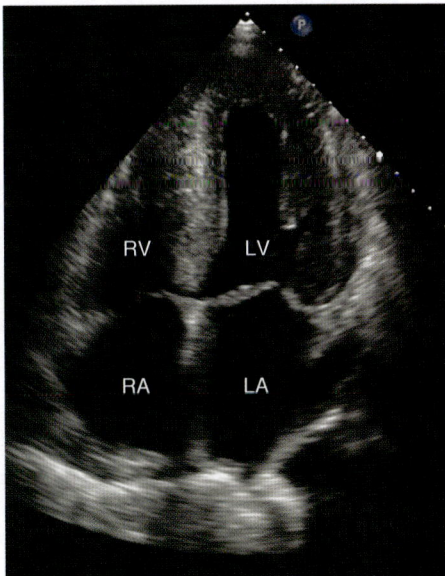
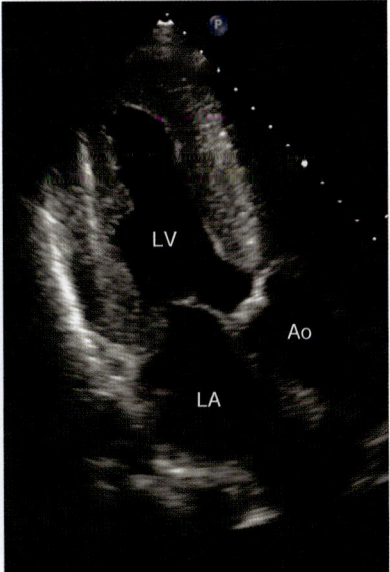

Fig. 9.25 Amyloidosis. Apical four-chamber *(left)* 2D echocardiographic images in a patient with a restrictive cardiomyopathy due to amyloidosis. Biventricular hypertrophy, biatrial enlargement, and both systolic and diastolic dysfunction of the LV are noted. Tissue Doppler imaging *(right)* shows severely reduced diastolic tissue Doppler velocities. *Ao,* Aorta.

Echocardiography usually cannot identify the cause of restrictive cardiomyopathy, but some features support a specific diagnosis (see Table 9.2). The classic "speckled" myocardium of amyloidosis is nonspecific, particularly with harmonic imaging. However, amyloid frequently also affects the valves, the conduction system, and the coronary microvasculature. Hemochromatosis results in conduction disease, in addition to a dilated or restrictive cardiomyopathy. Fabry disease is characterized by symmetric or asymmetric ventricular hypertrophy (which appears similar to hypertrophic cardiomyopathy), conduction defects, and, late in the disease, aortic root dilation. A hyperechoic endocardium helps distinguish Fabry disease from other causes of ventricular hypertrophy (Fig. 9.26). Sarcoidosis often causes conduction defects, and pericardial effusions are common. In hypereosinophilic syndrome, LV thrombus formation occurs in the absence of an underlying wall motion abnormality (particularly in the apex), thus resulting in gradual apical "obliteration" (as seen on angiography) or filling in of the apex with an echogenic mass (on echocardiography). Thrombus formation also occurs under the posterior mitral valve leaflet and leads to adherence of the posterior leaflet to the endocardium and significant mitral regurgitation. Heart disease related to radiation therapy results in a restrictive cardiomyopathy of both the LV and the RV and in accelerated calcific valve disease and coronary atherosclerosis of the segments within the radiation field.

Diastolic Function

The pattern of LV diastolic filling parallels the abnormalities in LV diastolic function in this disease. However, interpretation is complicated both by the numerous confounding factors that affect LV diastolic filling (see Chapter 7) and by temporal changes in diastolic filling as the disease progresses in an individual patient. Early in the disease course, impaired diastolic relaxation of the LV results in impaired early diastolic filling. The Doppler LV inflow curve shows reduced E velocity, increased A velocity, prolonged isovolumic relaxation time, and decreased early diastolic deceleration slope. The mitral annular tissue Doppler signal shows reduced E' and increased A' velocity (Fig. 9.27). The pulmonary vein flow curve shows a reduced diastolic filling phase and normal systolic filling phase, which results in a decreased ratio of systolic to diastolic pulmonary venous flow.

RA filling patterns, recorded in the hepatic vein (or superior vena cava), correspond to physical examination of the neck vein pulsations seen in patients

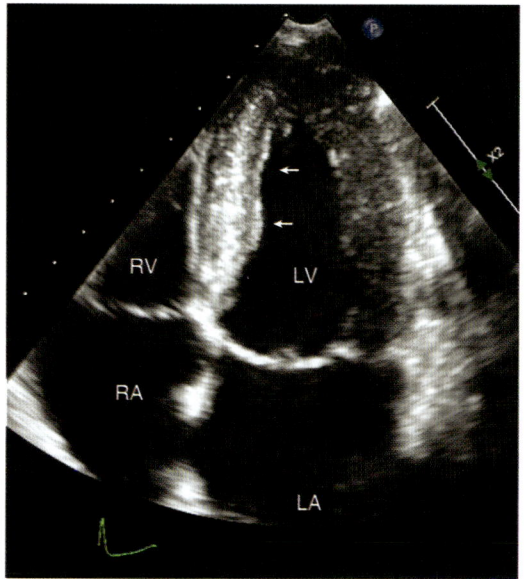

Fig. 9.26 ▶ **Fabry disease.** The apical four-chamber view in this patient with Fabry disease shows increased LV wall thickness with increased echodensity of the endocardium, particularly along the septum *(arrows)*.

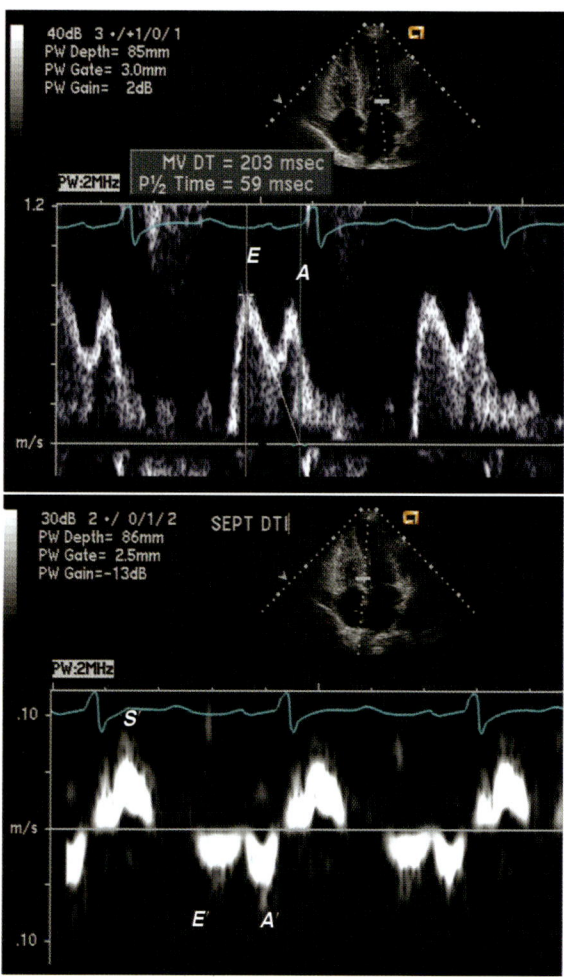

Fig. 9.27 Diastolic function in restrictive cardiomyopathy. LV diastolic filling in a patient with a restrictive cardiomyopathy shows pseudonormalization with an E velocity slightly greater than the A velocity *(top)*. This pattern is distinguished from normal by the tissue Doppler myocardial velocity *(bottom)* showing reduced early motion (E'), compared with the motion after atrial contraction (A').

with restrictive cardiomyopathy. Using this analogy, the hepatic vein flow pattern typically shows:

- A prominent reverse flow phase with atrial contraction (*a*-wave)
- A rapid filling curve in systole (*x*-descent)
- A blunted RA diastolic filling phase (diminished *v*-wave and *y*-descent)

These findings correspond to the pattern of RA pressure recordings at catheterization; the *x*-descent represents the "dip," and the blunted systolic filling phase represents the "plateau" of the dip-and-plateau pattern.

As the disease progresses, LA pressure rises, resulting in an increased pressure gradient from the LA to the LV at mitral valve opening. Along with reduced diastolic compliance of the LV, this increased mitral opening pressure leads to an increased *E* velocity and a rapid deceleration slope. The *A* velocity is reduced because of a combination of increased LV end-diastolic pressure and reduced atrial contractile function. Thus the pattern of diastolic filling in established restrictive cardiomyopathy (which may coincide with the initial clinical presentation) is similar to the "big *E*, little *A*" pattern seen in normal young individuals. However, this "pseudonormal" pattern of LV filling can be distinguished from normal by:

- The rapid early diastolic deceleration time (LV inflow)
- A reduced *E′* velocity (annular tissue velocity)
- An increased PV_a velocity and duration
- The patient's age, clinical presentation, and other associated echocardiographic findings

With a pseudonormal LV inflow pattern, mitral annular velocity shows a marked reduction in *E′* velocity with the ratio of transmitral *E* velocity to annular *E′* velocity corresponding to the elevation in LV end-diastolic pressure. In addition, pulmonary venous inflow in diastole is normal or increased as blood flows in a conduit from the pulmonary veins to LV. With atrial contraction, the increased resistance to LV filling results in an increase in the velocity and duration of the atrial flow reversal into the lower resistance pulmonary veins. Thus pulmonary venous flow shows an increased diastolic phase, a reduced systolic phase, and prominent *a*-wave flow reversal. This is in contrast to the normal pattern of nearly equal systolic and diastolic pulmonary venous inflow curves and a small *a*-wave.

Late in the disease course, a restrictive pattern of LV filling is seen with an increased *E* velocity and reduced *A* velocity, a steep early diastolic deceleration slope, and reduced isovolumic relaxation time.

Limitations and Technical Considerations

Differentiation between restrictive cardiomyopathy and constrictive pericarditis is problematic. Both have a similar clinical presentation, and both are characterized by preserved LV systolic function with impaired diastolic filling. Features that distinguish these two conditions include the patterns of atrial and ventricular diastolic filling, the presence or absence of pericardial thickening, and the degree of associated pulmonary hypertension. However, no single feature is diagnostic of either condition (see Table 10.4).

Attention to technical details is necessary in recording Doppler atrial and ventricular filling patterns, particularly attention to their relationship with the phase of respiration (see Chapter 7). Respiratory variation is assessed most reliably by using a respirometer to mark the onsets of inspiration and expiration. Before recording Doppler signals, 2D and color flow imaging is used to convince the sonographer that no significant respiratory variation exists in the angle between the ultrasound beam and direction of blood flow because respiratory changes in intercept angle could result in apparent changes in velocity, even under constant-flow conditions, due to the erroneous assumption that cosine θ remains 1 in the Doppler equation.

Clinical Utility

In a patient with symptoms of heart failure, a diagnosis of restrictive cardiomyopathy often is not suspected on clinical grounds. In some cases, echocardiographic findings may provide the first clues pointing toward this diagnostic possibility. In a patient with known restrictive cardiomyopathy, echocardiography can be used to follow disease progression. A meticulous examination with careful attention to technical details and with integration of imaging, Doppler, and clinical data allows differentiation between restrictive cardiomyopathy and constrictive pericarditis.

Alternate Approaches

Clinical history and laboratory tests are important in determining the cause of restrictive cardiomyopathy. Diagnostic evaluation also includes cardiac catheterization with measurement of intracardiac pressures at rest and with volume loading. Endomyocardial biopsy can be diagnostic, although sensitivity is low because of nonhomogeneous myocardial involvement in many of these conditions. Biopsy of noncardiac tissue may be diagnostic for amyloidosis. Chest computed tomographic imaging can exclude pericardial calcification or thickening. Cardiac magnetic resonance imaging can detect myocardial iron overload due to hemochromatosis or patchy late gadolinium enhancement with sarcoidosis and can distinguish myocardial involvement due to restrictive cardiomyopathy from constrictive pericarditis.

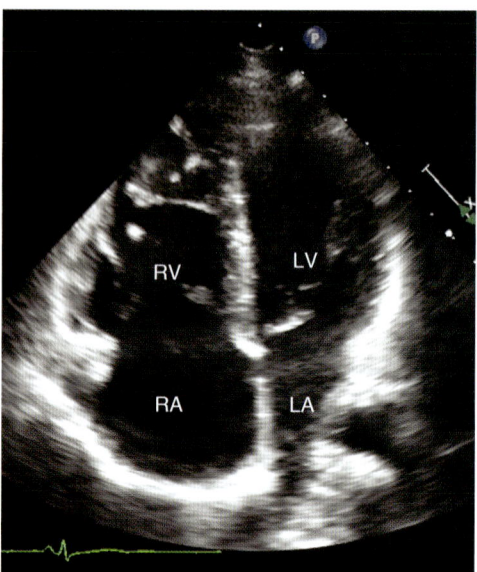

Fig. 9.28 ▶ **Arrhythmogenic right ventricular dysplasia.** In this patient with a history of resuscitated sudden death, the apical four-chamber view shows RV dilation and systolic dysfunction with an abnormal contour of the RV free wall.

OTHER CARDIOMYOPATHIES

Arrhythmogenic Right Ventricular Dysplasia

Arrhythmogenic RV dysplasia (ARVD) is a genetic form of cardiomyopathy that results in fibrofatty replacement of the RV wall and clinical manifestations of RV systolic dysfunction, arrhythmias, and sudden death. Echocardiographic findings include RV dilation and systolic dysfunction in the presence of a relatively normal LV and normal pulmonary pressures (Fig. 9.28). Prominent trabeculation of the RV, increased echogenicity of the moderator band, and small RV aneurysms also may be seen. However, echocardiographic findings are quite variable, and other imaging approaches, such as cardiac magnetic resonance imaging, are more accurate for this diagnosis.

Left Ventricular Noncompaction

Isolated LV noncompaction is a genetic cardiomyopathy characterized by decreased coronary flow reserve and a thickened, prominently trabeculated myocardium with deep recesses that communicate with the ventricular chamber (Fig. 9.29). A similar pattern of ventricular trabeculation is seen with secondary cardiomyopathies due to neuromuscular diseases and other conditions. Features of noncompaction overlap with the clinical presentation of dilated, hypertrophic, and restrictive cardiomyopathy. Noncompaction manifests clinically with heart failure,

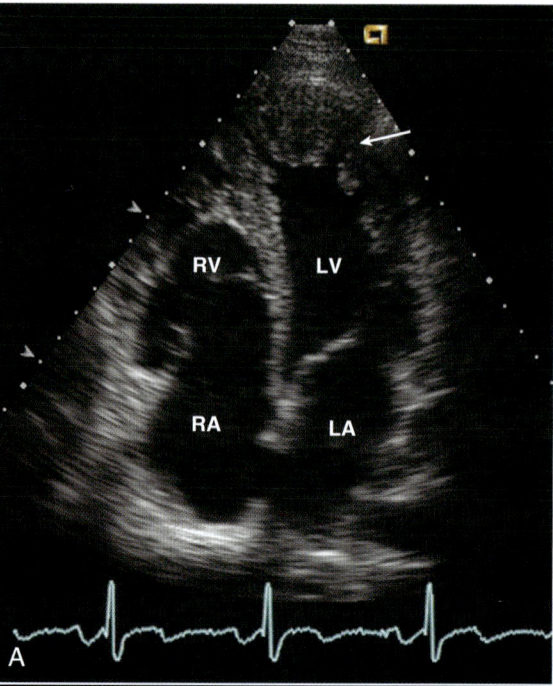

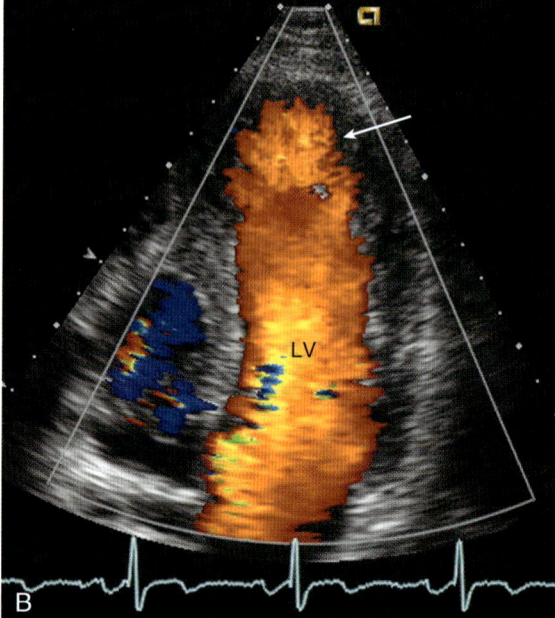

Fig. 9.29 ▶ **Left ventricular noncompaction.** The apical four-chamber view (A) shows the thick LV wall with deep trabecular recesses *(arrows)*. The color flow image (B) shows ventricular flow filling the trabeculated sections of the myocardium.

embolic events, and arrhythmias. Distinguishing echocardiographic features are hypokinesis and myocardial thickening localized to the apex, mid-lateral, and mid-inferior walls; a ratio of the thickness of the noncompacted to compacted myocardium at end-systole ≥2:1; and color Doppler showing flow extending into the trabecular recesses.

ADVANCED HEART FAILURE THERAPIES

Cardiac Resynchronization Therapy

Variability in the timing of myocardial contraction between different LV segments, or dyssynchrony, is evident on 2D imaging in many patients with heart failure; it can be quantitated with 3D wall motion analysis or with tissue Doppler or speckle tracking echocardiography. Dyssynchrony in the timing of RV and LV contraction also can be evaluated using M-mode or spectral Doppler approaches. It is plausible that measurement of mechanical dyssynchrony (rather than electrical dyssynchrony as seen on electrocardiography) should identify which patients might benefit from pacer therapy to resynchronize the pattern of contraction. However, clinical trials do not yet support the use of dyssynchrony measures; instead, resynchronization therapy is recommended in patients with heart failure and significant symptoms, a wide QRS (over 120 ms), and an LV ejection fraction 35% or less.

Left Ventricular Assist Devices

Mechanical support with an LV assist device (LVAD) (Fig. 9.30) can be used to maintain a normal cardiac output in patients with acute heart failure until myocardial recovery occurs or until the patient can receive a heart transplant. An LVAD also is used as destination therapy for long-term support

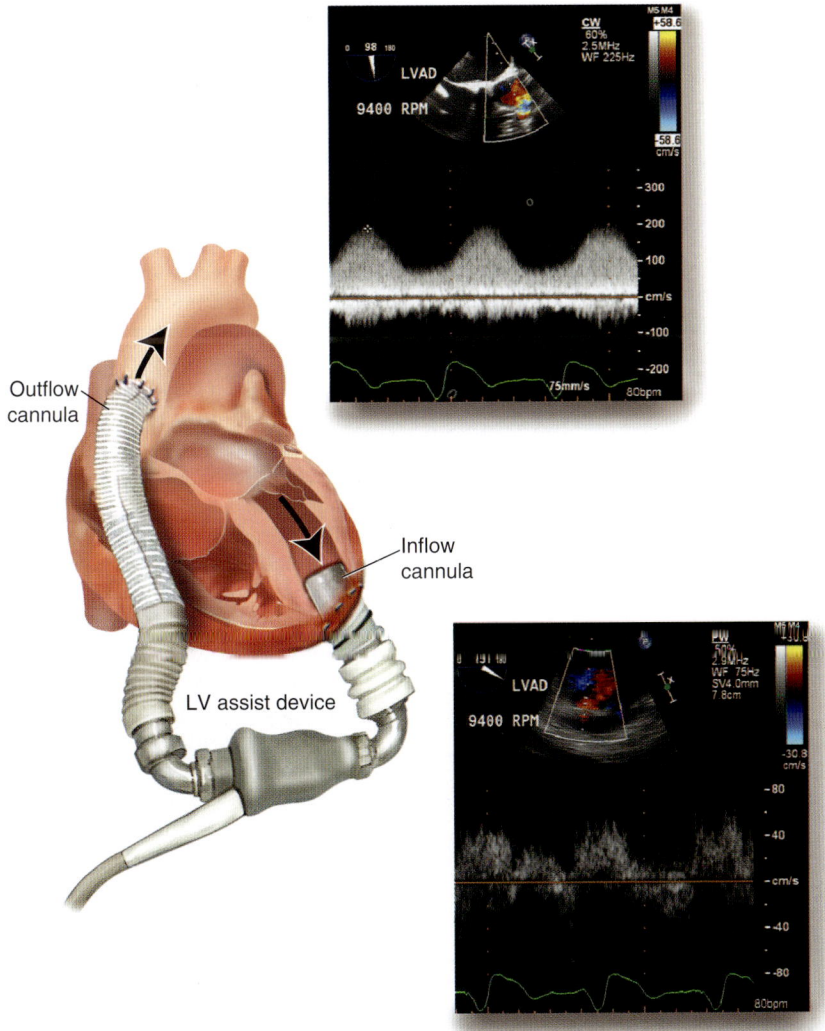

Fig. 9.30 **Left ventricular assist device.** Example of a continuous flow LV assist device with low-velocity inflow recorded from the apical cannula and outflow recorded in the ascending aorta. The aortic valve remains closed throughout systole on most beats with this type of LV assist device.

where recovery or transplantation is not likely to occur. Echocardiographic evaluation of patients with an LVAD is challenging, in part because current devices provide continuous rather than pulsatile flow, with blood intake into the device from a cannula at the LV apex, with blood pumped back into the ascending aorta. Imaging shows severe LV systolic dysfunction. In addition, the aortic valve may remain closed throughout the cardiac cycle because blood is pumped from the LV to the aorta without crossing the valve.

Flow patterns and expected velocity data vary among devices, but changes among studies often are most important in clinical decision making. In addition to standard imaging, as in any patient with heart failure, recommended parameters for echocardiographic evaluation of a patient with an LVAD include:

- Record LVAD type, mode, and pump speed.
- Measure LV dimensions and volumes in standard image planes.
- Record aortic valve motion with M-mode for several cardiac cycles to document aortic valve opening frequency and duration.
- Record LVAD inflow from the apical conduit using color and pulsed Doppler.
- Record LVAD outflow into the ascending aorta with color and pulsed Doppler.

Optimal images of the inflow and outflow cannulas often require oblique nonstandard image plans. Echocardiographic data are used to optimize LVAD flow parameters to avoid underfilling the device, thus causing either low forward flow rates and a dilated ventricle or excessively high flow rates, which can result in cannula obstruction due to a small LV chamber impinging on the inflow cannula orifice. Complications that can be detected include pericardial tamponade (often loculated), RV failure, and thrombus formation.

Total Artificial Heart

Echocardiographic evaluation of patients with a total artificial heart is limited because the pumping chambers of the artificial heart are plastic and do not allow acoustic access. On transthoracic imaging, RA filling pressures can be estimated from the appearance of the inferior vena cava, but other images usually cannot be obtained. On TEE imaging, views are limited to visualization of the RA and LA, along with the atrioventricular mechanical valves.

Cardiac Transplantation

Echocardiographic evaluation of a patient after cardiac transplantation typically is directed toward one of three goals: (1) assessment of cardiac anatomy and physiology prompted by a specific clinical problem, (2) the elusive goal of noninvasive diagnosis of early rejection of the transplanted heart, or (3) diagnosis of post-transplant coronary artery disease.

Cardiac Allograft Structure and Function

Common problems encountered in patients after cardiac transplantation include:

- Pericardial effusion, particularly early postoperatively
- RV systolic dysfunction due to inadequate myocardial preservation at the time of transplantation, persistently elevated pulmonary vascular resistance, or transplant rejection
- LV systolic dysfunction due to inadequate myocardial preservation, acute rejection early after transplantation, or superimposed coronary artery disease at a longer interval after transplantation

Primary valvular disease, of course, is uncommon because of screening of donor hearts before transplantation. However, mitral or tricuspid regurgitation secondary to ventricular dysfunction and annular dilation also is seen. Diastolic dysfunction is an early marker of rejection.

Typically, RV and LV size, wall thickness, and systolic function are normal in the absence of perioperative complications or rejection. However, abnormal septal motion, with anterior motion of the septum in systole with a slight decrease in the extent of systolic thickening of the septal myocardium, is the norm. Valvular anatomy and function are normal, with small amounts of mitral, tricuspid, and pulmonic regurgitation present with a prevalence similar to that in normal individuals. The suture lines in the aorta and pulmonary artery often are difficult to appreciate depending on the distance of the suture lines from the valve planes and the type of surgical procedure. A small pericardial effusion is seen early in the postoperative period but rarely persists beyond a few weeks. Pericardial effusions often are loculated because of postoperative pericardial adhesions, so examination in multiple tomographic planes from parasternal, apical, and subcostal windows is essential when this diagnosis is suspected. Some degree of persistent pulmonary hypertension may be present, as calculated from the velocity in the tricuspid regurgitant jet and estimates of RA pressure.

If the surgical approach included anastomoses of the normal and donor atrium, a normal echocardiogram after cardiac transplantation will show biatrial enlargement (Fig. 9.31), with a variably prominent ridge between the donor and recipient portions of both the RA and LA. The atrial suture line should not be mistaken for an abnormal atrial mass. When transplantation is performed with anastomosis of the superior and inferior vena cavae for the RA and a

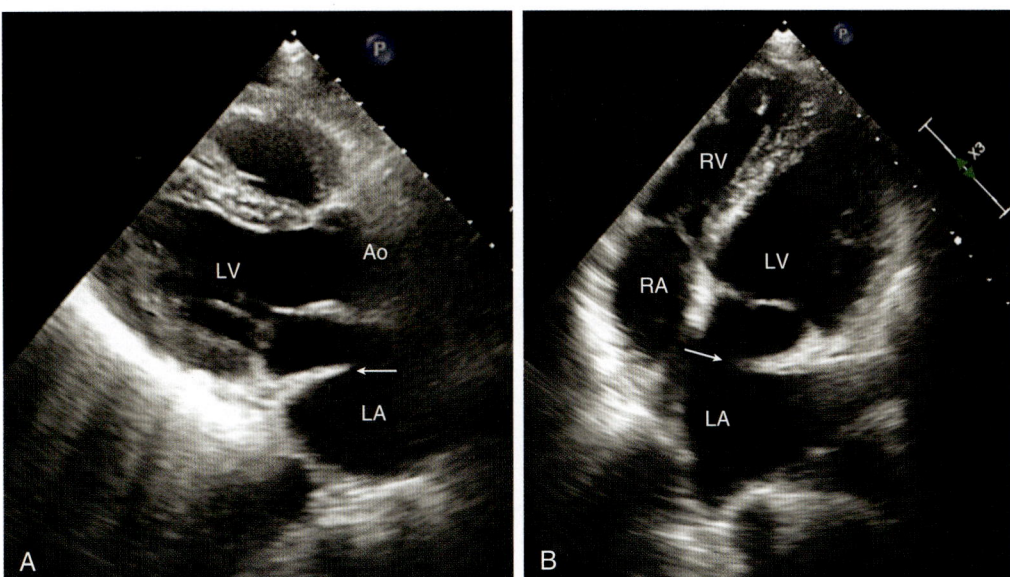

Fig. 9.31 Post–heart transplant image. Example of a heart transplant with a prominent anastomosis *(arrow)* between the severely dilated native LA and normal-size donor LA in a parasternal long-axis view (A) ▶ and an apical four-chamber view (B) ▶. Typically the residual native atrial size is smaller, with a less obvious bulge at the anastomosis. *Ao,* Aorta.

cuff of tissue with the pulmonary veins for the LA, little atrial enlargement occurs, and suture lines are less evident.

Acute Transplant Rejection

With acute, severe rejection, echocardiography shows increased LV mass, decreased systolic function, and an increase in the echogenicity of the myocardium. However, with mild or early rejection, echocardiographic changes are subtle and are not accurate or reproducible enough to allow adjustment of immunosuppressive medications in individual patients. Instead, proposed approaches to the diagnosis of early rejection have focused on measures of diastolic function, specifically measures of early diastolic relaxation. The Doppler changes in acute rejection include:

- Decreased pressure half-time (increased early diastolic deceleration slope)
- Decreased isovolumetric relaxation time
- Increased E velocity

Compared with the patient's own baseline study, a significant change (defined as >20% for E velocity and >15% for pressure half-time or isovolumic relaxation time) is consistent with rejection. Tissue Doppler measures are sensitive but not specific for the detection of rejection. In addition, many post-transplant patients have resting tachycardia, with E/A fusion, due to cardiac denervation. Some transplant centers have found these measures clinically useful, but most centers continue to rely on endomyocardial biopsy.

Post-Transplant Monitoring

As survival after cardiac transplantation has improved, increasing numbers of patients are seen with post-transplant coronary artery disease. Transplant coronary disease differs from typical atherosclerosis in that both epicardial vessels and the microvasculature are diffusely involved with an accelerated form of intimal hyperplasia. Echocardiographic exercise stress testing has a higher prevalence of false-negative results because of the diffuse disease process masking regional wall motion abnormalities. Dobutamine stress echocardiography is more accurate in this patient population and now is routine at many transplant centers. However, coronary angiography is needed for a definitive diagnosis, often with concurrent intravascular ultrasound examination of the coronary arteries.

Limitations, Technical Considerations, and Alternate Approaches

The standard method for the evaluation of transplant rejection remains transvenous endomyocardial biopsy. Some centers use echocardiographic (rather than fluoroscopic) guidance for this procedure. Because echocardiographic images are tomographic, any segment of the biopsy catheter going through the image plane will appear to be the "tip." Thus it is crucial to identify the open forceps at the tip for correct identification of the biopsy site. A subcostal window often is most practical because, with the patient supine, clear views of the RV and septum are obtained, and the sonographer is clear of the sterile field (usually the right internal jugular vein approach is used). In some cases, the apical views also are helpful.

HYPERTENSIVE HEART DISEASE

Basic Principles

Hypertensive heart disease is an end-organ consequence of systemic hypertension. Chronic systemic pressure overload results in LV hypertrophy to maintain normal wall stress. Initially diastolic function is impaired, whereas systolic function remains normal. With long-standing hypertension, systolic dysfunction and ventricular dilation can occur. Typical echocardiographic findings associated with chronic hypertension include:

- LV hypertrophy
- Diastolic dysfunction
- Ascending aortic dilation
- Aortic valve sclerosis
- Mitral annular calcification
- LA enlargement
- Atrial fibrillation

Echocardiographic Approach

Ventricular Hypertrophy

Standard imaging views demonstrate concentric LV hypertrophy with increased wall thickness and a nondilated chamber (Fig. 9.32). In contrast to hypertrophic cardiomyopathy, the pattern of hypertrophy is generally symmetric, including involvement of the basal posterior wall with an increased end-diastolic wall thickness (>11 mm). LV mass can be estimated from M-mode data, assuming hypertrophy is symmetric, but preferably is calculated from 2D data (see Chapter 6).

Diastolic Function

LV diastolic function is characterized by impaired early diastolic relaxation (Fig. 9.33). This results in a prolonged isovolumic relaxation time, reduced acceleration to a reduced E velocity, prolonged early diastolic deceleration slope, an increased A velocity, and an E/A ratio <1. When LV systolic dysfunction supervenes, the elevated LV end-diastolic pressure and elevated LA pressure result in "pseudonormalization" of this pattern with an enhanced E velocity (related to a higher mitral valve opening gradient) and reduced A velocity (due to the elevated LV end-diastolic pressure). Coexisting mitral regurgitation also can lead to a "paradoxical" higher E velocity despite impaired ventricular relaxation. Interestingly, in individuals with physiologic hypertrophy or "athlete's heart," diastolic dysfunction is not seen even when increased wall thickness is present. In pathologic hypertrophy (due to hypertension), diastolic dysfunction often is the first evidence of end-organ damage, usually antedating clear evidence of anatomic hypertrophy.

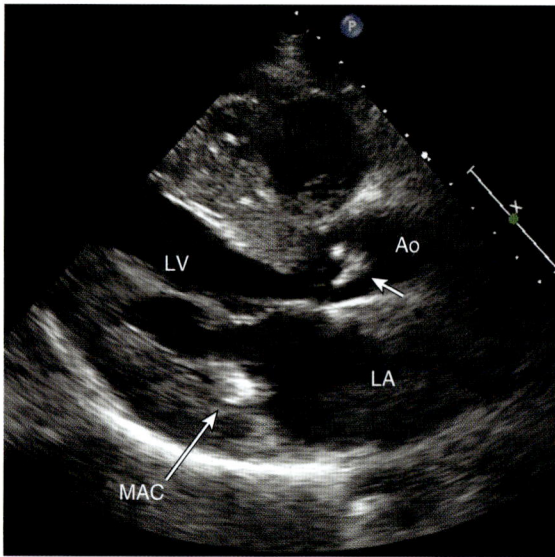

Fig. 9.32 **Hypertensive heart disease.** This parasternal long-axis view shows the typical echocardiographic findings with concentric LV hypertrophy, mitral annular calcification *(MAC)*, aortic valve sclerosis *(arrow)*, and increased echogenicity of the ascending aorta *(small arrow)*. Ao, Aorta.

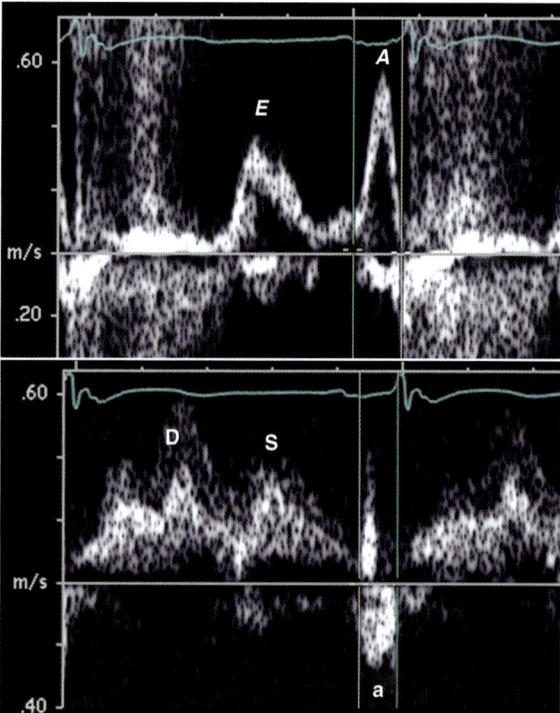

Fig. 9.33 **Diastolic dysfunction in hypertensive heart disease.** LV inflow *(top)* and pulmonary venous flow *(bottom)* in a patient with hypertension and concentric hypertrophy. Mild diastolic dysfunction is present with impaired relaxation as evidenced by the E/A ratio <1 and the prolonged deceleration time. However, LV end-diastolic pressure is normal with a low velocity and short duration of the pulmonary vein atrial reversal *(a)*.

Systolic Function

Typically, systolic function is preserved early in the disease course. Segmental wall motion abnormalities are not seen unless coexisting coronary artery disease is present. With a small, hypertrophied, normally functioning LV chamber, mid-cavity obliteration occurs at end-systole, with an associated Doppler velocity curve showing a brief, late systolic, high-velocity signal. The duration of this intracavity gradient is briefer than that seen with hypertrophic cardiomyopathy, the level of obstruction is mid-ventricular rather than subaortic, and systolic anterior motion of the mitral leaflets is not seen. Mid-cavity obliteration is exacerbated by hypovolemia or increased contractility.

Other Echocardiographic Findings

Dilation of the ascending aorta often is present in hypertensive patients and is associated with increased tortuosity of the ascending aorta, arch, and descending aorta. Increased irregular echogenicity of the aortic walls, representing atherosclerosis, also may be noted. In uncomplicated hypertension, the aortic annulus itself is not dilated. The aortic valve leaflets usually show sclerotic changes and associated mild aortic regurgitation. Mitral annular calcification frequently is present in patients with chronic hypertension and is one cause of mild to moderate mitral regurgitation in these patients. LA enlargement is due to a combination of a chronically elevated LV end-diastolic pressure and mitral regurgitation.

Limitations and Technical Considerations

LV mass determinations are dependent on optimal image quality with clear definition of endocardial and epicardial surfaces and on correct endocardial border tracing at end-diastole and end-systole. Differentiation between hypertensive heart disease and hypertrophic or restrictive heart disease is based on the pattern of hypertrophy, associated echocardiographic findings, and integration of the echocardiographic and clinical data.

Clinical Utility

Diagnosis and Prognosis

LV mass, measured by echocardiography, is a strong predictor of clinical outcome in patients with hypertension. In subjects with borderline hypertension, increased LV mass identifies a subgroup of patients with a poor prognosis without medical therapy. In patients with definite hypertension, the degree of LV hypertrophy reflects the chronic elevation of systemic pressure, in theory serving as an index of the temporally averaged blood pressure over long periods of time. Thus LV mass is a more accurate method for assessing the severity of hypertension than occasional blood pressure recordings in the physician's office or even 24-hour recordings of blood pressure. Changes in LV mass also are helpful for assessing the long-term effect of medical therapy.

Evaluation of Heart Failure Symptoms in a Patient With Hypertension

In a patient with chronic hypertension, heart failure symptoms may be due to diastolic or systolic LV dysfunction, superimposed coronary artery disease, or superimposed valvular disease. Early in the disease course, pathologic hypertrophy is associated with impaired early diastolic filling. Impaired ventricular filling leads to elevated LA pressures and pulmonary venous hypertension, resulting in dyspnea. Diagnosis of diastolic dysfunction with preserved systolic function can be made by echocardiography and has important clinical implications because the therapy for heart failure symptoms is quite different for diastolic versus systolic dysfunction.

Heart failure symptoms due to hypertension with preserved systolic function and severe LV hypertrophy have been termed *hypertensive hypertrophic cardiomyopathy*. This condition is characterized by normal to hyperdynamic systolic function, concentric hypertrophy, diastolic dysfunction, and a mid-ventricular late systolic gradient due to cavity obliteration (see Fig. 9.21). Strictly speaking, this combination of findings is not a "cardiomyopathy" and is not an inherited disorder but simply represents severe end-organ damage due to hypertension. However, awareness of this specific clinical picture results in consideration of this diagnosis in patients in whom hypertrophic or restrictive cardiomyopathy otherwise might be suspected.

With long-standing hypertension, impairment of LV contractility can occur, even in the absence of coexisting coronary artery disease. Physiologically, elevated afterload (as in valvular aortic stenosis) is the proximate cause of systolic dysfunction. However, systolic function does not always improve, even with aggressive antihypertensive therapy when systolic dysfunction is long-standing, a finding suggesting that irreversible changes in ventricular contractility have occurred. End-stage hypertensive heart disease has an echocardiographic appearance similar to end-stage dilated cardiomyopathy.

Alternate Approaches

The need for routine echocardiographic evaluation of patients with hypertension is controversial. Medical management based on intermittent office blood pressure measurements remains standard practice at most medical centers. When needed, estimates of the chronicity of blood pressure elevation can be obtained by 24-hour blood pressure monitors or evaluation of other end-organ damage (e.g., renal function, retinal examination). Although electrocardiographic estimates of LV hypertrophy are less accurate and precise than echocardiographic measurements, the cost differential between these diagnostic tests is substantial.

PULMONARY HEART DISEASE

Chronic Versus Acute Pulmonary Disease

Chronic pulmonary hypertension, whether due to intrinsic lung disease, recurrent pulmonary emboli, or primary pulmonary hypertension, results in a group of clinical signs and symptoms termed *cor pulmonale*. The underlying pathophysiology of this clinical syndrome is chronic pressure overload of the RV as it ejects into a high-resistance pulmonary vascular bed. Initially, compensatory hypertrophy occurs with preserved systolic function. Over time, contractility deteriorates, and RV dilation, moderate to severe tricuspid regurgitation, and consequent RA enlargement are seen (Fig. 9.34).

Acute pulmonary embolism also can affect right heart function because of the sudden onset of elevated pulmonary vascular resistance. Echocardiographic evaluation is helpful in assessing pulmonary artery pressures and RV function in patients with either chronic or acute pulmonary hypertension.

Echocardiographic Approach

Pulmonary Pressures

Standard approaches for the noninvasive evaluation of pulmonary pressures (PAP), as described in Chapter 6, are applicable to the patient with suspected or known pulmonary hypertension. The most reliable approach is to record the maximum tricuspid regurgitant jet velocity (V_{TR}) for calculation of the RV to RA systolic pressure difference (Fig. 9.35). Care is needed to interrogate the tricuspid regurgitant jet from multiple acoustic windows (apical, parasternal) with a systematic approach to transducer angulation to obtain a parallel intercept angle between the ultrasound beam and jet. RA pressure (RAP) is estimated from the size and respiratory variation in the inferior vena cava. Then pulmonary artery systolic pressure (in the absence of pulmonic stenosis) is calculated as:

$$\text{PAP} = 4V^2_{TR} + \text{RAP} \qquad \text{(Eq. 9.1)}$$

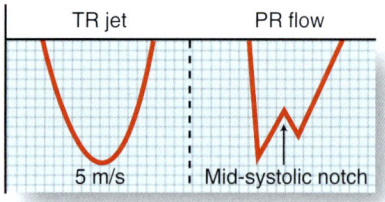

Diastolic pulmonary artery pressure can be estimated from the velocities in the pulmonic regurgitant Doppler curve. Pulmonary vascular resistance (PVR) can be estimated from the ratio of the tricuspid regurgitant jet velocity to the velocity time integral of RV outflow (VTI_{RVOT}), multiplied by 10 for conversion to Wood units (see Chapter 6):

$$\text{PVR(Wood units)} = 10(V_{TR}/VTI_{RVOT}) \qquad \text{(Eq. 9.2)}$$

Indirect signs of pulmonary hypertension often are seen that indicate the presence, but not the exact severity, of pulmonary hypertension. For example, an M-mode recording through the pulmonic valve shows a reduced *a*-wave and mid-systolic closure of the valve. This pattern has a reasonably high specificity (>90%) for detecting pulmonary hypertension but a low sensitivity (30% to 60%). This motion pattern is paralleled by the Doppler velocity curve, which shows an abrupt mid-systolic deceleration of flow (Fig. 9.36). Signs of RV pressure overload, including abnormal ventricular septal motion, also are valuable clues suggesting the presence of pulmonary hypertension.

Right Ventricular Pressure Overload

The response of the RV to chronic pressure overload consists of hypertrophy and dilation (Fig. 9.37). The increase in thickness of the RV free wall is best seen on the subcostal view. Ventricular septal motion is

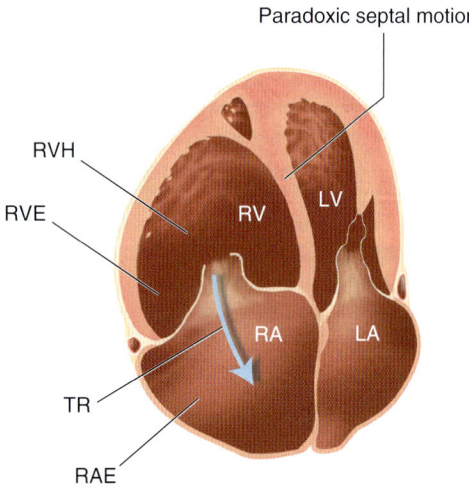

Fig. 9.34 Pulmonary heart disease. RV hypertrophy *(RVH)* and enlargement *(RVE)* are seen with paradoxical septal motion. Secondary tricuspid regurgitation *(TR)* and RA enlargement *(RAE)* are common. Elevated pulmonary artery pressures will be reflected in the high-velocity tricuspid regurgitant jet velocity and mid-systolic notching in the pulmonary artery velocity curve. *PR,* Pulmonic regurgitant.

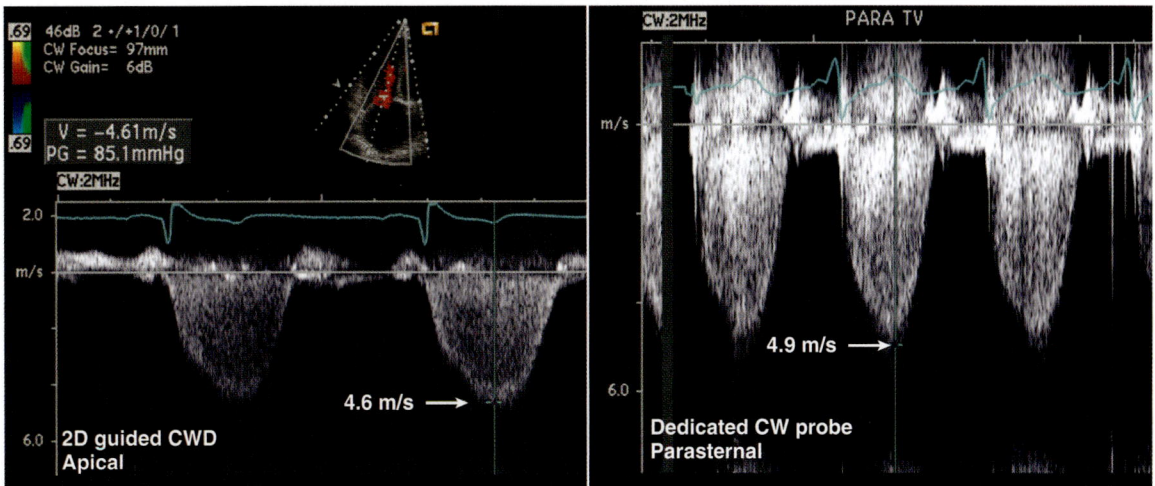

Fig. 9.35 Primary pulmonary hypertension. Tricuspid regurgitant jet in a patient with primary pulmonary hypertension. Using 2D and color-guided CW Doppler from the apex *(left)*, a clear signal is obtained, although signal strength is low, with a maximum jet of 4.6 m/s. The use of a dedicated CW probe *(right)* provides a stronger signal, and a higher jet velocity is obtained from a parasternal window. The maximum velocity of 4.9 m/s indicates an RV to RA pressure difference of 96 mmHg. RA pressure was elevated at 10 mmHg, so estimated pulmonary artery systolic pressure is 106 mmHg. Note the faint linear spread of the signal at peak of the curve *(see third beat in right panel)*. This faint signal is due to the transit time effect and should not be included in the velocity measurement

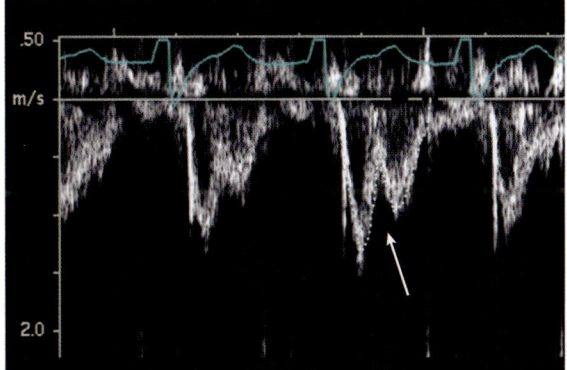

Fig. 9.36 Pulmonary artery velocity curve in pulmonary hypertension. The rapid acceleration (short time to peak velocity) and mid-systolic notching *(arrow)* are consistent with severe pulmonary hypertension.

abnormal or "paradoxical," with anterior motion of the septum during systole both on M-mode and 2D imaging. A rational explanation for this pattern of septal motion is based on the concept that the septum moves toward the center of mass of the heart during systole. With RV hypertrophy, the center of mass is shifted anteriorly, so the septum moves toward the center of the RV instead of the normal pattern of motion toward the center of the LV. On 2D imaging the curvature of the septum is reversed in both systole and in early to mid-diastole. In contrast, RV volume overload is characterized by diastolic flattening of the septum in late diastole with a normal curvature in systole, due to increased volume flow into the RV (compared with the LV) in diastole but normal ventricular pressures in systole (see Fig. 6.23).

With long-standing or acute pulmonary hypertension, RV systolic dysfunction can occur, with secondary dilation serving as a compensatory mechanism to maintain forward stroke volume. However, RV dilation leads to tricuspid regurgitation because of annular dilation and malalignment of the papillary muscles. This superimposed volume overload results in further RV dilation and more tricuspid regurgitation. RA dilation is due to both pressure (*v*-wave) and volume (tricuspid regurgitation) overload.

Secondary Tricuspid Regurgitation

Tricuspid regurgitation secondary to pulmonary hypertension, RV systolic dysfunction, or both can be evaluated with color Doppler flow imaging from parasternal, apical, and subcostal views. Severe regurgitation results in systolic flow reversal in the inferior vena cava and hepatic veins. Evaluation of tricuspid valve anatomy is needed to ensure that other causes of tricuspid regurgitation (e.g., vegetation, rheumatic, carcinoid, Ebstein anomaly) are not present.

The intensity of the CW Doppler tricuspid regurgitant jet relates to the severity of regurgitation, but the velocity relates to the RV to RA pressure difference. With acute tricuspid regurgitation, a rapid falloff in velocity in late systole is seen, consistent with an RA *v*-wave.

Limitations and Technical Considerations

The major limitation of echocardiography in the evaluation of cor pulmonale is poor ultrasound tissue penetration resulting in poor image quality and low Doppler signal strength. Hyperexpanded lungs obscure the

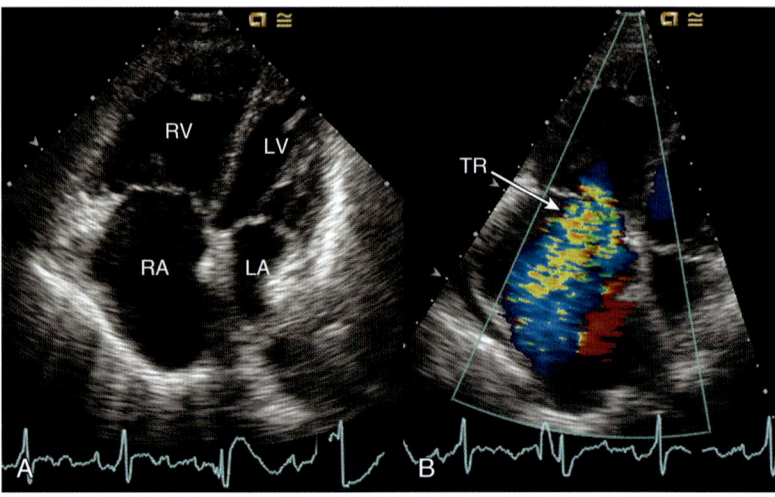

Fig. 9.37 ▶ **Cor pulmonale.** (A) Apical four-chamber view at end-diastole in a patient with chronic pulmonary disease and secondary pulmonary hypertension. RV enlargement, RV hypertrophy, paradoxical septal motion, and reduced systolic function of the RV are present. (B) Color Doppler shows severe tricuspid regurgitation *(TR)*.

standard acoustic windows in many patients with chronic lung disease. However, adequate image quality is obtained with current instruments in nearly all patients.

Assessment of the severity of pulmonary hypertension depends on obtaining a parallel intercept angle between the ultrasound beam and the tricuspid regurgitant jet. Underestimation of pulmonary artery pressures should be considered in all patients, especially when Doppler signal strength is suboptimal or when the Doppler data and clinical setting are discrepant. The absence of a recordable tricuspid regurgitant jet does not indicate normal pulmonary pressures. In this situation, the report indicates that the data are inadequate, and alternate diagnostic approaches should be considered. Overestimation of pulmonary pressures from the tricuspid regurgitant signal can be avoided by measuring the outer edge of the dark spectral envelope but avoiding the slight spectral broadening at peak velocity that results from the transit time effect.

Clinical Utility

In the patient with chronic lung disease and right heart failure, echocardiography allows the confirmation of a clinical diagnosis of cor pulmonale, assessment of the degree of pulmonary hypertension, and evaluation of RV size and systolic dysfunction.

In patients with primary pulmonary hypertension, echocardiography is essential in excluding other causes of pulmonary hypertension, such as an atrial septal defect or mitral regurgitation. In addition, noninvasive measurement of pulmonary pressure now is routinely used for evaluating changes in pulmonary pressures with medical therapy.

In the patient with an acute pulmonary embolus, imaging rarely shows a residual thrombus originating from or in transit through (from a deep vein thrombosis) the right heart. TEE imaging can demonstrate thrombus in the main, right, or left pulmonary artery. However, the sensitivity of echocardiography for the diagnosis of pulmonary embolism based on demonstrating a thrombus is low because the thrombus is lodged more distally in the pulmonary vasculature in most cases. In addition, adequate visualization of the pulmonary artery bifurcation is not possible in all patients because of interposition of the air-filled trachea and bronchi. Indirect signs of pulmonary embolism include:

- Elevated pulmonary artery pressures
- Evidence of acute RV pressure overload
- RV dilation and dysfunction
- Tricuspid regurgitation

Similar findings are seen in patients with chronic recurrent pulmonary emboli. The possibility of pulmonary embolism should be strongly considered in patients with these findings, even when a different working clinical diagnosis or "reason for echo" was entertained. Often patients in whom pulmonary embolism is subsequently diagnosed are initially referred for nonspecific indications including "chest pain," "dyspnea," or "heart failure."

Alternate Approaches

Cardiac catheterization allows direct measurement of RV and pulmonary artery pressures and calculation of pulmonary vascular resistance. RV size and systolic function can be evaluated by angiography.

Clinically, the standard approach for the diagnosis of pulmonary embolism is computed tomographic pulmonary angiography. When that procedure is not available, a radionuclide ventricular perfusion scan is appropriate. Pulmonary angiography with injection of contrast material directly into the main pulmonary artery is only rarely needed when results of other tests are inconclusive.

THE ECHO EXAM

Possible Diagnoses in a Patient Referred for "Heart Failure"	
Ischemic disease	
Valvular disease	
Hypertensive heart disease	
Cardiomyopathy	Dilated Hypertrophic Restrictive Other
Pericardial disease	Constriction Tamponade
Pulmonary heart disease	

Typical Cause of Increased Wall Thickness

	Hypertensive Heart Disease	Hypertrophic Cardiomyopathy	Restrictive Cardiomyopathy
LV hypertrophy	Present	Present	Present
Pattern of hypertrophy	Concentric	Asymmetric	Concentric
With clinical history of hypertension	Present	Absent	Absent
Outflow obstruction	Mid-ventricular cavity obliteration	Dynamic subaortic obstruction	Absent
RV hypertrophy	Absent	May be present	Present
Pulmonary hypertension	Mild	Mild	Moderate
LV systolic function	Normal initially but reduced late in disease course	Normal	Normal initially but reduced late in disease course
LV diastolic function	Abnormal	Abnormal	Abnormal

Cardiomyopathies: Typical Features

	Dilated	Hypertrophic	Restrictive	Athlete's Heart
LV systolic function	Moderately-severely ↓	Normal	Normal	Normal
LV diastolic function	May be abnormal	Abnormal	Abnormal	Normal
LV hypertrophy	↑ LV mass due to LV dilation with normal wall thickness	Asymmetric LV hypertrophy	Concentric LV hypertrophy	Normal wall thickness
Chamber dilation	All four chambers	LA and RA dilation if MR is present	LA and RA dilation	LV dilation
Outflow tract obstruction	Absent	Dynamic LV outflow tract obstruction in some patients	Absent	Absent
LV end-diastolic pressure	Elevated	Elevated	Elevated	Normal
Pulmonary artery pressures	Elevated	Elevated	Elevated	Normal

MR, Mitral regurgitation.

Echo Approach to the Cardiomyopathies

Modality	Echo Views and Flows	Measurements
Imaging	LV size and systolic function	LVEDV, LVESV
		Apical biplane EF
	Degree and pattern of LV hypertrophy	LV mass
	Evidence for dynamic outflow tract obstruction	SAM of the mitral valve
		Aortic valve mid-systolic closure
	RV size and systolic function	
	LA size	
Doppler echo	Associated valvular regurgitation	Measure vena contracta; quantitate if more than mild.
	LV diastolic function	Standard diastolic function evaluation with classification of severity and estimate of LVEDP
	LV systolic function	dP/dt from MR jet
		Calculation of cardiac output
	Pulmonary pressures	TR jet and IVC for PA systolic pressure
		Evaluate PR jet for PA diastolic pressure.
		Estimate pulmonary resistance.
	Color, pulsed, and CW Doppler to quantitate outflow obstruction	Maximum outflow tract gradient

EF, Ejection fraction; *ICV*, inferior vena cava; *LVEDP*, LV end-diastolic pressure; *LVEDV*, LV end-diastolic volume; *LVESV*, LV end-systolic volume; *MR*, mitral regurgitation; *PA*, pulmonary artery; *PR*, pulmonary regurgitation; *SAM*, systolic anterior motion; *TR*, tricuspid regurgitation.

SUGGESTED READING

1. Cheng RK, Masri SC: Dilated cardiomyopathy: the role of echocardiography in diagnosis and patient management. In Otto CM, editor: *The Practice of Clinical Echocardiography*, ed 5, Philadelphia, 2017, Elsevier, pp 483–504.
   Review of the echocardiographic approach to the patient with heart failure due to dilated cardiomyopathy. This chapter addresses both systolic and diastolic dysfunction and right and left heart failure. The effects of pharmacologic and mechanical therapies in heart failure also are discussed.

2. Benziger CP, do Carmo GA, Ribeiro AL: Chagas cardiomyopathy: clinical presentation and management in the Americas, *Cardiol Clin* 35(1):31–47, 2017.
   Chagas disease is endemic in Central and South America and is due to infection by the protozoan Trypanosoma cruzi. In the acute phase, a pericardial effusion is common. Chronic disease develops over several decades. In the asymptomatic phase, stress testing may be abnormal. As the disease progresses, apical aneurysms are common, but end-stage disease has an appearance similar to that of other causes of dilated cardiomyopathy.

3. Lyon AR, Bossone E, Schneider B, et al: Current state of knowledge on Takotsubo syndrome: a position statement from the Taskforce on Takotsubo Syndrome of the Heart Failure Association of the European Society of Cardiology, *Eur J Heart Fail* 18(1):8–27, 2016.
   This comprehensive review article describes the pathophysiology, clinical presentation, and diagnostic features of tako-tsubo syndrome. Compared with acute myocarditis, tako-tsubo syndrome occurs predominantly in women (90%) older than 50 years of age who present with chest pain, dyspnea, and palpitations but who have only a low to moderate troponin risk. Echocardiography shows typical "apical ballooning" and transient mitral regurgitation. The mortality rate is 4% to 5%, and 50% of patients have acute complications.

4. Woo A: Hypertrophic cardiomyopathy: echocardiography in diagnosis and management of patients. In Otto CM, editor: *The Practice of Clinical Echocardiography*, ed 5, Philadelphia, 2017, Elsevier, pp 505–533.
   This chapter details the echocardiographic findings in hypertrophic cardiomyopathy and correlates the echocardiographic data with clinical, genetic, and pathophysiologic aspects of the disease process.

5. Choudhury L, Rigolin VH, Bonow RO: Integrated imaging in hypertrophic cardiomyopathy, *Am J Cardiol* 119(2):328–339, 2017.
   Review of diagnostic imaging approaches in patients with hypertrophic cardiomyopathy. Detailed and clear illustration of 2D echo, CW Doppler, color Doppler, M-mode, and tissue Doppler imaging findings. Examples of findings on cardiac magnetic resonance imaging are also included. Helpful tables show the strengths of each modality and features that distinguish hypertrophic cardiomyopathy from athlete's heart, hypertensive heart disease, or an infiltrative disease.

6. Veselka J, Anavekar NS, Charron P: Hypertrophic obstructive cardiomyopathy, *Lancet* 389:1253–1267, 2017.
   This review provides a concise summary of the pathophysiology, clinical presentation, imaging findings and management options for hypertrophic cardiomyopathy.

7. Peteiro J, Bouzas-Mosquera A, Fernandez X, et al: Prognostic value of exercise echocardiography in patients with hypertrophic cardiomyopathy, *J Am Soc Echocardiogr* 25(2):182–189, 2012.
   In 239 patients with hypertrophic cardiomyopathy, 25% had LV outflow obstruction at rest, and 18% had provocable obstruction with exercise. In addition, wall motion abnormalities were seen with exercise in 8%. Adverse cardiac events at a mean follow-up of 4.2 years occurred in 8% of patients and included cardiac death, heart transplantation, appropriate defibrillator shocks, stroke, myocardial infarction, and hospitalization for heart failure. Multivariate predictors of outcome were LV wall thickness, rest wall motion score index, and exercise capacity, but not the presence of LV outflow obstruction.

8. Pelliccia A, Maron MS, Maron BJ: Assessment of left ventricular hypertrophy in a trained athlete: differential diagnosis of physiologic athlete's heart from pathologic hypertrophy, *Prog Cardiovasc Dis* 54(5):387–396, 2012.
   Athletes with physiologic hypertrophy can be distinguished from patients with pathologic hypertrophy based on LV geometry, family history, cardiac magnetic resonance imaging for myocardial fibrosis, LV diastolic function, and (in some cases) periods of deconditioning to alter LV mass.

9. Nagueh SF, Bierig SM, Budoff MJ, et al: American Society of Echocardiography clinical recommendations for multimodality cardiovascular imaging of patients with hypertrophic cardiomyopathy: endorsed by the American Society of Nuclear Cardiology, Society for Cardiovascular Magnetic Resonance, and Society of Cardiovascular Computed Tomography, *J Am Soc Echocardiogr* 24(5):473–498, 2011.
   A consensus statement with detailed information about the echocardiographic approach to diagnosis in patients with hypertrophic cardiomyopathy. Numerous illustrations and comparisons with other imaging modalities. Echocardiography is recommendation as the procedure of choice for evaluation of cardiac morphology, LV ejection fraction, outflow obstruction and LV diastolic dysfunction. Cardiac magnetic resonance imaging is recommended when echocardiography is suboptimal, with cardiac computed tomography as an alternative when cardiac magnetic resonance is contraindicated.

10. Naqvi TZ, Appleton CP: Restrictive cardiomyopathy: diagnosis and prognostic implications. In Otto CM, editor: *The Practice of Clinical Echocardiography*, ed 5, Philadelphia, 2017, Elsevier, pp 534–555
    Detailed discussion of the importance of echocardiography in the diagnosis, management, and evaluation of prognosis in patients with restrictive cardiomyopathies.

11. Redfield MM: Heart failure with preserved ejection fraction, *N Engl J Med* 375(19):1868–1877, 2016.
    Clear and concise, clinically oriented discussion of the diagnosis and management of heart failure with preserved ejection fraction. In a patient with heart failure symptoms, features on echocardiography include: (1) an ejection fraction greater than 50%; (2) LV hypertrophy, which is typical but not always present; (3) Doppler evidence for diastolic function, which is common but not independently diagnostic; (4) left atrial enlargement, which is typical; and (5) estimated pulmonary systolic pressure that is usually greater than 35 mmHg.

12. Falk RH, Alexander KM, Liao R, et al: AL (light-chain) cardiac amyloidosis: a review of diagnosis and therapy, *J Am Coll Cardiol* 68(12):1323–1341, 2016.
    Discussion of the pathophysiology of light chain amyloidosis followed by details of diagnosis and treatment. Typical echocardiographic findings are shown along with other types of diagnostic imaging.

13. Birnie DH, Nery PB, Ha AC, et al: Cardiac sarcoidosis, *J Am Coll Cardiol* 68(4):411–421, 2016.
    In patients with systemic sarcoidosis, clinical symptoms due to cardiac involvement occur in only about 5%, but asymptomatic cardiac involvement is present in up to 25% of patients. Cardiac sarcoidosis is characterized by conduction abnormalities, ventricular arrhythmias, and heart failure. Echocardiographic findings are nonspecific, including regional wall motion abnormalities that do not fit a typical pattern for coronary disease, basal interventricular thinning, LV diastolic and systolic dysfunction, and abnormal RV systolic function.

14. Towbin JA, Lorts A, Jefferies JL: Left ventricular non-compaction cardiomyopathy, *Lancet* 386(9995):813–825, 2015.
    Left ventricular noncompaction is a type of cardiomyopathy characterized by prominent LV trabeculation, often associated with other types of congenital heart disease, with a genetic pattern of inheritance in 30% to 50% of patients. Clinical symptoms include heart failure, arrhythmias, and embolic events. Both echocardiography and cardiac magnetic resonance imaging are helpful in making the diagnosis, with an end-diastolic ratio of noncompacted to compacted myocardium greater than 2:1 often considered diagnostic.

15. Wu AH, Kolias TJ: Cardiac transplantation: pretransplant and posttransplant evaluation. In Otto CM, editor: *The Practice of Clinical Echocardiography*, ed 5, Philadelphia, 2017, Elsevier, pp 577–595.
    The structure and function of the normal transplanted heart are reviewed, followed by a discussion of acute rejection and transplant vasculopathy.

16. Kirkpatrick JN: Echocardiography in mechanical circulatory support: normal findings, complications, and speed changes. In Otto CM, editor: *The Practice of Clinical Echocardiography*, ed 5, Philadelphia, 2017, Elsevier, pp 596–618.
    Current review of echocardiographic evaluation of LVADs including normal flow patterns and diagnosis of device dysfunction. The clinical utility of echocardiography in optimizing flow rates and in assessing ventricular recovery is also discussed. Different device types, echocardiographic findings, and indicators of device dysfunction are summarized in tables and figures.

17. Stainback RF, Estep JD, Agler DA, et al: American Society of Echocardiography. Echocardiography in the management of patients with left ventricular assist devices: recommendations from the American Society of Echocardiography, *J Am Soc Echocardiogr* 28(8):853–909, 2015.
    This document provides clear information on echocardiographic evaluation of LVADs. Numerous illustrations with a detailed table that summarizes recommendations. 93 references.

18. Celermajer DS, Playford D: Pulmonary hypertension: role of echocardiography in diagnosis and patient management. In Otto CM, editor: *The Practice of Clinical Echocardiography*, ed 5, Philadelphia, 2017, Elsevier, pp 633–650.
    This chapter provides a detailed review of the pathophysiologic response of the RV to chronic pressure overload and the effect of pulmonary disease on the right heart. Echocardiographic approaches with detailed illustrations are provided.

19. Marwick TH, Gillebert TC, Aurigemma G, et al: Recommendations on the use of echocardiography in adult hypertension: a report from the European Association of Cardiovascular Imaging (EACVI) and the American Society of Echocardiography (ASE), *J Am Soc Echocardiogr* 28(7):727–754, 2015.
    Detailed information about the cardiac changes seen with chronic hypertension, optimal approaches to measurement of LV mass, and differing pattern of LV hypertrophy. Recommendations for both clinical practice and research protocols are included.

10 Pericardial Disease

PERICARDIAL ANATOMY AND PHYSIOLOGY
PERICARDITIS
   Basic Principles
   Echocardiographic Approach
   Clinical Utility
PERICARDIAL EFFUSION
   Basic Principles
   Diagnosis of Pericardial Effusion
      Diffuse Effusion
      Loculated Effusion
      Distinguishing From Pleural Fluid
   Clinical Utility
PERICARDIAL TAMPONADE
   Echocardiographic Approach
      Right Atrial Systolic Collapse
      Right Ventricular Diastolic Collapse
      Reciprocal Changes in Ventricular Volumes
      Respiratory Variation in Diastolic Filling
      Tissue Doppler Early Diastolic Velocity
      Inferior Vena Cava Dilation
   Clinical Utility
      Diagnosis of Pericardial Tamponade
      Echo-Guided Pericardiocentesis
PERICARDIAL CONSTRICTION
   Basic Principles
   Echocardiographic Approach
      Imaging
      Doppler Examination
      Constrictive Pericarditis Versus Restrictive Cardiomyopathy
   Clinical Utility
THE ECHO EXAM
SUGGESTED READING

PERICARDIAL ANATOMY AND PHYSIOLOGY

The pericardium consists of two serous surfaces surrounding a closed, complex, saclike potential space. The visceral pericardium is continuous with the epicardial surface of the heart. The parietal pericardium is a dense but thin fibrous structure that is apposed to the pleural surfaces laterally and blends with the central tendon of the diaphragm inferiorly. Around the right and left ventricles (RV and LV) and the ventricular apex, the pericardial space is a simple ellipsoid structure conforming to the shape of the ventricles. Around the systemic and pulmonary venous inflows and around the great vessels, the parietal and visceral pericardia meet to close the "ends" of the sac—these areas often are referred to as *pericardial reflections*. The pericardial space encloses the right atrium (RA) and RA appendage anteriorly and laterally, with pericardial reflections around the superior and inferior vena cavae near their junction with the RA. Superiorly, the pericardium extends a short distance along the great vessels, with a small "pocket" of pericardium surrounding the great arteries posteriorly—the *transverse sinus*. The pericardial space extends laterally to the left atrium (LA), and a blind pocket of the pericardium extends posteriorly to the LA, between the four pulmonary veins—the *oblique sinus* (Fig. 10.1). The pericardial space normally contains a small amount (5 to 10 mL) of fluid that is detectable by echocardiography.

Anatomically, the pericardium isolates the heart from the rest of the mediastinum and from the lungs and pleural space, by serving as a barrier to infection and reducing friction with surrounding structures during contraction, rotation, and translation of the heart. In addition, the semirigid enclosure provided by the pericardium affects the pressure distribution to the cardiac chambers and mediates the interaction between RV and LV diastolic filling. The importance of the pericardium is most evident when it is affected by disease processes such as inflammation, thickening, or fluid accumulation.

PERICARDITIS

Basic Principles

Pericarditis is inflammation of the pericardium, and it can be due to a wide variety of causes, including bacterial or viral infection, trauma, uremia, and transmural myocardial infarction (Table 10.1). Clinically, the diagnosis of pericarditis is based on at least two of the four characteristic features:

- Typical chest pain
- Widespread ST elevation or PR depression on electrocardiography

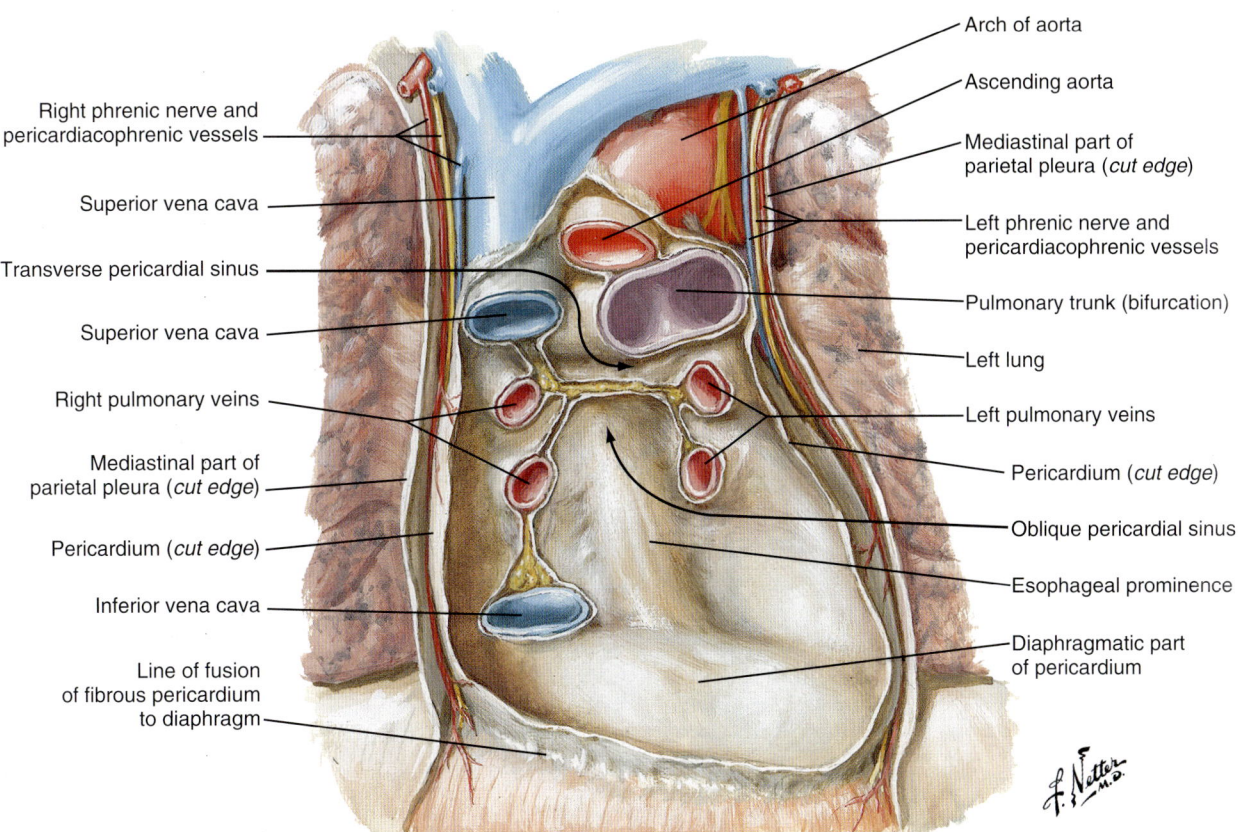

Fig. 10.1 Pericardial anatomy. The posterior wall of the pericardial sac after the heart has been removed by severing its continuity with the great arteries and veins and by cutting the two pericardial sleeves that surround the arteries and veins. Arrows indicate the transverse and oblique sinuses of the pericardium. *(From Netter FH: Atlas of Human Anatomy, Basel, Switzerland, 1989, Ciba-Geigy.)*

- Pericardial rub on auscultation
- New or increasing pericardial effusion

Although it is probable that most patients with pericarditis have a pericardial effusion at some point in the disease course, a pericardial effusion is not a necessary criterion for a diagnosis of pericarditis, nor does the presence of an effusion indicate a diagnosis of pericarditis. Interestingly, no correlation exists between the size of the pericardial effusion and the presence or absence of a pericardial "rub" on cardiac auscultation.

Echocardiographic Approach

In a patient with suspected pericarditis, the echocardiogram may show a pericardial effusion of any size or pericardial thickening with or without an effusion, or it may be entirely normal. A pericardial effusion is recognized as an echolucent space around the heart (Fig. 10.2).

Pericardial thickening is evidenced by increased echogenicity of the pericardium on two-dimensional (2D) imaging and as multiple parallel reflections posterior to the LV on M-mode recordings (Fig. 10.3). However, because the pericardium typically is the most echogenic structure in the image, it can be difficult to distinguish normal from thickened pericardium, and other imaging approaches, such as computed tomography (CT) or magnetic resonance (CMR), are more sensitive for this diagnosis.

Examination from several windows is needed when pericarditis is suspected because effusion or thickening can be localized and thus seen in only certain tomographic views. If a pericardial effusion is present, the possibility of tamponade physiology should be considered. If pericardial thickening is present, examination for evidence of constrictive physiology should be considered.

Clinical Utility

Pericarditis is a clinical diagnosis that cannot be made independently by echocardiography. The goal of the echocardiographic examination is to evaluate for pericardial effusion or thickening and to evaluate for tamponade physiology (Table 10.2).

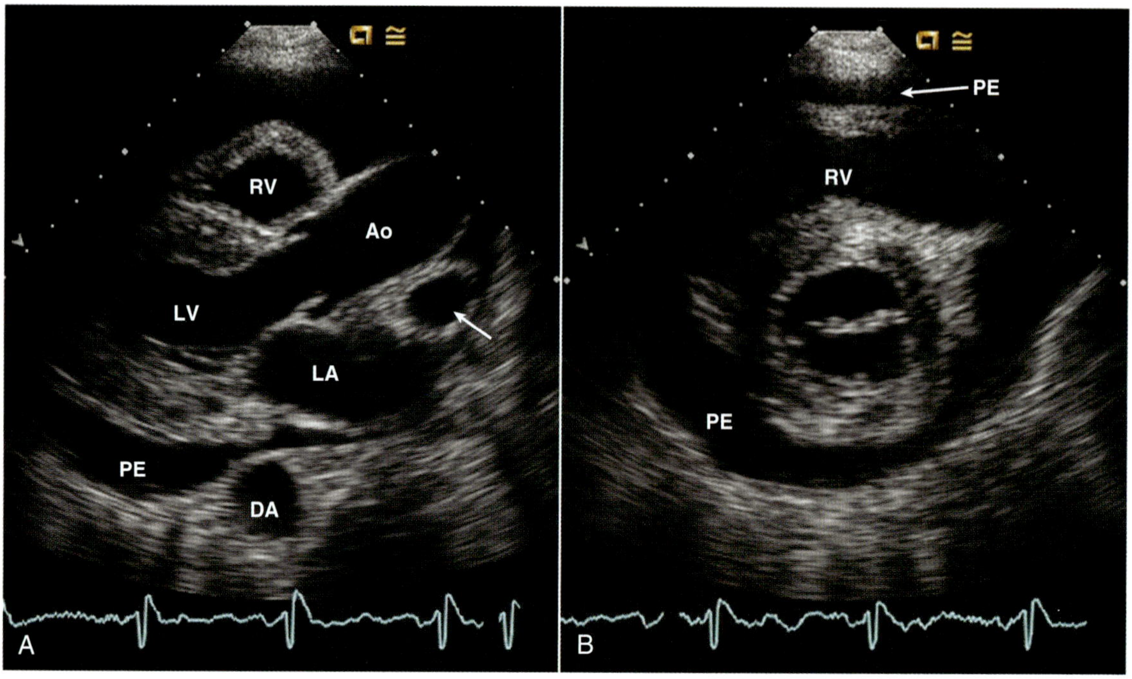

Fig. 10.2 Pericardial effusion on echocardiography. Parasternal long- and short-axis views of a moderate circumferential pericardial effusion *(PE)*. In the long-axis view (A) ▶ and short-axis view (B), ▶ the effusion tracks appear anterior to the descending aorta *(DA)* with a small amount of fluid posterior to the LA in the oblique sinus. Pericardial fluid in the transverse sinus (posterior to the aorta *[Ao]*) delineates the right pulmonary artery *(arrow)*, which is not usually seen in this view in adults. Pericardial fluid anterior to the RV is seen in both the long- and short-axis views.

TABLE 10.1	Causes of Pericardial Disease (With Examples)

Idiopathic

Infection

Viral
Bacterial (*Staphylococcus, pneumococcus,* tuberculosis)
Parasitic (*Echinococcus,* amebiasis, toxoplasmosis)

Neoplasia

Metastatic disease (e.g., lymphoma, melanoma)
Direct extension (e.g., lung carcinoma, breast carcinoma)
Primary cardiac malignancy

Inflammation

Post–myocardial infarction (e.g., Dressler syndrome)
Uremia
Systemic inflammatory diseases (e.g., lupus, scleroderma)
Post–cardiac surgery
Radiation

Intracardiac-Pericardial Communications

Blunt or penetrating chest trauma
Postcatheter procedures
Postinfarction LV rupture
Aortic dissection

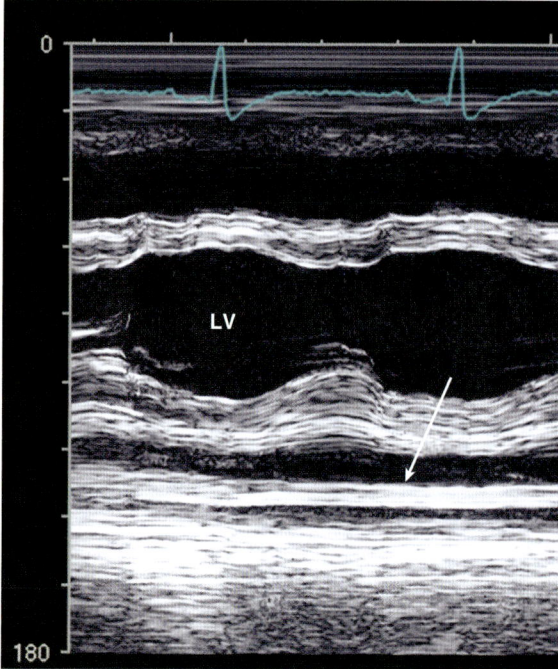

Fig. 10.3 Pericardial thickening on M-mode echocardiography. Multiple parallel dense echos *(arrow)* are seen posterior to the LV epicardium. This patient also has a small pericardial effusion, seen on M-mode as an echo-free space between the flat pericardium and the moving posterior wall.

TABLE 10.2 Pericardial Disease: Clinical-Echocardiographic Correlates

	Clinical Presentation	Echocardiographic Findings
Constrictive pericarditis	Dyspnea on exertion and signs of venous congestion (elevated venous pressure, ascites, and edema)	• Ventricular septal shift • Hepatic vein diastolic flow reversals in expiration • Preserved or increased medial E′ velocity, often with medial E′ > lateral E′ velocities • Respiratory variation in mitral E velocities • Plethora of the inferior vena cava • Decreased lateral longitudinal strain, as compared with medial
Pericardial effusion	Variable depending on cause; often asymptomatic and incidentally discovered	• Pericardial effusion size ranges from trivial to very large; location is circumferential or loculated; fluid echo-brightness varies with characteristics (transudative, exudative, or frankly bloody).
Tamponade	Variable; often nonspecific; includes hypotension, tachycardia, elevated venous pressure, and pulsus paradoxus	• Chamber collapse • Plethora of the inferior vena cava • Respiratory variation in right- and left-heart filling and venous flow patterns
Acute pericarditis	Characteristic chest pain and ECG changes; pericardial friction rub on auscultation	• Effusion is sometimes present and helps secure the diagnosis. • Ventricular regional wall motion abnormalities suggest associated myocarditis or an alternative diagnosis. • Tamponade or constrictive physiology can occur.

ECG, Electrocardiographic.
From Otto C, editor: *The Practice of Clinical Echocardiography*, ed 5, Philadelphia, 2017, Elsevier, Table 28-5.

PERICARDIAL EFFUSION

Basic Principles

A wide variety of disease processes can result in a pericardial effusion with a differential diagnosis similar to that for pericarditis (see Table 10.1). The physiologic consequences of fluid in the pericardial space depend both on the volume and the rate of fluid accumulation. A slowly expanding pericardial effusion can become quite large (>1000 mL) with little increase in pericardial pressure, whereas rapid accumulation of even a small volume of fluid (50 to 100 mL) can lead to a marked increase in pericardial pressure (Fig. 10.4).

Tamponade physiology occurs when the pressure in the pericardium exceeds the pressure in the cardiac chambers, thus resulting in impaired cardiac filling (Fig. 10.5). As pericardial pressure increases, filling of each cardiac chamber is sequentially impaired, with lower-pressure chambers (atria) affected before higher-pressure chambers (ventricles). The compressive effect of the pericardial fluid is seen most clearly in the phase of the cardiac cycle when pressure is lowest in that chamber—systole for the atrium, diastole for the ventricles. Filling pressures become elevated as a compensatory mechanism to maintain cardiac output. In fully developed tamponade, diastolic pressures in all four cardiac chambers are equal (and elevated) because of exposure of the entire heart to the elevated pericardial pressure.

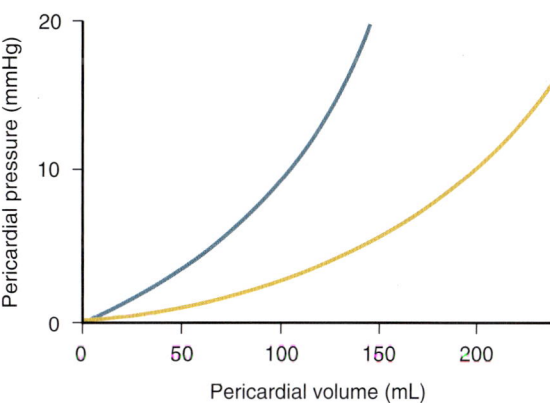

Fig. 10.4 Pericardial pressure versus pericardial volume. The graph shows an acute effusion (*blue line*, with a steep pressure-volume relationship) and a chronic effusion (*yellow line*, where large volumes lead to only mild pressure elevation).

Clinically, tamponade physiology manifests as low cardiac output symptoms, hypotension, and tachycardia. Jugular venous pressure is elevated and pulsus paradoxus (an inspiratory decline >10 mmHg in systemic blood pressure) is present on physical examination. The clinical finding of pulsus paradoxus is closely related to the echo findings of reciprocal respiratory changes in RV and LV filling and emptying.

Diagnosis of Pericardial Effusion

The sensitivity and specificity of echocardiography for detection of a pericardial effusion are very high (Table 10.3). Diagnosis continues to rely on 2D transthoracic echocardiographic imaging from multiple acoustic windows; transesophageal echocardiography (TEE) sometimes is helpful with loculated posterior effusions. Three-dimensional (3D) imaging is not needed routinely but occasionally is helpful in the diagnosis of loculated effusions or hematomas.

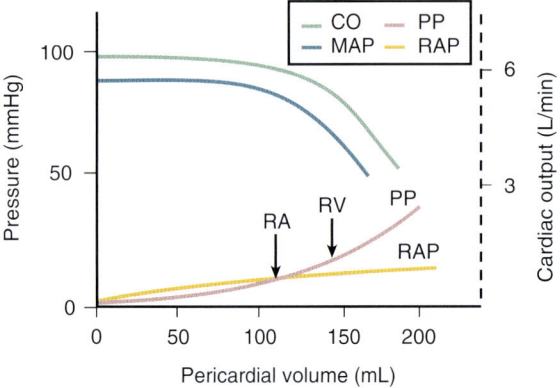

Fig. 10.5 Relationships among pericardial pressure, right atrial pressure, mean arterial pressure, and cardiac output. Note that when pericardial pressure *(PP)* exceeds RA pressure *(RAP)*, blood pressure (mean arterial pressure *[MAP]*) and cardiac output *(CO)* fall. When RV pressure is exceeded (at the arrow), cardiac output and mean arterial pressure fall further.

Diffuse Effusion

A pericardial effusion is recognized as an echolucent space adjacent to the cardiac structures. In the absence of prior pericardial disease or surgery, pericardial effusions usually are diffuse and symmetric with clear separation between the parietal and visceral pericardium (Fig. 10.6). A relatively echogenic area anteriorly, in the absence of a posterior effusion, most likely represents a pericardial fat pad. M-mode recordings are helpful, especially with a small effusion, showing the flat posterior pericardial echo reflection and the moving epicardial echo with separation between the two in both systole and diastole.

In the apical views, the lateral, medial, and apical extent of the effusion can be appreciated. In the apical four-chamber view, an isolated echo-free space superior to the RA most likely represents pleural fluid. The subcostal view demonstrates fluid between the diaphragm and RV and is particularly helpful in echo-guided pericardiocentesis.

The size of the pericardial effusion is considered to be small when the separation between the heart and the parietal pericardium is <0.5 cm, moderate when it is 0.5 to 2 cm, and large when it is >2 cm. More quantitative measures of the size of the pericardial effusion rarely are needed in the clinical setting.

In patients with recurrent or long-standing pericardial disease, fibrinous stranding within the fluid and on the epicardial surface of the heart often is seen. When a malignant effusion is suspected, it is difficult to distinguish this nonspecific finding from

TABLE 10.3	Echocardiographic Approach to Suspected Pericardial Disease	
	Views and Data Recording	**Interpretation**
2D imaging	• Parasternal long- and short-axis • Apical 4-chamber, 2-chamber, and long-axis • Subcostal 4-chamber and short-axis • Use respirometer if available.	• Multiple views are needed to define the extent and size of the effusion. • Chamber collapse and septal shift are helpful in diagnosis of tamponade physiology or constrictive pericarditis. • Loculated effusions are seen only in some views. • TEE is helpful for posterior loculated effusion.
M-mode	• Parasternal at mid-LV level	• Pericardial separation with flat posterior pericardial echos and normal motion of the posterior wall is diagnostic for an effusion.
Pulsed Doppler	• LV and RV inflow with respiration • Hepatic vein flow • Pulmonary vein flow • Use respirometer if available.	• Reciprocal respiratory changes in RV and LV filling are seen with tamponade or constriction. • Hepatic and pulmonary venous flows show prominent atrial reversal and reduced systolic flow in constriction.
Tissue Doppler imaging	• E' velocity at septal and lateral annulus	• Septal E' velocity is higher with constriction than restriction. • Septal E' > lateral E' velocity with constriction.
Speckle tracking strain imaging	• Apical longitudinal strain with bullet display	• Overall, global longitudinal strain is normal with constriction, but localized reduced strain at the basal lateral wall is typical.

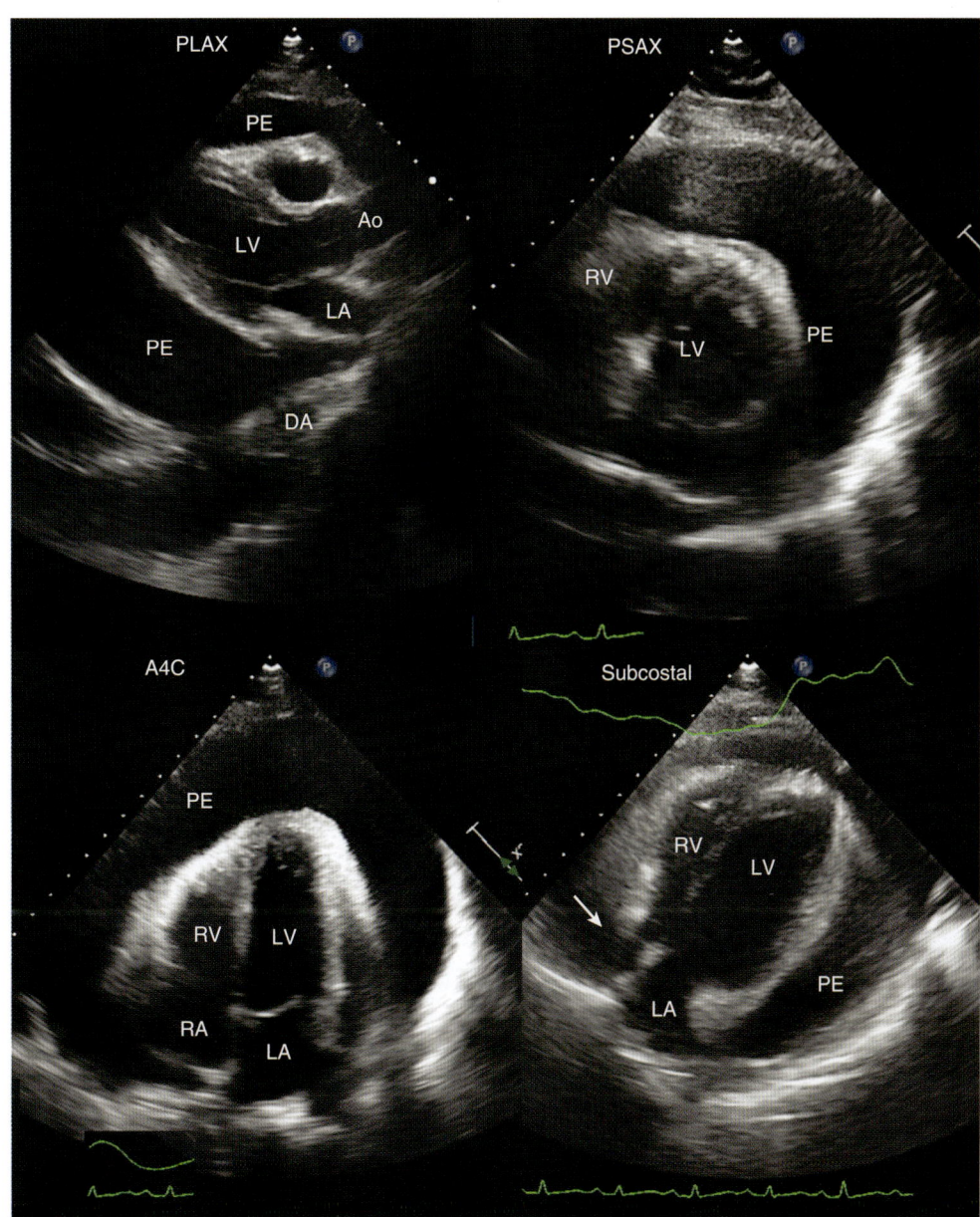

Fig. 10.6 Circumferential pericardial effusion. The echolucent effusion *(PE)* is seen in ▶ parasternal long-axis *(PLAX)*, ▶ short-axis *(PSAX)*, ▶ apical four-chamber *(A4C)*, and ▶ subcostal views in a patient early after mechanical aortic valve replacement. Note the shadowing and reverberations from the valve in the parasternal long-axis view. *Ao*, Aorta; *DA*, descending aorta.

metastatic disease. Features suggesting the latter include a nodular appearance, evidence of extension into the myocardium, and the appropriate clinical setting (Fig. 10.7).

Loculated Effusion

After surgical or percutaneous procedures, or in patients with recurrent pericardial disease, pericardial fluid often is *loculated* (Fig. 10.8). In this situation, the effusion is localized by adhesions to a small area of the pericardial space or consists of several separate areas of pericardial effusion, separated by adhesions. Recognition of a loculated effusion is especially important because hemodynamic compromise can occur with even a small, strategically located fluid collection. In addition, drainage of a loculated effusion is not always possible from a percutaneous approach.

Distinguishing From Pleural Fluid

To exclude the possibility of a loculated pericardial effusion reliably, echocardiographic evaluation requires examination from multiple acoustic windows. The

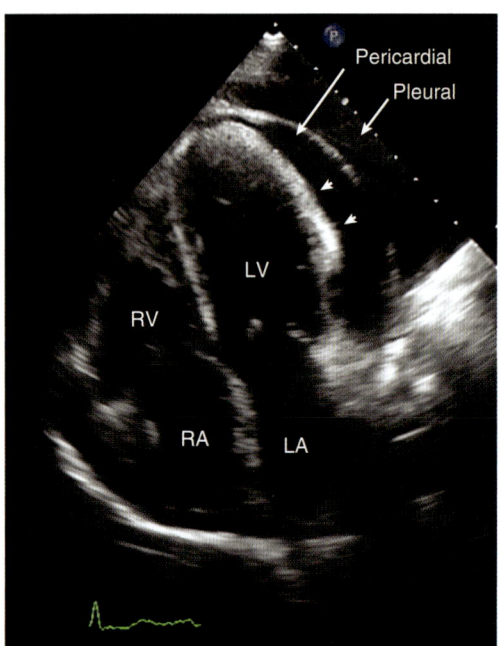

Fig. 10.7 ▶ **Malignant pericardial effusion.** Apical four-chamber view in a patient with metastatic lymphoma shows both a pericardial effusion lateral to the LV and pleural fluid. The irregular bright appearance along the lateral wall *(arrowheads)* is consistent with either adipose tissue or tumor involvement.

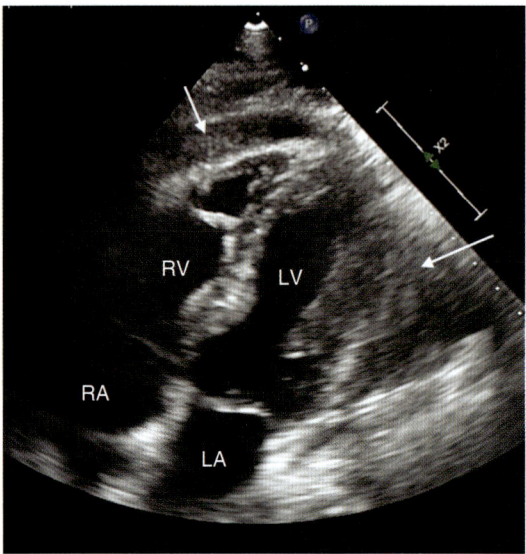

Fig. 10.8 ▶ **Pericardial hematoma.** In this subcostal four-chamber view, echogenic material is seen in the pericardial space anterior to the RV *(arrow)* and possibly lateral to the LV *(arrow)*, most consistent with hematoma after a percutaneous coronary procedure.

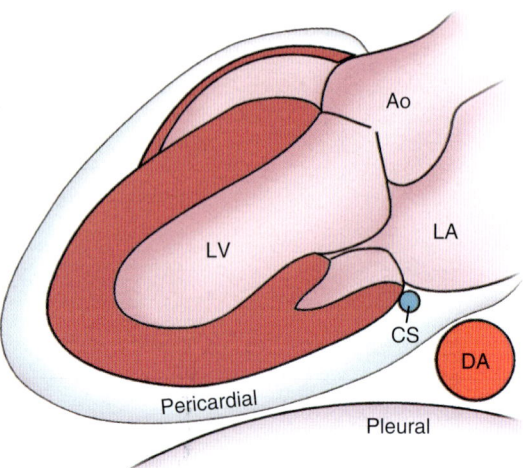

Fig. 10.9 ▶ **Pericardial versus pleural fluid.** Schematic diagram of the relationship between a pericardial effusion and the descending aorta *(DA)* compared with a left pleural effusion. Pericardial fluid tracks posterior to the LA in the oblique sinus of the pericardium, anterior to the descending aorta. *Ao,* Aorta; *CS,* coronary sinus.

parasternal approach demonstrates the extent of the fluid collection at the base of the heart in both long- and short-axis views. Note that pericardial fluid tracks posterior to the LA (in the oblique sinus), as well as posterior to the LV. Care should be taken that the coronary sinus or descending thoracic aorta is not mistaken for pericardial fluid. In fact, these structures can help in distinguishing pericardial from pleural fluid because a left pleural effusion extends posterolaterally to the descending aorta, whereas a pericardial effusion tracks anterior to the descending aorta (Fig. 10.9). When a large left pleural effusion is present, sometimes cardiac images can be obtained with the transducer on the patient's back (Fig. 10.10).

Clinical Utility

Echocardiography is very sensitive for the diagnosis of pericardial effusion, even when loculated, if care is taken to examine the heart in multiple tomographic planes from multiple acoustic windows. Loculated effusions can be difficult to assess in certain locations, particularly if they are localized to the atrial region, because the effusion itself may be mistaken for a normal cardiac chamber. TEE imaging better detects and defines the extent of loculated effusions after cardiac surgery, especially when the effusions are located posteriorly (Fig. 10.11).

Pericardial adipose tissue is common, especially anterior to the RV, and sometimes is mistaken for an effusion. Unlike pericardial fluid, adipose tissue exhibits a fine pattern of echogenicity, which helps with identification of this normal finding. A pericardial cyst is an uncommon congenital fluid filled sac, usually adjacent to the right heart. Pericardial cysts usually are missed on echocardiography and are better evaluated by chest CT or CMR. However, when present, they may be mistaken for a pericardial or pleural effusion (see Fig. 10.2).

The cause of the pericardial effusion is not always evident on echocardiographic examination. Irregular

Pericardial Disease | Chapter 10

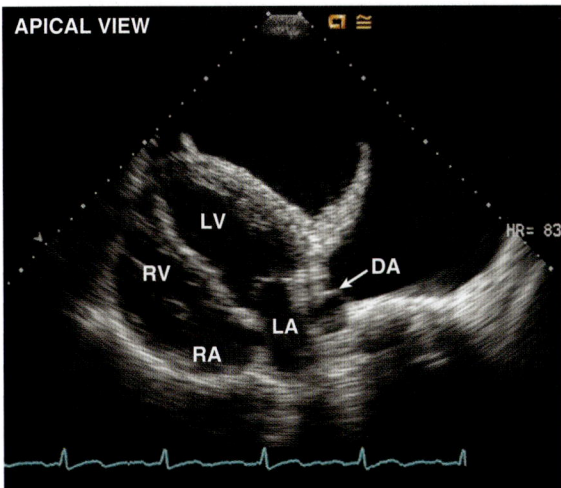

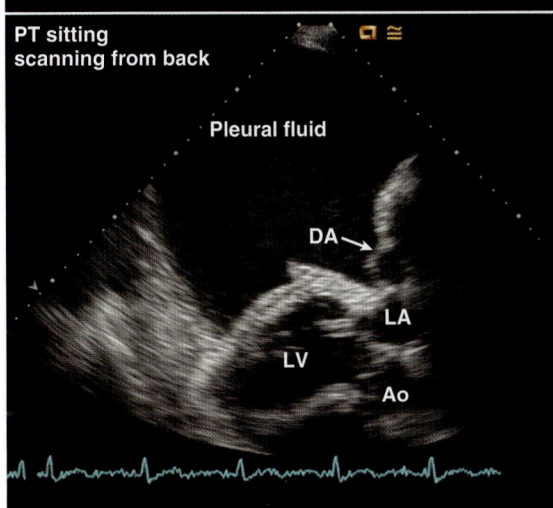

Fig. 10.10 Large pleural effusion. In a view with the transducer moved laterally from the apical position *(top)*, a large left pleural effusion is seen. This can be distinguished from pericardial fluid by the position of the descending aorta *(DA)*, by the presence of compressed lung, and by identification of both layers of the pericardium adjacent to the myocardium. Images also were obtained with the transducer on the patient's *(PT)* back *(bottom)*, thus demonstrating the relationship between the pleural fluid and the descending aorta. *Ao,* Aorta.

pericardial or epicardial masses in a patient with a known malignancy certainly raise the possibility of a malignant effusion, but this appearance can be mimicked by a fibrinous organization of a long-standing pericardial effusion. Masses adjacent to the cardiac structures (in the mediastinum) resulting in pericardial effusion can be missed by echocardiography. Wide-view tomographic imaging procedures, such as CT or CMR, are helpful in these cases.

Obviously, whether a pericardial effusion is infective or inflammatory in etiology cannot be determined by echocardiography. Depending on the associated clinical findings in each case, diagnostic pericardiocentesis, pericardial biopsy, or both will help establish the correct diagnosis.

With pericardial effusion due to aortic dissection or cardiac rupture (as a consequence of either myocardial infarction or a procedure), the entry site into the pericardium rarely can be detected, so a high level of suspicion is needed when these diagnoses are a possibility. The site of an LV rupture is "contained" by pericardial adhesions, resulting in formation of a pseudoaneurysm. A *pseudoaneurysm* is defined as a saccular structure communicating with the ventricle with walls composed of pericardium. In contrast, the walls of a "true" aneurysm are composed of thinned, scarred myocardium (see Fig. 8.27).

PERICARDIAL TAMPONADE

The term *pericardial tamponade* is defined as hemodynamic compromise—hypotension and/or decreased cardiac output—due to compression of the cardiac chambers by fluid in the pericardial space.

Echocardiographic Approach

When cardiac tamponade occurs with a diffuse, moderate to large pericardial effusion, the associated physiologic changes are evident on echocardiographic and Doppler examination (Fig. 10.12), including:

- RA systolic collapse for greater than one-third of systole
- RV diastolic collapse
- Reciprocal respiratory changes in RV and LV volumes (septal shifting)
- Reciprocal respiratory changes (>25%) in RV and LV filling
- Reduced early diastolic tissue Doppler velocity
- Severe dilation of the inferior vena cava

Right Atrial Systolic Collapse

When intrapericardial pressure exceeds RA systolic pressure (lowest point of the atrial pressure curve), inversion or collapse of the RA free wall occurs. Because the RA free wall is a thin, flexible structure, brief RA wall inversion can occur in the absence of tamponade physiology. However, the longer the duration of RA inversion relative to the cycle length, the greater is the likelihood of cardiac tamponade. Inversion for greater than one third of systole has a sensitivity of 94% and a specificity of 100% for the diagnosis of tamponade. Careful frame-by-frame 2D-image analysis is needed for this evaluation (Fig. 10.13).

Right Ventricular Diastolic Collapse

RV diastolic collapse occurs when intrapericardial pressure exceeds RV diastolic pressure *and* when the

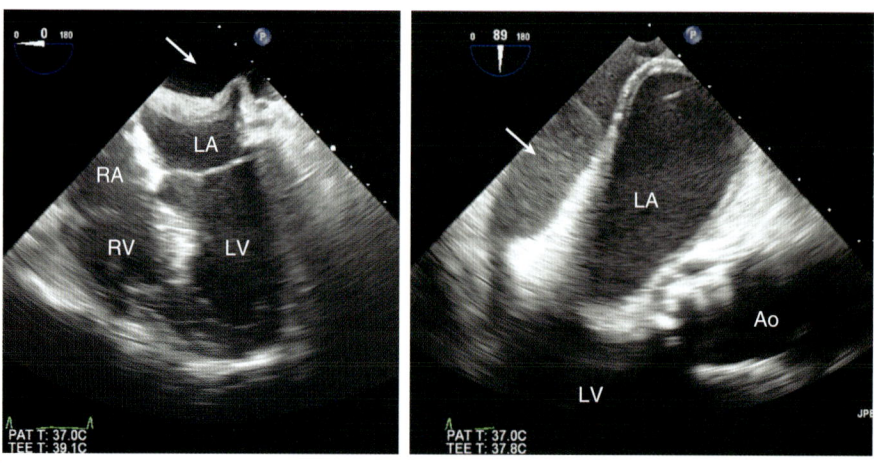

Fig. 10.11 ▶ ▶ **Transesophageal echocardiography imaging of loculated effusion.** In this patient with hypotension early after surgical aortic valve and root replacement, no pericardial fluid is noted around the RV or LV, but the TEE four-chamber and long-axis views show pericardial fluid posterior to the left atrium with compression of the left atrial wall resulting in tamponade physiology. *Ao,* Aorta.

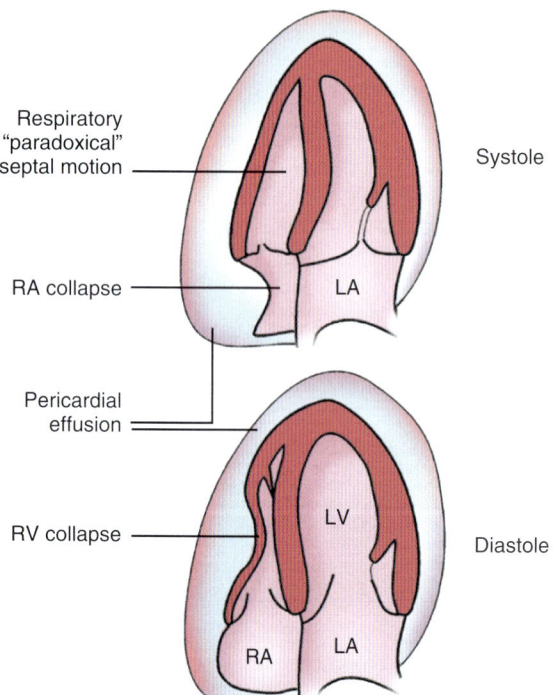

Fig. 10.12 2D echo findings with tamponade physiology.

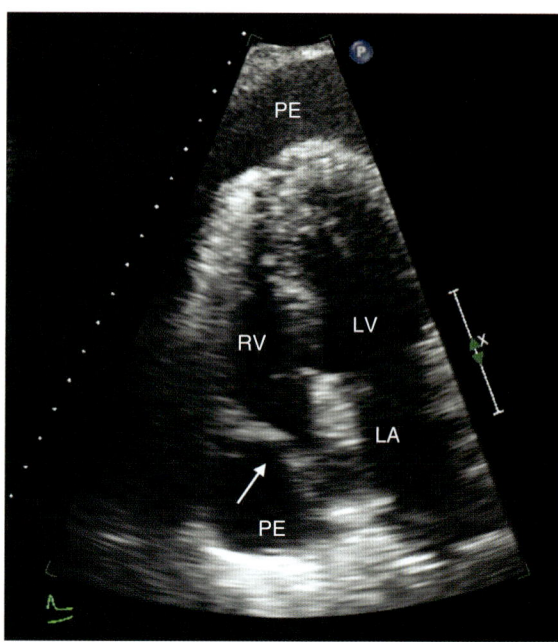

Fig. 10.13 ▶ **Right atrial systolic collapse.** Apical four-chamber view showing systolic collapse on the RA free wall *(arrow)* in a patient with clinical tamponade physiology. *PE,* Pericardial effusion.

RV free wall is normal in thickness and compliance. The presence of RV hypertrophy or infiltrative diseases of the myocardium allows development of a pressure gradient between the pericardial space and the RV chamber without inversion of the normal contour of the free wall. RV diastolic collapse is best appreciated in the parasternal long-axis view or from a subcostal window. If the timing of RV wall motion is not clear on 2D imaging, an M-mode recording through the RV free wall is helpful. The presence of RV diastolic collapse is somewhat less sensitive (60% to 90%) but more specific (85% to 100%) than brief RA systolic collapse for diagnosing tamponade physiology (Fig. 10.14).

Reciprocal Changes in Ventricular Volumes

Reciprocal respiratory variation in RV and LV volumes and consequent septal shifting are seen on 2D imaging when tamponade is present. In the apical four-chamber view, an increase in RV volume with inspiration (shift in septal motion toward the LV in diastole and toward the RV in systole) and a decrease during expiration (normalization of septal motion) can be appreciated.

Pericardial Disease | Chapter 10

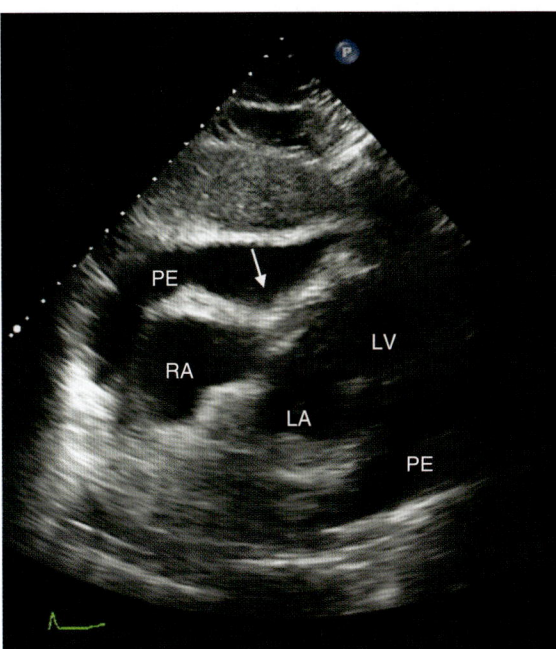

Fig. 10.14 ▶ **Right ventricular diastolic collapse.** In the same patient as in Fig. 10.13, the subcostal four-chamber view shows the pericardial effusion *(PE)* with compression (or collapse) of the RV *(arrows)* in diastole.

This pattern of motion corresponds to the physical finding of pulsus paradoxus. The proposed explanation for this observation is that total pericardial volume (heart chambers plus pericardial fluid) is fixed in tamponade; thus as intrathoracic pressure becomes more negative during inspiration, enhanced RV filling limits LV diastolic filling. This pattern reverses during expiration.

Respiratory Variation in Diastolic Filling

Doppler recordings of RV and LV diastolic filling in patients with tamponade physiology show a pattern that parallels the changes in ventricular volumes. With inspiration, the RV early diastolic filling velocity is augmented, whereas LV diastolic filling diminishes (Figs. 10.15 and 10.16). In addition, the flow velocity integral in the pulmonary artery increases with inspiration, whereas the aortic flow velocity integral decreases. In the acutely ill patient, these changes can be difficult to demonstrate in part because of respiratory changes in the intercept angle between the Doppler beam and the flow of interest, thus causing artifactual apparent velocity changes. Differentiating the normal respiratory variation in diastolic filling from the

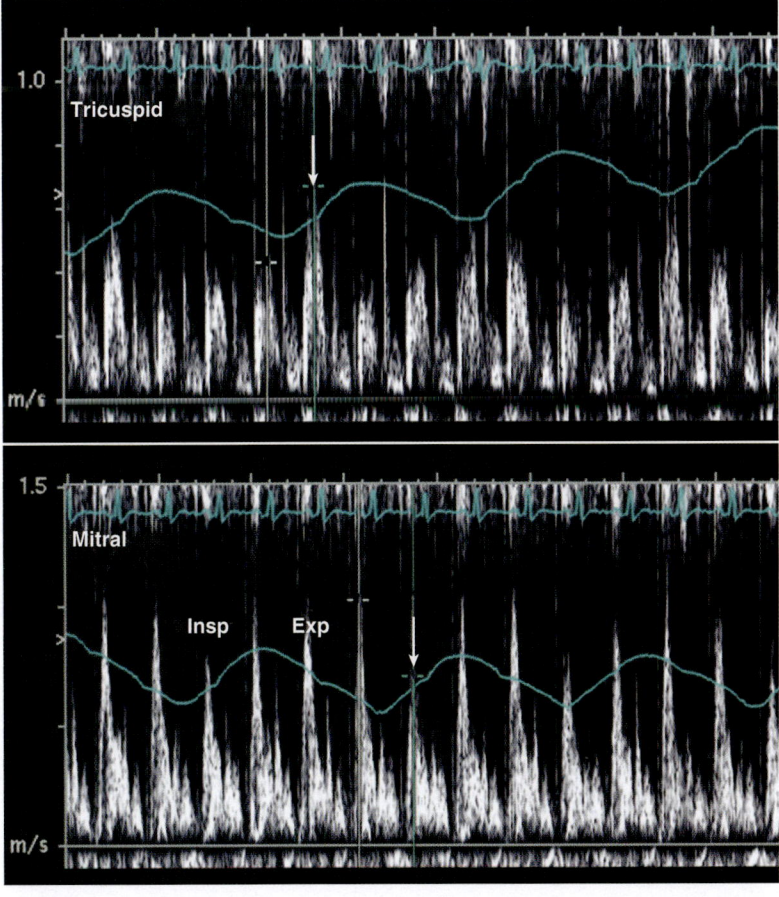

Fig. 10.15 Reciprocal respiratory variation in right ventricular and left ventricular filling. Doppler recording of LV inflow with superimposed respirometer tracing in a patient with tamponade showing increased tricuspid flow and decreased mitral flow *(arrows)* on the first beat after inspiration *(Insp)*, reflecting the reciprocal respiratory changes in RV and LV diastolic filling. *Exp,* Expiration.

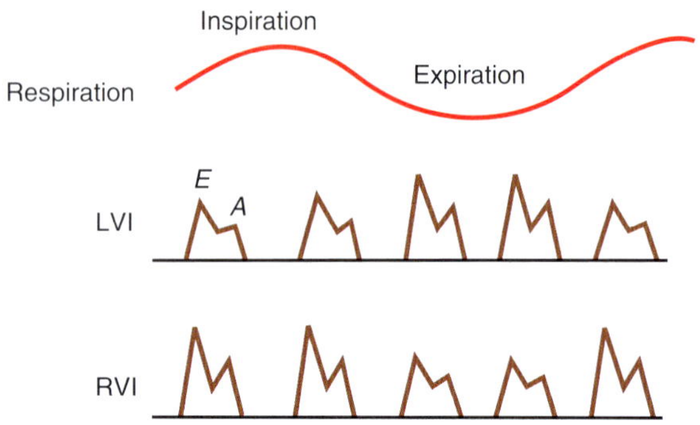

Fig. 10.16 Right ventricular and left ventricular inflow with tamponade physiology. Schematic diagram of LV and RV diastolic inflow (*RVI* and *LVI*) Doppler curves with tamponade physiology showing enhanced RV (and reduced LV) diastolic filling with inspiration and a reversal of this pattern during expiration.

excessive variation (>25%) seen in tamponade may be subtle in borderline cases. Tamponade physiology is not an all-or-none phenomenon; hemodynamic impairment is more evident as the degree of pericardial compression (pericardial pressure) increases.

Tissue Doppler Early Diastolic Velocity

The early diastolic mitral annular tissue Doppler velocity *(E′)* is reduced when tamponade is present and returns to normal after pericardiocentesis, likely reflecting changes in cardiac output. However, respiratory variation is not seen, and the sensitivity and specificity of this finding have not been evaluated.

Inferior Vena Cava Dilation

Inferior vena cava plethora, a dilated inferior vena cava with <50% inspiratory reduction in diameter near the inferior vena cava–RA junction, also is a sensitive (97%), albeit nonspecific (40%), indicator of tamponade physiology. This simple finding reflects the elevated RA pressure seen in tamponade.

Clinical Utility
Diagnosis of Pericardial Tamponade

In evaluating a patient for cardiac tamponade, it is essential to remember that tamponade is a clinical and hemodynamic diagnosis. Furthermore, varying degrees of tamponade physiology are possible. The most important finding on echocardiography in a patient with suspected pericardial tamponade is whether or not a pericardial effusion is present. The absence of a pericardial effusion *excludes* the diagnosis, but again care must be taken that a loculated effusion is not missed. Only rarely does tamponade physiology result from other mediastinal contents under pressure (e.g., air due to barotrauma or a compressive mass). Conversely, in a patient with convincing clinical evidence for tamponade, the presence of a moderate to large pericardial effusion on echocardiography *confirms* the diagnosis; further evaluation with Doppler is not needed and should not delay appropriate intervention.

In intermediate cases, either when the diagnosis has not been considered or when clinical evidence is equivocal, 2D findings of chamber collapse and inferior vena cava plethora in addition to Doppler findings showing marked respiratory variation in RV and LV filling are helpful, in conjunction with the clinical data (see Table B.10). Another approach to making this diagnosis is right heart catheterization showing depressed cardiac output and equalization of RA, RV diastolic, and pulmonary artery wedge pressures.

Echo-Guided Pericardiocentesis

The success rate without complications of percutaneous needle pericardiocentesis can be enhanced by using echocardiographic guidance. With the patient in the position planned for the procedure, the optimal transcutaneous approach is identified based on the location of the effusion, the distance from the chest wall to the pericardium, and the absence of intervening structures. The transducer angle and pericardial depth are noted, and the transducer position is marked before preparing the site for the procedure. After the procedure, the residual amount of pericardial fluid is assessed using standard tomographic views (Fig. 10.17). If monitoring during the procedure is needed, an acoustic window that allows visualization of the effusion but does not compromise the sterile field is identified. (Alternatively, a sterile sleeve is used for the transducer.) Note that with *tomographic* imaging it is difficult to identify the *tip* of the needle because any segment of the needle passing through the image plane appears to be the tip. The source of error is minimized by scanning in both superior-inferior and lateral-medial directions during the procedure or using 3D imaging. Confirmation that the needle tip is in the pericardial space can be made by injecting a small amount of agitated sterile saline solution through the needle to achieve an echo-contrast effect.

PERICARDIAL CONSTRICTION
Basic Principles

In constrictive pericarditis, the serous surfaces of the visceral and parietal pericardium are adherent, thickened, and fibrotic, with resultant loss of the pericardial space and impairment of diastolic ventricular filling. Pericardial constriction can occur after repeated episodes of pericarditis, after cardiac surgery, after radiation therapy, and from a variety of other causes. The diagnosis often is delayed because clinical symptoms are nonspecific—fatigue and malaise due to low cardiac output—and physical findings either

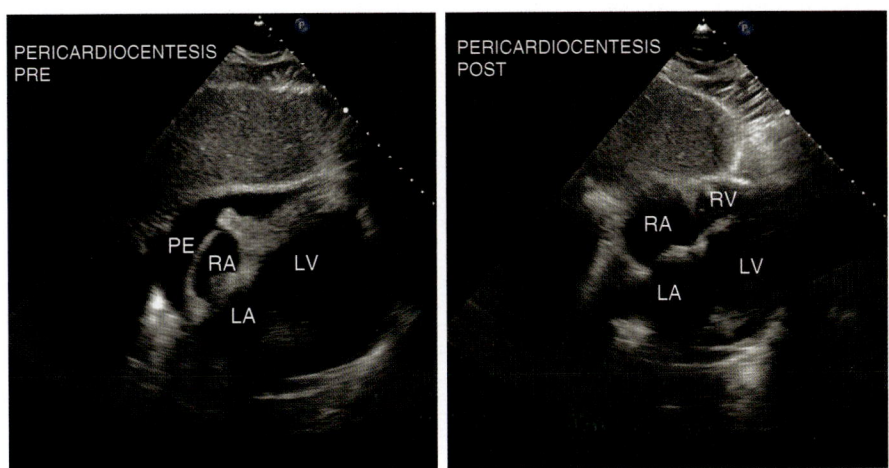

Fig. 10.17 Pericardiocentesis. Subcostal four-chamber view recorded in the catheterization laboratory immediately before and after pericardiocentesis with removal of 700 mL of fluid. On the pre-pericardiocentesis image *(left)*, ▶ a large pericardial effusion *(PE)*, a small ventricular chamber, and RA collapse are seen. The post-pericardiocentesis image *(right)* ▶ shows the absence of an effusion, an increase in RV and LV volumes, and a normal contour of the RA wall.

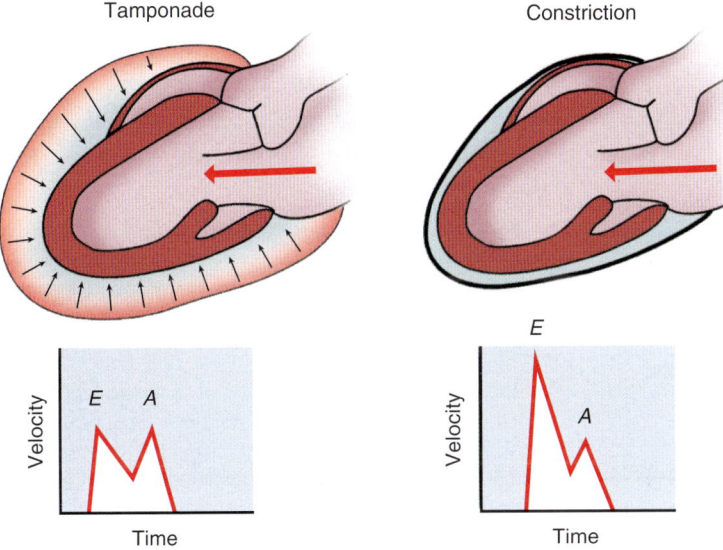

Fig. 10.18 Pericardial tamponade compared with pericardial constriction. With tamponade, diastolic filling is impaired in both early and late diastole because of the elevated pericardial pressures "compressing" the heart. With constriction, early diastolic filling is rapid but ends abruptly when the volume limits of the rigid pericardial space are reached.

are subtle (elevated jugular venous pressure, distant heart sounds) or occur only late in the disease course (ascites and peripheral edema).

The physiology of constrictive pericarditis is characterized by impaired diastolic cardiac filling due to the abnormal pericardium surrounding the cardiac structures, which act like a rigid "box" (Fig. 10.18). Early diastolic filling is rapid, with an abrupt cessation of ventricular filling as diastolic pressure rises—when the "box" is "full." Pressure tracings (Fig. 10.19) typically show:

- A brief, rapid fall of ventricular pressure in early diastole followed by
- A high mid-diastolic pressure plateau (*dip-plateau* or *square root sign*)
- A rapid fall in RA pressure with the onset of ventricular filling (*y*-descent)
- Only modest elevation of RV and pulmonary artery systolic pressures
- An RV diastolic pressure plateau that is one third or more of systolic pressure
- Equalization of diastolic pressures in the RV and LV even after volume loading

Echocardiographic Approach

Echocardiographic evaluation of the patient with possible constrictive pericarditis requires careful integration of imaging and Doppler data. In addition to standard imaging planes, Doppler flow, and tissue Doppler data, additional recordings of ventricular

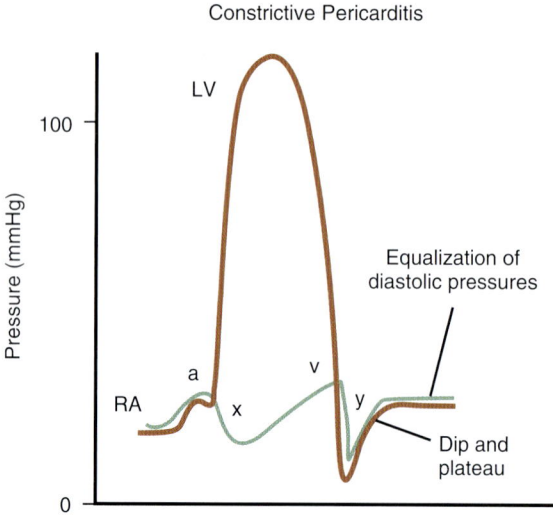

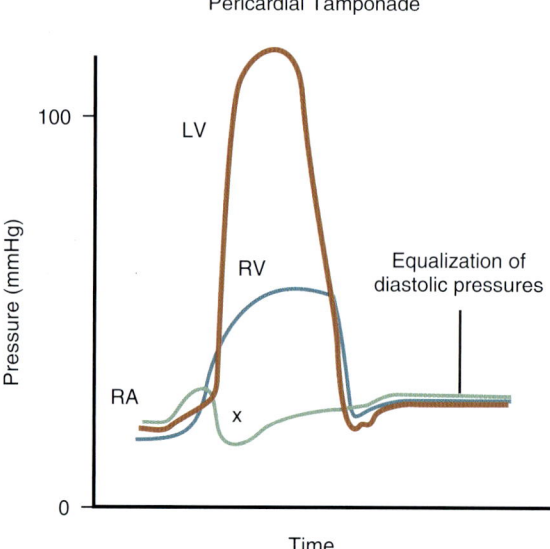

Fig. 10.19 Typical pressure tracings in tamponade and constriction.

and atrial inflows are needed at lower sweep speeds (to show more sequential beats on the saved images) with a respirometer tracing or other annotation of the respiratory phase.

Imaging

Typically, LV wall thickness, internal dimensions, and systolic function are normal in the patient with constrictive pericarditis. LA enlargement is seen because of chronic LA pressure elevation. Pericardial thickening is evident on 2D imaging as increased echogenicity in the region of the pericardium (Fig. 10.20). Careful examination from several acoustic windows is needed because the spatial distribution of pericardial thickening often is asymmetric.

M-mode imaging still is helpful for the diagnosis of pericardial thickening on transthoracic imaging. From the parasternal approach, an M-mode recording shows multiple echo-densities, posterior to the LV epicardium, moving parallel with each other; they persist even at a low-gain setting. High time resolution M-mode recordings also demonstrate abrupt posterior motion of the ventricular septum in early diastole, with flat motion in mid-diastole and abrupt anterior motion following atrial contraction. This pattern of motion appears to be due to initial rapid RV diastolic filling followed by both equalization of filling of the RV and LV as the "plateau" phase of the pressure curve is reached and increased RV filling after atrial contraction. The LV posterior wall endocardium shows little posterior motion during diastole (<2 mm from early to late diastole) because of the impairment of diastolic filling resulting in a "flat" pattern of diastolic posterior wall motion.

On subcostal views, the inferior vena cava and hepatic veins are dilated, reflecting the elevated RA pressure.

Doppler Examination

The Doppler findings in constrictive pericarditis reflect the abnormal hemodynamics in this condition (Figs. 10.21 and 10.22), including:

- Characteristic patterns of RA and LA filling
- Respiratory variation in LV and RV filling
- Respiratory variation in the isovolumic relaxation time (IVRT)
- Tissue Doppler S' >8 cm/s and E' >8 cm/s

Pulsed Doppler recordings of hepatic vein flow (from a subcostal approach) measure RA filling and show a prominent a-wave and a deep y-descent (Fig. 10.23) in addition to a marked increase in flow velocities with inspiration. Similarly, pulsed Doppler recordings of pulmonary vein flow (transthoracic apical four-chamber view or TEE approach) indicate LA filling and again show a prominent a-wave, prominent y-descent, a prominent diastolic filling phase, and blunting of the systolic phase of atrial filling.

Both RV and LV diastolic filling show a high E velocity, reflecting rapid early diastolic filling due to the initial high atrial to ventricular pressure difference. As LV pressure rises, filling abruptly ceases, reflected in a short deceleration time of the E velocity curve. Little ventricular filling occurs in late diastole because of the elevated LV diastolic pressure (the "plateau") and the constrictive effect of the thickened pericardium. Doppler recordings of ventricular inflow thus show a very small A velocity following atrial contraction.

Marked reciprocal respiratory variations in RV and LV diastolic inflow velocities are seen because of the differing effects of changes in intrapleural

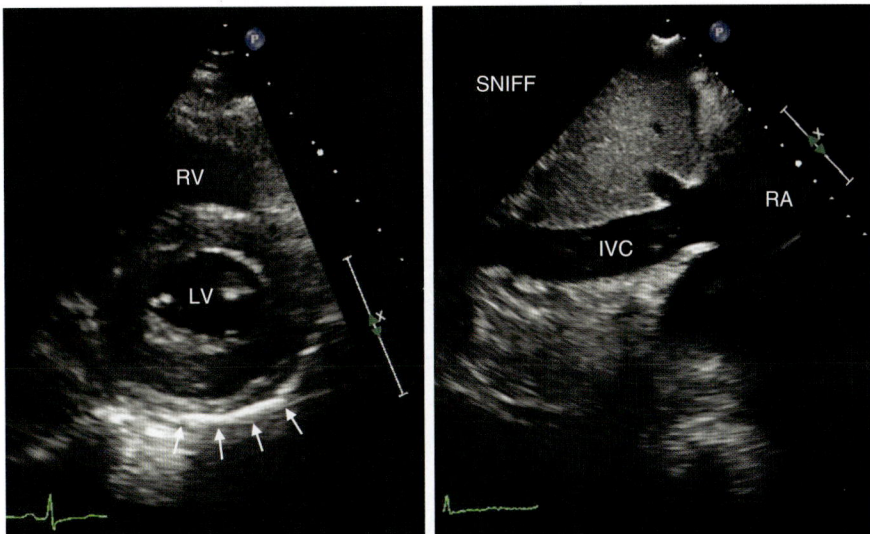

Fig. 10.20 ▶ ▶ **Constrictive pericarditis.** In the parasternal short-axis view, thickened pericardium *(arrows)* and a small effusion are seen posterior to the LV. The subcostal view shows a dilated inferior vena cava *(IVC)* with no respiratory change in diameter.

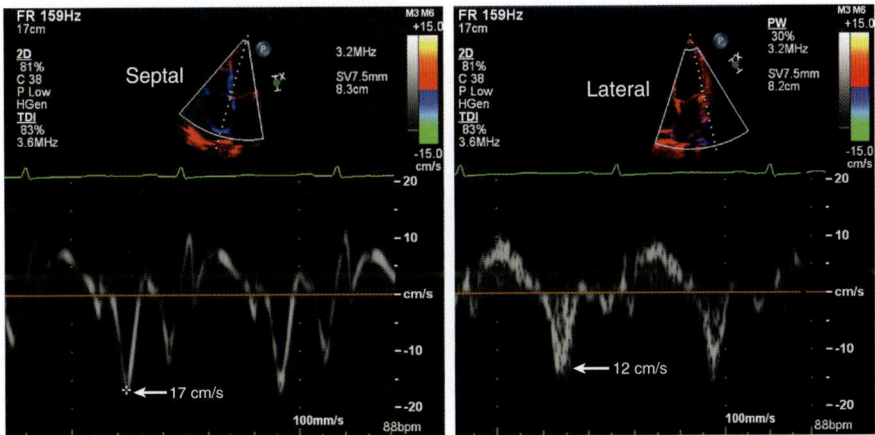

Fig. 10.21 Tissue Doppler annular motion with constrictive pericarditis. With constrictive pericarditis the typical pattern of a higher E′ velocity at the septum compared to the lateral wall is reversed. As in this example, septal annular E′ velocity is 17 cm/s compared with a lateral annular E′ velocity of 12 cm/s, an imaging finding sometimes called "annulus reversus." The likely explanation for this finding is restriction diastolic expansion of the lateral LV wall by the adherence pericardium with a compensatory increase in septal motion as the LV fills in early diastole.

pressure on filling of the two ventricles (Fig. 10.24). With inspiration, intrapleural pressure becomes more negative, resulting in augmentation of RV diastolic filling and inflow velocity. In contrast, LV filling velocities *decrease* with inspiration and *increase* with expiration. Although similar directional changes in filling velocities occur in normal individuals, the respiratory changes are much greater (variation >25%) in patients with constrictive pericarditis.

The LV isovolumic relaxation time—measured from the aortic closure to the mitral opening click on Doppler recordings—increases by a mean of 20% with inspiration in patients with constrictive pericarditis. Tissue Doppler findings in constrictive pericarditis include an increased early diastolic velocity *(E′)*, consistent with rapid early diastolic filling.

Constrictive Pericarditis Versus Restrictive Cardiomyopathy

Even though the hemodynamic features of pericardial tamponade and pericardial constriction have some similarities, differentiating between these two diagnoses usually is straightforward based on the presence or absence of a pericardial effusion (Table 10.4). Differentiating between constrictive pericarditis and a restrictive cardiomyopathy is more difficult. Both are characterized by clinical signs and symptoms of elevated venous pressure and low cardiac output, and both show a normal-sized LV chamber with normal systolic function on 2D echocardiography. Pericardial thickening frequently is difficult to appreciate, and other 2D and M-mode findings do not reliably differentiate

Fig. 10.22 Doppler flow patterns in constrictive pericarditis versus those in restrictive cardiomyopathy. In a patient with constrictive pericarditis, LV inflow *(LVI)* shows respiratory variation, an elevated *E* velocity with a steep deceleration time, and a small A velocity; tissue Doppler imaging *(TDI)* shows an *E′* greater than 8 cm/s; and pulmonary vein *(PV)* inflow shows a ratio of systolic *(S)* to diastolic *(D)* flow of about 1. In contrast, with restrictive cardiomyopathy, little respiratory variation occurs, *E′* is reduced, and the pulmonary S/D ratio is reduced. Δ, Change.

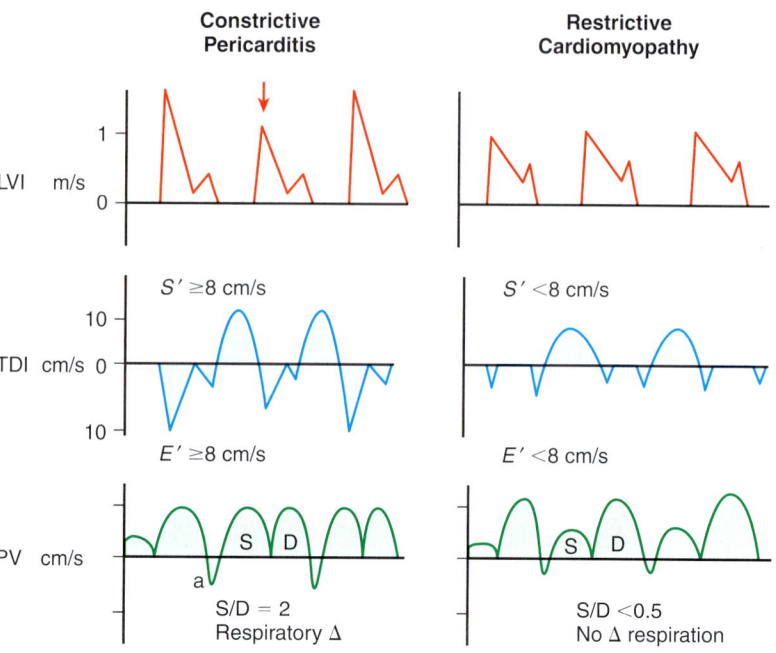

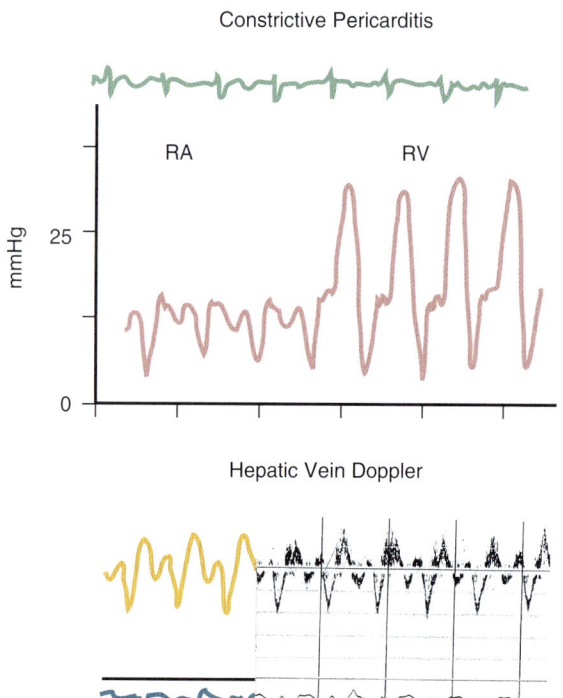

Fig. 10.23 Pressure tracing and hepatic vein flow in a patient with constrictive pericarditis. Note the prominent *a*-wave, flat diastolic segment, and prominent *y*-descent, all consistent with the "square root sign" or dip and plateau in the pressure tracings.

between these two diagnoses. Doppler findings that favor constrictive pericarditis over restrictive cardiomyopathy include (1) reciprocal respiratory changes in ventricular volumes and filling parameters with a 25% or greater difference in maximum *E* velocity from expiration to inspiration and (2) normal or only mildly elevated pulmonary pressures. The relative difference in the *E′* tissue Doppler velocity also is helpful. With restrictive cardiomyopathy, the septal *E′* velocity is lower than the lateral *E′* velocity (e.g., the normal pattern). With constrictive pericarditis, this pattern is reversed with a higher septal compared with lateral *E′* velocity, often called "annulus reversus" due to tethering of the lateral wall by the adherent pericardium. However, Doppler data are not absolutely accurate because of overlap among groups in the Doppler findings and because of differing hemodynamics in patients with restrictive cardiomyopathy depending on disease stage (see Chapter 9).

Studies suggest that newer approaches, such as speckle tracking echocardiography, may be useful in differentiating constrictive pericarditis from restrictive cardiomyopathy (Fig. 10.25).

Clinical Utility

The diagnosis of pericardial constriction remains problematic, with no single diagnostic feature on echocardiographic or Doppler examination. However, the conjunction of several findings in a patient in whom the level of clinical suspicion is high increases the likelihood of this diagnosis and is definitive in some cases (see Table B.11). Conversely, the echo and Doppler findings sometimes provide the first clues to this diagnosis in a patient in whom it was not previously considered, for example, a patient presenting with ascites and no prior cardiac history.

TEE is more accurate than transthoracic echocardiography for the diagnosis of pericardial thickening,

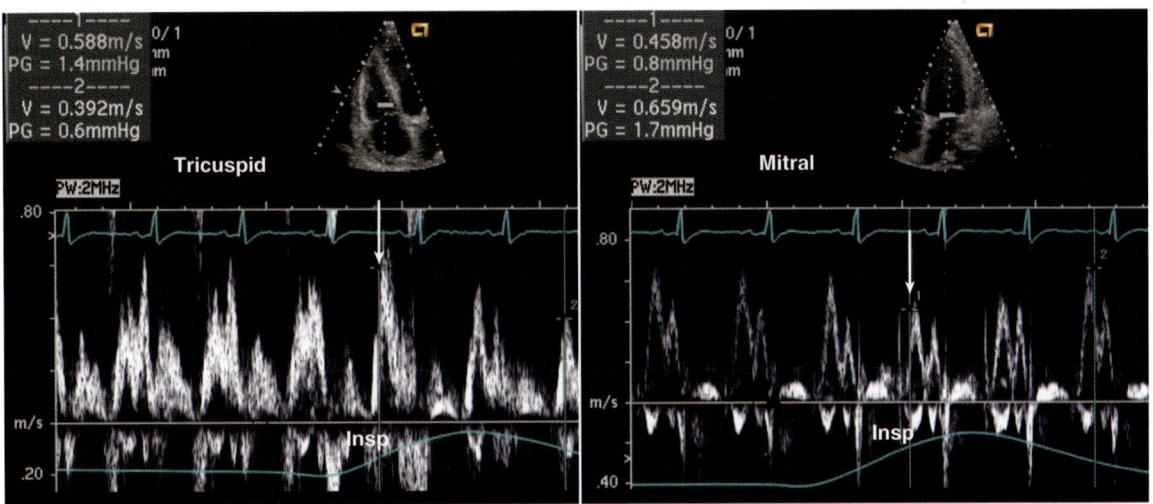

Fig. 10.24 Respiratory variation in right ventricular and left ventricular diastolic filling in constrictive pericarditis. An increase in tricuspid flow and a decrease in mitral flow velocities are noted on the first beat after inspiration *(Insp, arrows)*, with the decrease greater than 25% compared with the maximum velocities.

TABLE 10.4	Comparison of Pericardial Tamponade, Constriction, and Restrictive Cardiomyopathy		
	Pericardial Tamponade	**Constrictive Pericarditis**	**Restrictive Cardiomyopathy**
Hemodynamics			
RA pressure	↑	↑	↑
RV/LV filling pressures	↑, RV = LV	↑, RV = LV	↑, LV > RV
Pulmonary artery pressures	Normal	Mild elevation (35–40 mmHg systolic)	Moderate to severe elevation (≥60 mmHg systolic)
RV diastolic pressure plateau		> ⅓ peak RV pressure	> ⅓ peak RV pressure
Radionuclide diastolic filling		Rapid early filling, impaired late filling	Impaired early filling
2D echo	Moderate to large PE Inferior vena cava plethora	Pericardial thickening without effusion	LV hypertrophy Normal systolic function
	Small ventricular chambers RV diastolic and RA systolic collapse	Respiratory ventricular septal shift	No respiratory change in septal motion
Doppler echo	Reciprocal respiratory changes in RV and LV filling	E > a on LV inflow Prominent y-descent in hepatic vein Pulmonary venous flow = prominent a-wave, reduced systolic phase Respiratory variation in IVRT and in E velocity	(1) Early in disease e < A on LV inflow (2) Late in disease E > a (3) Constant IVRT (4) Absence of significant respiratory variation
Tissue Doppler	↓ E' without respiratory variation	↑ E' Lateral E' < septal E'	E' <8 cm/s with S' <8 cm/s Lateral E' > septal E'
Longitudinal systolic strain		Normal	Globally decreased
Other diagnostic tests	Therapeutic/diagnostic pericardiocentesis	CT or CMR for pericardial thickening	Endomyocardial biopsy

CMR, Cardiac magnetic resonance imaging; *CT,* computed tomography; *IVRT,* isovolumic relaxation time; *PE,* pericardial effusion.

Fig. 10.25 Strain imaging in constriction. Longitudinal systolic strain (speckle tracking) "bull's-eye" map in a patient with constrictive pericarditis. Global average longitudinal systolic strain is nearly normal (−17.8%). Lateral *(LAT)* strain is prominently reduced compared with septal *(SEPT)* strain because of the tethering effects of the diseased pericardium. *A2C,* Apical two-chamber; *A4C,* apical four-chamber; *ANT,* Anterior; *INF,* inferior; *POST,* posterior. *(From Otto CM, editor:* The Practice of Clinical Echocardiography, *ed 5, Philadelphia, 2017, Fig. 28.10.)*

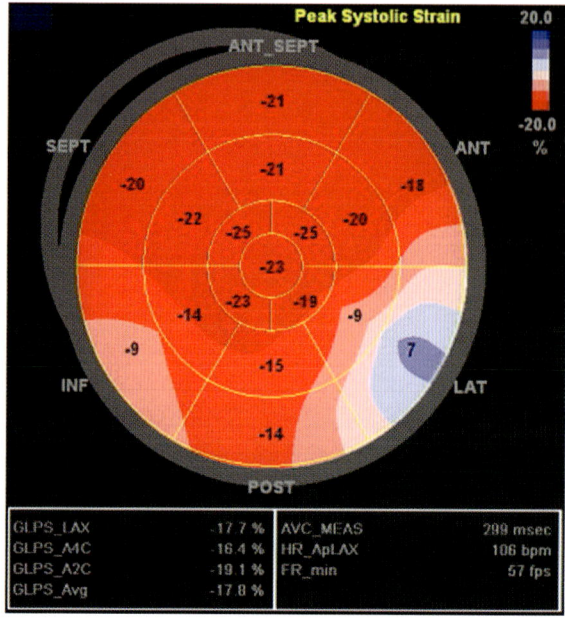

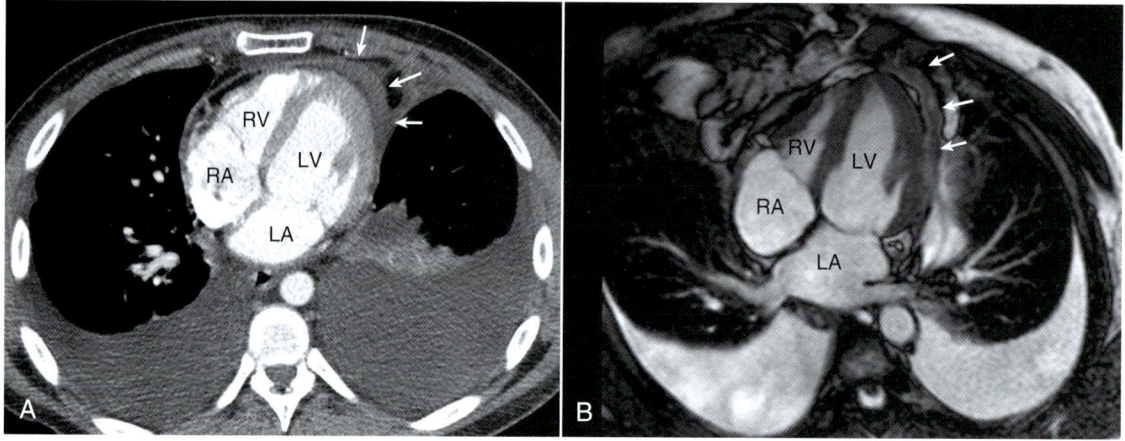

Fig. 10.26 Computed tomography and cardiac magnetic resonance imaging for pericardial thickening. In a 32-year-old man who received radiation therapy 15 years ago, chest computed tomography (A) shows thickening of the pericardium *(arrows)* and bilateral pleural effusion. (B) In the same patient, a similar cardiac magnetic resonance view shows pericardial thickening as a low-signal band *(arrows)* at the apex and around the lateral LV wall, anterior to the RV.

with a sensitivity of 95% and specificity of 86%. However, CT or CMR scanning is more definitive for the detection of pericardial thickening and calcification, especially when they are asymmetric (Fig. 10.26). Endomyocardial biopsy occasionally confirms a diagnosis of restrictive cardiomyopathy due to an infiltrative process. Right- and left-sided heart catheterization shows equalization of diastolic pressure in the four cardiac chambers when constrictive pericarditis is present.

Differentiation between constrictive pericarditis and restrictive cardiomyopathy is further complicated by the concurrent presence of both conditions in some patients, for example, in patients with radiation-induced heart disease. Similarly, although constrictive pericarditis typically occurs in the absence of a pericardial effusion, some patients have an overlap condition with a clinical presentation consistent with effusive-constrictive pericarditis.

THE ECHO EXAM

Pericardial Disease

Pericardial Effusion

Views
- Parasternal
- Apical
- Subcostal

Distinguish from pleural fluid

Size
- Small (<0.5 cm)
- Moderate (0.5–2.0 cm)
- Large (>2.0 cm)

Diffuse versus loculated

Evaluate for tamponade physiology if moderate or large

TEE if needed, especially in postoperative patients

Pericardial Tamponade

Clinical findings
- Low cardiac output
- Elevated venous pressures
- Pulsus paradoxus
- Hypotension

2D-echo
- Moderate to large pericardial effusion
- RA systolic collapse (duration greater than one third of systole)
- RV diastolic collapse
- Reciprocal respiratory changes in RV and LV volumes
- Inferior vena cava plethora

Doppler
- Respiratory variation in RV and LV diastolic filling
- Increased RV filling on first beat after inspiration
- Decreased LV filling on first beat after inspiration

Constrictive Pericarditis

Imaging
- Pericardial thickening
- Normal LV size and systolic function
- LA enlargement
- Flattened diastolic wall motion
- Abrupt posterior motion of the ventricular septum in early diastole
- Dilated inferior vena cava and hepatic veins

Doppler
- Prominent y-descent on hepatic vein or superior vena cava flow pattern
- LV inflow showing prominent E velocity with a rapid early diastolic deceleration slope and a small or absent A velocity
- Increase in LV IVRT by >20% on first beat after inspiration
- Respiratory variations in RV and LV diastolic filling (difference >25%) with inspiratory ↑RV ↓LV filling with inspiration
- Tissue Doppler ↑ E′ >8 cm/s with S′ >8 cm/s
- Annulus reversus with septal E′ > lateral E′
- Pulmonary venous flow showing prominent a-wave and blunting of systolic phase

LV Pseudoaneurysm

- Abrupt transition from normal myocardium to aneurysm
- Acute angle between myocardium and aneurysm
- Narrow neck
- Ratio of neck diameter to aneurysm diameter <0.5
- Often lined with thrombus

IVRT, Isovolumic relaxation time.

SUGGESTED READING

General

1. Welch TD: Pericardial disease. In Otto CM, editor: *The Practice of Clinical Echocardiography*, 5th ed, Philadelphia, 2017, Elsevier, pp 556–576.
   Detailed chapter on pericardial disease with discussions of anatomy and physiology, pathophysiology of constriction and tamponade, a practical echocardiographic approach, and numerous illustrations of echocardiographic findings. 89 references.

2. Klein AL, Abbara S, Agler DA, et al: American Society of Echocardiography clinical recommendations for multimodality cardiovascular imaging of patients with pericardial disease: endorsed by the Society for Cardiovascular Magnetic Resonance and Society of Cardiovascular Computed Tomography, *J Am Soc Echocardiogr* 26(9):965–1012, 2013.
   Consensus document with a textbook-style summary of pericardial anatomy, pathophysiology, and each type of pericardial disease. In addition to pericarditis, effusion, and tamponade, detailed information is provided about rarer diagnoses such as effusive-constrictive pericarditis, pericardial masses, pericardial cysts, and congenital absence of the pericardium. Detailed echo protocols are provided in an appendix. 63 pages. 58 figures plus 49 supplemental figures, 215 references.

3. Adler Y, Charron P, Imazio M, et al: 2015 ESC guidelines for the diagnosis and management of pericardial diseases: the Task Force for the Diagnosis and Management of Pericardial Diseases of the European Society of Cardiology (ESC) endorsed by: the European Association for Cardio-Thoracic Surgery (EACTS), *Eur Heart J* 36:2921, 2015.
   The section on diagnosis in these guidelines emphasizes that TTE is the "first-line imaging test in patients with suspected pericardial disease." Additional standard testing includes markers of inflammation (e.g., C-reactive protein levels), standard blood tests, electrocardiography, and chest radiography. CT and CMR imaging also

are helpful, particularly for diagnosis of pericardial thickening.

4. Rodriguez ER, Tan CD: Structure and anatomy of the human pericardium, *Prog Cardiovasc Dis* 59(4):327–340, 2017.
   Detailed review of pericardial anatomy with anatomic illustrations and histologic correlation.

5. Hoit BD: Pathophysiology of the pericardium, *Prog Cardiovasc Dis* 59(4):341–348, 2017.
   Both cardiac tamponade and pericardial constriction result in elevated and equalized filling pressures in the atria and ventricles, septal shift with respiration, and reduced cardiac output. However, early diastolic filling is reduced in tamponade but increased with constriction. With cardiac tamponade the pericardial space continues to transmit respiratory changes in thoracic pressure that result in an inspiratory increase in venous return. With pericardial constriction, intrathoracic pressure changes are not transmitted to the cardiac chambers, so no respiratory increase in venous return occurs.

6. Verhaert D, Gabriel RS, Johnston D, et al: The role of multimodality imaging in the management of pericardial disease, *Circ Cardiovasc Imaging* 3:333, 2010.
   Concise, well-illustrated review of different imaging modalities for pericardial disease with a useful flow chart to guide diagnostic testing.

Pericarditis

7. Imazio M, Gaita F: Diagnosis and treatment of pericarditis, *Heart* 101(14):1159–1168, 2015.
   Pericarditis may be due to a wide range of causes including viral infection, inflammatory diseases, pericardial injury, and cancer (especially lung cancer, breast cancer, and lymphoma), but most cases have no identifiable cause (i.e., idiopathic). Diagnosis is based on clinical features, with echocardiography to evaluate for effusion and tamponade physiology. The review summarizes the etiology, presentation, and management of pericarditis.

8. Cremer PC, Kumar A, Kontzias A, et al: Complicated pericarditis: understanding risk factors and pathophysiology to inform imaging and treatment, *J Am Coll Cardiol* 68(21):2311–2328, 2016.
   In this review, the authors suggest that risk factors for development of complicated pericarditis are use of early high-dose corticosteroids, failure to use colchicine, and an elevated high-sensitivity C-reactive protein level. Therapies that reduce inflammation prevent recurrent episodes and increase the likelihood of disease resolution. CMR imaging of inflammation may be helpful in monitoring therapy.

9. Imazio M: Pericardial involvement in systemic inflammatory diseases, *Heart* 97(22):1882–1892, 2011.
   Pericardial involvement is common in patients with a systemic inflammatory disease; it usually reflects systemic disease activity, effusion size often is larger than that seen with idiopathic pericarditis, and the effusion may be the first sign of the systemic inflammatory disease. An emerging cause of pericarditis is autoinflammatory disease, caused by mutations in genes involved in regulation or activation of the inflammatory response, such as familial Mediterranean fever and the tumor necrosis factor receptor-1 associated periodic syndrome (TRAPS).

Pericardial Effusion

10. Vakamudi S, Ho N, Cremer PC: Pericardial effusions: causes, diagnosis, and management, *Prog Cardiovasc Dis* 59(4):380–388, 2017.
    Nicely illustrated review of the presentation, diagnosis, and management of pericardial effusion.

11. Veress G, Feng D, Oh JK: Echocardiography in pericardial diseases: new developments, *Heart Fail Rev* 18(3):267–275, 2013.
    Concise review summarizing developments in the echocardiographic evaluation of pericardial disease. Includes a discussion of the role of tissue Doppler imaging with examples of E and E′ changes with constrictive pericarditis. Speckle tracking echocardiography also can be used to demonstrate abnormal longitudinal mechanics in patients with restrictive cardiomyopathy, whereas abnormal circumferential deformation, torsion, and untwisting are seen in patients with constrictive pericarditis.

Pericardial Tamponade

12. Chandraratna PA, Mohar DS, Sidarous PF: Role of echocardiography in the treatment of cardiac tamponade, *Echocardiography* 31(7):899–910, 2014.
    Provides an explanation of the pathophysiology of tamponade and includes illustrations and flow charts for use of echocardiography to guide removal of pericardial fluid.

13. Refaat MM, Katz WE: Neoplastic pericardial effusion, *Clin Cardiol* 34(10):593–598, 2011.
    Neoplastic pericardial effusions occur with direct extension or metastatic spread of the underlying malignant disease. Oncology patients also may have effusions due to opportunistic infection, complications of radiation therapy, or toxicity of chemotherapy. Management depends on the patient's prognosis and clinical presentation, with therapeutic options including pericardiocentesis, sclerotherapy, balloon pericardiotomy, and surgical intervention.

Pericardial Constriction

14. Welch TD, Ling LH, Espinosa RE, et al: Echocardiographic diagnosis of constrictive pericarditis: Mayo Clinic criteria, *Circ Cardiovasc Imaging* 7:526, 2014.
    In a study of 130 patients with surgically confirmed constrictive pericarditis, the three echocardiographic variables independently associated with constriction were 2D or M-mode evidence of ventricular septal shift, septal annular tissue Doppler E′ velocity 9 cm/s or greater, and a hepatic vein pulsed Doppler diastolic reversal ratio (reversal velocity divided by forward velocity in diastole) of 0.79 or higher. The combination of septal shift and one of the other factors was most accurate for diagnosing constriction, with a sensitivity of 87% and a specificity of 91%. Although specificity increased to 97% when all three factors are present, sensitivity fell to 64%.

15. Miranda WR, Oh JK: Constrictive pericarditis: a practical clinical approach, *Prog Cardiovasc Dis* 59(4):369–379, 2017.
    Practical approach to echocardiographic evaluation of the patient with suspected constrictive pericarditis including flow charts, hemodynamic tracings, and echocardiographic images.

16. Coylewright M, Welch TD, Nishimura RA: Mechanism of septal bounce in constrictive pericarditis: a simultaneous cardiac catheterisation and echocardiographic study, *Heart* 99(18):1376, 2013.
    Short case report showing the correlation between direct pressure measurements in the LV and RV and the pattern of septal motion on echocardiography.

17. Butz T, Piper C, Langer C, et al: Diagnostic superiority of a combined assessment of the systolic and early diastolic mitral annular velocities by tissue Doppler imaging for the differentiation of restrictive cardiomyopathy from constrictive pericarditis, *Clin Res Cardiol* 99(4):207–215, 2010.
    In 26 patients with restrictive cardiomyopathy due to amyloidosis, compared with 34 patients with constrictive pericarditis, tissue Doppler septal annular velocities were lower for both: (1) systolic

longitudinal velocity (S') (4.1 ± 1.5 vs. 7.3 ± 2.1 cm/s; P < 0.001) and (2) early diastolic longitudinal velocity (E') (4.1 ± 1.6 vs. 12.9 ± 4.9 cm/s; P < 0.001). The combined use of an averaged (septal and lateral annular) S' cutoff value <8 cm/s plus an E' cutoff value <8 cm/s had a 93% sensitivity rate and an 88% specificity rate for the diagnosis of restrictive cardiomyopathy.

18. Choi JH, Choi JO, Ryu DR, et al: Mitral and tricuspid annular velocities in constrictive pericarditis and restrictive cardiomyopathy: correlation with pericardial thickness on computed tomography, *JACC Cardiovasc Imaging* 4(6):567–575, 2011.
    In 37 patients with constrictive pericarditis, the ratio of lateral and septal E' was significantly lower (0.94 ± 0.17) in patients with constrictive pericarditis compared with 35 patients with restrictive cardiomyopathy (1.35 ± 0.31; P < 0.001) or 70 normal controls (1.36 ± 0.24; P < 0.001).

Other

19. Kim MJ, Kim HK, Jung JH, et al: Echocardiographic diagnosis of total or left congenital pericardial absence with positional change, *Heart* 103(15):1203–1209, 2017.
    In 11 patients with congenital absence of the pericardium confirmed by CT or CMR imaging, echocardiography shows dynamic alterations in cardiac position with changes in patient positioning that are not seen with other cardiac conditions. In brief, when the patient is in a left lateral decubitus position, the cardiac apex is dorsally displaced at end-diastole at end-diastole and swings anteriorly in systole. This unique cardiac movement is not observed when the patient lies in the right lateral decubitus position because the heart is now positioned more anteriorly in the thorax, a position that limits further anterior motion in systole.

20. Heidenreich PA, Kapoor JR: Radiation induced heart disease: systemic disorders in heart disease, *Heart* 95(3):252–258, 2009.
    Detailed review of the late effects of radiation therapy on the heart. Acute pericarditis is less common with current radiation protocols, but it still occurs in about 5% of patients. However, about 20% of patients develop evidence of constrictive pericarditis, typically in the 10 years after mediastinal irradiation. Radiation also can lead to myocardial fibrosis, particularly that of the RV, with resultant diastolic and systolic dysfunction, and is associated with conduction system disease, premature calcific valve disease, and early coronary atherosclerosis.

21. Tower-Rader A, Kwon D: Pericardial masses, cysts and diverticula: a comprehensive review using multimodality imaging, *Prog Cardiovasc Dis* 59(4):389–397, 2017.
    Pericardial masses, cysts, and diverticula are quite rare and thus may be confusing when seen on echocardiography. Pericardial tumors sometimes appear circumferentially, mimicking a pericardial hematoma, and other times they are nodular or irregular in shape and location, depending on tumor type and the pattern of disease spread. A benign congenital outpouching of the pericardium is seen as a circumscribed echolucent area adjacent to the pericardium on echocardiography and is defined as a cyst (no communication with pericardial space) or diverticulum.

11 Valvular Stenosis

BASIC PRINCIPLES
  Approach to the Evaluation of Valvular Stenosis
  Fluid Dynamics of Valvular Stenosis
    High-Velocity Jet
    Relationship Between Pressure Gradient and Velocity
    Distal Flow Disturbance
    Proximal Flow Patterns
AORTIC STENOSIS
  Diagnostic Imaging of the Aortic Valve
    Calcific Aortic Stenosis
    Bicuspid Aortic Valve
    Rheumatic Aortic Stenosis
    Congenital Aortic Stenosis
    Differential Diagnosis
  Quantitation of Aortic Stenosis Severity
    Maximum Aortic Jet Velocity
    Pressure Gradients
    Continuity Equation Valve Area
    Other Measures
  Coexisting Valvular Disease
  Response of the Left Ventricle
  Clinical Applications
    Decisions About Timing of Intervention
    Disease Progression and Prognosis in Asymptomatic Aortic Stenosis
  Evaluation of Low Flow Aortic Stenosis
    Aortic Stenosis With Left Ventricular Systolic Dysfunction
    Low Flow Aortic Stenosis With a Normal LV Ejection Fraction

MITRAL STENOSIS
  Diagnostic Imaging of the Mitral Valve
    Rheumatic Disease
    Mitral Annular Calcification
    Differential Diagnosis
  Quantitation of Mitral Stenosis Severity
    Pressure Gradients
    Mitral Valve Area
    Technical Considerations and Potential Pitfalls
  Consequences of Mitral Stenosis
    Left Ventricular Response
    Left Atrial Enlargement and Thrombus
    Pulmonary Hypertension
    Mitral Regurgitation
    Other Coexisting Valvular Disease
  Clinical Applications in Specific Patient Populations
    Disease Stages, Hemodynamic Progression, and Timing of Intervention
    Patients Undergoing Balloon Mitral Commissurotomy

TRICUSPID STENOSIS

PULMONIC STENOSIS

THE ECHO EXAM

SUGGESTED READING

BASIC PRINCIPLES

Approach to the Evaluation of Valvular Stenosis

Narrowing, or stenosis, of a cardiac valve can be due to a congenitally abnormal valve, a postinflammatory process (e.g., rheumatic), or age-related calcification. As the degree of valve opening decreases, the increasing obstruction to blood flow results in an increased flow velocity and pressure gradient across the valve. In isolated valve stenosis, clinical symptoms typically occur when the valve orifice is reduced to one quarter its normal size. In mixed stenosis and regurgitation, symptoms can occur when each lesion, if isolated, would be considered only moderate in severity.

Secondary changes in patients with valvular stenosis include the response of the specific cardiac chambers affected by pressure overload. The ventricular response to pressure overload is hypertrophy; the atrial response is dilation. Chronic pressure overload also can lead to irreversible changes in other upstream cardiac chambers and in the pulmonary vascular bed (e.g., in mitral stenosis).

Complete echocardiographic evaluation of the patient with valvular stenosis includes:

- Imaging of the valve to define the cause of stenosis
- Quantitation of stenosis severity
- Evaluation of coexisting valvular lesions
- Assessment of left ventricular (LV) systolic function
- The response to chronic pressure overload of other upstream cardiac chambers and the pulmonary vascular bed

This echocardiographic evaluation then is integrated with pertinent clinical data for a complete evaluation of the patient.

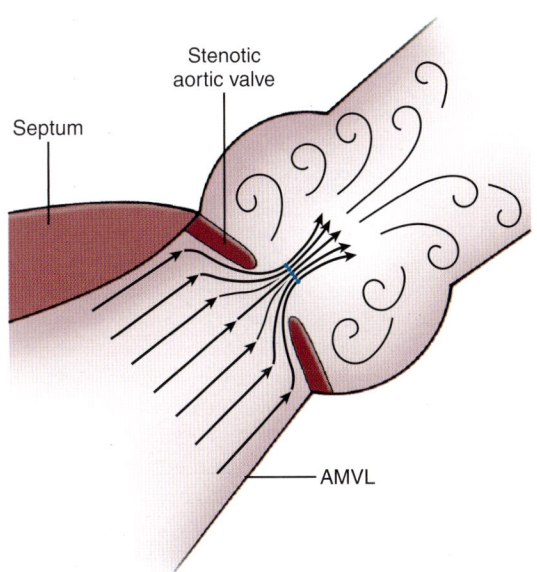

Fig. 11.1 Fluid dynamics of the stenotic aortic valve. The LV outflow tract is bounded by the septum and anterior mitral valve leaflet *(AMVL)*. As LV outflow tract flow accelerates and converges, a relatively flat velocity profile occurs proximal to the stenotic valve, as indicated by the *arrowheads*. Flow accelerates in a spatially small zone adjacent to the valve as blood enters the narrowed orifice. In the stenotic orifice, a high-velocity laminar jet is formed with the narrowest flow stream (vena contracta, indicated by the *blue line*) occurring downstream from the orifice. Beyond the jet, flow is disturbed, with blood cells moving in multiple directions and velocities. *(Reprinted with permission from Judge KW, Otto CM: Doppler echocardiographic evaluation of aortic stenosis, Cardiol Clin 8:203, 1990.)*

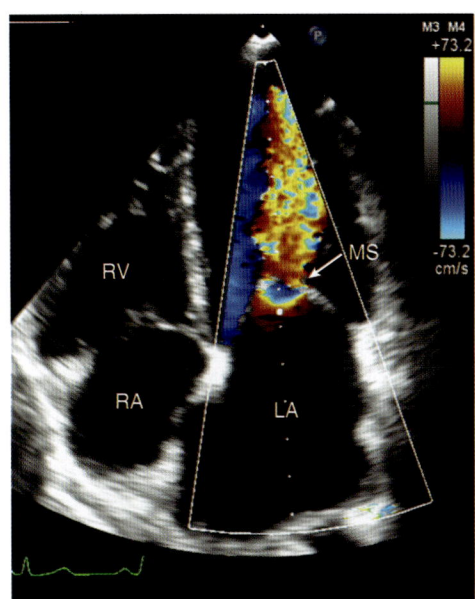

Fig. 11.2 ▶ **Mitral stenosis (MS) jet on color flow imaging.** The apical four-chamber view shows a long jet directed toward the LV apex with a proximal isovelocity surface area on the LA side of the valve.

Fluid Dynamics of Valvular Stenosis

High-Velocity Jet

The fluid dynamics of a stenotic valve are characterized by the formation of a laminar, high-velocity jet in the narrowed orifice. The flow profile in cross section at the origin of the jet is relatively blunt (or flat) and remains blunt as the jet reaches its narrowest cross-sectional area in the vena contracta, slightly downstream from the anatomic orifice (Fig. 11.1). Thus, the narrowest cross-sectional area of flow (physiologic orifice area) is smaller than the anatomic orifice area. The magnitude of the difference between physiologic and anatomic area depends on orifice geometry and the Reynolds number (a descriptor of the inertial and shear stress properties of the fluid). The ratio of the physiologic to anatomic orifice area is known as the *discharge coefficient*.

The length of the high-velocity jet also is dependent on orifice geometry and can be variable in the clinical setting with, for example, a very short jet across a deformed, irregular, calcified aortic valve and a longer jet across a smoothly tapering, symmetric, rheumatic mitral valve or a congenitally stenotic semilunar valve (Fig. 11.2).

Relationship Between Pressure Gradient and Velocity

The pressure gradient across the stenotic valve is related to the velocity in the jet, according to the unsteady Bernoulli equation:

$$\Delta P = \tfrac{1}{2}\rho(v_2^2 - v_1^2) + \rho(dv/dt)dx + R(v) \quad \text{(Eq. 11.1)}$$

$$\underbrace{\phantom{\tfrac{1}{2}\rho(v_2^2 - v_1^2)}}_{\text{Convective acceleration}} \; \underbrace{}_{\text{Local acceleration}} \; \underbrace{}_{\text{Viscous resistance}}$$

where ΔP is the pressure gradient across the stenosis (mmHg), ρ is the mass density of blood (1.06×10^3 kg/m^3), v_2 is velocity in the stenotic jet, v_1 is the velocity proximal to the stenosis, $(dv/dt)dx$ is the time-varying velocity at each distance along the flowstream, and R is a constant describing the viscous losses for that fluid and orifice.

Historically, Daniel Bernoulli first described this equation in 1738 from studies of steady water flow in rigid tubes. The concepts were later expanded and refined by Euler. Of note, these equations may not be strictly applicable to pulsatile blood flow in compliant chambers and vessels, although clinical studies have shown that remarkably accurate pressure gradient predictions can be made with this approach. This equation was first applied to Doppler data by Holen in 1976 for stenotic mitral valves and by Hatle in 1979 for stenotic aortic valves.

By eliminating the terms for viscous losses and acceleration, substituting known values for the mass density of blood, and adding a conversion factor for measuring velocity in units of meters per second (m/s) and pressure gradient in millimeters of mercury (mmHg), the Bernoulli equation can be reduced to:

$$\Delta P = 4\,(v_2^2 - v_1^2) \qquad \text{(Eq. 11.2)}$$

If the proximal velocity is less than 1 m/s, as is commonly the case for stenotic valves, it becomes even smaller when squared (e.g., $[0.8]^2 = 0.64$). Thus, the proximal velocity often can be ignored in the clinical setting so that:

$$\Delta P = 4\,v^2 \qquad \text{(Eq. 11.3)}$$

This simplified Bernoulli equation allows highly accurate and reproducible calculation of maximum pressure gradients (from maximum velocity) and mean pressure gradients (by integrating the instantaneous pressure difference over the flow period).

Distal Flow Disturbance

Distal to the stenotic jet, the flowstream becomes disorganized, with multiple blood flow velocities and directions, although fully developed turbulence, as strictly defined in fluid dynamic terms, may not occur. The distance that this flow disturbance propagates downstream is related to stenosis severity. In addition, the *presence* of a downstream flow disturbance can be extremely useful in defining the exact anatomic site of obstruction, for example, allowing differentiation of subvalvular outflow obstruction (flow disturbance on the ventricular side of the valve) from valvular obstruction (flow disturbance only distal to the valve) (Fig. 11.3).

Proximal Flow Patterns

Proximal to a stenotic valve, flow is smooth and organized (laminar) with a normal flow velocity. The spatial flow velocity profile proximal to a stenotic valve depends on valve anatomy, inlet geometry, and the degree of flow acceleration. For example, in calcific aortic stenosis, the acceleration of blood flow by ventricular systole, coupled with a tapering outflow tract geometry, results in a relatively uniform flow velocity (a "flat" flow profile) across the outflow tract just proximal to the stenotic valve. Immediately adjacent to the valve orifice, acceleration occurs as flow converges to form the high-velocity jet, but this region of proximal acceleration is spatially small. The flow profile differs slightly for congenital aortic stenosis in that the proximal acceleration region under the domed leaflets in systole is larger than that of calcific stenosis. However, proximal flow patterns are similar regardless of disease etiology in that a relatively flat velocity profile is present at the aortic annulus.

In contrast, the flow pattern proximal to the stenotic mitral valve is quite different (Fig. 11.4). Here, the left atrial (LA) to LV pressure gradient drives flow passively from the large inlet chamber (the LA) abruptly across the stenotic orifice. Proximal flow acceleration is prominent over a large region of the LA. The three-dimensional (3D) velocity profile is curved; that is, flow velocities are faster adjacent to and in the center of a line continuous with the jet direction through the narrowed orifice and slower at increasing radial distances from the valve orifice. The proximal velocity profile of an atrioventricular valve thus is hemielliptical, unlike the more flattened velocity profile proximal to a stenotic semilunar valve. Any 3D surface area proximal to a narrowed orifice at which all the blood velocities are equal can be referred to as a *proximal isovelocity surface area* (PISA).

The clinical importance of these flow patterns is that stroke volume can be calculated proximally to

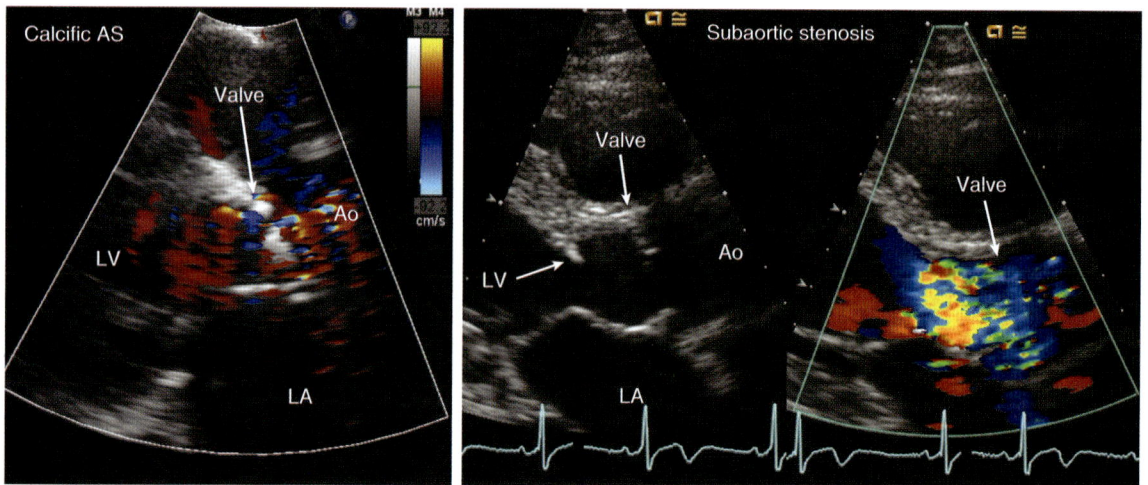

Fig. 11.3 Level of outflow obstruction. Color flow imaging in calcific valvular aortic stenosis *(AS)* in a parasternal long-axis view ▶ *(left)* with the poststenotic flow disturbance identifying the site of obstruction at the valvular level. In contrast, in a patient with subaortic stenosis ▶ ▶ *(right)*, flow acceleration occurs proximal to the valve. A membrane is not seen on these images but was demonstrated on TEE. *Ao,* Aorta.

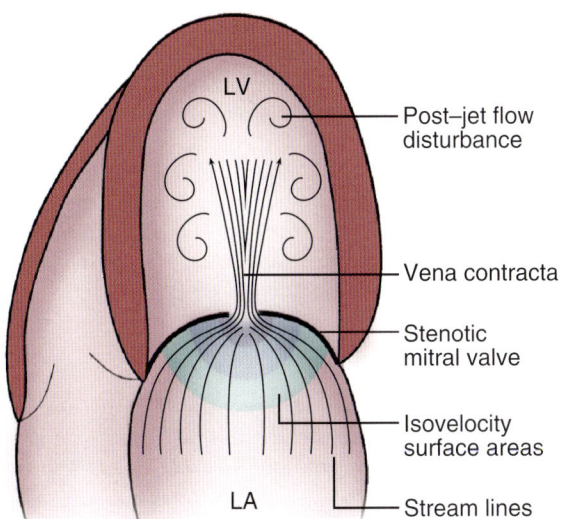

Fig. 11.4 Fluid dynamics of rheumatic mitral stenosis. The stream lines of flow accelerate as they approach the stenotic orifice, with several curved proximal isovelocity surface areas indicated. The mitral stenosis jet is long, with the post–jet flow disturbance occurring adjacent and distal to the laminar jet.

a stenotic valve based on knowledge of the cross-sectional area of flow and the spatial mean flow velocity over the period of flow, as described in Chapter 6. This concept applies to the flat flow profile proximal to a stenotic aortic valve (used in the continuity equation), to the proximal flow patterns seen in mitral stenosis, and to the proximal isovelocity surface areas seen with regurgitant lesions (see Chapter 12).

AORTIC STENOSIS

Diagnostic Imaging of the Aortic Valve

Aortic valve stenosis (Fig. 11.5) in adults most often is due to:

- Calcific stenosis of a trileaflet or congenital bicuspid valve
- Congenital valve disease (bicuspid or unicuspid)
- Rheumatic valve disease

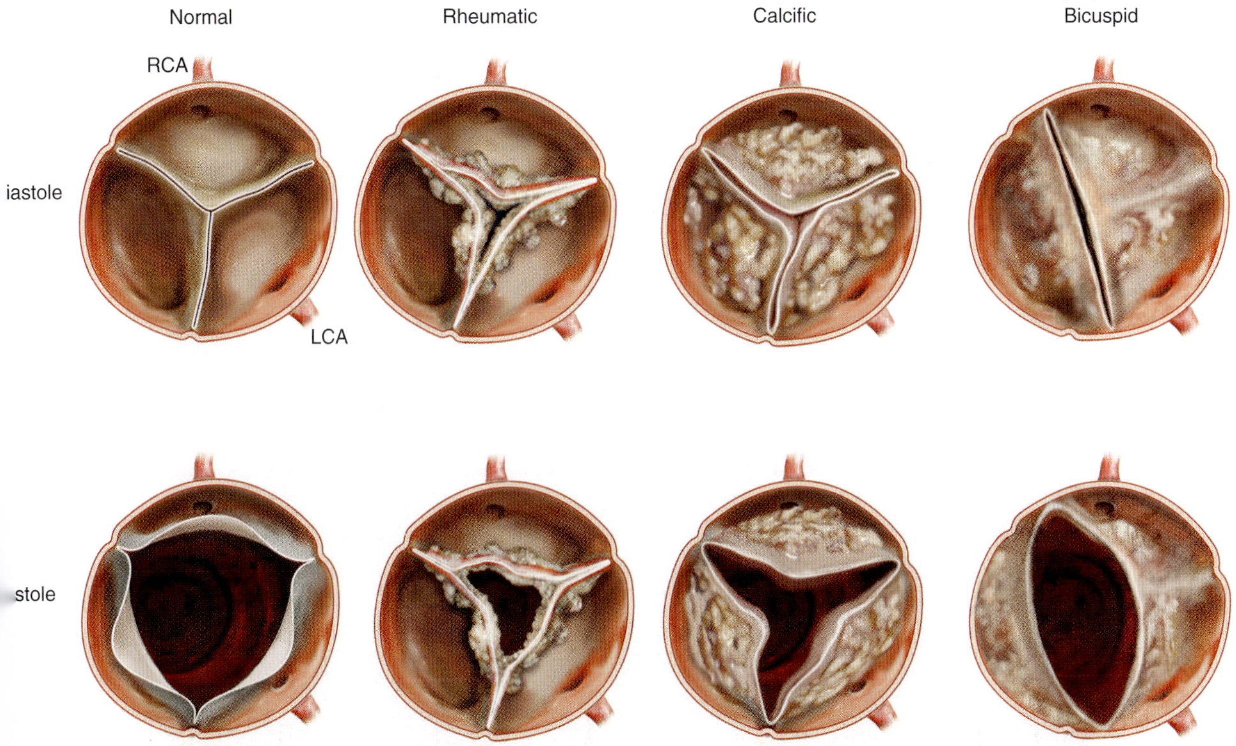

Fig. 11.5 Causes of aortic stenosis. This illustration shows the aortic valve viewed from above in a TTE parasternal short-axis image orientation in diastole *(top)* and systole *(bottom)* for a normal valve *(left)* and the three main causes of aortic stenosis. The diagnostic features of rheumatic stenosis are commissural fusion and mitral valve involvement, with the characteristic triangular aortic valve opening in systole. Calcific aortic stenosis is characterized by fibrocalcific masses on the aortic side of the leaflet that result in increased leaflet stiffness without commissural fusion, with a stellate shaped orifice in systole. Often, shadowing and reverberations limit image quality. With a congenital bicuspid valve, two commissures and two leaflets (with a raphe are present between the fused right and left coronary cusps in this example) with an elliptical shape of the open valve in systole. A unicuspid valve (not shown here) has only one commissure with a teardrop-shaped systolic opening. *LCA,* Left coronary artery; *RCA,* right coronary artery. *(From Jander N, Minners J: Aortic stenosis: disease severity, progression and timing of intervention. In Otto CM, editor: The Practice of Clinical Echocardiography, ed 5, Philadelphia, 2017, Elsevier, Fig. 15-1.)*

Calcific Aortic Stenosis

About 25% of all adults older than 65 years of age have aortic valve "sclerosis"—focal areas of increased echogenicity, typically at the base of the valve leaflets, without significant obstruction to LV outflow. About 10% to 15% of these patients have progressive leaflet thickening over several years that results in significant obstruction to LV outflow and typically manifests at 70 to 85 years of age. When obstruction is present, imaging shows a marked increase in echogenicity of the leaflets consistent with calcific disease and reduced systolic opening. Direct measurement of valve area on short-axis two-dimensional (2D) or 3D imaging is possible in some patients either with excellent transthoracic (TTE) images or from a transesophageal echocardiographic (TEE) approach. However, directly planimetered aortic valve areas should be interpreted with caution because of the complex anatomy of the orifice and calcific shadowing and reverberation, even with 3D imaging. It is critical to ensure that the narrowest orifice of the valve is visualized and nonplanar geometry is considered. Even when carefully performed, direct measurement of valve area on imaging reflects anatomic valve area, whereas Doppler data provide functional valve area (Fig. 11.6).

Bicuspid Aortic Valve

A congenital bicuspid valve accounts for two thirds of cases of severe aortic stenosis in adults younger than 70 years of age and one third of cases in those

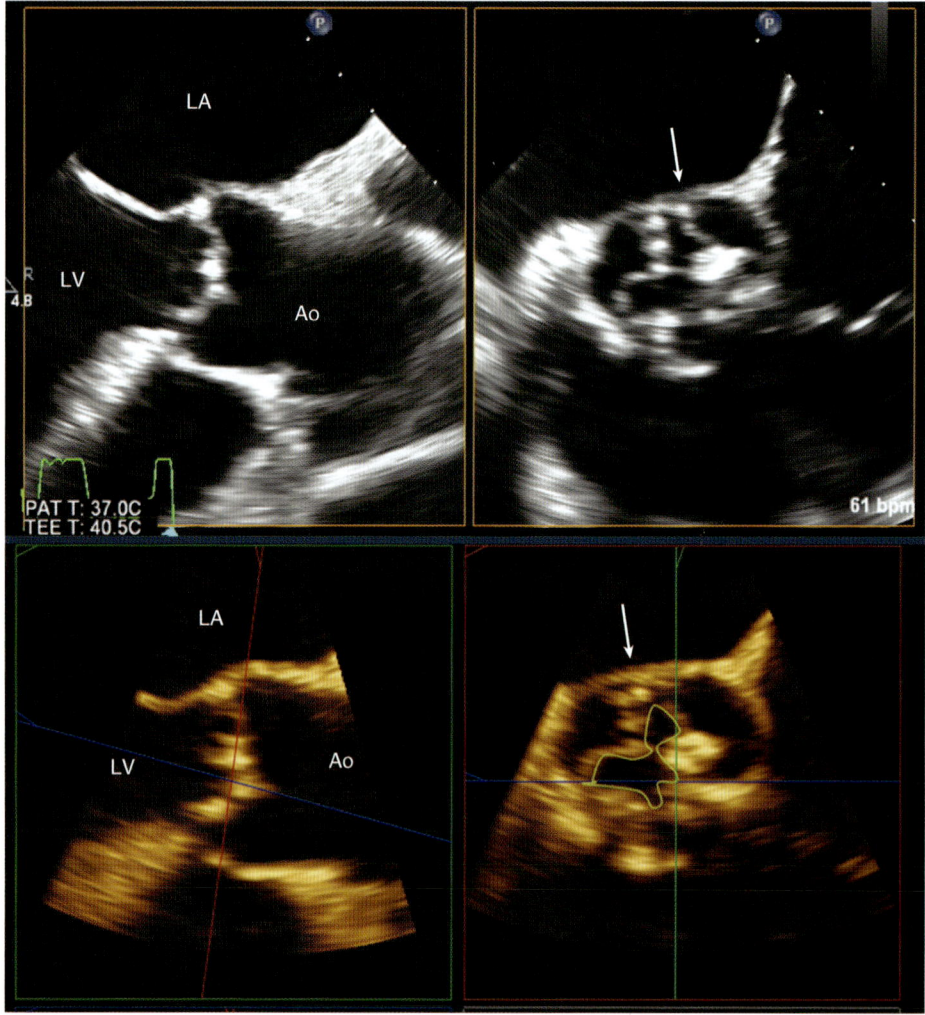

Fig. 11.6 2D ▶ **and 3D** ▶ ▶ **transesophageal echocardiography of calcific aortic stenosis.** Biplane 2D TEE views *(top)* of calcific aortic stenosis in long-axis *(left)* and short-axis *(right)* views show moderate leaflet calcification with a prominent area on the left coronary cusp. A volumetric 3D acquisition *(bottom)* has been formatted in corresponding long-axis and short-axis views. Planimetered aortic valve area *(arrows)* was measured at 1.2 cm² in this patient that corresponded to an aortic jet velocity of 3.4 m/s. Planimetry, even from 3D images, is not routinely recommended due to reverberations and shadowing by valve calcification, as in this example. *Ao,* Aorta.

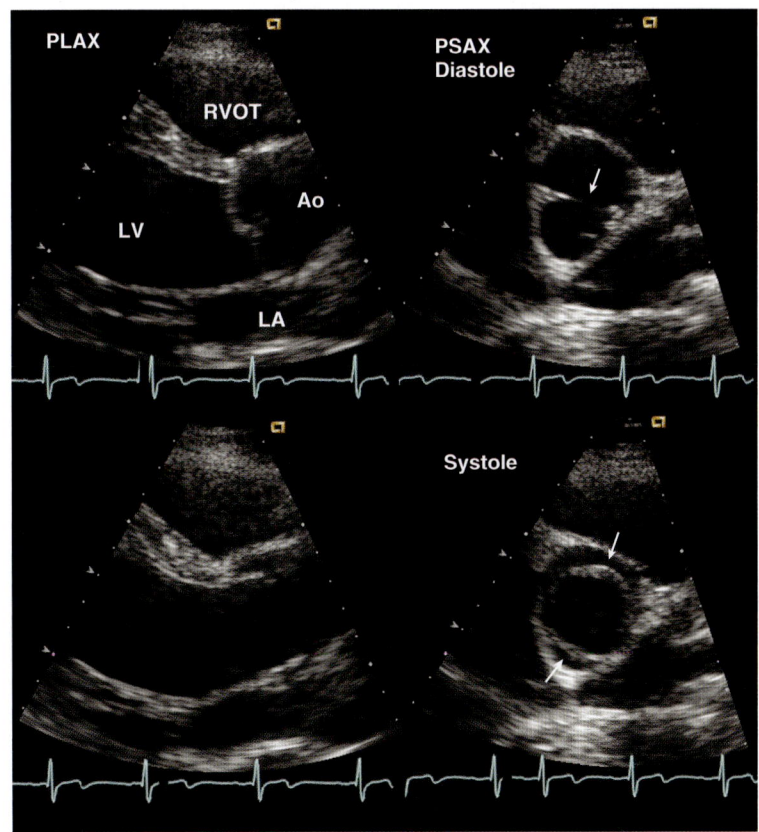

Fig. 11.7 Bicuspid aortic valve. Diastolic ▶ *(top)* and systolic ▶ *(bottom)* frames in a parasternal long-axis (PLAX) view show diastolic sagging and systolic doming of the leaflets. In the parasternal short-axis (PSAX) view, only two leaflets *(arrows)* are seen to open in systole with the commissures at 4 o'clock and 10 o'clock positions. *Ao*, Aorta; *RVOT*, RV outflow tract.

older than 70 years of age. Secondary calcification of a bicuspid aortic valve can be difficult to distinguish from calcification of a trileaflet valve once stenosis becomes severe; however, earlier in the disease course, a bicuspid valve can be identified on 2D parasternal short-axis views by demonstrating only two open leaflets in systole (Fig. 11.7). Long-axis views show systolic bowing of the leaflets into the aorta, thus resulting in a "domelike" appearance. M-mode recordings may help in identifying a bicuspid valve if an eccentric closure line is present but can be misleading in terms of the degree of leaflet separation if the M-mode recording is taken through the base, rather than the tips, of the bowed leaflets. Similarly, planimetry of valve area may be erroneous if the image plane is not aligned with the narrowest point at the leaflet tips. The 3D imaging is helpful in the identification of bicuspid valve anatomy when the diagnosis is not clear.

The most common bicuspid valve phenotype (seen in 70% to 80% of patients) is a larger anterior leaflet with the valve opening along an anterolateral-posteromedial closure line due to congenital fusion of the right and left coronary cusps (Fig. 11.8). A larger rightward leaflet with the closure line running anteriorly to posteriorly due to congenital fusion of the right and noncoronary cusps accounts for about 20% to 30% of cases. Fusion of the noncoronary and left coronary cusps, with a medial-lateral closure line, is least common. Many bicuspid valves have a

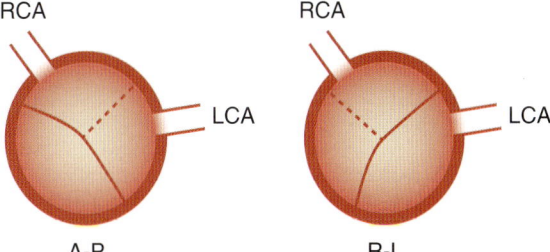

Fig. 11.8 Bicuspid valve classification. Schematic diagram of the different bicuspid aortic valve phenotypes drawn in an orientation similar to a TTE parasternal short-axis view. Positions of the right coronary artery *(RCA)* and left coronary artery *(LCA)* ostia are shown. The *A-P* phenotype shows anterior-posterior leaflet orientation with fusion of the right and left coronary cusps. The *R-L* phenotype shows right and left leaflet orientation with fusion of the right and noncoronary cusps. A raphe *(dotted line)* may or may not be present. (From Schaefer BM, Lewin MB, Stout KK, et al: Usefulness of bicuspid aortic valve phenotype to predict elastic properties of the ascending aorta, Am J Cardiol 99:686–690, 2007.)

raphe in the larger leaflet, so the closed valve in diastole appears trileaflet; accurate identification of the number of aortic valve leaflets can be made only in systole. Doppler interrogation of the aortic valve should be performed whenever a bicuspid valve is suspected to evaluate for stenosis, regurgitation, or both. Bicuspid aortic valve disease often is associated with dilation of the aortic sinuses and ascending aorta, with the pattern and severity of aortic dilation related to valve morphology.

Rheumatic Aortic Stenosis

In about 30% of patients with mitral stenosis, rheumatic disease also affects the aortic valve. 2D and 3D imaging shows increased echogenicity along the leaflet edges, commissural fusion, and systolic doming of the aortic leaflets. Often, superimposed calcific changes make recognition of rheumatic aortic valve disease challenging. Rheumatic valvular disease preferentially involves the mitral valve, so a rheumatic cause is likely when aortic disease occurs concurrently with typical rheumatic mitral valve changes.

Congenital Aortic Stenosis

Congenital aortic stenosis usually is diagnosed in childhood, but some patients may not become symptomatic until young adulthood or may have restenosis after surgical valvotomy performed in childhood or adolescence. These patients most often have a unicuspid valve with a single eccentric orifice and prominent systolic doming.

Differential Diagnosis

The differential diagnosis of LV outflow obstruction includes:

- Fixed subvalvular obstruction (a subaortic membrane or a muscular subaortic stenosis)
- Dynamic subaortic obstruction (hypertrophic cardiomyopathy)
- Supravalvular stenosis

In a patient with a clinical diagnosis of valvular aortic stenosis, the echocardiographic study should demonstrate whether the obstruction is, in fact, valvular or whether one of these other diagnoses accounts for the clinical presentation (Fig. 11.9).

A subaortic membrane should be suspected in young adults when the valve anatomy is not clearly stenotic yet Doppler examination reveals a high transaortic pressure gradient. Because the membrane may be poorly depicted on a TTE study, TEE imaging should be considered when this diagnosis is suspected (see Fig. 17.1). The spatial orientation of the jet and the shape of the continuous-wave (CW) Doppler velocity curve are similar for fixed obstructions, whether subvalvular, supravalvular, or valvular, but careful pulsed Doppler or color flow imaging allows localization of the level of obstruction by detection of the poststenotic flow disturbance and site of increase in flow velocity.

In dynamic outflow obstruction, the timing and shape of the late-peaking CW Doppler velocity curve are distinctive. In addition, the degree of obstruction changes dramatically with provocative maneuvers, as detailed in Chapter 9. In the occasional patient with both subvalvular *and* valvular obstruction, high-pulse repetition frequency Doppler ultrasound can be helpful in defining the maximum velocities at each site of obstruction.

Quantitation of Aortic Stenosis Severity

The severity of valvular aortic stenosis can be determined accurately using equations derived from our understanding of the fluid dynamics of a stenotic valve. Standard evaluation of stenosis severity includes:

- Maximum aortic jet velocity
- Mean transaortic pressure gradient
- Continuity equation valve area

Maximum Aortic Jet Velocity

Transvalvular velocity is the key measure in the evaluation of a patient with aortic valve stenosis. Aortic jet velocity alone is the strongest predictor of clinical outcome, the most reliable and reproducible measure for serial follow-up studies, and a key element in decision making about the timing of valve replacement. Because of the high velocities seen in aortic stenosis (usually 3 to 6 m/s), CW Doppler ultrasound is needed for optimal recording of the aortic jet signal. Examination should include use of a nonimaging, dedicated CW Doppler transducer because the smaller "footprint" of the dedicated transducer allows optimal positioning and angulation of the ultrasound beam, and signal-to-noise ratio is higher compared with a combined imaging and Doppler transducer.

Accurate measurement of aortic velocity requires a parallel intercept angle between the direction of the jet and the ultrasound beam. With a parallel alignment, cosine θ equals 1 and thus can be ignored in the Doppler equation (see Chapter 1). However, any deviation from a parallel intercept angle results in an underestimation of jet velocity. Although intercept angles within 15° of parallel will result in an error in velocity of 5% or less, an intercept angle of 30° will result in a measured velocity of 4.3 m/s when the actual velocity is 5 m/s. Underestimation of velocity, which is squared in the Bernoulli equation, results in an even larger error in calculated pressure gradient.

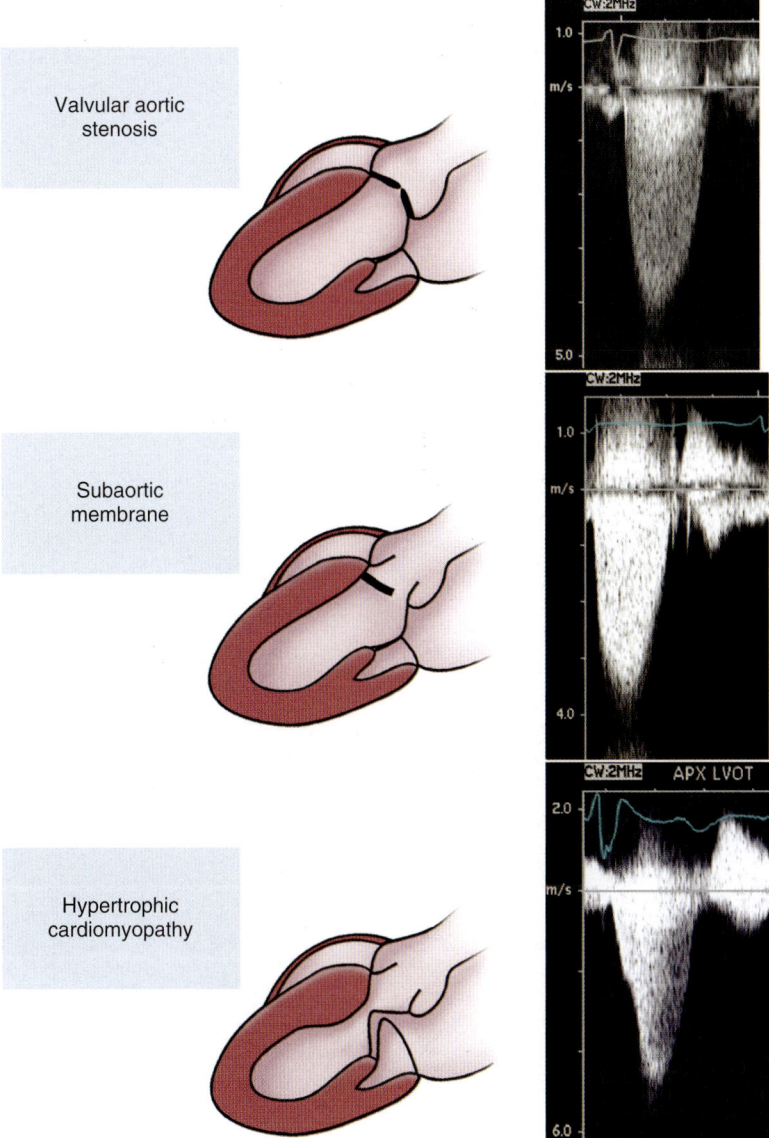

Fig. 11.9 Different types of left ventricular outflow obstruction. Examples of the shape of the CW Doppler velocity curve in valvular aortic stenosis, fixed subvalvular obstruction due to a subaortic membrane, and dynamic obstruction due to hypertrophic cardiomyopathy. Note that the CW curves for subvalvular and valvular aortic stenosis are similar, although coarse fluttering of the valve with subvalvular obstruction results in a "rough" appearance of the systolic velocity curve. These can be distinguished by 2D and color flow imaging. The shape of the curve with dynamic obstruction is distinctly different, with the velocity peaking in late systole.

The direction of the aortic jet often is eccentric relative to both the plane of the aortic valve and the long axis of the aorta and rarely can be predicted from images of valve anatomy or by color flow Doppler imaging. Pragmatically, the solution to the problem of aligning the ultrasound beam parallel to an aortic jet of unknown direction is to perform a careful search from several acoustic windows with optimal patient positioning and multiple transducer angulations. The highest-velocity signal obtained then is assumed to represent the most parallel intercept angle. At a minimum, the aortic jet should be interrogated from an apical approach with the patient in a steep left lateral decubitus position on an examination bed with an apical cutout, from a high right parasternal position with the patient in a right lateral decubitus position, and from the suprasternal notch with the patient supine and the neck extended. In some cases, the highest-velocity signal may be recorded from a subcostal or left parasternal window. Even with a careful examination, the possibility of underestimation of jet velocity because of a nonparallel intercept angle should always be considered.

When the CW beam is aligned with the aortic jet, a smooth velocity curve is seen with a well-defined peak velocity and spectral darkening along the outer edge of the velocity curve. Audibly, the signal is high frequency and tonal. The spectral recording should be made with an appropriate velocity scale (about 1 m/s higher than the observed maximum jet velocity),

TABLE 11.1 Other High-Velocity Systolic Jets That May Be Mistaken for Aortic Stenosis

Subaortic obstruction (fixed or dynamic)
Mitral regurgitation
Tricuspid regurgitation
Ventricular septal defect
Pulmonic or branch pulmonary artery stenosis
Peripheral vascular stenosis (e.g., subclavian artery)

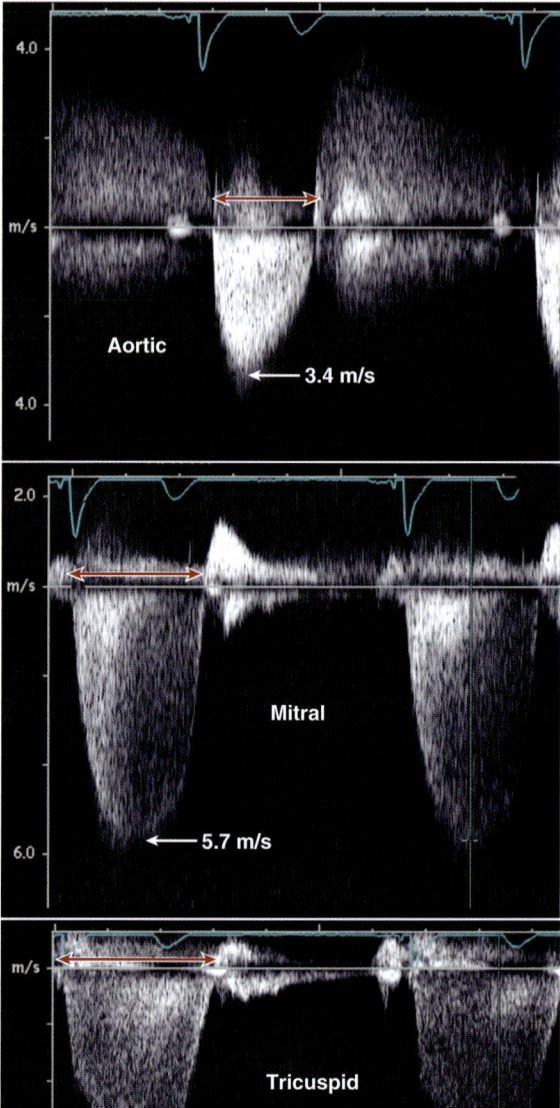

wall filters set at a high level, and gain adjustment to provide clear definition of the peak signal. Maximum velocity is measured at the edge of the dark spectral envelope. The velocity-time integral is measured by digitizing the velocity curve over systole.

Care is needed to identify the origin of the high-velocity jet correctly. Other high-velocity systolic jets (Table 11.1 and Fig. 11.10) may be mistaken for aortic stenosis if inadequate attention is paid to timing, shape, and associated diastolic flow curves. In some cases, 2D-"guided" CW Doppler may be helpful in the correct identification of the jet, followed by recording with a nonimaging transducer for optimal signal quality.

Pressure Gradients

Maximum transaortic pressure gradient (ΔP_{max}) can be calculated from the maximum aortic jet velocity (V_{max}) by using the simplified Bernoulli equation:

$$\Delta P_{max} = 4 V_{max}^2 \quad \text{(Eq. 11.4)}$$

Mean pressure gradient (ΔP_{mean}) can be calculated by digitally tracing the aortic jet velocity curve (where $v_1, \ldots, v_n$ are instantaneous velocities) and then averaging the instantaneous gradients over the systolic ejection period:

$$\Delta P_{mean} = \frac{(4v_1^2 + 4v_2^2 + 4v_3^2 + \cdots + 4v_n^2)}{n} \quad \text{(Eq. 11.5)}$$

With native aortic valve stenosis, the transaortic pressure gradient correlates closely and linearly with the maximum transaortic gradient, so the mean gradient can be approximated from published regression equations as:

$$\Delta P_{mean} = 2.4(V_{max})^2 \quad \text{(Eq. 11.6)}$$

With careful attention to technical details, Doppler-determined pressure gradients are accurate, as has been demonstrated in numerous in vitro and animal models and in clinical studies (see Appendix B, Table B.12). Although Doppler maximum gradients correspond to maximum instantaneous gradients by catheter measurement, and Doppler mean gradients correspond to catheter-measured mean gradients,

Fig. 11.10 Correct identification of the aortic jet. From an apical approach, three different high-velocity systolic jets directed away from the transducer were recorded in this patient with moderate aortic stenosis, mild mitral regurgitation, and severe pulmonary hypertension. These three flow signals can be differentiated based on timing *(red arrows)*, shape, and associated diastolic flow signals.

neither Doppler gradient correlates with the peak-to-peak gradient reported at catheterization. In fact, peak aortic and peak LV pressures do not occur simultaneously, so none of the instantaneous velocities recorded with Doppler ultrasound are strictly comparable with this invasive measurement. Potential confusion about Doppler pressure gradient data in an individual patient can be avoided by comparing only mean gradients (Fig. 11.11) or by simply

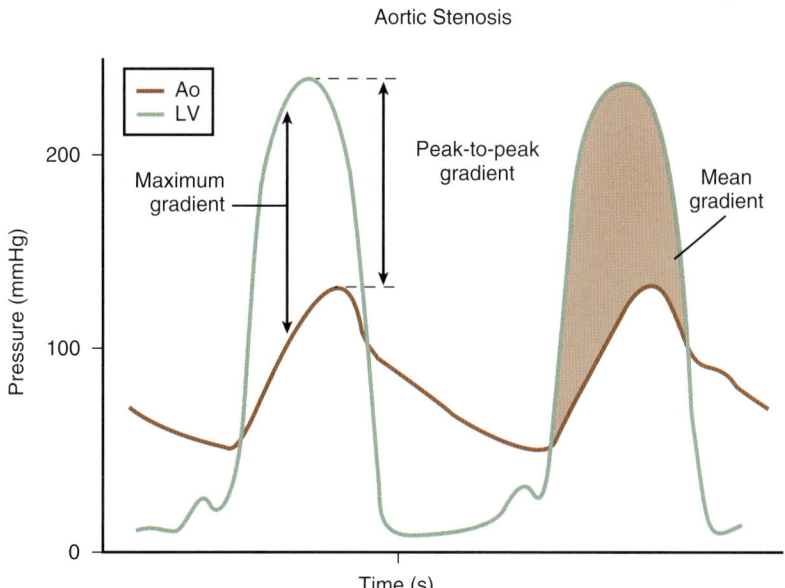

Fig. 11.11 **Left ventricular and aortic pressures in aortic valve stenosis.** LV and aortic *(Ao)* pressures were measured directly with fluid-filled catheters in a patient with severe valvular aortic stenosis. Note that the maximum instantaneous gradient is greater than the peak-to-peak gradient. Mean gradient is indicated by the *shaded area*.

recognizing that aortic velocity alone is the strongest predictor of clinical outcome.

Physiologic changes in pressure gradient should be taken into consideration when comparing nonsimultaneous data recordings and inpatient management decisions. Pressure gradients depend on volume flow rate in addition to the degree of valve narrowing, so in an individual patient the pressure gradient rises when transaortic stroke volume increases (e.g., anxiety, exercise) and falls when stroke volume decreases (e.g., sedation, hypovolemia).

The dependence of pressure gradients on volume flow rate can lead to erroneous conclusions about stenosis severity in adult patients with either a chronically elevated or depressed transaortic stroke volume. For example, a patient with coexisting aortic regurgitation has a high transaortic pressure gradient with only a moderate degree of valve narrowing. Conversely, a patient with LV systolic dysfunction or coexisting mitral regurgitation may have a low transaortic pressure gradient despite severe aortic stenosis. These coexisting conditions are common in adults with valvular aortic stenosis, so determination of the stenotic orifice area is essential for complete evaluation of disease severity.

Continuity Equation Valve Area

Aortic valve area can be calculated based on the principle of continuity of flow (Fig. 11.12). Specifically, the stroke volume (SV) just proximal to the aortic valve in the LV outflow tract (SV_{LVOT}) and that in the stenotic aortic valve orifice (SV_{Ao}) are equal:

$$SV_{LVOT} = SV_{Ao} \quad \text{(Eq. 11.7)}$$

If flow is laminar with a spatially flat velocity profile,

$$SV = CSA \times VTI \quad \text{(Eq. 11.8)}$$

where CSA is the cross-sectional area of flow (cm^2), SV is stroke volume (cm^3), and VTI is the velocity-time integral (cm). Because flow both proximal to and in the aortic jet itself is laminar with a reasonably flat velocity profile,

$$CSA_{LVOT} \times VTI_{LVOT} = CSA_{Ao} \times VTI_{Ao} \quad \text{(Eq. 11.9)}$$

All the variables in this equation can be measured with 2D or Doppler echo except CSA_{Ao}, which is the stenotic aortic valve area (AVA) itself. Rearranging the equation,

$$AVA = (CSA_{LVOT} \times VTI_{LVOT})/VTI_{Ao} \quad \text{(Eq. 11.10)}$$

Thus, the measurements needed to calculate valve area with the continuity equation (Fig. 11.13) are as follows:

- LV outflow tract (or aortic annulus) diameter
- LV outflow tract VTI
- Aortic jet VTI

LV outflow tract diameter, measured on a 2D parasternal long-axis mid-systolic image, is used to calculate a circular outflow tract cross-sectional area (CSA). The velocity-time integral in the outflow tract is recorded with pulsed Doppler from an apical approach. The velocity-time integral in the aortic stenosis jet is recorded with CW Doppler ultrasound from the window that yields the highest velocity signal.

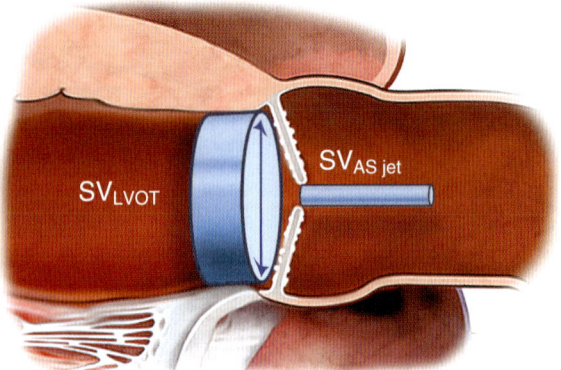

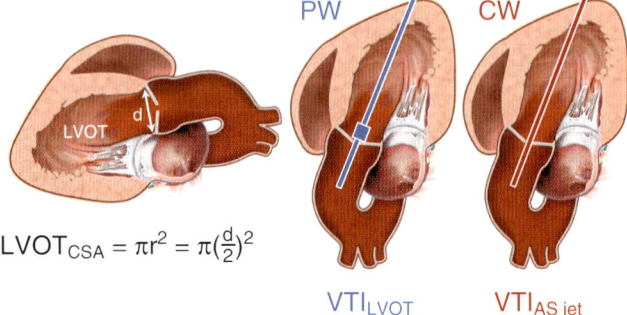

Fig. 11.12 Continuity equation aortic valve area. The continuity equation is based on the concept that volume flow during ejection is equal in the proximal LV outflow tract *(LVOT)* and in the narrowed aortic valve orifice. Calculation of aortic valve area *(AVA)* requires measurement of LVOT diameter *(d)* from a parasternal long-axis view for estimating circular cross-sectional area *(CSA)* and pulsed wave *(PW)* Doppler recording of the LVOT velocity-time integral *(VTI)* from an apical approach to calculate transaortic stroke volume *(SV)*. The aortic stenosis jet *(AS_{jet})* signal is recorded with CW Doppler from whichever window gives the highest maximum velocity.

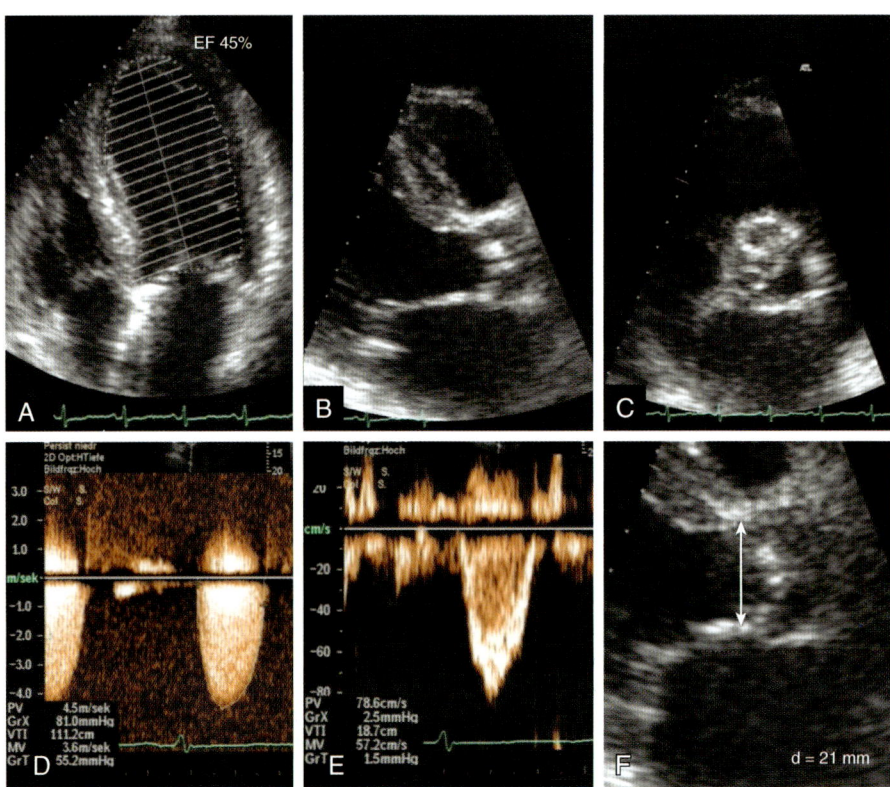

Fig. 11.13. Assessment of aortic stenosis severity. (A) Assessment of LV function by ejection fraction *(EF)*. (B) Long-axis view to assess morphology, degree of calcification, and opening movement ▶. (C) Short-axis view to assess morphology and number of cusps further ▶. (D) CW Doppler to measure peak velocity, mean gradient, and aortic velocity time integral *(VTI)*. (E) Pulsed-wave Doppler to measure prestenotic velocity and velocity time integral in the LV outflow tract. (F) LV outflow tract diameter *(d)* in zoom modus to calculate LV outflow tract area. Images show a severely stenosed calcified tricuspid aortic valve with mean gradient of 55 mmHg, calculated aortic valve area of 0.6 cm², and reduced ejection fraction of 45%. *(From Jander N, Minners J: Aortic stenosis: disease severity, progression and timing of intervention. In Otto CM, editor:* The Practice of Clinical Echocardiography, *ed 5, Philadelphia, 2017, Elsevier, Fig. 15-4.)*

For clinical use, the continuity equation can be simplified by substituting maximum velocities (V) for velocity-time integrals. Because the shape and timing of outflow tract and aortic jet velocity curves are similar, their ratios are nearly identical:

$$\text{VTI}_{\text{LVOT}}/\text{VTI}_{\text{Ao}} \cong V_{\text{LVOT}}/V_{\text{Ao}} \quad \text{(Eq. 11.11)}$$

The simplified continuity equation, then, is:

$$\text{AVA} = \text{CSA}_{\text{LVOT}} \times (V_{\text{LVOT}}/V_{\text{Ao}}) \quad \text{(Eq. 11.12)}$$

POTENTIAL PITFALLS. Continuity equation valve areas have been well validated in comparison with Gorlin formula valve areas calculated from invasive measurements of pressure gradient and cardiac output (see Appendix B, Table B.13). Some of the discrepancies between Doppler echo and invasive measurements of valve area are due to measurement variability for the invasive data and to limitations of the Gorlin formula itself. However, technical considerations in recording the Doppler and 2D echo data and the measurement variability of the noninvasive technique also are important (Tables 11.2 and 11.3). Each laboratory should confirm the accuracy of its data by comparison with those of an experienced echocardiography laboratory or with other diagnostic tests.

OUTFLOW TRACT DIAMETER. LV outflow tract diameter is measured in mid-systole, immediately adjacent to the aortic valve leaflets, from the white-black interface of the septal endocardial echo to the white-black interface at the base of the anterior mitral leaflet. A parasternal long-axis view provides the most accurate measurement because it depends on the axial (rather than lateral) resolution of the ultrasound beam. For calculation of aortic valve area, outflow tract cross-sectional area (CSA) is assumed to be circular so that:

$$\text{CSA}_{\text{LVOT}} = \pi(D/2)^2 \quad \text{(Eq. 11.13)}$$

Note that small errors in outflow tract diameter measurement may lead to large errors in calculated cross-sectional area. Furthermore, of the measurements made for evaluating aortic stenosis severity, outflow tract diameter shows the greatest intraobserver and interobserver variability. Several measurements should be averaged to minimize this potential source of error.

Outflow tract diameter must be measured in each patient for accurate valve area calculations. Although women tend to have smaller outflow tracts than men and outflow diameter correlates to body size when people of all ages from infancy to adulthood are considered, in the adult population the relationship between sex or body size (either body surface area, height, or weight) and outflow tract diameter is weak. Conversely, outflow tract diameter tends to remain constant in a given adult patient over time. Apparent differences in diameter at follow-up visits are more

TABLE 11.2 Pitfalls in Echocardiographic Evaluations of Aortic Stenosis

Technical

Acoustic access
Intercept angle between aortic stenosis jet and ultrasound beam
Outflow tract diameter imaging
Respiratory motion
Learning-curve effect

Interpretation

Identification of flow signal origin (AS vs. MR)
Beat-to-beat variability (AF, PVCs)
Intraobserver and interobserver measurement variability
Calculation errors

Physiology

Interim changes in heart rate or stroke volume
Dependence of velocity and ΔP on volume flow rate
Progression of AS severity

Low Flow Low Gradient AS

When EF <50%, assess changes in velocity and valve area with increased flow rates
When EF normal, index AVA to body size, calculated stroke volume index, consider other measures

AF, Atrial fibrillation; *AS*, aortic stenosis; *AVA*, aortic valve area; *EF*, ejection fraction; *MR*, mitral regurgitation; *ΔP*, pressure gradient; *PVCs*, premature ventricular contractions.

TABLE 11.3 Possible Causes of Discrepancies in Measures of Aortic Stenosis Severity

Severe AS by Velocity or Gradient But Not by Valve Area (AS Velocity >4 m/s and AVA >1.0 cm²)

LVOT diameter overestimated
LVOT velocity recorded too close to valve
High transaortic flow rate due to:
- Moderate to severe aortic regurgitation
- High output state
- Large body size

Severe AS by Valve Area But Not by Velocity or Gradient (AS Velocity ≤4 m/s and AVA ≤1.0 cm²)

LVOT diameter underestimated
LVOT velocity recorded too far from valve
Small body size
Low transaortic flow volume due to:
- Low ejection fraction
- Small ventricular chamber
- Moderate to severe mitral regurgitation
- Moderate to severe mitral stenosis
- Low output, low gradient severe AS

AS, Aortic stenosis; *AVA*, aortic valve area; *LVOT*, LV outflow tract.

likely to represent measurement error than an actual interval anatomic change.

Recent 3D imaging approaches show that the LV outflow tract is not exactly circular, so outflow tract diameter or aortic annulus measurements is not used for determining the correct transcatheter prosthetic valve size; 3D analysis of multidetector cardiac computed tomographic images is recommended for sizing of transcatheter valves. However, a circular assumption remains reasonable for valve area calculations used in clinical decision making.

OUTFLOW TRACT VELOCITY. The outflow tract systolic velocity signal is recorded from an apical approach using pulsed Doppler echo. Either an anteriorly angulated four-chamber view or an apical long-axis view can be used. A sample volume 2 to 3 mm in length is positioned just proximal to the region of acceleration into the stenotic jet. Correct positioning is ensured by starting with the sample volume in the jet and slowly repositioning it apically until a smooth velocity curve with a well-defined peak velocity and little spectral broadening is seen. The presence of an aortic valve closing (but not opening) click indicates that the sample volume is immediately adjacent to the valve. A transducer position is chosen initially that indicates a parallel alignment between the ultrasound beam and the long axis of the outflow tract on 2D imaging. Then, transducer position and angulation are adjusted, based on the audible Doppler signal and the velocity curve, to record the highest-velocity signal proximal to the flow acceleration region. In addition, the sample volume is moved laterally across the outflow tract in each apical view to document a flat flow velocity profile.

The rationale for this protocol for sample volume positioning is that the outflow tract diameter and velocity signals need to be recorded *at the same* anatomic site for accurate transaortic stroke volume calculations. Necessarily, these two recordings are made nonsimultaneously from different acoustic windows because of the need for a parallel orientation between the Doppler beam and the direction of blood flow for accurate velocity measurement versus a perpendicular orientation between the 2D echo beam and the outflow tract for accurate diameter measurement. Measuring both immediately adjacent to the stenotic valve provides a reference point that ensures that both measurements are made at the same spatial location.

The maximum outflow tract velocity is measured at the edge of the most intense spectral signal. The time-velocity integral is measured by tracing the modal velocity of the systolic flow curve. Wall filters are set low enough that the systolic ejection period is clearly defined.

Other Measures

Several other measures of aortic stenosis severity have been proposed, including stroke work loss, recovered pressure gradient, energy loss index, valvulo-arterial impedance, aortic valve resistance, and projected valve area at normal flow rate. As discussed in the American Society of Echocardiography and European Association of Echocardiography guidelines (see Suggested Reading 1), these measures may be useful in research studies but are rarely needed in clinical practice.

One simple measure that may be useful clinically, especially when image quality for measurement of LV outflow tract diameter is suboptimal, is the velocity ratio, which, in effect, is "indexed" for body size. Obviously, normal valve area is dependent on body size—infants and children have smaller valve areas than adults, and large adults are expected to have larger valve areas than small adults. One way to take the effect of body size into account is to "index" valve area by dividing it by body surface area (BSA):

$$\text{Aortic valve index} = \text{AVA/BSA} \quad \text{(Eq. 11.14)}$$

An alternate approach is to define the "normal" valve area for that individual as the cross-sectional area of the outflow tract. Then, the increase in velocity from outflow tract to aortic jet reflects stenosis severity regardless of body size. If the:

$$\text{"Normal" AVA} = \text{CSA}_{\text{LVOT}} \text{ and}$$
$$\text{Actual AVA} \cong \text{"Normal" AVA} \times V_{\text{LVOT}}/V_{\text{Ao}},$$
$$\text{then Actual AVA/"Normal" AVA} \cong V_{\text{LVOT}}/V_{\text{Ao}}$$
$$\text{(Eq. 11.15)}$$

A velocity ratio that is near 1 indicates little obstruction, a velocity ratio of 0.5 indicates a valve area that is one half normal, and a velocity ratio of 0.25 indicates a valve area reduced to one fourth its normal value.

Coexisting Valvular Disease

Most (approximately 80%) patients with predominant aortic stenosis also have aortic regurgitation, most often mild or moderate in severity. The degree of regurgitation can be evaluated as described in Chapter 12. Although coexisting aortic regurgitation results in an increase in the transaortic pressure gradient (because of increased transaortic volume flow), valve area calculations are accurate because the stroke volume in the continuity equation still represents transaortic stroke volume.

Coexisting mitral regurgitation also is common because of mitral annular calcification in adults with calcific aortic stenosis and can be evaluated as described in Chapter 12. Particular attention should be directed toward aortic valve area calculations when mitral regurgitation is present. Otherwise, severe aortic stenosis may be missed if the transaortic pressure

ECHO MATH: Aortic Stenosis Severity

Example

A 79-year-old man experiences dyspnea on exertion and is noted to have a 3/6 systolic murmur at the base, radiating to the carotids with a single S_2 and a diminished carotid upstrokes.

Echocardiography shows a calcified aortic valve with:

Aortic jet velocity (V_{max})	4.5 m/s
Velocity-time integral (VTI_{AS})	83 cm
Mean gradient	46 mmHg
LV outflow tract diameter ($LVOT_D$)	2.4 cm
LVOT velocity (V_{LVOT})	0.9 m/s
Velocity-time integral (VTI_{LVOT})	16 cm

The *maximum jet velocity* of 4.5 m/s indicates severe stenosis, which is confirmed by calculation of maximum and mean pressure gradients.

Maximum pressure gradient is calculated from maximum aortic jet velocity (V_{max}) as:

$$\Delta P_{max} = 4(V_{max})^2 = 4(4.5)^2 = 81 \text{ mmHg}$$

Mean pressure gradient is calculated by tracing the outer edge of the CW Doppler velocity curve, with the echo instrument calculating and then averaging instantaneous pressure gradients over the systolic ejection period. The simplified method for the estimation of mean gradient is:

$$\Delta P\ 2.4(V_{max})^2 = 2.4(4.5)^2 = 49 \text{ mmHg}$$

To correct for transvalvular volume flow rate, the velocity ratio and valve area are calculated:

Velocity ratio is:

$$V_{LVOT}/V_{max} = 1.1/4.5 = 0.24$$

Aortic valve area is:

$$AVA = (CSA_{LVOT} \times VTI_{LVOT})/VTI_{AS\text{-}Jet}$$

Where cross-sectional area (CSA) of the LVOT is:

$$CSA_{LVOT} = \pi(LVOT_D/2)^2 = 3.14(2.4/2)^2 = 4.5 \text{ cm}^2$$

Thus:

$$AVA = (4.5 \text{ cm}^2 \times 16 \text{ cm})/83 \text{ cm} = 0.87 \text{ cm}^2$$

Simplified formula for valve area is:

$$AVA = (CSA_{LVOT} \times V_{LVOT})/V_{max}$$

Thus:

$$AVA = (4.5 \text{ cm}^2 \times 0.9 \text{ cm/s})/4.5 \text{ cm/s} = 0.9 \text{ cm}^2$$

This mean gradient (>40 mmHg), velocity ratio (<0.25), and valve area (<1.0 cm^2) are all consistent with severe stenosis.

---

gradient is low because of low transaortic volume flow.

Patients with rheumatic aortic stenosis may have significant mitral stenosis, mitral regurgitation, or mixed mitral disease. Evaluation of aortic stenosis severity is unaffected by these coexisting lesions, other than the aforementioned potential for a low transaortic pressure gradient, if the transaortic volume flow rate is depressed.

Response of the Left Ventricle

The LV response to the chronic pressure overload of valvular aortic stenosis is concentric hypertrophy—an increase in LV mass due to increased wall thickness without chamber dilation. Hypertrophy tends to normalize LV wall stress, because:

$$\text{Wall stress} \cong (R/Th) \times P \quad \text{(Eq. 11.16)}$$

where R is ventricular radius, Th is wall thickness, and P is LV pressure. The relative wall thickness (the ratio of wall thickness to radius) is a useful and simple measure of the degree of hypertrophy. LV mass (which can be indexed for body size) can be calculated from tracings of endocardium and epicardium at end-diastole, as described in Chapter 6.

In aortic stenosis, LV systolic function tends to be preserved until late in the disease course. When LV systolic dysfunction does occur, it may be due to the increased afterload of outflow obstruction and thus is reversible after valve replacement. Ventricular systolic function can be evaluated qualitatively or quantitatively, as described in Chapter 6. Even a qualitative evaluation has significant prognostic implications in unoperated adults with aortic stenosis.

Clinical Applications

Decisions About Timing of Intervention

Doppler echocardiography is the diagnostic test of choice for adults with suspected aortic stenosis. A complete echocardiographic examination includes the evaluation of stenosis severity, assessment of LV systolic function, and evaluation of coexisting valvular lesions. Aortic stenosis severity is classified as Stage A to D based on valve anatomy, clinical symptoms, hemodynamics, and LV systolic function (Table 11.4). Stage A disease (at risk of aortic stenosis) includes aortic sclerosis, defined as the presence of irregular focal thickening of the aortic valve leaflets without obstruction to outflow (a jet velocity <2.0 m/s). When aortic sclerosis is present, further evaluation of stenosis severity is not needed, but repeat evaluation in 3 to 5 years is appropriate because many of these patients progress to significant valve obstruction.

When Stage B or Stage C aortic stenosis is present, a complete evaluation of disease severity and periodic follow-up is recommended (Fig. 11.14). As usual, caution is needed to ensure that the jet velocity measurement

TABLE 11.4 Stages of Valvular Aortic Stenosis

Stage	Definition	Valve Anatomy	Valve Hemodynamics	Hemodynamic Consequences	Symptoms
A	At risk of AS	• Bicuspid aortic valve (or other congenital valve anomaly) • Aortic valve sclerosis	• Aortic V_{max} <2 m/s	• None	• None
B	Progressive AS	• Mild to moderate leaflet calcification of a bicuspid or trileaflet valve with some reduction in systolic motion or • Rheumatic valve changes with commissural fusion	• Mild AS: • Aortic V_{max} 2.0–2.9 m/s or mean ΔP <20 mmHg • Moderate AS: • Aortic V_{max} 3.0–3.9 m/s or mean ΔP 20–39 mmHg	• Early LV diastolic dysfunction may be present • Normal LVEF	• None
C: Asymptomatic Severe AS					
C1	Asymptomatic severe AS	• Severe leaflet calcification or congenital stenosis with severely reduced leaflet opening	• Aortic V_{max} ≥4 m/s or mean ΔP ≥40 mmHg • AVA typically ≤1.0 cm^2 (or AVAi ≤0.6 cm^2/m^2). • Very severe AS is an aortic V_{max} ≥5 m/s or mean ΔP ≥60 mmHg.	• LV diastolic dysfunction • Mild LV hypertrophy • Normal LVEF	• None: Exercise testing is reasonable to confirm symptom status.
C2	Asymptomatic severe AS with LV dysfunction	• Severe leaflet calcification or congenital stenosis with severely reduced leaflet opening	• Aortic V_{max} ≥4 m/s or mean ΔP ≥40 mmHg • AVA typically ≤1.0 cm^2 (or AVAi ≤0.6 cm^2/m^2)	• LVEF <50%	• None
D: Symptomatic Severe AS					
D1	Symptomatic severe high gradient AS	• Severe leaflet calcification or congenital stenosis with severely reduced leaflet opening	• Aortic V_{max} ≥4 m/s or mean ΔP ≥40 mmHg • AVA typically ≤1.0 cm^2 (or AVAi ≤0.6 cm^2/m^2) but may be larger with mixed AS/AR	• LV diastolic dysfunction • LV hypertrophy • Pulmonary hypertension may be present.	• Exertional dyspnea or decreased exercise tolerance • Exertional angina • Exertional syncope or presyncope
D2	Symptomatic severe low flow/low gradient AS with reduced LVEF	• Severe leaflet calcification with severely reduced leaflet motion	• AVA ≤1.0 cm^2 with resting aortic V_{max} <4 m/s or mean ΔP <40 mmHg • Dobutamine stress echocardiography shows AVA ≤1.0 cm^2 with V_{max} ≥4 m/s at any flow rate.	• LV diastolic dysfunction • LV hypertrophy • LVEF <50%	• HF • Angina • Syncope or presyncope
D3	Symptomatic severe low gradient AS with normal LVEF or paradoxical low flow severe AS	• Severe leaflet calcification with severely reduced leaflet motion	• AVA ≤1.0 cm^2 with aortic V_{max} <4 m/s or mean ΔP <40 mmHg • Indexed AVA ≤0.6 cm^2/m^2 and stroke volume index <35 mL/m^2 • Measured when patient is normotensive (systolic BP <140 mmHg)	• Increased LV relative wall thickness • Small LV chamber with low stroke volume • Restrictive diastolic filling • LVEF ≥50%	• HF • Angina • Syncope or presyncope

AR, Aortic regurgitation; *AS*, aortic stenosis; *AVA*, aortic valve area; *AVAi*, aortic valve area indexed to body surface area; *BP*, blood pressure; *HF*, heart failure; *LVEF*, LV ejection fraction; *ΔP*, pressure gradient; and V_{max}, maximum aortic velocity.
From Nishimura RA, Otto CM, Bonow RO, et al: AHA/ACC guideline for the management of patients with valvular heart disease: executive summary. A report of the American College of Cardiology/American Heart Association Task Force on Practice Guidelines. *Circulation* 129:2440–2492, 2014.

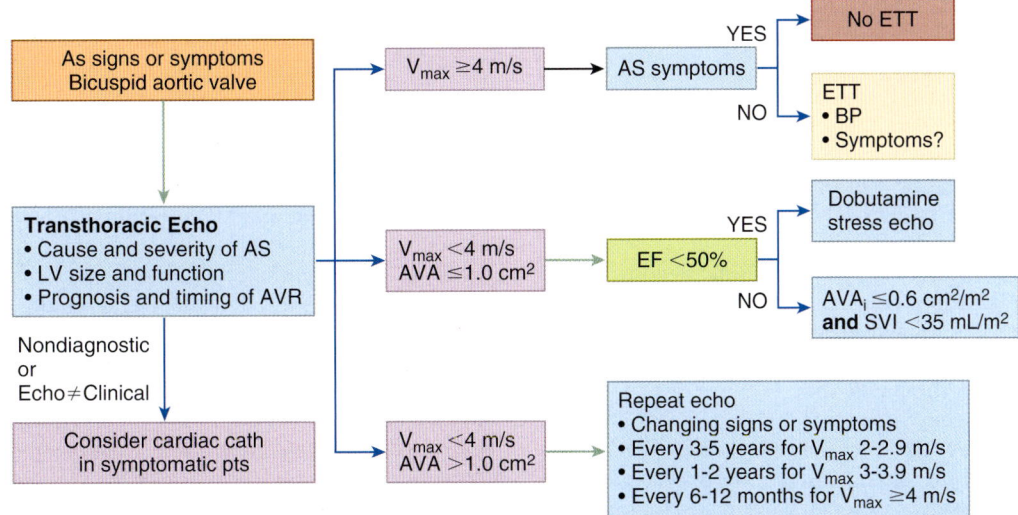

Fig. 11.14 Recommendations for next steps in adults with aortic stenosis. Echocardiography is the standard approach for diagnosis and quantitation of aortic valve disease and often is the only diagnostic test needed for clinical decision making. However, exercise testing *(ETT)* may be helpful in patients with severe asymptomatic aortic stenosis *(AS)*, dobutamine stress echocardiography is helpful when ejection fraction *(EF)* is reduced and measurement of stroke volume index *(SVI)* and indexed valve area is appropriate when low gradient severe AS is a clinical concern. In patients with mild to moderate AS, recommendations for periodic imaging should be included in the echo report. *AVA*, Aortic valve area; *AVAi*, indexed AVA; *AVR*, aortic valve replacement; *BP*, blood pressure; *Vmax*, maximum velocity.

is accurate—a nonparallel intercept angle between the aortic jet and the Doppler beam can result in an underestimation of jet velocity and the erroneous conclusion that severe stenosis is not present.

Severe symptomatic aortic stenosis is classified into three subcategories based on aortic velocity, mean gradient, valve area, and transaortic stroke volume index. Severe stenosis is present when aortic velocity is greater than 4 m/s, regardless of valve area. An apparent discrepancy in measures of stenosis severity when velocity is greater than 4 m/s most likely is due to measurement error (particularly LV outflow tract diameter), a large body size, or concurrent aortic regurgitation. A very high aortic velocity (>5 m/s) indicates very severe aortic stenosis.

When aortic jet velocity is between 3 and 4 m/s, calculations of valve area are essential; although most of these patients have only moderate stenosis, some have severe stenosis with a low transaortic stroke volume (see later). Identification of severe stenosis is critical because valve replacement is appropriate when symptoms are present and obstruction is severe. The role of echocardiography in evaluation of the patient before transcatheter aortic valve implantation is discussed in Chapter 18.

Disease Progression and Prognosis in Asymptomatic Aortic Stenosis

In observing individual patients over time, the reproducibility of a technique, in addition to its accuracy, is important. Reproducibility of Doppler echo data includes:

- Recording variability (e.g., intercept angle, wall filters, signal strength, acoustic window)
- Measurement variability (e.g., identification of the maximum velocity, outflow tract diameter)
- Physiologic variability (e.g., interim changes in heart rate, stroke volume, or pressure gradient)

Aortic jet maximum velocity measurement is reproducible with an intraobserver variability of 3.2% and an interobserver variability of 3.1%. Outflow tract velocity, recorded by two experienced sonographers, also is reproducible with intraobserver and interobserver variability of 3% and 3.9%, respectively. Measurement of outflow tract diameter shows the greatest variability, with intraobserver and interobserver mean coefficients of variation of 5.1% and 7.9%, respectively. These variabilities indicate that, for values at the middle of the range, a change greater than measurement variability is greater than 0.2 m/s for maximum jet velocity, greater than 0.1 m/s for outflow tract velocity, greater than 0.2 cm for outflow tract diameter, and greater than 0.15 cm^2 for aortic valve area.

Doppler echo has been used to follow disease progression in asymptomatic adults with valvular aortic stenosis. Several observations from these studies are noteworthy. First, prognosis depends on the presence or absence of clinical symptoms rather than on numeric measures of hemodynamic severity alone. Significant overlap occurs in all measures of hemodynamic severity between symptomatic and asymptomatic adults, and it is not unusual to see asymptomatic individuals with a jet velocity greater than 4 m/s. Second, the rate of hemodynamic progression is variable from patient to patient. On average, jet velocity increases by 0.3 m/s per year, mean pressure gradient increases by about 7 mmHg per year, and valve area decreases by about 0.1 cm^2 per year. Third, although hemodynamic progression may manifest as an increase in aortic jet velocity (and transaortic pressure gradient), disease progression can occur with no change in jet velocity if the patient has a concurrent decrease in transaortic volume flow rate.

In patients with asymptomatic aortic stenosis, clinical outcome is highly dependent on Doppler jet velocity. In those with an initial jet velocity less than 3 m/s, the rate of symptom onset requiring valve replacement is 8% per year, compared with 17% per year for those with a jet velocity between 3 and 4 m/s and 40% per year for those with a jet velocity greater than 4 m/s. Based on these data, periodic echocardiography is appropriate, even in clinically stable patients, at intervals of 1 year or less with severe stenosis, every 1 to 2 years with moderate stenosis, and at intervals of 3 years or longer with mild stenosis.

Evaluation of Low Flow Aortic Stenosis
Aortic Stenosis With Left Ventricular Systolic Dysfunction

When aortic velocity is less than 4.0 m/s but valve area is less than 1.0 cm^2, the possibility of "low gradient, low output" aortic stenosis must be considered. When LV systolic dysfunction is present (ejection fraction <50%), aortic valve opening may be reduced due to the low flow rate across as the valve with only mild or moderate valve disease. For example, with an LV assist device, the aortic valve opens very little because little flow occurs across the valve. Conversely, severe valve stenosis may be present with a low gradient due to the low volume flow rate. The diagnostic problem is distinguishing stiff leaflets that cannot open from relatively normal leaflets that could open if volume flow rate was normal.

The first steps in evaluation or the patient with low output, low gradient aortic stenosis with LV systolic dysfunction are evaluation for other causes of LV dysfunction, assessment of aortic valve anatomy (e.g., a bicuspid valve) and leaflet calcification, consideration of the therapeutic options and comorbidities, and observation of the patient's response to medical therapy. If severe stenosis remains a concern, the next step is low-dose dobutamine stress echocardiography. Under direct physician supervision, aortic jet velocity, mean gradient, and continuity equation valve area are measured at baseline and with gradually increasing doses of dobutamine, up to a maximum dose of 20 μg/kg/min (Figs. 11.15 and 11.16). A significant increase in valve area with an increase in transaortic volume flow rate reflects flexible leaflets (mild to moderate

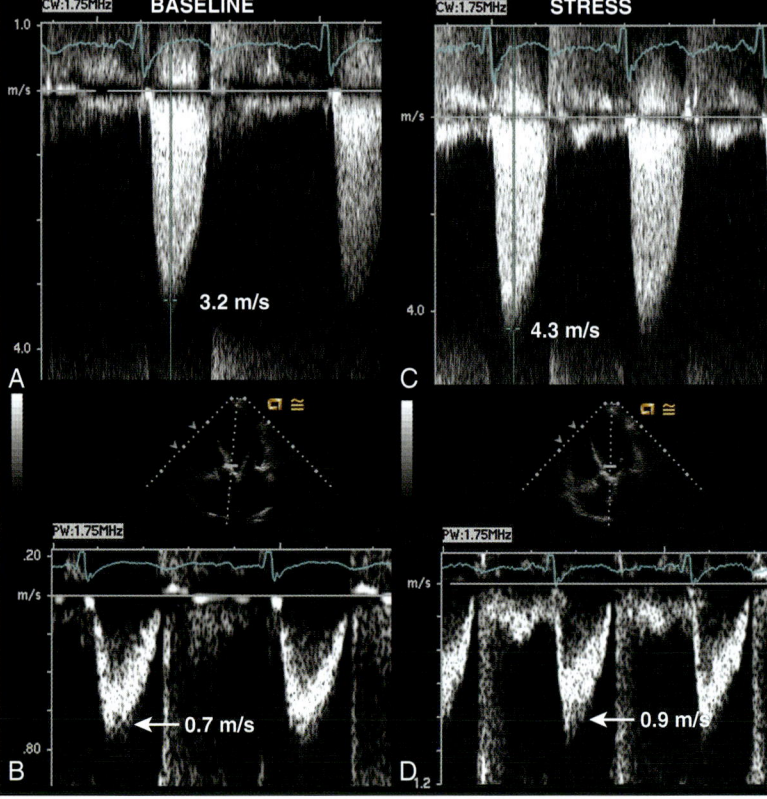

Fig. 11.15 Dobutamine stress echocardiography for the evaluation of low output, low gradient aortic stenosis. Dobutamine stress echocardiography in this 84-year-old man with calcific valve disease shows (A) a resting aortic velocity of 3.2 m/s and a mean gradient of 26 mmHg, and (B) LV outflow velocity of 0.7 m/s and a valve area of 0.8 cm^2. With dobutamine infusion at a maximum dose of 15 μg/kg/min, his heart rate increased from 74 to 95 beats/min from rest to stress, and his blood pressure fell slightly from 132/74 mmHg at rest to 116/58 mmHg at peak stress. Doppler data recorded at peak dose showed (C) an aortic velocity of 4.3 m/s and a mean gradient of 47 mmHg, and (D) LV outflow velocity of 0.9 m/s and a valve area of 0.8 cm^2. These findings are consistent with true severe AS. *(From Otto CM, Owens DS: Stress testing for structural heart disease. In Gillam LD, Otto CM, editors: Advanced Approaches in Echocardiography: Practical Echocardiography Series, Philadelphia, 2012, Saunders, Fig. 11-7.)*

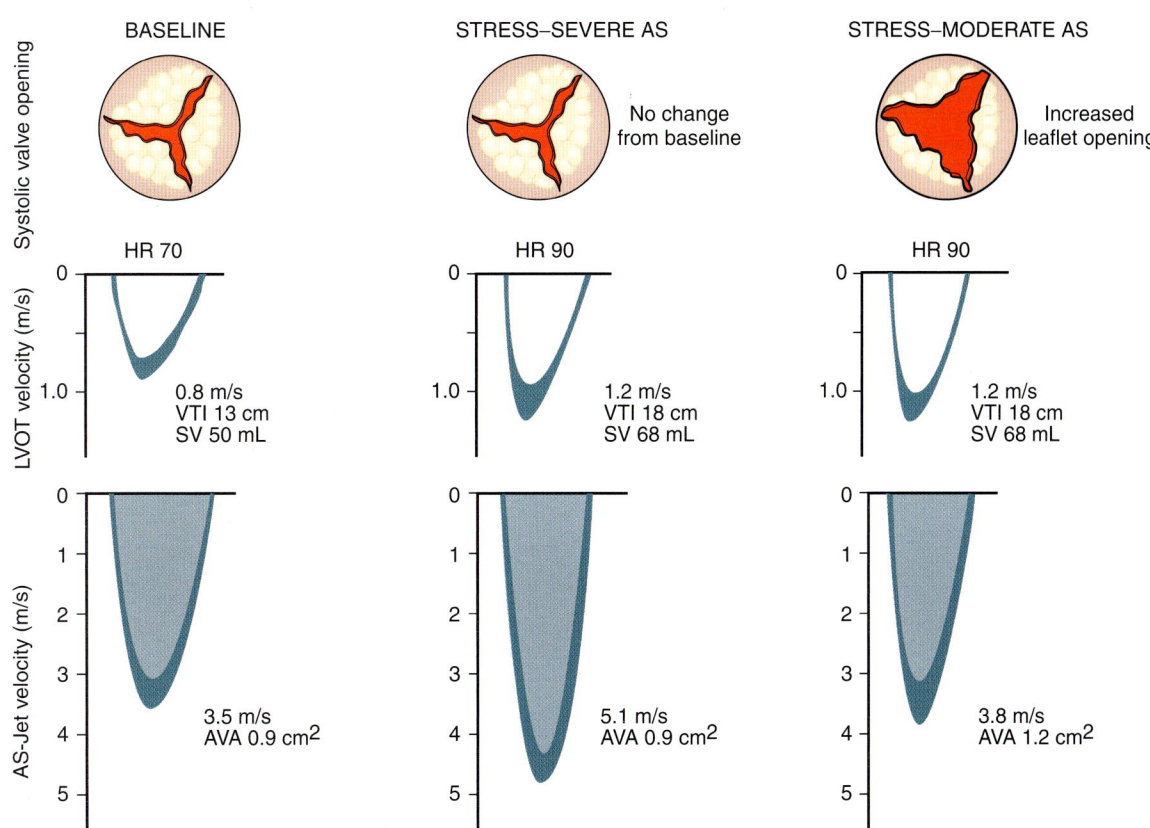

Fig. 11.16 Low output, low gradient aortic stenosis. Changes in aortic valve opening and Doppler flows with dobutamine stress echocardiography for low output, low gradient aortic stenosis *(AS)*. The baseline data show a hypothetical patient with an ejection fraction of 35% and limited aortic valve systolic opening, an aortic jet velocity *(AS-jet)* of 3.5 m/s, and an aortic valve area *(AVA)* of 0.9 cm². If true severe AS is present *(middle panel)*, as EF increases from 35% to 45%, the transaortic flow rate increases but the aortic opening is fixed, resulting in a marked increase in aortic velocity (and pressure gradient) with no change in valve area. In a patient with the same baseline data but "pseudosevere AS," the increase in EF and transaortic stroke volume *(SV)* "push" the aortic leaflets to open more so a smaller increase in aortic velocity occurs in association with an increase in AVA. Current diagnostic testing relies on Doppler data with dobutamine stress testing because direct imaging of valve anatomy is not adequate for visualization of the exact systolic orifice. *HR,* Heart rate; *LVOT,* LV outflow tract; *VTI,* velocity-time integral. *(From Otto CM, Owens DS: Stress testing for structural heart disease. In Gillam LD, Otto CM, editors:* Advanced Approaches in Echocardiography: Practical Echocardiography Series, *Philadelphia, 2012, Saunders, Fig. 11-6.)*

stenosis), whereas a fixed valve area indicates stiff leaflets that cannot open any further. Stress findings consistent with severe stenosis (Stage D2) are a jet velocity greater than 4.0 m/s or a mean gradient greater than 40 mmHg with a simultaneous valve area less than 1.0 cm² at any flow rate. Lack of contractile reserve—the failure of transaortic volume flow rate or LV ejection fraction to increase by at least 20% with dobutamine—is a poor prognostic sign.

Low Flow Aortic Stenosis With a Normal LV Ejection Fraction

Even when LV ejection fraction is normal, the volume of transaortic flow may be small if the ventricular size is small—for example, in older women or hypertensive patients. Sometimes called "paradoxical" low flow aortic stenosis, Stage D3 aortic stenosis is characterized by severe aortic leaflet thickening and calcification, a valve area less than 1.0 cm² with an indexed valve area less than 0.6 cm²/m², and a stroke volume index less than 35 mL/m² with an ejection fraction greater than 50%. However, the diagnosis of Stage D3 severe aortic stenosis remains problematic and can be made only if other potential causes of symptoms have been treated or excluded. Dobutamine stress echocardiography is generally not recommended in this patient subgroup because LV systolic function is normal and LV volumes are small, both of which limit any potential increase in stroke volume. A more detailed discussion of this problem can be found in the Suggested Reading list.

MITRAL STENOSIS

Echocardiography in the patient with mitral stenosis includes evaluation of:

- Valve anatomy, mobility, and calcification
- Mean transmitral pressure gradient
- Mitral valve area by 2D or 3D imaging
- Doppler pressure half-time valve area
- Pulmonary artery pressures
- Coexisting mitral regurgitation

Diagnostic Imaging of the Mitral Valve
Rheumatic Disease

Rheumatic disease predominantly affects the mitral valve and is nearly always the cause of mitral stenosis. Rheumatic valvular disease is characterized by commissural fusion, which results in bowing or doming of the valve leaflets in diastole (Fig. 11.17). The base and mid-sections of the leaflets move toward the ventricular apex, whereas the motion of the leaflet tips is restricted because of fusion of the anterior and posterior leaflets along the medial and lateral commissures. Thickening at the leaflet tips occurs frequently, but the remainder of the leaflets can show variable degrees of thickening, calcification, or both. If the base and mid-portions of the leaflets are relatively thin, leaflet mobility is normal other than the fused commissures. The rheumatic process also typically affects the subvalvular region with fusion, shortening, fibrosis, and calcification of the mitral chordae.

In rheumatic mitral stenosis, 2D and 3D echo allows for detailed evaluation of mitral valve morphology, including assessment of leaflet thickness, leaflet mobility, the degree of calcification, and the extent of subvalvular involvement on TTE parasternal and apical views (Fig. 11.18). If TTE images are suboptimal, TEE imaging may be needed for the evaluation of mitral valve anatomy, although definition of subvalvular disease may be limited because of shadows and reverberations from calcification of the mitral valve and annulus. 3D imaging is helpful for the visualization of valve anatomy and is recommended for measurement of valve orifice area.

Mitral Annular Calcification

Mitral annular calcification is a common finding on echocardiography in older adults. Mild annular calcification appears as an isolated area of calcification on the LV side of the posterior annulus, near the base of the posterior mitral leaflet. In more severe mitral annular calcification, increased echogenicity is seen in a hemielliptical pattern involving the entire posterior annulus The area of fibrous continuity between the anterior mitral leaflet and the aortic root is involved in some patients with concurrent calcific aortic stenosis and severe mitral annular calcification.

The echocardiographic finding of mitral annular calcification, like that of aortic valve sclerosis, indicates a higher risk of adverse cardiovascular outcomes,

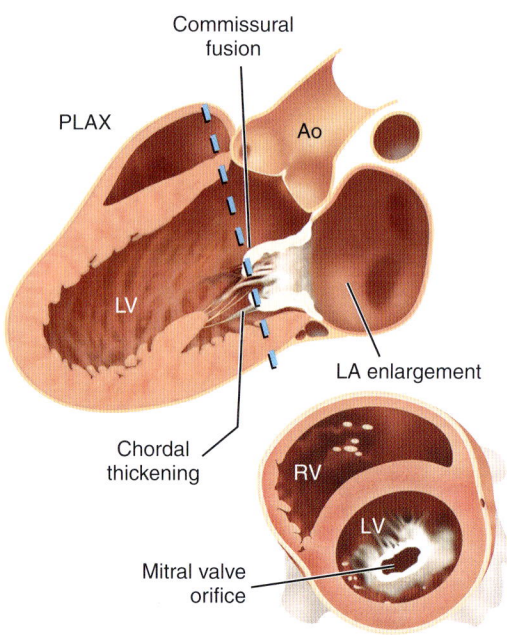

Fig. 11.17 2D echo findings in mitral stenosis. In the parasternal long-axis view *(PLAX)*, commissural fusion with diastolic doming of the mitral leaflets is seen in addition to chordal thickening and fusion. In a parasternal short-axis view *(PSAX)*, at the mitral valve orifice level, the area of opening can be directly traced on the image. The plane of the short-axis view is indicated by a *dashed line* on the long-axis image. *Ao,* Aorta.

even when valve function is relatively normal. Mitral annular calcification may result in mild to moderate mitral regurgitation due to increased rigidity of the mitral annulus. Occasionally, the calcification extends into the base of the mitral leaflets themselves, thus resulting in functional mitral stenosis due to narrowing of the diastolic flow area (Fig. 11.19). Calcific mitral stenosis can be distinguished from rheumatic disease by careful imaging techniques that demonstrate thin and mobile mitral leaflet tips without commissural fusion.

Differential Diagnosis

In patients referred for echocardiography with suspected mitral stenosis, the initial differential diagnosis includes other causes of pulmonary congestion. Standard echo Doppler evaluation will reveal whether LV systolic dysfunction, aortic valve disease, or mitral regurgitation is present. The possibility of diastolic LV dysfunction also should be considered. The rare case of an atrial myxoma or other atrial tumor obstructing LV inflow, thus mimicking the clinical presentation of mitral stenosis, can easily be diagnosed by 2D imaging (see Chapter 15). Rarely, a patient

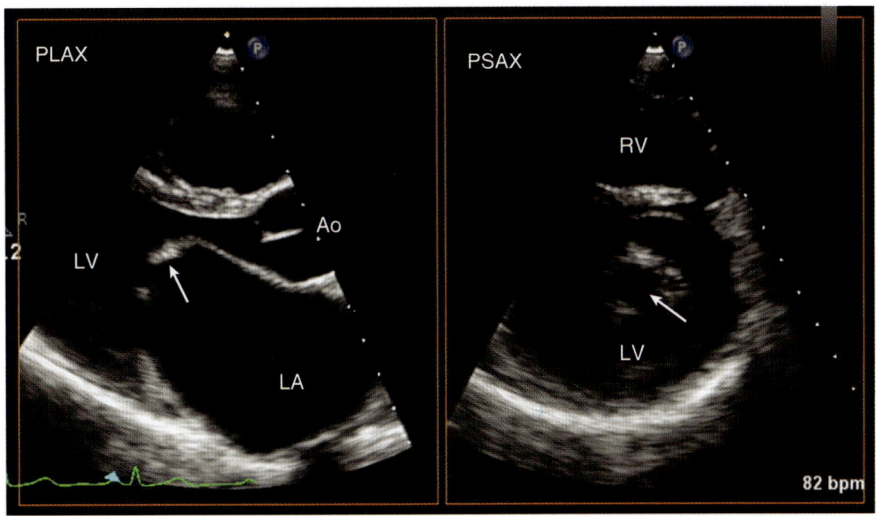

Fig. 11.18 **Rheumatic mitral stenosis.** Simultaneous biplane imaging in parasternal long-axis *(PLAX)* and short-axis *(PSAX)* views shows the typical finding in rheumatic mitral stenosis. The long-axis view *(left)* shows "doming" of the anterior mitral leaflet *(arrow)* due to commissural fusion,. This patient has minimal chordal thickening and fusion. LA enlargement is present. The short-axis view *(right)* better demonstrates commissural fusion and allows for accurate planimetry of the mitral orifice area if care is taken to identify the smallest opening by scanning slowly from the apex toward the base. 3D imaging for measurement of mitral orifice area is recommended when possible to ensure that the smallest area at the tip of the leaflets is visualized. *Ao,* Aorta.

with mild obstruction due to cor triatriatum may present as an adult.

Quantitation of Mitral Stenosis Severity
Pressure Gradients

The mean diastolic transmitral pressure gradient (Fig. 11.20) can be determined from the transmitral velocity curve using the simplified Bernoulli equation:

$$\text{Mean mitral } \Delta P = \frac{4v_1^2 + 4v_2^2 + 4v_3^4 + \cdots + 4v_n^2}{n}$$

(Eq. 11.17)

With severe stenosis, the mean pressure gradient may be as high as 20 to 30 mmHg, but often it is only 5 to 15 mmHg. The variability in pressure gradients in severe mitral stenosis is due to the dependence of pressure gradients on the volume flow rate in addition to valve area. Severe mitral stenosis may be associated with a low stroke volume (due to the limitation of LV diastolic filling), resulting in a relatively low mean gradient. If volume flow rate increases, for example, with exercise, an increase in transmitral gradient is seen. Thus, calculation of valve area, considering both pressure gradient and volume flow rate, is particularly important in quantitation of mitral stenosis severity.

Mitral Valve Area

Direct Imaging of Valve Area. Compared with valvular aortic stenosis, the 3D anatomy of rheumatic mitral stenosis is simpler, with a planar elliptical orifice that is relatively constant in position in mid-diastole (Fig. 11.21). Thus, 2D- or 3D-guided short-axis imaging of the diastolic orifice allows direct planimetry of valve area. This approach has been well validated compared with measurement of valve area at surgery and in comparison with catheterization-determined valve areas. Because the shape of the mitral valve inflow region is similar to a funnel, with the narrowest cross-sectional area at the leaflet tips, if 2D imaging is used, it is important that the scan start apically, slowly moving the image plane toward the mitral valve to identify the smallest orifice. With a low overall gain setting, the inner edge of the black-white interface is traced. The 3D imaging allows more reliable planimetry of mitral valve area when 3D guidance is used to align the image in the plane of the minimal orifice at the leaflet tips. The degree and asymmetry of commissural fusion at baseline and after intervention also is best evaluated by 3D imaging (Figs. 11.22 and 11.23).

Pressure Half-Time Valve Area. Calculation of mitral valve area by the pressure half-time ($T\frac{1}{2}$) method is based on the concept that the *rate* of pressure decline across the stenotic mitral orifice is determined by the cross-sectional area of the orifice: the smaller the orifice, the slower the rate of pressure decline (Figs. 11.24 and 11.25). The influence of LA and LV compliance on the rate of pressure decline is assumed to be negligible, an assumption that is not always warranted, especially immediately after percutaneous commissurotomy.

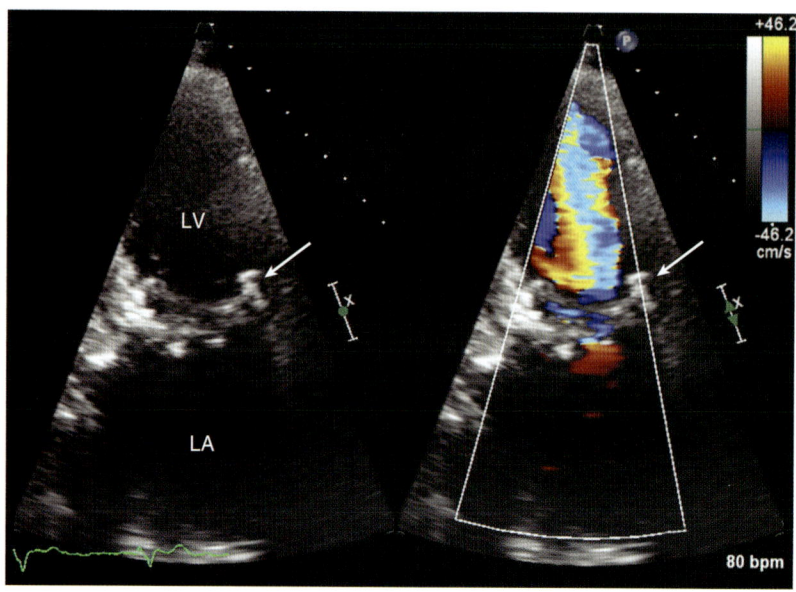

Fig. 11.19 ▶ **Severe mitral annular calcification.** In this older adult patient, severe mitral annular calcification *(arrows)* is present with involvement of the mitral leaflets by the calcific process seen in the apical view with a narrow antegrade flow jet on color Doppler.

Fig. 11.20 Doppler velocities with severe mitral annular calcification. Transmitral flow curve in the same patient as in Fig. 11.19. Using this velocity curve, pressure gradients can be calculated with the Bernoulli equation, and valve area can be calculated by the pressure half-time method. Note the well-defined maximal velocity and the clearly defined, linear deceleration slope. An *A* velocity is not seen because atrial fibrillation is present. Mitral regurgitation *(MR)* also is seen. *MS,* Mitral stenosis.

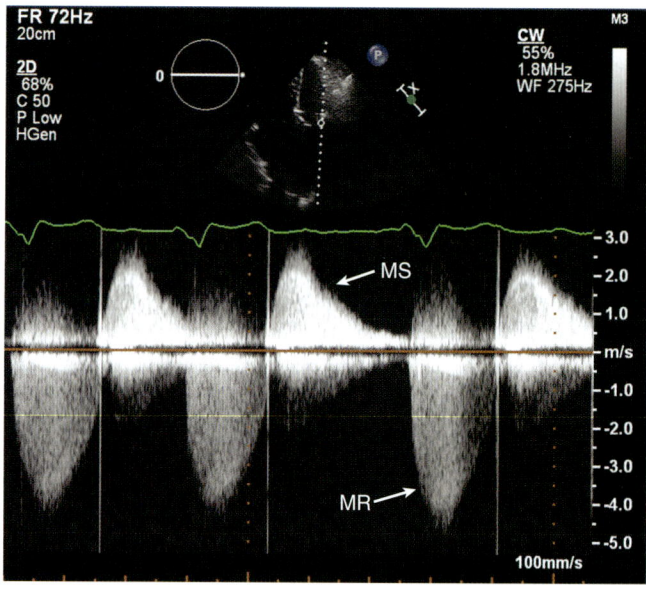

The pressure half-time is defined as the time interval (in milliseconds) between the maximum early-diastolic transmitral pressure gradient and the time point at which the pressure gradient is half the maximum value. Initially, the pressure half-time concept was evaluated using invasive measurements of LA and LV pressure, which demonstrated that pressure half-time is constant for a given individual, even with exercise-induced changes in volume flow rate, a finding suggesting that this measurement is a constant measure of stenosis severity for a given valve area.

This concept then was adapted to transmitral Doppler flow velocity curves. Given the quadratic relationship between velocity and pressure gradients, the half-time is determined from a Doppler spectral velocity curve as the time interval from the maximum mitral velocity (V_{max}) to the point where the velocity has fallen to V_{max}. Initial studies comparing Doppler half-time data with invasively determined Gorlin valve areas found a linear relationship, with a half-time of approximately 220 ms corresponding to a valve area of 1 cm^2. The empirical formula:

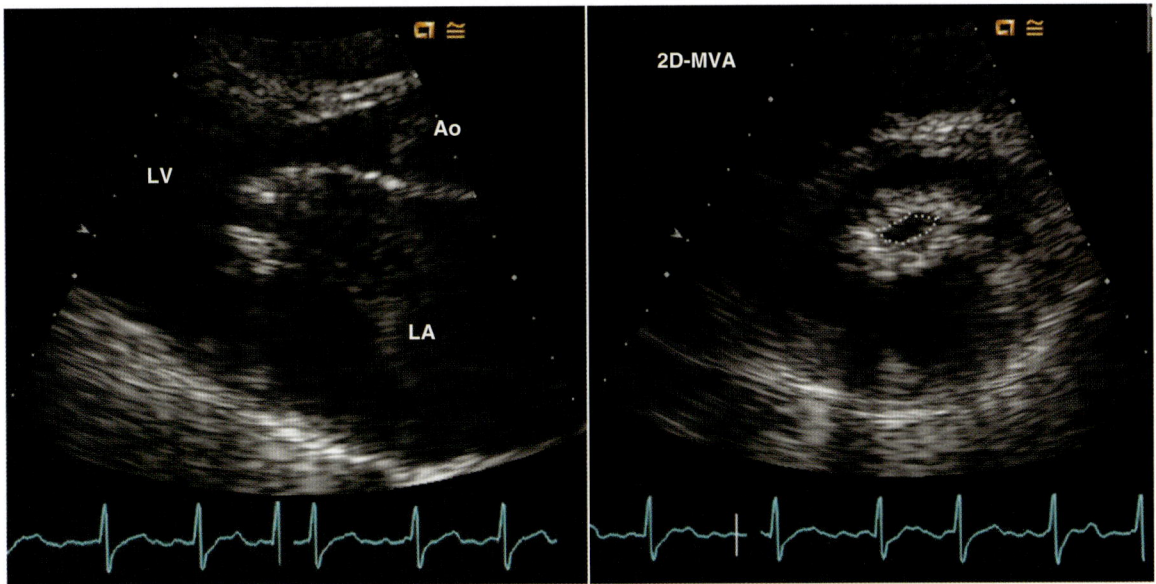

Fig. 11.21 2D transthoracic planimetry of mitral valve area. Long-axis ▶ *(left)* and short-axis ▶ *(right)* views show thickened and calcified leaflet tips. Note the diastolic doming and severe commissural fusion. Mitral valve area *(MVA)* by 2D planimetry is 0.6 cm². In addition, severe LA enlargement is present. *Ao,* Aorta.

$$MVA = 220/T\frac{1}{2} \quad \text{(Eq. 11.18)}$$

was proposed and has been shown to correlate well with invasive valve areas in several clinical studies (see Appendix B, Table B.14).

CONTINUITY EQUATION MITRAL VALVE AREA. The continuity principle for the calculation of valve area also can be applied to the mitral orifice:

$$MVA = \text{Transmitral SV}/VTI_{MSjet} \quad \text{(Eq. 11.19)}$$

where SV is stroke volume (cm³), VTI is the velocity-time integral (cm) in the mitral stenosis jet, and MVA (cm²) is the mitral valve area.

Stroke volume can be determined from the LV outflow tract cross-sectional area and velocity-time integral (in the absence of aortic or mitral regurgitation) or from the pulmonary artery diameter and velocity-time integral. Note that stroke volume measured at either of these sites will represent transmitral volume flow accurately only if no significant mitral regurgitation is present.

In theory, transmitral volume flow rate can be calculated accurately in mitral stenosis even when mitral regurgitation is present using the proximal isovelocity surface area method. The color Doppler flow parameters are adjusted to demonstrate a well-defined hemispherical aliasing surface area on the LA side of the mitral orifice. The velocity at this location equals the Nyquist limit (the "aliasing" velocity). The cross-sectional area of the aliased boundary is calculated as the surface area of a hemisphere with diameter measured from the color flow image. Multiplying cross-sectional area by the known velocity yields the volume flow rate, which then is used in conjunction with the transmitral velocity-time interval in the continuity equation. One difficulty with this approach is that the volume flow rate must be integrated over the diastolic filling period; a single color image yields only the volume flow rate at one time point in diastole. Because of this problem, the proximal isovelocity method has not been widely applied in mitral stenosis.

Technical Considerations and Potential Pitfalls

As for any intracardiac blood flow, accurate pressure gradient calculations depend on accurate velocity measurements, which require a near-parallel intercept angle between the direction of blood flow and the Doppler beam (Table 11.5). The mitral stenosis jet nearly always can be recorded from an apical approach, but careful transducer positioning and angulation are needed to record an optimal signal. Color flow imaging may be helpful in defining the jet direction in a given tomographic plane. Depending on the maximum jet velocity, the velocity curve can be recorded with conventional pulsed, high-pulse repetition frequency, or CW Doppler ultrasound. Pulsed Doppler recordings may show better definition of the maximum velocity and early-diastolic slope than CW Doppler recordings because of a better signal-to-noise ratio.

Direct planimetry of mitral valve area is best done using a 3D volumetric data set. Although historically, measurement on 2D short-axis images was well validated, this approach requires meticulous scanning to

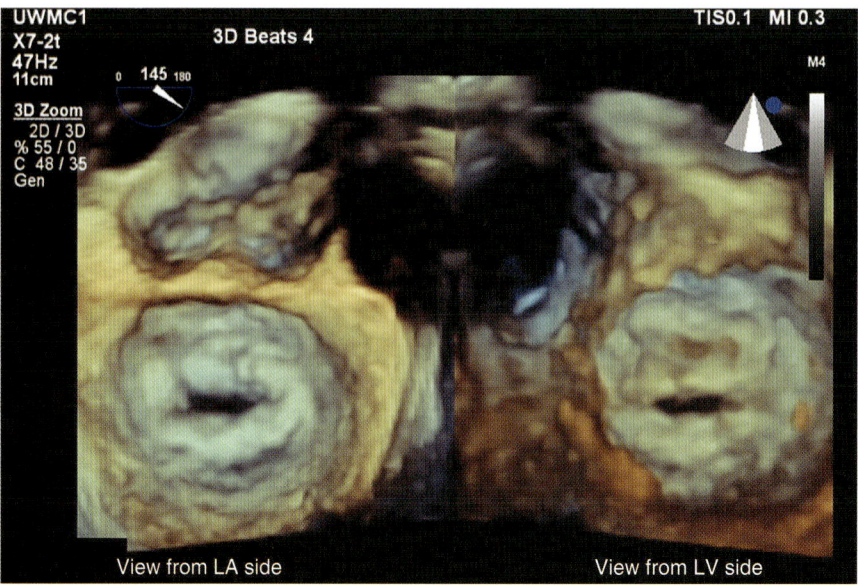

Fig. 11.22 ▶ **3D imaging of rheumatic mitral stenosis.** 3D TEE imaging of a stenotic mitral valve viewed from the LA side *(left)* is oriented with the aortic valve *(Ao)* at the top of the image. Symetric commissural fusion of the medial and lateral commissures between the anterior and posterior leaflets is seen. Rotating the 3D view to the LV side of the valve confirms fusion of the both commissures.

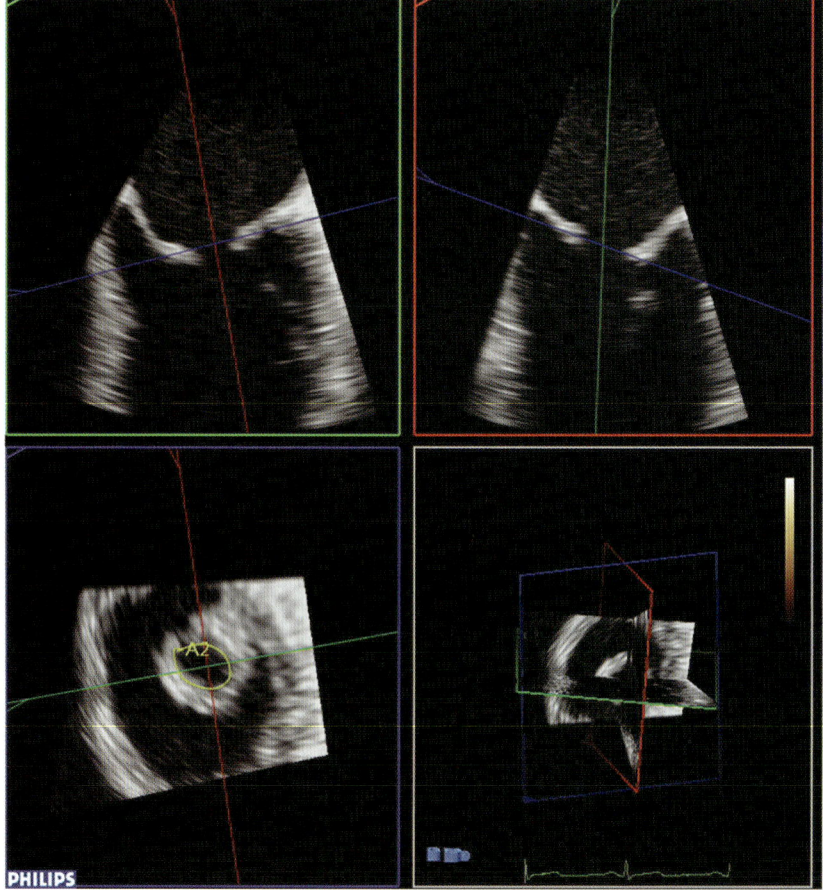

Fig. 11.23 **3D planimetry of valve area in rheumatic mitral stenosis.** A full-volume 3D acquisition on TEE imaging was used to obtain a short-axis view of the orifice at the leaflet tips *(lower left)* by adjusting the red, blue, and green image planes in orthogonal views. Valve area *(A2)* is measured at 1.15 cm^2 in this 36-year-old man with recurrent pulmonary edema.

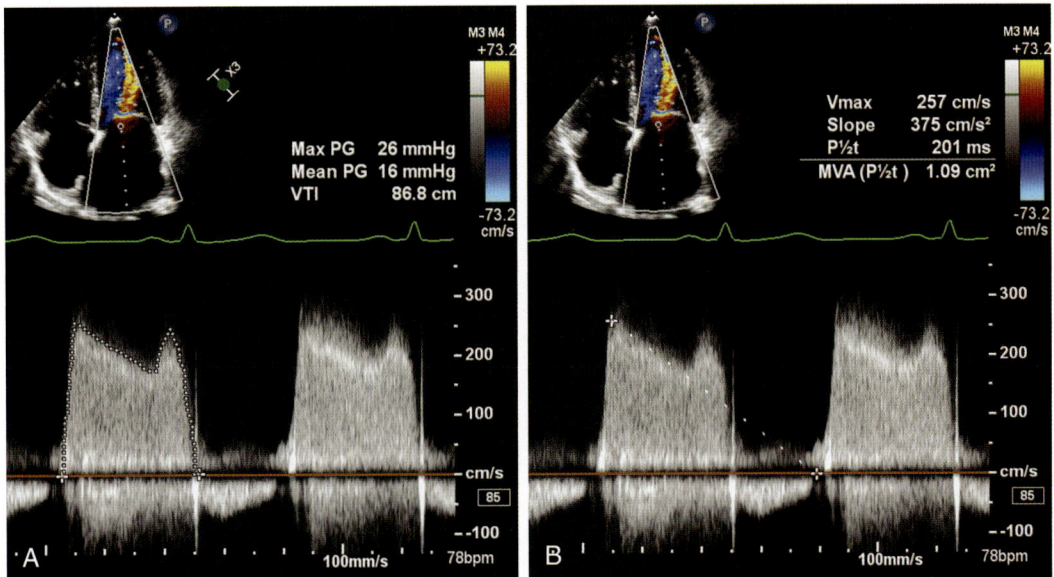

Fig. 11.24 Pressure gradient and pressure half-time in severe mitral stenosis. In this patient with mitral stenosis, (A) the pulsed Doppler LV inflow curve is traced to measure the mean diastolic pressure gradient *(PG)* of 16 mmHg. (B) A line drawn from the peak early diastolic velocity *(Vmax)* along the slope of the early deceleration curve provides the pressure half-time *(P½t)* of 201 ms, indicating a valve area of 1.1 cm². The pressure half-time of 302 ms corresponds to a valve area of 0.7 cm². The patient is in sinus rhythm, so an *A* velocity is seen in late diastole.

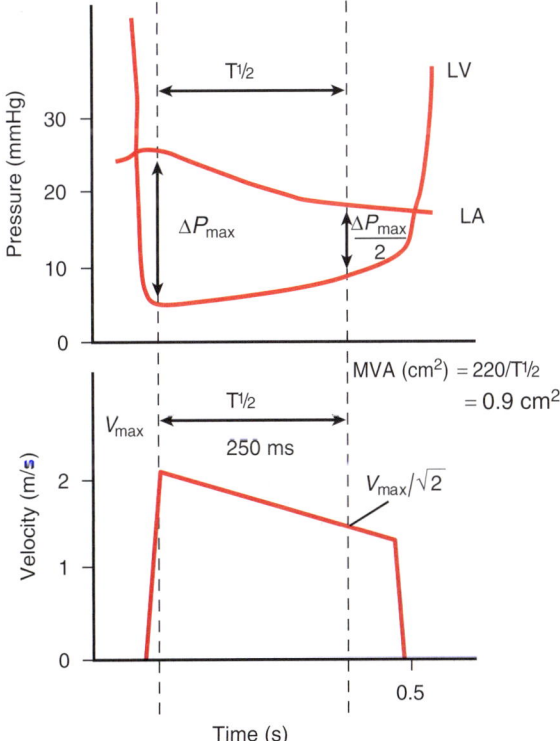

Fig. 11.25 Relationship between left atrial and left ventricular pressures and the Doppler velocity curve in mitral stenosis. Maximum velocity *(Vmax)* and the diastolic slope are identified as shown, yielding a pressure half-time *(T½)* of 226 ms, corresponding to a mitral valve area *(MVA)* of 1 cm². No *A* velocity is noted because atrial fibrillation is present. ΔP_{max}, Maximum pressure gradient.

obtain the correct image plane at the leaflet tips. With both 2D and 3 D approaches, definition of valve area may be difficult if image quality is poor, if extensive distortion of valve anatomy is present, or if calcification results in shadowing and reverberations. Valve area can be underestimated if gain settings are too high and can be overestimated if the smallest area at the leaflet tips is not recorded. Low gain settings and careful measurement from a 3D volume or 2D scanning in a short-axis plane from the apex toward the base can help avoid these potential problems.

Pressure half-time valve area calculations have significant limitations in certain clinical settings. When coexisting aortic regurgitation is present, LV filling occurs both antegrade across the mitral valve and retrograde across the aortic valve. This may result in a more rapid rise in LV diastolic pressure than if there were no aortic regurgitation, thus resulting in a shorter half-time measurement. Conversely, if severe aortic regurgitation impairs mitral leaflet opening, functional mitral stenosis may be superimposed on anatomic mitral stenosis, with lengthening of the half-time measurement. In clinical practice, if rheumatic mitral stenosis is present with only mild to moderate aortic regurgitation, the half-time method remains a useful approach for the evaluation of stenosis severity. If aortic regurgitation is severe or if the mitral valve anatomy is atypical, the potential influence of coexisting lesions should be considered.

A major assumption of the half-time method is that LA and LV compliances do not significantly

TABLE 11.5	Pitfalls in the Evaluation of Mitral Stenosis Severity

Pressure Gradient

Intercept angle between mitral stenosis jet and ultrasound beam
Beat-to-beat variability in atrial fibrillation
Dependence on transvalvular volume flow rate (e.g., exercise, coexisting mitral regurgitation)

2D or 3D Valve Area

Image orientation
Tomographic plane
2D gain settings
Intraobserver and interobserver variability in planimetry of orifice
Poor acoustic access
Deformed valve anatomy after commissurotomy

$T\frac{1}{2}$ Valve Area

Definition of V_{max} and early-diastolic slope
Nonlinear early-diastolic velocity slope
Sinus rhythm with A-wave superimposed on early-diastolic slope
Influence of coexisting aortic regurgitation
Changing LV and LA compliances immediately after commissurotomy

Continuity Equation Mitral Valve Area

Accurate measurement of transmitral stroke volume

V_{max}, Maximum velocity; $T\frac{1}{2}$, half-time.

affect the rate of pressure gradient decline across the stenotic orifice. Although this assumption appears to be warranted in clinically stable patients, it is *not* justified in the period immediately after balloon mitral commissurotomy. After relief of mitral stenosis, the fall in LA pressure and the increase in LV filling are accompanied by directionally opposite changes in LA and LV compliance. During the 24 to 72 hours after the procedure, equilibrium has not been reached, and the pressure half-time may not be an accurate reflection of orifice area. After this adjustment period, compliances stabilize, and the pressure half-time method again provides useful information.

Even under physiologically stable conditions, accurate pressure half-time measurements require careful recording of the mitral stenosis velocity curve. It is important that the intercept angle be parallel to flow and *constant* throughout diastole to avoid artifactual distortion in the shape of the curve. The maximum early-diastolic velocity and the early-diastolic deceleration slope should be well defined. In addition, pressure half-times are most easily and reproducibly measured if the deceleration slope is linear. If a linear slope cannot be obtained even after careful adjustment of transducer position and angulation, the half-time measurement should be made using the mid-diastolic slope of the curve.

In atrial fibrillation, several beats are averaged because mean gradient will vary with the RR interval. Although the half-time will be relatively constant despite variation in the length of diastole, only beats in which the diastolic filling period is long enough to show the early-diastolic slope clearly are appropriate for measurement. Although the pressure half-time method is accurate when sinus rhythm is present, the increase in velocity due to atrial contraction may obscure the early-diastolic slope, particularly at high heart rates, so half-time measurements may not be possible unless a slow heart rate allows clear definition of the mid-diastolic slope.

Continuity equation mitral valve area determinations are most accurate in patients without significant coexisting mitral regurgitation. In this subgroup, continuity equation mitral valve area calculations provide a useful alternative to the pressure half-time method, especially in situations of altered chamber compliances. The accuracy of the continuity equation method, as in aortic stenosis, depends on a parallel intercept angle between the mitral stenotic jet and the ultrasound beam and a careful stroke volume calculation from diameter and velocity recordings. Accurate pulmonary artery diameter measurement for stroke volume calculations can be difficult in adult patients because of poor acoustic access. LV outflow tract diameter nearly always can be depicted reliably. However, many patients with mitral stenosis have some degree of coexisting aortic or mitral regurgitation so that transaortic stroke volume does not equal transmitral stroke volume.

Consequences of Mitral Stenosis

Left Ventricular Response

The LV in mitral stenosis is small with normal wall thickness and normal systolic function, although diastolic function is impaired because of the restriction of flow across the mitral orifice. The presence of LV dilation suggests that significant coexisting mitral or aortic regurgitation or primary myocardial dysfunction (cardiomyopathy or ischemic disease) is present.

Left Atrial Enlargement and Thrombus

Chronic pressure overload of mitral stenosis leads to gradual enlargement of the LA. LA size can become extremely large in long-standing severe mitral stenosis. In conjunction with a low volume flow rate due to the stenotic valve, LA enlargement results in stasis of blood flow and thrombus formation. Thrombi are located preferentially in the LA appendage but also can occur in the body of the atrium as a protruding thrombus or as a laminated thrombus along the atrial wall or interatrial septum (Fig. 11.26). LA thrombi are most common when atrial fibrillation is present but may occur even in sinus rhythm.

TTE echo has a high specificity for the detection of an LA thrombus (i.e., if it is visualized, it most likely is a real finding), but the sensitivity is less than 50%, so many are missed. In part, this relates to the difficulty of imaging the LA appendage in adults. Sometimes the LA appendage can be visualized in a laterally angulated parasternal short-axis view at the aortic valve level or from an apical two-chamber view angulated slightly superiorly; however, often the atrial appendage cannot be visualized at all. When the atrial appendage is seen, image quality usually is too poor to allow a reliable exclusion of an atrial thrombus because of poor ultrasound tissue penetration in addition to beam-width artifact at the depth of the LA from surface imaging.

TEE has a high sensitivity (about 99%) and specificity (about 99%) for the detection of an LA thrombus. The LA appendage can be depicted well in multiple image planes by using a multiplane probe. In addition, the higher transducer frequencies (5 to 7 MHz) and lower imaging depths result in high-resolution images. Although a thrombus in the appendage often protrudes into the chamber, laminated thrombi in the body of the atrium may be more difficult to recognize, especially along the interatrial septum.

Pulmonary Hypertension

In mitral stenosis, increased LA pressure results in pulmonary venous hypertension and consequent pulmonary artery hypertension. Initially, the increase in pulmonary artery pressure is "passive"—the pressure difference across the pulmonary bed (pulmonary artery minus LA pressure) is normal. In this situation, although pulmonary pressures are elevated, pulmonary vascular resistance is normal, and pulmonary pressures will fall toward normal after relief of mitral stenosis. With long-standing pulmonary venous hypertension, irreversible changes in the pulmonary vascular bed occur, leading to elevated pulmonary vascular resistance and persistent pulmonary hypertension after relief of mitral stenosis. Pulmonary pressures and resistance should be evaluated in all patients with mitral stenosis, as described in Chapter 6.

Exercise testing to evaluate the change in pulmonary pressure from rest to exercise may be considered when symptoms are greater than expected for the degree of stenosis. Pulmonary pressures are calculated from the tricuspid regurgitant jet measured at rest and immediately after exercise. Rapid data acquisition after exercise is essential for an accurate estimation of the maximum exercise change.

Mitral Regurgitation

Some degree of coexisting mitral regurgitation is common in patients with mitral stenosis. Mitral regurgitant severity can be evaluated using standard techniques (see Chapter 12), and it is an important factor in deciding on appropriate therapy. For example, significant mitral regurgitation is a contraindication to surgical or percutaneous commissurotomy. Coexisting mitral regurgitation elevates the transmitral pressure gradient (due to increased

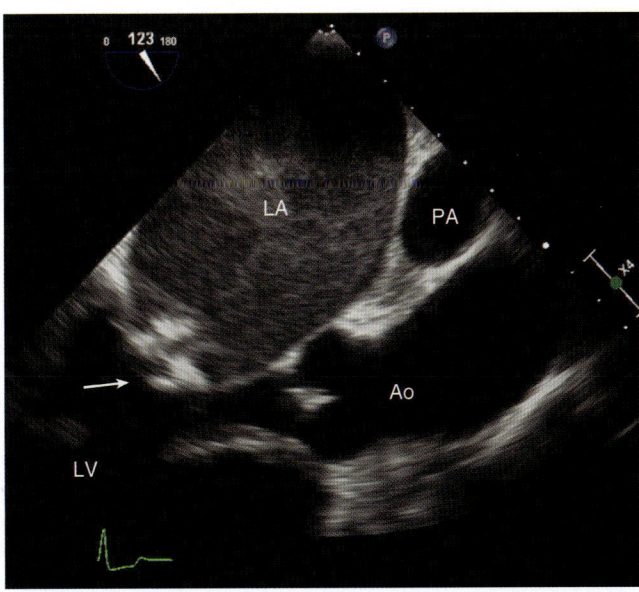

Fig. 11.26 **Spontaneous LA contrast.** On this TEE image, swirling spontaneous contrast is seen in the enlarged LA of a patient with severe mitral stenosis. The severely calcified rheumatic mitral valve is seen *(arrow)*. *Ao,* Aorta.

transmitral volume flow rate), but both 2D echo and pressure half-time valve area measurements remain accurate.

ECHO MATH: Mitral Stenosis Severity

Example

A 26-year-old pregnant woman presents with dyspnea and is noted to have a diastolic murmur at the apex. Echocardiography shows rheumatic mitral stenosis with:

MVA_{2D}	$0.8\ cm^2$
Mean ΔP	5 mmHg
$T\frac{1}{2}$	260 ms
Mitral valve morphology score	
Leaflet thickness	2
Mobility	1
Calcification	1
Subvalvular	2
TOTAL	6
Tricuspid regurgitant jet velocity	3.1 m/s
Estimated RA pressure	10 mmHg
Mitral regurgitation	Mild

Mean pressure gradient is calculated by tracing the outer edge of the CW Doppler velocity curve, with the echo instrument calculating and then averaging instantaneous pressure gradients over the systolic ejection period.

Doppler mitral valve area ($MVA_{Doppler}$) is calculated as:

$$MVA_{Doppler} = 220/T\frac{1}{2} = 220/260 = 0.85\ cm^2$$

The 2D mitral valve area and the pressure half-time valve area show reasonable agreement, and both are consistent with severe mitral stenosis.

Pulmonary artery pressure (PAP) is:

$$PAP = 4(V_{TR})^2 + RAP = 4(3.1)^2 + 10\ mmHg = 48\ mmHg$$

Pulmonary pressure is moderately elevated consistent with a secondary response to severe mitral stenosis.

The mitral morphology score is low, and only mild mitral regurgitation is present, which indicates a high likelihood of immediate and long-term success with balloon mitral valvuloplasty. TEE is needed just before mitral valvuloplasty to evaluate for LA thrombus.

Other Coexisting Valvular Disease

The rheumatic disease process also can affect the aortic valve (second in frequency to the mitral valve) and, less commonly, the tricuspid valve. Aortic valve involvement may result in stenosis, regurgitation, or both, which can be evaluated with appropriate 2D and Doppler echo techniques. Evaluation of aortic regurgitation by color flow imaging may be complicated in the presence of mitral stenosis because of merging of the two diastolic flow disturbances in the LV. Imaging the aortic regurgitant jet in short axis just proximal to the aortic valve and using other Doppler methods for the evaluation of regurgitant severity will prevent this potential problem.

Rheumatic tricuspid stenosis may be difficult to appreciate on 2D imaging. Doppler flow patterns are similar to those seen in mitral stenosis, and the same quantitative methods for the evaluation of stenosis severity can be applied. Even in the absence of rheumatic involvement of the tricuspid valve, significant tricuspid regurgitation is common (due to pulmonary hypertension and annular dilation) in patients with mitral stenosis. Careful evaluation of tricuspid regurgitation severity is especially important preoperatively in case tricuspid annuloplasty is needed at the time of mitral valve surgery.

Clinical Applications in Specific Patient Populations

Disease Stages, Hemodynamic Progression, and Timing of Intervention

Echo Doppler is the standard clinical method for making the diagnosis and defining the stage of disease in patients with valvular mitral stenosis (Table 11.6). Disease progression can be followed and the timing of intervention can be determined using Doppler echo and clinical data alone. Evaluation by cardiac catheterization rarely is needed.

Patients Undergoing Balloon Mitral Commissurotomy

In the potential candidate for percutaneous balloon mitral commissurotomy, echo Doppler evaluation of mitral valve morphology is important in patient selection both in terms of predicted hemodynamic results and in terms of the risk of procedural complications. Mitral valve morphology may be described by a qualitative assessment, an additive scoring system (Tables 11.7 and 11.8), or quantitative measurements of leaflet mobility. Whatever approach is used, the important features to consider are leaflet mobility, leaflet thickness, leaflet and commissural calcification, and subvalvular involvement (Fig. 11.27). In general, the best hemodynamic results are seen with thin, mobile leaflets that have commissural fusion but little calcification or subchordal thickening. However, some patients with relatively unfavorable morphology do

TABLE 11.6 Stages of Mitral Stenosis

Stage	Definition	Valve Anatomy	Valve Hemodynamics	Hemodynamic Consequences	Symptoms
A	At risk of MS	• Mild valve doming during diastole	• Normal transmitral flow velocity	• None	• None
B	Progressive MS	• Rheumatic valve changes with commissural fusion and diastolic doming of the mitral valve leaflets • Planimetered MVA >1.5 cm^2	• Increased transmitral flow velocities • MVA >1.5 cm^2 • Diastolic pressure half-time <150 ms	• Mild to moderate LA enlargement • Normal pulmonary pressure at rest	• None
C	Asymptomatic severe MS	• Rheumatic valve changes with commissural fusion and diastolic doming of the mitral valve leaflets • Planimetered MVA ≤1.5 cm^2 • (MVA ≤1.0 cm^2 with very severe MS)	• MVA ≤1.5 cm^2 • (MVA ≤1.0 cm^2 with very severe MS) • Diastolic pressure half-time ≤150 ms • (Diastolic pressure half-time ≥220 ms with very severe MS)	• Severe LA enlargement • Elevated PASP >30 mmHg	• None
D	Symptomatic severe MS	• Rheumatic valve changes with commissural fusion and diastolic doming of the mitral valve leaflets • Planimetered MVA ≤1.5 cm^2	• MVA ≤1.5 cm^2 • (MVA ≤1.0 cm^2 with very severe MS) • Diastolic pressure half-time ≥150 ms • (Diastolic pressure half-time ≥220 ms with very severe MS)	• Severe LA enlargement • Elevated PASP >30 mmHg	• Decreased exercise tolerance • Exertional dyspnea

The transmitral mean pressure gradient should be obtained to further determine the hemodynamic effect of the MS and is usually >5 to 10 mmHg in severe MS; however, due to the variability of the mean pressure gradient with heart rate and forward flow, it has not been included in the criteria for severity.
MS, Mitral stenosis; *MVA*, mitral valve area; *PASP*, pulmonary artery systolic pressure.
From Nishimura RA, Otto CM, Bonow RO, et al: AHA/ACC guideline for the management of patients with valvular heart disease: executive summary. A report of the American College of Cardiology/American Heart Association Task Force on Practice Guidelines. *Circulation* 129:2440–2492, 2014.

---

have relief of mitral stenosis with percutaneous commissurotomy. It is noteworthy that patients with the most heavily calcified and deformed valves (and the most severe stenosis) are more likely to have procedure-related morbidity and mortality.

Another factor to consider in this patient population is the degree of coexisting mitral regurgitation because percutaneous commissurotomy is contradicted if moderate or severe regurgitation is present. In addition, because any LA thrombi may be dislodged by the catheters during the procedure, TEE typically is used to evaluate for an LA thrombus before the procedure. During the procedure, catheter and balloon position, hemodynamic results, LA thrombus, and procedural complications may be monitored using TEE or intracardiac echocardiographic imaging (Fig. 11.28). 3D echocardiography allows for a more reliable assessment of commissural opening during balloon commissurotomy (Fig. 11.29).

After percutaneous commissurotomy, Doppler allows the identification of complications, permits assessment of hemodynamic results, and provides a baseline for future disease progression. Potential complications include (1) an increase in the severity of mitral regurgitation and (2) the presence of an atrial septal defect (usually small) at the transseptal catheter puncture site. Hemodynamic results can be evaluated with standard echo Doppler techniques, again with an awareness of the potential inaccuracies in the half-time method in the immediate postcommissurotomy period. Doppler evaluation of postprocedure pulmonary artery systolic pressure also can be helpful. Predictors of long-term outcome after balloon mitral commissurotomy include mitral valve area, severity of mitral regurgitation, and the mitral morphology score.

TRICUSPID STENOSIS

Tricuspid stenosis is uncommon in adult patients; in nearly all cases, it is due to rheumatic disease in association with rheumatic mitral involvement.

TABLE 11.7 Mitral Valve Morphology by 2D Echocardiography

Grade*	Mobility	Thickening	Calcification	Subvalvular Thickening
1	Highly mobile valve with only leaflet tips restricted	Leaflets near normal in thickness (4–5 mm)	A single area of increased echo brightness	Minimal thickening just below the mitral leaflets
2	Leaflet mid and base portions have normal mobility.	Mid-leaflets normal, considerable thickening of margins (5–8 mm)	Scattered areas of brightness confined to leaflet margins	Thickening of chordal structures extending to one third of the chordal length
3	Valve continues to move forward in diastole, mainly from the base.	Thickening extending through the entire leaflet (5–8 mm)	Brightness extending into the mid portions of the leaflets	Thickening extended to distal third of the chords
4	No or minimal forward movement of the leaflets occurs in diastole.	Considerable thickening of all leaflet tissue (>8–10 mm)	Extensive brightness throughout much of leaflet tissue	Extensive thickening and shortening of all chordal structures extending down to papillary muscles

*The total echocardiographic score is derived from an analysis of mitral leaflet mobility, valvular and subvalvular thickening, and calcification, each of which is graded from 0 to 4 according to the foregoing criteria. This gives a total score of 0 to 16.
From Wilkins GT, Weyman AE, Abascal VM, et al: Percutaneous balloon dilatation of the mitral valve: an analysis of echocardiographic variables related to outcome and the mechanism of dilatation, *Br Heart J* 60:299–308, 1988.

TABLE 11.8 The French Three-Group Grading of Mitral Valve Anatomy

Echocardiographic Group	Mitral Valve Anatomy
Group 1	Pliable, noncalcified anterior mitral leaflet and mild subvalvular disease (i.e., thin chordae ≥10 mm long)
Group 2	Pliable noncalcified anterior mitral leaflet and severe subvalvular disease (i.e., thickened chordae <10 mm long)
Group 3	Calcification of mitral valve of any extent, as assessed by fluoroscopy, whatever the state of subvalvular apparatus

Reprinted from Iung B, Cormier B, Discimetiere P, et al: Functional results 5 years after successful percutaneous mitral commissurotomy in a series of 528 patients and analysis of predictive factors, *J Am Coll Cardiol* 27:407–414, 1996, with permission from the American College of Cardiology Foundation.

Carcinoid heart disease affects both tricuspid and pulmonic valves and can lead either to stenosis or to regurgitation. Right atrial (RA) tumors, large vegetations, or a large atrial thrombus (which may have embolized from the venous bed) can obstruct right ventricular (RV) inflow and mimic tricuspid stenosis.

2D echo images show thickening and shortening of the tricuspid valve leaflets (Fig. 11.30). Commissural fusion and diastolic bowing indicate rheumatic disease. Doppler recordings of the transvalvular flow velocity allow for the calculation of mean gradient and pressure half-time valve area, as described for the mitral valve.

PULMONIC STENOSIS

Pulmonic stenosis in adults is most often due to congenital disease, either residual stenosis after reparative surgery in childhood or clinically insignificant obstruction. Pulmonic stenosis may occur in conjunction with other congenital lesions such as ventricular inversion (congenitally corrected transposition of the great arteries) or tetralogy of Fallot.

2D echo imaging of the pulmonic valve shows thickened leaflets with systolic bowing. On Doppler interrogation, the antegrade velocity is increased with corresponding maximum and mean pressure gradients

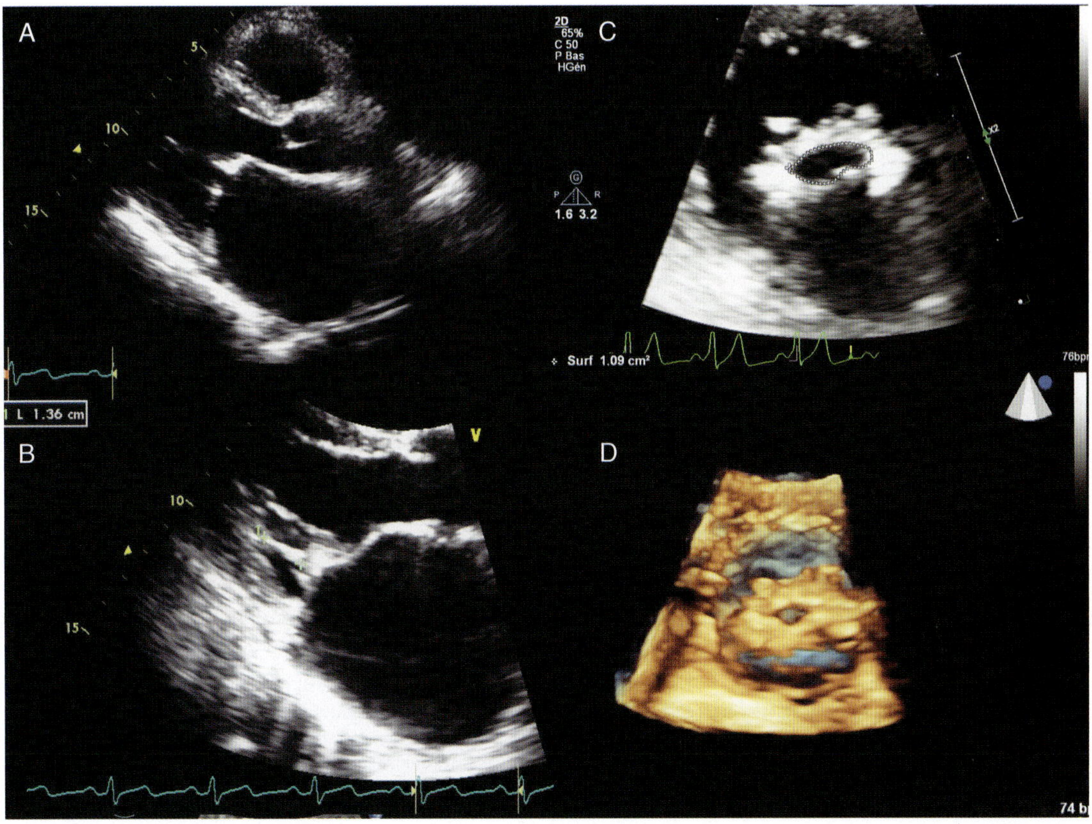

Fig. 11.27 Mitral valve morphology. TTE. ▶ (A) Parasternal long-axis view showing a thickened, noncalcified, and pliable valve. (B) Parasternal long-axis view showing moderate impairment of the subvalvular apparatus (length of chordae 13.6 mm) as shown by *cross-marks*. ▶ (C) Parasternal short-axis view showing thickening of the leaflet tips and fusion of both commissures with the valve orifice area traced as shown by the *dotted line*. ▶ (D) 3D parasternal short-axis view showing valve thickening and fusion of both commissures. *(From Otto CM, editor:* The Practice of Clinical Echocardiography, *ed 5, Philadelphia, 2017, Elsevier, Fig. 21-2.)*

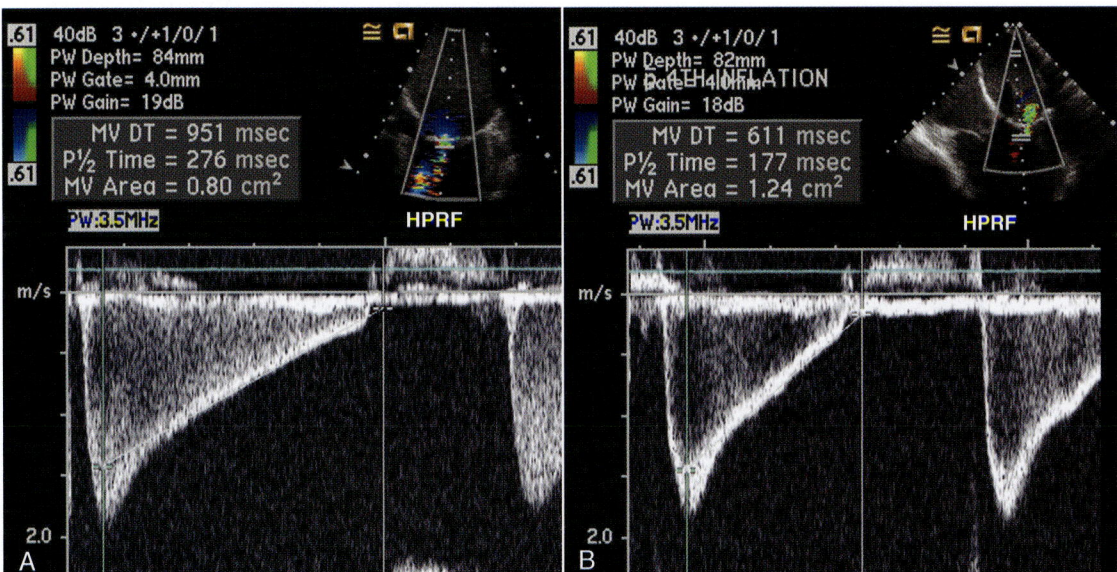

Fig. 11.28 Transesophageal mitral valve hemodynamics during balloon commissurotomy. Doppler velocity curves across the stenotic mitral valve before (A) and after (B) percutaneous mitral valvuloplasty were recorded from a TEE approach Pressure half-time decreased from 276 to 177 ms, indicating an increase in valve area from 0.8 to 1.2 cm². This is a suboptimal increase in valve area, but color flow also showed an increase in mitral regurgitant severity, which limited further dilation. Note that the pressure half-time is measured from the linear mid-diastolic segment of the flow signal, extrapolating back to the onset of flow, ignoring the early-diastolic short steep deceleration.

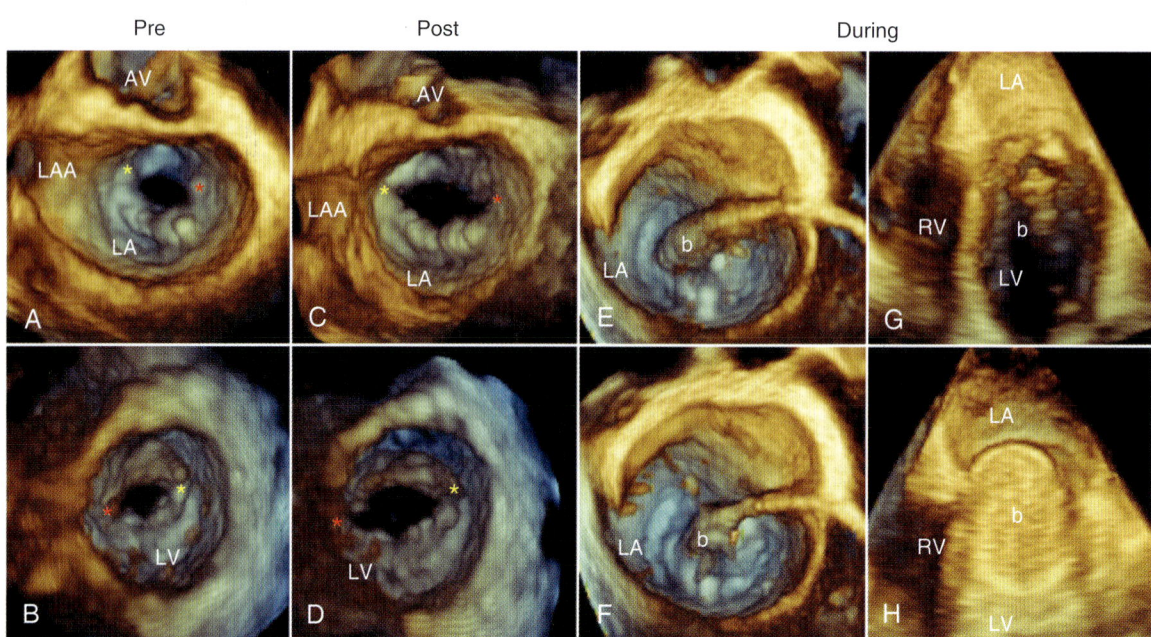

Fig. 11.29 3D transesophageal-guided mitral valve balloon valvuloplasty. (A) and (B) The stenotic mitral valve orifice in a patient with severe mitral stenosis before mitral valve balloon valvuloplasty. ▶ (A) The mitral valve as seen from the LA. ▶ (B) The stenotic mitral valve as seen from the LV. The *red asterisk* points to the fused posteromedial commissure; the *yellow asterisk* points to the fused anterolateral commissure. ▶ (C) and (D) The commissural splitting produced by the balloon valvuloplasty. Note the significant enlargement of the mitral valve area and the splitting of the commissures. (E) to (H) 3D TEE images obtained during mitral valve balloon valvuloplasty guidance. In (E) the deflated balloon *(b)* has been advanced through the interatrial septum and is directed to the mitral orifice. In (F) the deflated balloon has been advanced through the mitral orifice into the LV. In (G) the deflated balloon is seen along the long axis of the LV. In (H) the inflated balloon is seen in its longitudinal cross section stretching and splitting the mitral valve commissures. *AV,* Aortic valve; *LAA,* LA appendage. *(From Salcedo EE, Carroll JD: Echocardiographic guidance of structural heart disease interventions. In Otto CM, editor:* The Practice of Clinical Echocardiography, *ed 4, Philadelphia, 2012, Saunders, Fig. 5-10.)*

via the Bernoulli equation (Fig. 11.31). Pulmonic valve area is not usually calculated, but the continuity equation principle can be applied in this situation, by using an appropriate intracardiac location for stroke volume determination. Differentiation of valvular pulmonic stenosis from subvalvular or supravalvular obstruction can be difficult by 2D echo. Careful examinations with color flow and conventional pulsed Doppler can be very helpful in defining the site of the poststenotic flow disturbance (and thus the site of obstruction).

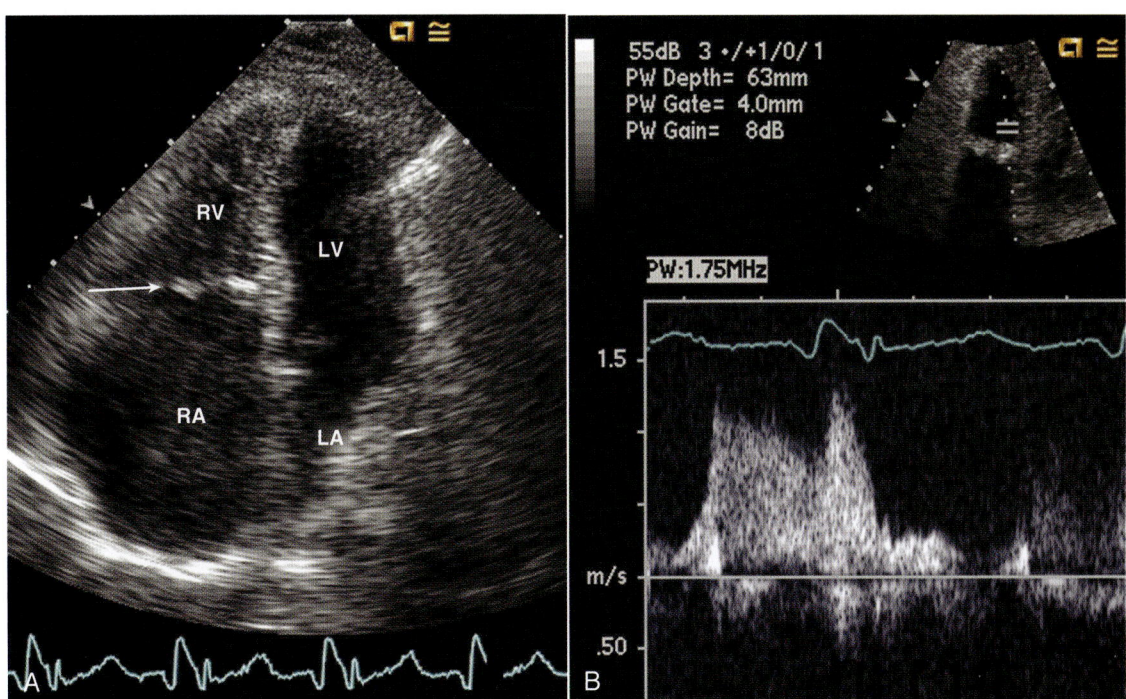

Fig. 11.30 Rheumatic tricuspid stenosis. In the apical four-chamber view (A), thickened valve leaflets *(arrow)* and RA enlargement are seen. (B) The Doppler RV inflow velocity shows a slightly high mean gradient and prolonged deceleration time.

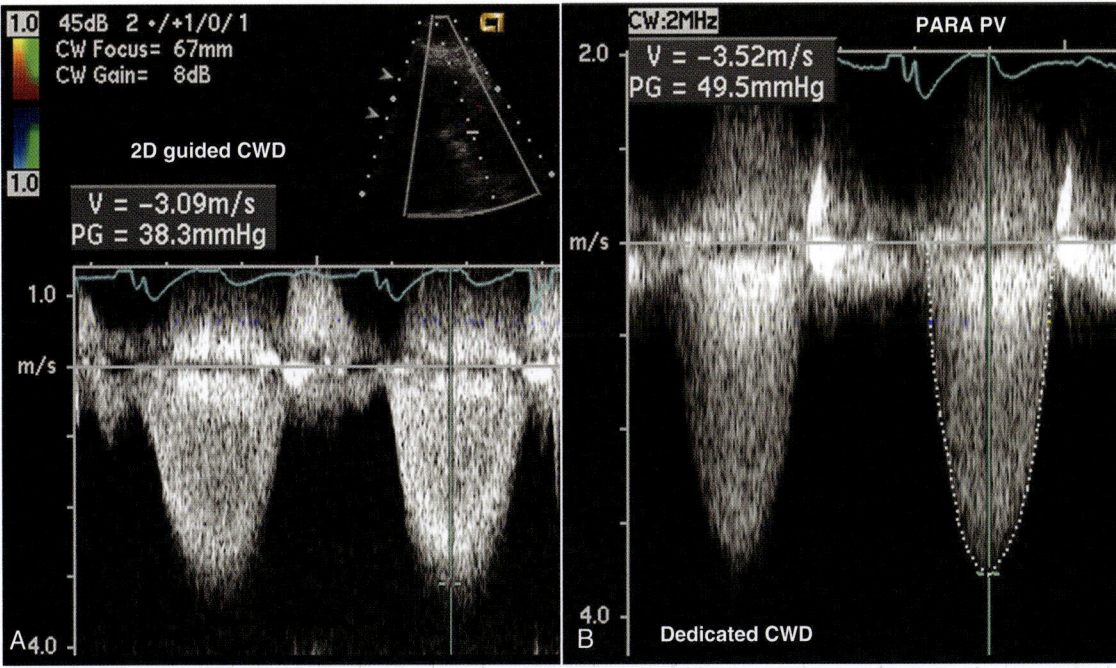

Fig. 11.31 Pulmonic valve stenosis. In this 26-year-old woman with repaired tetralogy of Fallot, a 2D-guided CW Doppler image from the parasternal window in an RV outflow view (A) shows a maximum velocity of 3.1 m/s. However, with a dedicated CW Doppler transducer (B), a velocity of 3.5 m/s was recorded because the smaller transducer can be angled to be more parallel to the jet and the nonimaging transducer has a better Doppler signal-to-noise ratio.

THE ECHO EXAM

Aortic Stenosis: Key Measures

Parameter	Key Measures	Clinical Decision Thresholds
Valve anatomy	Calcific Bicuspid (2 leaflets in systole) Rheumatic	
Stenosis severity	Jet velocity (V_{max})	≥4 m/s (severe) ≥5 m/s (very severe)
	Mean pressure gradient (ΔP_{mean})	≥40 mmHg
	LVOT/AS velocity ratio	≤0.25
	Aortic valve area (AVA)	<1.0 cm^2 <0.6 cm^2/m^2
Stroke volume	Stroke volume index	<35 mL/m^2
Rate of progression	Annual changes in V_{max} on serial studies	≥0.3 m/s/yr
Coexisting aortic regurgitation	Qualitative evaluation of severity	
LV response	LV hypertrophy LV dimensions or volumes LV ejection fraction	<50%
Other findings	Pulmonary pressures Mitral regurgitation	

LVOT, LV outflow tract.

Technical Details for Quantitation of Aortic Stenosis Severity

Components	Modality	View	Recording	Measurements
LVOT diameter $LVOT_D$	2D	Parasternal long-axis	Adjust depth, optimize endocardial definition, zoom mode.	Inner edge to inner edge of LVOT, parallel and adjacent to aortic valve, mid-systole
LVOT flow V_{LVOT} VTI_{LVOT}	Pulsed Doppler	Apical 4-chamber (anteriorly angulated)	Sample volume 2–3 mm, envelope of flow with defined peak, start with sample volume at valve and move apically.	Trace modal velocity of spectral velocity curve.
AS jet V_{max} $VTI_{AS\text{-}jet}$	CW Doppler	Apical, SSN, other	Examination from multiple windows, careful positioning, and transducer angulation to obtain highest-velocity signal	Measure maximum velocities at edge of intense velocity signal.
Pressure gradient		$\Delta P_{max} = 4(V_{max})^2$		
Continuity equation		AVA (cm^2) = [π($LVOT_D$ / 2)^2 × VTI_{LVOT}] / $VTI_{AS\text{-}jet}$		
Simplified continuity equation		AVA (cm^2) = [π($LVOT_D$ / 2)^2 × V_{LVOT}] / $V_{AS\text{-}jet}$		
Velocity ratio		Velocity ratio = V_{LVOT} / $V_{AS\text{-}jet}$		
Stroke volume index		SV_i = [π($LVOT_D$ / 2)^2 × VTI_{LVOT}] / BSA		

AS, Aortic stenosis; *AVA*, aortic valve area; *BSA*, body surface area; *LVOT*, LV outflow tract; *SSN*, suprasternal notch; *V*, velocity; *VTI*, velocity-time integral.

Mitral Stenosis: Key Measures

Parameter	Key Measures	Clinical Decision Thresholds
Valve anatomy	Valve thickness and mobility Calcification Commissural fusion Subvalvular involvement	
Stenosis severity	2D or 3D valve area	MVA ≤1.5 cm^2 (severe) MVA ≤1.0 cm^2 (very severe)
	Mean pressure gradient Pressure half-time valve area	Variable depending on flow rate ≥150 ms (severe) ≥220 ms (very severe)
LA	Size (dimension or volume) TEE for thrombus before transcatheter balloon commissurotomy	
Coexisting mitral regurgitation	Qualitative and quantitative evaluation of severity	
Pulmonary vasculature	Pulmonary systolic pressure RV size and function	>30 mmHg
Other findings	Aortic valve involvement LV size and systolic function	

MVA, Mitral valve area.

Technical Details for Quantitation of Mitral Stenosis Severity

Parameter	Modality	View	Recording	Measurements
2D planimetry of valve area MVA$_{2D}$	2D	Parasternal short-axis	Scan from apex to base to identify minimal valve area	Planimetry of inner edge of dark-light interface
2D planimetry of valve area MVA$_{3D}$	3D full-volume acquisition	TTE or TEE	Acquire full volume of mitral valve with analysis in x, y, z planes after acquisition.	Adjust image planes to obtain planar view of mitral orifice at leaflet tips. Trace white-black interface.
Mean gradient Mean ΔP	Pulsed (HPRF) or CW Doppler	Apical 4-chamber or long-axis	Align Doppler beam parallel to MS jet. Adjust angle to obtain smooth envelope, clear peak, and linear deceleration slope.	Trace maximum velocity of spectral velocity curve
Pressure half-time ($T\frac{1}{2}$)	Pulsed (HPRF) or CW Doppler	Apical 4-chamber or long-axis	Same as mean gradient. Adjust scale so velocity curve fills the screen. HPRF Doppler often has less noise than CW Doppler signal.	Place line from maximum velocity along mid-diastolic linear slope. MVA = 220 / $T\frac{1}{2}$

HPRF, High pulse repetition frequency; *MVA*, mitral valve area.

SUGGESTED READING

Guidelines

1. Baumgartner H, Hung J, Bermejo J, et al: Recommendations on the echocardiographic assessment of aortic valve stenosis: a focused update from the European Association of Cardiovascular Imaging and the American Society of Echocardiography, *J Am Soc Echocardiogr* 30:372–392, 2017.
   This consensus document updates recommendations for echocardiographic assessment of aortic stenosis severity. Additional details on evaluation of low flow, low gradient aortic stenosis are provided.

2. Baumgartner H, Hung J, Bermejo J, et al: Echocardiographic assessment of valve stenosis: recommendations for clinical practice. From the European Society of Echocardiography and American Society of Echocardiography, *J Am Soc Echocardiogr* 22:1–23, 2009.
   The original consensus document reviews approaches to the evaluation of mitral valve stenosis. Recommendations are provided for which measurements to use in clinical practice along with details on data acquisition and measurements. Tables summarize the formulas with advantages and limitations of each. A comprehensive list of references is included.

3. Nishimura RA, Otto CM, Bonow RO, et al: 2017 AHA/ACC focused update of the 2014 AHA/ACC guideline for the management of patients with valvular heart disease: a report of the American College of Cardiology/American Heart Association Task Force on Clinical Practice Guidelines, *Circulation* 135:e1159–e1195, 2017.
   These detailed guidelines (plus the original 2014 document) for management of adults with valvular heart disease include definitions of hemodynamic severity for valve stenosis and valve regurgitation as shown in the tables for stages of aortic and mitral stenosis.

Aortic Stenosis

4. Jander N, Minners J: Aortic stenosis: Disease severity, progression, timing of intervention and role in monitoring transcatheter valve implantation. In Otto CM, editor: *The Practice of Clinical Echocardiography*, ed 5, Philadelphia, 2017, Elsevier, pp 261–287.
   Advanced discussion of the echocardiographic approach to the evaluation of aortic stenosis severity with a review of the impact of echocardiographic findings on the clinical decision-making process. Topics covered include stress echocardiography for the detection of symptom onset and evaluation of low output aortic stenosis, other measures of stenosis severity, and the role of echocardiography in following progressive disease. Echocardiographic monitoring of transcatheter aortic valve implantation is reviewed.

5. Otto CM, Prendergast B: Aortic-valve stenosis—from patients at risk to severe valve obstruction, *N Engl J Med* 371(8):744–756, 2014.
   A concise overview of the causes, disease progression, outcomes and treatment of aortic stenosis including discussion of disease stages and diagnostic testing.

6. Linefsky J, Otto CM: Aortic stenosis: clinical presentation, disease stages and timing of intervention. In Otto CM, Bonow RO, editors: *Valvular Heart Disease*, ed 5, Philadelphia, 2018, Elsevier, (Chapter 9).
   Comprehensive chapter on the diagnosis and disease stages of aortic valve disease. Additional chapters in this book address transcatheter aortic valve implantation, including a chapter dedicated to imaging guidance before and during transcatheter valve implantation.

7. Braverman AC, Cheng A: Bicuspid aortic valve disease and associated aortic disease. In Otto CM, Bonow RO, editors: *Valvular Heart Disease*, ed 5, Philadelphia, 2018, Elsevier, (Chapter 11).
   Bicuspid aortic valve disease is present in about 1% of the population, and most of these patients will require aortic valve replacement during their lifetime. A bicuspid valve accounts for about 50% of all aortic valve replacements. Associated dilation of the aortic sinuses and ascending aorta is common and requires careful evaluation by echocardiography and other imaging approaches.

8. Lindman BR, Clavel MA, Mathieu P, et al: Calcific aortic stenosis, *Nat Rev Dis Primers* 2:16006, 2016.
   Review article covering all aspects of calcific aortic valve disease from epidemiology and pathophysiology to medical and surgical management. A useful overview to put the role of echocardiography in perspective.

9. Lindman B, Bonow B, Otto CM: Current management of calcific aortic stenosis, *Circ Res* 113:223–237, 2013.
   Review of the current data on the clinical evaluation of aortic stenosis, including the role of echocardiography, with an emphasis on risk stratification in the asymptomatic patient to optimize timing of valve replacement. Recommendations on clinical and echocardiographic follow-up and on the timing of aortic valve replacement.

10. Clavel MA, Burwash IG, Pibarot P: Cardiac imaging for assessing low-gradient severe aortic stenosis, *JACC Cardiovasc Imaging* 10(2):185–202, 2017.
    Detailed discussion of the approach to diagnosis in patients who suspected low flow, low gradient aortic stenosis. The recommended steps in evaluation are (1) confirm the accuracy of the standard echo measurements for aortic stenosis severity, (2) identify whether low gradient is related to a low or normal ejection fraction, (3) consider dobutamine stress echocardiography or computed tomographic calcium scoring, and (4) consider whether valve replacement would result in a larger valve area and lower gradient than the current severity of native valve disease.

Mitral Stenosis

11. Iung B, Vahanian A: Mitral stenosis: patient selection, hemodynamic results, complications and long-term outcomes with balloon mitral commissurotomy. In Otto CM, editor: *The Practice of Clinical Echocardiography*, ed 5, Philadelphia, 2017, Elsevier, pp 395–415.
    Review of the use of echocardiography in patient selection, prediction of hemodynamic results, the diagnosis of complications, and long-term outcome after mitral valvotomy. Research applications and alternate approaches are also discussed.

12. Iung B, Vahanian A: Mitral stenosis. In Otto CM, Bonow RO, editors: *Valvular Heart Disease*, ed 5, Philadelphia, 2018, Elsevier, (Chapter 16).
    Chapter providing an overview of mitral stenosis including clinical presentation, diagnosis, natural history and management. The role of echocardiography in predicting outcomes and in selection of patients for transcatheter procedures is discussed in detail.

13. Dreyfus J, Brochet E, Lepage L, et al: Real-time 3D transoesophageal measurement of the mitral valve area in patients with mitral stenosis, *Eur J Echocardiogr* 12(10):750–755, 2011.
    In 80 patients referred to echocardiography for the evaluation of mitral stenosis, valve area by standard 2D TTE imaging correlated well with 3D TEE valve area and showed no significant difference when the 2D study was performed and interpreted

by an experienced operator. The 3D valve area by an inexperienced operator also correlated with the 2D valve area measured by the experienced operator. The authors conclude that 3D TEE mitral valve area is similar to 2D TTE valve area, so 3D TEE is most helpful when TTE images are poor or when operators are less experienced in making this measurement.

Tricuspid Stenosis

14. Bruce CJ, Connolly HM: Right sided valve disease in adults. In Otto CM, editor: *The Practice of Clinical Echocardiography*, ed 5, Philadelphia, 2017, Elsevier, pp 651–676.
Advanced discussion for echocardiographers of tricuspid and pulmonic valve disease in adults. Technical details of echocardiographic image acquisition and measurement are provided with numerous example and anatomic correlation.

15. Lin G: Diseases of the tricuspid valve. In Otto CM, Bonow RO, editors: *Valvular Heart Disease*, ed 5, Philadelphia, 2018, Elsevier, (Chapter 23).
Book chapter on the clinical presentation, diagnosis, and management of tricuspid valve disease.

16. Kelly MC, Jennings R, Heron M: Treatment of trivalvular rheumatic heart disease: why it matters where we live, *BMJ Case Rep* 2014:2014.
Case example of rheumatic tricuspid valve disease in a patient with rheumatic aortic and mitral valve involvement. Concise discussion of presentation of multivalve involvement with rheumatic heart disease.

Pulmonic Stenosis

17. Kim Y: Pulmonic valve disease in adults. In Otto CM, Bonow RO, editors: *Valvular Heart Disease*, ed 5, Philadelphia, 2018, Elsevier, (Chapter 24).
Pulmonic valve disease in adults usually is congenital in etiology, either isolated pulmonic valve disease or, more commonly, in patients with surgical repair for tetralogy of Fallot. This chapter summarizes the clinical presentation, diagnosis, imaging approach, and clinical management.

12 Valvular Regurgitation

BASIC PRINCIPLES
    Etiology of Valvular Regurgitation
    Fluid Dynamics of Valvular Regurgitation
    Volume Overload
    Detection of Valvular Regurgitation
    Valvular Regurgitation in Normal Individuals

APPROACHES TO QUANTITATION OF REGURGITANT SEVERITY
    Color Doppler Imaging
        Jet Size and Shape
        Vena Contracta
        Proximal Flow Convergence
    CW Doppler Approach
    Distal Flow Reversals
    Volume Flow at Two Intracardiac Sites
    Limitations and Alternate Approaches

AORTIC REGURGITATION
    Diagnostic Imaging of the Valve Apparatus
    Left Ventricular Response
    Indirect Signs of Aortic Regurgitation
    Evaluation of Aortic Regurgitant Severity
        Screening Examination
        Vena Contracta
        Aortic Flow Reversal
        CW Doppler
        Regurgitant Volume and Fraction
    Clinical Utility
        Diagnostic Utility for Aortic Regurgitation
        Timing of Surgical Intervention for Chronic Asymptomatic Aortic Regurgitation

MITRAL REGURGITATION
    Diagnostic Imaging of the Mitral Valve Apparatus
    Response of the Left Ventricle, Left Atrium, and Pulmonary Vasculature
    Evaluation of Mitral Regurgitant Severity
        Screening Examination
        Vena Contracta
        Proximal Isovelocity Surface Area
        Regurgitation Volume and Orifice Area
        Pulmonary Vein Flow Reversal
    Clinical Utility
        Diagnosis and Severity of Mitral Regurgitation
        Clinical Follow-Up and Timing of Intervention
        Decision Making Concerning Type of Intervention

TRICUSPID REGURGITATION
    Diagnostic Imaging of the Tricuspid Valve Apparatus
    Right Ventricular and Right Atrial Dilation
    Evaluation of Tricuspid Regurgitation Severity
    Clinical Utility

PULMONIC REGURGITATION

THE ECHO EXAM

SUGGESTED READING

Echocardiographic evaluation of the patient with valvular regurgitation includes an assessment of valve anatomy, the severity of regurgitation, chamber dilation due to the imposed volume overload, ventricular function, and the degree of pulmonary hypertension. In some cases, the clinical significance of valvular regurgitation is related to the *presence* of abnormal regurgitation, regardless of severity. For example, the detection of aortic regurgitation (AR) in a patient with chest pain and an enlarged aorta heightens the suspicion of aortic dissection. In other situations (e.g., mitral valve prolapse), the *severity* of regurgitation is an essential factor in clinical decision making regarding surgical intervention. In chronic regurgitation due to primary valve disease, regurgitant severity and the *response of the left ventricle (LV) to chronic volume overload* are the most important factors in deciding on the timing of valve surgery.

BASIC PRINCIPLES

Etiology of Valvular Regurgitation

Valvular regurgitation is due to congenital or acquired abnormalities of the valve leaflets or to abnormalities of the associated supporting structures. For example, dilation of the ascending aorta or sinuses can result in AR even with anatomically normal valve leaflets. Similarly, LV dilation can result in mitral regurgitation (MR) even with normal valve leaflets and chordae. Echocardiographic examinations allow definition of the etiology of valvular regurgitation in most cases. Even when a single definite cause is not evident, the differential diagnosis of the etiology of regurgitation often can be narrowed to the few most likely possibilities. The examination also provides clues to whether regurgitation is acute or chronic in duration.

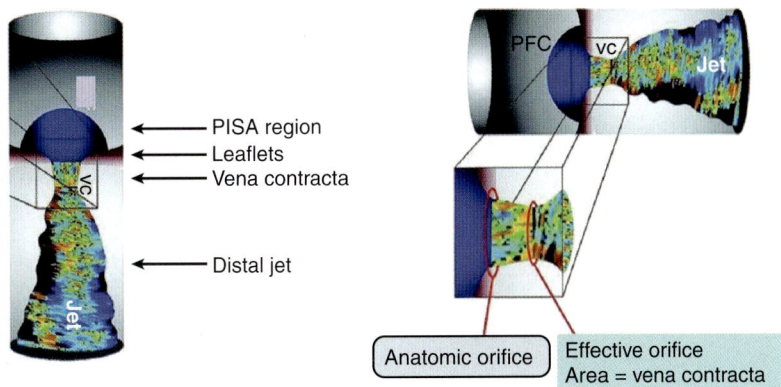

Fig. 12.1 The three components of a regurgitant jet. The proximal isovelocity surface area *(PISA)* region, also referred to as the proximal flow convergence *(PFC)* region, the vena contracta *(VC)*, and the distal jet. The effective regurgitant orifice area is the orifice area defined by the narrowest regurgitant flow stream and typically occurs distal to the anatomic orifice defined by the valve leaflets. *(Adapted from Roberts BJ, Grayburn P: Color flow imaging of the vena contracta in mitral regurgitation: technical considerations, J Am Soc Echocardiogr 16:1002–1006, 2003.)*

When transthoracic echocardiographic images are not diagnostic for the evaluation of aortic or mitral valve anatomy and the etiology of regurgitation, transesophageal echocardiographic (TEE) imaging is appropriate if needed for clinical decision making. With diseases of the aorta, visualization of the ascending aorta often is suboptimal on transthoracic imaging, so TEE, computer tomographic imaging, or cardiac magnetic resonance imaging typically is needed to define the extent and severity of disease fully.

Fluid Dynamics of Valvular Regurgitation

The fluid dynamics of a regurgitant valve (Fig. 12.1) are, in many ways, similar to the fluid dynamics of a stenotic valve and are characterized by:

- Regurgitant orifice area (ROA)
- High-velocity regurgitant jet
- Proximal flow convergence region
- Downstream flow disturbance
- Increased antegrade flow volume

Even though the anatomy of inadequate valve closure is quite complex, the valve can be thought of as having a regurgitant orifice, which in simple physiologic terms is characterized by a high-velocity laminar jet (Table 12.1). The instantaneous velocity in this jet *(v)* is related to the instantaneous pressure difference (ΔP) across the valve, as stated in the simplified Bernoulli equation: $\Delta P = 4v^2$. Recording this high-velocity jet with continuous-wave (CW) Doppler allows assessment of the time course of the difference in pressure between the two chambers on either side of the valve.

On the upstream side of the regurgitant valve, flow acceleration proximal to the regurgitant orifice is present, and a proximal isovelocity surface area (PISA) can be defined, similar to that seen on the left atrial (LA) side of the stenotic mitral valve. The proximal isovelocity surface area, multiplied by

TABLE 12.1 Relationship Between Fluid Dynamics of Valvular Regurgitation and Diagnostic Approach

Fluid Dynamic Characteristic	Diagnostic Approach
Conservation of mass through the regurgitant orifice	Continuity equation for regurgitant orifice area
High-velocity jet in regurgitant orifice	Pressure-velocity relationship of CW Doppler curve
Proximal flow convergence	Proximal isovelocity surface area
Downstream flow disturbance	Jet area in chamber receiving regurgitant flow
Increased volume flow across valve	Stroke volume across regurgitant minus competent valve

the aliasing velocity, provides a method for quantitative evaluation of regurgitant stroke volume. The narrowest segment of the regurgitant jet, the vena contracta, occurs just distal to the regurgitant orifice, with vena contracta diameter reflecting regurgitant orifice area.

As the high-velocity jet enters the chamber receiving the regurgitant flow, the flow pattern becomes disturbed with nonlaminar flow, multiple blood flow velocities, and multiple blood flow directions. The *size* of the downstream regurgitant flow disturbance is affected by both physiologic and technical factors and thus is less useful for the quantitation of regurgitant severity (Table 12.2). In addition, the *shape* and *direction* of the regurgitant jet are affected by the anatomy and orientation of the regurgitation orifice, the driving

TABLE 12.2	Factors That Affect Regurgitant Jet Size and Shape
Physiologic	
Regurgitant volume	
Driving pressure	
Size and shape of regurgitant orifice	
Receiving chamber constraint	
Wall impingement	
Timing relative to the cardiac cycle	
Influence of coexisting jets or flow streams	
Technical	
Ultrasound system gain	
Nyquist limit (pulse repetition frequency)	
Transducer frequency	
Frame rate	
Image plane	
Depth	
Signal strength	

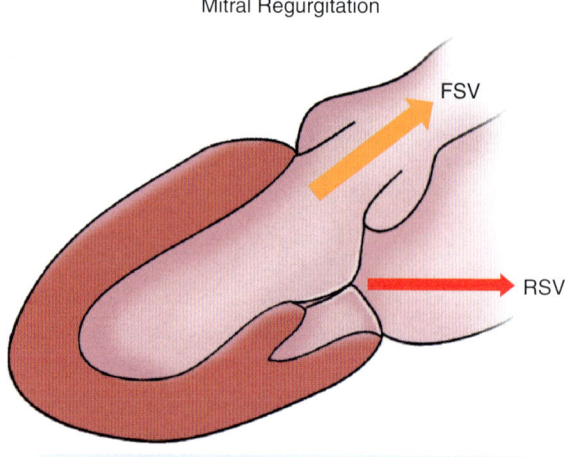

Fig. 12.2 Total, forward, and regurgitant stroke volume. When mitral regurgitation is present, total stroke volume *(total SV)* is the sum of the regurgitant stroke volume *(RSV)* and forward stroke volume *(FSV)*.

force across the valve, and the size and compliance of the receiving chamber. Jets are "pulled" toward adjacent walls (e.g., MR in the LA) if within a critical distance from the wall at the entry site and also are "pulled" toward other flowstreams (e.g., AR and mitral stenosis). Eccentric jets that adhere to the wall of the chamber have a smaller color jet area on two-dimensional (2D) color flow imaging (and a smaller three-dimensional [3D] volume) because entrainment of additional fluid elements into the jet occurs on only one side instead of on all sides, as with a central jet.

Volume Overload

In patients with a regurgitant valve, the term *total stroke volume* refers to the total volume of blood pumped by the ventricle on a single beat. *Forward stroke volume* is the amount of blood delivered to the peripheral circulation, and *regurgitant volume* is the amount of backflow across the abnormal valve (Fig. 12.2).

Chronic valvular regurgitation results in progressive volume overload of the ventricle. Volume overload of the LV results in chamber dilation with normal wall thickness so that total LV mass is increased. An important clinical feature of chronic LV volume overload is that an irreversible decrease in systolic function can occur in the absence of symptoms. In fact, an irreversible decrease in contractility can occur despite a normal ejection fraction because of the altered loading conditions of the ventricle when regurgitation is present.

Serial echocardiographic evaluation of LV size and systolic function is a standard method of clinical evaluation, but two factors potentially limit the reliability of this approach. First, suboptimal image quality or recording techniques results in erroneous measurements. Care is needed to ensure that the dimensions are measured perpendicular to the long and short axes of the LV, and instrument settings must be adjusted for optimal endocardial definition. Accurate tracing of endocardial borders for the calculation of ventricular volumes depends on clear endocardial definition, standard image planes without foreshortening of the long axis of the ventricle, and a trained and experienced individual tracing the borders at end-diastole and end-systole. With 2D imaging, left-sided contrast enhancement is recommended for accurate measurement of LV volumes and ejection fraction if endocardial definition is suboptimal. Calculation of LV volumes from a 3D volume acquisition avoids apical foreshortening or geometric assumptions and now is recommended whenever possible (see Chapter 6).

Second, the reproducibility of LV measurements must be considered. Overall reproducibility includes variation in *recording* the data, variation in *measuring* the data, and *physiologic* variation (e.g., heart rate and loading conditions) that affect the measurement. These sources of measurement variability affect all imaging approaches. When comparing serial studies, it is advisable to compare measurements on side-by-side images and to consider the limits of measurement variability for each approach. With 2D-guided M-mode measurements, an interval change of greater than 8 mm in end-systolic or end-diastolic dimensions represents a definite clinical change. Using 2D echocardiography, a change in ventricular volume or a change in ejection fraction greater than 10% on serial studies performed in the same laboratory indicates a significant change. 3D volumes have lower variability in recording and measuring data but are still subject to physiologic variability.

Detection of Valvular Regurgitation

Valvular regurgitation can be detected with:

- Color flow imaging
- CW Doppler ultrasound

Although anatomic imaging provides detailed information about the valve apparatus and ventricular function, it provides only indirect evidence for the presence or absence of valvular regurgitation. The finding of an anatomically abnormal mitral valve in the presence of LA and LV dilation suggests that MR may be present, but Doppler examination is necessary for direct confirmation or exclusion of the diagnosis. Although a few M-mode findings have been shown to be specific for diagnosing valvular regurgitation (e.g., high-frequency fluttering of the anterior mitral leaflet in AR), these findings are not sensitive enough to exclude valve dysfunction reliably.

With color flow imaging, detection of regurgitation is based on identification of the flow disturbance downstream from the regurgitant orifice. When instrument settings and examination technique are optimal, color flow imaging is extremely sensitive (>90%) and specific (nearly 100%) for the detection of valvular regurgitation as compared with angiography. In fact, color flow imaging is so sensitive that regurgitation often is detected that is not audible by auscultation. These cases most often are true-positive results, as evidenced by angiographic confirmation. False-positive results can occur with color flow imaging when the origin or timing of the flow signal is mistaken. For example, normal pulmonary venous inflow into the LA sometimes is mistaken for MR. False-negative results occur when signal strength is low because of poor acoustic access or attenuation due to the depth of interrogation. False-negative results also occur if color flow processing parameters are set incorrectly or if the examiner fails to evaluate the valve in more than one tomographic plane. Additional parameters important in the detection of valvular regurgitation with color flow imaging include frame rate, Nyquist limit, color gain, and color velocity-variance display.

CW Doppler detection of valvular regurgitation is based on the identification of the high-velocity jet through the regurgitant orifice. An advantage of CW Doppler is that beam width is broad at the level of the valves when recorded from an apical approach. Identification of the regurgitant signal uses the velocity, shape, timing, and associated antegrade flow signal to identify the origin of the signal correctly (Fig. 12.3).

Valvular Regurgitation in Normal Individuals

A small degree of regurgitation, often termed *physiologic*, is present in a high percentage of otherwise normal individuals (Fig. 12.4). Typically, physiologic regurgitation is:

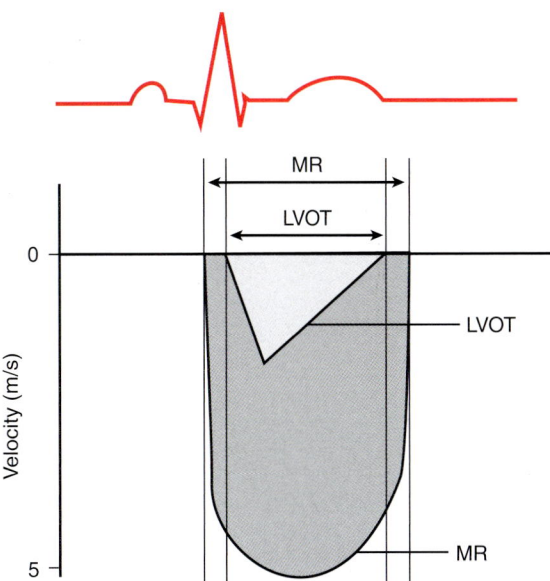

Fig. 12.3 Relative timing of mitral regurgitation and left ventricular outflow tract flow signals. Mitral regurgitation *(MR)* extends from the onset of isovolumic contraction to the end of isovolumic relaxation. LV outflow is shorter, occurring only during ejection. *LVOT,* LV outflow tract.

- Spatially restricted to the area immediately adjacent to valve closure
- Short in duration
- Represents only a small regurgitant volume

With a meticulous search for valve regurgitation, MR can be detected in 70% to 80%, tricuspid regurgitation in 80% to 90%, and pulmonic regurgitation in 70% to 80% of normal individuals. This small degree of regurgitation is normal and has no adverse clinical implications. AR is found in only a small percentage (5%) of young individuals with an otherwise normal echocardiographic study, but the prevalence of detectable AR increases with age. The clinical significance of a small amount of AR is unknown.

APPROACHES TO QUANTITATION OF REGURGITANT SEVERITY

The severity of valvular regurgitation typically is described using semiquantitative measures as mild, moderate, or severe (Table 12.3). The size of the color Doppler jet is not accurate for the evaluation of regurgitant severity. Instead, semiquantitative measures include:

- Vena contracta width
- CW Doppler signal strength compared with antegrade flow
- Pressure half-time (for AR)
- Distal flow reversals

Fig. 12.4 ▶ **Normal mitral regurgitation.** Example of "physiologic" mitral regurgitation recorded with color *(left)* and CW *(right)* Doppler in a normal individual. The color flow signal is localized to a small region adjacent to the valve coaptation point, and the intensity of the CW Doppler signal is low compared with antegrade flow with an incomplete waveform seen only in early systole. *Ao,* Aorta; *MV,* mitral valve.

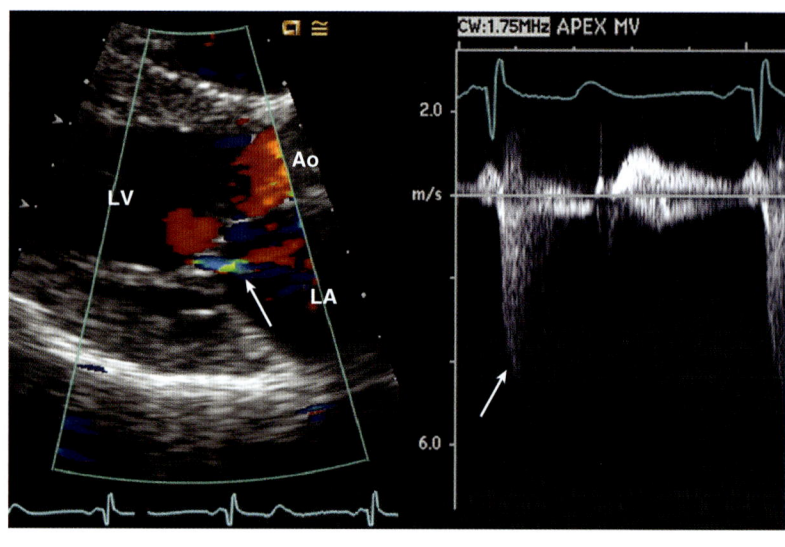

TABLE 12.3 Doppler Evaluation of Valvular Regurgitation

Method	Doppler Parameters	Limitations	Correlation With Other Imaging Modalities
Color flow imaging	• Jet origin • Jet direction • Jet size	• Variation with technical and physiologic factors	• LV or aortic angiography • CMR flow visualization
CW Doppler	• Signal intensity • Shape of velocity curve	• Qualitative	• Invasive hemodynamics • CMR velocity data
Vena contracta width	• Width of jet origin	• Small values, careful measurement needed	• CMR flow visualization
Proximal isovelocity surface area (PISA)	• Calculation of RVol and ROA	• Less accurate with eccentric jets • Peak values only	• CMR flow visualization
Volume flow at two sites	• Calculation of RVol and ROA	• Tedious	• Invasive RVol and RF • CMR measurement of volume flow rates. • CMR LV and RV stroke volumes
Distal flow reversals	• Pulmonary vein (MR), aorta (AR) or hepatic vein (TR)	• Qualitative, affected by filing pressures, AF	• None

AF, Atrial fibrillation; *AR,* aortic regurgitation; *CMR,* cardiac magnetic resonance; *MR,* mitral regurgitation; *RF,* regurgitant fraction; *ROA,* regurgitant orifice area; *RVol,* regurgitant volume; *TR,* tricuspid regurgitation.

In addition, several quantitative measures (see Appendix B, Table B.15) of regurgitant severity have been well validated, including:

- Regurgitant volume
- Regurgitant fraction
- Regurgitant orifice area

Regurgitant volume (RVol) is the retrograde volume flow rate across the valve, expressed either as an instantaneous flow rate in milliliters per second or (more correctly) averaged over the cardiac cycle in milliliters per beat. Regurgitant volume can be calculated by three different approaches:

- PISA flow rate
- Antegrade volume flow across the regurgitant valve minus the flow across a competent valve
- Total LV stroke volume (SV_{total}) measured from LV volumes minus Doppler forward stroke volume

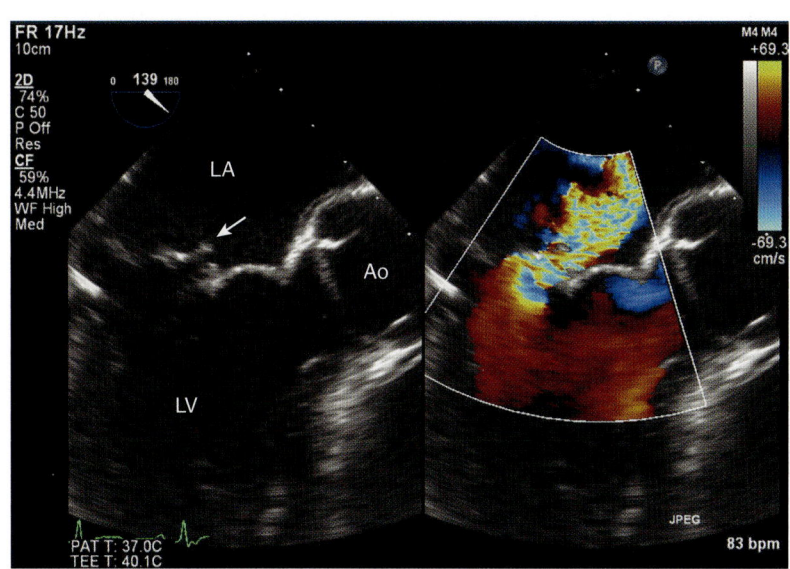

Fig. 12.5 Anteriorly directed mitral regurgitation on transesophageal echocardiography. The long-axis TEE view shows a partial flail posterior mitral leaflet *(arrow)*. The anteriorly directed jet seen on color Doppler *(right)* confirms that mitral regurgitation is due to isolated posterior leaflet dysfunction, and the width of the jet as it crosses the mitral valve, the vena contracta, is consistent with severe regurgitation. Ao, Aorta.

Regurgitant fraction (RF) is:

$$RF = RVol/SV_{total} \quad \text{(Eq. 12.1)}$$

Regurgitant orifice area (ROA) is calculated, using the continuity equation, from regurgitant volume and the velocity-time integral of the regurgitant jet (VTI_{RJ}). Because the regurgitant volumes (RVol) proximal to and *in* the regurgitant orifice are equal,

$$RVol = ROA \times VTI_{RJ} \quad \text{(Eq. 12.2)}$$

solving for regurgitant orifice area gives

$$ROA = RVol/VTI_{RJ} \quad \text{(Eq. 12.3)}$$

with RVol in cm^3, VTI_{RJ} in cm, and ROA in cm^2.

Color Doppler Imaging

Jet Size and Shape

In the past, regurgitant severity often was graded based on the size of the flow disturbance in the chamber receiving the regurgitant jet on a 1+ (mild) to 4+ (severe) scale. However, this grading system is quite inaccurate, particularly when regurgitation is more than mild, with substantial overlap in jet areas between patients with moderate and severe regurgitation. Color flow "mapping" also is subject to marked variability due to gain and other instrument settings, as well as physiologic variability. Thus, the area or length of a regurgitant jet is an unreliable indicator of disease severity and should not be used in patient management.

Color flow imaging of the regurgitant jet does remain clinically useful for the detection of valve regurgitation, for evaluation of the timing of flow, and for insights into the cause of regurgitation (Figs. 12.5 and 12.6). Because color flow imaging basically is pulsed Doppler ultrasound with somewhat different

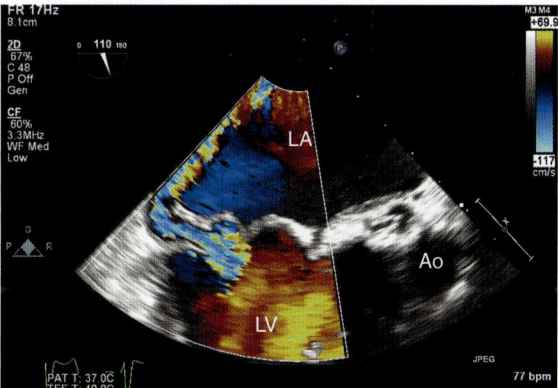

Fig. 12.6 Posteriorly directed mitral regurgitation on transesophageal echocardiography. With a partial flail anterior mitral leaflet, the regurgitant jet is posteriorly directed (opposite the affected leaflet) as seen on this TEE long-axis view. Vena contracta width is consistent with severe mitral regurgitation. Ao, Aorta.

signal processing and display formats, it is important to remember that signal aliasing still occurs. However, the usefulness of flow imaging depends on the timing and spatial location of the Doppler signals and *not* absolute blood flow velocity. Thus, signal aliasing does not limit the utility of flow imaging and, in fact, enhances the appreciation of abnormal flow patterns. In addition, flow imaging can be performed from windows where the intercept angle between the ultrasound beam and the direction of regurgitant flow is nonparallel. These windows often allow a shorter distance from the transducer to the flow region of interest, thereby resulting in a better signal-to-noise ratio. For example, AR is best evaluated from the parasternal approach (Fig. 12.7). Although the direction of an AR jet in the parasternal long-axis view is nearly perpendicular to the ultrasound beam, multiple flow

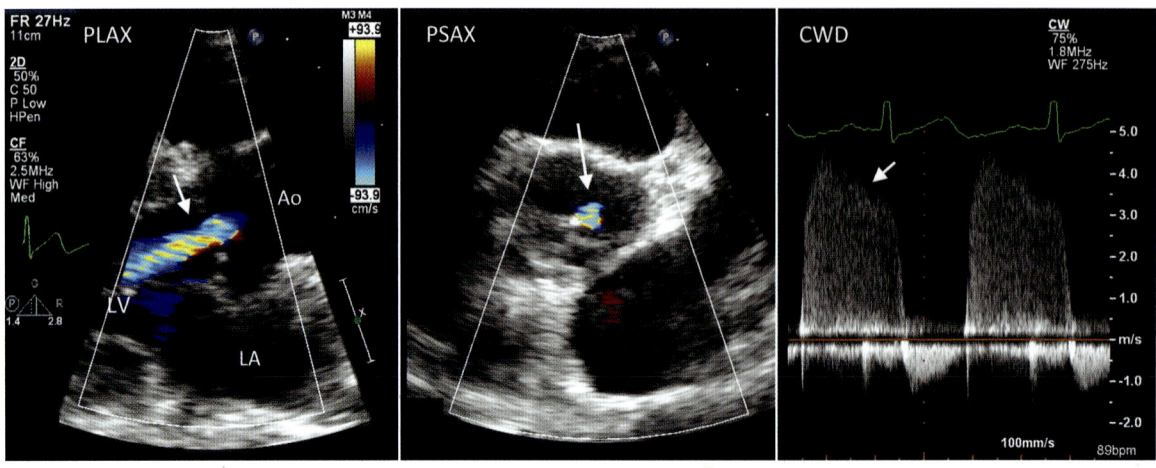

Fig. 12.7 Mild aortic regurgitation. In a zoomed parasternal long-axis view *(PLAX, left),* ▶ a narrow jet of aortic regurgitation (AR) is seen with a vena contracta width *(arrow)* of 3 mm. The parasternal short-axis view *(PSAX, center)* ▶ just beneath the valve plane confirms a small central jet *(arrow)* of regurgitation. CW Doppler *(CWD, right)* shows a faint diastolic signal *(arrow)*, compared with antegrade systolic flow, with a velocity and waveform typical for AR. *Ao,* Aorta.

directions within the jet allow detection of the diastolic flow disturbance. Of course, an accurate blood velocity determination cannot be made both because of the nonparallel intercept angle and because the velocity exceeds the Nyquist limit of the pulsed Doppler mode.

The appearance of a regurgitant jet with color flow imaging will vary depending on the ultrasound system, transducer frequency, and specific instrument settings. Correct visual interpretation depends on experience with a particular instrument and knowledge of the influence of instrument settings on the visual display. On most systems, a "variance" color scale results in a green regurgitant signal superimposed on the normal red-blue flow patterns. A "velocity" scale results in a mosaic of red, blue, and white pixels in the regurgitant jet. Because the goal of this application is to identify the location and timing of abnormal flow signals in a tomographic format, the exact color scale used is not particularly important as long as it displays the boundaries of the flow disturbance accurately.

Given the physics of pulsed Doppler color flow imaging, it is self-evident that an abnormal color pattern is not synonymous with abnormal flow. An abnormal color pattern can be seen even with normal intracardiac flow patterns; for example, the normal antegrade flow velocity of laminar flow across the aortic valve exceeds the Nyquist limit, resulting in aliasing and an "abnormal" color pattern. Conversely, abnormal flow signals do not demonstrate variance or a mosaic pattern if the flow velocities are within the Nyquist limit for that interrogation depth. For example, the low velocities seen in pulmonic regurgitation result in a uniform color display even though the flow pattern is abnormal. Interpretation of the color images will be most consistent from study to study if instrument settings and flow maps are standardized for each laboratory.

Recommended instrument settings for color flow imaging are:

- Nyquist limit at the maximum for the imaging depth (60 to 80 cm/s)
- Color gain setting just below random speckle from nonmoving targets
- Maximum frame rate (e.g., narrow sector, decrease depth)
- Consistent color velocity-variance display scale

Evaluation of the exact timing of a flow signal in relation both to valve closing and to the QRS complex can be helpful in correct identification of the signal. With color flow imaging, temporal resolution is sacrificed for spatial resolution because frame rates are far lower than the sampling rate of pulsed or CW Doppler. Simultaneous recording of an electrocardiographic lead is essential for frame-by-frame analysis of the color flow images to verify the timing of the disturbance.

Vena Contracta

The vena contracta, the narrowest diameter of the flowstream, reflects the diameter of the regurgitant orifice with the advantages that it is independent of volume flow rate and driving pressure and that it is relatively unaffected by instrument settings. However, because vena contracta diameters have a narrow range of values, care is needed to obtain adequate images for measurement. To optimize both temporal and spatial resolution, the recommended approach to measurement of vena contracta is to use a view:

- Perpendicular to jet width
- Zoom mode
- Narrow sector
- Minimum depth

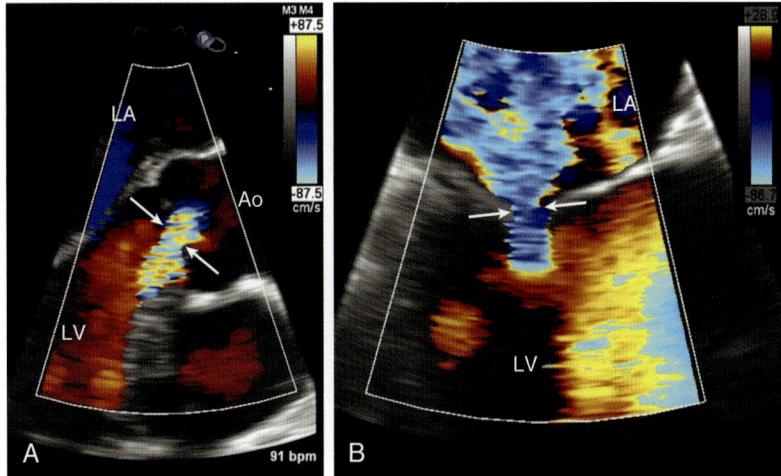

Fig. 12.8 Vena contracta measurement. (A) An eccentric aortic regurgitant jet is seen in a TEE long-axis view. ▶ The long-axis view allows for the identification of the proximal flow convergence region and the downstream jet expansion, with the vena contracta identified as the narrowest segment joining them. Vena contracta width is measured perpendicular to the flow direction *(arrows)*. (B) On TEE imaging in a four-chamber view, vena contracta width of a mitral regurgitant jet *(right)* measured as the narrow neck between the proximal isovelocity surface area and flow expansion in the LA. ▶ A view perpendicular to the jet direction is not feasible on TEE, but the image is still recorded using a narrow sector width and zoom mode to improve measurement precision.

Angulation out of the standard image planes is needed to depict both the proximal acceleration region and downstream flow expansion for accurate identification of the vena contracta (Fig. 12.8).

Vena contracta diameter varies with dynamic changes in regurgitant orifice area, for example, with late-systolic MR due to mitral valve prolapse. However, vena contracta width remains accurate in the setting of acute regurgitation, whereas jet area is misleading. The 3D visualization of vena contracta area shows promise, particularly for nonsymmetrical regurgitant orifices, but this technique is limited by low frame rates, and it can be challenging to acquire adequate-quality 3D color images, even with TEE imaging (Fig. 12.9).

Proximal Flow Convergence

Color flow imaging allows for the calculation of the retrograde volume flow rate based on measurement of the flow convergence region proximal to the regurgitant orifice. Acceleration of flow occurs proximal to the valve plane with, in concept, a series of isovelocity "surfaces" leading to the high-velocity jet in the regurgitant orifice. Immediately adjacent to the orifice, these surfaces are small with higher flow velocities; at increasing distances from the orifice, areas are larger and velocities are lower. Based on the principle of volume flow calculation by Doppler techniques, the volume flow rate (in this case, regurgitant flow) for a PISA, when averaged over the temporal flow period (Fig. 12.10), is

Regurgitant flow rate = PISA × Aliasing velocity

(Eq. 12.4)

The velocity of the PISA can be determined from the color flow image as the aliasing velocity where a distinct red-blue interface is seen (Fig. 12.11). At this interface, the velocity is known, being equivalent to the Nyquist limit on the velocity color scale. The size of the PISA can be maximized to allow more accurate regurgitant flow rate calculations using a zoomed image with the Doppler velocity baseline shifted so that the aliasing velocity is 30 to 40 cm/s in the direction of flow.

The shape of the isovelocity surface proximal to a regurgitant valve typically is hemispherical, with a tendency toward a hemielliptical shape closer to the orifice. Assuming a hemispherical shape, the PISA is calculated from measurements of the distance from the aliasing velocity to the regurgitant orifice as the surface area of a hemisphere:

$$\text{PISA} = 2\pi r^2 \quad \text{(Eq. 12.5)}$$

Note that the PISA method for calculating regurgitant volume is analogous to calculation of stroke volume proximal to a stenotic valve. The differences between these approaches are (1) the differing shapes of the proximal velocity stream lines; (2) the use of color flow, rather than pulsed Doppler, to measure velocity at a given location; and (3) the need for temporal averaging when color data from single images are used.

The PISA method can be combined with the velocity-time integral of CW Doppler flow through the regurgitant orifice to calculate regurgitant orifice area using Eq. 12.3. Instead of averaging PISA over the duration of flow, most clinicians calculate the

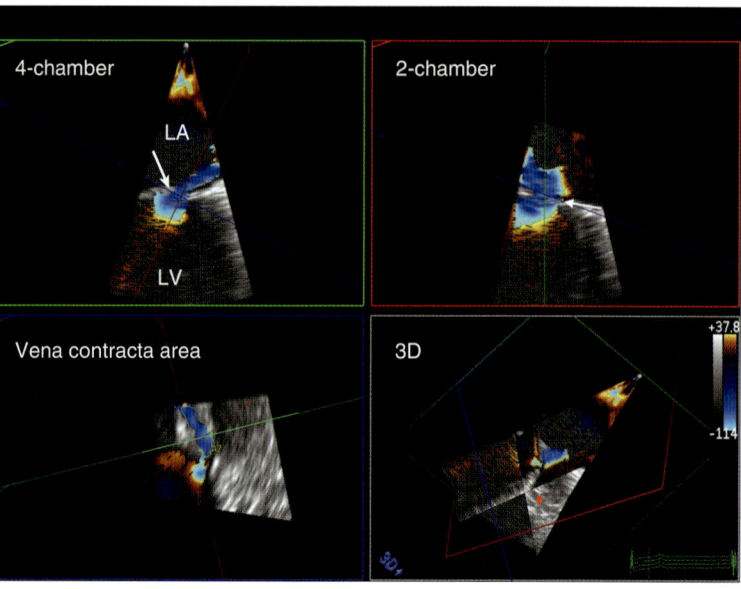

Fig. 12.9 3D color Doppler vena contracta imaging. A 3D volume acquisition of the mitral regurgitant jet using color Doppler flow imaging is then cropped to show a view equivalent to a four-chamber view *(upper left)* with the vena contracta indicated by the *arrow*. The color boxes and lines match so that the red line in the four-chamber view corresponds to the image plane shown in the red box in the two-chamber view *(upper right)*, and so on. These image planes are iteratively adjusted to obtain a short-axis view of vena contracta area *(lower left)*, which is equivalent to regurgitant orifice area, measuring 0.6 cm² in this example. The 3D rendition in *the lower right* shows the orientation of the three image planes relative to each other. 3D color Doppler has the advantage of allowing visualization of the regurgitant flow area, but slow frame rates are a major disadvantage.

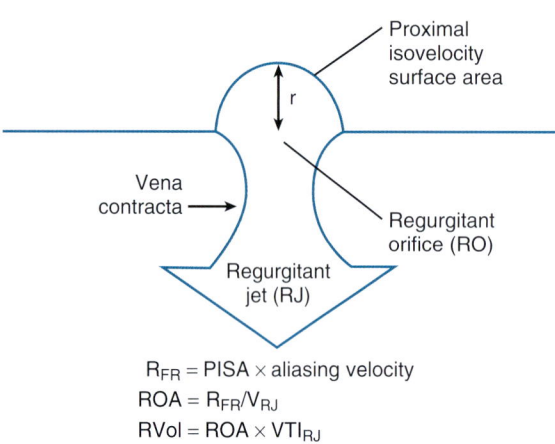

R_{FR} = PISA × aliasing velocity
ROA = R_{FR}/V_{RJ}
RVol = ROA × VTI_{RJ}

Fig. 12.10 Proximal isovelocity surface area concept. Proximal to a regurgitant orifice, flow accelerates, resulting in concentric proximal isovelocity surface areas *(PISAs)*. The radius *(r)* is used to calculate the PISA. The color Doppler aliasing velocity is used to calculate the instantaneous regurgitant flow rate *(R_{FR})* based on the aliasing velocity. Regurgitant orifice area *(ROA)* is estimated by dividing the flow rate *(R_{FP})* by the maximum velocity of the regurgitant jet *(V_{RJ})*. Regurgitant volume *(RVol)* then is calculated by multiplying regurgitant orifice area by the velocity-time integral *(VTI)* of the regurgitant jet.

maximum instantaneous regurgitant orifice area (ROA_{max} in cm²) based on the maximum regurgitant flow rate (R_{FR} in milliliters per second) combined with maximum MR jet velocity (V_{MR} in centimeters per second):

$$ROA_{max} = R_{FR}/V_{MR} \quad \text{(Eq. 12.6)}$$

This approach assumes that R_{FR} and V_{MR} occur at the same time point in the cardiac cycle. The PISA should be recorded in a view parallel to the flowstream, typically an apical four-chamber view for MR, using a narrow sector and zoom mode, with the aliasing velocity adjusted to optimize visualization of a hemispherical aliasing boundary. If the PISA is hemielliptical or if the valve is nonplanar, an alternate approach should be used or appropriate corrections should be made in the calculations.

CW Doppler Approach

Several types of information regarding the severity of valvular regurgitation can be derived from the spectral display of the CW Doppler signal:

- Signal intensity relative to antegrade flow
- Antegrade flow velocity
- Time course (shape) of velocity curve

First, signal intensity is proportional to the number of blood cells contributing to the regurgitant signal. Because the ultrasound beam is relatively broad and signals from the entire length of the beam are recorded, much of the regurgitant jet can be encompassed in the beam with appropriate adjustment of beam direction. It is particularly helpful to compare the intensity of the regurgitant signal with antegrade flow across the same valve as a qualitative estimate of regurgitant severity (see Fig. 12.11). A weak signal reflects mild regurgitation, whereas a signal nearly equal in intensity to antegrade flow reflects severe regurgitation. Moderate regurgitation has intermediate signal strength relative to antegrade flow.

Second, the associated antegrade velocity across the regurgitant valve provides useful information. Regurgitation results in an increase in the antegrade volume flow rate across the valve, which is reflected in an increase in the antegrade velocity across the valve. The greater the severity of regurgitation, the

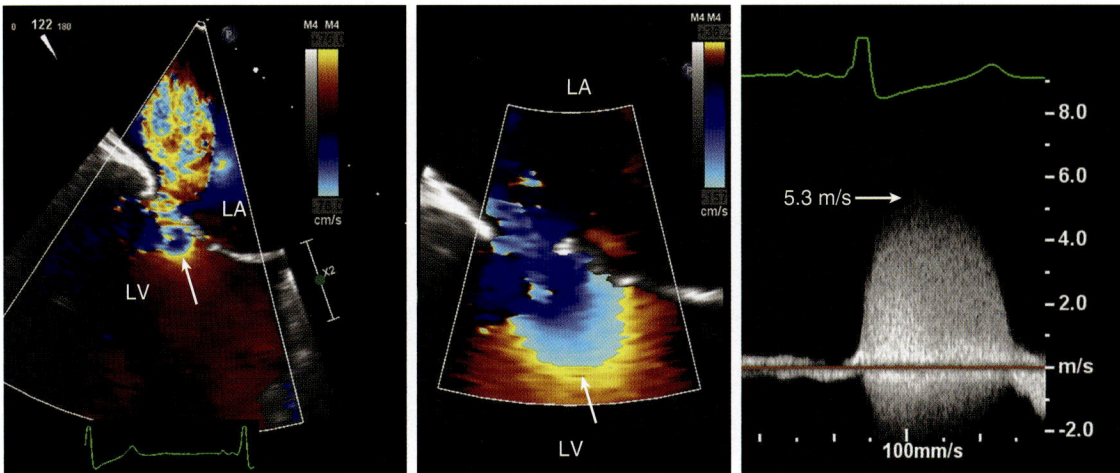

Fig. 12.11 Proximal isovelocity surface area imaging. TEE imaging in a long-axis *(left)* ▶ view shows mitral regurgitation with the color Doppler parameters at the default for that depth (aliasing velocity 76 cm/s in both directions). A proximal isovelocity surface area (PISA) is seen *(arrow)*, but the shape is not hemispherical, and accurate measurement is problematic. In the same image plane *(center)* ▶, zoom mode is used to focus on the proximal jet geometry. The PISA *(arrow)* is optimized by (1) decreasing the depth, narrowing the sector, using the zoom mode and (2) moving the zero baseline of the velocity color scale (no variance) to an aliasing velocity of 30 to 40 cm/s in the direction of regurgitant flow (toward the transducer on TEE). The PISA radius of 1.1 cm (surface area = $2\pi r^2$ = 7.6 cm^2) at an aliasing velocity of 36 cm/s indicates an instantaneous regurgitant flow rate of 273 mL/s. On CW Doppler *(right)*, the maximum mitral regurgitant jet velocity is 5.3 m/s, so regurgitant orifice area is 0.52 cm^2, consistent with severe mitral regurgitation. This is the same patient as Fig. 12.9.

higher is the antegrade velocity. Of course, the possibility of coexisting valvular stenosis also must be considered.

Third, the shape of the velocity curve depends on the time-varying pressure gradient across the regurgitant valve. Each instantaneous velocity is related to the instantaneous pressure gradient across the valve, as stated in the Bernoulli equation. Normal LV systolic pressure is 100 to 140 mmHg, and normal LA pressure is 5 to 15 mmHg, so the LV to LA pressure difference in systole is 85 to 135 mmHg. Thus, the MR velocity curve typically shows a maximum velocity of 5 to 6 m/s. When ventricular function is normal, rapid acceleration to peak velocity occurs, with a maintained high velocity in systole and with rapid deceleration before diastolic opening of the mitral valve. An increase in end-systolic LA pressure *(v-wave)* results in a late-systolic decline in the instantaneous pressure gradient and in the instantaneous velocity (Fig. 12.12).

Similarly, the shape of the AR velocity curve depends on the time course of the diastolic pressure difference across the aortic valve. When LV end-diastolic pressure is low and aortic end-diastolic pressure is normal or mildly reduced, a large pressure difference (and high velocity) across the valve is present throughout diastole with a slow rate of pressure decline (Fig. 12.13). Acute or severe regurgitation results in more rapid equalization of LV and aortic pressures with a more rapid velocity decline in diastole.

The utility of the CW Doppler curve depends, in large part, on technical factors in data recording in addition to correct data interpretation. The high-velocity regurgitant signal is optimized by:

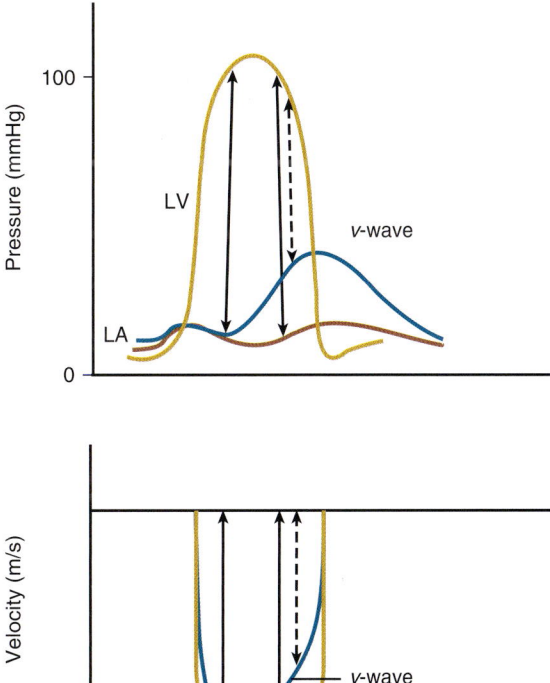

Fig. 12.12 Pressure-velocity relationships for mitral regurgitation. LV and LA pressures and the Doppler velocity curve in chronic *(yellow lines)* and acute *(blue lines)* mitral regurgitation are shown. Note that the shape of the velocity curve reflects the shape of the pressure difference between the LV and the LA so that a late systolic rise in LA pressure *(v-wave)* is seen as a more rapid decrease in velocity in late systole on the Doppler curve.

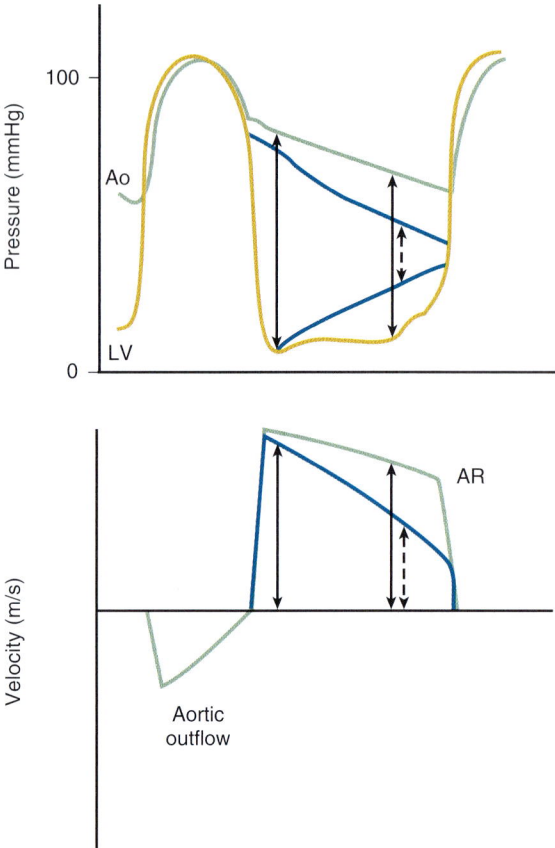

Fig. 12.13 Pressure-velocity relationships for aortic regurgitation. LV and central aortic *(Ao)* pressures and the corresponding Doppler velocity curve are shown for chronic *(green)* and acute *(blue)* aortic regurgitation *(AR)*. Again, the shape of the velocity curve is related to the instantaneous pressure differences across the valve, as stated in the Bernoulli equation. With acute AR, aortic pressure falls more rapidly and ventricular diastolic pressure rises more rapidly, resulting in a steeper deceleration slope on the Doppler curve.

- Sweep speed of spectral display at 100 mm/s
- Velocity range adjusted so that signal of interest fits but fills the screen
- High-pass ("wall") filter set at the maximum level
- Gain and dynamic range adjusted to show dark outer edge of the velocity curve
- Examination from multiple acoustic windows
- Adjustment of transducer position and angulation

Optimal patient positioning, examination from multiple windows, and transducer angulation are needed to ensure a near-parallel intercept angle between the direction of the ultrasound beam and the regurgitant jet to avoid underestimation of velocities. Use of a dedicated, small CW transducer often facilitates the examination and provides a better signal-to-noise ratio than 2D-guided CW Doppler. In addition, the 2D image often distracts the examiner from searching for the highest-velocity signal. Color flow imaging is of limited value for locating the best CW signal because it provides only 2D information; jet direction in the elevation plane remains unknown. Temporal factors also affect data quality, and caution is needed in interpreting the shape of the velocity curve if jet direction (and thus the Doppler-jet intercept angle) varies during the regurgitant flow period.

Distal Flow Reversals

When atrioventricular valve regurgitation is severe enough that a significant volume of blood is displaced by the regurgitant jet, flow reversal is seen in the veins entering the atrium. With severe tricuspid regurgitation, the normal pattern of systolic inflow into the right atrium (RA) from the superior and inferior vena cavae is reversed. This can be demonstrated with a pulsed Doppler sample volume positioned in the central hepatic vein (Fig. 12.14). Severe MR results in reversal of the normal patterns of systolic inflow into the LA from the pulmonary veins. This usually is difficult to demonstrate on a transthoracic study because of signal attenuation at the depth of the pulmonary vein but is easily recorded from a TEE approach (Fig. 12.15). Systolic flow reversal in the pulmonary veins (for MR) or in the hepatic veins (for tricuspid regurgitation) is only useful when sinus rhythm is present because normal venous inflow patterns often are abnormal with other cardiac rhythms, such as atrial fibrillation.

Regurgitation of a semilunar valve results in reversal of flow in the associated great vessel as blood flows from the great vessel across the incompetent valve into the ventricle. The distance from the valve plane that this flow reversal extends in the great vessel is proportional to regurgitant volume. For example, with severe AR, holodiastolic flow reversal is seen in the proximal abdominal aorta. With moderate regurgitation, holodiastolic flow reversal extends only to the descending thoracic aorta.

Volume Flow at Two Intracardiac Sites

Regurgitant stroke volume can be calculated using 2D diameter measurements in conjunction with pulsed Doppler flow velocities at two intracardiac sites. Total stroke volume is calculated from antegrade flow across the regurgitant valve as the cross-sectional area of flow times the velocity-time integral of transvalvular flow. Forward stroke volume is calculated as antegrade flow across a different (and nonregurgitant) valve (Fig. 12.16).

For example, with AR, transaortic stroke volume (SV) represents total LV stroke volume and can be calculated as:

$$SV_{total} = CSA_{LVOT} \times VTI_{LVOT} \quad \text{(Eq. 12.7)}$$

where CSA is cross-sectional area, VTI is the velocity-time integral, and LVOT is the LV outflow tract. Forward stroke volume is represented by LV inflow across the mitral annulus (MA), because the amount of blood filling

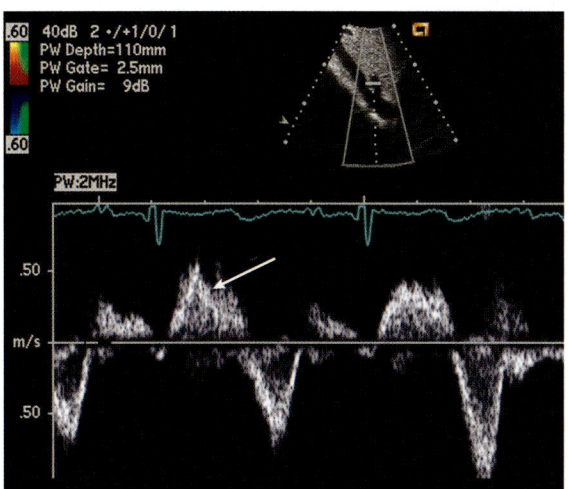

Fig. 12.14 Hepatic vein systolic flow reversal with severe tricuspid regurgitation and normal sinus rhythm. With the sample volume positioned in the central hepatic vein from a subcostal approach, systolic *(arrow)* flow reversal in the hepatic vein velocity curve is seen when severe tricuspid regurgitation is present. Forward flow into the RA in diastole also is seen.

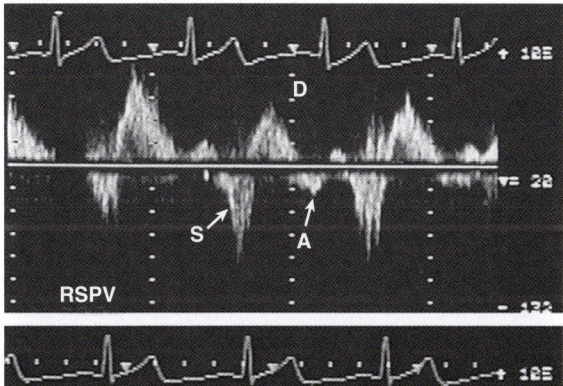

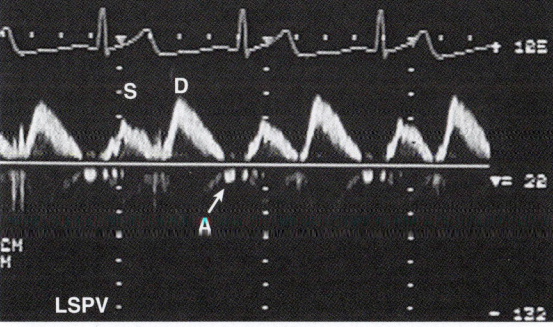

Fig. 12.15 Pulmonary vein systolic flow reversal with severe mitral regurgitation and normal sinus rhythm. Systolic flow reversal *(S)* in the right superior pulmonary vein *(RSPV)* Doppler velocity curve *(top)* and blunting of systolic flow in the left superior pulmonary vein *(LSPV, bottom)* are seen on TEE imaging in a patient with an eccentric, anteromedially directed regurgitant jet. *A,* Atrial reversal; *D,* diastolic flow.

the ventricle equals the amount of blood delivered to the body on each beat, and can be calculated as:

$$SV_{forward} = CSA_{MA} \times VTI_{MA} \quad \text{(Eq. 12.8)}$$

With AR, alternate sites for the measurement of forward stroke volume are the pulmonary artery

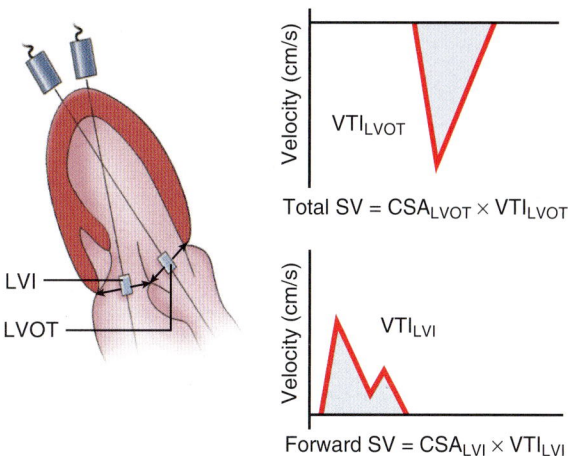

Fig. 12.16 Concept of volume flow measurement across a regurgitant versus normal valve. Calculation of aortic regurgitant stroke volume *(Regurg. SV)* by measurement of transvalvular volume flow rate at two intracardiac sites is illustrated. Transaortic flow, representing total stroke volume, is calculated from the cross-sectional area *(CSA)* and velocity-time integral *(VTI)* of the LV outflow tract *(LVOT)*. Transmitral flow, representing forward stroke volume, is calculated from the cross-sectional area and velocity-time integral of LV inflow *(LVI)* across the mitral annulus. Regurgitant stroke volume is the difference between total and forward stroke volume.

and right ventricular (RV) inflow region. Regurgitant volume is calculated as:

$$RVol = SV_{total} - SV_{forward} \quad \text{(Eq. 12.9)}$$

Regurgitant fraction and regurgitant orifice area then are calculated with Eqs. 12.1 and 12.3. Alternatively, total stroke volume can be derived from 2D or 3D imaging of the LV with identification of endocardial borders at end-diastole and end-systole.

Calculation of regurgitant volume and regurgitant fraction from volume flow at two intracardiac sites has been shown to be accurate in animal models and in selected patient series. However, small errors in diameter measurement lead to large errors in cross-sectional area calculations because of the quadratic relationship between the two ($CSA = \pi r^2$). Other potential pitfalls in volume flow measurement are discussed in detail in Chapter 6. This method clearly can provide accurate quantitation of regurgitant severity when image quality is excellent; in other cases, it is helpful to compare the antegrade velocity-time integral (or peak velocity) for the regurgitant valve with the antegrade flow across a competent valve as an indicator of their relative stroke volumes.

Limitations and Alternate Approaches

Echocardiography is the clinical standard for the evaluation of valvular regurgitation. The diagnostic value of the echocardiographic study is increased when

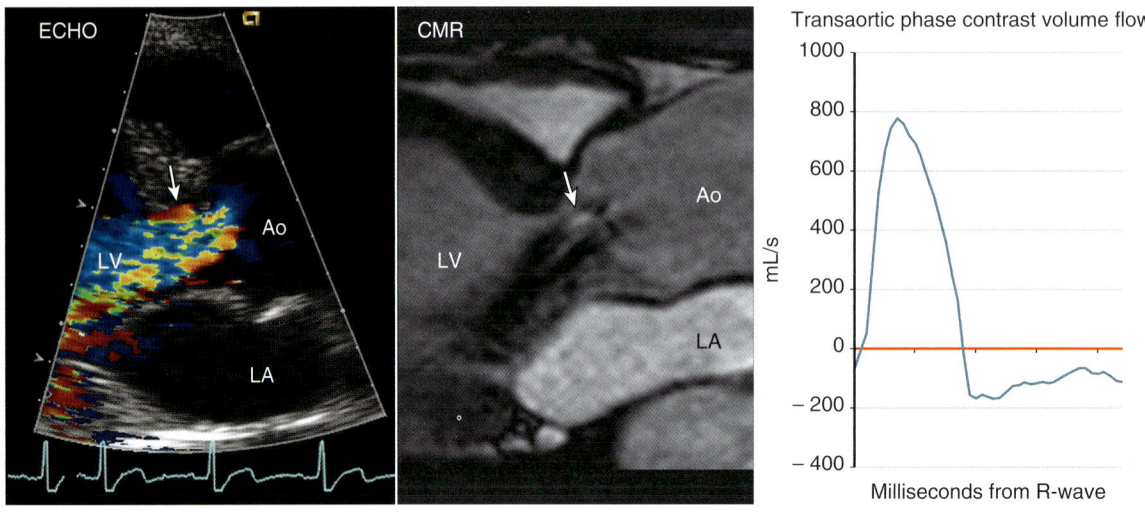

Fig. 12.17 Cardiac magnetic resonance imaging for quantitation of aortic regurgitation. Severe aortic regurgitation (AR; *arrows*) due to a bicuspid aortic valve is seen on Doppler color flow imaging *(left)* and on cardiac magnetic resonance *(CMR)* imaging *(center)*. The regurgitant flow appears as a black void in the lighter LV chamber using this pulse sequence. The CMR transaortic volume flow rate curve *(right)* allows quantitation of AR severity, where the area under the systolic curve represents total stroke volume and the area under the diastolic curve measures regurgitant volume. *Ao,* Aorta.

the interpretation integrates data from several potential measures of regurgitant severity into a summary statement. Rather than being redundant, the different approaches to regurgitant severity serve as cross-checks on one another. Errors or limitations of one approach will be recognized when other approaches, with better data quality, show discrepant results. Current guidelines recommend an integrative approach to evaluation of regurgitant severity based on multiple quantitative and semiquantitative measurements, as well as consideration of valve anatomy, LV size, and systolic function and pulmonary pressures. Because valvular regurgitant is dynamic and varies with loading conditions, it is essential to record blood pressure at the time of the echocardiographic examination.

When transthoracic data are suboptimal, TEE is the next step. If further data are needed for clinical decision making, other approaches can be considered. Cardiac magnetic resonance imaging provides quantitative measures of ventricular size and systolic function and of regurgitant volume and fraction (Fig. 12.17), and it is more reproducible than echocardiography for quantitation of AR. Cardiac catheterization can be used to measure intracardiac pressures, angiographic visualization of regurgitation, and calculation of quantitative measures of regurgitant severity.

AORTIC REGURGITATION

The echocardiographic approach to the patient with AR includes not only evaluation of the presence of regurgitation but also the etiology and severity of regurgitation along with effects of the regurgitant lesion on ventricular size and function.

Diagnostic Imaging of the Valve Apparatus

AR is due either to abnormalities of the aorta or to abnormalities of the leaflets themselves (Table 12.4). The disease processes that cause valvular aortic stenosis *(congenital bicuspid valve, calcific valve disease,* and *rheumatic disease)* also can result in AR because of alterations in leaflet flexibility or shape leading to inadequate diastolic coaptation of the leaflets. The imaging findings for these diagnoses are discussed in Chapter 11.

Other diseases that cause AR include *myxomatous valve disease*, which can affect the aortic valve in addition to the mitral valve. The leaflets are thickened and redundant on 2D or 3D imaging with slight sagging of the leaflets into the LV outflow tract in diastole. The normal hemicylindrical configuration of each leaflet in diastole is distorted so that the short-axis view intersects the center of the leaflet *en face*, thus resulting in the false appearance of an ill-defined echogenic "mass."

Endocarditis results in AR either by leaflet perforation due to the infectious process or to deformity of diastolic leaflet closure resulting from the presence of a vegetation (Fig. 12.18). Less common abnormalities of the aortic valve leaflets leading to AR include congenital leaflet fenestrations, nonbacterial thrombotic endocarditis (e.g., systemic lupus erythematosus), infiltrative diseases (e.g., amyloidosis), systemic inflammatory diseases (e.g., ankylosing spondylitis), mucopolysaccharidosis, and glycogen storage diseases.

Abnormalities of the aorta can result in AR, even when the leaflets themselves are normal, by alterations in the geometry of the structures supporting the leaflets.

TABLE 12.4 Aortic Regurgitation: Clinical Echocardiographic Correlation

	Chronic Primary AR	Chronic AR Due to Aortic Disease	Acute AR
Causes (examples)	• Bicuspid aortic valve • Rheumatic valve disease • Calcific valve disease • Systemic inflammatory disease	• Marfan syndrome • Familial aortic aneurysm • Hypertensive disease • Aortitis	• Endocarditis • Aortic dissection • Blunt chest trauma
Clinical presentation and disease course	• Asymptomatic diastolic murmur • Slow disease progression over many years leads to dyspnea and decreased exercise capacity.	• Diastolic murmur on exam or AR on echocardiography in a patient with aortic disease	• New-onset heart failure • Pulmonary edema • Cardiogenic shock
LV response	• Progressive severe LV dilation • Some develop irreversible contractile dysfunction without symptoms. • EF remains normal until late in disease course but is not an accurate marker for myocardial dysfunction.	• LV dilation depending on AR severity	• Normal LV size with normal EF • Severely elevated LV filling pressures • Reduced forward cardiac output
Valve anatomy	• Bicuspid aortic valve with two leaflets • Commissural fusion and mitral valve involvement with rheumatic disease • Concurrent stenosis with calcific disease	• Normal aortic leaflet anatomy with stretched leaflets and central regurgitation • Dilation of aortic sinuses or ascending aorta • Effacement of the sinotubular junction is typical for Marfan syndrome.	• Perforated or flail aortic valve leaflet with endocarditis and valve destruction • Paravalvular abscess may be present. • Aortic dissection flap resulting in flail leaflet, undermining of commissural support or distortion of valve anatomy
Key Doppler findings	• Vena contracta measurement • CW Doppler signal • Flow reversal in the descending aorta	• Vena contracta measurement • CW Doppler signal • Flow reversal in the descending aorta	• Color Doppler with wide vena contracta • Dense CW Doppler signal with steep deceleration slope • Holodiastolic flow reversal in the descending aorta
Definition of severe AR	• Vena contracta width >0.6 cm • Holodiastolic flow reversal in the proximal abdominal aorta • Regurgitant volume >60 mL • Regurgitant fraction >50% • ROA >0.3 cm²	• Vena contracta width >0.6 cm • Holodiastolic flow reversal in the proximal abdominal aorta • Regurgitant volume >60 mL • Regurgitant fraction >50% • ROA >0.3 cm²	• Qualitative signs of severe AR are adequate for clinical decision making because therapy is directed at the underlying disease process.
Indications for intervention with severe AR*	• Symptom onset • LVESD >50 mm • LVEF <55%	• Timing of intervention often depends on the severity of aortic dilation and cause of disease, rather than AR severity.	• Urgent surgical intervention for ascending aortic dissection • Early surgery for endocarditis complicated by acute severe aortic regurgitation
Options for intervention	• Surgical aortic valve replacement • Aortic valve repair is possible in selected cases.	• Replacement of the aortic sinuses and ascending aorta with "sparing" of the aortic valve, which is positioned inside the prosthetic conduit (David procedure) • Bentall procedure with a prosthetic valve-conduit replacement of the aortic valve and root (with coronary reimplantation)	• Aortic root replacement for aortic dissection • In some cases, the valve can be resuspended at the sinotubular junction. • Aortic valve replacement

*Major accepted indications for intervention; guidelines should be consulted for other indications and more details.
AR, Aortic regurgitation; *EF*, ejection fraction; *LVEF*, LV ejection fraction; *LVESD*, LV end-systolic dimension; *ROA*, regurgitant orifice area.

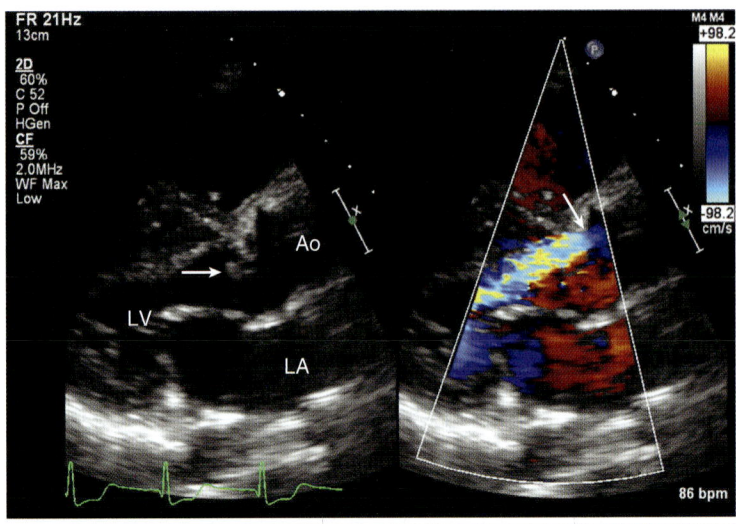

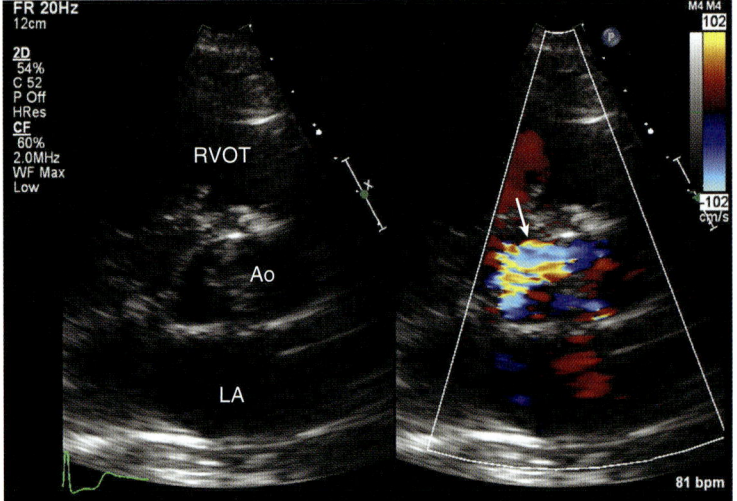

Fig. 12.18 Acute aortic regurgitation. 2D imaging of the aortic valve in long-axis *(top)* ▶ and short-axis *(bottom)* ▶ views shows a valvular vegetation consistent with endocarditis. Color Doppler *(right)* shows a wide jet of aortic regurgitation (vena contracta 6 mm; *arrow*) adjacent to the vegetation, suggestive of perforation or destruction of the right coronary cusp. *Ao,* Aorta; *RVOT,* RV outflow tract.

The aortic annulus is not a discrete planar ring of fibrous tissue but rather a complex, crown-shaped structure where the leaflets attach to the aortic valve with the three "points" of the crown at the commissures and the three lowest points at the midsection of each leaflet. Dilation of this area at the base of the aorta—often termed *annular dilation*—results in AR because of inadequate coaptation of the stretched leaflets. Note that adjacent leaflets normally overlap (apposition zone), so mild degrees of annular dilation do not result in valvular incompetence. Annular dilation has a variety of causes, including *chronic hypertension, cystic medial necrosis,* or *Marfan syndrome.* Marfan syndrome is characterized by effacement of the normal sinotubular junction with dilation of the annulus and sinuses of Valsalva (see Chapter 16). In cystic medial necrosis, the sinotubular junction usually is identifiable, although dilation typically involves the sinuses in addition to the ascending aorta. *Bicuspid aortic valve disease* often is associated with significant dilation of the aortic sinuses and ascending aorta. AR due to *syphilitic aortitis* is rare in the United States. When present, it typically is characterized by extensive calcification of the dilated ascending aorta. *Aortic dissection* can result in AR either by annular dilation leading to inadequate coaptation or by the false channel of the dissection undermining the aortic annulus and resulting in a flail leaflet (see Chapter 16).

The *differential diagnosis* for the echocardiographer in the evaluation of a patient referred for suspected AR depends on the specific indications for the examination. If a diastolic murmur has been noted on auscultation, differential diagnoses include pulmonic regurgitation, mitral or tricuspid stenosis, and (rarely) a coronary arteriovenous fistula. In some cases, only the diastolic portion of a continuous murmur (e.g., a patent ductus arteriosus) is appreciated on auscultation. If AR is suspected because of a concern for aortic dissection, the differential diagnosis should focus on examination of the ascending aorta.

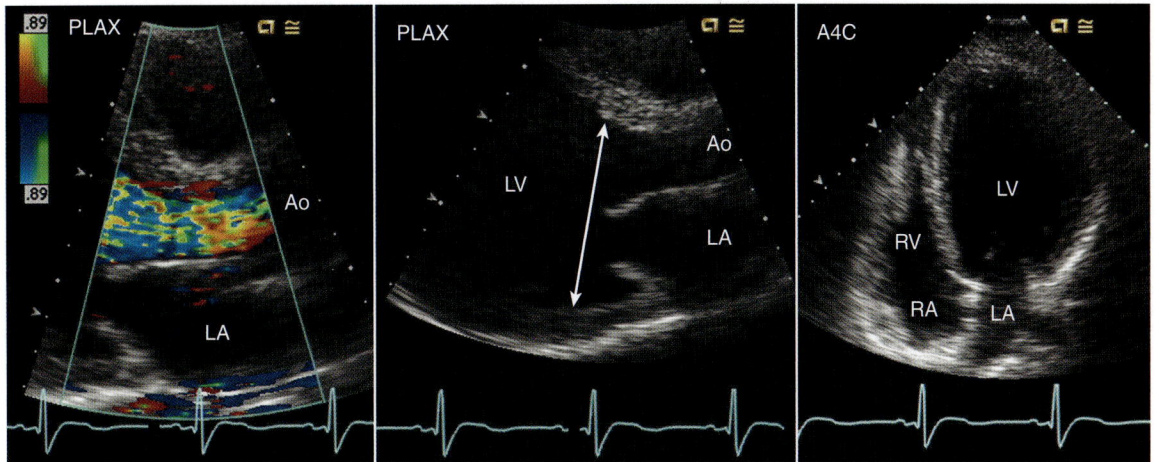

Fig. 12.19 ▶ ▶ ▶ **Left ventricle dilation and increased sphericity with chronic severe aortic regurgitation.** In a young woman with severe aortic regurgitation *(AR, left)*, significant compensatory LV dilation is seen. The parasternal long-axis view *(PLAX)* shows moderate LV dilation at the base *(arrow)*, but further dilation and increased sphericity of the LV is seen in the apical four-chamber view *(A4C)*, with the typical appearance of LV dilation due to AR. *Ao,* Aorta.

Left Ventricular Response

When exposed to chronic volume overload from AR, the LV progressively dilates and becomes more spherical (Fig. 12.19). Initially, LV systolic function remains normal. With chronic gradually increasing AR, the LV remains compliant in diastole, so end-diastolic pressure remains normal. Typically, LV size slowly increases over a period of years without impairment of systolic function. However, LV systolic dysfunction eventually occurs in the presence of hemodynamically significant chronic volume overload, and in some individuals, irreversible LV systolic dysfunction supervenes even in the absence of clinical symptoms.

In contrast to chronic regurgitation, in acute AR, the short interval from the onset of volume overload to clinical presentation means that significant LV dilation has not yet occurred. The physiologic differences between acute and chronic AR are reflected both in the 2D echocardiographic findings and in the Doppler examination.

Indirect Signs of Aortic Regurgitation

In addition to anatomic abnormalities of the aortic valve and the secondary LV dilation that occurs in response to volume overload, several indirect signs of AR are recognized (Fig. 12.20):

- Increased *E*-point septal separation (EPSS)
- High-frequency fluttering of the anterior mitral leaflet
- Reversed diastolic curvature of the anterior mitral leaflet
- Jet lesion on septum or mitral valve

If the regurgitant jet impinges on the anterior mitral valve leaflet, it causes impaired leaflet opening, resulting in an increased distance between the maximal anterior motion of the mitral valve in early diastole (the *E* point) and the most posterior motion of the interventricular septum (e.g., increased *E*-point septal separation). High-frequency fluttering of the anterior mitral valve leaflet resulting from impingement of the regurgitant jet also is seen on M-mode recording (with its high sampling rate), though it is rarely seen on 2D imaging (because of the relatively low frame rate).

On 2D long- and short-axis imaging, when AR is present the anterior mitral leaflet atypically appears curved in diastole, with the concavity toward the ventricular septum with the region of abnormal curvature corresponding to the direction of the regurgitant jet. In short-axis views, a discrete area of reversed curvature corresponding to the spatial location of the regurgitant jet often is seen. This contrasts with the normal linear appearance of the anterior leaflet in diastole in long-axis views and the normal diastolic curvature toward the ventricular septum in the short-axis view. This observation is sometimes called *reverse doming* because the curvature of the anterior leaflet is the opposite of that seen in rheumatic mitral stenosis. With chronic regurgitation, the focal blood flow disturbance impinging on the septum or anterior mitral leaflet results in a raised fibrotic lesion—identifiable by the pathologist post mortem as a jet lesion—which appears as an area of increased echogenicity on 2D imaging.

Although none of these indirect signs of AR provides quantitative data, their presence on a point of care limited study suggests a previously unsuspected diagnosis and should prompt a complete Doppler examination. Recognition of the impact of AR on mitral leaflet motion and the appearance of jet lesions avoids misinterpretation of these findings.

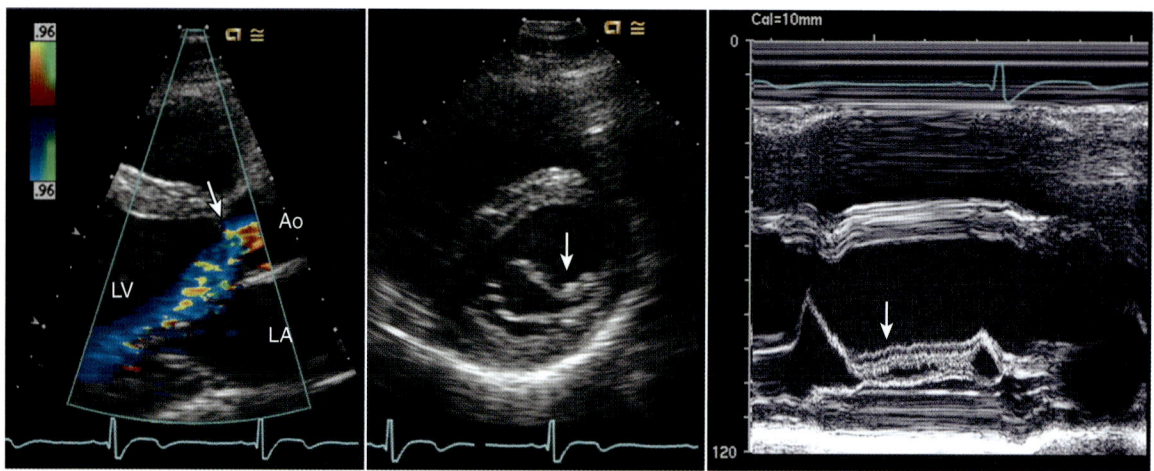

Fig. 12.20 Other imaging findings with severe aortic regurgitation. In this young man with a bicuspid aortic valve and asymptomatic aortic regurgitation (AR), color Doppler imaging in a parasternal long-axis view *(left)* ▶ shows a vena contracta width of 7 mm, consistent with severe regurgitation. In the 2D short-axis view *(center)*, ▶ reverse doming of the mitral leaflet *(arrow)* is seen due to impingement by the AR jet. The M-mode tracing *(right)* shows increased E-point septal separation and high-frequency fluttering of the anterior mitral leaflet *(arrow)*. *Ao,* Aorta.

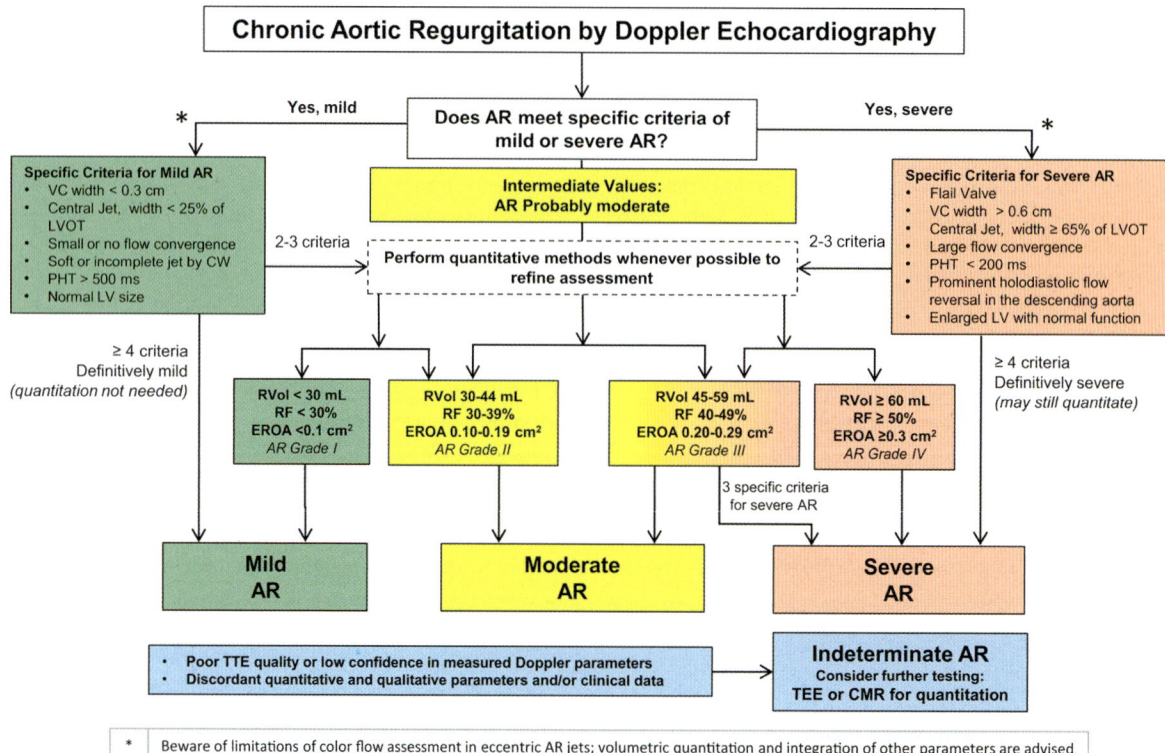

Fig. 12.21 Algorithm for the integration of multiple parameters of aortic regurgitant severity. Good-quality echocardiographic imaging and complete data acquisition are assumed. If imaging is technically difficult, consider TEE or cardiac magnetic resonance *(CMR)*. Aortic regurgitation *(AR)* severity often is indeterminate due to poor image quality, technical issues with data, internal inconsistency among echo findings, or discordance with clinical findings. *EROA,* Estimated regurgitant orifice area; *LVOT,* LV outflow tract; *PHT,* Pressure half-time; *RF,* regurgitant fraction; *RVol,* regurgitant volume; *VC,* vena contracta. (From Zoghbi WA, Adams D, et al: Recommendations for noninvasive evaluation of native valvular regurgitation: a report from the American Society of Echocardiography developed in collaboration with the Society for Cardiovascular Magnetic Resonance, J Am Soc Echocardiogr 30(4):303–371, Fig. 25.)

Evaluation of Aortic Regurgitant Severity

Screening Examination

Screening for AR with color flow imaging and CW Doppler ultrasound is part of a routine echocardiographic examination (Fig. 12.21). Parasternal views in both long and short axis are helpful and allow identification of the exact origin of the regurgitant jet in addition to assessment of its width and cross-sectional area. Mild AR fills only a small

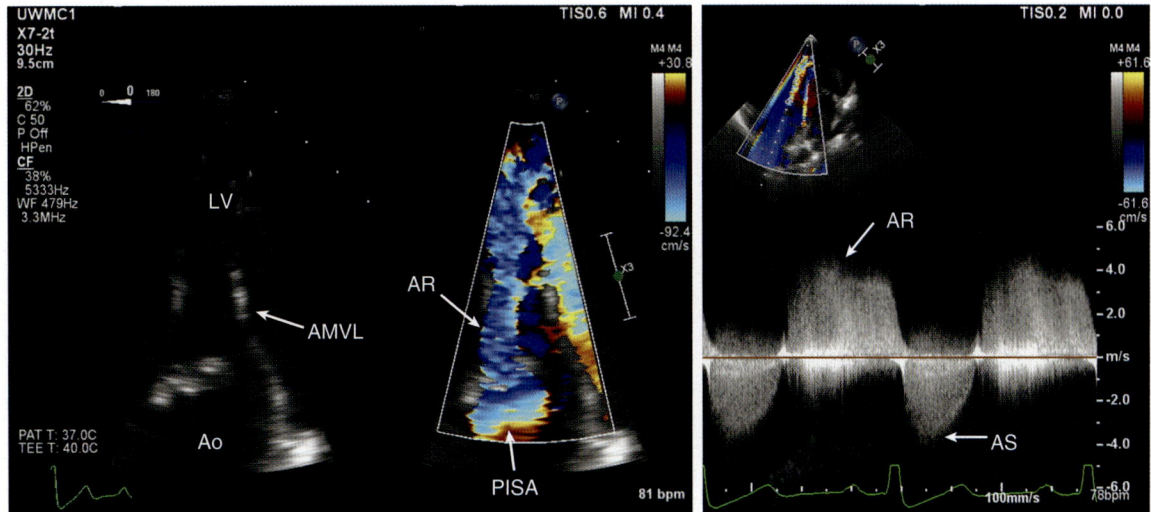

Fig. 12.22 ▶ **Severe aortic regurgitation.** In this 23-year-old patient with a bicuspid aortic valve and acute endocarditis, the TEE transgastric anteriorly angulated apical four-chamber view *(left)* shows a broad jet of aortic regurgitation *(AR)* with a proximal isovelocity surface area *(PISA)* on the aortic side of the valve. CW Doppler *(right)* shows a dense diastolic flow signal of AR with an increased antegrade flow velocity indicating at least moderate aortic stenosis *(AS)*. *AMVL,* Anterior mitral valve leaflet; *Ao,* Aorta.

area of the LV outflow tract (see Fig. 12.7), whereas moderate to severe regurgitation fills a larger percentage of the outflow tract diameter or area (Fig. 12.22). Eccentric jets traverse the outflow tract obliquely, a feature that makes measurement of jet size more difficult. A central jet that fills less than 25% of the outflow tract is consistent with mild regurgitation.

CW Doppler is used to record the antegrade aortic velocity signal from an apical approach, with careful angulation to identify an AR signal, if present. A weak or absent diastolic signal confirms that significant regurgitation is not present.

Vena Contracta

If the screening examination suggests more than mild AR, the next step is measurement of the vena contracta width, followed by further quantitation of regurgitant severity if needed for clinical decision making.

The vena contracta is visualized using color flow imaging in a parasternal long-axis view in the zoom mode, with a narrow sector, to optimize temporal and spatial resolution. Careful angulation medially and laterally from the long-axis plane is needed to identify the narrowest segment of the regurgitant jet clearly (see Fig. 12.7). A vena contracta width less than 0.3 cm is consistent with mild regurgitation, and no further evaluation is needed. A wider vena contracta width or poor data quality will prompt further evaluation of regurgitant severity. With eccentric jets, diameter is measured perpendicularly to the long axis of the jet, not the long axis of the outflow tract.

Aortic Flow Reversal

With severe AR, holodiastolic flow reversal is seen in the proximal abdominal aorta, recorded from the subcostal window (Fig. 12.23). This observation is analogous to the physical examination finding of diastolic reversal in the femoral arteries (Duroziez sign). Holodiastolic flow reversal in the abdominal aorta is sensitive (100%) and specific (97%) for diagnosing severe AR. False-positive results may be due to the presence of a patent ductus arteriosus, where the diastolic flow is from aorta to pulmonary artery rather than to the LV. More proximal holodiastolic flow reversal, in the descending thoracic aorta, also is sensitive for detection of severe AR but is less specific; it is also seen in some subjects with only moderate regurgitation.

CW Doppler

The CW Doppler spectral recording of AR has its onset at aortic valve closure (during isovolumic relaxation) with a rapid increase in velocity to a maximum of 3 to 5 m/s, followed by a gradual decline in velocity during diastole. The velocity abruptly decelerates during isovolumic contraction and reaches baseline at aortic valve opening. The intensity of the signal, relative to antegrade velocity, is an indicator of regurgitant severity. In moderate or severe AR, the signal can easily be recorded throughout diastole, whereas mild AR often is not holodiastolic; instead, a recordable signal is seen only at the beginning or end of diastole. This observation is due to low signal strength or variation in jet direction during diastole resulting in significant intercept angle changes.

Fig. 12.23 ▶ **Holodiastolic flow reversal in the aorta.** Doppler velocity curve in the proximal abdominal aorta from a transthoracic subcostal window shows holodiastolic flow reversal consistent with severe aortic regurgitation. Note that diastolic flow is seen below the baseline throughout diastole, whereas the normal aortic flow pattern is brief reversal in early and late diastole with no or low velocity forward flow in mid-diastole.

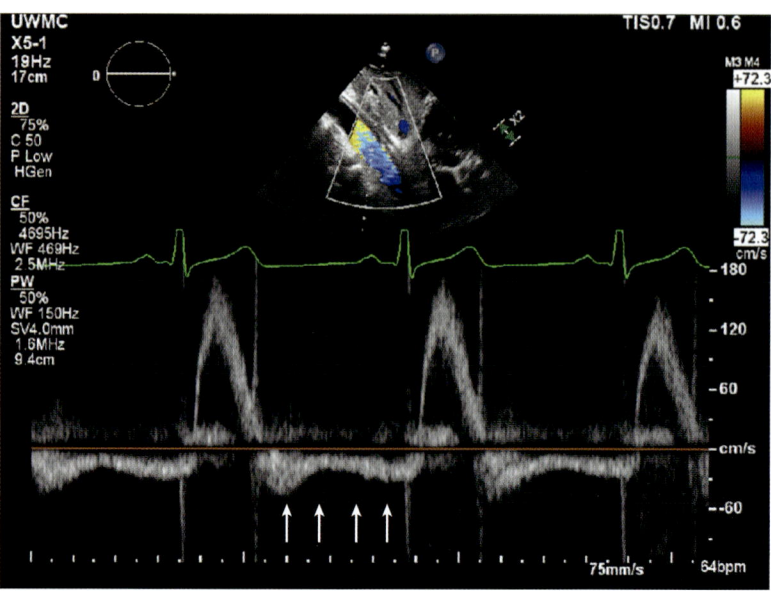

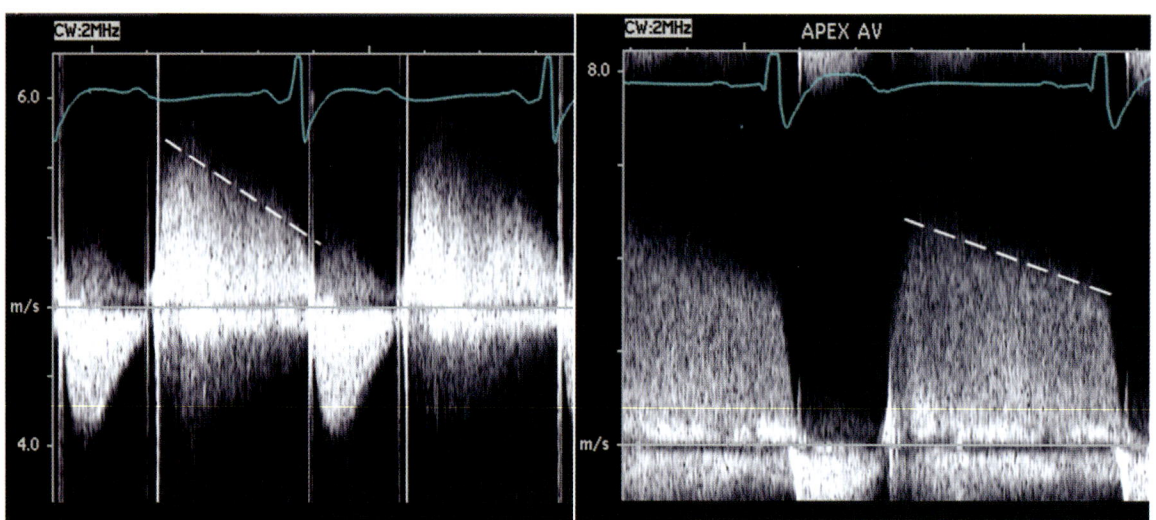

Fig. 12.24 Continuous-wave Doppler with acute versus chronic aortic regurgitation. CW Doppler recording in two patients, one with acute aortic regurgitation (AR) due to aortic dissection *(left)* and one with chronic regurgitation due to calcific aortic valve disease *(right)*, showing the differences in the deceleration slope in these clinical situations.

The shape of the CW Doppler time-velocity curve depends on the time-varying instantaneous pressure gradient across the valve in diastole, thus reflecting both the severity and the chronicity of regurgitation. Chronic, severe AR results in an increased aortic pulse pressure with a low end-diastolic aortic pressure. The rapid rate of decline in aortic pressure is reflected in a more rapid decline in the Doppler velocity—that is, a steeper diastolic deceleration slope even if end-diastolic LV pressure remains low (Fig. 12.24). Thus, the diastolic deceleration slope provides a semiquantitative measure of AR severity. A flat slope (pressure half-time >500 ms) is consistent with mild regurgitation, and a steep slope (pressure half-time <200 ms) indicates severe regurgitation.

However, in addition to AR severity, other factors that affect either LV or aortic diastolic pressure also affect the course of the pressure difference (and velocity) across the regurgitant valve. With *acute* regurgitation, even if only moderate in severity, LV compliance has not yet adapted, as occurs in response to chronic volume overload, so a significant increase in end-diastolic pressure is seen. In extreme cases, aortic and LV end-diastolic pressures equalize at end-diastole, resulting in a triangular CW velocity signal with a linear deceleration slope from maximum velocity to the baseline. Other factors that affect LV diastolic pressure (e.g., systolic dysfunction, ischemia) or aortic diastolic pressure (e.g., sepsis, patent ductus arteriosus) also will affect the shape of the AR velocity curve.

The CW signal for AR usually is best recorded from an apical window to obtain a parallel intercept angle between the jet and the blood flow direction. Occasionally, an eccentric jet, directed either anteriorly or posteriorly, is best recorded from a parasternal approach. If signal strength from the suprasternal notch is adequate, a signal similar to that recorded from the apex (but, of course, inverted) is seen.

Regurgitant Volume and Fraction

It is rarely possible to image a measurable proximal isovelocity surface area for the quantitation of AR severity. Instead, AR volume and fraction can be calculated as the difference between transaortic and transmitral volume flow. Alternately, both forward and total stroke volume can be calculated in the proximal

The vena contracta width indicates more than mild AR, but this could be moderate or severe.

Holodiastolic flow reversal in the proximal abdominal aorta would be consistent with severe AR. Flow reversal in the descending thoracic aorta indicates at least moderate AR but is less specific for severe AR.

CW Doppler signal density indicates at least moderate AR and a deceleration slope >3 m/s^2, but <5 m/s^2 is also consistent with moderate or severe AR.

Next, regurgitant volume (RVol), regurgitant fraction (RF), and regurgitant orifice area (ROA) are calculated.

Using the LVOT and mitral annulus diameters (MA$_D$), the circular cross-sectional areas (CSA) of flow are calculated:

$$CSA_{LVOT} = \pi(LVOT_D/2)^2 = 3.14(2.7/2)^2 = 6.2\ cm^2$$

$$CSA_{MA} = \pi(MA_D/2)^2 = 3.14(3.1/2)^2 = 7.5\ cm^2$$

Stroke volume (SV) across each valve (cm^3 = mL), then is:

$$SV_{LVOT} = (CSA_{LVOT} \times VTI_{LVOT})$$
$$= 6.2\ cm^2 \times 24\ cm = 149\ cm^3$$

$$SV_{MA} = (CSA_{MA} \times VTI_{MA}) = 7.5\ cm^2 \times 12\ cm = 91\ cm^3$$

Regurgitant volume (RVol) is calculated from transaortic flow (TSV, total stroke volume) and transmitral flow (FSV, forward stroke volume), as:

$$RVol = TSV - FSV = 149\ mL - 91\ mL = 58\ mL$$

Regurgitant fraction (RF) is:

$$RVol = RSV/TSV \times 100\%$$
$$= 58\ mL/149\ mL \times 100\% = 39\%$$

Regurgitant orifice area (ROA) is:

$$VTI_{AR} = 58\ cm^3/204\ cm = 0.28\ cm^2$$

The RVol, RF, and ROA all are consistent with moderate (but nearly severe) AR.

ECHO MATH: Aortic Regurgitation Severity

Example
A 37-year-old man presents with an asymptomatic diastolic murmur. Echocardiography shows a bicuspid aortic valve with more than mild AR with:

Vena contracta width	5 mm
Descending aorta	Holodiastolic flow reversal in descending thoracic, but not proximal abdominal, aorta
CW Doppler	AR signal less dense than antegrade flow
	VTI$_{AR}$ = 150 cm
LVOT diameter (LVOT$_D$)	2.8 cm
VTI$_{LVOT}$	24 cm
Mitral annulus (MA) diameter	3.1 cm
VTI$_{MA}$	12 cm

---

descending thoracic aorta with total flow measured in systole and regurgitant flow in diastole. Because significant AR results in systolic expansion of the aorta, the antegrade flow velocity integral must be multiplied by the systolic cross-sectional area. Similarly, the flow velocity integral of the reversed flow in diastole is multiplied by the diastolic cross-sectional area. Either 2D short-axis imaging or an M-mode image through the aortic arch can be used for the measurement of systolic and diastolic cross-sectional areas. Note that this quantitative approach is the logical extension of the semiquantitative approach, which relies on the *presence* and spatial extent of holodiastolic flow reversal in the aorta in patients with AR.

TABLE 12.5 Stages of Chronic Aortic Regurgitation

Stage	Definition	Valve Anatomy	Valve Hemodynamics	Hemodynamic Consequences	Symptoms
A	At risk of AR	• Bicuspid aortic valve (or other congenital valve anomaly) • Aortic valve sclerosis • Diseases of the aortic sinuses or ascending aorta • History of rheumatic fever or known rheumatic heart disease • IE	• AR severity: none or trace	• None	• None

B	Progressive AR	• Mild to moderate calcification of a trileaflet valve bicuspid aortic valve (or other congenital valve anomaly)
		• Dilated aortic sinuses
		• Rheumatic valve changes
		• Previous IE
			• **Mild AR:**
			  • Jet width <25% of LVOT
			  • Vena contracta <0.3 cm
			  • RVol <30 mL/beat
			  • RF <30%
			  • ERO <0.10 cm^2
			  • Angiography grade 1+
			• **Moderate AR:**
			  • Jet width 25%–64% of LVOT
			  • Vena contracta 0.3–0.6 cm
			  • RVol 30–59 mL/beat
			  • RF 30%–49%
			  • ERO 0.10–0.29 cm^2
			  • Angiography grade 2+
				• Normal LV systolic function
				• Normal LV volume or mild LV dilation
					• None

C	Asymptomatic severe AR	• Calcific aortic valve disease
		• Bicuspid valve (or other congenital abnormality)
		• Dilated aortic sinuses or ascending aorta
		• Rheumatic valve changes
		• IE with abnormal leaflet closure or perforation
			• **Severe AR:**
			  • Jet width ≥65% of LVOT
			  • Vena contracta >0.6 cm
			  • Holodiastolic flow reversal in the proximal abdominal aorta
			  • RVol ≥60 mL/beat
			  • RF ≥50%
			  • ERO ≥0.3 cm^2
			  • Angiography grade 3+ to 4+
			  • In addition, diagnosis of chronic severe AR requires evidence of LV dilation
				• **C1:** Normal LVEF (≥50%) and mild to moderate LV dilation (LVESD ≤50 mm)
				• **C2:** Abnormal LV systolic function with depressed LVEF (<50%) or severe LV dilation (LVESD >50 mm or indexed LVESD >25 mm/m^2)
					• None; exercise testing is reasonable to confirm symptom status.

D	Symptomatic severe AR	• Calcific valve disease
		• Bicuspid valve (or other congenital abnormality)
		• Dilated aortic sinuses or ascending aorta
		• Rheumatic valve changes
		• Previous IE with abnormal leaflet closure or perforation
			• **Severe AR:**
			  • Doppler jet width ≥65% of LVOT
			  • Vena contracta >0.6 cm
			  • Holodiastolic flow reversal in the proximal abdominal aorta
			  • RVol ≥60 mL/beat
			  • RF ≥50%
			  • ERO ≥0.3 cm^2
			  • Angiography grade 3+ to 4+
			  • In addition, diagnosis of chronic severe AR requires evidence of LV dilation.
				• Symptomatic severe AR may occur with normal systolic function (LVEF ≥50%), mild to moderate LV dysfunction (LVEF 40% to 50%), or severe LV dysfunction (LVEF <40%).
				• Moderate to severe LV dilation is present.
					• Exertional dyspnea or angina or more severe HF symptoms

AR, Aortic regurgitation; *ERO*, effective regurgitant orifice; *HF*, heart failure; *IE*, infective endocarditis; *LVEF*, LV ejection fraction; *LVESD*, LV end-systolic dimension; *LVOT*, LV outflow tract; *RF*, regurgitant fraction; *RVol*, regurgitant volume.
From Nishimura RA, Otto CM, Bonow RO, et al: AHA/ACC guideline for the management of patients with valvular heart disease: executive summary. A report of the American College of Cardiology/American Heart Association Task Force on Practice Guidelines, *Circulation* 129(23):2440–2492, 2014.

Clinical Utility

Diagnostic Utility for Aortic Regurgitation

Echocardiography is an essential component in defining the disease stage in adults with AR, ranging from those at risk of progressive disease to those with severe valve dysfunction (Table 12.5). Echocardiography has a high sensitivity and specificity for detection of AR and also provides information on the etiology of valve disease, associated conditions, and the degree of LV dilation. If AR is detected in the course of an echocardiogram ordered for some other indication, it is incumbent on the echocardiographer to search carefully for the cause of regurgitation because this may be the first clue that aortic dilation or a disease process affecting the aortic leaflets is present.

Timing of Surgical Intervention for Chronic Asymptomatic Aortic Regurgitation

Most patients with severe AR undergo intervention for symptoms, but some benefit from valve replacement even in the absence of symptoms. Optimal timing of surgical intervention is challenging because measures of LV systolic function depend on loading conditions, which are altered by the presence of valvular regurgitation. Periodic echocardiography is recommended in the asymptomatic patient with significant regurgitation to measure changes in LV size and systolic function. Clinical guidelines recommend surgical intervention for progressive LV dilation (end-systolic dimension >50 mm, LV end-diastolic dimension >65 mm) or other evidence of decreased systolic function (LV ejection fraction <50%). Although current guidelines for the timing of intervention rely on studies using only linear measurements of LV size; given the improved accuracy and reproducibility of 3D echocardiographic LV volumes, it is hoped that future studies will allow us to replace linear dimensions with end-systolic volume indexes in clinical decision making.

MITRAL REGURGITATION

Diagnostic Imaging of the Mitral Valve Apparatus

Functionally, the mitral valve apparatus consists of several components:

- LA wall
- Mitral annulus
- Anterior and posterior leaflets
- Chordae
- Papillary muscles
- LV myocardium underlying the papillary muscles

Dysfunction or altered anatomy of any one of these components can result in MR (Fig. 12.25).

Mitral annular dilation is associated with either LA or LV dilation and results in MR because of incomplete leaflet coaptation. The normal mitral apparatus is a saddle-shaped ellipse with its most apical points seen in the apical four-chamber view and its most basal points seen in the long-axis view. As with the aortic valve, the mitral leaflets have a normal area of overlap (or apposition), so some degree of mitral annular dilation is tolerated without significant regurgitation.

The mitral annulus area normally is smaller in systole than in diastole. Increased rigidity of the annulus, as seen with *mitral annular calcification*, impairs systolic contraction of the annulus and leads to MR. Mitral annular calcification has a typical appearance on 2D imaging as an area of increased echogenicity on the LV side of the annulus immediately adjacent to the attachment point of the posterior leaflet. Acoustic shadowing, due to the presence of calcium, is seen. In short-axis views, the annular calcium may be focal or extensive, involving the entire U-shaped posterior annulus. The region of anterior mitral leaflet-posterior aortic wall continuity is involved only rarely. Mitral annular calcification is commonly seen in older adult patients and in younger patients with renal failure or hypertension (see Fig. 11.19).

Diseases of the mitral valve leaflets include myxomatous disease, rheumatic disease, endocarditis, Marfan syndrome, and rare disorders such as infiltrative diseases (e.g., amyloid, sarcoid, or mucopolysaccharidosis) and systemic inflammatory disorders (e.g., systemic lupus erythematosus, or rheumatoid arthritis). *Myxomatous* mitral valve disease is characterized by thickened, redundant leaflets and chordae with excessive motion and sagging of portions of the leaflets into the LA in systole (Figs. 12.26 and 12.27). The severity of disease is variable, ranging from mitral valve prolapse, with only minimal displacement of the leaflets into the LA in systole, to severe involvement

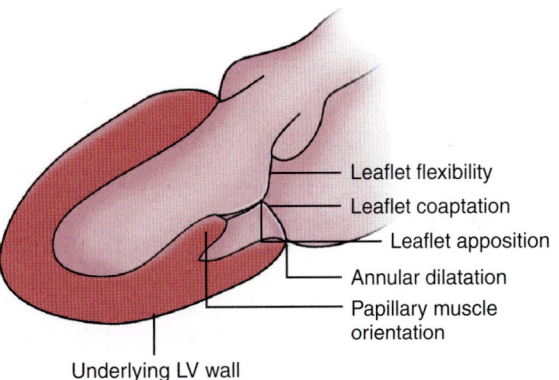

Fig. 12.25 Causes of mitral regurgitation. Schematic diagram illustrating how abnormalities of any part of the complex mitral valve apparatus can result in mitral regurgitation.

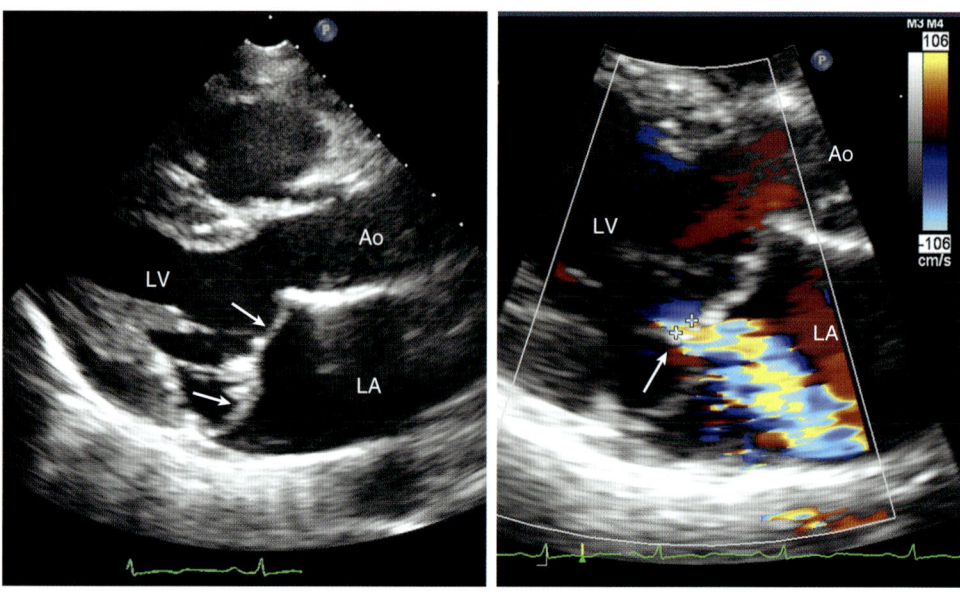

Fig. 12.26 Mitral valve prolapse. In a young woman with mitral valve prolapse, in the parasternal long-axis view *(left)*, ▶ an end-systolic image shows sagging of both mitral leaflets *(arrows)* into the left atrium in systole with both leaflets behind the plane of the annulus. The leaflets also are diffusely thickened and redundant. Color Doppler *(right)* ▶ shows a central jet of mitral regurgitation with a vena contracta width *(arrow)* of 4 mm. *Ao,* Aorta.

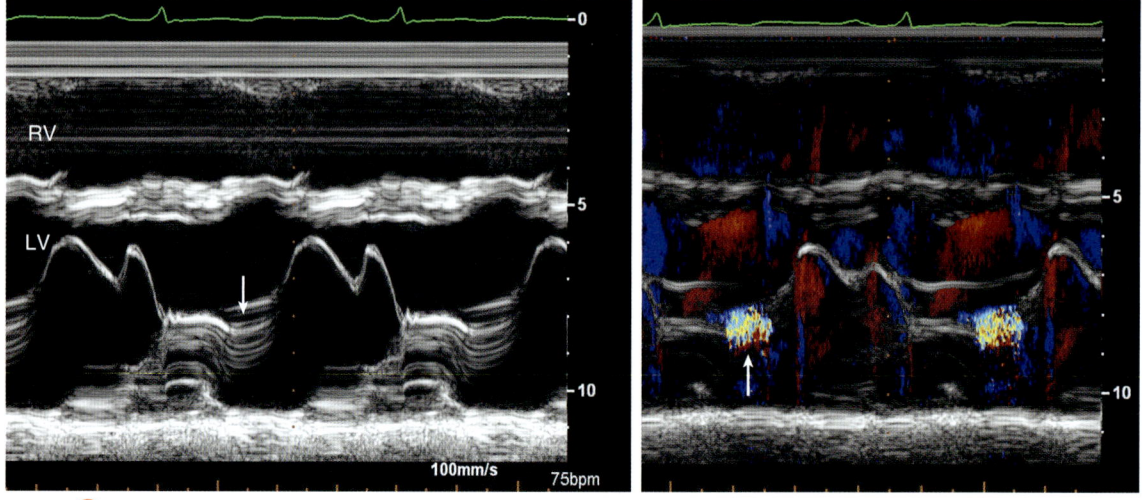

Fig. 12.27 ▶ **M-mode findings in mitral prolapse.** In the same patient as Fig. 12.26, an M-mode recording *(left)* of the mitral valve shows late systolic posterior motion of the leaflets *(arrow).* Color M-mode shows a late systolic mitral regurgitation signal *(arrow).*

of both leaflets by myxomatous disease with frankly prolapsed or flail leaflet segments. *Chordal disruption* or *elongation* leads to MR because of inadequate tensile support of the closed leaflets in systole. Chordal elongation results in severe bowing of the leaflet, or leaflet segment, into the LA, with the tip of the leaflet still directed toward the ventricular apex. With chordal rupture, a flail segment of the leaflet is present such that the leaflet is displaced into the LA in systole, with the tip of the leaflet pointing away from the ventricular apex (Fig. 12.28). 3D TEE imaging of the mitral valve is particularly important for the evaluation of myxomatous mitral valve disease. Precise delineation of the involved segments of the anterior and posterior leaflets improves communication with other physicians caring for the patient and allows optimal planning of the surgical approach to valve repair (Fig. 12.29). Acute MR due to chordal rupture typically manifests as acute pulmonary edema (Fig. 12.30).

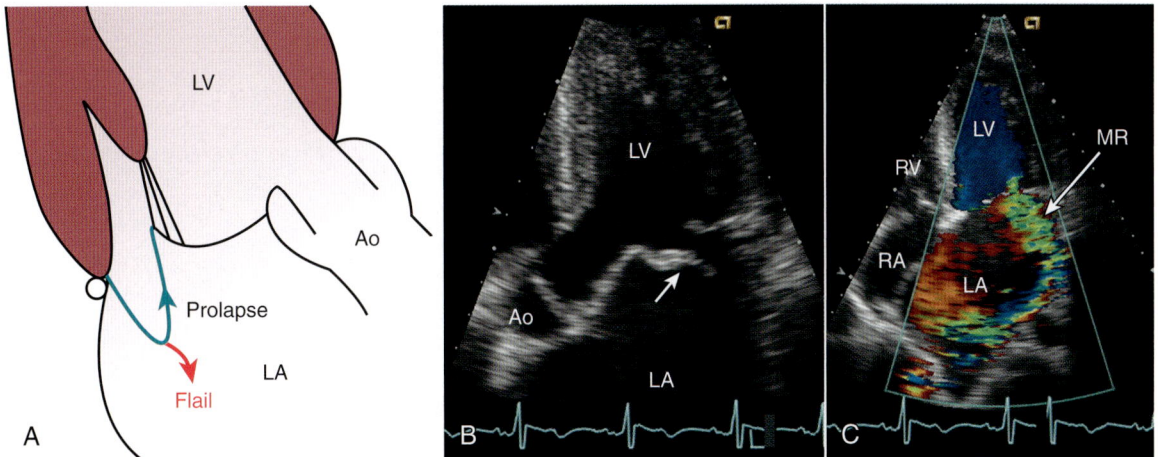

Fig. 12.28 Flail mitral valve leaflet. The term *prolapse* of the mitral leaflet indicates that the chordal connections of the leaflet to the papillary muscle are intact so that, regardless of the severity of prolapse, the tip of the leaflet still points toward the LV apex. (A) With chordal rupture, the mitral leaflet segment becomes "flail," and the tip of the flail segment points toward the roof of the LA. (B) ▶ In an apical four-chamber view, a partial flail anterior mitral leaflet *(arrow)* is seen in a young man with myxomatous mitral valve disease. Note that the tip of the flail segment points away from the LV apex *(middle)*. (C) ▶ Color Doppler imaging demonstrates an eccentric posterior and laterally directed jet of mitral regurgitation *(MR, arrow)*. The online video shows a flail posterior mitral leaflet in a different patient. *Ao*, Aorta.

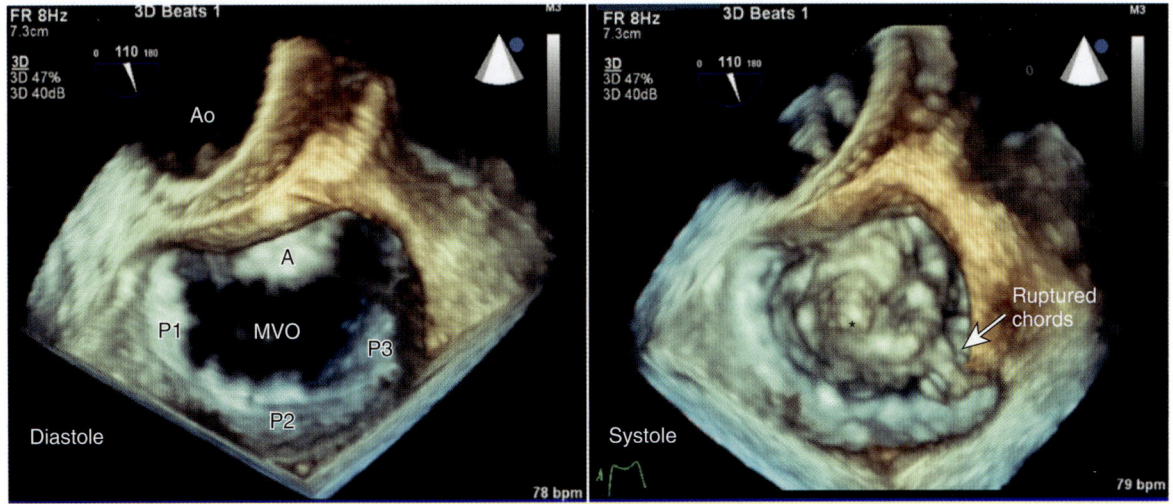

Fig. 12.29 ▶ ▶ **3D mitral valve.** In the surgeon's view of the mitral valve from the LA side of the valve (with the aortic valve and aorta *(Ao)* at the top of the image), in diastole the anterior leaflet and posterior leaflet (with P1, P2, and P3 scallops) are seen in the open position with the normal mitral valve orifice *(MVO)*. In systole, severe prolapse of the anterior leaflet *(A)* is seen, particularly one bulging section *(asterisk)*, and a flail segment with two small ruptured chords *(arrow)* is well visualized, resulting in severe posteriorly directed mitral regurgitation (see Fig. 12.6). This patient also has a bileaflet mechanical aortic prosthesis; the open leaflets can be seen in the systolic image.

Rheumatic MR, like rheumatic mitral stenosis, is characterized by some degree of commissural fusion, but chordal fusion and shortening are more prominent. *Endocarditis* results in MR by leaflet destruction, perforation, or deformity. *Marfan syndrome* is associated with a long, redundant anterior leaflet that sags into the LA in systole. Infiltrative diseases result in irregular leaflet thickening and inadequate coaptation. *Age-related degenerative changes* in the mitral leaflets often are seen (with or without associated mitral annular calcification) and appear as irregular areas of thickening and increased echogenicity of the mitral leaflets.

Ischemic MR may be due to regional LV dysfunction with abnormal contraction of the papillary muscle or underlying ventricular wall. In patients with a myocardial infarction, myocardial scarring results in MR at rest. In patients with normal resting myocardial function but inducible ischemia with stress, MR may be intermittent. Ischemic MR is characterized by restricted leaflet motion, with tethering of valve

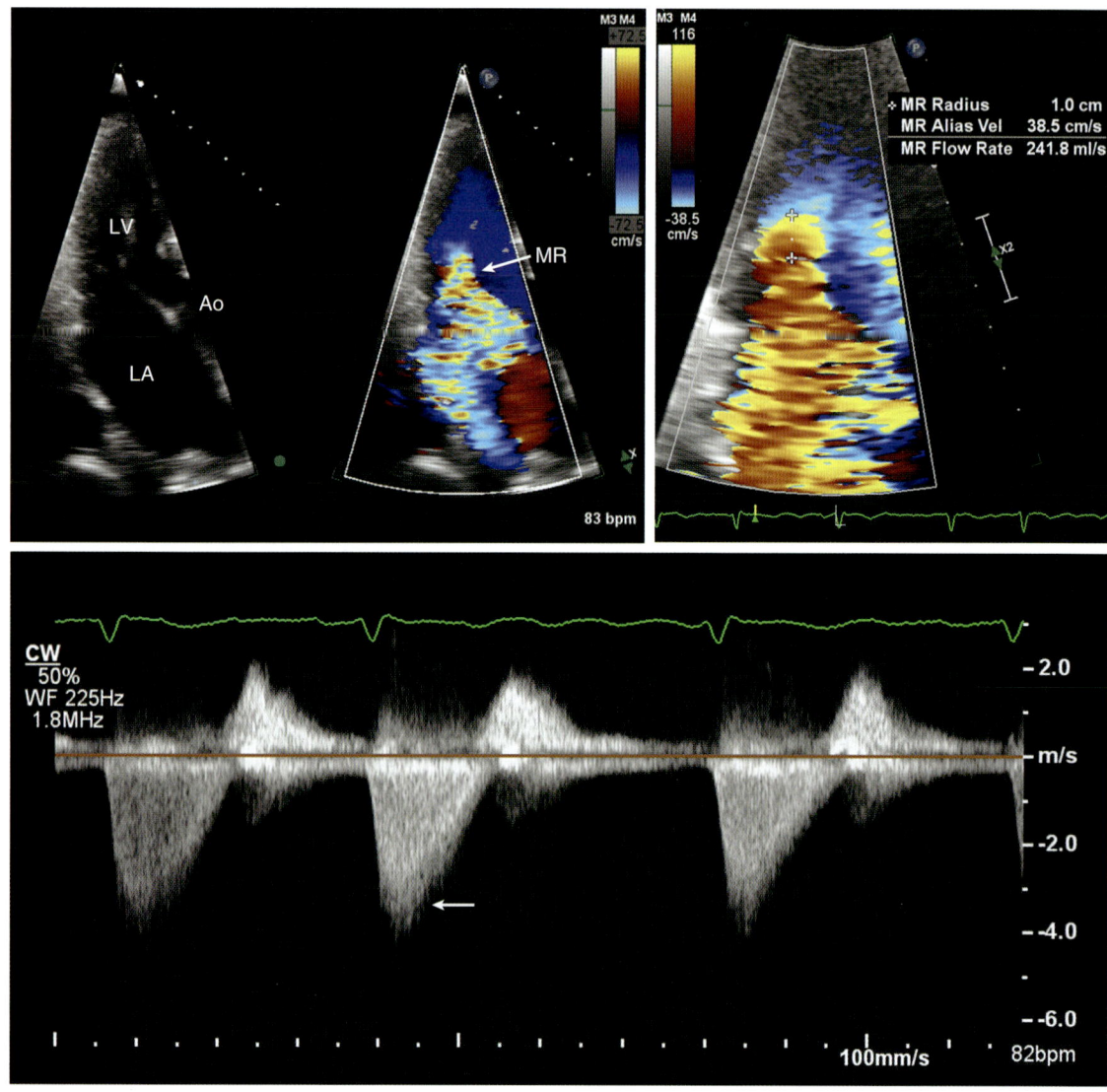

Fig. 12.30 **Acute mitral regurgitation.** This 73-year-old man presents with pulmonary edema. In the transthoracic apical long-axis view, mitral regurgitation (MR) is seen with a wide vena contracta and large jet area *(top left)*. ▶ The proximal isovelocity surface area *(top right)* ▶ is measured as 1.0 cm after zooming the image, adjusting the color Doppler zero baseline to 39 cm/s away from the transducer, thus yielding an instantaneous regurgitant flow rate of 242 mL/s. The CW Doppler peak velocity is 3.6 m/s *(bottom)*, so the effective regurgitant orifice area is 0.67 cm², indicating very severe mitral regurgitation. The CW Doppler signal *(bottom)* has a triangular shape, indicating a rapid rise in LA pressure during systole due to acute regurgitation. The low peak velocity reflects a low systolic blood pressure and high LA pressure with an LV to LA systolic pressure difference of only 52 mmHg. *Ao,* Aorta.

closure resulting in the appearance of "tenting" or tethering of the mitral valve in systole (Figs. 12.31 and 12.32).

Papillary muscle rupture can occur as a complication of acute myocardial infarction. If the entire papillary muscle is disconnected from the underlying LV wall, few patients will survive because of acute, severe MR. Echocardiographic evaluation in those who do survive shows a mass (the ruptured papillary muscle) attached to flail segments of anterior and posterior leaflets (because each papillary muscle attaches to both leaflets) (see Fig. 2.6). The ruptured papillary muscle head is seen in the LA in systole and in the LV in diastole (see Fig. 8.24). Severe MR is present on Doppler examination. Partial rupture of a papillary muscle, defined as rupture of one of several "heads" or as partial disconnection of the base of the papillary muscle, is seen more often than complete rupture because patients are more likely to survive long enough to undergo diagnostic evaluation. In this situation, the echocardiogram shows a thin, attenuated, excessively mobile papillary muscle and, if one head has ruptured, a mass attached to the leaflet with prolapse into the LA in systole.

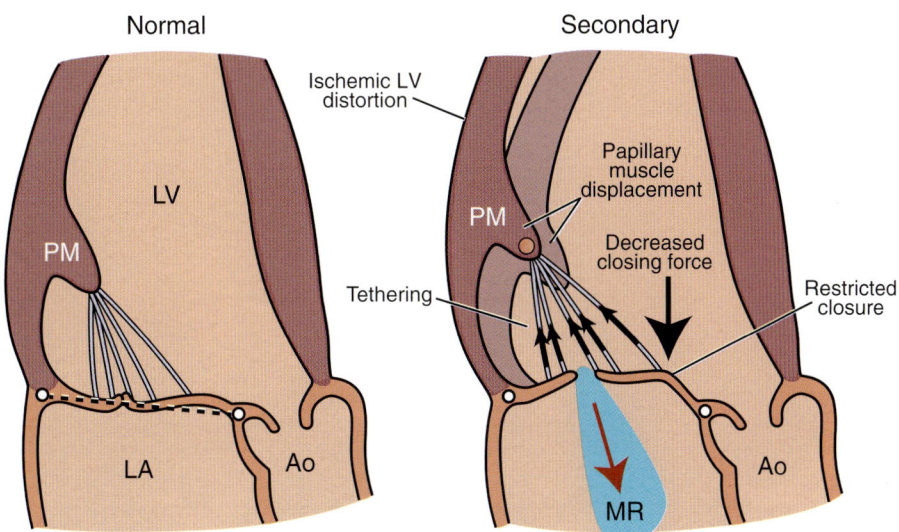

Fig. 12.31 Mechanism of secondary mitral regurgitation. These diagrams illustrate the normal forces contributing to a competent mitral valve *(left)* and the changes that result in secondary mitral regurgitation *(MR, right)*. The normal angle between the papillary muscle *(PM)* and mitral annulus *(dashed line)* determines the tethering effect of the mitral chords. Diseases that displace the papillary muscle or distort the LV shape (e.g., ischemic disease) adversely affect this normal tethering mechanism, thus resulting in decreased closing force and restricted closure. *Ao,* Aorta. Dilation of the mitral annulus further contributes to inadequate leaflet closure. *(From Hung J, Delling F, Capoulade R: Mitral regurgitation: valve anatomy, regurgitant severity and timing of intervention. In Otto CM, editor:* The Practice of Clinical Echocardiography, *ed 5, Philadelphia, 2017, Elsevier, pp 322–342, Fig. 18 10.)*

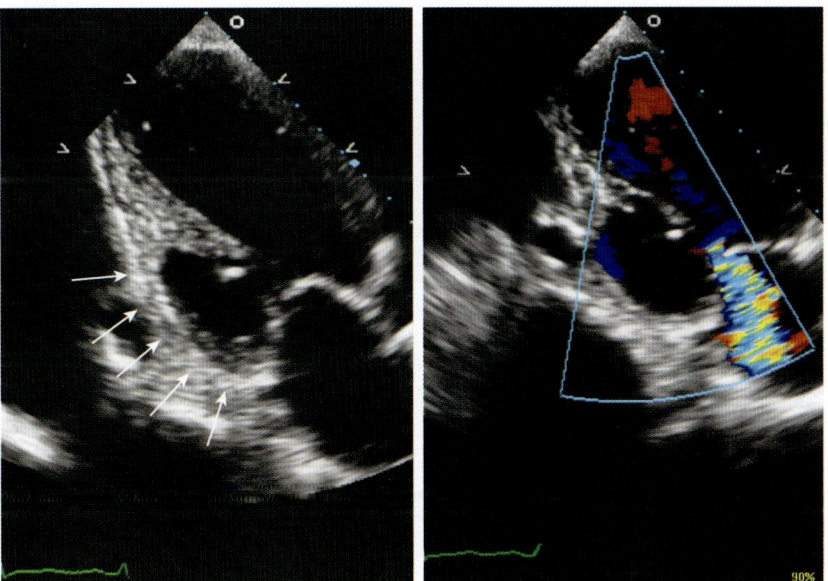

Fig. 12.32 Ischemic mitral regurgitation. In this patient with coronary artery disease, an inferior basal aneurysm *(left; arrows)* results in distortion of the LV wall that leads to mitral leaflet tethering and restricted closure with development of secondary mitral regurgitation *(right)*. *(From Hung J., Delling F, Capoulade R: Mitral regurgitation: valve anatomy, regurgitant severity and timing of intervention. In Otto CM, editor:* The Practice of Clinical Echocardiography, *ed 5, Philadelphia, 2017, Elsevier, pp 322–342, Fig. 18-11.)*

MR due to LV dilation and systolic dysfunction, in patients with normal valve leaflets and chordae, often is called *functional MR* (Fig. 12.33). The mechanism of functional MR remains controversial, with some studies suggesting abnormal orientation of the papillary muscles and others suggesting annular dilation.

Obviously, although MR due to conditions with unique anatomic features can be reliably diagnosed by echocardiographic imaging (rheumatic or myxomatous disease), considerable overlap exists in the anatomic features of other conditions (degenerative versus infiltrative leaflet abnormalities). In some cases, it is difficult to determine whether MR is the cause or consequence of ventricular dilation and systolic dysfunction. When the cause is unclear, the echocardiographer can describe the valve anatomy and indicate possible reasons for the findings even though the specific tissue diagnosis remains unknown.

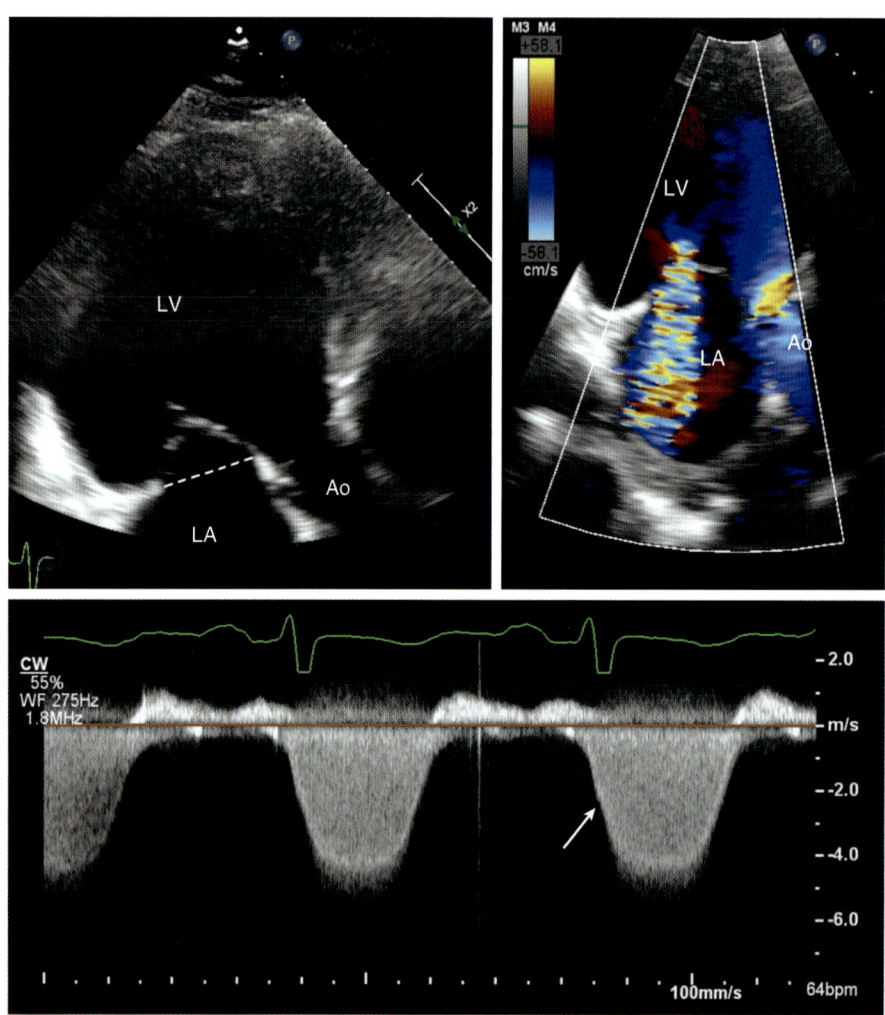

Fig. 12.33 Secondary mitral regurgitation. In this patient with dilated cardiomyopathy (LV ejection fraction 23%), the apical long-axis view *(upper left)* ▶ shows severe LV dilation with "tenting" of the mitral leaflets with the end-systolic valve closure on the LV size of the mitral annulus *(dashed line)*. Color Doppler *(upper right)* ▶ shows central mitral regurgitation. CW Doppler *(bottom)* shows a moderately dense signal compared with antegrade flow with a slow rate of increase in velocity in early systole *(arrow)*, thus reflecting a reduced LV dP/dt. *Ao*, Aorta.

Response of the Left Ventricle, Left Atrium, and Pulmonary Vasculature

MR results in LV volume overload because of the increase in total LV stroke volume as blood is ejected both forward into the aorta and retrograde across the mitral valve. With acute MR, the LV empties more completely (i.e., ejection fraction increases), such that forward cardiac output is maintained. With compensated chronic regurgitation, LV diastolic volume increases and ejection fraction is normal, such that end-systolic volume is within the normal range or only mildly increased (Fig. 12.34). Although it may seem that afterload is decreased in patients with MR due to ejection into the low-pressure LA, the effect of decreased ejection force is counterbalanced by increased ventricular chamber size without an increase in wall thickness. Thus, with chronic MR, afterload is normal and ejection fraction typically is in the normal range (not increased). Quantitation of LV size and systolic function is a primary focus on serial studies in patients with chronic MR and is a key element in clinical decision making.

With chronic regurgitation, progressive LV dilation eventually occurs as the regurgitant volume (and thus total LV stroke volume) increases. As with AR, an irreversible decline in LV contractility can occur in the absence of symptoms. The LA gradually dilates to accommodate the regurgitant volume while maintaining a normal pressure because of an increase in compliance (i.e., the LA pressure-volume relationship is shifted downward and to the right). With acute MR, the regurgitant volume is delivered into a small, noncompliant LA, resulting in a significant increase in pressure and a *v*-wave in the LA pressure curve.

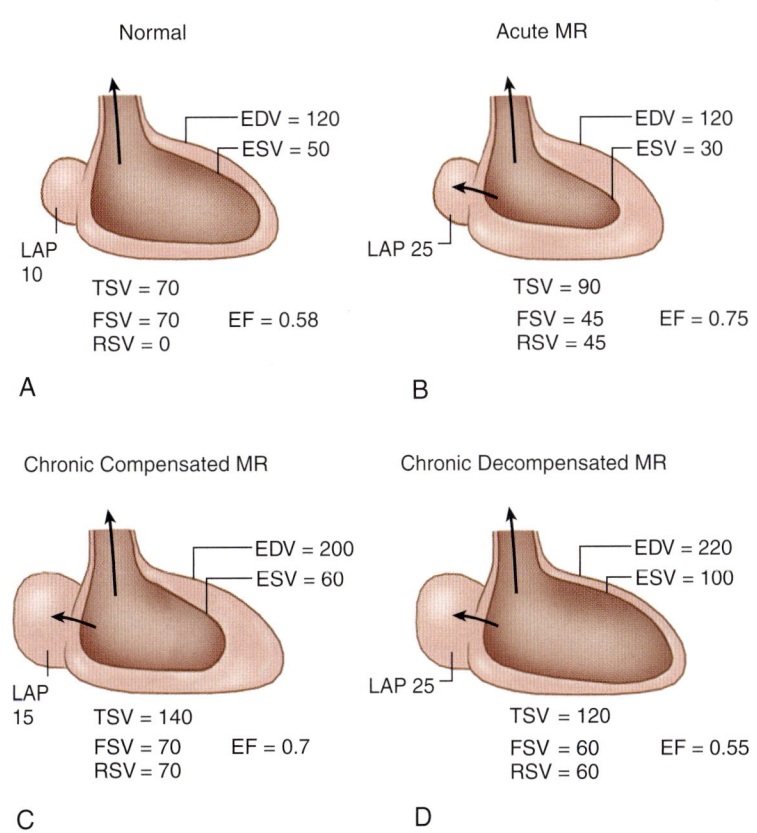

Fig. 12.34 Left ventricle response in mitral regurgitation. Three phases of mitral regurgitation *(MR)* compared with normal physiology. (A) Normal physiology. (B) In acute MR, an increase in preload and a decrease in afterload cause an increase in end-diastolic volume *(EDV)* and a decrease in end-systolic volume *(ESV)*, producing an increase in total stroke volume *(TSV)*. However, forward stroke volume *(FSV)* is diminished because 50% of the TSV regurgitates as the regurgitant stroke volume *(RSV)*, resulting in an increase in LA pressure *(LAP)*. (C) In the chronic compensated phase, eccentric hypertrophy has developed, and EDV is now increased substantially. Afterload has returned to normal as the radius term of the Laplace relationship increases with the increase in EDV. Normal muscle function and a large increase in EDV permit a substantial increase in TSV from the acute phase. This, in turn, permits a normal FSV. LA enlargement now accommodates the regurgitant volume at a lower LA pressure. Ejection fraction *(EF)* remains greater than normal. (D) In the chronic decompensated phase, muscle dysfunction has developed, impairing EF and diminishing both TSV and FSV. The EF, although still "normal," has decreased to 0.55, and LA pressure is elevated again because less volume is ejected during systole, thus causing a higher ESV. *(From Carabello BA: Progress in mitral and AR,* Curr Probl Cardiol *28:553, 2003.)*

Pulmonary artery pressure increases passively in response to both the chronic, mildly elevated LA pressure seen with chronic MR and the sudden, severe elevation seen with acute regurgitation. When LA pressure is chronically elevated, pulmonary vascular resistance increases. Echocardiographic evaluation of pulmonary artery pressures is a basic component of the exam in patients with MR (see Chapter 6).

Evaluation of Mitral Regurgitant Severity
Screening Examination

The basic screening examination for MR includes color flow imaging and CW Doppler ultrasound (Fig. 12.35). Color Doppler imaging allows the detection of the presence of MR and separates mild regurgitation from moderate to severe disease. The shape and direction of the jet are helpful in diagnosis; an eccentric jet suggests pathologic regurgitation and provides clues to the mechanism of regurgitation. Abnormalities of the posterior leaflet tend to result in an anteriorly directed jet, whereas anterior leaflet and papillary muscle dysfunction tend to result in a posteriorly directed jet. Dilation of the LV or mitral annulus results in a central, symmetric regurgitant jet. In addition to parasternal long- and short-axis views, apical four-chamber and long-axis views are useful because they are nearly orthogonal to each other. However, signal attenuation at the depth of the LA limits the utility of apical views if ultrasound penetration is suboptimal. A central jet with an area less than 4.0 cm^2 or less than 20% of the LA area in a nonoblique view is consistent with mild MR.

The CW Doppler spectral recording of MR shows a rapid increase in velocity during isovolumic

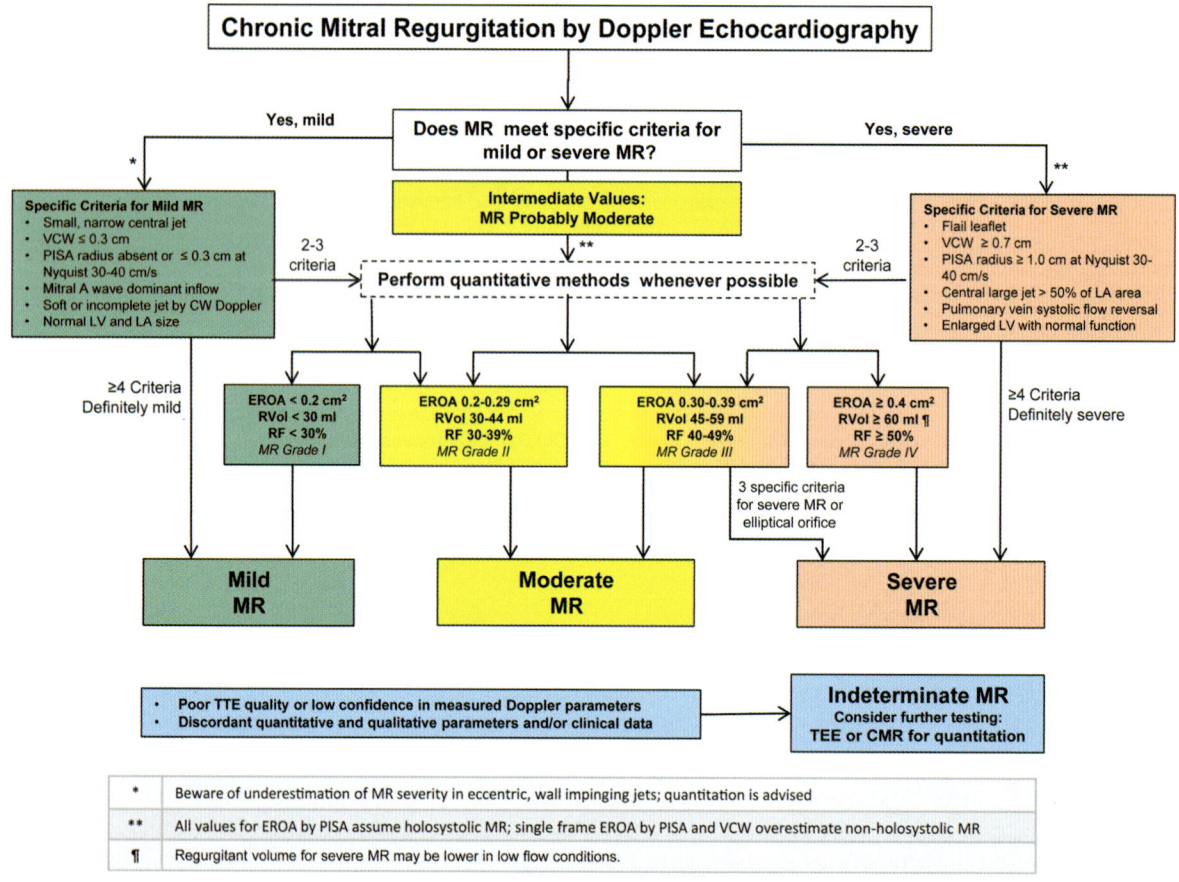

Fig. 12.35 Algorithm for the integration of multiple parameters of mitral regurgitation severity. Good-quality echocardiographic imaging and complete data acquisition are assumed. If imaging is technically difficult, consider TEE or cardiac magnetic resonance *(CMR)*. Mitral regurgitation *(MR)* severity often is indeterminate due to poor image quality, technical issues with data, internal inconsistency among echo findings, or discordance with clinical findings. *EROA*, Estimated regurgitant orifice area; *PISA*, Proximal isovelocity surface area; *RF*, regurgitant fraction; *RVol*, regurgitant volume; *VCW*, vena contracta width. (From Zoghbi WA, Adams D, Bonow RO, et al: Recommendations for noninvasive evaluation of native valvular regurgitation: a report from the American Society of Echocardiography developed in collaboration with the Society for Cardiovascular Magnetic Resonance, J Am Soc Echocardiogr 30(4):303–371, Fig. 18.)

contraction (proportional to the rate of rise in LV pressure or *dP/dt*) from baseline to a maximum velocity of 5 to 6 m/s. The velocity stays high throughout systole with a curve paralleling the rise and fall of LV pressure when LA pressure is normal. During isovolumic relaxation, the velocity rapidly returns to baseline. Signal intensity of the MR signal, in comparison with antegrade flow, is related to MR severity. In addition, significant regurgitation is associated with an increase in the antegrade velocity because of increased transmitral volume flow.

With acute MR (Table 12.6), an increase in LA pressure during late systole—a *v*-wave—usually is present because of a steep pressure-volume relationship of the nondilated LA. In this situation, the pressure gradient between the LV and LA is high initially but then begins to equalize in late systole as LA pressure rises. The corresponding Doppler velocity curve shows a high initial velocity with a more rapid fall in velocity in mid-systole to late systole. This pattern of Doppler velocities also is termed a *v*-wave (see Fig. 12.30).

Vena Contracta

Vena contracta diameter should be measured if color Doppler imaging shows an eccentric or large jet or if CW Doppler suggests more than mild MR. In patients with MR, vena contracta width is optimally visualized in a parasternal long-axis or short-axis view, although apical views may be used if parasternal images are inadequate. MR vena contracta measurements ideally are made with:

- Transthoracic parasternal or TEE 120° long-axis view
- Visualization of the narrow neck between the proximal acceleration and distal jet expansion
- Zoom mode
- Measurement perpendicular to the direction of flow

A vena contracta width greater than 0.3 cm indicates that further quantitation of regurgitant severity is needed.

TABLE 12.6 Mitral Regurgitation: Clinical Echocardiographic Correlation

	Chronic Primary MR	Chronic Secondary MR	Acute MR
Causes (examples)	• Mitral valve prolapse • Rheumatic valve disease	• Dilated cardiomyopathy • Chronic ischemic disease	• Endocarditis • Chordal rupture • Papillary muscle rupture or dysfunction
Clinical presentation and disease course	• Asymptomatic systolic murmur • Slow disease progression over many years leads to dyspnea and decreased exercise capacity.	• Systolic murmur on exam and MR on echocardiography in a patient with chronic heart failure	• New-onset heart failure • Pulmonary edema • Cardiogenic shock
LV response	• Mild LV dilation • Some develop irreversible contractile dysfunction without symptoms. • EF remains normal until late in the disease course but is not an accurate marker for myocardial dysfunction.	• LV dilation and dysfunction are due to the underlying disease process. • Evaluation of dynamic mitral valve anatomy allows diagnosis of functional MR.	• Normal LV size with normal EF • Elevated LV filling pressures • Reduced forward cardiac output
Valve anatomy	• Typical findings for mitral prolapse or other cause of MR • TEE provides improved image quality. • 3D imaging is helpful in most cases.	• Tethering of mitral leaflets • Annular dilation • Normal leaflet thickness and anatomy	• Mitral leaflet perforation or inadequate coaptation due to valve destruction • Flail chord or leaflet segment • TEE may be needed for diagnosis.
Key Doppler findings	• Vena contracta measurement • CW Doppler signal • Quantitation of regurgitant severity • Calculation of PA systolic pressure (exercise testing may be needed)	• Vena contracta measurement • CW Doppler signal • Quantitation of regurgitant severity • Calculation of PA systolic pressure	• Color Doppler with wide vena contracta • Dense CW Doppler signal with "v-wave"
Definition of severe MR	• Vena contracta width ≥0.7 cm • Regurgitant volume ≥60 mL • Regurgitant fraction ≥50% • Regurgitant orifice area ≥0.4 cm^2	• Vena contracta width ≥0.7 cm • Regurgitant volume ≥60 mL • Regurgitant fraction ≥50% • Regurgitant orifice area ≥0.4 cm^2	• Qualitative signs of severe MR are adequate for clinical decision making.
Indications for intervention with severe MR*	• Symptom onset • LVESD ≥40 mm • LVEF ≤60% • Valve repairability affects timing of intervention.	• Persistent severe MR causing symptoms despite optimal heart failure therapy	• Urgent surgical intervention usually is needed, except for some coronary disease cases where revascularization may decrease MR severity.
Options for intervention	• Surgical mitral valve repair (preferred) • Mitral valve replacement	• Medical therapy for heart failure • Cardiac resynchronization therapy • Surgical mitral valve replacement at time of other heart surgery • Transcatheter mitral clip†	• Treat underlying disease process (e.g., coronary disease, endocarditis). • Stabilize in ICU with IABP. • Urgent surgical valve repair or replacement

*Major accepted indications for intervention; guidelines should be consulted for other indications and more details.
†Investigational device in the United States.
EF, Ejection fraction; *IABP*, intra-aortic balloon pump; *ICU*, intensive care unit; *LVEF*, LV ejection fraction; *LVESD*, LV end-systolic dimension; *MR*, mitral regurgitation; *PA*, pulmonary artery.

Proximal Isovelocity Surface Area

With a central regurgitant jet, regurgitant volume and orifice area can be calculated by the PISA approach. Optimal visualization of PISA on transthoracic imaging (see Fig. 12.10) typically requires:

- Apical four-chamber or long-axis view
- Narrow sector width
- Zoom mode
- Aliasing velocity set at 30 to 40 cm/s in the direction of blood flow
- Simultaneous 2D imaging to show leaflet closure plane
- Radius measured from aliasing velocity to valve closure plane.

The PISA also can be imaged from a TEE approach or with 3D color Doppler imaging. With each of these approaches, the aliasing velocity is adjusted to 30 to 40 cm/s by shifting the color Doppler baseline to provide a clearly identified hemispherical PISA. Underestimation of regurgitation occurs if the PISA appears flattened; overestimation occurs if the PISA is oval. Instantaneous regurgitant volume flow rate is calculated as indicated in Eq. 12.4. The maximum velocity of the MR jet on CW Doppler recording is then used in Eq. 12.6 to determine regurgitant orifice area. In patients with regurgitation only in late systole, rather than holosystolic, this approach overestimates regurgitant severity (Fig. 12.36).

Evaluation of regurgitant severity is complex when multiple jets are present along the leaflet coaptation line (Fig. 12.37). The 3D visualization of vena contracta and PISA shows promise for more reliable quantitation of regurgitant severity, but this approach currently is time consuming, requires considerable experience, and is limited by low frame rates.

Regurgitation Volume and Orifice Area

The proximal isovelocity surface area approach is less accurate with eccentric jets or when the isovelocity surface area is not hemispherical. In these situations, quantitation of MR by pulsed Doppler volume flow rates is more appropriate. Regurgitant volume across the mitral valve ($RVol_{mitral}$) can be calculated from total LV stroke volume measured across the mitral valve (SV_{mitral}) minus forward stroke volume measured in the LV outflow tract (SV_{LVOT}) (Fig. 12.38):

$$RVol_{mitral} = SV_{mitral} - SV_{LVOT} \quad \text{(Eq. 12.10)}$$

Alternate sites for the measurement of forward stroke volume are the tricuspid valve and the pulmonary artery. The regurgitant orifice area then can be calculated using this regurgitant volume and the velocity-time integral of the CW Doppler MR jet (see Eq. 12.3).

Pulmonary Vein Flow Reversal

As the MR jet enters the LA, it necessarily displaces blood that was already in the chamber. When severe regurgitation is present, systolic flow reversal in the pulmonary veins is seen in some patients. On transthoracic imaging, the flow pattern in the right inferior pulmonary vein can be recorded from the apical four-chamber view in most patients, although the signal-to-noise ratio is suboptimal at this depth in some adult patients. On TEE, the flow pattern in all four pulmonary veins can be recorded, which is

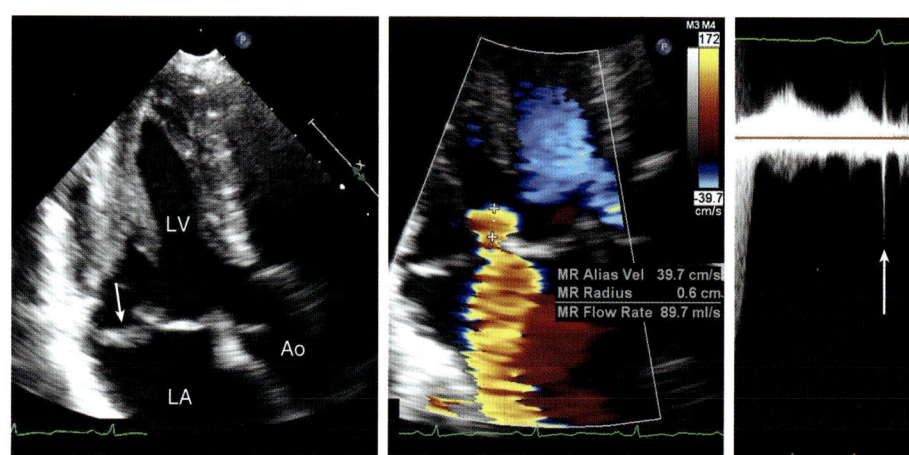

Fig. 12.36 **Late systolic mitral valve prolapse.** This young woman with posterior leaflet prolapse *(left)* has only late systolic mitral regurgitation *(MR)* when color images are viewed frame by frame. Late systolic regurgitant orifice area is calculated as 0.16 cm² from the proximal isovelocity surface area diameter (0.6 cm *cross marks in center*), aliasing velocity (40 cm/s), and maximum velocity on CW Doppler (5.4 m/s). However, this calculation overestimates regurgitant severity because regurgitation only occurs in the last half of systole, as shown by the delay between onset of systole *(arrow)* and the Doppler flow signal on the CW Doppler tracing *(right)*. Using the CW Doppler velocity-time integral, regurgitant volume is only 12 mL, and effective regurgitant orifice area averaged over systolic is even smaller than calculated. *Ao*, Aorta.

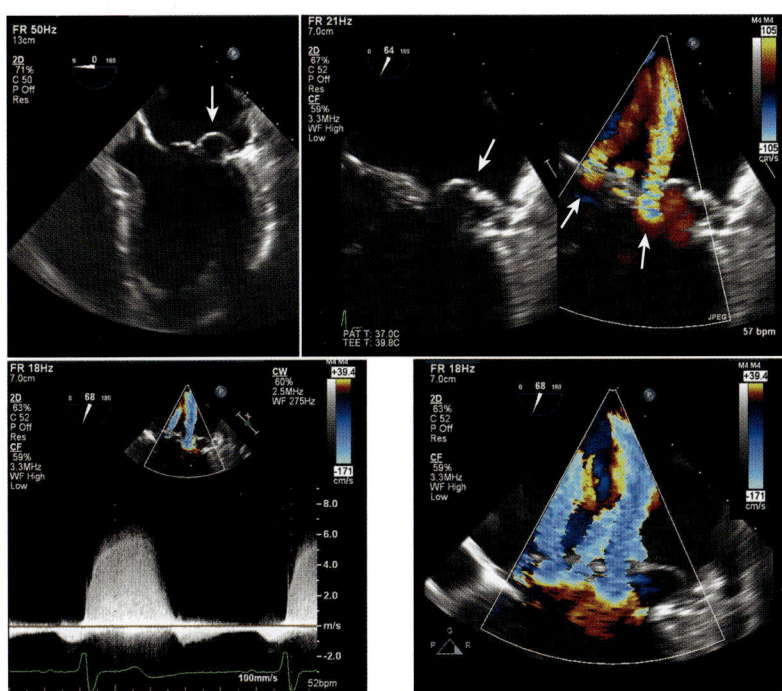

Fig. 12.37 Multiple mitral regurgitant jets on transesophageal echocardiography. In this 64-year-old man with an asymptomatic systolic murmur, TTE showed an LV end-systolic dimension of 46 mm, an ejection fraction of 53%, and moderate to severe mitral regurgitation (MR). TEE imaging shows prolapse of the P2 segment of the posterior leaflet *(arrow)* in the four-chamber view *(upper left)*. In the two-chamber plane, prolapse of P1 also is seen, and color Doppler shows three MR jets both laterally and medially *(upper right)*. The CW Doppler signal *(lower left)* and proximal isovelocity surface area (PISA) measurements *(lower right)* were used to quantitate regurgitant severity. Using the PISA from the MR jet between P1 and the anterior leaflet, effective regurgitant orifice area is calculated as 0.4 cm². Given multiple jets, overall regurgitation is even more severe.

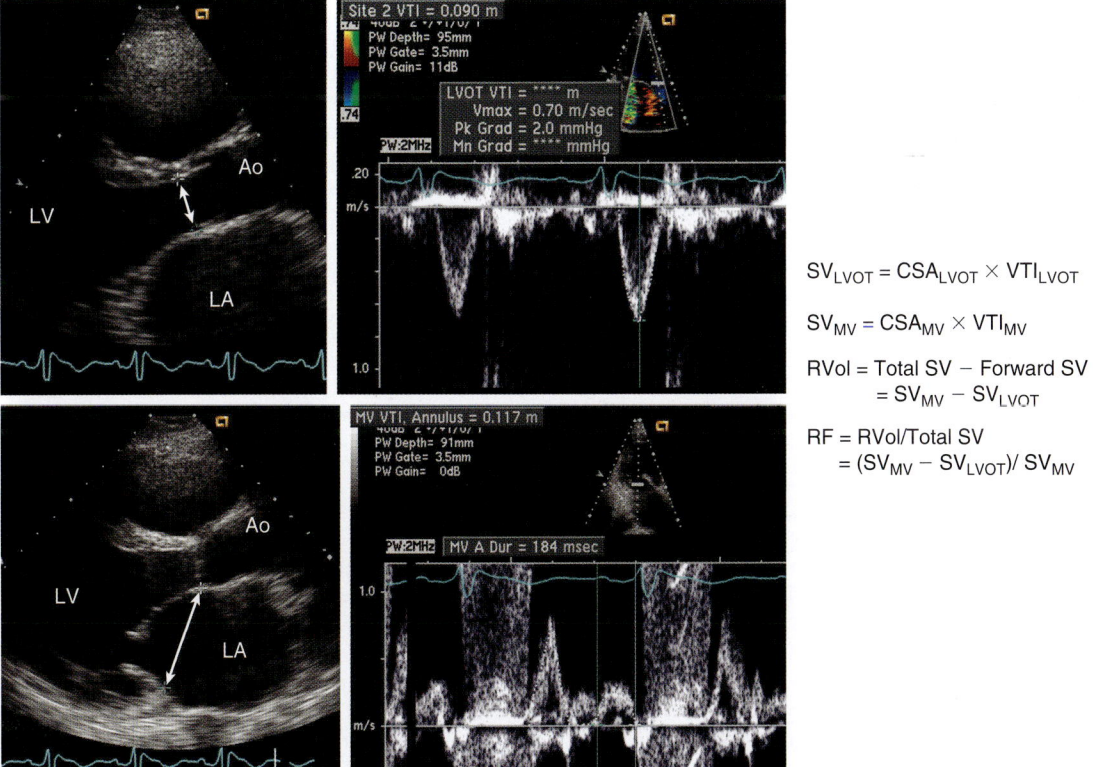

$SV_{LVOT} = CSA_{LVOT} \times VTI_{LVOT}$

$SV_{MV} = CSA_{MV} \times VTI_{MV}$

$RVol = \text{Total SV} - \text{Forward SV}$
$= SV_{MV} - SV_{LVOT}$

$RF = RVol/\text{Total SV}$
$= (SV_{MV} - SV_{LVOT})/SV_{MV}$

Fig. 12.38 Quantitative evaluation of mitral regurgitant severity by calculation of transmitral and transaortic volume flow rates. Mitral annulus diameter (4.5 cm) and the velocity-time integral *(VTI)* of flow across the mitral annulus (11.7 cm) are used to calculate total stroke volume *(SV)* at 186 mL. Forward SV is determined from the cross-sectional area *(CSA;* 2.5 cm²) and VTI integral of the LV outflow tract (LVOT) flow (10.5 cm) as 67 mL. Regurgitant volume *(RVol)* is 119 mL, and regurgitant fraction *(RF)* is 64%. *Ao,* Aorta.

particularly helpful with an eccentric regurgitant jet because the pattern of systolic flow reversal is not always uniform.

False-negative results (e.g., a normal pulmonary vein flow pattern despite severe regurgitation) occur when the LA is severely enlarged and compliant, so that all the excess volume is contained in the LA without displacement into the pulmonary veins. False-positive results (e.g., blunted or reversed systolic pulmonary vein flow when regurgitation is *not* severe) occur when an eccentric jet is directed into a pulmonary vein, thereby causing flow reversal in one vein even when regurgitation is not severe. False-positive results also are seen in patients who are not in sinus rhythm because the normal pattern of systolic atrial filling partly depends on the preceding emptying of the atrium due to atrial contraction. Other physiologic factors that affect the atrial inflow patterns include respiratory phase, cardiac rhythm, atrial and venous compliance, ventricular diastolic filling, and age. Thus, although the presence and severity of venous systolic flow reversal are useful adjuncts in the evaluation of atrioventricular valve regurgitant severity *in patients in sinus rhythm*, they certainly is not pathognomonic findings.

Clinical Utility

Diagnosis and Severity of Mitral Regurgitation

Echocardiography is the clinical standard for diagnosis and clinical decision making in patients with MR. The first step in assessment is evaluation of valve anatomy and motion, as well as LV size and systolic function, to determine the cause of regurgitation, most importantly whether valve dysfunction is due to primary leaflet disease or is secondary to LV dilation and systolic dysfunction. Disease stage then is defined based on clinical and imaging parameters for primary and secondary MR, as shown in Tables 12.7 and 12.8.

The vena contracta width indicates severe MR.

CW Doppler signal density indicates moderate-to-severe MR, and the absence of a v-wave suggests a chronic disease process. The dP/dt is <1000 mmHg/s, consistent with decreased LV contractility.

Color flow indicates a central jet, so the proximal isovelocity surface area (PISA) method can be used to quantitate regurgitant severity.

The PISA is calculated from the radius (r) measurement as:

$$PISA = 2\pi r^2 = 2\pi(1.0\ cm)^2 = 6.3\ cm^2$$

The maximum instantaneous regurgitant flow rate (R_{FR}) is calculated from PISA and the aliasing velocity ($V_{aliasing}$) as:

$$R_{FR} = PISA \times V_{aliasing} = 6.3\ cm \times 30\ cm/s = 189\ cm^3/s$$

Maximum regurgitant orifice area (instantaneous) then is calculated from the R_{FR} and MR jet velocity (where 4.6 m/s = 460 cm/s):

$$ROA_{max} = R_{FR}/V_{MR} = (189\ cm^3/s)/460\ cm/s = 041\ cm^2$$

Regurgitant volume over the systolic flow period can be estimated as:

$$RVol = ROA \times VTI_{MR}$$
$$= 0.41\ cm^2 \times 130\ cm = 53\ cm^3\ or\ mL$$

This ROA and regurgitant volume is consistent with moderate MR.

If the jet is eccentric, quantitation may be performed using transaortic (forward) stroke volume and transmitral (total) stroke volume calculations, as illustrated for AR.

Clinical Follow-Up and Timing of Intervention

Sequential echocardiographic studies can be used to follow asymptomatic patients with MR. Although regurgitation severity and valve anatomy provide the impetus for follow-up, the most important variables on serial studies are LV size and systolic function. Current data suggest that, in adults with *severe primary* MR, evidence of progressive ventricular dilation, an end-systolic dimension 40 mm or greater, or any reduction in LV systolic function (ejection fraction 60% or less) should prompt consideration of surgical intervention, regardless of the symptomatic status of the patient, to prevent irreversible ventricular dysfunction postoperatively.

ECHO MATH: Mitral Regurgitation Severity

Example

A 52-year-old man with dilated cardiomyopathy presents with worsening heart failure symptoms. Echocardiography shows a dilated LV with an ejection fraction of 32% and a central jet of MR with:

Vena contracta width	8 mm
CW Doppler	MR signal as dense as antegrade flow with no evidence for a v-wave
	dP/dt = 840 mmHg/s
	V_{MR} = 4.6 m/s
	VTI_{MR} = 130 cm
PISA radius	1.2 cm
Aliasing velocity	30 cm/s
Right superior pulmonary vein	Systolic flow reversal

TABLE 12.7 Stages of *Primary* Mitral Regurgitaion

Grade	Definition	Valve Anatomy	Valve Hemodynamics*	Hemodynamic Consequences	Symptoms
A	At risk of MR	• Mild mitral valve prolapse with normal coaptation • Mild valve thickening and leaflet restriction	• No MR jet or small central jet area <20% LA on Doppler • Small vena contracta <0.3 cm	• None	• None
B	Progressive MR	• Severe mitral valve prolapse with normal coaptation • Rheumatic valve changes with leaflet restriction and loss of central coaptation • Prior IE	• Central jet MR 20%–40% LA or late systolic eccentric jet MR • Vena contracta <0.7 cm • Regurgitant volume <60 mL • Regurgitant fraction <50% • ERO <0.40 cm^2 • Angiographic grade 1–2+	• Mild LA enlargement • No LV enlargement • Normal pulmonary pressure	• None
C	Asymptomatic severe MR	• Severe mitral valve prolapse with loss of coaptation or flail leaflet • Rheumatic valve changes with leaflet restriction and loss of central coaptation • Prior IE • Thickening of leaflets with radiation heart disease	• Central jet MR >40% LA or holosystolic eccentric jet MR • Vena contracta ≥0.7 cm • Regurgitant volume ≥60 mL • Regurgitant fraction ≥50% • ERO ≥0.40 cm^2 • Angiographic grade 3–4+	• Moderate or severe LA enlargement • LV enlargement • Pulmonary hypertension may be present at rest or with exercise • **C1:** LVEF >60% and LVESD <40 mm • **C2:** LVEF ≤60% and LVESD ≥40 mm	• None
D	Symptomatic severe MR	• Severe mitral valve prolapse with loss of coaptation or flail leaflet • Rheumatic valve changes with leaflet restriction and loss of central coaptation • Prior IE • Thickening of leaflets with radiation heart disease	• Central jet MR >40% LA or holosystolic eccentric jet MR • Vena contracta ≥0.7 cm • Regurgitant volume ≥60 mL • Regurgitant fraction ≥50% • ERO ≥0.40 cm^2 • Angiographic grade 3–4+	• Moderate or severe LA enlargement • LV enlargement • Pulmonary hypertension present	• Decreased exercise tolerance • Exertional dyspnea

*Several valve hemodynamic criteria are provided for assessment of MR severity, but not all criteria for each category will be present in each patient. Categorization of MR severity as mild, moderate, or severe depends on data quality and integration of these parameters in conjunction with other clinical evidence.
ERO, Effective regurgitant orifice; *IE*, infective endocarditis; *LVEF*, LV ejection fraction; *LVESD*, LV end-systolic dimension; *MR*, mitral regurgitation.
From Nishimura RA, Otto CM, Bonow RO, et al: AHA/ACC guideline for the management of patients with valvular heart disease: executive summary. A report of the American College of Cardiology/American Heart Association Task Force on Practice Guidelines. *Circulation* 129(23):2440–2492, 2014.

TABLE 12.8 Stages of *Secondary* Mitral Regurgitation

Grade	Definition	Valve Anatomy	Valve Hemodynamics*	Associated Cardiac Findings	Symptoms
A	At risk of MR	• Normal valve leaflets, chords, and annulus in a patient with coronary disease or cardiomyopathy	• No MR jet or small central jet area <20% LA on Doppler • Small vena contracta <0.30 cm	• Normal or mildly dilated LV size with fixed (infarction) or inducible (ischemia) regional wall motion abnormalities • Primary myocardial disease with LV dilation and systolic dysfunction	• Symptoms due to coronary ischemia or HF may be present that respond to revascularization and appropriate medical therapy
B	Progressive MR	• Regional wall motion abnormalities with mild tethering of mitral leaflet • Annular dilation with mild loss of central coaptation of the mitral leaflets	• ERO <0.40 cm²† • Regurgitant volume <60 mL • Regurgitant fraction <50%	• Regional wall motion abnormalities with reduced LV systolic function • LV dilation and systolic dysfunction due to primary myocardial disease	• Symptoms due to coronary ischemia or HF may be present that respond to revascularization and appropriate medical therapy
C	Asymptomatic severe MR	• Regional wall motion abnormalities and/or LV dilation with severe tethering of mitral leaflet • Annular dilation with severe loss of central coaptation of the mitral leaflets	• ERO ≥0.40 cm²† • Regurgitant volume ≥60 mL • Regurgitant fraction ≥50%	• Regional wall motion abnormalities with reduced LV systolic function • LV dilation and systolic dysfunction due to primary myocardial disease	• Symptoms due to coronary ischemia or HF may be present that respond to revascularization and appropriate medical therapy
D	Symptomatic severe MR	• Regional wall motion abnormalities and/or LV dilation with severe tethering of mitral leaflet • Annular dilation with severe loss of central coaptation of the mitral leaflets	• ERO ≥0.40 cm²† • Regurgitant volume ≥60 mL • Regurgitant fraction ≥50%	• Regional wall motion abnormalities with reduced LV systolic function • LV dilation and systolic dysfunction due to primary myocardial disease	• HF symptoms due to MR persist even after revascularization and optimization of medical therapy • Decreased exercise tolerance • Exertional dyspnea

*Several valve hemodynamic criteria are provided for assessment of MR severity, but not all criteria for each category will be present in each patient. Categorization of MR severity as mild, moderate, or severe depends on data quality and integration of these parameters in conjunction with other clinical evidence.
†The measurement of the proximal isovelocity surface area by 2D TTE in patients with secondary MR underestimates the true ERO due to the crescentic shape of the proximal convergence.
ERO, Effective regurgitant orifice; *HF*, heart failure; *MR*, mitral regurgitation.
From Nishimura RA, Otto CM, Bonow RO, et al: 2017 AHA/ACC focused update of the 2014 AHA/ACC guideline for the management of patients with valvular heart disease: a report of the American College of Cardiology/American Heart Association Task Force on Clinical Practice Guidelines, *Circulation* 135(25):e.1159–e.1195, 2017.

Decision Making Concerning Type of Intervention

Once the decision has been made that relief of MR is needed, the echocardiographic images are invaluable in considering whether mitral valve repair or reconstruction is possible or whether valve anatomy is amenable to a transcatheter procedure. 3D TEE imaging is essential for complete visualization of valve anatomy and measurements specific to each procedure (see Chapter 18). Before any procedure, images are reviewed with the heart valve team, including the surgeon and interventional cardiologist, focusing on the exact cause of MR, the degree of annular dilation, the relative involvement of anterior and posterior leaflets, the chordal and papillary muscle structural integrity, and overall ventricular size and systolic function. Typically, posterior leaflet prolapse and annular dilation are most amenable to surgical repair, whereas more complex or extensive disease requires more complex procedures with a lower likelihood of successful repair. Intraprocedural monitoring for surgical or transcatheter mitral valve procedures is discussed in Chapter 18.

TRICUSPID REGURGITATION

Diagnostic Imaging of the Tricuspid Valve Apparatus

Tricuspid regurgitation occurs with abnormalities of the supporting structures (annulus, RV) or the leaflets themselves. Tricuspid regurgitation secondary to *annular dilation* often is due either to primary RV dilation and systolic dysfunction or to *pulmonary hypertension*. Left-sided heart disease leading to pulmonary hypertension—especially mitral stenosis or regurgitation—often results in significant tricuspid regurgitation, presumably based on RV dilation and systolic dysfunction.

Abnormalities of the tricuspid valve leaflets also are a cause of tricuspid regurgitation. *Rheumatic disease* involves the tricuspid valve in approximately 20% to 30% of cases, nearly always occurring in conjunction with mitral and aortic valve involvement. Rheumatic tricuspid disease typically is mild and is difficult to appreciate on 2D echocardiography unless careful attention is directed toward imaging the valve leaflets and searching for evidence of commissural fusion. Rheumatic tricuspid regurgitation is more common than rheumatic tricuspid stenosis.

Carcinoid heart disease is a rare condition, but the echocardiographic findings are pathognomonic. Carcinoid heart disease (seen with metastatic carcinoid tumor to the liver) is characterized by thickened, shortened, and immobile tricuspid valve leaflets with resultant tricuspid regurgitation or, less often, tricuspid valve stenosis (see Fig. 15.10). The pulmonic valve also may be involved. *Endocarditis* may involve the tricuspid valve, which results in tricuspid regurgitation, and is most common in patients with a history of intravenous drug abuse.

Ebstein anomaly of the tricuspid valve is a congenital abnormality in which one or more leaflets of the tricuspid valve are displaced from the tricuspid annulus toward the ventricular apex (see Figs. 17.9 and 17.10). Most often, the septal leaflet is involved, either in isolation or in association with apical displacement of posterior and anterior leaflets. The degree of apical displacement is extremely variable. Although the normal tricuspid valve insertion plane is slightly more apical than the mitral valve attachment plane, Ebstein anomaly should be considered when the separation between mitral and tricuspid valve planes is greater than 1 cm. The portion of the RV excluded from the pumping chamber is said to be *atrialized* because it effectively functions as part of the RA. The RA appears severely enlarged because of "atrialization" of the base of the ventricle *plus* dilatation of the atrium as a result of tricuspid regurgitation. RV enlargement is also seen if significant tricuspid regurgitation is present.

Right Ventricular and Right Atrial Dilation

Hemodynamically significant tricuspid regurgitation results in progressive RV and RA enlargement due to volume overload. This dilation complicates an assessment of the cause of regurgitation because the dilation itself further increases regurgitant severity.

RV volume overload is associated with a pattern of abnormal septal motion characterized on M-mode recording by posterior motion of the septum in diastole (because RV filling exceeds LV filling) and anterior motion of the septum in systole, often referred to as *paradoxical septal motion*. On 2D short-axis imaging, the ventricular septum appears "flattened" in diastole as the increased transtricuspid stroke volume fills the RV. In systole, the ventricular septum moves toward the center of gravity of the heart (normally toward the middle of the LV), which is the midline of the RV if severe RV dilation is present.

The differential diagnosis of RV dilation and paradoxical septal motion includes other causes of RV volume overload, such as an atrial septal defect or a partial anomalous pulmonary venous return; RV dilation also is due to pressure overload resulting from pulmonic valve disease or to pulmonary hypertension caused by either left-sided heart disease or intrinsic lung disease.

Evaluation of Tricuspid Regurgitation Severity

Tricuspid regurgitation is best evaluated by integrating multiple parameters (Fig. 12.39):

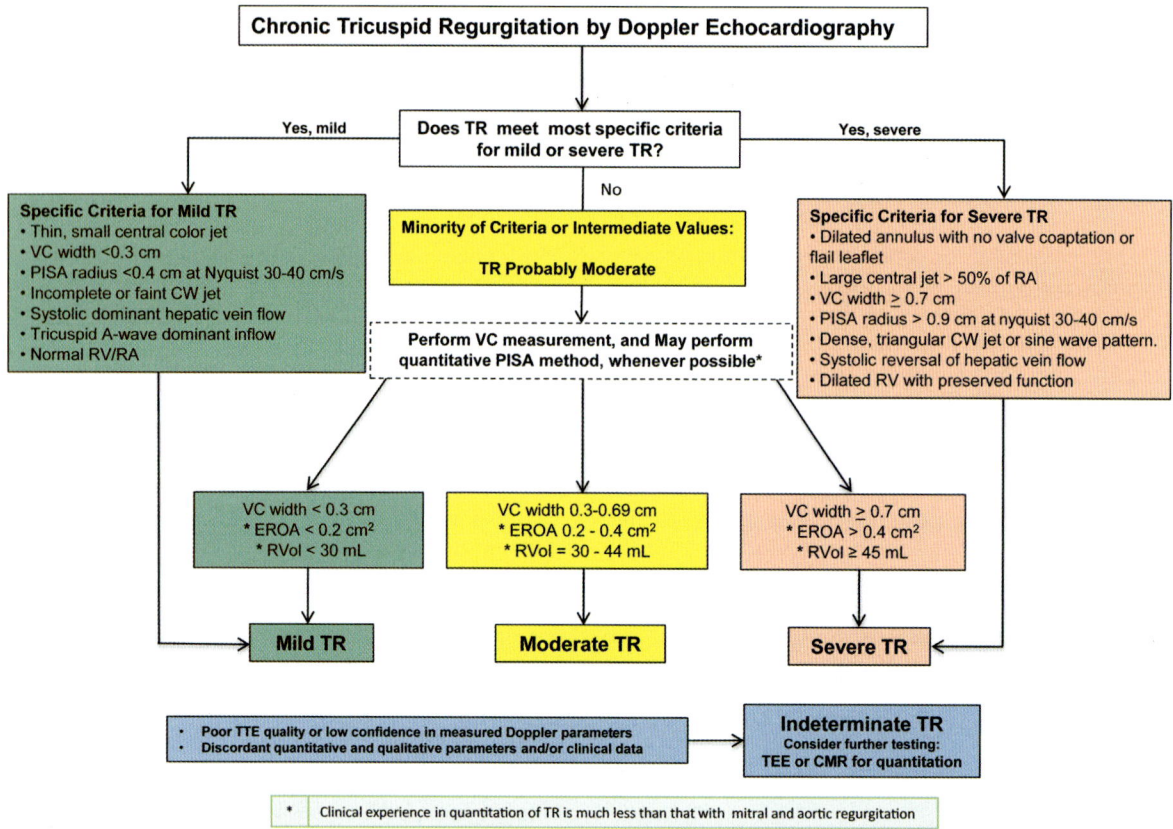

Fig. 12.39 **Algorithm for the integration of multiple parameters of tricuspid regurgitation severity.** Good-quality echocardiographic imaging and complete data acquisition are assumed. If imaging is technically difficult, consider TEE or cardiac magnetic resonance (*CMR*). Tricuspid regurgitation (*TR*) severity often is indeterminate due to poor image quality, technical issues with data, internal inconsistency among echo findings, or discordance with clinical findings. *EROA*, Estimated regurgitant orifice area; *PISA*, proximal isovelocity surface area; *RF*, regurgitant fraction; *RVol*, regurgitant volume; *VC*, vena contracta. (From Zoghbi WA, Adams D, Bonow RO, et al: Recommendations for noninvasive evaluation of native valvular regurgitation: a report from the American Society of Echocardiography developed in collaboration with the Society for Cardiovascular Magnetic Resonance, J Am Soc Echocardiogr, 30(4):303–371, Fig. 31.)

- Color Doppler with a thin small jet indicates mild tricuspid regurgitation versus a large central jet filling >50% of the RA, which indicates severe tricuspid regurgitation.
- Vena contracta width <0.3 cm indicates mild tricuspid regurgitation versus ≥0.7 cm indicates severe tricuspid regurgitation.
- CW Doppler shows an incomplete or faint signal with mild tricuspid regurgitation but a dense triangular signal with severe tricuspid regurgitation.
- PISA radius <0.4 cm is seen with mild tricuspid regurgitation versus >0.9 cm with severe tricuspid regurgitation at a color Doppler Nyquist limit of 30–40 cm/s.
- Hepatic vein flow in systole is normal with mild tricuspid regurgitation but reversed with severe tricuspid regurgitation.

Useful views for evaluating tricuspid regurgitation include a parasternal short-axis view, the RV inflow view, and the apical four-chamber view. Mild to moderate tricuspid regurgitation often is directed along the interatrial septum and must be distinguished from normal caval inflow or from atrial septal defect flow. If needed for clinical decision making, regurgitant volume and orifice area can be calculated by the proximal isovelocity surface area or pulsed Doppler methods.

Severe tricuspid regurgitation results in systolic flow reversal in the inferior and superior vena cavae, analogous to the physical finding of a systolic pulsation in the neck veins. Inferior vena caval flow is best recorded in the central hepatic vein, which provides a flow channel with no venous valves between the recording site and the RA and a parallel intercept angle to the ultrasound beam from the subcostal approach (see Fig. 12.14). As with pulmonary vein flow reversal for severe MR, hepatic vein systolic flow reversal is specific for severe tricuspid regurgitation *only when sinus rhythm is present*. Normal systolic filling of the RA partly depends on the preceding phase of emptying with atrial contraction, so loss of atrial contraction affects the pattern of flow in systole.

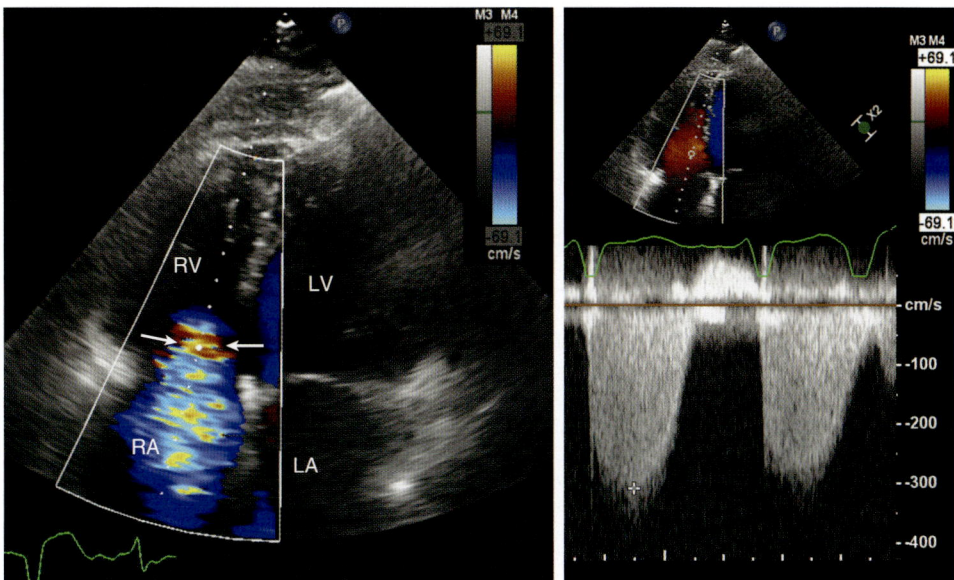

Fig. 12.40 Severe tricuspid regurgitation with high right ventricular systolic pressure. In a patient with a dilated cardiomyopathy and moderate pulmonary hypertension, color Doppler flow imaging *(left)* shows tricuspid regurgitation due to annular dilation with a vena contracta of 8 mm *(arrows)*. CW Doppler *(right)* shows a dense signal with a peak velocity about 3 m/s, indicating an RA to RV systolic pressure difference of 36 mmHg.

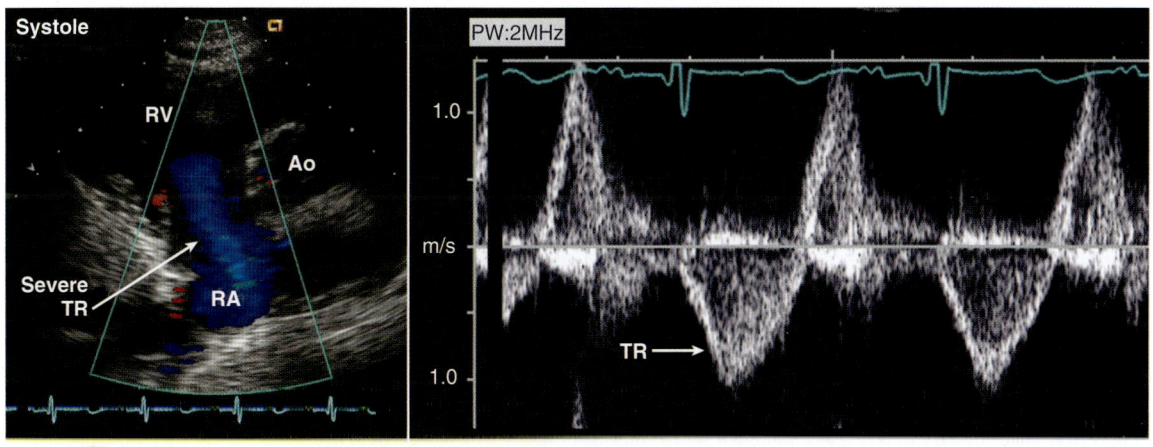

Fig. 12.41 Severe tricuspid regurgitation with low right ventricular systolic pressure. Severe tricuspid regurgitation *(TR)* with normal RV and pulmonary systolic pressures is characterized by low velocity laminar flow on color flow imaging *(left)* and on pulsed Doppler *(right)*. Velocities are low because little pressure difference exists between the RA and RV in systole. *Ao,* Aorta.

The maximum velocity of the tricuspid regurgitant jet reflects the maximum pressure difference across the tricuspid valve and *not* the severity of regurgitation. Severe regurgitation with a normal RV systolic pressure (as seen with tricuspid valve endocarditis) has a low maximum velocity (Figs. 12.40 and 12.41). Mild tricuspid regurgitation in the presence of pulmonary hypertension (as seen with primary pulmonary hypertension) has a high maximum velocity. However, the *intensity* of the CW signals relative to the antegrade flow signal intensity does relate to regurgitant severity. In addition, the shape of the velocity-time curve indicates the time course of the instantaneous pressure differences across the valve; an RA *v*-wave seen in acute regurgitation results in a more rapid decline in velocity in late systole similar to that seen in acute MR.

Clinical Utility

Doppler echocardiography is the standard clinical approach for the evaluation of tricuspid regurgitation. Evaluation of tricuspid regurgitant severity is particularly important in the patient undergoing mitral valve surgery (Table 12.9). Many of these patients have significant coexisting tricuspid regurgitation, and clinical symptoms often persist postoperatively if this condition is not recognized and treated (with tricuspid annuloplasty) at the time of surgery.

TABLE 12.9 Stages of Tricuspid Regurgitation

Stage	Definition	Primary TR Valve Anatomy	Secondary TR	Valve Hemodynamics*	Hemodynamic Consequences
A	At risk of TR	• Mild rheumatic change • Mild prolapse • Other (e.g., IE with vegetation, early carcinoid deposition, radiation) • Intra-annular RV pacemaker or ICD lead • After cardiac transplantation (biopsy related)	• Normal • Early annular dilation	• No or trace TR	• None
B	Progressive TR	• Progressive leaflet deterioration/destruction • Moderate to severe prolapse, limited chordal rupture	• Early annular dilation • Moderate leaflet tethering	• Central jet area <5.0 cm² (mild) or 5–10 cm² (moderate) • Vena contracta <0.70 cm • CW jet density and contour: soft and parabolic • Hepatic vein flow: systolic dominance (mild) or blunted (moderate)	• No RV enlargement • No or mild RA enlargement • No or mild IVC enlargement with normal respirophasic variation • Normal RA pressure
C	Asymptomatic, severe TR	• Flail or anatomically abnormal leaflets	• Severe annular dilation (>40 mm or 21 mm/m²) • Marked leaflet tethering	• Central jet area >10.0 cm² • Vena contracta width >0.7 cm • CW jet density and contour: dense, triangular with early peak • Hepatic vein flow: systolic reversal	• RV, RA, IVC dilated with decreased IVC respirophasic variation • Elevated RA pressure with "c-V" wave • Diastolic interventricular septal flattening may be present.
D	Symptomatic severe TR	• Flail or anatomically abnormal leaflets	• Severe annular dilation (>40 mm or >21 mm/m²) • Marked leaflet tethering	• Central jet area >10.0 cm² • Vena contracta width >0.70 cm • CW jet density and contour: dense, triangular with early peak • Hepatic vein flow: systolic reversal	• RV, RA, IVC dilated with decreased IVC respirophasic variation • Elevated RA pressure with "c-V" wave • Diastolic interventricular septal flattening • Reduced RV systolic function in late phase

*Several valve hemodynamic criteria are provided for assessment of severity of TR, but not all criteria for each category will necessarily be present in every patient. Categorization of severity of TR as mild, moderate, or severe also depends on image quality and integration of these parameters with clinical findings.
ICD, Implantable cardioverter-defibrillator; *IE*, infective endocarditis; *IVC*, inferior vena cava; *TR*, tricuspid regurgitation.
Modified from Nishimura RA, Otto CM, Bonow RO, et al: AHA/ACC guideline for the management of patients with valvular heart disease: executive summary. A report of the American College of Cardiology/American Heart Association Task Force on Practice Guidelines, *Circulation* 129(23):2440–2492, 2014.

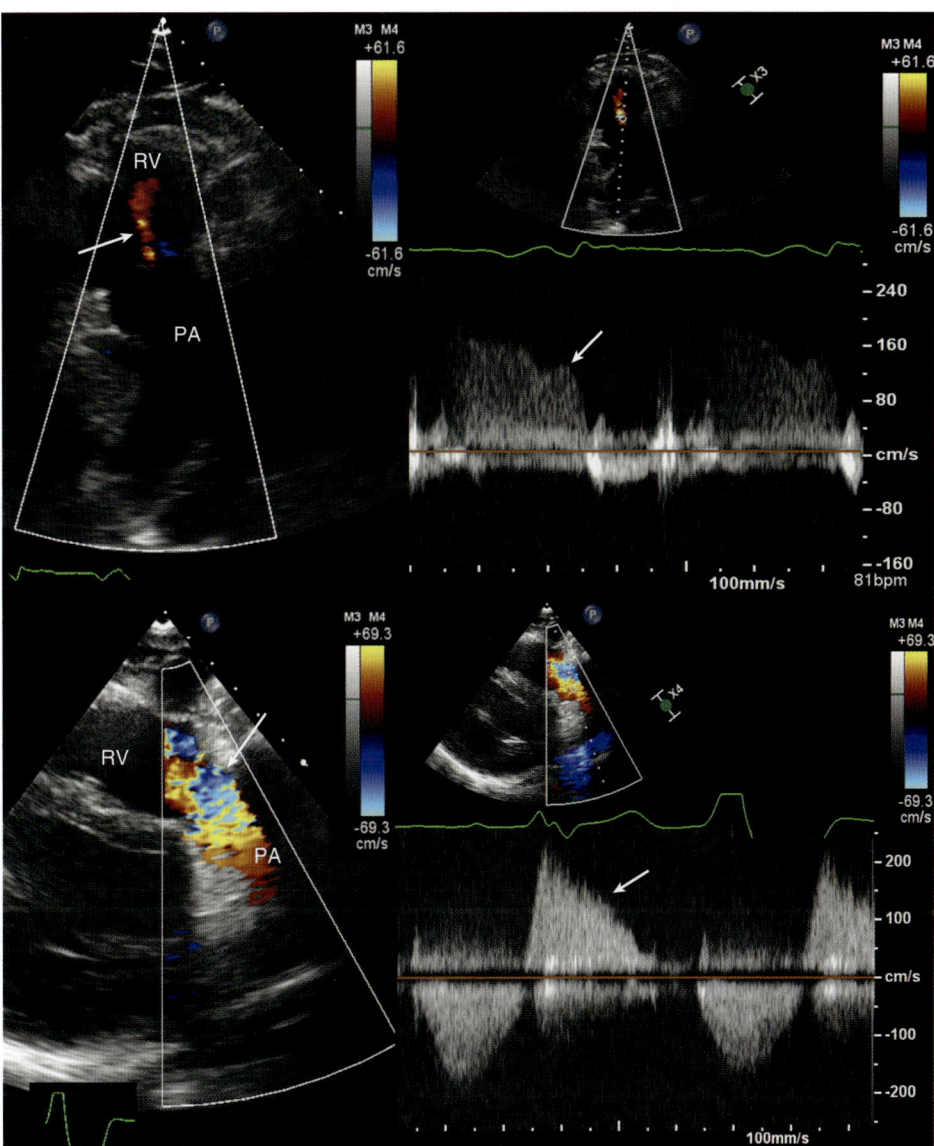

Fig. 12.42 **Mild versus severe pulmonic valve regurgitation.** Color Doppler flow imaging in an RV outflow view *(left)* show a small narrow jet of mild pulmonic regurgitation *(top left)* ▶ compared with a wide jet that fills the RV outflow tract with severe regurgitation *(bottom left)* ▶. With mild regurgitation, the pulsed Doppler velocity curve *(upper right)* shows a faint diastolic signal with a flat deceleration slope with an end-diastolic velocity *(arrow)* only slightly less than in early diastole *(arrow)*. With severe pulmonic regurgitation *(lower right)*, the diastolic flow curve is equal in density to antegrade flow with a steep deceleration slope *(arrow)* reaching the baseline before end-diastole. *PA,* Pulmonary artery.

In patients undergoing tricuspid valve repair or surgery for endocarditis, intraoperative TEE can be used to optimize the surgical approach and assess the functional consequences of the repair procedure.

PULMONIC REGURGITATION

Pulmonic regurgitation most often is an incidental benign finding, with a small amount of diastolic backflow across the pulmonic valve seen in most normal individuals (Fig. 12.42). Pathologic pulmonic regurgitation usually is a result of congenital pulmonic valve disease, either untreated mild disease or residual regurgitation after pulmonic valve surgery. The most common cause of significant pulmonic regurgitation in adults is previous surgery for tetralogy of Fallot. Acquired pulmonic regurgitation is rare and is the result of endocarditis, carcinoid syndrome, or myxomatous valve disease.

Evaluation of pulmonic valve anatomy is limited in adult patients by poor acoustic access. With congenital disease, thickened, deformed leaflets are seen. In endocarditis, a valvular vegetation may be identified, although the pulmonic valve is involved least often. Carcinoid syndrome results in shortening

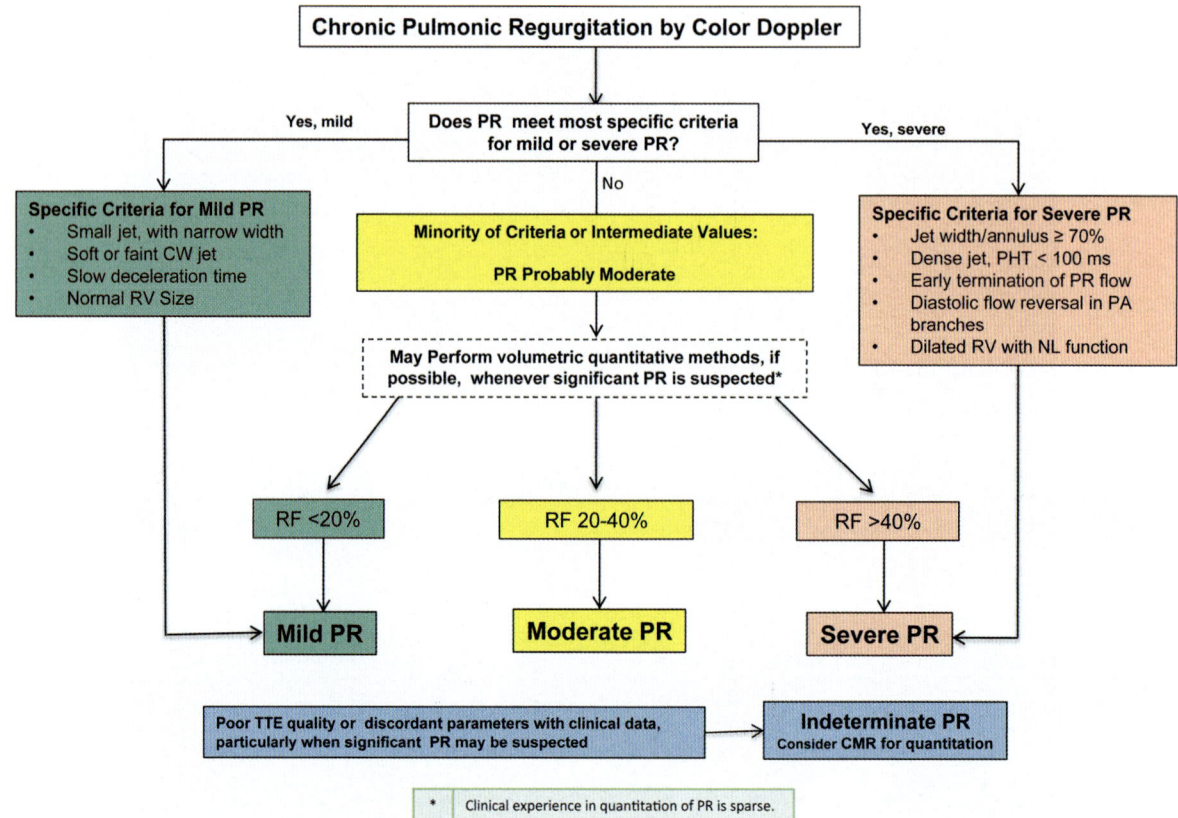

Fig. 12.43 **Algorithm for the integration of multiple parameters of pulmonic regurgitation severity.** Good-quality echocardiographic imaging and complete data acquisition are assumed. If imaging is technically difficult, consider cardiac magnetic resonance *(CMR)* or TEE. Pulmonic regurgitation *(PR)* severity often is indeterminate due to poor image quality, technical issues with data, internal inconsistency among echo findings, or discordance with clinical findings. *NL,* Normal; *PA,* pulmonary artery; *PHT,* pressure half-time; *RF,* regurgitant fraction. (From Zoghbi WA, Adams D, Bonow RO, et al: Recommendations for noninvasive evaluation of native valvular regurgitation: a report from the American Society of Echocardiography developed in collaboration with the Society for Cardiovascular Magnetic Resonance, J Am Soc Echocardiogr 30(4):303–371, Fig. 35.)

and thickening of the pulmonic valve leaflet, similar to the involvement of the tricuspid valve, leading to stenosis, regurgitation, or both. Myxomatous valve disease is rare, resulting in thickening, redundancy, and systemic sagging of the pulmonic valve leaflets.

Mild pulmonic regurgitation is characterized by a narrow jet on color Doppler imaging. The CW Doppler signal is much less dense than the antegrade flow signal, and the diastolic slope is relatively flat. Severe pulmonic regurgitation shows a wide color jet (at least 70% of outflow tract width); the CW Doppler signal is almost equal in density to antegrade flow with a steep diastolic deceleration, often reaching the zero baseline before the end of diastole (Fig. 12.43). The color Doppler signal with severe pulmonic regurgitation often shows a uniform color (without variance) because the velocity of regurgitation is low and less than the Nyquist limit. Holodiastolic flow reversal is present in the main pulmonary artery when significant regurgitation is present and must be distinguished from diastolic flow reversal due to a patent ductus arteriosus.

In adults, evaluation of pulmonic regurgitation is of most importance in patients with uncorrected or residual congenital heart disease (see Fig. 17.29). In these patients, the severity of pulmonic regurgitation is a factor in deciding whether to perform further surgical procedures and in the specific design of the surgical procedure.

The velocity in the pulmonic regurgitant curve reflects the pulmonary artery to RV diastolic pressure difference. The instantaneous end-diastolic pulmonary artery to RV gradient (calculated as $4v^2$) can be added to an estimate of RV diastolic pressure (from inferior vena cava size and respiratory variation) to provide an estimate of diastolic pulmonary artery pressure. This approach to the estimation of pulmonary artery pressure complements systolic pressure estimation from the tricuspid regurgitant jet and serves as an internal validity check when both can be recorded accurately.

THE ECHO EXAM: VALVE REGURGITATION

Aortic Regurgitation: Echo Approach

Parameter	Key Measures	Clinical Decision Thresholds
Cause	Valve abnormality Dilated aorta	
Severity of regurgitation	Vena contracta width Descending aorta holosystolic flow reversal CW Doppler deceleration slope Calculation of RVol, RF, and ROA	>0.6 cm PHT <200 ms RVol ≥60 mL RF ≥50% ROA ≥0.3 cm^2
Coexisting aortic stenosis	Aortic jet velocity	
LV response	LV dimensions or volumes LV ejection fraction dP/dt	LVESD >50 mm LVEF <50%
Other findings	Dilation of sinuses or ascending aorta Aortic coarctation (with bicuspid valve)	>45, 50, or 55 mm depending on specific diagnosis (see Chapter 16)

LVEF, LV ejection fraction; *LVESD*, LV end-systolic dimension; *PHT*, pressure half-time; *RF*, regurgitant fraction; *ROA*, regurgitant orifice area; *RVol*, regurgitant volume.

Quantitation of Aortic Regurgitation Severity

Parameter	Modality	View	Recording	Measurements and Calculations
Vena contracta width	Color flow imaging	Parasternal long-axis	Angulate, decrease depth, narrow sector, zoom.	Narrowest segment of regurgitant jet between proximal flow convergence and distal jet expansion
Descending aortic diastolic flow reversal	Pulsed Doppler	Subcostal and SSN	Sample volume 2–3 mm; decrease wall filters, adjust scale.	Evidence for holodiastolic flow reversal
CW Doppler signal (intensity, slope, VTI)	CW Doppler	Apical	Careful positioning and transducer angulation to obtain clear signal	Compare signal intensity of retrograde flow with antegrade flow, measure slope along edge of dense signal.
Volume flow at 2 sites (RVol, RF, ROA)	2D and pulsed Doppler	Parasternal (2D) and apical	LVOT diameter and VTI Mitral annulus diameter and VTI	TSV = SV$_{LVOT}$ = (CSA$_{LVOT}$ × VTI$_{LVOT}$) FSV = SV$_{MA}$ = (CSA$_{MA}$ × VTI$_{MA}$) RVol = TSV − FSV ROA = RSV / VTI$_{AR}$

AR, Aortic regurgitation; *CSA*, cross-sectional area; *FSV*, forward stroke volume; *LVOT*, LV outflow tract; *MA*, mitral annulus; *RF*, regurgitant fraction; *ROA*, regurgitant orifice area; *RSV*, regurgitant stroke volume; *SSN*, suprasternal notch; *RVol*, regurgitant volume; *SV*, stroke volume; *TSV*, total stroke volume; *VTI*, velocity-time integral.

Mitral Regurgitation: Echo Approach

Parameter	Key Measures	Clinical Decision Thresholds
Cause	Primary valve disease Secondary (functional)	
Severity of regurgitation	Vena contracta width Jet direction (central, eccentric) CW Doppler signal Calculation of RVol, RF, and ROA Pulmonary vein flow reversal	≥0.7 cm ROA ≥0.4 cm^2 RVol ≥60 mL RF ≥50%
LV response	LV dimensions or volumes LV ejection fraction dP/dt	LVESD ≥40 mm LVEF ≤60%
Pulmonary vasculature	Pulmonary systolic pressure RV size and systolic function	
Other findings	LA size	

LVEF, LV ejection fraction; *LVESD*, LV end-systolic dimension; *RF*, regurgitant fraction; *ROA*, regurgitant orifice area; *RVol*, regurgitant volume.

Quantitation of Mitral Regurgitation Severity

Parameter	Modality	View(s)	Recording	Measurements and Calculations
Vena contracta width	Color flow imaging	Parasternal long-axis	Angulate, decrease depth, narrow sector, zoom.	Narrowest segment proximal flow convergence and distal jet expansion
Color flow imaging	Color flow imaging	Parasternal and apical	Narrow sector; decrease depth.	Central vs. eccentric, anterior vs. posterior
CW Doppler signal	CW Doppler	Apical	Careful positioning and transducer angulation to obtain clear signal	Compare signal intensity of retrograde with antegrade flow.
Proximal isovelocity surface area	Color flow imaging	Apical 4-chamber or apical long-axis	Decrease depth, narrow sector, zoom, adjust aliasing velocity. Adjust aliasing velocity so PISA is hemispherical.	PISA= $2\pi r^2$ R_{FR} = PISA × $V_{aliasing}$ ROA_{max} = R_{FR} / V_{MR} RV = ROA × VTI_{MR}
Volume flow at 2 sites	2D and pulsed Doppler	Parasternal (2D) and apical	LVOT diameter and VTI Mitral annulus diameter and VTI	TSV = SV_{MA} = (CSA_{MA} × VTI_{MA}) FSV = SV_{LVOT} = (CSA_{LVOT} × VTI_{LVOT}) RVol = TSV − FSV ROA = RSV / VTI_{AR}
2D LV total and Doppler LVOT forward SV	2D and pulsed Doppler	Parasternal (2D) and apical	LVOT diameter and VTI Apical biplane LV volumes	TSV = EDV − ESV (on 2D LV volumes) FSV= SV_{LVOT} = (CSA_{LVOT} × VTI_{LVOT}) RVol = TSV − FSV ROA = RSV / VTI_{AR}
Pulmonary vein systolic flow reversal	Pulsed Doppler	Apical 4-chamber on TTE or TEE	Pulmonary vein flow in all 4 veins	Qualitative systolic flow reversal

AR, Aortic regurgitation; *CSA*, cross-sectional area; *EDV*, end-diastolic volume; *ESV*, end-systolic volume; *FSV*, forward stroke volume; *LVOT*, LV outflow tract; *MA*, mitral annulus; *max*, maximum; *MR*, mitral regurgitation; *PISA*, proximal isovelocity surface area; *RF*, regurgitant fraction; R_{FR}, regurgitant flow rate; *ROA*, regurgitant orifice area; *RSV*, regurgitant stroke volume; *RVol*, regurgitant volume; *SSN*, suprasternal notch; *RVol*, regurgitant volume; *SV*, stroke volume; *TSV*, total stroke volume; *VTI*, velocity-time integral.

Tricuspid Regurgitation: Echo Approach

Parameter	Key Measures	Clinical Decision Thresholds
Cause	Primary valve disease Secondary (functional)	
Severity of regurgitation	Vena contracta width PISA radius CW Doppler signal Calculation of RVol, RF, and ROA Hepatic vein systolic flow reversal (NSR)	≥0.7 cm >0.9 cm (aliasing velocity 30–40 cm/s) Dense, triangular shape ROA >0.4 cm^2 RVol ≥45 mL
Right ventricle	RV size	Dilated with preserved function

PISA, Proximal isovelocity surface area; *RF*, regurgitant fraction; *ROA*, regurgitant orifice area; *RVol*, regurgitant volume.

Pulmonic Regurgitation: Echo Approach

Parameter	Key Measures	Clinical Decision Thresholds
Valve anatomy	Valve abnormality	
Severity of regurgitation	Jet width/annulus Early termination of PR flow Diastolic flow reversal in PR branches Calculation of RF	≥70% PHT <100 ms RF >40%
Coexisting pulmonic stenosis	Pulmonic systolic velocity	
RV response	RV size RV systolic function	

PHT, Pressure half-time; *PR*, pulmonic regurgitant; *RF*, regurgitant fraction.

SUGGESTED READING

General

1. Zoghbi WA, Adams D, Bonow RO, et al: Recommendations for noninvasive evaluation of native valvular regurgitation: a report from the American Society of Echocardiography developed in collaboration with the Society for Cardiovascular Magnetic Resonance, *J Am Soc Echocardiogr* 30(4):303–371, 2017.
   Clear recommendations and detailed description of methods for the quantitation of valvular regurgitation by echocardiography. Essential reading for all echocardiographers.

2. Otto CM, Schwaegler RG, Freeman RV: Valve regurgitation. In *Echocardiography Review Guide*, ed 3, Philadelphia, 2016, Elsevier.
   This review guide summarizes basic principles, provides additional examples of images and Doppler data, reviews technical aspects of data acquisition and measurement, and demonstrates calculations for the quantitation of regurgitant severity. Self-assessment questions with explanations of the answers are also provided.

3. Stout KK, Verrier ED: Acute valvular regurgitation, *Circulation* 119:3232–3241, 2009.
   Acute valvular regurgitation often is initially missed because the clinical presentation mimics an acute pulmonary process. The echocardiographer should be alert to this possible diagnosis and be aware of the differences compared to chronic regurgitation on imaging and Doppler studies. When TTE data are suggestive but not diagnostic, TEE imaging is appropriate. Management often includes urgent surgical intervention.

Mitral Regurgitation

4. Hung J, Delling F, Capoulade R: Mitral regurgitation: valve anatomy, regurgitant severity and timing of intervention. In Otto CM, editor: *The Practice of Clinical Echocardiography*, ed 5, Philadelphia, 2017, Elsevier, pp 651–676.
   Book chapter that provides advanced-level discussion of mechanisms of MR and approaches to the quantitation of regurgitant severity. Gives additional details and illustrations of the PISA approach, tips for optimal imaging, and potential pitfalls. 3D imaging of the PISA and vena contracta may be useful when MR is moderate to severe.

5. Zamorano JL, Fernández-Golfin C, González-Gómez A: Quantification of mitral regurgitation by echocardiography, *Heart* 101(2):146–154, 2015.
   Educational article on the echocardiographic approach to quantitation of MR including color Doppler vena contracta width, PISA method, and volumetric methods. The role of 3D TEE for both anatomy and regurgitant severity is emphasized. A flow chart provides a simple clinical approach to patient evaluation.

6. Topilsky Y, Michelena H, Bichara V, et al: Mitral valve prolapse with mid-late systolic mitral regurgitation: pitfalls of evaluation and clinical outcome compared with holosystolic regurgitation, *Circulation* 125(13):1643–1651, 2012.
   In a comparison of 111 patients with late-systolic MR and 90 patients with holosystolic MR due to mitral valve prolapse, despite similar effective regurgitant orifice areas, late systolic MR was associated with a lower regurgitant volume and fewer adverse clinical outcomes. This study emphasizes the importance of considering the timing of MR and evaluating regurgitation volume, in addition to the regurgitant orifice area.
7. Gaasch WH, Shah SP, Labib SB, et al: Impedance to retrograde and forward flow in chronic mitral regurgitation and the physiology of a double outlet ventricle, *Heart* 103(8):581–585, 2017.
   A mathematical model of the left ventricular and chronic MR, with validation in a small group of patients, shows that impedance to backflow across the small regurgitant orifice of the mitral valve is greater than the impedance to forward flow out the aortic valve as long as regurgitant fraction is <58%. This contradicts the traditional notion that MR is a "low afterload state" and suggests that better measures of LV stress shortening are needed in disease management.
8. Carabello BA: A tragedy of modern cardiology: using ejection fraction to gauge left ventricular function in mitral regurgitation, *Heart* 103(8): 570–571, 2017.
   Short editorial discussing the myth of a low impedance pathway in patients with chronic MR and the need for better measures of LV contractile function.
9. Asgar AW, Mack MJ, Stone GW: Secondary mitral regurgitation in heart failure: pathophysiology, prognosis, and therapeutic considerations, *J Am Coll Cardiol* 65(12):1231–1248, 2015.
   Secondary MR in patients with primary LV systolic dysfunction is associated with adverse clinical outcomes, but management remains controversial. This review summarizes medical therapy, cardiac resynchronization therapy, and the indications for interventions to reduce MR severity, including transcatheter and surgical approaches.
10. Henri C, Piérard LA, Lancellotti P, et al: Exercise testing and stress imaging in valvular heart disease, *Can J Cardiol* 30(9):1012–1026, 2014.
    Stress testing can be helpful in all types of valvular heart disease to ensure patients are asymptomatic and to measure the blood pressure response to exercise. Supine bicycle exercise echocardiography in patients with primary MR shows an increase in MR severity (increase of regurgitant orifice area ≥10 mm^2 and regurgitant volume ≥15 mL) and development of pulmonary hypertension (systolic pressure >60 mmHg in about one half of patients with only moderate MR at rest. Exercise-induced pulmonary hypertension indicates a higher risk of adverse outcome.

Aortic Regurgitation

11. Evangelista A, Gay LG: Aortic valve regurgitation: quantitation of disease severity and timing of surgical intervention. In Otto CM, editor: *The Practice of Clinical Echocardiography*, ed 5, Philadelphia, 2017, Elsevier, pp 303–321.
    Detailed textbook chapter on echocardiographic evaluation of the mechanism and severity of AR. The utility of vena contracta width, aortic diastolic flow reversal, and CW Doppler signal density relative to antegrade flow is discussed. The importance of evaluating aortic dimensions in adults with AR is emphasized.
12. Bonow RO, Leon MB, Doshi D, et al: Management strategies and future challenges for aortic valve disease, *Lancet* 387(10025):1312–1323, 2016.
    This review discusses AR (as well as aortic stenosis). Adults with chronic AR are at risk of developing irreversible LV systolic dysfunction even in the absence of symptoms, a situation that necessities periodic imaging. Transcatheter options are limited, and most patients require surgical aortic valve replacement once symptoms, LV systolic dysfunction, or other indications for intervention are present. In some cases, surgical valve repair or reimplantation of the native valve within a prosthetic aortic graft is possible.
13. Michelena HI, Prakash SK, Della Corte A, et al: Bicuspid aortic valve: identifying knowledge gaps and rising to the challenge from the International Bicuspid Aortic Valve Consortium (BAVCon), *Circulation* 129(25):2691–2704, 2014.
    A comprehensive review of bicuspid aortic valve anatomy, associated aortopathy, natural history imaging approach and future challenges.

Tricuspid and Pulmonic Regurgitation

14. Bruce CJ, Connolly H: Right sided valve disease in adults. In Otto CM, editor: *The Practice of Clinical Echocardiography*, ed 5, Philadelphia, 2017, Elsevier, pp 322–323.
    Clinical and echocardiographic features of tricuspid and pulmonic valve disease in adults are summarized. Excellent pathologic and imaging illustrations.
15. Rodés-Cabau J, Taramasso M, O'Gara PT: Diagnosis and treatment of tricuspid valve disease: current and future perspectives, *Lancet* 388(10058): 2431–2442, 2016.
    Review of the clinical presentation, imaging findings and management of primary and secondary tricuspid regurgitation. Diagrams show surgical approach. Potential role of novel transcatheter approaches also is presented.

Alternate Approaches

16. Krieger EV, Lee J, Branch KR, et al: Quantitation of mitral regurgitation with cardiac magnetic resonance imaging: a systematic review, *Heart* 102(23):1864–1870, 2016, 2016.
    MR can be quantitated in four different ways by cardiac magnetic resonance imaging: (1) the difference between total LV stroke volume measured by tracing LV images and forward stroke volume measures by velocity-encoded ascending aortic data, (2) the difference between anatomic LV and RV stroke volume, (3) the difference between total inflow across the mitral valve and forward flow across the aortic valve, and (4) direct measurement of regurgitant flow acorss the mitral valve. The details of each method are presented, including consolidated data on reproducibility and clinical validity.
17. Harris AW, Krieger EV, Kim M, et al: Cardiac magnetic resonance imaging versus transthoracic echocardiography for prediction of outcomes in chronic aortic or mitral regurgitation, *Am J Cardiol* 119(7):1074–1081, 2017.

In 29 subjects with chronic AR, cardiac magnetic resonance imaging was more predictive than echocardiography of valve surgery or cardiac hospitalization over a mean follow-up of 4.4 years. In in 22 patients with chronic MR, the 2 methods performed similarly. For AR, a cardiac magnetic resonance–derived regurgitant volume >50 mL identified those at high risk, with 50% undergoing valve surgery versus 0% for those with regurgitant volume ≤50 mL, and was more strongly associated with outcomes than regurgitant volume by TTE (P < 0.05). For MR, 6.8% of patients with regurgitant volume by TTE ≤30 mL developed the primary end point versus 70% in those with regurgitant volume >30 mL.

13 Prosthetic Valves

BASIC PRINCIPLES
   Types of Prosthetic Valves
      Bioprosthetic Valves
      Homograft Valves
      Mechanical Valves
      Valved Conduits
   Mechanisms of Prosthetic Valve Dysfunction
      Primary Structural Failure
      Thromboembolic Complications
      Endocarditis
   Technical Aspects of Echo Evaluation

ECHOCARDIOGRAPHIC APPROACH
   Imaging
      Bioprosthetic Valves
      Mechanical Valves
      Microcavitation
      Valved Conduits
   Normal Doppler Findings
      Prosthetic Valve "Clicks"
      Antegrade Flow Patterns and Velocities
      Normal Regurgitation

Prosthetic Valve Stenosis
   Pressure Gradients
   Valve Areas
Prosthetic Valve Regurgitation
   Detection
   Severity and Etiology
Other Echocardiographic Findings

LIMITATIONS AND ALTERNATE APPROACHES

CLINICAL UTILITY
   Baseline Prosthetic Valve Function
   Prosthetic Valve Stenosis
   Transcatheter Valve Implantation
   Patient-Prosthesis Mismatch
   Prosthetic Valve Regurgitation
   Prosthetic Valve Endocarditis
   Prosthetic Valve Thrombosis

THE ECHO EXAM

SUGGESTED READING

Echocardiographic evaluation of prosthetic valves is similar, in many respects, to the evaluation of native valve disease. However, some important differences exist. First, several types of prosthetic valves are available, with differing fluid dynamics for each basic design and differing flow velocities for each valve size. Second, the mechanisms of valve dysfunction are somewhat different from those for native valve disease. Third, the technical aspects of imaging artificial devices—specifically, the problem of acoustic shadowing—significantly affect the diagnostic approach when prosthetic valve dysfunction is suspected (Table 13.1).

Echocardiographers frequently are asked to evaluate prosthetic valve function because of the increasing number of prosthetic valves implanted annually and the greater longevity of patients with prosthetic valves. Both an understanding of the basic approach to echocardiographic evaluation (as outlined in this chapter) and detailed knowledge of the specific flow dynamic for the size and type of prosthesis in an individual patient are needed for appropriate patient management.

BASIC PRINCIPLES

Types of Prosthetic Valves

The three basic types of prosthetic valves (Figs. 13.1 and 13.2) are:

- Tissue valves, or bioprostheses
- Homograft valves
- Mechanical valves

Bioprosthetic heart valves are implanted either surgically or by a transcatheter approach.

Bioprosthetic Valves

Tissue valves are composed of three biologic leaflets with an anatomic structure similar to that of the native aortic valve. With stented prosthetic valves, the leaflets (typically porcine), or pericardium (usually bovine or equine) shaped to mimic normal leaflets, are mounted on a cloth-covered rigid support that functions as the crown-shaped aortic annulus with a raised "stent" at each of the three commissures (Fig. 13.3). Variations in the support structure and leaflet

TABLE 13.1 Prosthetic Valves: Clinical Echocardiographic Correlates

	Mechanical AVR	Surgical Bioprosthetic AVR	Transcatheter Bioprosthetic AVR	Mechanical MVR	Bioprosthetic MVR
Fluid dynamics	Complex fluid dynamics depending on valve type	Central orifice, laminar flow, blunt flow profile	Central orifice, laminar flow, blunt flow profile	Complex fluid dynamics depending on valve type	Central orifice, laminar flow, blunt flow profile
Echo imaging	Shadowing and reverberations limit valve imaging.	Echogenic sewing ring and 3 struts Trileaflet porcine or pericardial tissue similar to that of a native aortic valve	Increased echogenicity of aortic sinuses and annulus due to supporting stent Biologic valve leaflets appear similar to a native aortic valve	Shadowing and reverberations limit valve imaging on TTE. Valve occluder motion well seen on TEE	Stented valve, flow directed toward septum Trileaflet porcine or pericardial tissue similar to that of a native aortic valve
Normal Doppler findings	Antegrade velocity <3 m/s with triangular flow curve Mild eccentric AR due to occluder closure	Antegrade velocity <3 m/s with triangular flow curve No to trace central AR	Antegrade velocity <3 m/s with triangular flow curve Mild valvular or paravalvular AR	Antegrade velocity <1.9 m/s with short T½ Mild eccentric MR due to occluder closure	Antegrade velocity <1.9 m/s with short T½ No to trace central MR
Advantages/ disadvantages	Excellent long-term durability Requires long-term anticoagulation	Variable durability, longer in older patients Does not require anticoagulation	Unknown long-term durability Currently recommended in higher-risk patients Does not require anticoagulation	Excellent long-term durability Requires long-term anticoagulation	Variable durability, longer in older patients Does not require anticoagulation (unless needed for AF)
Complications	Valve thrombosis Pannus Paravalvular AR Endocarditis	Leaflet degeneration Stenosis Regurgitation Pannus Paravalvular AR Endocarditis	Leaflet degeneration Stenosis Regurgitation Pannus Paravalvular AR Endocarditis	Valve thrombosis Pannus Paravalvular MR Endocarditis	Leaflet degeneration Stenosis Regurgitation Pannus Paravalvular MR Endocarditis
Echo follow-up (in addition to annual clinical evaluation)	Baseline postop Changing signs or symptoms	Baseline postop Changing signs or symptoms Annual exams starting 5 years after implantation	Baseline postop Changing signs or symptoms Annual exams recommended at this time	Baseline postop Changing signs or symptoms	Baseline postop Changing signs or symptoms Annual exams starting 5 years after implantation

AF, Atrial fibrillation; *AR*, aortic regurgitation; *AVR*, aortic valve replacement; *MR*, mitral regurgitation; *MVR*, mitral valve replacement; *postop*, postoperative.

types abound in commercially available valves; some include anticalcification treatments. "Stentless" tissue valves also have been developed that use a flexible cuff of fabric or tissue, instead of rigid stents, to support the valve leaflets. Stentless valves often are implanted as part of a composite tissue valve and aortic root.

In the past, bioprosthetic valves were implanted only surgically using cardiopulmonary bypass to support the circulation while the valve was implanted. Now, specially designed bioprosthetic valves can be implanted by a transcatheter approach with the tissue leaflets mounted on a compressible stent (Fig. 13.4).

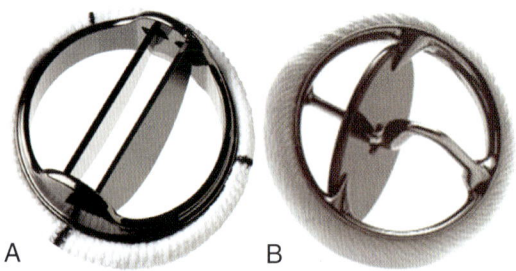

Fig. 13.1 Examples of mechanical valve types. (A) bileaflet valve (St. Jude Medical Regent valve). (B) Tilting-disk valve (Medtronic-Hall valve). Images of other specific valve types can be found using an Internet search. (A, Copyright St. Jude Medical Inc., St. Paul, Minn. B, Copyright Medtronic, Inc., Minneapolis, Minn.)

Homograft Valves

Homograft valves are cryopreserved human aortic or pulmonic valves harvested at autopsy. Typically, the valve and great vessel are preserved as a block, to be trimmed appropriately at the time of implantation in the aortic or pulmonic position. Whereas the fluid dynamics of a homograft are similar to those of a native valve, flow velocities are slightly higher and valve areas are slightly smaller than for a normal native valve because of the space occupied by the homograft annulus in the patient's outflow tract. Because of late severe tissue calcification with homograft valves, the approach usually is reserved for adults with complex aortic root abscesses.

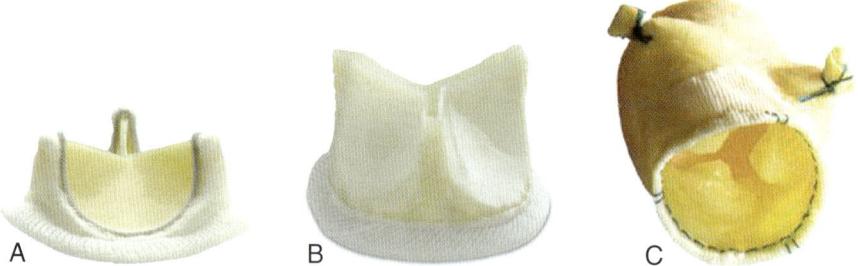

Fig. 13.2 Examples of surgical tissue valve prostheses. Carpentier-Edwards Perimount aortic valve (A), St. Jude Trifecta valve (B), and Medtronic stentless freestyle valve (C). (A, Copyright Edwards Lifesciences, LLC, Irving, Calif. B, Copyright St. Jude Medical, Inc., St. Paul, Minn. C, Copyright Medtronic, Inc., Minneapolis, Minn.)

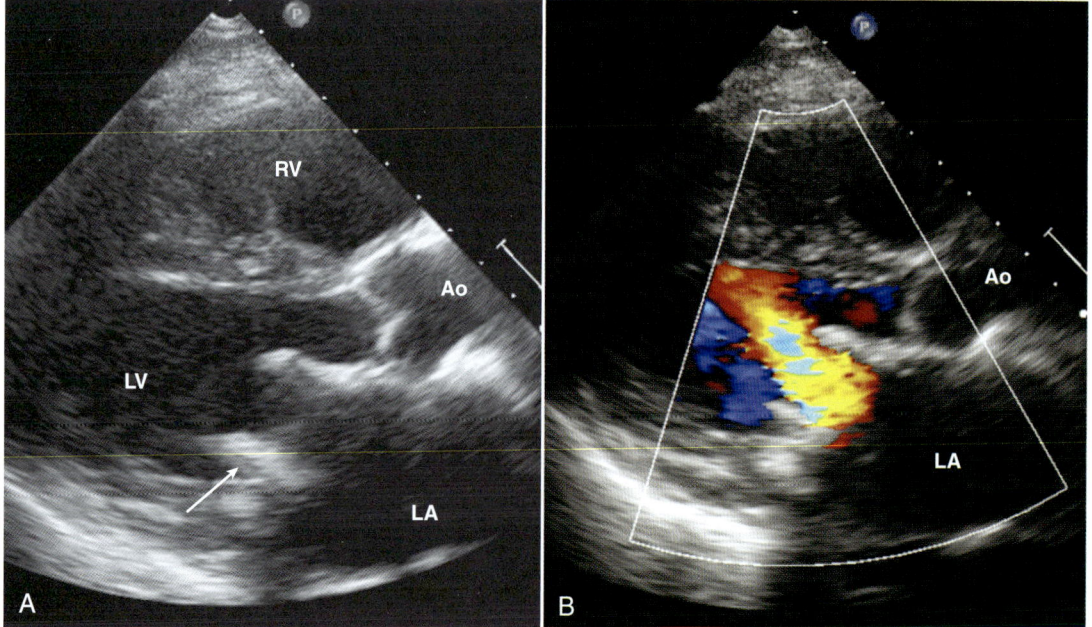

Fig. 13.3 Bioprosthetic mitral valve. Parasternal long-axis view of a stented mitral bioprosthetic valve. (A) ▶ The valve struts *(arrow)* protrude into the ventricular chamber, with antegrade flow seen with color Doppler (B) ▶ directed toward the ventricular septum. *Ao,* Aorta.

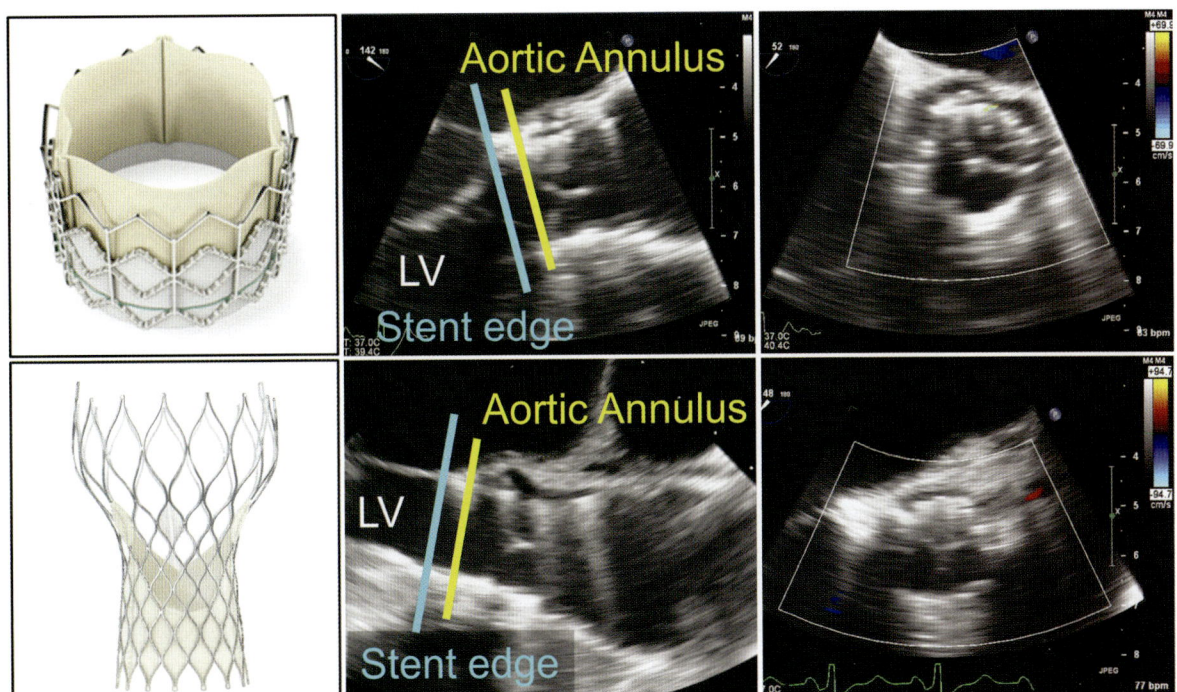

Fig. 13.4 **Transcatheter aortic valve bioprosthesis.** First-generation balloon-expandable transcatheter aortic valve *(top)* ▶ are implanted with the edge of the stent 2 to 4 mm below the aortic annulus, bringing the cusps at the level of native aortic leaflets. Self-expanding transcatheter aortic valves *(bottom)* ▶ are implanted slightly lower (3 to 6 mm below annulus), but the prosthetic cusps are in a supra-annular position. Patients in this example have no or trace periprosthetic regurgitation. Knowledge of the appropriate position is essential for diagnosing transcatheter aortic valve migration and malposition. TEE images. *(From Pislaru SV, Nkomo VT, Sandhu GS. Assessment of prosthetic valve function after TAVR, JACC Cardiovasc Imaging 9[2]:193–206, 2016.)*

Mechanical Valves

Various mechanical valves currently are available. In addition, several other types of valves, which were implanted in the past, are still in situ in some patients. The two basic types of currently implanted mechanical valves are:

- A bileaflet valve in which two semicircular disks hinge open to form two large lateral orifices and a smaller central orifice (Figs. 13.5 and 13.6)
- A tilting-disk valve in which a single circular disk opens at an angle to the annulus plane, being constrained in its motion by a smaller "cage," a central strut, or a slanted slot in the valve ring

In the past, ball-cage mechanical valves also were used and are still occasionally encountered. With a ball-cage valve, a spherical occluder is contained by a metal "cage" when the valve is open and fills the orifice in the closed position.

Valved Conduits

Valved conduits are used in congenital heart surgery and in ascending aortic repairs when both a new passageway for blood flow and a valve are needed. Conduits are constructed from biologic (e.g., a homograft) or artificial (e.g., various types of fabric) material, either with a stented tissue or a mechanical valve. Fluid dynamics similar to those for a valve implanted in the native annulus. A stentless valve in root prosthesis also can be used in this situation.

Mechanisms of Prosthetic Valve Dysfunction

The types of disease processes that affect prosthetic valves are distinctly different from those seen with native valvular heart disease and can be classified into three groups:

- Structural failure
- Thromboembolic complications
- Endocarditis

Primary Structural Failure

Failure of a bioprosthetic valve to open or close properly (mechanical failure) usually is the result of slowly progressive tissue degeneration with fibrocalcific changes of the leaflets, a process that results in

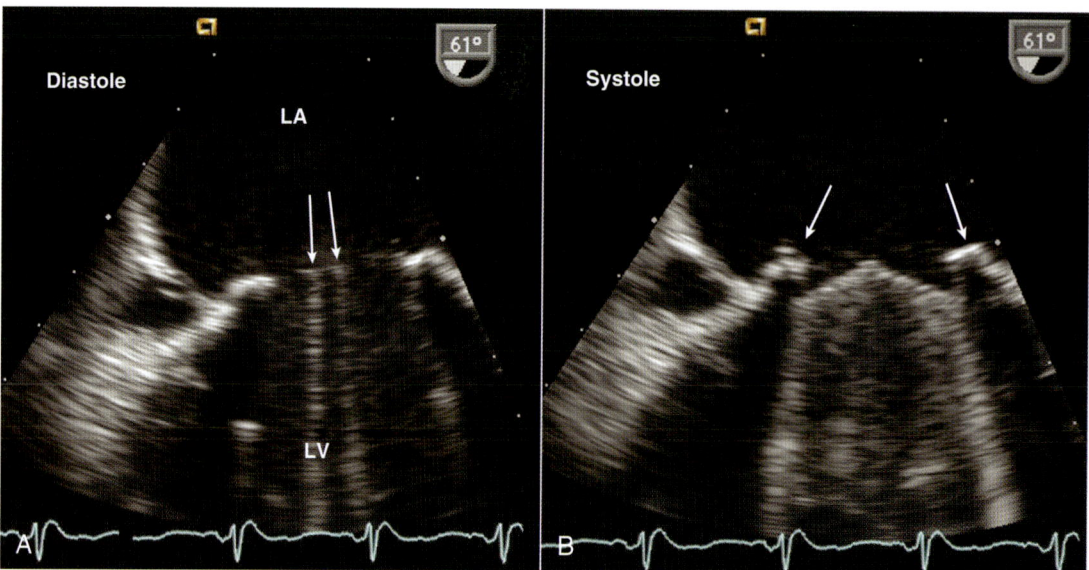

Fig. 13.5 ▶ **Bileaflet mitral valve prosthesis.** TEE images. (A) The sewing ring and two parallel open leaflets *(arrows)* in diastole. (B) In systole, the two leaflets close with a slightly obtuse closure angle with reverberations from the leaflets and shadowing from the sewing ring *(arrows)* obscuring the LV side of the valve.

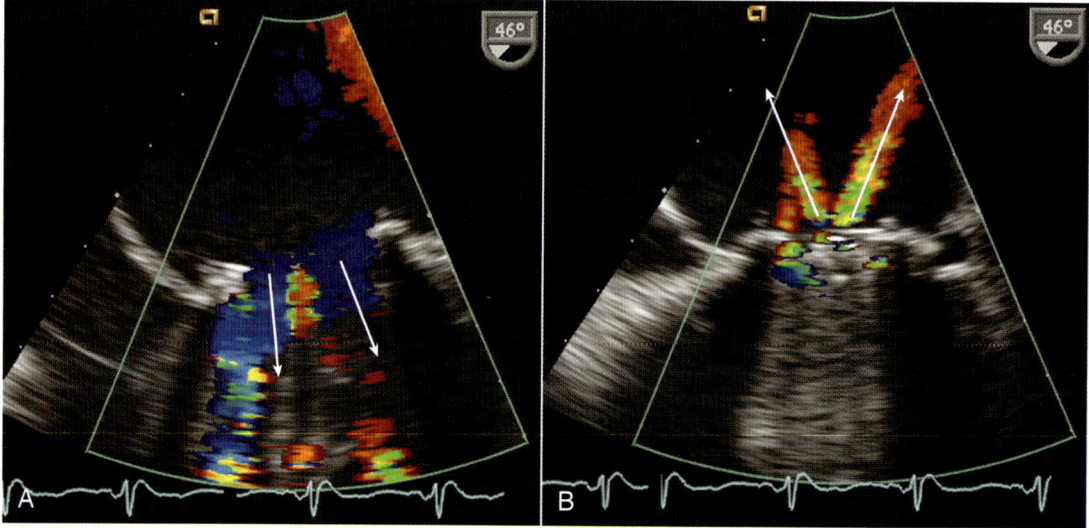

Fig. 13.6 ▶ **Normal Doppler color flow patterns with a bileaflet mitral valve prosthesis.** (A) In diastole, antegrade flow is seen across the valve with two large lateral orifices *(arrows)* and a small central orifice, which appears red because of local flow acceleration. (B) In systole, two normal jets of regurgitation *(arrows)* are seen.

increased resistance to opening (stenosis) or failure to coapt during valve closure (regurgitation). Typically, failure of tissue valves occurs 10 or more years after valve implantation. Acute bioprosthetic valve stenosis is rare. Acute bioprosthetic regurgitation can occur with a leaflet tear, usually adjacent to a region of calcification.

Failure of a mechanical valve can occur because of faulty design or wear and tear of the prosthetic material resulting in disk escape or incomplete valve closure. However, these complications were seen only with older-generation valves. Current-generation mechanical valves are reliable and very durable. More often, mechanical valve stenosis or regurgitation is due to thrombus formation or pannus ingrowth around the valve, thus impairing disk excursion or closure.

With both bioprosthetic and mechanical valves, paravalvular regurgitation can occur around the sewing ring because of loss of suture material postoperatively; this is most often related to fibrocalcific disease in the valve annulus. The new onset of paravalvular regurgitation late after surgery raises the possibility of an infectious process (endocarditis) resulting in valve dehiscence.

Thromboembolic Complications

Prosthetic valves, particularly mechanical valves, are prone to thrombus formation with consequent systemic embolic events or valve dysfunction. Echocardiographic evaluation for prosthetic valve thrombus is limited, except with very large masses, because of shadowing and reverberations. In addition, clinical events may be associated with clots smaller than the limits of clinical ultrasound resolution. Thus, echocardiography cannot exclude the possibility of thrombus on a prosthetic valve; in patients with embolic events, the prosthetic valve itself is a potential source of embolus.

Endocarditis

Infection of a valve prosthesis is a serious clinical problem, so suspected endocarditis is a frequent indication for echocardiography in patients with prosthetic valves. Endocarditis on a bioprosthesis may result in vegetations similar to those seen on a native valve. However, with a mechanical valve, the infection often is paravalvular, and no discrete vegetation may be present.

Technical Aspects of Echo Evaluation

Evaluating prosthetic valves by echocardiography has two major challenges. The normal fluid dynamics of the prosthetic valve must be distinguished from prosthetic valve dysfunction. However, the most technically limiting aspect of the echocardiographic evaluation of prosthetic valves is the problem of acoustic shadowing. The sewing rings of both surgical bioprosthetic and mechanical valves, the supporting stent of transcatheter valves, and the occluders of mechanical valves all are strong echo reflectors, resulting in acoustic shadows and reverberations (Fig. 13.7). These reverberations and shadows obscure the motion of the valve structures and block detection of imaging and Doppler abnormalities in the acoustic shadow region. During the examination, considerable effort is directed toward using windows and views that avoid these imaging artifacts. Transesophageal echocardiography (TEE) is particularly useful in the evaluation of prosthetic mitral valves because it provides acoustic access from the left atrial (LA) side of the valve. Three-dimensional (3D) imaging often is helpful, although acoustic shadowing and reverberations still limit optimal valve visualization.

ECHOCARDIOGRAPHIC APPROACH

Imaging

Bioprosthetic Valves

Stented tissue prosthetic valves have a trileaflet structure similar to that of a native aortic valve. An M-mode recording through the leaflets shows the typical "boxlike" opening in systole (for the aortic position) or diastole (for the mitral position), as is seen with a normal native aortic valve. However, with conventional valve designs, the echogenic sewing ring and struts limit visualization of the leaflets, with the specific ultrasound appearance of the supporting structures depending on the specific model (Fig. 13.8). When examining a patient with an unfamiliar valve type, a quick look online at valve photographs can be helpful. *Stentless bioprosthetic valves* have an echocardiographic appearance very similar to that of a native aortic valve, other than increased echogenicity in the aortic root in the early postoperative period. This valve is best identified by reviewing the chart or asking the patient about any cardiac surgical procedures before beginning the study.

Transcatheter valves (see Fig. 13.4) in the aortic or pulmonic position appear similar to normal native valves, with three thin valve leaflets. However, increased echogenicity or thickness of the para-annular region is evidence. Some transcatheter aortic valves have a longer supporting cage that extends into the left ventricular (LV) outflow tract or ascending aorta. Transcatheter mitral valves have a supporting cylindrical cage that extends into the LV chamber, with a variable appearance depending on specific valve type.

Aortic homografts appear similar to native aortic valves except for some increased thickness in the LV outflow tract and the ascending aorta at the proximal and distal suture sites. Typically, the homograft is implanted using the mini-root technique with the homograft replacing a segment of the native aorta. This approach necessitates reimplantation of the coronary arteries. In the past, the aortic homograft sometimes was positioned inside the patient's native aorta with appropriate trimming to maintain patency of the coronary ostia. In patients with endocarditis, the attached anterior mitral leaflet of the homograft is an option for patching a ventricular septal defect or abscess cavity. The echocardiographic appearance of a homograft is very similar to that of a native aortic valve, except for the associated surgical changes. Standard parasternal long- and short-axis image planes provide optimal visualization of valve leaflet anatomy and motion.

Improved images of prosthetic tissue valves can be obtained from a TEE approach, particularly for valves in the mitral position, because the ultrasound beam has a perpendicular orientation to the leaflets with no intervening structures from this approach. With aortic valve prostheses, TEE imaging is less rewarding because the posterior part of the sewing ring shadows the valve leaflets. When images of the leaflets themselves are suboptimal, Doppler data can provide valuable information.

The longevity of bioprosthesis valves typically is limited by slowly progressive tissue failure with

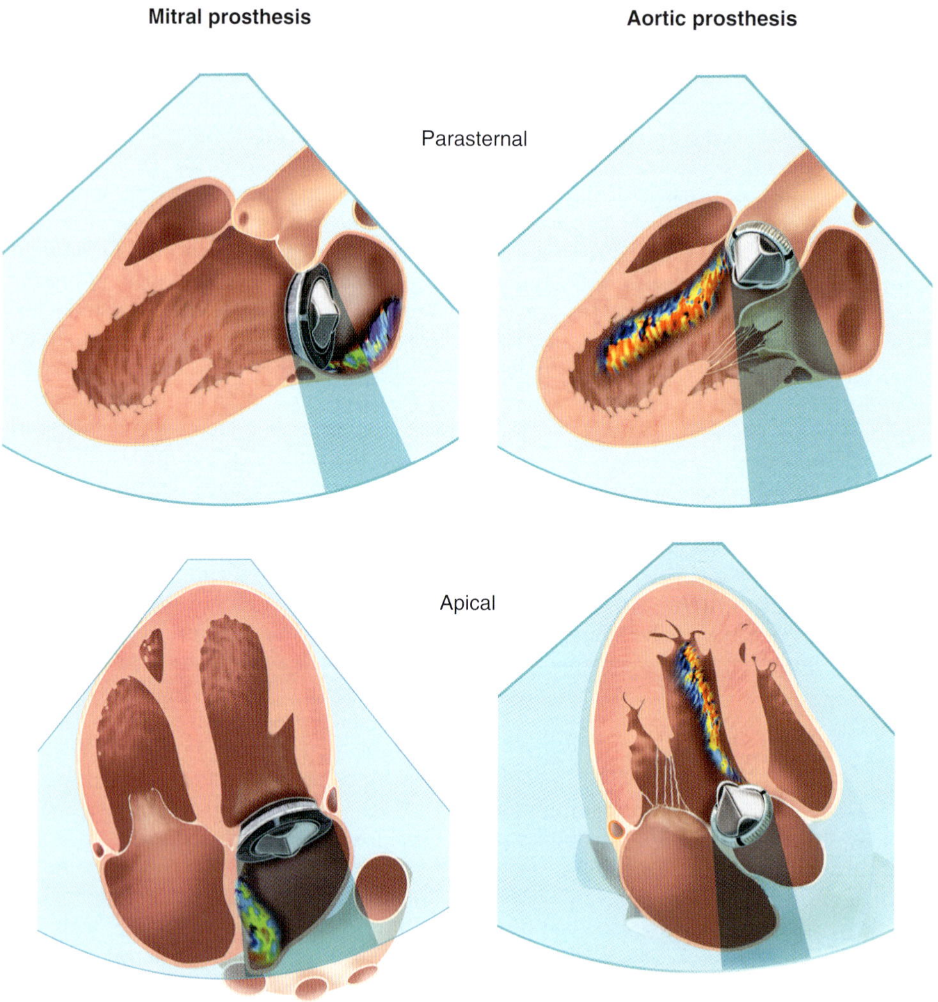

Mitral prosthesis   Aortic prosthesis

Parasternal

Apical

Fig. 13.7 Acoustic shadowing on transthoracic echocardiography and transesophageal echocardiography with prosthetic valves. Effect of mechanical prosthetic valve position and echocardiographic imaging view on shadowing and masking of a regurgitation jet by Doppler. A higher effect from TTE imaging is seen on prostheses in the mitral position compared with the aortic position. *(Modified from Zoghbi WA, Chambers JB, Dumesnil JG, et al: Recommendations for evaluation of prosthetic valves with echocardiography and Doppler ultrasound: a report from the American Society of Echocardiography's Guidelines and Standards Committee and the Task Force on Prosthetic Valves, J Am Soc Echocardiogr 22[9]:975–1014, 2009.)*

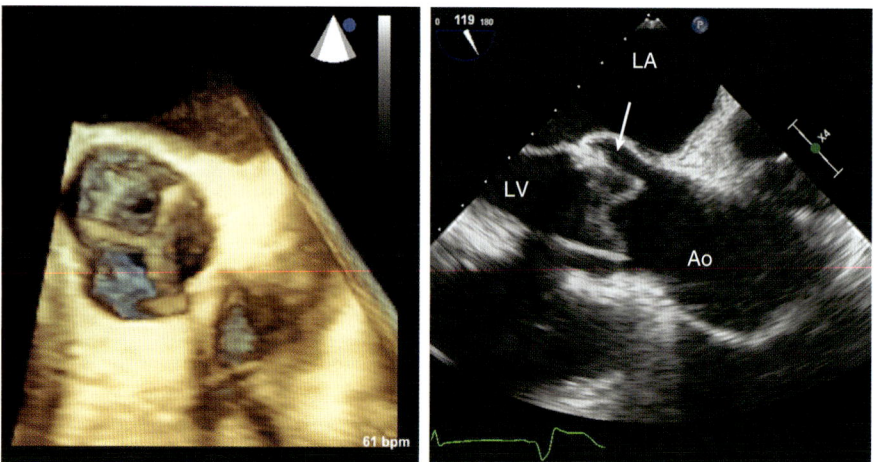

Fig. 13.8 Bioprosthetic aortic valve. TEE 3D view of a normal stented aortic valve replacement viewed from the aorta *(left)*. ▶ The three struts *are* located in the positions of the native valve commissures. The 2D long-axis view *(right)* ▶ shows the position and height of the valve relative to the aortic annulus. *Ao,* Aorta.

fibrocalcific changes resulting in leaflet deformity (leading to regurgitation), increased stiffness (leading to stenosis), or both. Echocardiographically, increased echogenicity and irregularity of the leaflets are typical, although images of the leaflets often are suboptimal because of shadowing and reverberation.

Mechanical Valves

Ultrasound imaging of mechanical valves from a transthoracic echocardiographic (TTE) approach is frustrating because of severe reverberations and acoustic shadowing. Although imaging provides clues to the type of valve prostheses (e.g., "low-profile" bileaflet or tilting-disk valve vs. "high-profile" ball-cage valve), obviously it is simpler to ascertain the exact valve type and size from the patient's medical record or valve identification card. Assessing motion of the valve occluder often is difficult. For example, the leading edge of a tilting-disk valve results in a strong reverberation across the image that obscures motion of the disk itself. In addition, an oblique image plane often is obtained relative to the prosthetic valve because orientation of the prosthesis within the annulus is not standard. With a tomographic plane perpendicular to the open bileaflet valve, the two leaflets can be identified clearly; this is an image plane that is best identified on multiplane TEE imaging or by using 3D volumetric imaging (Fig. 13.9).

Technical limitations make the identification of prosthetic valve endocarditis or thrombosis problematic because the abnormalities may be obscured by reverberations or hidden by acoustic shadowing. TEE imaging can be helpful in identifying thrombus or infected vegetations on the atrial side of a mitral prosthesis because the TEE approach avoids "masking" of the LA by the prosthetic valve from transthoracic parasternal and apical windows. In a patient with a mechanical aortic valve, the subaortic region can be evaluated well from a transthoracic approach from parasternal and apical windows. In this situation, TEE images are less helpful because of shadowing of the outflow tract by the posterior aspect of the prosthesis.

Microcavitation

An incidental finding in some patients with a mechanical prosthetic valve is the phenomenon of *spontaneous contrast*. This phenomenon is similar to the spontaneous LA contrast seen in patients with an enlarged LA and low-velocity flow, which has been reported to be associated with a high propensity for thrombus formation. However, with a prosthetic valve, only a few bright mobile echogenic particles are seen downstream from the valve, even in the absence of a low flow state. The presumed mechanism of prosthetic valve spontaneous contrast is microcavitation due to impact of the occluder against the sewing ring.

Valved Conduits

Ultrasound imaging of a bioprosthetic or mechanical valve in a conduit (e.g., right ventricular [RV] to pulmonary artery) is difficult because of ultrasound attenuation by the conduit prosthetic material. Stenosis in a valved conduit can occur as a result of either stenosis of the valve prosthesis or fibrotic ingrowth along the length of the conduit. In addition, residual or progressive stenosis at the proximal or distal anastomosis site can occur. Imaging the narrowing in the conduit often is difficult, but a careful Doppler examination allows detection of the abnormal flow velocities. CW Doppler is used to assess the maximum flow velocity, whereas pulsed Doppler or color flow

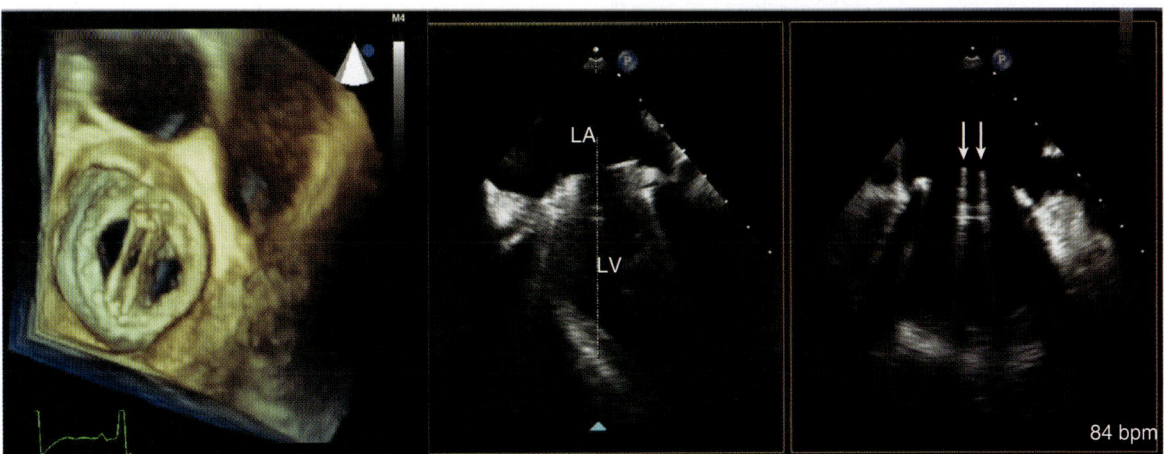

Fig. 13.9 3D imaging of a bileaflet mechanical mitral prosthesis. On the diastolic 3D *(left)* ▶ TEE image, looking from the LA side of the valve, the two open valve occluders are well seen. The 2D biplane images *(right)* ▶ in systole show the open valve occluders *(arrows)* with the narrow central and two larger lateral orifices typical of this valve type.

imaging is used to localize the level of obstruction along the length of the conduit.

Normal Doppler Findings

Prosthetic Valve "Clicks"

The motion of the occluder of a mechanical valve (or the tissue leaflets of a biologic valve) creates a brief, intense Doppler signal that appears as a dark, narrow band of short duration on the spectral display (Fig. 13.10). Audibly, this signal is similar to the valve "click" appreciated on auscultation. However, unlike in auscultation, usually both opening and closing valve clicks are noted on spectral Doppler analysis. The Doppler signals associated with valve opening and closing are similar to those seen with native valves but are of greater intensity. The motion of the occluder also results in color flow artifacts, with color signals covering large areas of the image that are inconsistent from beat to beat.

Antegrade Flow Patterns and Velocities

Bioprosthetic valves have a flow profile similar to that of a native aortic valve, with three leaflets that open to a circular orifice (in systole in the aortic position or in diastole in the mitral position), providing laminar antegrade flow with a relatively blunt flow profile. In the mitral position, the orientation of the bioprosthesis results in the inflow stream being directed anteriorly and medially toward the ventricular septum in most patients instead of toward the ventricular apex, as is seen for normal native valves. This results in a reversed vortex of blood flow in mid-diastole, as seen in an apical four-chamber view.

Flow profiles of different mechanical valves vary substantially, and none is analogous to flow across a normal native valve. Bileaflet mechanical valves have complex fluid dynamics that affect the Doppler echocardiographic evaluation of these valves. With the leaflets open, two large lateral valve orifices with a small, narrow central slit-like orifice are present. The flow velocity profile shows three peaks corresponding to these three orifices, with higher velocities in the center of each orifice. The local acceleration forces within the narrow central orifice result in localized high-pressure gradients in this region of the valve, which often are substantially higher than the overall pressure gradient across the valve (Fig. 13.11).

The fluid dynamics of a tilting-disk valve are characterized by two orifices in the open position, one larger than the other (major vs. minor), with an asymmetric flow profile as blood accelerates along the tilted surface of the open disk. Subtle variations in this flow pattern depend on the shape of the disk (convex vs. concave surface), in addition to the sewing ring design.

With a ball-cage valve in the open position, blood flows across the sewing ring and around the ball occluder on all sides. When the valve closes, a small amount of regurgitation is seen circumferentially around the ball as it seats in the sewing ring.

Prosthetic valve normal velocities, pressure gradients, and valve areas depend on the valve type, size, and position. However, compared with a normal native valve, all prosthetic valves are inherently stenotic to some extent. Specifically, the expected antegrade velocities and pressure gradients across a normally functioning prosthetic valve are higher than the corresponding values for a native valve. Similarly, the effective orifice area of a prosthetic valve is smaller

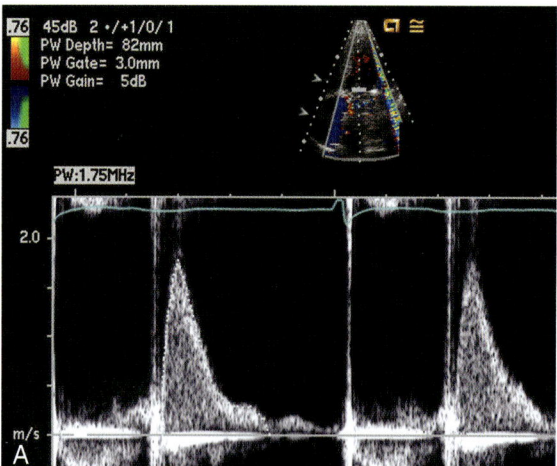
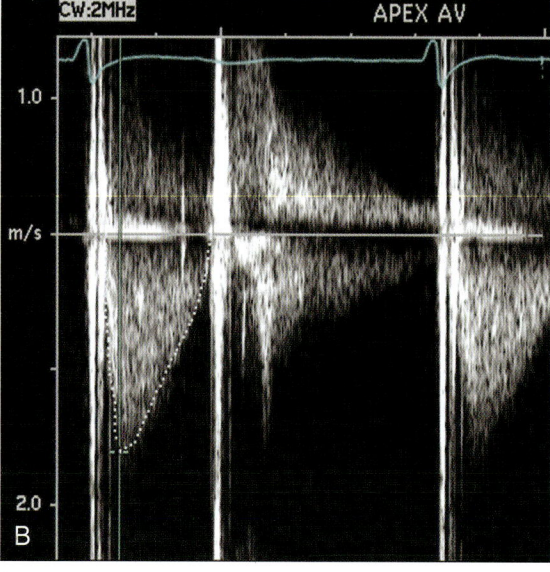

Fig. 13.10 Normal mechanical valve Doppler flows. In this patient with both aortic and mitral valve replacement, the mechanical mitral valve prosthesis (A) antegrade velocity is increased (compared with that of a native valve), but pressure half-time is steep, indicating no significant stenosis. The mechanical aortic valve *(AV)* prosthesis (B) antegrade velocity also is slightly increased compared with a native valve, but the triangular shape indicates a normal flow pattern. Prominent valve clicks are seen on both tracings.

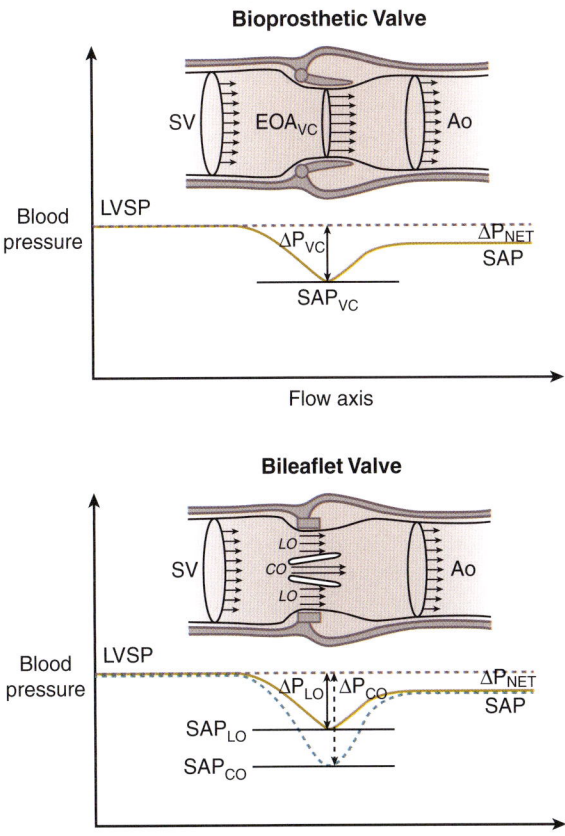

Fig. 13.11 Prosthetic aortic valve hemodynamics. Schematic representation of velocity and pressure changes from the LV outflow tract to the ascending aorta *(Ao)* in the presence of a stented bioprosthesis and a bileaflet mechanical valve illustrating the phenomenon of pressure recovery. Because of pressure recovery, velocities are lower and systolic arterial pressure *(SAP)* is higher at the distal aorta than at the level of the vena contracta *(VC)*. This is further exaggerated in the case of a bileaflet valve, in which the velocity is higher in the central orifice *(CO)*, and thus pressure drop is higher at that level. Doppler gradients are estimated from maximal velocity at the level of the vena contracta and represent the maximal pressure drop, whereas invasive estimations of gradients usually reflect net pressure difference *(ΔP)* between LV systolic pressure *(LVSP)* and ascending aorta. *EOA*, Effective orifice area; *LO*, lateral orifice; *SV*, stroke volume in LV outflow tract. *(From Zoghbi WA, Chambers JB, Dumesnil JG, et al. Recommendations for evaluation of prosthetic valves with echocardiography and Doppler ultrasound: a report from the American Society of Echocardiography's Guidelines and Standards Committee and the Task Force on Prosthetic Valves, J Am Soc Echocardiogr 22[9]:975–1014, 2009.)*

prosthetic valves are shown in Appendix A, Tables A.6 and A.7.

However, valve hemodynamics are also affected by patient characteristics such as body size, transvalvular volume flow, heart rate, and other clinical factors. Current guidelines recommend an echocardiogram within 3 months of valve implantation that then serves as the new baseline for each individual patient. This approach facilitates the detection of changes in prosthetic valve function over time, with each patient serving as his or her own control. Sometimes the implanted valve is relatively small for the patient's body size, resulting in *patient-prosthesis mismatch*, with baseline hemodynamics consistent with stenosis (i.e., high velocity, small valve area) despite normal valve function. A postoperative baseline study helps distinguish patient-prosthesis mismatch from progressive stenosis due to mechanical valve failure.

Normal Regurgitation

Normal prosthetic valve function implies a small degree of valvular regurgitation in virtually all mechanical valves and in a high percentage (30% to 50%) of bioprosthetic valves. The spatial patterns of regurgitation correspond to the fluid dynamics of each valve type. Bioprosthetic valves typically have a small amount of central regurgitation.

When a bileaflet valve closes, two criss-cross jets of regurgitation are seen in the plane parallel to the leaflet opening plane (see Fig. 13.6). In the perpendicular plane, two smaller diverging regurgitant jets are seen. With a tilting-disk valve, regurgitation occurs at the closure line, with the major regurgitant jet directed away from the sewing ring at the edge of the major orifice. With a single-disk valve and a central strut (e.g., Medtronic-Hall, Medtronic, Inc., Minneapolis, Minn.), a small central jet of regurgitation also occurs around the central hole of the disk, as might be expected. The orientation of the prosthetic valve in the annulus can be variable, depending on surgical preference, so that the open disk position and the orientation of the regurgitant jet vary correspondingly, often with additional small regurgitant jets circumferentially around the annulus. However, the total volume of regurgitation is small with normal prosthetic valve function.

On a transthoracic study, it is difficult to separate normal from pathologic prosthetic regurgitation, especially for the mitral position. On color flow imaging, normal prosthetic regurgitation tends to be a uniform color with little variance, whereas pathologic regurgitation shows aliasing and variance with a "confetti-like" appearance of the flow pattern. On a CW Doppler examination, normal prosthetic regurgitation has a low signal strength and persists through only part of the cardiac cycle. On TEE imaging, the

than the orifice area of a normal native valve. In general, larger valve sizes have lower velocities and gradients and larger effective orifice areas. Mitral prostheses have lower velocities and gradients compared with aortic prostheses because valve sizes are larger and passive transcavitary flow from the atrium into the ventricle in diastole occurs with a lower pressure gradient compared with active ejection and a higher LV-to-aortic pressure gradient in systole for aortic prostheses. Expected normal velocities, pressure gradients, and valve areas for several commonly seen normal patterns of prosthetic regurgitation for each valve type can be identified, keeping in mind that normal regurgitation tends to be relatively uniform in color, even though the jet area appears relatively large. Physiologic regurgitation originates within the sewing ring with typical patterns for each valve type. Pathologic regurgitation is characterized by:

- An eccentric or large jet
- Marked variance on the color flow display
- A jet that often originates around the valve sewing ring (paravalvular)
- Visualization of a proximal flow acceleration region on the LV side of the mitral valve

Prosthetic Valve Stenosis
Pressure Gradients

The principles applied to the evaluation of native valve stenosis also have been used for suspected stenosis of prosthetic valves. From a CW Doppler recording of the antegrade velocity across the valve, obtained at a parallel intercept angle, maximum instantaneous and mean pressure gradients can be calculated using the Bernoulli Eq. ($4v^2$). Although the maximum velocity across a prosthetic valve is higher than that for a native valve, the shape of the velocity curve is triangular (in contrast to the rounded contour seen in aortic stenosis). Thus, the calculated mean gradient typically is less for a prosthetic valve than for a native valve with the same maximum antegrade velocity (see Fig. 13.10).

Maximum and mean pressure gradients across bioprosthetic valves calculated by Doppler echo compare well with directly measured pressure gradients (see Appendix B, Table B.16). The situation is more complex for mechanical valves because of the differing fluid dynamics of each type of prosthesis. In theory, the pressure gradient across a given degree of stenosis will be identical whether the stenosis consists of a single orifice or multiple orifices, with the Bernoulli relationship being valid for each orifice. Thus, a maximum pressure gradient of 36 mmHg will correspond to a single or multiple 3 m/s jets across the valve. However, although this theory holds true when local acceleration and viscous forces can be ignored, local higher-pressure gradients do occur with some valve types. This phenomenon has been studied most thoroughly for the bileaflet valve.

With the valve leaflets open, the bileaflet valve has a narrow, slitlike central orifice flanked by two larger semicircular orifices (see Fig. 13.11). The walls of this narrow central orifice are formed by the parallel valve disks, which are nearly perpendicular to the sewing ring of the valve. Within this narrow central flow stream, acceleration forces result in a localized high-pressure gradient (and corresponding high velocity) with rapid pressure recovery distal to the valve.

Therefore the pressure difference measured between the upstream side of the valve and this central orifice is greater than the pressure difference between the upstream and downstream sides of the valve. Because CW Doppler ultrasound records the highest velocity along the length of the ultrasound beam, this higher localized velocity is recorded. Although this high localized gradient is measured correctly, the gradient of interest is the upstream-to-downstream valve gradient. This explains the observation that, even though the correlation between Doppler and invasive pressure gradient measurements is high, the slope of the regression line indicates that the Doppler approach consistently "overestimates" the overall transvalvular gradient. This overestimation is large enough that an erroneous diagnosis of severe stenosis may be made if the phenomenon of pressure recovery is not recognized.

Interestingly, the overestimation of pressure gradients across bileaflet valves becomes less significant in the presence of prosthetic valve stenosis. The proposed mechanism for this observation is a gradual reduction in the size of the central orifice as leaflet opening is reduced. Clinically, this poses a problem in that a high velocity across a bileaflet valve could represent overestimation of the pressure gradient with normal valve function or a correct estimate of a high gradient with a stenotic valve. Again, a baseline study in the postoperative period provides a standard of comparison when subsequent valve dysfunction is suspected.

Valve Areas

Even when accurately measured, the physiologic limitation of transvalvular velocities across prosthetic valves is that velocities vary with volume flow rate for a given orifice area. A normally functioning valve prosthesis in an individual patient has:

- A high transvalvular velocity if cardiac output is elevated (e.g., with exercise, anemia, or fever)
- A low transvalvular velocity if cardiac output is depressed (e.g., LV dysfunction)

For these reasons, a flow-independent measure of prosthetic valve function is more useful clinically.

AORTIC. Bioprosthetic aortic valves have fluid dynamics similar to those of native aortic valves, and it is logical to assume that continuity equation valve area calculations are valid in this situation (Fig. 13.12). In fact, direct comparisons of Doppler echo (prosthetic aortic valve area [AVA_{prost}]) and invasive valve areas in patients with suspected stenosis of bioprosthetic aortic valves have shown a reasonable correlation. As for a native aortic valve, the components of the continuity equation are the LV outflow tract velocity-time integral (VTI_{LVOT}), the LV outflow tract cross-sectional area (CSA_{LVOT}), and the aortic jet

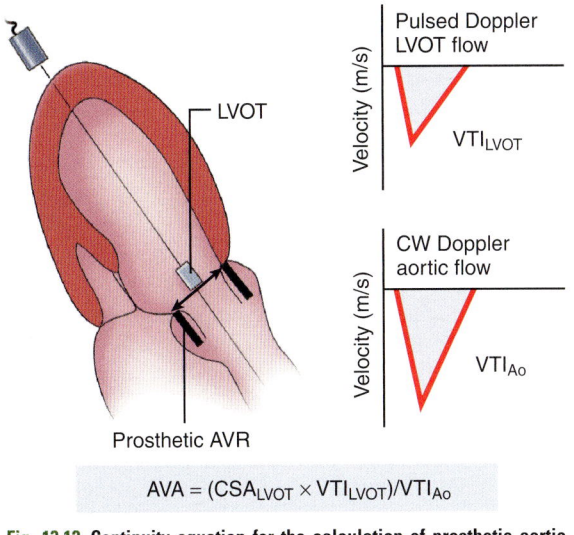

Fig. 13.12 Continuity equation for the calculation of prosthetic aortic valve area. LV outflow tract *(LVOT)* flow is recorded from an apical approach using pulsed Doppler with the sample volume positioned just proximal to the prosthetic valve. LVOT diameter is measured from a parasternal long-axis view for calculation of a circular cross-sectional area *(CSA)* of flow. CW Doppler is used to record the flow signal across the prosthetic valve from whichever window yields the highest velocity jet. *Ao,* Aorta; *AVR,* aortic valve replacement; *AVA,* aortic valve area; *VTI,* velocity-time integral.

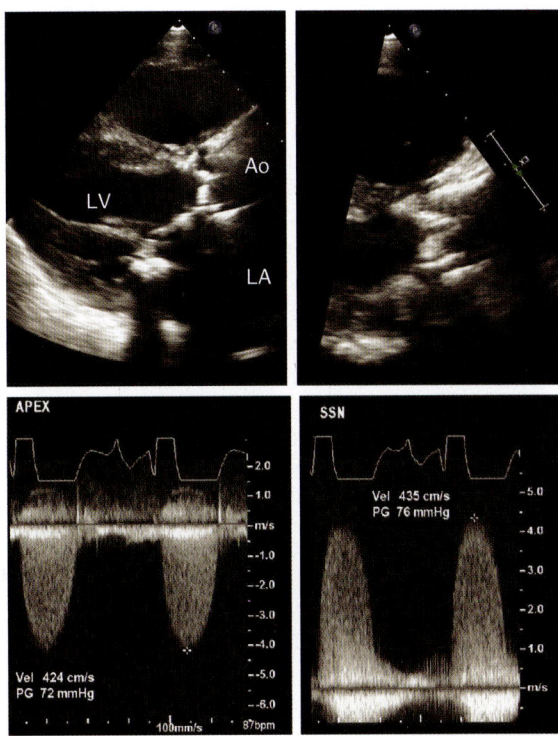

Fig. 13.13 ▶▶ **Bioprosthetic aortic valve stenosis.** In this patient with bioprosthetic aortic valve stenosis, the severely calcified valve leaflets are seen in the long-axis view and in a zoomed image for measurement of outflow tract diameter. Mitral annular calcification also is present. Transvalvular velocity is 4.2 m/s from the apex and 4.4 m/s from the suprasternal notch *(SSN)* approach, consistent with severe prosthetic valve stenosis. Severe stenosis is confirmed by the increased acceleration time and the rounded shape of the velocity curve. *Ao,* Aorta; *PG,* pressure gradient; *Vel,* velocity.

velocity-time integral (VTI_{Ao}). The continuity equation, then, is:

$$AVA_{prost} = (CSA_{LVOT} \times VTI_{LVOT})/VTI_{Ao} \quad \text{(Eq. 13.1)}$$

LV outflow tract velocity is recorded from an apical approach using pulsed Doppler echo with the sample volume positioned proximal to the prosthetic valve, thereby avoiding the small region of flow acceleration immediately adjacent to the valve. Aortic jet velocity is recorded with CW Doppler from whichever window gives the highest velocity signal, as for native valve stenosis. LV outflow tract diameter is measured in a parasternal long-axis view in mid-systole from the septal endocardium to the anterior mitral leaflet parallel to and immediately adjacent to the aortic valve (Fig. 13.13). Direct measurement of outflow tract diameter is preferable to the use of the implanted prosthetic valve size, because valve size relates to the external diameter of the sewing ring, not the effective diameter of the subvalvular flow region. A circular cross-sectional LV outflow tract area is calculated as $\pi(D/2)^2$ from this diameter measurement.

The use of the continuity equation for mechanical aortic valves is more problematic. Presumably, if the transvalvular velocity-time integral is an accurate reflection of transvalvular volume flow rate, then calculated valve areas should be accurate. Remember that the continuity equation assumes a flat flow velocity profile in the stenotic orifice (or vena contracta), as well as proximal to the valve. Clearly, this assumption is not true for bileaflet valves. The local high velocities in the central orifice will result in a significant error in measurement of volume flow rate across the valve orifice, with a consequent underestimation of valve area. However, for tilting-disk valves, limited data suggest that the continuity equation is reasonably accurate, despite complex fluid dynamics, because the CW velocity signal provides an approximation of the spatial mean flow velocity across the valve (see Appendix B, Table B.17).

Another approach to the evaluation of suspected prosthetic aortic valve stenosis is to measure the "step-up" in velocity across the valve. The ratio of the outflow tract velocity to the aortic jet velocity reflects the degree of stenosis—if no obstruction is present, these velocities will be nearly equal with a ratio close to 1; as the degree of narrowing increases, the aortic jet velocity will increase with no change in outflow tract velocity, thus resulting in a progressive decline in the velocity ratio. Because all prosthetic valves are inherently stenotic to some degree, the "normal" velocity ratio across an aortic prosthesis ranges from 0.35 to 0.50, compared with 0.75 to 0.90 for a normal native aortic valve.

The velocity ratio has several advantages because it:

- Takes volume flow rate into account
- Does not require an outflow tract diameter measurement
- Is easily measured and reproducible
- Serves as a baseline "normal" value for comparison on follow-up studies

Some investigators advocate measuring the velocity ratio with increases in flow rate (e.g., with exercise) to increase specificity for excluding prosthetic valve stenosis. Pragmatically, even if Doppler velocities and continuity equation valve areas overestimate the degree of prosthetic valve stenosis, in an individual patient a *change* in velocity or valve area is valuable in clinical management decisions (Table 13.2).

MITRAL. Prosthetic mitral valve areas can be estimated using the pressure half-time approach, as for native mitral valve stenosis. The expected normal half-time for a prosthetic valve is longer than that of a native valve, with the specific value depending on valve type and size. For bioprosthetic mitral valves, valve area can be estimated from the same formula as for native valves:

$$MVA = 220/T\tfrac{1}{2} \quad \text{(Eq. 13.2)}$$

where the pressure half-time ($T\tfrac{1}{2}$) is measured in milliseconds, as described in Chapter 11.

Somewhat surprisingly, the empirical constant 220 also appears to provide a reasonable approximation of mitral valve area for mechanical prostheses. With a bileaflet valve, the higher localized velocities in the central slitlike orifice affect the accuracy of pressure gradient calculations. However, the pressure half-time measurement is less affected because it depends on the *time course* of the velocity decline relative to the maximum velocity rather than on the velocities themselves.

Continuity equation valve area also can be calculated for a mitral prosthesis (in the absence of mitral

TABLE 13.2 Prosthetic Stenosis and Regurgitation: Findings Suggestive of Significant Valve Dysfunction With Stented Bioprosthetic and Mechanical Valves

	Severe Stenosis	Severe Regurgitation
AVR	V_{max} >4 m/s Mean ΔP >35 mmHg Velocity ratio <0.25 Rounded, late peaking velocity curve shape EOA <0.8 cm^2	LV dilation AR jet width ≥65% of LVOT diameter CW Doppler signal dense with $T\tfrac{1}{2}$ <200 ms Holodiastolic flow reversal in DA RVol >60 mL RF >50%
MVR	V_{max} >2.5 m/s Mean ΔP >10 mmHg $T\tfrac{1}{2}$ >200 ms VTI_{mitral}/VTI_{LVOT} >2.5 EOA <1.0 cm^2	LV dilation Large central MR jet or variable size wall-impinging jet Large PISA with vena contracta ≥0.6 cm CW Doppler signal dense with triangular shape Pulmonary vein systolic flow reversal Pulmonary hypertension (esp. if new) RVol ≥60 mL, RF ≥50%, EROA ≥0.50 cm^2
PVR	V_{max} >3 m/s (or >2 m/s with a homograft) with a progressive increase in velocity on serial studies	RV dilation Jet width >50% of pulmonic annulus CW Doppler signal dense, steep deceleration; flow ends in mid-diastole to late diastole. Diastolic flow reversal in pulmonary artery RF >50%
TVR	V_{max} >1.7 m/s Mean ΔP ≥6 mmHg $T\tfrac{1}{2}$ ≥230 ms	TR jet area >10 cm^2 Vena contracta width >0.7 cm CW Doppler signal dense with triangular shape Holosystolic flow reversal in hepatic veins Severe RA dilation

AR, Aortic regurgitation; *AVR*, aortic valve replacement; *DA*, descending aorta; *EOA*, effective orifice area; *EROA*, effective regurgitant orifice area; *LVOT*, LV outflow tract; *mean* ΔP, mean transvalvular pressure gradient; *MR*, mitral regurgitation; *MVR*, mitral valve replacement; *PISA*, proximal isovelocity surface area; *PVR*, pulmonary vascular resistance; *RF*, regurgitant fraction; *RVol*, regurgitant volume; $T\tfrac{1}{2}$, half-time; *TR*, tricuspid regurgitation; *TVR*, tricuspid valve replacement; V_{max}, maximum antegrade transvalvular velocity; *VTI*, velocity-time integral.
Summarized and modified from Zoghbi WA, Chambers JB, Dumesnil JG, et al: Recommendations for evaluation of prosthetic valves with echocardiography and Doppler ultrasound: a report from the American Society of Echocardiography's Guidelines and Standards Committee and the Task Force on Prosthetic Valves, *J Am Soc Echocardiogr* 22(9):975–1014, 2009.

regurgitation) by using the antegrade stroke volume across the aortic or pulmonic valve in the equation.

The antegrade velocity curve across a mitral bioprosthesis is recorded from an apical approach using pulsed, high pulse repetition frequency, or CW Doppler ultrasound. Care in positioning the transducer is needed because inflow often is directed obliquely into the ventricular chamber. Some echocardiographers find it helpful to use the color flow image to aid in alignment of the Doppler beam parallel to the inflow stream. In many patients, after mitral valve replacement, the inflow stream is directed anteriorly and medially toward the ventricular septum. In these patients, a low parasternal window may provide an optimal intercept angle for recording antegrade velocity. As for native mitral valve stenosis, Doppler acquisition parameters are adjusted to show a smooth velocity deceleration slope and a band of velocity signals along the edge of the curve.

Prosthetic Valve Regurgitation

Detection

The echocardiographic approaches described for the evaluation of native valve regurgitation in Chapter 12 also apply to the evaluation of prosthetic valve regurgitation. The major differences between native or prosthetic valves are:

- The prosthetic valve has a higher antegrade velocity.
- The degree of normal prosthetic regurgitation is greater than the trivial amounts of native valve regurgitation seen in normal individuals.
- Acoustic shadowing, reverberations, and beamwidth artifact make the evaluation of a prosthetic valve more difficult.

These differences decrease the sensitivity of transthoracic echocardiography for the detection of prosthetic regurgitation, so TEE imaging is needed more frequently.

Transthoracic color Doppler flow imaging for the detection of prosthetic valve regurgitation can be helpful, particularly if a view in which the ultrasound beam has access to the chamber receiving the regurgitant flow without first traversing the valve prosthesis can be obtained. For the aortic valve, both parasternal and apical views are helpful because the ultrasound signal reaches the LV outflow tract region without intercepting the valve prosthesis, thereby avoiding the problem of acoustic shadowing. For the mitral valve, the parasternal approach is helpful if a view in which the LA side of the valve is not shadowed by the valve prosthesis can be obtained. Apical views often are limited because of acoustic shadowing, but occasionally, a paraprosthetic jet can be identified from this approach. In addition to acoustic shadowing, color artifacts are prominent in patients with prosthetic valves, and these artifacts further obscure the detection of abnormal flow signals.

CW Doppler also is helpful for the detection of prosthetic regurgitation, with the advantage of a wide beam size at the depth of a prosthetic valve and a high signal-to-noise ratio, enhancing the likelihood that a weaker signal or eccentric jet (i.e., paraprosthetic regurgitation) will be identified (Fig. 13.14). The timing of the presumed regurgitant signal is extremely important for correct identification of the origin of the Doppler signal. Many laboratories find it helpful to examine the prosthetic valve with CW Doppler

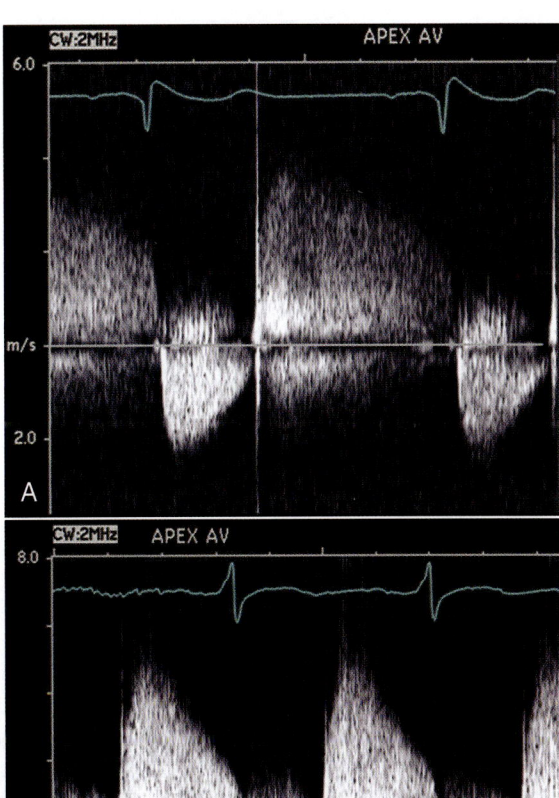

Fig. 13.14 Continuous-wave Doppler prosthetic aortic regurgitation. (A) The CW Doppler signal in this patient with a bioprosthetic aortic valve *(AV)* shows mild aortic regurgitation. (B) One year later, the patient had new heart failure symptoms (now 11 years after valve replacement). The CW Doppler signal now shows severe aortic regurgitation with a dense signal compared with antegrade flow and a steep deceleration time. The antegrade velocity is higher because of increased transaortic volume flow. Direct inspection at surgery showed a cusp tear adjacent to an area of calcification.

starting with the ultrasound beam aligned in the flow direction of the valve and then slowly scanning in progressively larger circles to identify any potential paraprosthetic jets (Fig. 13.15).

Because of the problems of acoustic shadowing and reverberations, even the most carefully performed transthoracic examinations have a low sensitivity for the detection and quantitation of prosthetic regurgitation. Especially for the mitral position, the TEE approach provides both improved image quality and the opportunity to interrogate the valve from the LA side—that is, the acoustic shadow now will obscure the LV rather than the LA. Thus, when prosthetic mitral valve regurgitation is suspected, a TEE study is recommended (Fig. 13.16). A transthoracic study showing prosthetic regurgitation can be clinically useful (high positive predictive value) but rarely allows for accurate quantitation of mitral regurgitant severity. A transthoracic study that does not show prosthetic regurgitation does not exclude this possibility (low negative predictive value).

Severity and Etiology

When prosthetic regurgitation is detected, the first step is deciding whether "normal" or pathologic prosthetic regurgitation is present. Although the normal backflow across the valve represents a small volume of blood, the color jets on TEE imaging can be fairly large in area. Distinguishing features are the characteristic pattern for each valve type, a uniform color pattern rather than the mosaic flow disturbance seen with pathologic regurgitation, and the absence of other features (increased antegrade velocity, chamber sizes and function, pulmonary hypertension) to suggest significant regurgitation.

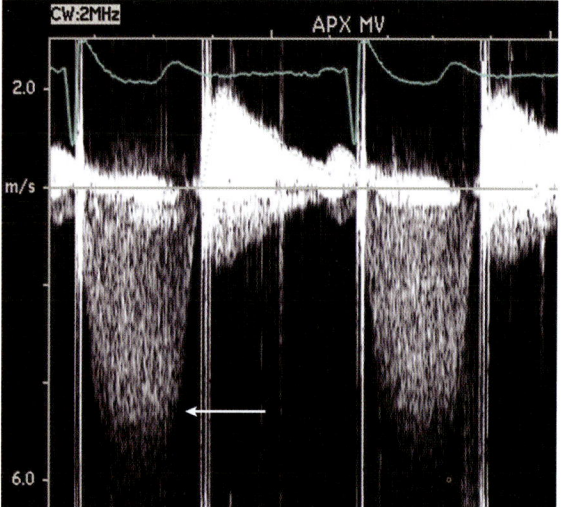

Fig. 13.15 Continuous-wave Doppler prosthetic mitral regurgitation. CW Doppler recording of mechanical prosthetic mitral regurgitation obtained from an apical *(APX)* window. The regurgitant signal *(arrow)* starts immediately after the mitral closure click and continues up to the onset of antegrade flow across the prosthesis in diastole. The signal is not as dense as antegrade flow, thus suggesting that regurgitation is not severe. However, TEE is preferred for evaluation of regurgitant severity of a mechanical mitral valve *(MV)* because shadowing often results in underestimation from the TTE approach.

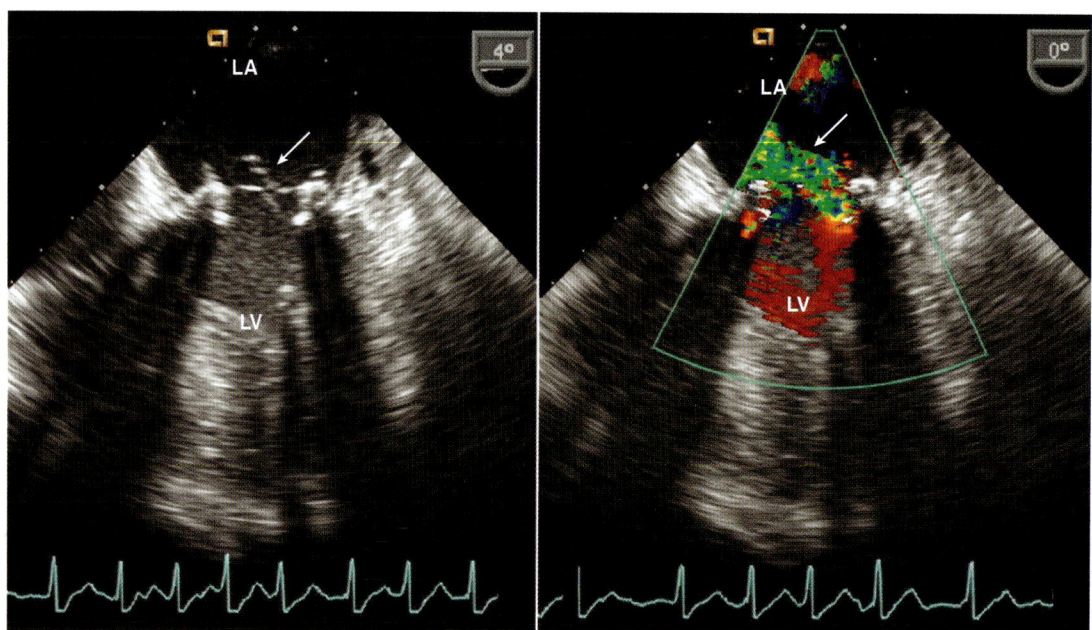

Fig. 13.16 Bioprosthetic valve structural failure. TEE echocardiography showing a stented tissue mitral valve prosthesis with a flail leaflet *(arrow)*, due to endocarditis, on 2D imaging *(left)*. Color flow shows an eccentric jet of regurgitation through the valve with a wide vena contracta, consistent with severe prosthetic regurgitation *(right)*.

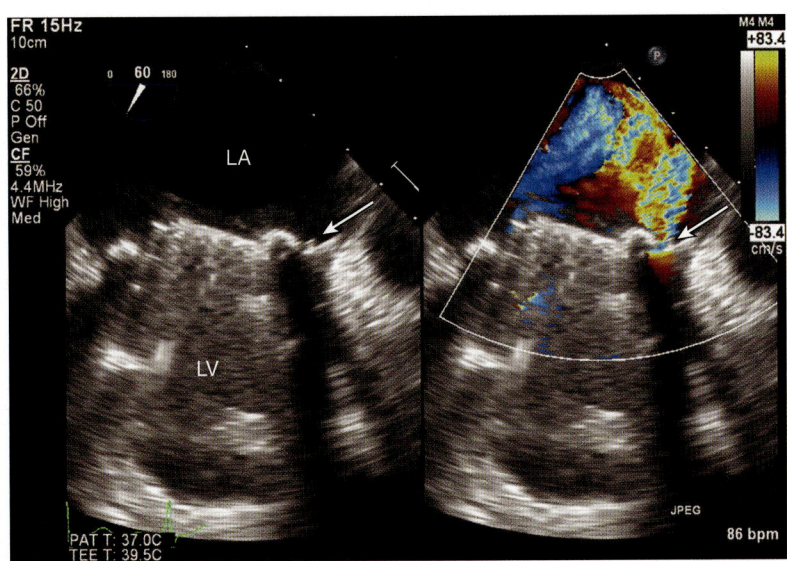

Fig. 13.17 ▶ **Paravalvular mitral regurgitation.** TEE imaging *(left)* in this patient with a mechanical mitral prosthesis shows an area of discontinuity *(arrow)* along the anterior sewing ring in a TEE two-chamber view, with *(right)* color Doppler demonstrating severe paravalvular regurgitation *(arrow)* with a wide vena contracta and large eccentric jet. Reverberations from the valve obscure the LV.

Pathologic regurgitation of surgical bioprosthetic valves most often is due to degenerative changes of the leaflets (see Fig. 13.16). This process can be slowly progressive, with gradually increasing severity of a central regurgitant stream, or it can occur abruptly, with cusp rupture adjacent to a fibrocalcific nodule. The cause of mechanical valves regurgitation most often is incomplete closure resulting from pannus ingrowth around the sewing ring or from thrombus formation. With transcatheter aortic valve implantation, paravalvular regurgitation can occur immediately after valve implantation, likely due to undersizing of the prosthesis or to calcification from the native valve preventing a fully circular deployment, thus allowing flow around the valve stent or supporting cage (Fig. 13.17).

Paraprosthetic regurgitation also can occur with mechanical valves or surgically implanted bioprosthetic valves. Immediately after implantation, a small degree of paraprosthetic regurgitation is normal on intraoperative TEE echocardiography and usually does not have long-term adverse clinical consequences. However, more severe or persistent paravalvular regurgitation is likely to cause symptoms. The cause of paraprosthetic regurgitation most often is a scarred and/or calcified annulus resulting in disruption of the sutures securing the valve or a paravalvular abscess with tissue destruction. Distinguishing prosthetic from paraprosthetic regurgitation is difficult on transthoracic imaging; in most cases, TEE is needed (Fig. 13.18). The regurgitant jet originates externally from the sewing ring, with an eccentric jet extending into the receiving chamber. A single or multiple paraprosthetic jet or jets may be present. Color flow imaging shows proximal flow acceleration (on the LV side of the mitral valve) into the regurgitant orifice that facilitates identification of the paraprosthetic origin of the signal. 3D TEE is useful for procedural guidance for transcatheter closure of paravalvular leaks (see Chapter 18).

Although evaluation of prosthetic regurgitation follows the same principles as for native valve disease, quantitation can be challenging. Qualitative measures remain clinically helpful, including:

- The shape, origin, and orientation of the regurgitant jet
- The circumferential extent of the diastolic flow disturbance around a transcatheter valve
- Vena contracta diameter (if visualized)
- The intensity and shape of the CW Doppler signal
- Evidence for distal flow reversals (e.g., descending aorta diastolic flow in aortic regurgitation)
- The antegrade velocity across the prosthetic valve
- Estimated pulmonary pressures (particularly with mitral regurgitation)

Calculations of regurgitant volume and orifice area are more difficult because calculation of antegrade flow rates across a prosthetic valve is challenging and jets are usually eccentric, thereby limiting the proximal isovelocity surface area (PISA) approach. Signs of severe prosthetic regurgitation are helpful in some clinical situations (see Table 13.2). However, the presence of pathologic prosthetic regurgitation and its clinical consequences (e.g., hemolysis, heart failure)

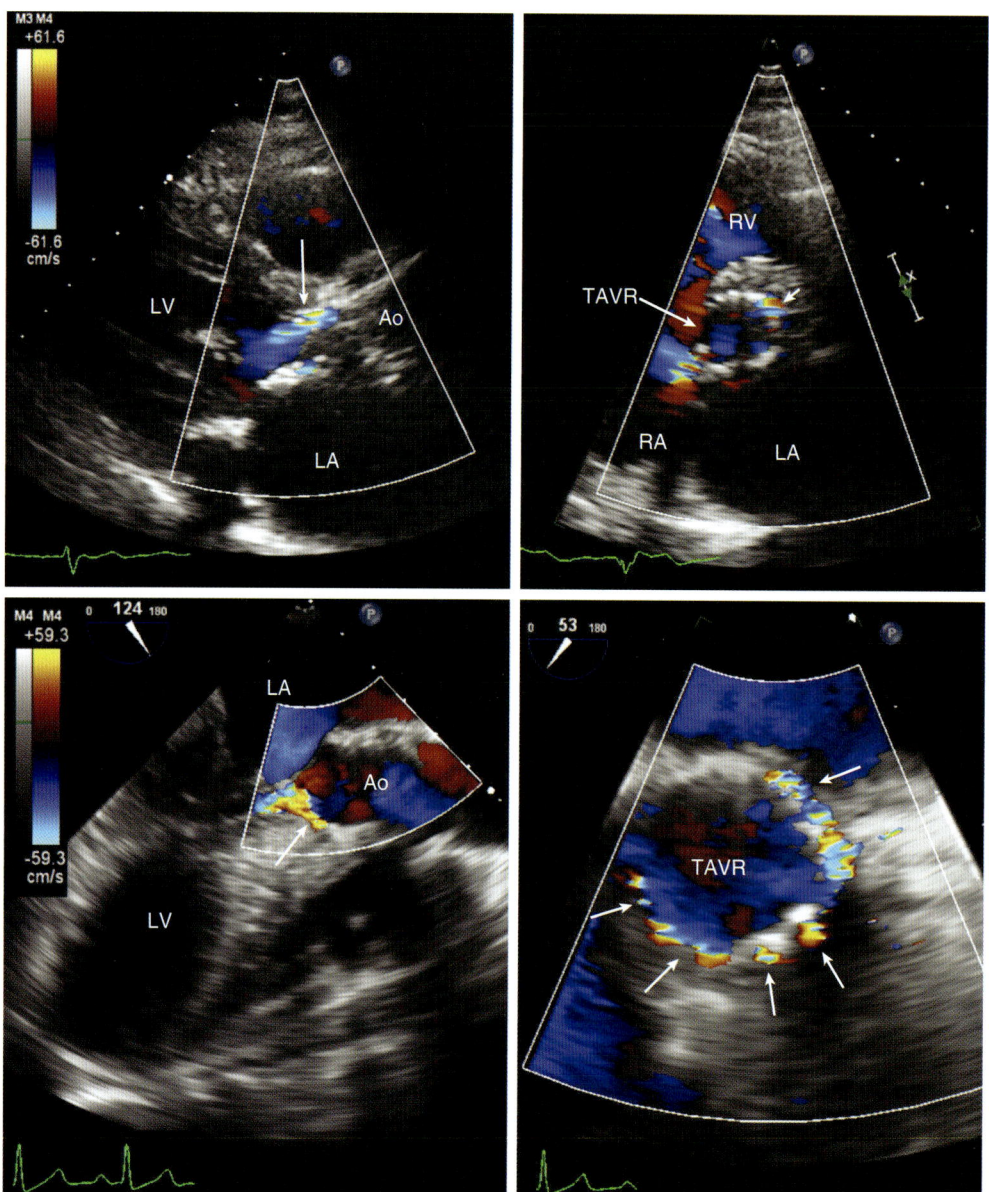

Fig. 13.18 Paravalvular regurgitation after transcatheter aortic valve replacement. Paravalvular regurgitation after transcatheter aortic valve replacement (TAVR) with a balloon-expandable valve in two different patients. In the first patient *(top)*, the TEE long-axis *(left)* and short-axis *(right)* views show a small anterior lateral *(arrows)* jet of aortic regurgitation. In the second patient *(bottom)*, the TEE long-axis view *(left)* shows a small anterior jet of aortic regurgitation *(arrow)*, but a zoomed short-axis view *(right)* of the valve shows multiple jets *(arrows)* around the valve stent consistent with moderate to severe paravalvular regurgitation. CW Doppler and flow in the descending thoracic aorta also were used to grade regurgitant severity. *Ao,* Aorta.

often is more important than exact measures of severity.

Other Echocardiographic Findings

In addition to direct imaging or Doppler evaluation of regurgitation, several other findings on the echocardiographic examination are integrated in the overall interpretation of prosthetic valve function. These include:

- LV size, hypertrophy, and systolic function
- Antegrade prosthetic valve flow velocity
- Pulmonary artery pressures

For example, persistent LV hypertrophy after aortic valve replacement for aortic stenosis raises the possibility of prosthetic valve stenosis or patient-prosthesis mismatch. In other cases, LV dilation is due to aortic or mitral prosthetic regurgitation with resultant volume overload. A hyperdynamic (but previously normal) LV may indicate prosthetic mitral regurgitation. Although it is difficult to separate persistent postoperative abnormalities from new pathologic findings in some patients, a change between examinations is of concern.

An increase in antegrade velocity may be due to increased volume flow because of prosthetic regurgitation rather than prosthetic stenosis. In this case, although the calculated gradient will be higher, the valve area will be unchanged. Alternatively, an increased flow velocity across the prosthetic valve may be due to a high cardiac output state (e.g., fever, anemia, or anxiety). In this situation, antegrade velocities across the other cardiac valves will be increased proportionately.

Although pulmonary hypertension can persist after successful mitral valve surgery, *recurrent* pulmonary hypertension (after an initial postoperative decline) often is due to prosthetic valve dysfunction.

LIMITATIONS AND ALTERNATE APPROACHES

The major limitation of transthoracic echocardiography for the evaluation of prosthetic valves is technical, specifically reverberations, artifacts, and acoustic shadowing. The last of these problems can be circumvented to some extent with the TEE approach by casting the shadow in the opposite direction. Reverberations and other ultrasound artifacts remain problems with both approaches.

Other limitations are overestimation of transvalvular pressure gradients with bileaflet mechanical valves, limited validation of valve area calculations for mechanical valves, and the problem of differentiating "normal" from pathologic prosthetic valve regurgitation.

Importantly, the same factors that can lead to errors in the evaluation of native valves also are significant limitations in the evaluation of prosthetic valves. Most notably, these factors include ultrasound tissue penetration, Doppler intercept angle assumptions, accurate diameter measurement, correct image orientation, and correct identification of the origin of Doppler signals.

When the echocardiographic examination finding is negative or when the examination yields results discordant with other clinical findings, other diagnostic procedures are appropriate. Cardiac computed tomographic imaging allows the evaluation of mechanical valve occluder motion and now is recommended instead of fluoroscopy for this indication. Cardiac computed tomography also is the most accurate approach for the evaluation of pannus formation and paravalvular thrombus. Cardiac magnetic resonance imaging also is helpful, although artifact from metallic valve components limits visualization of valve structures. Cardiac catheterization can be performed with direct measurement of intracardiac pressures to confirm the pressure gradient across the valve and measure pulmonary artery pressures. Angiographic evaluation (LV for mitral regurgitation, aortic root for aortic regurgitation) is helpful in evaluating prosthetic regurgitation on a semiquantitative (0 to 4+) scale.

CLINICAL UTILITY

Baseline Prosthetic Valve Function After Implantation

A baseline echocardiographic examination after implantation of a prosthetic valve is recommended in all patients. Wide variability exists in normal antegrade velocities and in the degree of "normal" regurgitation across prosthetic valves even for a given size, type, and position. Establishing baseline Doppler findings in each patient soon after implantation serves as a reference point in case prosthetic valve dysfunction is suspected in the future. Approximately 6 to 8 weeks postoperatively is a reasonable time to obtain this baseline study, because by then the patient has recovered from surgery, is returning to cardiology follow-up, and has a stable hemodynamic status with a normal cardiac output. This timing of the examination also allows an initial evaluation of regression of LV hypertrophy or dilation, recovery of LV systolic function, changes in pulmonary artery pressures, and other long-term effects of the valve surgery.

Prosthetic Valve Stenosis

Echocardiography is the initial diagnostic approach to the evaluation of suspected prosthetic valve stenosis (Figs. 13.19 and 13.20). The antegrade velocity and mean gradient across the prosthetic valve, particularly in comparison with previous data in that patient, may be diagnostic. Valve area can be calculated by the continuity equation for valves in the aortic (Fig. 13.21) position and by the pressure half-time method for valves in the mitral (Fig. 13.22) or tricuspid position (Fig. 13.23). Despite the overestimation of the average transvalvular gradient that occurs with Doppler evaluation of bileaflet mechanical valves, this approach still is helpful in assessing changes over time in an individual patient.

The differential diagnosis of an increased antegrade velocity across the valve includes a high cardiac output state or coexisting valvular regurgitation, in addition to prosthetic valve stenosis. A significant prosthetic or paraprosthetic regurgitant jet can increase the antegrade volume flow rate across the valve

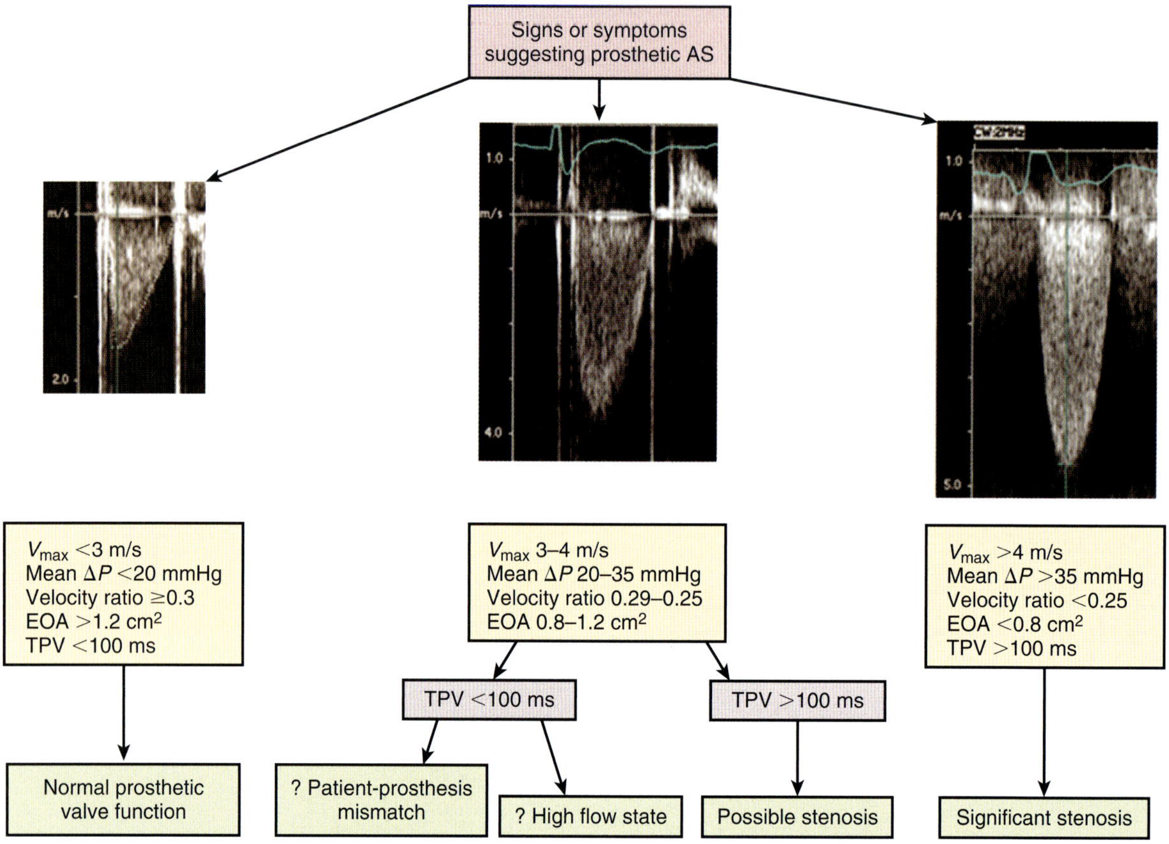

Fig. 13.19 Approach to evaluation of prosthetic aortic stenosis. A practical approach to the evaluation of possible prosthetic aortic stenosis (AS) is to start with standard measures of stenosis severity including antegrade velocity (V_{max}), mean pressure gradient (ΔP), effective orifice area (EOA), and the ratio of LV outflow to aortic velocity. Although normal values for each valve type and size should be referenced, the simple break points of 3 and 4 m/s are a quick first step. In those with intermediate measures of stenosis severity, the shape of the velocity curve can be helpful with a triangular shape (short time to peak velocity [TPV]) suggesting normal valve function and a rounded waveform (longer TPV) suggesting significant stenosis. *(This approach is abstracted from Zoghbi WA, Chambers JB, Dumesnil JG, et al: Recommendations for evaluation of prosthetic valves with echocardiography and Doppler ultrasound: a report from the American Society of Echocardiography's Guidelines and Standards Committee and the Task Force on Prosthetic Valves, J Am Soc Echocardiogr 22[9]:975–1014, 2009.)*

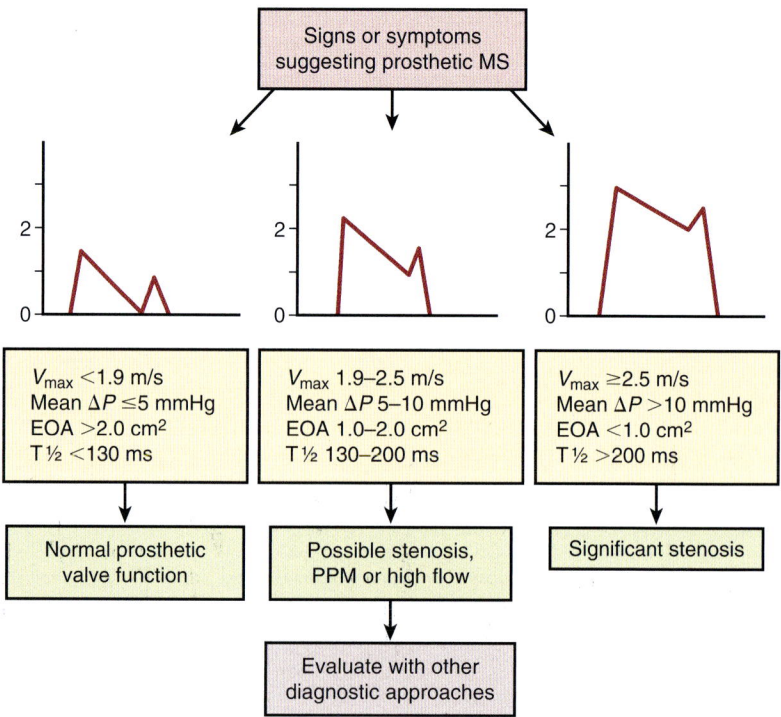

Fig. 13.20 Approach to the evaluation of prosthetic mitral stenosis. A practical approach to the evaluation of possible prosthetic mitral stenosis (MS) is to start with standard measures of stenosis severity, including antegrade velocity (V_{max}), mean pressure gradient (ΔP), effective orifice area (EOA), and the pressure half-time ($T\frac{1}{2}$). Although normal values for each valve type and size should be referenced, these simple break points are a quick first step. In patients with intermediate measures of stenosis severity, the differential diagnosis includes significant stenosis, patient-prosthesis mismatch (PPM), and a high flow state. In this setting, additional diagnostic evaluation, such as computed tomographic imaging or cardiac catheterization, may be needed. *(This approach is abstracted from Zoghbi WA, Chambers JB, Dumesnil JG, et al: Recommendations for evaluation of prosthetic valves with echocardiography and Doppler ultrasound: a report from the American Society of Echocardiography's Guidelines and Standards Committee and the Task Force on Prosthetic Valves, J Am Soc Echocardiogr 22[9]:975–1014, 2009.)*

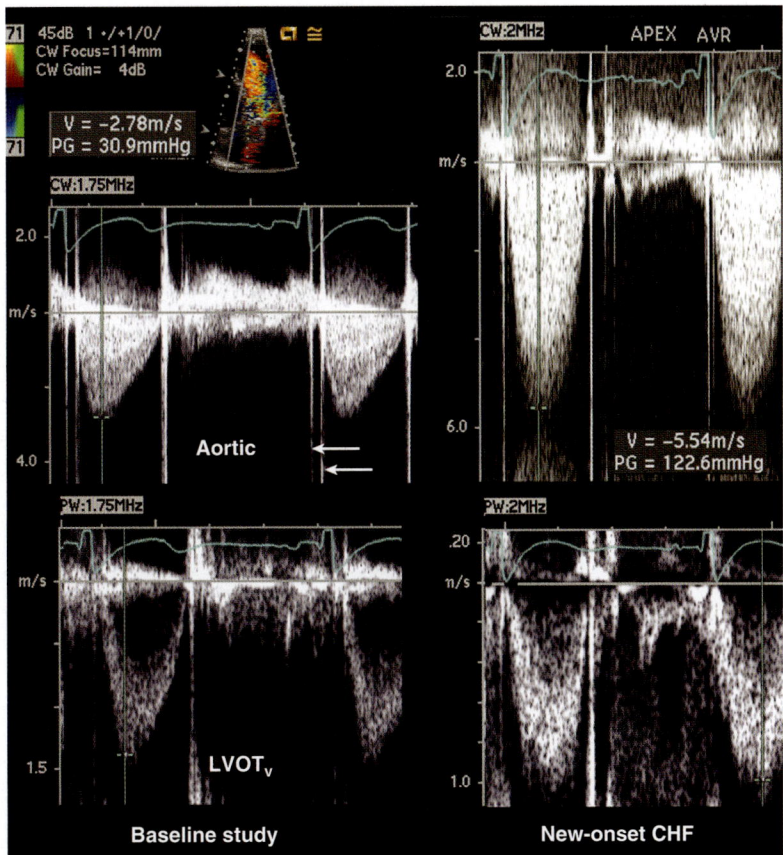

Fig. 13.21 **Mechanical aortic valve thrombosis.** This 56-year-old man with a mechanical aortic valve replacement *(AVR)* presented with heart failure and noncompliance with anticoagulation. 2D transthoracic imaging showed reverberations and shadowing from the prosthesis, with poor visualization of occluder motion. However, Doppler data were diagnostic, with the CW Doppler signal of transaortic flow increasing from a baseline of 2.8 m/s (maximum gradient 31 mmHg) to 5.5 m/s (maximum gradient 123 mmHg), concurrent with a decline in the LV outflow tract *(LVOT)* velocity *(V)* and consistent with a decreased cardiac output. This patient has a mechanical mitral valve as well, as indicated by the two prosthetic valve clicks *(arrows)*. *CHF,* Congestive heart failure; *PG,* pressure gradient.

substantially, thus resulting in a high velocity and a high transvalvular gradient. Valve area, however, remains relatively normal.

With careful examination techniques, the antegrade velocity across the prosthetic valve can be recorded in nearly all patients. When signal strength is suboptimal, invasive evaluation may be required. This is most likely for the evaluation of a prosthetic valve in a conduit (typically RV or right atrium [RA] to pulmonary artery). In this situation, the valve is difficult to image because of shadowing by the vascular graft, and it is difficult to obtain a window where the Doppler beam is parallel to flow across the prosthetic valve.

Transcatheter Valve Implantation

Echocardiographic evaluation is a standard component in evaluation of patients undergoing transcatheter valve implantation to assess the severity of disease before the procedure (Fig. 13.24) and to assess for complications and hemodynamics results after valve implantation (Fig. 13.25). Transcatheter aortic valve implantation now is routinely performed for treatment of severe symptomatic aortic stenosis, particularly in older adults and those at high risk for a surgical procedure. In addition to a baseline postimplantation study, routine annual imaging is recommended to evaluate valve function and any associated abnormalities (Table 13.3).

Fig. 13.22 Bioprosthetic mitral stenosis. In the TEE four chamber view *(left)* ▶ the bioprosthetic mitral valve leaflets are thick *(arrow)*, with video images showing reduced motion. Color Doppler *(right)* ▶ demonstrates a narrow antegrade flow stream in diastole with a proximal acceleration region *(arrow)*. CW Doppler *(bottom)* allows quantitation of mitral stenosis severity based on the mean pressure gradient and pressure half-time *(PHT)*.

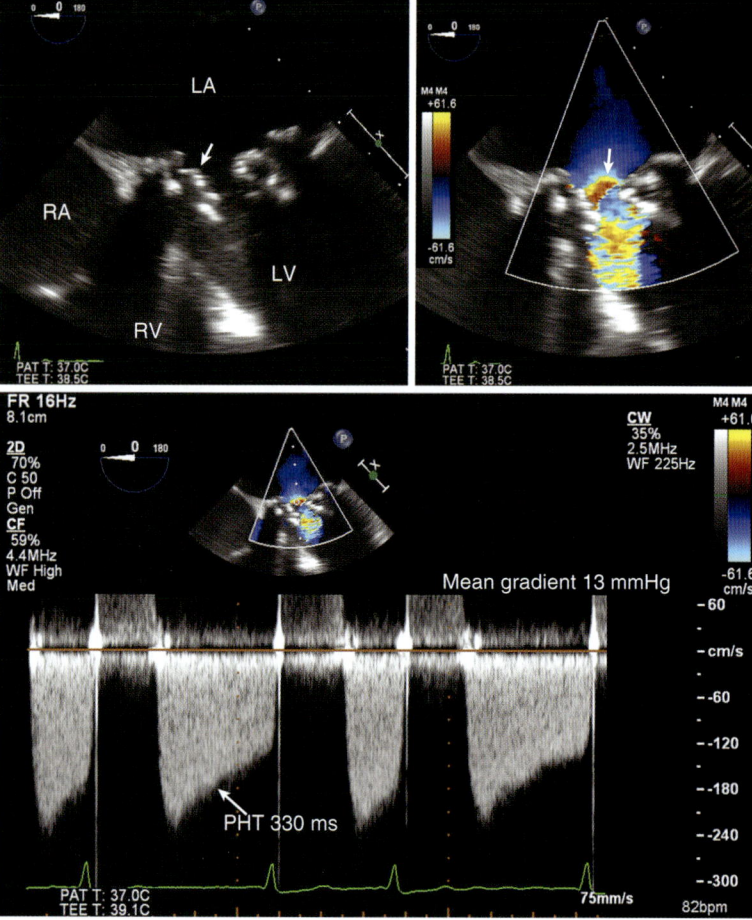

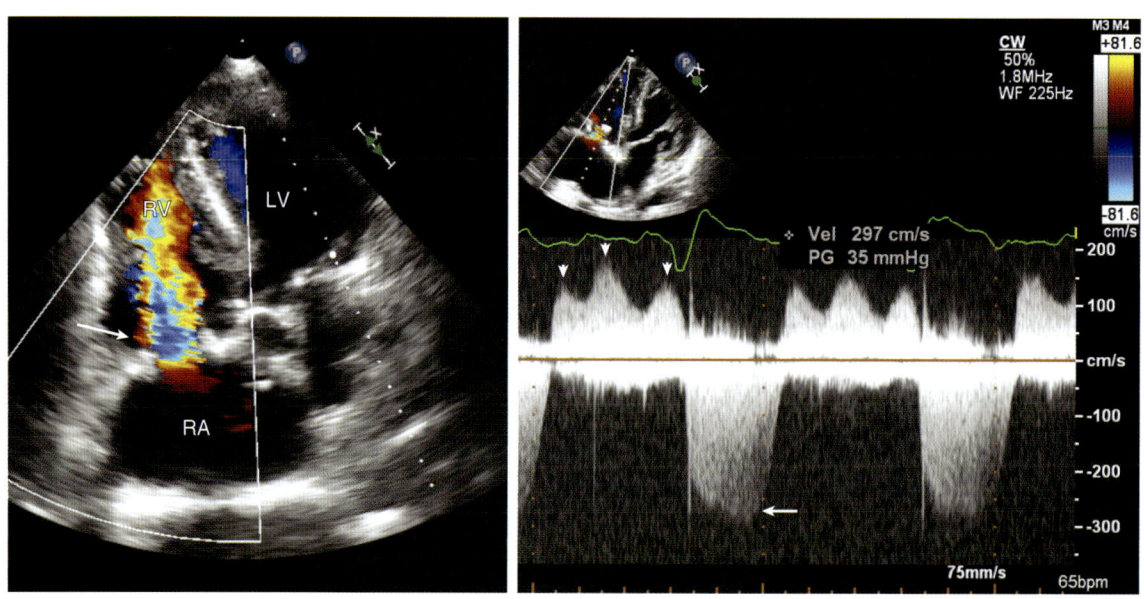

Fig. 13.23 Bioprosthetic tricuspid valve stenosis. A 36-year-old man with a previous tricuspid valve replacement for Ebstein anomaly and chronic heart failure due to LV systolic dysfunction presented with an acute exacerbation of his heart failure symptoms. Color Doppler *(left)* ▶ of the bioprosthetic tricuspid valve suggests mimal stenosis with a color flow stream filling the annulus area. CW Doppler *(right)* shows a moderately dense tricuspid regurgitation signal with a velocity *(Vel)* of 3 m/s *(arrow)* indicating only mild pulmonary hypertension. In diastole, the pressure gradient *(PG)* is minimally elevated, but the flow curve shows repeated peaks in diastole *(arrowheads)* consistent with atrial flutter.

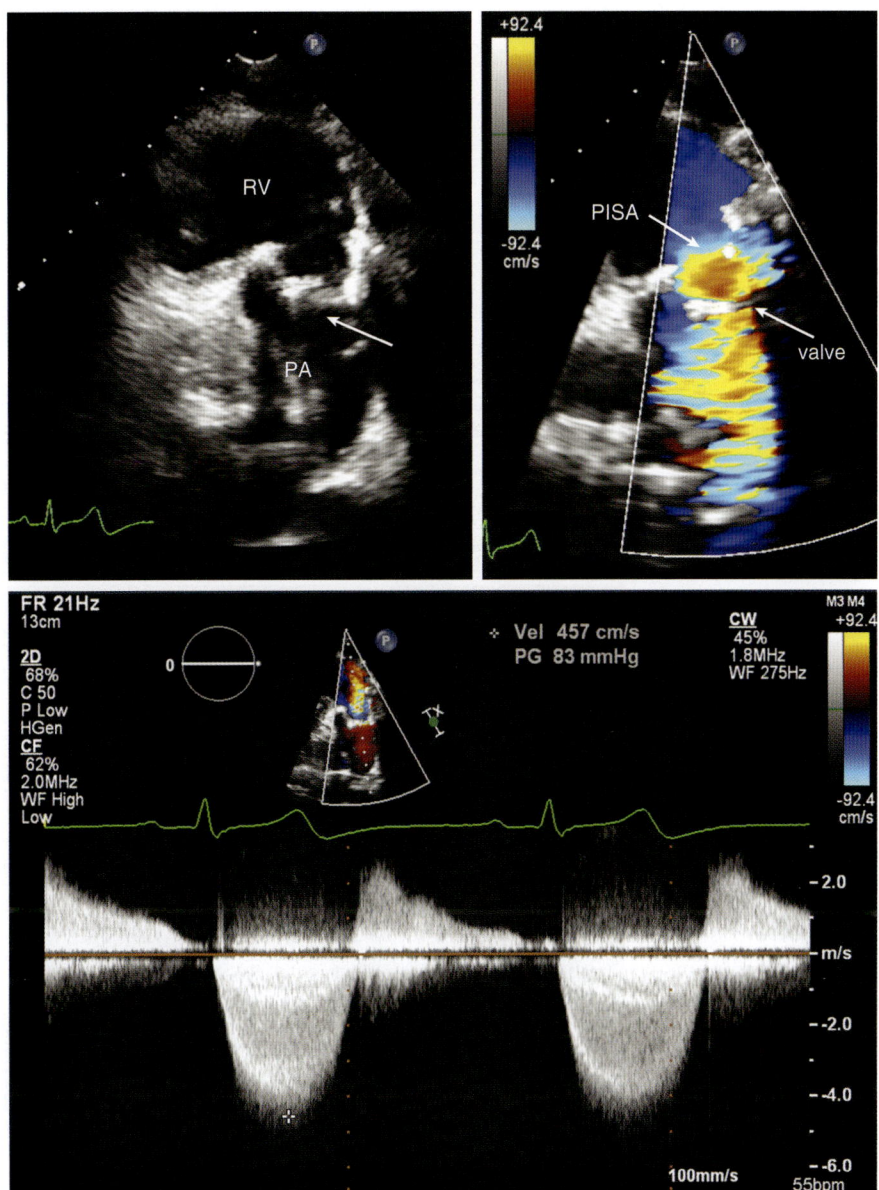

Fig. 13.24 **Bioprosthetic pulmonic valve stenosis.** In this 34-year-old man with tetralogy of Fallot repair in childhood, the bioprosthetic pulmonic valve is calcified *(arrow)* and relatively immobile on 2D imaging *(upper left)*. ▶ Color Doppler *(upper right)* ▶ shows flow acceleration on the RV side of the valve with a flow disturbance that begins at the valve level. CW Doppler *(bottom)* shows an antegrade velocity of 4.5 m/s, consistent with severe stenosis. Coexisting pulmonic regurgitation is seen on the CW Doppler tracing. *PA*, Pulmonary artery; *PG*, pressure gradient, *PISA*, proximal isovelocity surface area; *Vel*, velocity.

Patient-Prosthesis Mismatch

In some patients, the size of the prosthetic aortic valve that can be implanted results in inadequate blood flow to meet the metabolic demands of the patient, even when the prosthetic valve itself is functioning normally. This situation, called patient-prosthesis mismatch, as previously noted, is defined as an indexed effective orifice area ≤0.85 cm^2/m^2 and is a predictor of a high transvalvular gradient, persistent ventricular hypertrophy, and an increased rate of cardiac events after aortic valve replacement. The impact of a relatively small valve area is most noticeable with severe patient-prosthesis mismatch, defined as an orifice area 0.65 cm^2/m^2. Patient-prosthesis mismatch can be avoided by choosing a valve prosthesis that will have an adequate indexed orifice area, based on the patient's body size and annular dimension. In some cases, annular enlargement or other approaches should be considered to allow implantation of an appropriately sized valve or avoidance of a prosthetic valve.

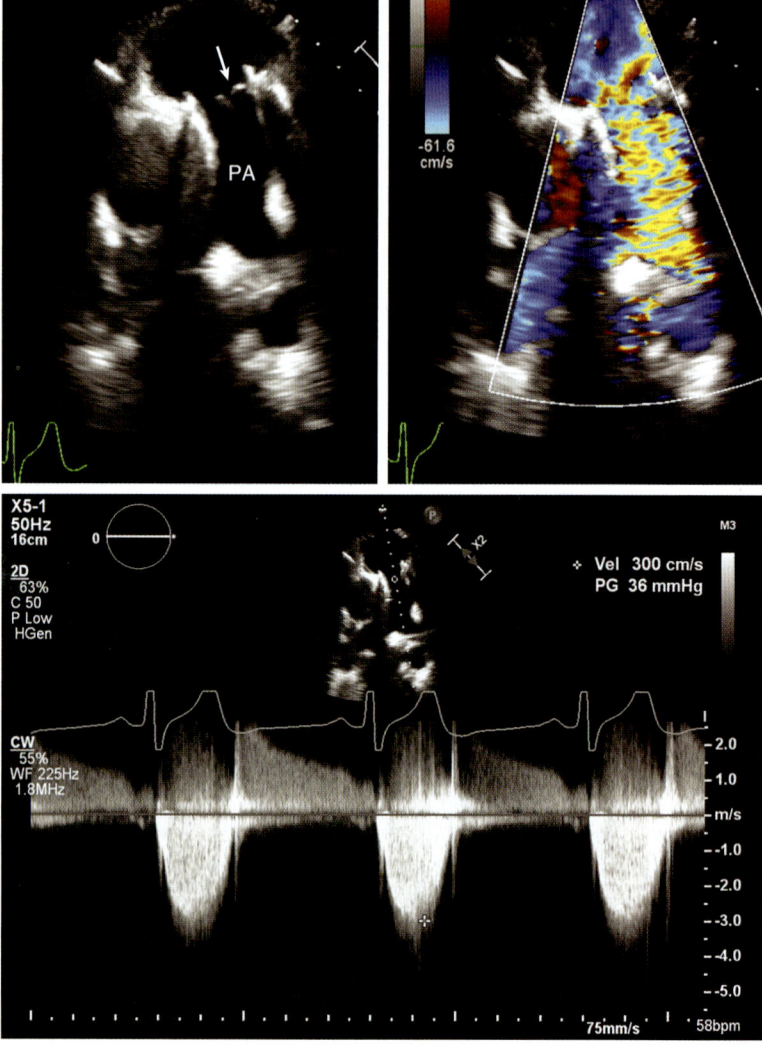

Fig. 13.25 Transcatheter pulmonic valve-in-valve prosthesis. In the same patient as Fig. 13.24, a transcatheter pulmonic valve replacement was placed within the old surgical bioprosthetic valve. On 2D imaging *(upper left)* ▶ the valve leaflets now are thin *(arrow)* with normal systolic opening. Color Doppler *(upper right)* ▶ still shows signal aliasing in the RV outflow tract and pulmonary artery *(PA)* with CW Doppler *(bottom)* showing a velocity *(Vel)* of 3.0 m/s across the transcatheter valve *(bottom)*. However, the velocity of flow proximal to the pulmonic valve was 2.6 m/s, so these findings are consistent with normal valve function and a high cardiac output. *PG,* Pressure gradient.

Prosthetic Valve Regurgitation

Transthoracic echocardiography is accurate for the diagnosis of aortic prosthetic valve regurgitation and for the differentiation of normal from pathologic regurgitation (Figs. 13.26 and 13.27). However, because of acoustic shadowing, the sensitivity for the detection of mitral prosthetic regurgitation is lower, and it is more difficult to distinguish normal from pathologic regurgitation. TEE echocardiography imaging is needed when this diagnosis is suspected on clinical grounds. TEE echocardiography has a high accuracy for detection of prosthetic regurgitation and reliably distinguishes transprosthetic from paraprosthetic regurgitation.

Prosthetic Valve Endocarditis

Detection of valvular vegetations on prosthetic valves is difficult with transthoracic echocardiography because of reverberations and acoustic shadowing (Fig. 13.28). Features that may increase the suspicion of prosthetic valve endocarditis on a transthoracic echocardiographic examination include Doppler evidence of valve dysfunction (either regurgitation due to incomplete closure or stenosis due to an infected pannus on the inflow surface of the valve), evidence of valve instability (i.e., "rocking"), an unexplained increase in pulmonary artery pressures, or an interval change in chamber dimensions. Prosthetic valve endocarditis often involves the sewing ring and annulus, resulting in formation

TABLE 13.3 Echo Evaluation After Transcatheter Aortic Valve Implantation

Key Data	Imaging Approach	Possible Abnormalities
Prosthetic valve anatomy	2D and 3D imaging in long- and short-axis views on TTE or TEE Position of valve stent Leaflet appearance and motion	Valve positioned too low or too high relative to aortic annulus Thickened leaflets, valve thrombosis, restricted leaflet motion
Transvalvular flow patterns	Color Doppler in long- and short-axis views of prosthetic valve for visualization of systolic and diastolic flow across valve	Detection of paravalvular regurgitation Describe the extent of paravalvular regurgitation around the valve circumference. Valvular regurgitation
Prosthetic valve hemodynamics	CW Doppler is best recorded on TTE from the apical window. Antegrade valve velocity and VTI for calculation of mean gradient and aortic valve area Detection of AR and measurement of AR pressure half-time	Increased velocity and reduced valve area with patient-prosthesis mismatch, valve thrombosis, or valve obstruction. A change from previous studies suggests valve thrombosis. Paravalvular regurgitation is associated with adverse clinical outcomes.
Transvalvular volume flow rate	Pulsed Doppler LV outflow tract peak velocity and VTI are recorded from apical view for calculation of stroke volume and valve area.	Low stroke volume index
LV anatomy and systolic function	3D or 2D biplane imaging is used for qualitative evaluation of LV global and regional function and LV hypertrophy. Calculation of ejection fraction, LV diastolic and systolic volumes	Global LV systolic dysfunction with reduced ejection fraction Regional wall motion abnormalities may be old, due to coexisting coronary disease, or new due to procedural complication. LV hypertrophy due to chronic pressure overload resulting in small LV volumes and a low stroke volume index
LV diastolic function	Multiple Doppler parameters (see Chapter 7)	Diastolic dysfunction contributes to persistent symptoms after TAVI.
Mitral valve anatomy and function	2D and 3D imaging of mitral valve anatomy and motion Color and CW Doppler evaluation for mitral stenosis and/or mitral regurgitation	Mitral annular calcification and degenerative leaflet changes, resulting in mitral regurgitation are common in patients undergoing TAVI. Quantitation of MR severity (see Chapter 12) is helpful for clinical decision making. Rarely the TAVI valve impinges on anterior mitral leaflet motion.
Pulmonary pressures	Estimate pulmonary pressure based on tricuspid regurgitation velocity and inferior vena cava diameter.	Elevated pulmonary pressures are common in patients undergoing TAVI and contribute to symptoms.
RV size and systolic function	2D imaging of RV size and systolic function with measurement of TAPSE and other parameters	RV systolic dysfunction may be due to pulmonary hypertension or primary myocardial disease.
Pericardium	Evaluate for pericardial effusion in multiple views.	Pericardial effusion after the procedure should be reported promptly to the interventional cardiology team.

AR, Aortic regurgitation; *MR*, mitral regurgitation; *TAPSE*, tricuspid annular plane systolic excursion; *TAVI*, transcatheter aortic valve implantation; *VTI*, velocity-time integral.

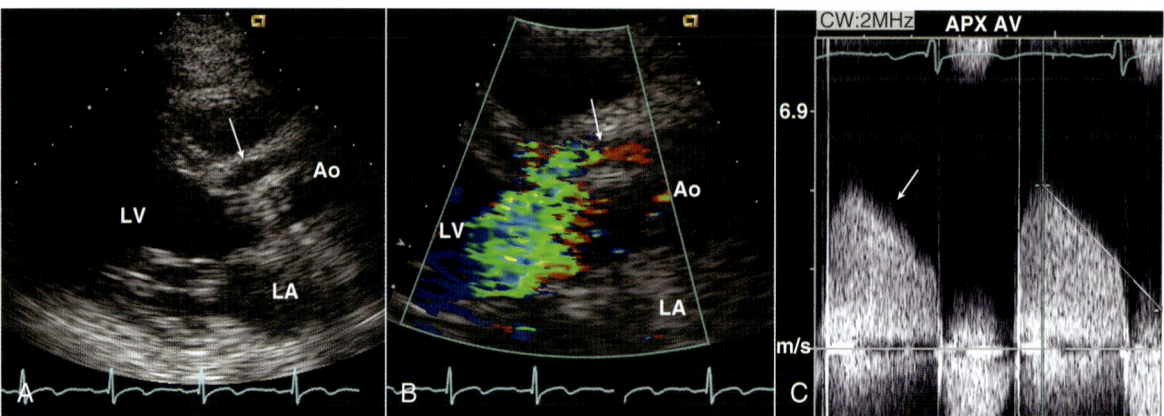

Fig. 13.26 Paravalvular aortic regurgitation on transthoracic echocardiography. (A) ▶ A parasternal long-axis view shows an echo-free space *(arrow)* anterior to a mechanical aortic valve replacement. (B) ▶ Color Doppler shows a diastolic flow disturbance originating in this space *(arrow)* with flow into the LV chamber. (C) CW Doppler confirms that this flow is aortic regurgitation, showing the typical timing and velocity curve *(arrow)* with a density and slope consistent with severe regurgitation. *Ao,* Aorta.

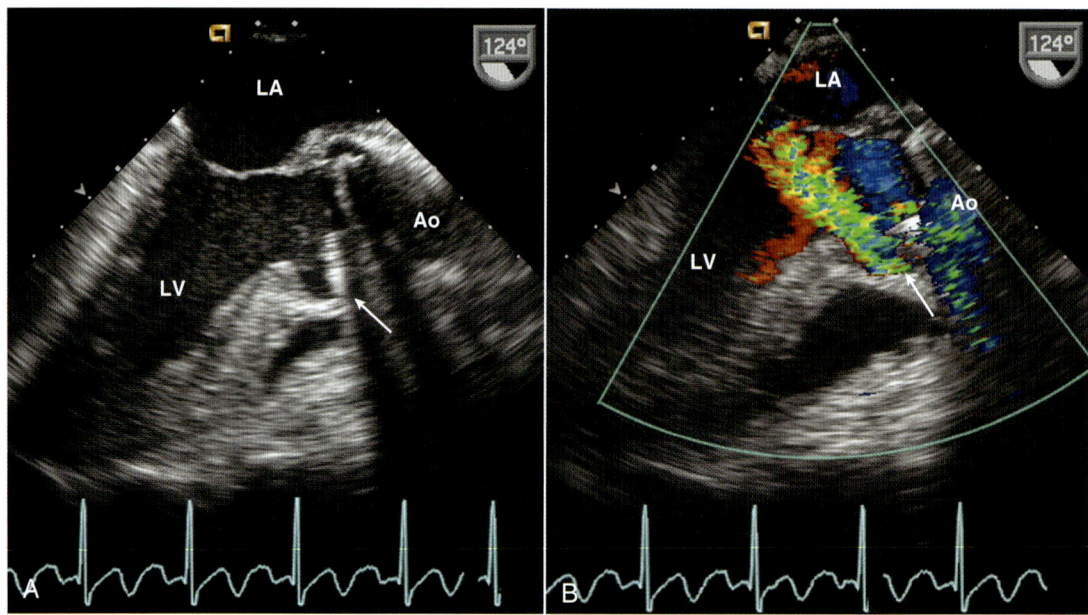

Fig. 13.27 ▶▶ Paravalvular aortic regurgitation on transesophageal echocardiography. (A) In the same patient as in Fig. 13.27, TEE provides better definition of the area of valve dehiscence adjacent to the septum *(arrow)*. The TEE probe has been positioned so that the shadows from the valve prosthesis do not obscure the area of interest. (B) Color Doppler shows aortic regurgitation originating from this site.

of a paravalvular abscess ("ring" abscess) rather than the typical vegetation seen with native valve infection. Identification of an abscess is limited on TTE echocardiography.

Thus, given the technical and pathologic peculiarities of the evaluation of suspected prosthetic valve endocarditis, TEE imaging is needed in the majority of these patients. TEE echocardiography has a high sensitivity for the detection of prosthetic valve endocarditis, abscess formation, or both. As for native valve endocarditis (see Chapter 14), cardiac abscesses may be echo dense or relatively echo free. Persistent infection also may result in an aneurysm instead of an abscess cavity (Fig. 13.29).

Prosthetic Valve Thrombosis

In patients with embolic events presumed secondary to prosthetic valve thrombosis, even TEE echocardiographic results may be negative if the thrombi are small or if a new thrombus has not formed since the embolic event. When thrombi are documented on TEE echocardiography, this finding may be important in patient management. However, an

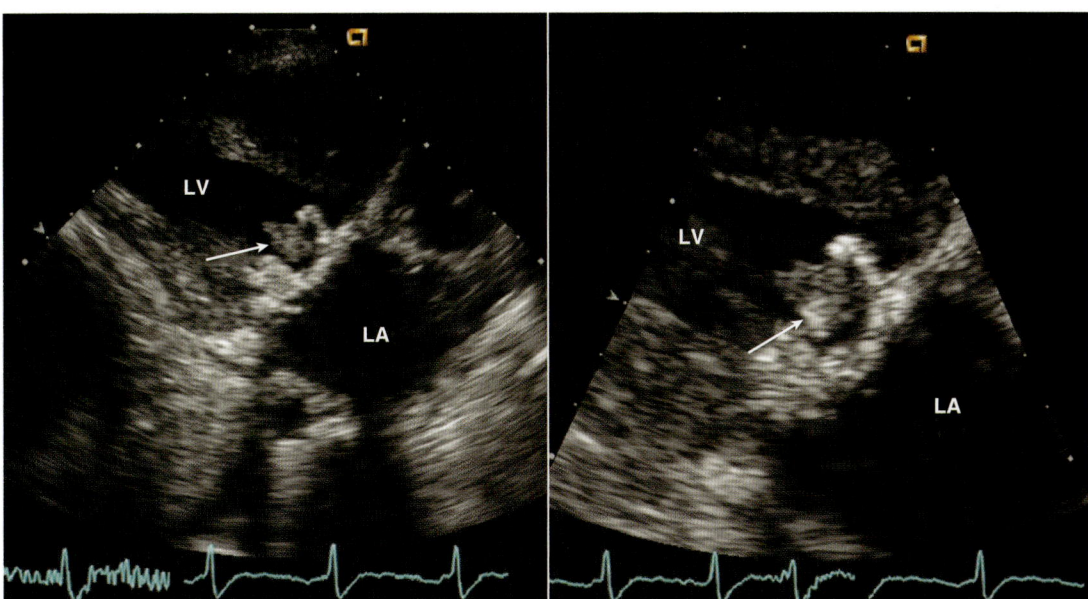

Fig. 13.28 Bioprosthetic mitral valve endocarditis. *(Left)* Although TTE images often are nondiagnostic for prosthetic valve endocarditis, the large valvular vegetation on the stented tissue mitral prosthesis in this patient is obvious *(arrow)* in a low parasternal long-axis view. In the image on the right, the depth has been decreased to improve image resolution, which allows the vegetation within the struts of the prosthetic valve to be seen.

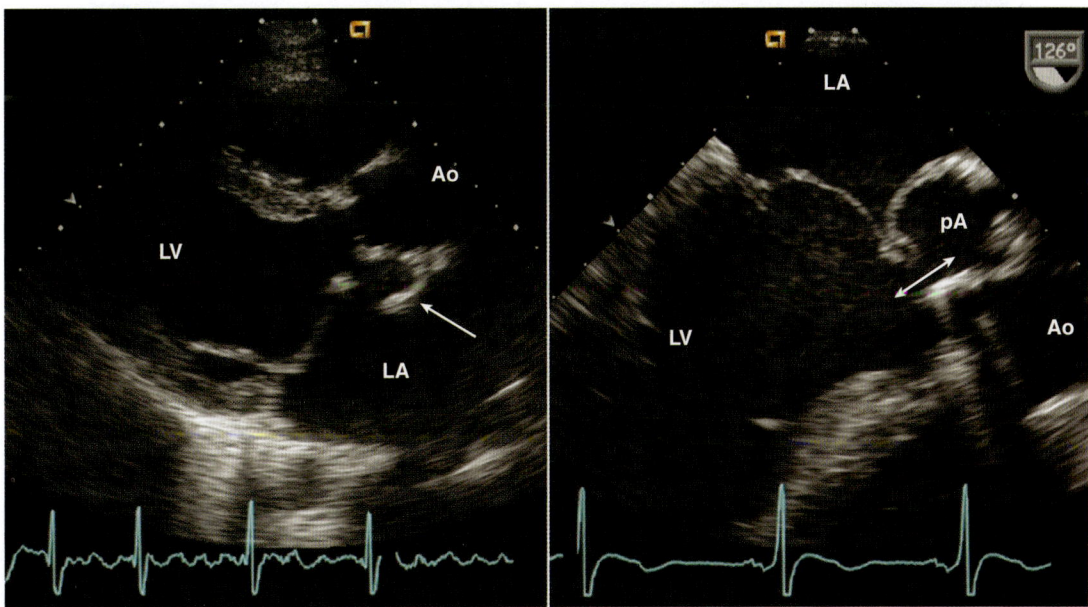

Fig. 13.29 Aneurysm of the mitral aortic intravalvular fibrosa. In a 28-year-old man with a mechanical aortic valve replacement, the TTE long-axis image *(left)* shows a pseudoaneurysm between the posterior aspect of the aortic prosthesis and the base of the anterior mitral leaflet *(arrow)*. The corresponding TEE image *(right)* shows the narrow neck of the pseudoaneurysm *(pA; double arrow)*. Doppler color flow imaging showed flow into the pseudoaneurysm from the LV in systole (with flow back into the LV) and the associated collapse of the pseudoaneurysm in diastole. *Ao,* Aorta.

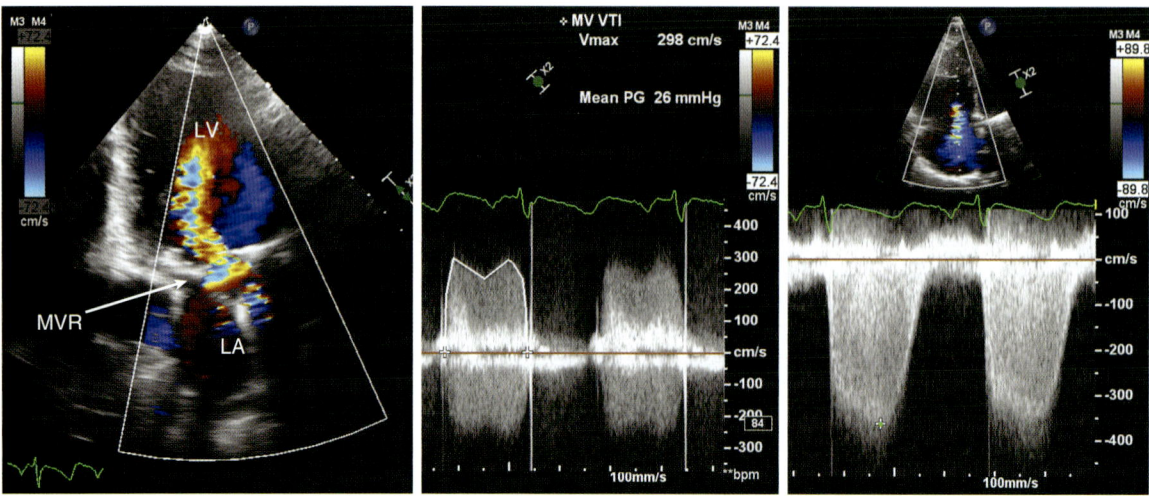

Fig. 13.30 ▶ **Mechanical mitral valve thrombosis on transthoracic echocardiography imaging.** This pregnant woman with a bileaflet mechanical mitral valve *(MV)* presented with acute heart failure. TTE shows a narrow inflow stream on color Doppler in an apical two-chamber view *(left)*. The CW Doppler mean transmitral gradient *(PG; center)* is markedly elevated at 26 mmHg with a prolonged pressure half-time. The CW Doppler signal of the tricuspid regurgitant jet *(right)* shows a peak velocity *(Vmax)* of 3.6 m/s. Estimated RA pressure was 10 mmHg, so that estimated pulmonary systolic pressure is 46 mmHg. Her previous echocardiograms had shown a transmitral gradient of 4 to 5 mmHg and normal pulmonary pressures. Thus, these findings suggest prosthetic valve stenosis, likely due to acute thrombosis. *MVR,* Mitral valve replacement; *VTI,* velocity-time integral.

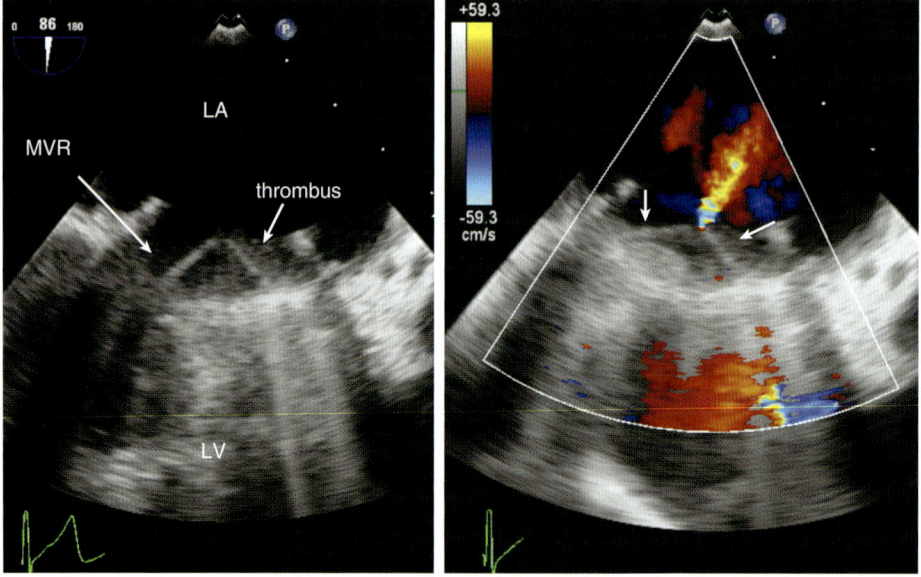

Fig. 13.31 Transesophageal echocardiography mechanical mitral valve thrombosis. In the same patient as Fig. 13.30, TEE imaging shows the prosthetic mitral valve replacement *(MVR)* in diastole *(left)* ▶ and systole *(right)* ▶ with normal motion of one of the valve occluders *(arrows)*. The other occluder is immobile with hazy echo densities filling the normal valve orifice consistent with thrombosis, which was confirmed at surgery.

embolic event in a patient with a prosthetic valve (especially mechanical) presumably is related to the presence of a prosthetic valve, even if TEE echocardiography is negative. Thus, the potential clinical implications of the study results should be considered *before* the examination. If the treatment and subsequent management would be the same whether or not a thrombus is documented, then TEE echocardiography is not necessary. If documentation of a thrombus or exclusion of other possible abnormalities would affect patient management, then TEE echocardiography examination is appropriate. Because infected pannus due to prosthetic valve endocarditis cannot be differentiated from thrombus on ultrasound imaging, careful clinical and bacteriologic correlation is needed whenever an abnormal valve-associated mass is observed (Figs. 13.30 and 13.31).

Prosthetic Valves | Chapter 13   397

THE ECHO EXAM

Transthoracic Evaluation of Prosthetic Valves

Components	Modality	View	Recording	Measurements
Antegrade flow velocity	Pulsed or CW Doppler	Apical	• Antegrade transmitral or transaortic velocity	• Peak velocity (compare with normal values for valve type and size)

Measures of valve stenosis	Pulsed and CW Doppler	Apical	• Careful positioning to obtain highest-velocity signal across prosthetic valve
			• LV outflow velocity proximal to aortic valve
			• Annular diameter
				• Maximum velocity and mean gradient
				• Aortic valve prostheses
				  • Continuity equation valve area (central flow)
				  • Ratio of LVOT to aortic velocity
				  • Acceleration time
				  • Shape of CW Doppler curve
				• Mitral valve
				  • Continuity equation valve area
				  • Pressure half-time

Valve regurgitation	Color imaging and CW Doppler	Parasternal, apical, SSN	• Jet origin, direction, and size on color Doppler • CW Doppler of each valve • Pulmonary vein flow • Descending aorta flow	• Vena contracta width • Paravalvular regurgitation extent around valve • Intensity of CW Doppler signal • Pulmonary vein systolic flow reversal (MR) • Descending aorta flow reversal (AR)
Pulmonary pressures	CW Doppler	RV inflow and apical	• TR jet velocity • IVC size and variation	• Calculate PAP as $4v^2$ of TR jet plus estimated RA pressure.
LV	2D or 3D imaging	Apical	• Apical biplane images of LV or 3D volumetric data set	• 3D or biplane LV volumes and ejection fraction

AR, Aortic regurgitation; *IVC*, inferior vena cava; *LVOT*, LV outflow tract; *MR*, mitral regurgitation; *PAP*, pulmonary artery pressure; *SSN*, Suprasternal notch; *TR*, tricuspid regurgitation.

TEE Evaluation of Prosthetic Valves

Components	Modality	View	Recording	Limitations
Valve imaging	2D and 3D echo	High esophageal	• Mitral valve in high esophageal 4-chamber view • Aortic valve in high esophageal long- and short-axis views	• Aortic valve prosthesis shadows anterior segments of the aortic valve. • With both aortic and mitral prostheses, the aortic shadow obscures the mitral prosthesis.
Antegrade flow velocity	Pulsed or CW Doppler	High esophageal or transgastric apical	• Antegrade transmitral or transaortic velocity	• Alignment of Doppler beam with transaortic valve flow is problematic; compare with TTE data
Measures of valve stenosis	Pulsed and CW Doppler	High esophageal or transgastric apical	• Careful positioning to obtain highest-velocity signal	• Maximum velocity • Mean gradient • Aortic valves: ratio of LVOT to aortic velocity (alignment often suboptimal) • Mitral valve: pressure half-time

Continued

Basic Principles—cont'd				
Components	**Modality**	**View**	**Recording**	**Limitations**
Valve regurgitation	Color imaging and CW Doppler	High esophageal with rotational scan	• Document origin of jet and proximal flow acceleration, and jet size and direction.	• Measure vena contracta, record pulmonary venous flow pattern, search carefully for eccentric jets.
Pulmonary pressures	CW Doppler	RV inflow and apical	• TR jet velocity • IVC size and variation	• Calculate PAP as $4v^2$ of TR jet plus estimated RA pressure. • Difficult to align Doppler beam parallel to TR jet; correlate with TTE data.

IVC, Inferior vena cava; *LVOT*, LV outflow tract; *PAP*, pulmonary artery pressure; *TR*, tricuspid regurgitation.

SUGGESTED READING

Guidelines

1. Zoghbi WA, Chambers JB, Dumesnil JG, et al: Recommendations for evaluation of prosthetic valves with echocardiography and Doppler ultrasound: a report from the American Society of Echocardiography's Guidelines and Standards Committee and the Task Force on Prosthetic Valves, *J Am Soc Echocardiogr* 22(9):975–1014, 2009.
   Detailed consensus document with recommendations for echocardiographic evaluation of prosthetic valves. Tables provide definitions for mild, moderate, and severe prosthetic stenosis and regurgitation. Online supplements provide tables for normal values for each valve type and size in addition to video images of typical findings. An extensive list of references is provided. Essential reading.

2. Lancellotti P, Pibarot P, Chambers J, et al: 2016 Recommendations for the imaging assessment of prosthetic heart valves: a report from the European Association of Cardiovascular Imaging endorsed by the Chinese Society of Echocardiography, *Eur Heart J Cardiovasc Imaging* 17:589–590, 2016.
   Recommendations for use of echocardiography for evaluation of prosthetic heart valve function, timing of routine monitoring, and diagnosis of patient-prosthesis mismatch. Includes details of prosthetic valve models and types, advantages, and limitations of different imaging modalities, in addition to echocardiographic evaluation.

Prosthetic Valve Hemodynamics

3. Yoganathan AP, Raghav V: Fluid dynamics of prosthetic valves. In Otto CM, editor: *The Practice of Clinical Echocardiography*, 5th ed, Philadelphia, 2017, Elsevier, pp 433–454.
   Review of the basic principles of fluid dynamics and the application of fluid dynamics to the evaluation of prosthetic heart valves. Extensive tables summarize in vitro data for each valve type and size. Illustrations show the flow patterns for each valve type. Mathematical descriptions of fluid dynamics are included.

4. O'Gara PT: Prosthetic heart valves. In Otto CM, Bonow RO, editors: *Valvular Heart Disease*, 4th ed, Philadelphia, 2013, Elsevier, pp 420–438.
   Clinical review of prosthetic heart valves with sections on hemodynamics and long-term outcome for each valve type, medical management of patients with prosthetic valves, and evaluation and treatment of prosthetic valve dysfunction.

5. Chambers JB: The echocardiography of replacement heart valves, *Echo Res Pract* 3(3):R35–R43, 2016.
   Concise review of the echocardiographic approach to evaluation of prosthetic heart valves with numerous images and videos. Includes summary of guidelines. Free access.

Surgical Prosthetic Valve Dysfunction

6. Mahjoub H, Dahou A, Dumesnil JG, et al: Echocardiographic recognition and quantitation of prosthetic valve dysfunction. In Otto CM, editor: *The Practice of Clinical Echocardiography*, 5th ed, Philadelphia, 2017, Elsevier, pp 455–482.
   Advanced-level review and discussion of echocardiographic evaluation of prosthetic valve dysfunction. Numerous tables summarize normal values for prosthetic valves and findings reported with abnormal valve function. Excellent photographs and echocardiographic images of each valve type. Complications reviewed include mechanical failure, thrombosis, endocarditis, patient-prosthesis mismatch, prosthetic stenosis, and regurgitation.

7. Dumesnil J, Pibarot P: Doppler echocardiographic evaluation of prosthetic valve function, *Heart* 98:69–78, 2012.
   Detailed text and elegant illustrations highlight echocardiographic evaluation of prosthetic valve dysfunction. An algorithm for the evaluation of high prosthetic valve gradients is provided, emphasizing importance of indexed effective orifice area. Causes of apparent high Doppler velocities with a bileaflet mechanical valve include a central jet artifact, occult mitral regurgitation, a high flow state, significant prosthetic aortic regurgitation, technical error, and prosthetic valve stenosis.

8. Bach DS: Echo/Doppler evaluation of hemodynamics after aortic valve replacement: principles of interrogation and evaluation of high gradients, *JACC Cardiovasc Imaging* 3:296–304, 2010.
   Focused discussion of causes of a high Doppler velocity after aortic valve replacement. Possible causes include mistaking an mitral regurgitant jet for LV outflow, overtracing the Doppler spectral signal, a high flow state (e.g., fever, anemia, hyperthyroid, aortic regurgitation), and the pressure recovery phenomenon. Causes of prosthetic valve obstruction include biologic leaflet calcification; thrombus, pannus, or

vegetation preventing normal occluder motion; subvalvular or supravalvular obstruction; and patient-prosthesis mismatch.

9. Oxorn DC, Otto CM: Surgical prosthetic valves. In Oxorn DC, Otto CM, editors: *Intraoperative and Interventional Echocardiography: Atlas of Transesophageal Imaging*, Philadelphia., 2017, Elsevier, pp 149–204.

    This print and digital atlas chapter includes 20 cases of prosthetic valve dysfunction requiring surgical intervention. Echocardiographic images and videos are accompanied by surgical views and pathological correlation.

Transcatheter Aortic Valves

10. Bloomfield GS, Gillam LD, Hahn RT, et al: A practical guide to multimodality imaging of transcatheter aortic valve replacement, *JACC Cardiovasc Imaging* 5(4):441–455, 2012.

    This review of the approach to imaging the patient being considered for transcatheter aortic valve implantation is essential reading. The 3D anatomy of the aortic valve is reviewed, the measurements needed for clinical decision making (especially aortic annulus diameter) are described, and the findings that might preclude transcatheter aortic valve implantation are summarized. The role of other imaging modalities is presented with excellent illustrations of the typical findings.

11. Pislaru SV, Nkomo VT, Sandhu GS: Assessment of prosthetic valve function after TAVR, *JACC Cardiovasc Imaging.* 9(2):193–206, 2016.

    Systematic review of the approach to echocardiographic evaluation of balloon-expandable and self-expanding bioprosthetic transcatheter aortic valves. Imaging should address valve position and leaflet motion, color Doppler for aortic regurgitation, CW Doppler for transaortic velocity, gradient and calculation of effective valve area, and assessment of LV size and systolic function. Complications with transcatheter valves that might be detected on echocardiography including malposition, thrombosis, obstruction, and paravalvular regurgitation. 16 figures and 15 online videos. An excellent introduction for centers doing transcatheter valve implantation.

12. Otto CM, Kumbhani DJ, Alexander KP, et al: 2017 ACC expert consensus decision pathway for transcatheter aortic valve replacement in the management of adults with aortic stenosis: a report of the American College of Cardiology Task Force on Clinical Expert Consensus Documents, *J Am Coll Cardiol* 69:1313–1346, 2017.

    Detailed checklist for management of patients undergoing transcatheter valve implantation, including key elements of imaging by echocardiography and other modalities before, during, and after the procedure. An essential reference for every echocardiography laboratory.

14 Endocarditis

BASIC PRINCIPLES

ECHOCARDIOGRAPHIC APPROACH
  Valvular Vegetations
    Transthoracic Echocardiography
    Transesophageal Imaging
    Diagnostic Accuracy
  Valve Dysfunction
  Paravalvular Abscess and Intracardiac Fistula
  Other Echocardiographic Findings

LIMITATIONS AND TECHNICAL CONSIDERATIONS
  Active Versus Healed Vegetations
  Nonbacterial Thrombotic Endocarditis

  Diagnosis With Underlying Valve Disease
  Prosthetic Valves and Intracardiac Devices

CLINICAL UTILITY
  Suspected Endocarditis
  Known Endocarditis
  Alternate Approaches

THE ECHO EXAM

SUGGESTED READING

Echocardiography is an essential component of the evaluation of a patient with infective endocarditis. In combination with clinical and bacteriologic data, the echocardiographic finding of a valvular vegetation allows for an accurate diagnosis of endocarditis. In addition, echocardiographic assessment of the degree of valve dysfunction and detection of complications, such as a paravalvular abscess or fistula, are needed for optimal patient care.

Although transthoracic echocardiography (TTE) is adequate in some cases, transesophageal echocardiography (TEE) imaging is more sensitive and specific, both for the detection of valvular vegetations and for the detection of complications. Furthermore, demonstration of normal valve anatomy and function on TEE imaging reliably excludes endocarditis in patients in whom this diagnosis is suspected.

BASIC PRINCIPLES

The diagnosis of endocarditis is most secure with pathologic confirmation of a valvular vegetation with active infection, local tissue destruction, and/or paravalvular abscess formation. In the clinical setting, endocarditis is diagnosed based on a combination of echocardiographic, laboratory, and physical examination findings, as detailed in Table 14.1. The major criteria for the diagnosis of endocarditis are persistent bacteremia with typical organisms and echocardiographic evidence of endocardial involvement. Minor criteria include less specific bacteriologic and echocardiographic findings, factors predisposing to endocarditis (e.g., preexisting valve disease or intravenous drug use), vascular events (e.g., pulmonary or systemic emboli), immunologic phenomena (e.g., glomerulonephritis), and signs of systemic infection (e.g., fever).

The goals of echocardiography in a patient with a diagnosis of infective endocarditis are to evaluate the:

- Presence, location, size, and number of valvular vegetations
- Dysfunction of the affected valve(s), especially valvular regurgitation
- Underlying anatomy of the affected valve(s) and any coincident valvular disease
- Impact of valvular dysfunction on left ventricle (LV) size and systolic function
- Other complications of endocarditis (e.g., paravalvular abscess, pericardial effusion)

In addition, echocardiographic findings provide prognostic data on the anticipated clinical course, the risk of systemic embolization, and the indications for and timing of surgical intervention.

In a patient with a low likelihood of endocarditis on clinical grounds, an echocardiogram often is requested to "rule out" endocarditis. In this setting, the goals of the echocardiographic examination are:

- The identification of any valvular vegetations
- The assessment of valve anatomy and function with respect to anatomic or physiologic factors that increase the likelihood of endocarditis (e.g., bicuspid aortic valve, mitral valve prolapse)

If an abnormality is identified, complete evaluation is directed toward the goals listed for clinical endocarditis. If no vegetations are identified on transthoracic imaging, additional imaging studies still are often needed, depending on the clinical situation.

TABLE 14.1 Duke Criteria for Infective Endocarditis With European Society of Cardiology 2015 Modification

Pathologic Criteria

Microorganisms: demonstrated by culture of histology in a vegetation, *or* in a vegetation that has embolized, *or* in an intracardiac abscess

Pathologic lesions: vegetation or intracardiac abscess present, confirmed by histology showing active endocarditis

Clinical Criteria

Definite endocarditis:	2 major criteria *or* 1 major and 3 minor criteria *or* 5 minor criteria
Possible endocarditis:	1 major plus 1 minor *or* 3 minor criteria
Rejected endocarditis:	Firm alternate diagnosis Resolution of symptoms with antibiotic Rx ≤4 days No pathologic evidence of endocarditis at surgery with antibiotic Rx ≤4 days Does not meet criteria for possible endocarditis

Major Criteria

Positive Blood Culture for Infective Endocarditis

- Typical microorganism for infective endocarditis from two separate blood cultures: viridans streptococci,* *Streptococcus gallolyticus* (*S. bovis*), HACEK group, *Staphylococcus aureus*; or community-acquired enterococci, in the absence of a primary focus; *or*
- Persistently positive blood culture, defined as recovery of a microorganism consistent with infective endocarditis from:
  - At least 2 blood cultures drawn more than 12 hours apart, *or*
  - All of 3 or a majority of 4 or more separate blood cultures, with first and last drawn at least 1 hour apart
- Positive blood culture for *Coxiella burnetii* or anti–phase 1 IgG antibody titer >1:800

Evidence of Endocardial Involvement

- Positive echocardiogram for infective endocarditis
  - Vegetation,
  - Abscess, pseudoaneurysm, intracardiac fistula,
  - Valvular perforation or aneurysm,
  - New partial dehiscence of prosthetic valve, *or*
- Abnormal activity around the site of prosthetic valve implantation detected by ^{18}F-FDG PET/CT (>3 months after implantation) or radiolabeled leucocytes with SPECT/CT
- Definite paravalvular lesions by cardiac CT

Minor Criteria

- Predisposition: predisposing heart condition *or* injection drug use
- Fever >38.0° C (100.4° F)
- Vascular phenomena including those detected by imaging: major arterial emboli, septic pulmonary infarcts, mycotic aneurysm, intracranial hemorrhage, conjunctival hemorrhages, Janeway lesions
- Immunologic phenomena: glomerulonephritis, Osler nodes, Roth spots, rheumatoid factor
- Microbiologic evidence: positive blood culture but not meeting major criterion as noted previously[†] *or* serologic evidence of active infection with organism consistent with infective endocarditis

*Including nutritional variant strains.
[†]Excluding single positive cultures for coagulase-negative staphylococci and organisms that do not cause endocarditis.
CT, Computed tomography; ^{18}F-FDG, 18-fluorine–fluorodeoxyglucose; HACEK, Haemophilus spp., Actinobacillus actinomycetemcomitans, Cardiobacterium hominis; Eikenella spp., and Kingella kingae; IgG, immunoglobulin G; PET, positron emission tomography; SPECT, single photon emission computed tomography.
From Habib G, Lancellotti P, Antunes MJ, et al: 2015 ESC guidelines for the management of infective endocarditis. *Eur Heart J* 21;36(44):3075–3128, 2015, as adapted from Li JS, Sexton DJ, Mick N, et al: Proposed modification to the Duke criteria for the diagnosis of infective endocarditis. *Clin Infect Dis* 30:633–638, 2000.

Chapter 14 | Endocarditis

ECHOCARDIOGRAPHIC APPROACH

Valvular Vegetations

Transthoracic Echocardiography

On echocardiographic imaging, features typical features of a valvular vegetation (Table 14.2) are:

- An abnormal echogenic, irregular mass, usually attached to a valve
- Site of attachment on the upstream side of the valve leaflet
- A pattern of motion that is dependent on, but more chaotic than, normal valve motion

For example, an aortic valve vegetation is attached to the LV side of the valve leaflet but shows motion in excess of normal valve excursion with rapid oscillations in diastole (best appreciated on M-mode recordings). Typically, an aortic valve vegetation prolapses into the LV outflow tract in diastole and extends into the aortic root in systole (Fig. 14.1). A mitral valve vegetation is attached on the atrial side of the valve, prolapses into the left atrium (LA) in systole, and moves into the LV, beyond the normal range of mitral valve opening, in diastole (Fig. 14.2), again with rapid motion independent of normal leaflet motion.

Valvular vegetations vary in size from so small as to be undetectable with current imaging techniques to greater than 3 cm in length. Vegetations can be attached at any area of the leaflet, although lesions at the coaptation line are most common. More than one valve can be involved, either by direct extension of infection or as a separate process, thus emphasizing the caveat that each valve requires careful examination even if a vegetation has been identified on another valve. In most but not all cases, endocarditis occurs on a previously abnormal valve.

Multiple acoustic windows and two-dimensional (2D) or three-dimensional (3D) views are needed for the detection of a valvular vegetation. Because the vegetation is a focal structure, it is seen only in certain tomographic planes. 3D imaging often improves visualization of vegetations on transthoracic echocardiography in some patients, depending on image quality, but it has the disadvantage of lower spatial resolution and slower frame rates.

With 2D imaging, slow scanning between the standard image planes—for example, between the parasternal long-axis view and the right ventricular (RV) inflow view—increases the likelihood of identifying a valvular vegetation. Orthogonal views further ensure that all segments of the valve leaflets are examined. In a patient with suspected endocarditis, a complete examination is needed with scanning from parasternal, apical, subcostal, and suprasternal notch views for careful evaluation of each valve. The reported sensitivity of transthoracic imaging for the detection of valvular vegetations ranges from less than 50% to as high as 90% (see Appendix B, Table B.18).

AORTIC VALVE. Aortic valve vegetations most often are detected in parasternal long- and short-axis views. Careful angulation from medial to lateral in the long-axis plane and from inferior to superior in the short-axis plane is needed because vegetations often are eccentrically located. Image quality is optimized by use of a minimum depth setting and adjustment of gain and processing parameters. An echogenic mass attached to the ventricular side of the leaflet with independent motion and prolapse into the outflow tract in diastole is diagnostic for a valvular vegetation (Fig. 14.3). Rapid oscillating motion is best appreciated on an M-mode recording.

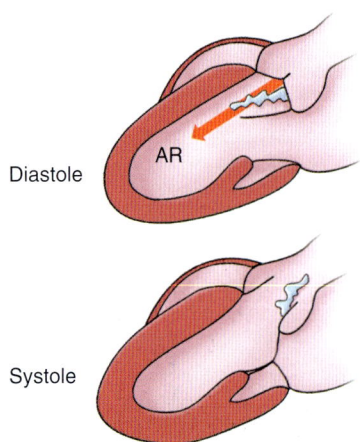

Fig. 14.1 Schematic diagram of an aortic valve vegetation. An irregularly shaped mobile mass is attached to the ventricular side of the leaflet with prolapse into the LV outflow tract in diastole. *AR,* Aortic regurgitation.

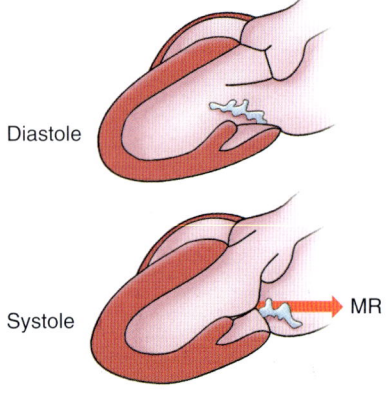

Fig. 14.2 Schematic diagram of a mitral valve vegetation. An irregularly shaped mobile mass is attached to the atrial side of the leaflet with prolapse into the LA in systole. *MR,* Mitral regurgitation.

TABLE 14.2 Diagnosis of Endocarditis: Echocardiographic-Clinical Correlates

	Definition	Exam Points	Diagnostic Value	Limitations
Valvular vegetations	Mass attached to leaflet with independent motion	Use multiple acoustic windows and image planes. Angle between standard views. Use a high-frequency transducer and zoom mode.	Vegetations have high specificity for diagnosis of endocarditis. TEE is more sensitive than TTE for detection of vegetations.	Noninfective masses, healed vegetations, and artifacts may be mistaken for a vegetation.
Leaflet destruction	New or worsening valve regurgitation	Use standard Doppler approaches for detection and quantitation of valve dysfunction.	Valve dysfunction in association with a vegetation is diagnostic for endocarditis.	Other causes of valve dysfunction must be considered. With prosthetic mitral valve, TEE is essential for evaluation of valve function when endocarditis is suspected.
Abscess	Infected area adjacent to valve, usually in the aortic or mitral annulus	Use multiple acoustic windows and image planes. Angle between standard views. Use zoom mode.	TEE is much more sensitive than TTE for detection of paravalvular abscess.	Cardiac abscesses may be echolucent or echodense.
Aneurysm or pseudoaneurysm	Localized dilation of a valve leaflet, aortic sinus, or aortic-mitral intervalvular fibrosa (aneurysm) or a contained rupture (pseudoaneurysm)	Look for an abnormal contour of valve leaflets, aortic sinuses, or a space between the base on the anterior mitral leaflet and aortic root. Examine the paraaortic region for excess echodensity. Use color Doppler to examine flow in these regions.	Echo findings of aneurysm or pseudoaneurysm are accurate and can be used for clinical decision making.	TEE often is needed for accurate diagnosis.
Fistula	Abnormal communication between cardiac chambers or great vessels	An aortic paravalvular abscess can rupture into the LA, RA, or RV outflow tract.	Color Doppler detection of abnormal flow combined with pulsed and CW Doppler to define flow hemodynamics is diagnostic for a fistula	The full extent of tissue destruction is difficult to assess with imaging approaches.
Prosthetic valve dehiscence	Detachment (partial) of the prosthetic valve from the annular tissue	Look for excess motion ("rocking") of the prosthetic valve (>20°).	Valve dehiscence usually is accompanied by severe paravalvular regurgitation.	Valve "rocking" is diagnostic but rarely seen.

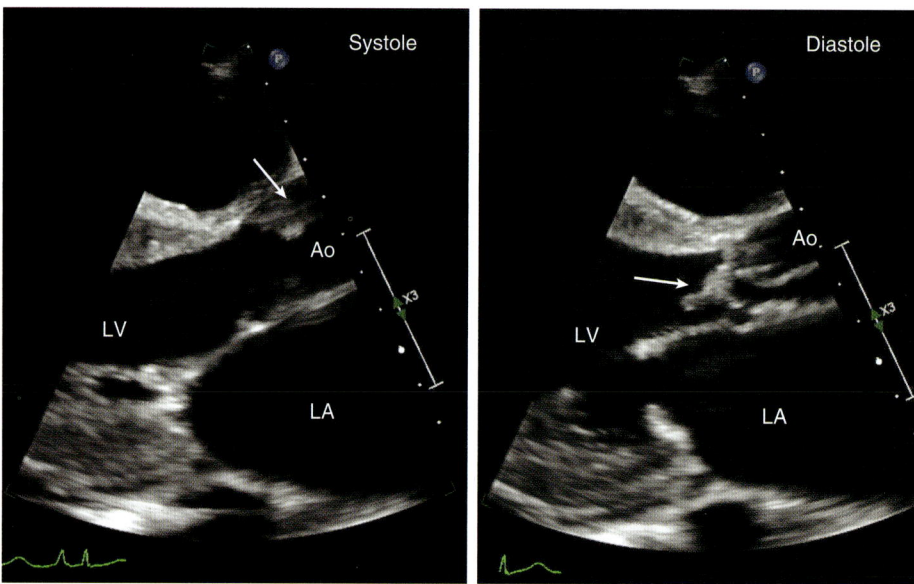

Fig. 14.3 ▶ **Aortic valve vegetation.** In a TTE parasternal long-axis view, a large echodensity *(arrow)* is seen in the aorta *(Ao)* attached to the anterior aortic valve leaflet in systole with prolapse into the LV outflow tract in diastole. In addition to moving with the leaflet, the mass showed rapid oscillating motion typical of a vegetation.

Less typically, a vegetation is attached to the aortic side of the leaflet or shows little independent motion. A definitive diagnosis is more difficult if the underlying valve anatomy is abnormal. For example, a vegetation on a calcified aortic valve may be difficult to diagnose because of shadowing and reverberations by the leaflet calcification. In these cases, the findings of independent motion and prolapse into the LV in diastole are particularly helpful signs. Recent changes compared with previous echocardiograms increase the likelihood of valve infection; stable findings compared with previous studies decrease the likelihood of an acute process.

Findings that may be mistaken for an aortic valve vegetation include beam-width artifact related to a calcified nodule, a prosthetic valve, the normal leaflet apposition zone, or the normal leaflet thickening at the central coaptation region (the nodule of Arantius). Occasionally, a linear echo representing a normal variant called a *Lambl excrescence* is seen. These small fibroelastic protrusions from the ventricular side of the leaflet closure zone occur with increasing frequency with age and are present in a high percentage of patients (Fig. 14.4).

An aortic valve vegetation also may be seen in apical views, both from an anteriorly angulated four-chamber view and from an apical long-axis view. The finding of an abnormality in both parasternal and apical views decreases the likelihood of an ultrasound artifact because the relationship of the ultrasound beam and the aortic valve is entirely different from these two windows. Aortic valve vegetations typically are accompanied by new or worsening aortic regurgitation (Fig. 14.5).

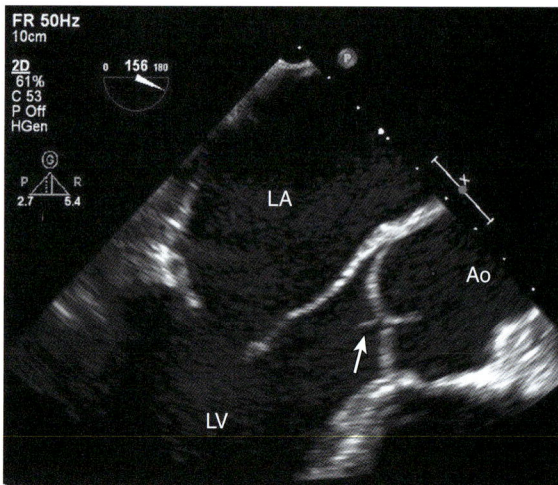

Fig. 14.4 ▶ **Lambl excrescence.** TEE long-axis view showing a thin, linear echodensity *(arrow)* at the aortic closure line that may be mistaken for a valvular vegetation. *Ao,* Aorta.

MITRAL VALVE. Mitral valve vegetations typically are located on the atrial side of the leaflets. Diagnostic features include rapid independent motion, prolapse into the LA in systole, and functional evidence of valve dysfunction. Parasternal long- and short-axis views with careful scanning across the valve apparatus in both image planes allow assessment of the presence, size, and location of any vegetations (Fig. 14.6). Apical four-chamber, two-chamber, and long-axis views again are helpful both in visualizing valve and vegetation anatomy and in distinguishing a true valve mass from an ultrasound artifact.

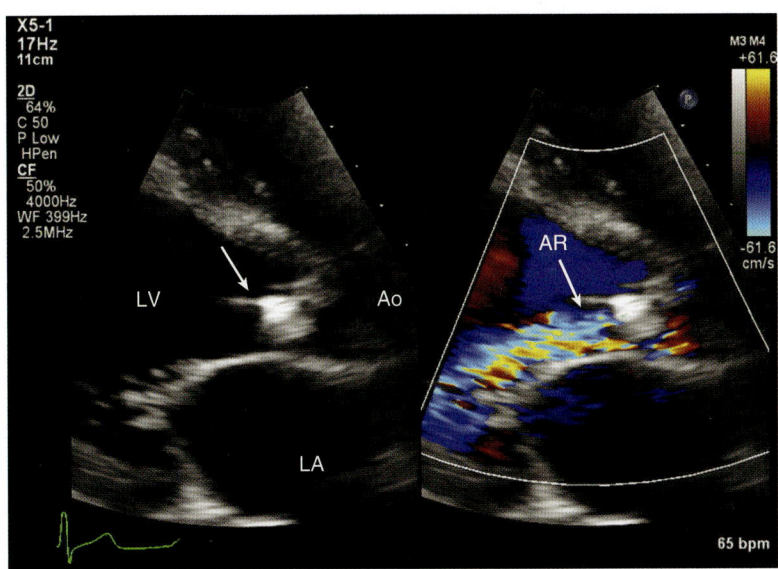

Fig. 14.5 **Aortic valve vegetation and regurgitation.** In a TTE apical long-axis view *(left)*, a large aortic valve vegetation is seen prolapsing into the LV outflow tract in diastole. The color Doppler image *(right)* shows a broad jet of aortic regurgitation *(AR, arrow)* around the vegetation. *Ao,* Aorta.

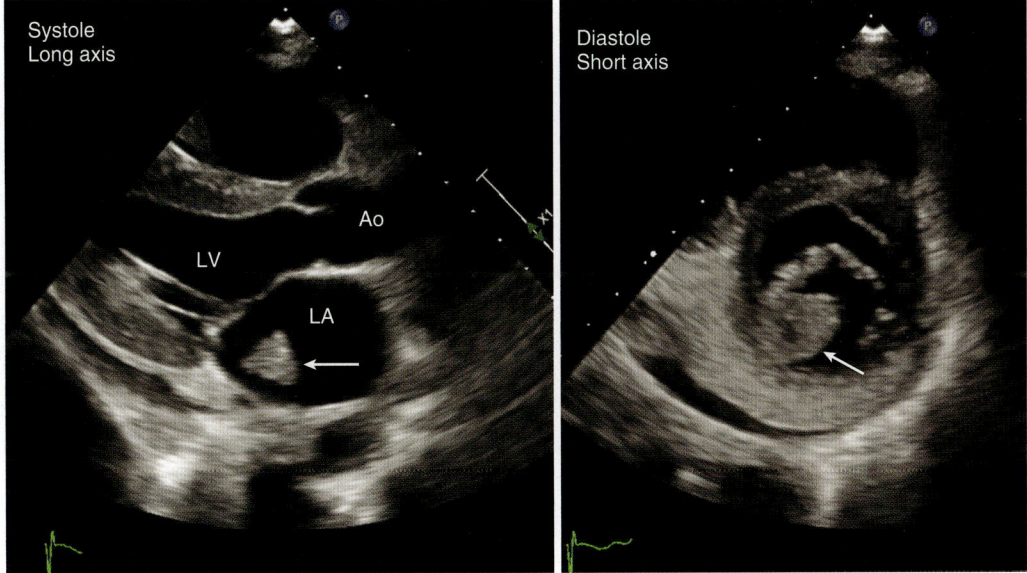

Fig. 14.6 **Mitral valve vegetation.** Typical-appearing mitral valve vegetations *(arrow)* seen in the parasternal long-axis view in systole that are prolapsed into the LA *(left)*. In a short-axis diastolic view *(right)*, the mass *(arrow)* is attached to the medial aspect of both the anterior and posterior leaflets. A small pericardial effusion also is present. *Ao,* Aorta.

As for the aortic valve, beam-width artifacts can be mistaken for a vegetation. A particular artifact to be aware of is the appearance of a "mass" on the atrial side of the anterior mitral leaflet in the apical four-chamber view due to beam-width artifact from a calcified or prosthetic aortic valve. Other types of mitral valve pathology that are difficult to distinguish from a valvular vegetation include a severely myxomatous leaflet, a partial flail leaflet, and a ruptured papillary muscle. Again, comparison with previous studies helps differentiate an acute process from chronic underlying valve disease. Endocarditis also can occur on an anatomically normal valve (Fig. 14.7). With mitral valve endocarditis, mitral regurgitation often, but not invariably, is present.

TRICUSPID VALVE. Tricuspid valve endocarditis occurs most often in intravenous drug users and is associated with large vegetations due to *Staphylococcus aureus* infection. The RV inflow view often is diagnostic, showing a large, mobile mass of echoes attached to the atrial side of the leaflet with prolapse into the right atrium (RA) in systole (Fig. 14.8). Given the range of excursion and mobility of these vegetations, it is not surprising that septic pulmonary

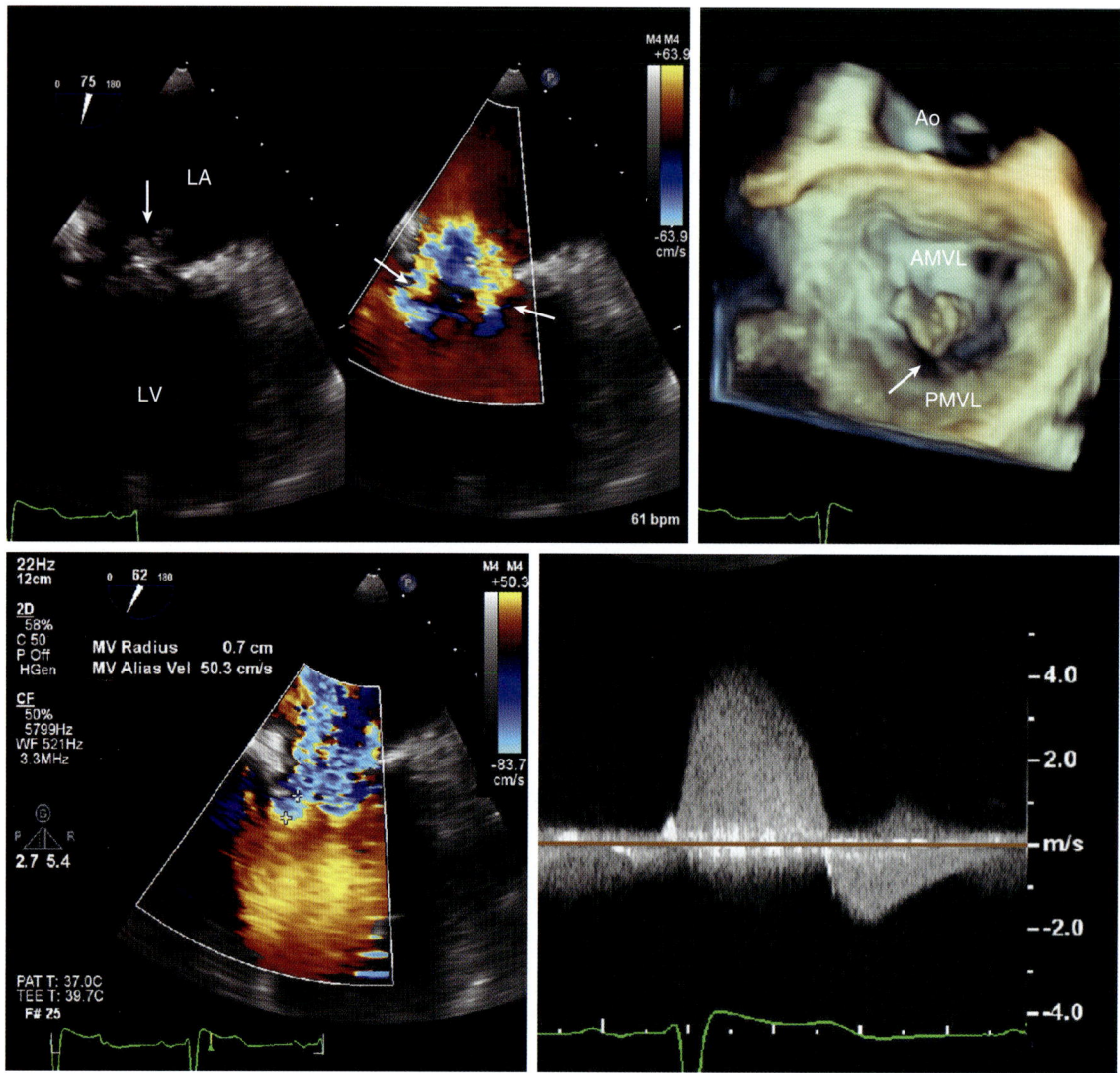

Fig. 14.7 Transesophageal echocardiography imaging of a mitral valve vegetation. TEE imaging in a two-chamber view *(top left)* shows an irregularly shaped mass *(arrow)* attached to the left atrial side of the mitral valve *(MV)* in systole. Color Doppler *(top center)* shows two jets of mitral regurgitation around the vegetation. ▶ The 3D image better demonstrates the attachment of the vegetation *(arrows)* to the center of the anterior mitral valve leaflet *(AMVL)* with the posterior mitral valve leaflet *(PMVL)* seen inferiorly. In the *bottom* images, color Doppler *(bottom left)* has been optimized to show the proximal velocity surgical area with CW Doppler *(bottom right)* showing the high-velocity systolic signal. ▶ Although more than one regurgitant jet is present, the calculated size of the larger regurgitant orifice is 0.39 cm², thus regurgitant is severe. *Ao*, Aorta; *Vel*, velocity.

emboli are frequent complications of tricuspid valve endocarditis. The apical and subcostal four-chamber views allow further evaluation of the presence and extent of tricuspid valve infection. Assessment of tricuspid regurgitant severity and consequent RA and RV dilation also can be performed from these windows.

PACER LEAD INFECTIONS. Infections of intracardiac devices, particularly pacer or defibrillator leads in the right side of the heart, have become increasingly common because of the greater number of patients with these devices. Accurate diagnosis of lead infection is important because therapy typically requires removal of the pacer leads and pacemaker, in addition to prolonged antibiotics. Small fibrinous strands are common on pacer leads, and small thrombi also may be seen. No definitive findings have been identified that distinguish an infected from noninfected pacer lead mass, so infection must be assumed to present when blood culture results are positive. Pacer lead vegetations resemble valvular vegetations—a mobile mass attached to the pacer lead with independent motion. Some pacer lead infections can be diagnosed on transthoracic imaging, but TEE is much more sensitive for this diagnosis and is recommended when this diagnosis is of concern.

Endocarditis | Chapter 14

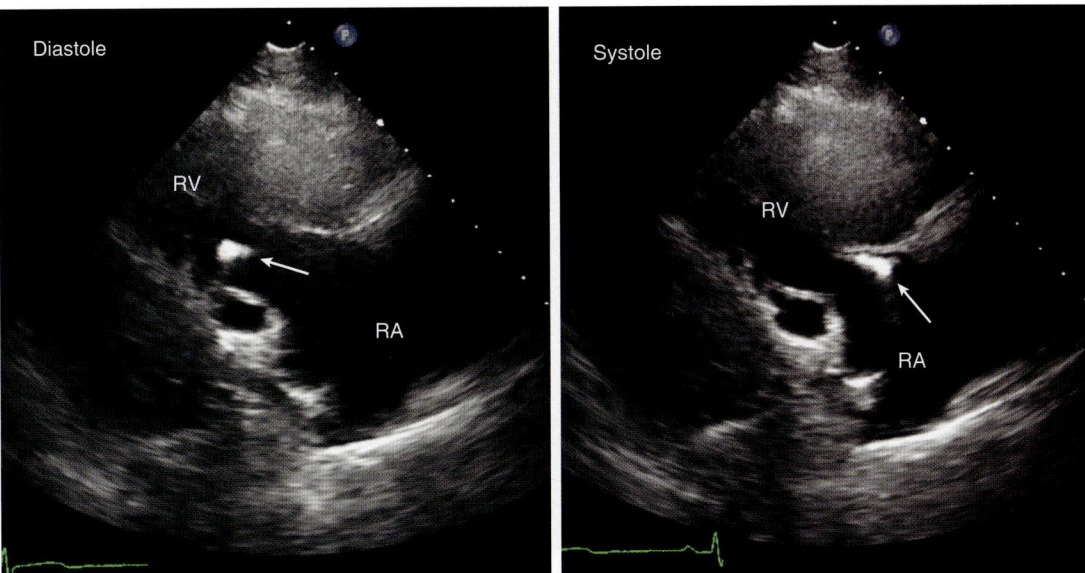

Fig. 14.8 **Tricuspid valve vegetation.** TTE imaging in an RV inflow view of a patient with a history of intravenous drug use and a remote history of tricuspid valve endocarditis. In diastole *(left)*, a bright echodense mass *(arrow)* is seen attached to the valve leaflet. In systole, this mass prolapses into the RA with incomplete tricuspid valve closure resulting in severe tricuspid regurgitation. These findings are consistent with healed endocarditis, although blood cultures were obtained to exclude active infection.

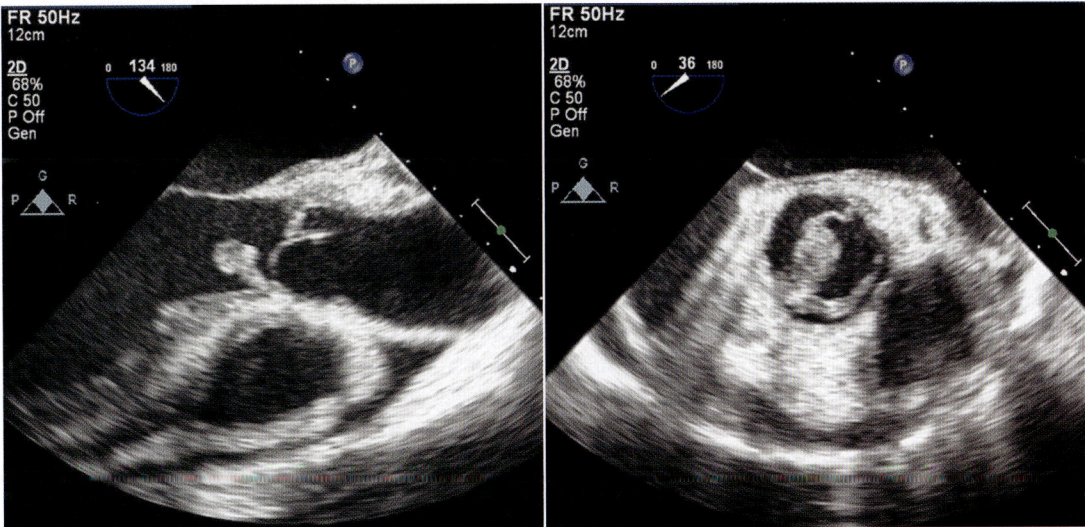

Fig. 14.9 **Transesophageal echocardiography aortic valve vegetation.** In the same patient as in Fig. 14.8, the TEE long-axis view *(left)* shows the attachment of the vegetation at the base of the aortic valve. The short-axis view *(right)* shows that the underlying anatomy is a bicuspid valve with an additional vegetation *(short arrow)* attached to the more posterior valve leaflets. The increased echodensity posterior to the aortic valve in the long-axis views raises concern for paravalvular abscess.

Transesophageal Imaging

From the TEE approach, the aortic valve is examined in multiple 2D image planes, including standard long-axis (typically at approximately 120° rotation) and short-axis (about 45° rotation) views. As with transthoracic imaging, careful scanning from medial to lateral in the long-axis view and from superior to inferior in the short-axis view is needed to evaluate valve anatomy fully and to achieve a high sensitivity for the detection of valvular vegetations (Figs. 14.9 and 14.10). When the image plane is oblique, an en face view of the aortic leaflet may be mistaken for an aortic valve mass. Evaluation in more than one image plane and assessment of the pattern of motion (rapid oscillating independent motion versus motion *with* the valve) avoid this potential error. Image quality is enhanced by the use of a higher-frequency transducer

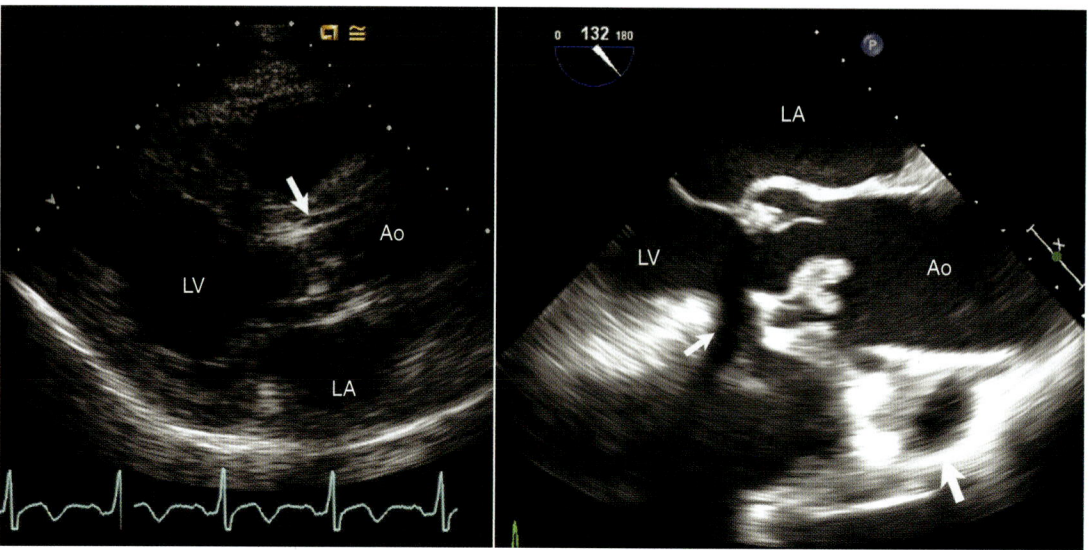

Fig. 14.10 Fungal endocarditis. TTE *(left)* ▶ and TEE *(right)* ▶▶ imaging in a patient with fungal endocarditis. The unusual-appearing valvular vegetation *(arrow)* is seen on TTE imaging but is better defined on TEE imaging, with a dense spherical mass with some small attached areas of independent motion *(arrows)*. *Ao,* Aorta.

and magnification of the area of interest, but small, normal variants of valve anatomy should not be interpreted as abnormalities. Sometimes the aortic valve can be evaluated from a transgastric apical view; however, image quality often is no better than from a transthoracic approach because of the distance from the transducer to the aortic valve. 3D imaging of the aortic valve with a full-volume acquisition to view both the aortic and ventricular sides of the valve is helpful, although it is limited by lower resolution and slower frame rates than those with 2D imaging.

The mitral valve is well seen from a high esophageal position. Because the mitral valve plane is perpendicular to the ultrasound beam from this approach, excellent 2D images can be obtained in multiple views by slowly rotating the multiplane transducer from 0° to 180°. Particular attention should be paid to standard four-chamber (at 0°), two-chamber (at 60°), and long-axis (at 120°) views. The degree of mitral regurgitation can be assessed with color flow imaging in these same views. Given the distance of the mitral valve from the chest wall in both parasternal and apical transthoracic views, TEE imaging often provides dramatically better images and important clinical data (Fig. 14.11). 3D imaging of the mitral valve is particularly helpful because the orientation of the valve to the TEE probe allows acquisition of high-quality 3D datasets that provide 3D views of the left atrial side of the valve. These images help localize the size and attachment site of the vegetations and allow identification of leaflet perforation (see Fig. 14.11).

The tricuspid valve is seen in the TEE four-chamber view and from a transgastric approach. Because the tricuspid valve lies closer to the chest wall than the mitral valve, transthoracic imaging often is diagnostic. TEE imaging is most valuable in these patients for the detection of left-sided valve involvement. TEE also may be diagnostic when infection of a pacer lead is suspected (Fig. 14.12). Again, 3D imaging is particularly valuable for defining the spatial relationship of the vegetation to the pacer lead.

Diagnostic Accuracy

Numerous studies have evaluated the sensitivity of echocardiography for the diagnosis of valvular vegetation by comparing the echo findings with subsequent surgical or autopsy findings. Fewer data are available on specificity because most studies include only subjects with a definite diagnosis of endocarditis. Thus, the study group has no subjects without the disease. Second, when surgical or autopsy inspection of the valve is the standard of reference, only patients who are sick enough to need surgery or who have died are included in the study group. Direct inspection of valves that appeared normal on echocardiography rarely is available.

A few studies (see Appendix B, Table B.18) have circumvented these study design problems by including all patients with *suspected* endocarditis (some have the disease and some do not) and using clinical outcome rather than direct valve inspection as the standard of reference. All these studies demonstrate a high specificity of transthoracic echocardiography (93% to 98%) and TEE (100%) imaging in excluding the diagnosis of endocarditis.

The specificity of echocardiography depends on distinguishing a valvular vegetation from other intracardiac masses and from ultrasound artifacts.

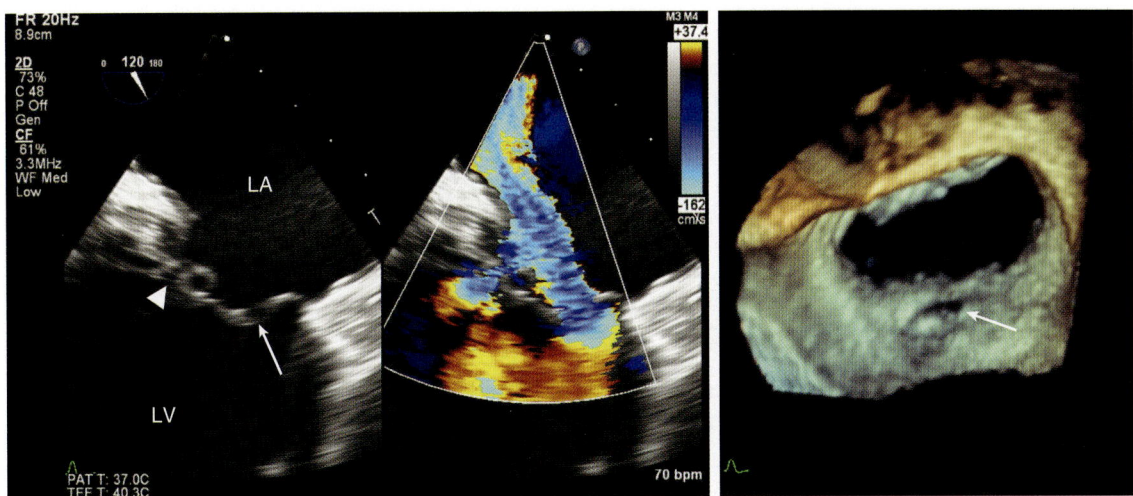

Fig. 14.11 Mitral leaflet perforation. TEE echocardiography in a in a 28-year-old man with systemic embolic events and blood culture results positive for *Staphylococcus aureus*. A view midway between a two-chamber and long-axis view *(left)* ▶ shows an apparent discontinuity in the mitral leaflet *(arrow)*, distant from the normal coaptation plane *(arrowhead)*. Color flow Doppler *(center)* ▶ shows a large eccentric jet of severe mitral regurgitation that goes through the base of the anterior leaflet, consistent with leaflet perforation due to infective endocarditis, as well as a smaller jet at the coaptation plane. The 3D image of the mitral valve from the left atrial size *(right)* ▶ better demonstrates the location and size of the posterior leaflet perforation *(arrow)*.

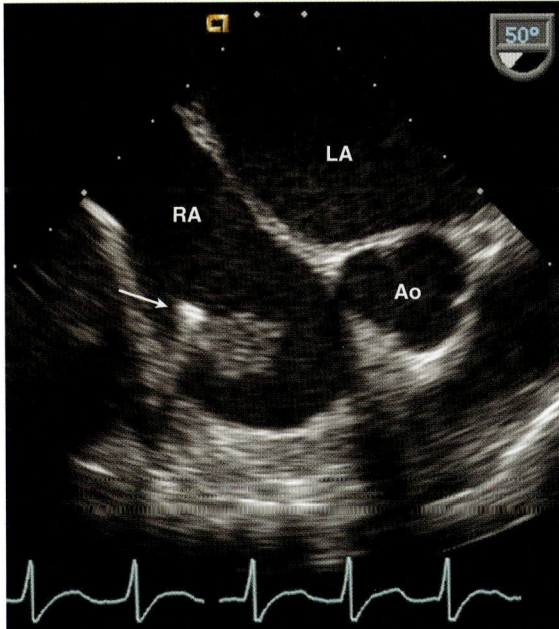

Fig. 14.12 ▶ **Pacer lead infection.** In a TEE short-axis view, a pacer lead *(arrow)* is seen in the RA with an attached mobile echodensity consistent with thrombus or vegetation. Ao, Aorta.

Echocardiographic findings that might be mistaken for a vegetation include:

- Papillary fibroelastoma
- Myxomatous mitral valve disease
- Nonbacterial thrombotic endocarditis
- Systemic lupus erythematosus
- Thrombus (especially with prosthetic valves)
- Beam-width artifact
- Normal valve variants such as a Lambl excrescence or nodule of Arantius

Valve Dysfunction

Valve leaflet destruction by the infectious process and distortion of leaflet closure by the vegetation typically result in valvular regurgitation. Regurgitation can occur at the closure line or through a perforation in the leaflet itself. The degree of regurgitation varies from none to mild, moderate, or severe. Assessment of valvular regurgitation in endocarditis is performed using the pulsed, color flow, and continuous-wave (CW) Doppler approaches described in Chapter 12, with careful attention to the features that distinguish acute from chronic regurgitation. Because endocarditis often affects a previously abnormal valve, acute regurgitation superimposed on chronic regurgitation results in mixed findings on echocardiography.

Valve stenosis due to endocarditis is rare. Occasionally, a large vegetation partially obstructs the orifice of the open valve and causes some degree of functional stenosis.

Although 90% of patients with endocarditis have a new murmur, approximately 10% do not, and a few have no regurgitation detectable on Doppler examination. This is most likely to occur if the vegetation is located at the base of the leaflet, thus resulting in little distortion of leaflet closure. Echocardiographic recognition of the diagnosis in this subgroup is all the more important in that endocarditis often is not suspected clinically, with the echocardiogram ordered for other reasons.

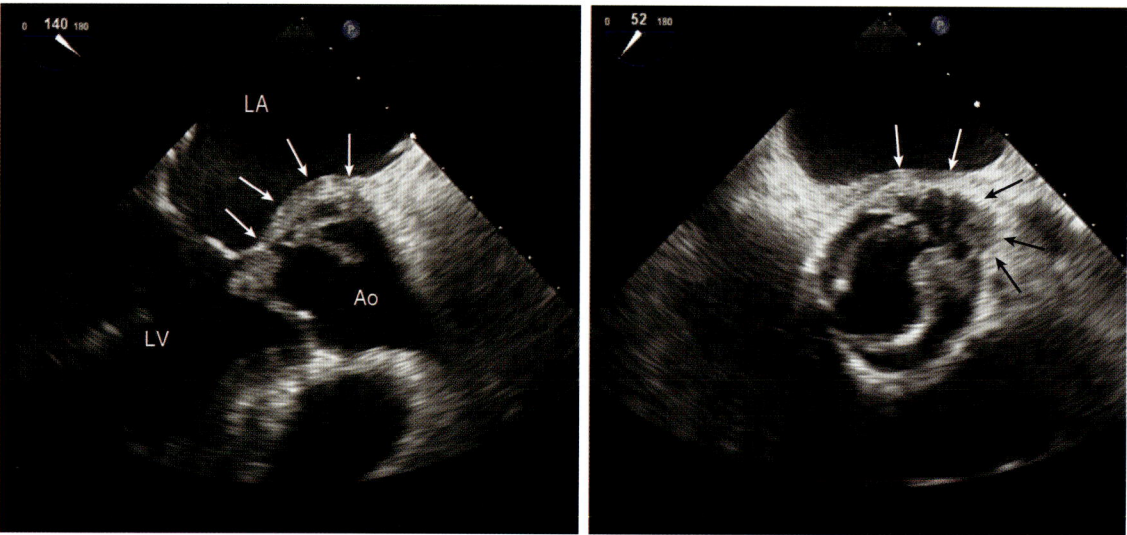

Fig. 14.13 Paravalvular abscess. In addition to a valvular vegetation, the TEE long-axis image *(left)* ▶ in a patient with aortic valve endocarditis shows thickening of the posterior aortic wall and irregular areas of echolucency and echodensity in the aortic annulus and sinuses *(arrows)*. The short-axis view *(right)* ▶ shows a congenital bicuspid aortic valve with thickening, dilation, and irregularity of the aortic sinus. At surgery, a paravalvular abscess was present. *Ao,* Aorta.

Paravalvular Abscess and Intracardiac Fistula

Unlike abscesses elsewhere in the body, a cardiac abscess is either echolucent or echodense on ultrasound examination. Typically, abscesses occur in the valve annulus adjacent to the infected leaflet tissue and are more common with aortic than with mitral valve endocarditis. For the diagnosis of an aortic annular abscess, findings include increased echogenicity, an echolucent area in the base of the septum, or increased thickness of the posterior aortic root (Fig. 14.13). Involvement of the aortic annulus can extend into the contiguous anterior mitral valve leaflet with evidence of increased thickness of the leaflet tissue, a valvular vegetation, and/or leaflet perforation. A sinus of Valsalva aneurysm occurs when the aortic wall is infected, which is diagnosed based on a dilated and distorted aortic sinus, even in the absence of rupture. In effect, this represents an abscess that is in direct communication with the bloodstream.

Rupture of an aortic annular abscess results in different complications depending on the exact site of rupture. The region of the noncoronary cusp ruptures into the RV outflow tract either in the sinus of Valsalva (an aortic-to-RV connection) or from the LV outflow tract through the septum into the RV (a ventricular septal defect). An aortic-to-RV fistula shows both systolic and diastolic left-to-right flow on Doppler interrogation, whereas a ventricular septal defect shows predominantly systolic flow. Rupture also can occur from the LV into the mitral-aortic intervalvular fibrosa with flow into and out of the abscess cavity from the LV outflow tract (Fig. 14.14).

The right coronary sinus region ruptures into the RV or RA, often with involvement of the adjacent septal leaflet of the tricuspid valve. Again, rupture can occur either from the aorta or from the LV outflow tract into the right side of the heart. Note that a small segment of ventricular septum (the atrioventricular septum) actually separates the LV from the *RA,* so that a ventriculoatrial communication is possible. The left coronary sinus of the aortic valve ruptures into the LA or RA, sometimes with extension of infection directly into the interatrial septum (Figs. 14.15 and 14.16).

A mitral annular abscess appears as increased thickening and echogenicity in the posterior aspect of the mitral annulus. Infection can extend into the basal segments of the ventricular myocardium or into the pericardial space. Again, identification often is difficult on echocardiographic imaging, and the diagnosis should be pursued with TEE echocardiography when suspected on clinical grounds. An unusual complication of mitral valve endocarditis is a persistent contour abnormality, in effect a pseudoaneurysm of the valve leaflet, which persists even after the infection is treated.

Tricuspid valve endocarditis can be associated with a ring abscess, again manifested as increased thickening and echogenicity in the annulus region.

Diagnosis of paravalvular abscess by transthoracic imaging has a markedly lower sensitivity and specificity (Appendix B, Table B.19) compared with TEE imaging because of poor ultrasound tissue penetration resulting in suboptimal image quality. A high index of suspicion is needed by the echocardiographer, and subtle abnormalities suggesting a valve abscess should not be ignored. However, even with careful imaging from

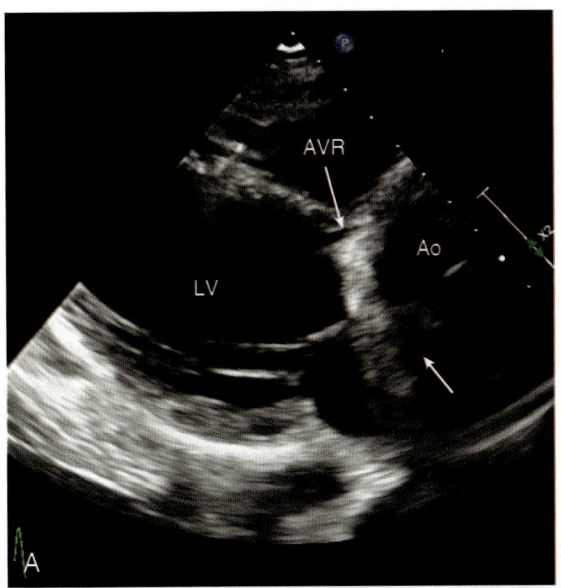

Fig. 14.14 Aneurysm of the mitral-aortic intervalvular fibrosa. (A) ▶ In this patient with a mechanical aortic valve replacement *(AVR)*, TTE shows shadowing and reverberations from the prosthetic valve in this parasternal long-axis image. However, real-time images suggested an abnormal echodensity on the LA size of the aortic valve in the region indicated by the *arrow*, thus prompting a TEE study. (B) ▶ and (C) ▶ In the same patient as in A, TEE long-axis images demonstrate an aortic root abscess and complex pseudoaneurysm of the aortic-mitral intravalvular fibrosa. The posterior aortic wall is markedly thickened *(between arrowheads)* consistent with an aneurysm, but an echo-free space *(asterisk)* is also present between the aortic valve prosthesis and the aortic wall. This contained space is a pseudoaneurysm due to rupture of the fibrous tissue between the aortic and mitral valves. The pseudoaneurysm communicates with the LV but not the aorta *(Ao)*. In diastole, blood flows from the pseudoaneurysm back into the LV, but in this case also into the LA across a perforation in the pseudoaneurysm *(arrow)*. Systolic images (C) show flow from the LV into the pseudoaneurysm *(arrow)*, in addition to mitral regurgitation *(MR)*.

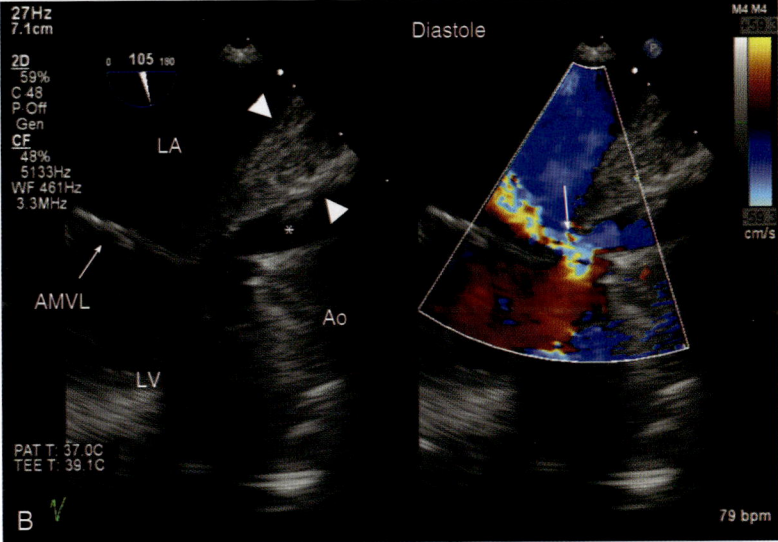

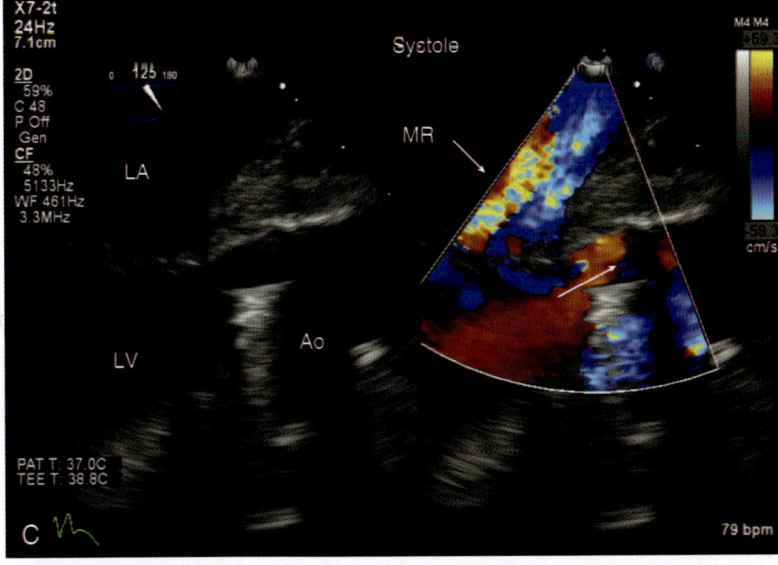

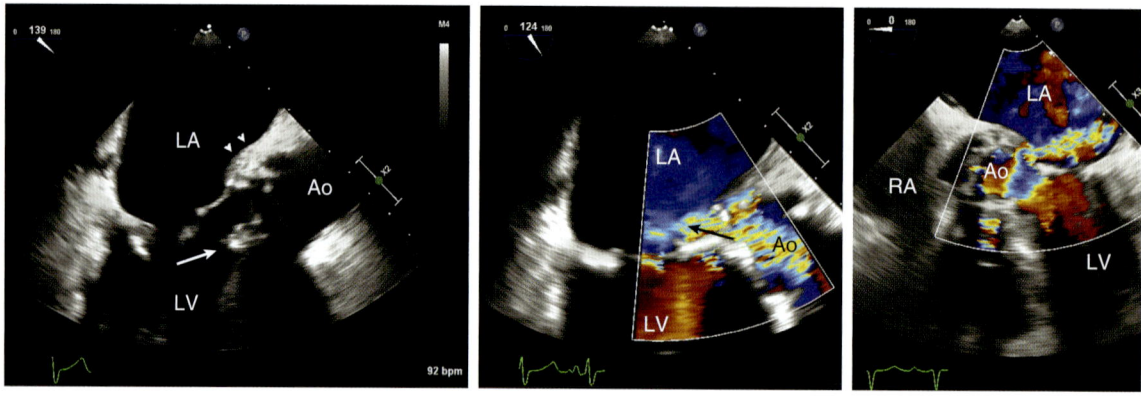

Fig. 14.15 Bioprosthetic annular abscess with fistula from aorta to left atrium. TEE long-axis views in a patent with endocarditis of a bioprosthetic aortic valve show an aortic valve vegetation *(arrow)* and thickening of the posterior aortic wall *(arrowheads)* consistent with a paravalvular abscess *(left).* ▶ Color Doppler in long-axis *(center)* ▶ and short-axis *(right)* ▶ views show both systolic and diastolic flow from the aortic sinus into the LA across a small perforation in the paravalvular abscess. *Ao,* Aorta.

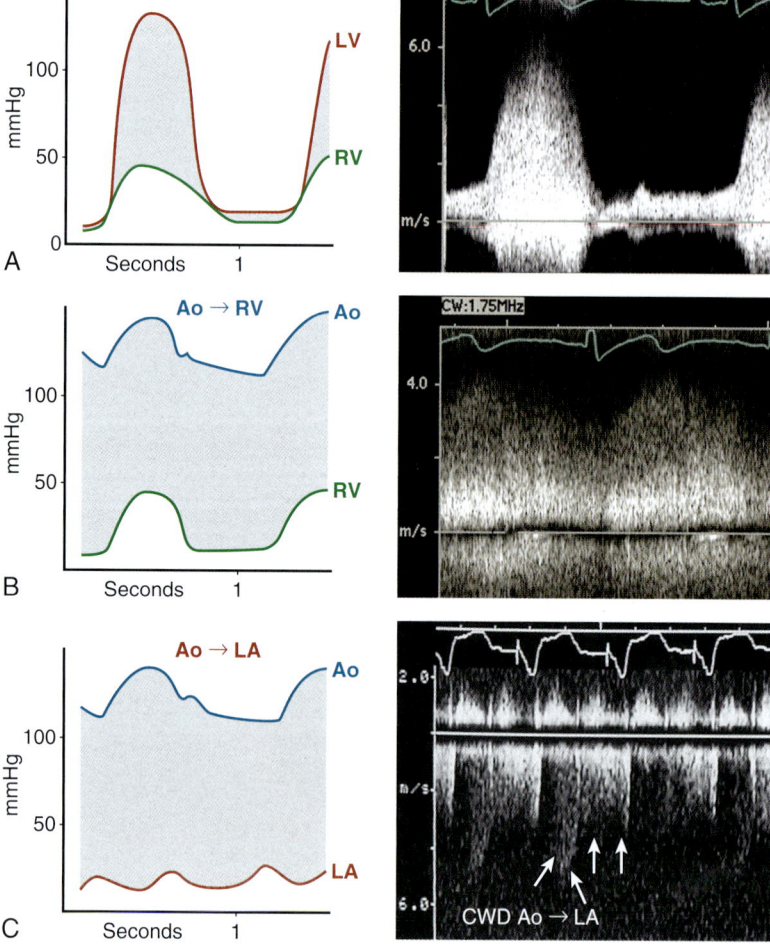

Fig. 14.16 Doppler flows with intracardiac fistulas. The velocity, timing, and shape of the CW Doppler curve can be used to determine the origin of an abnormal flow pattern seen on color Doppler in patients with endocarditis and extensive tissue destruction. The pressure tracings *(left)* and corresponding Doppler recordings *(right)* show the following: (A) A ventricular septal defect results in high-velocity left-to-right flow from the LV to RV in systole with an ejection-type curve. Persistent low velocity diastolic left-to-right flow is seen if LV diastolic pressure exceeds RV diastolic pressure. (B) A fistula from the aorta to the RV outflow tract due to a ruptured aortic annular abscess results in high-velocity flow in systole and diastole that reflects the large pressure difference between the aorta *(Ao)* and the RV. Velocity decreases slightly in systole as the pressure gradient diminishes due to RV contraction. (C) With a fistula from the aorta to the LA, very high-velocity, continuous systolic and diastolic flow is seen consistent with the high pressure difference between these chambers throughout the cardiac cycle.

several acoustic windows in multiple tomographic planes, a definite diagnosis is not always possible. TEE imaging is especially important in patients with prosthetic valve endocarditis because paravalvular abscesses are common, and shadowing and reverberations from the valve prosthesis compromise the examination (see Chapter 13).

The superior image quality of TEE is associated with a higher sensitivity (87%) and specificity (96%) for the diagnosis of a paravalvular abscess. In addition to 2D findings of abnormal areas of increased echogenicity or abnormal echolucent areas adjacent to the valve, color flow imaging and conventional pulsed Doppler may allow demonstration of flow into and out of these abnormal areas consistent with an abscess that partially communicates with the bloodstream.

Other Echocardiographic Findings

In addition to direct assessment of valvular disease, the examination includes an evaluation of cardiac chamber size and function. Acute aortic regurgitation results in only mild LV dilation, but a subacute or acute course superimposed on mild to moderate chronic disease results in significant ventricular dilation. Severe valve destruction often results in a flail leaflet (see Fig. 13.16). Mitral regurgitation results in LA and LV enlargement. LV systolic dysfunction is atypical but may be present due to long-standing valvular disease or secondary to the acute infectious process. Pulmonary pressures often are elevated because of mitral regurgitation, directly resulting in an elevated LA pressure, or because of aortic regurgitation with a high end-diastolic LV pressure. A small pericardial effusion often is seen in patients with endocarditis. A larger effusion raises the concern of purulent pericarditis due to direct extension from a paravalvular abscess.

LIMITATIONS AND TECHNICAL CONSIDERATIONS

Active Versus Healed Vegetations

Sequential echocardiographic studies in a patient undergoing effective treatment for endocarditis typically show a gradual reduction in size, a decrease in mobility, and an increase in echogenicity of the valvular vegetation. Sometimes vegetations either abruptly "disappear" from the heart because of embolization; thus, a patient with active endocarditis may have no visible vegetation if recent embolization has occurred. A persistent vegetation with no change in size or echodensity raises concern for inadequate treatment or ongoing infection; however, some patients have vegetations evident long after the acute episode. The diagnosis of endocarditis is based on a combination of microbiological, clinical (e.g., fevers, systemic emboli, new murmur, and peripheral manifestation of endocarditis), and imaging findings, as detailed in Table 14.1. Obviously, echocardiography provides no information regarding the causative organism. Although certain causal agents (e.g., fungal endocarditis, *Haemophilus influenzae*) are associated with larger vegetations, this observation is not diagnostically useful in an individual patient.

Nonbacterial Thrombotic Endocarditis

The echocardiographic appearance of nonbacterial thrombotic endocarditis, typically seen in patients with malignant disease or systemic lupus erythematosus, is somewhat similar to that of infectious endocarditis, but the vegetations tend to be smaller, are located near the leaflet base, show variable echodensity, and have less independent motion. However, none of these differences are independently diagnostic, so differentiation of infective from nonbacterial thrombotic endocarditis depends on clinical and bacteriologic correlation (Fig. 14.17).

Diagnosis With Underlying Valve Disease

Endocarditis most often occurs on a previously abnormal valve because the local flow disturbance increases the likelihood of bacterial deposition. When the underlying disease is anatomically straightforward, such as a bicuspid aortic valve, this poses little problem in diagnosing superimposed valvular vegetations. Often, however, the presence of an abnormal valve makes exclusion or confirmation of a valvular vegetation more difficult. For example, with calcific aortic stenosis, the irregular areas of increased echogenicity on the valve leaflets could represent a vegetation or chronic fibrocalcific changes. Findings of independent rapid

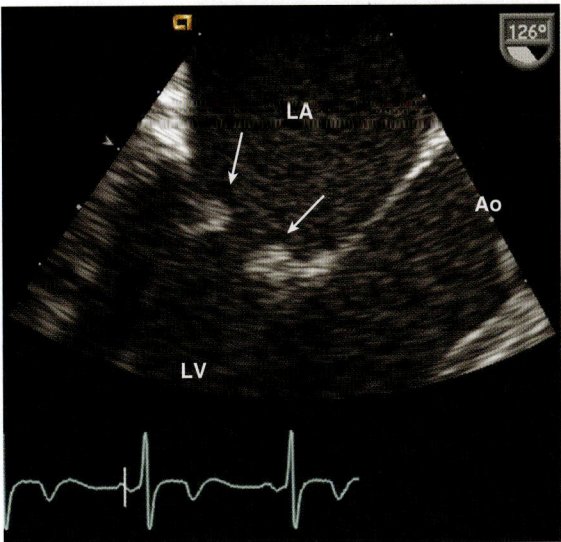

Fig. 14.17 **Nonbacterial thrombotic endocarditis.** TEE in a 49-year-old woman with systemic lupus erythematosus shows mitral valve masses *(arrows)* consistent with nonbacterial thrombotic endocarditis. *Ao,* Aorta.

motion and prolapse into the outflow tract in diastole increase the likelihood of a vegetation, but the absence of these findings does not allow for a definite conclusion on the absence of a vegetation.

Another example is myxomatous mitral valve disease, in which an independently mobile mass of echoes attached to the leaflet and prolapsing into the LA in systole could represent either a valvular vegetation or a flail leaflet segment and attached chordae. When underlying valve disease is present, the improved 2D and 3D images obtained by the TEE approach may increase the certainty of diagnosis.

Prosthetic Valves and Intracardiac Devices

Evaluation of prosthetic valves for suspected endocarditis is problematic for two reasons. First, infection often involves the area around the sewing ring of the prosthetic valve, rather than resulting in a discrete valvular vegetation. Second, reverberations and shadowing by the prosthesis limit the ability of echocardiography to detect abnormalities. This is a particular problem with transthoracic imaging of mitral prostheses, in which the LA side of the valve is "masked" by the prosthesis so that neither the paravalvular infection in the mitral annulus nor the resulting valvular incompetence can be detected (see Chapter 13). Acoustic shadowing is less of a problem with aortic valve prostheses because aortic regurgitation can be evaluated from both apical and parasternal windows without "masking" by the valve prosthesis. However, because the anterior part of the valve prosthesis shadows the more posterior portions, images of the valve leaflets may be suboptimal.

With suspected prosthetic valve endocarditis, the transthoracic examination provides clues that suggest the diagnosis even when definitive findings are not present. For example, if color flow imaging is non-diagnostic because of shadowing and color flow artifacts, CW Doppler evidence for prosthetic valve regurgitation suggests infection with leaflet or annular destruction (Fig. 14.18). Care is needed in the

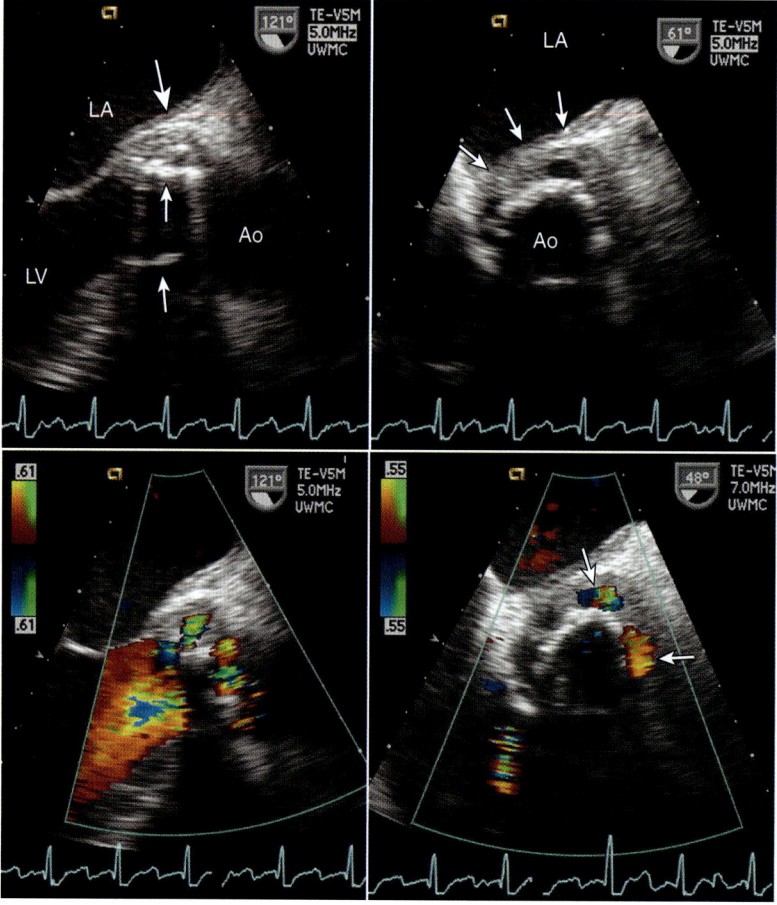

Fig. 14.18 Bioprosthetic valve annular abscess. TEE images of a stented bioprosthetic aortic valve show the valve struts *(small arrows)* in the long-axis view *(top left)*. In both the long-axis view and the short-axis view *(top right)*, thickening is seen posterior to the prosthetic valve with echolucent areas *(arrows)*. Color Doppler *(bottom)* shows turbulent flow in these echolucent areas consistent with partial valve dehiscence and communication with the LV chamber. *Ao,* Aorta.

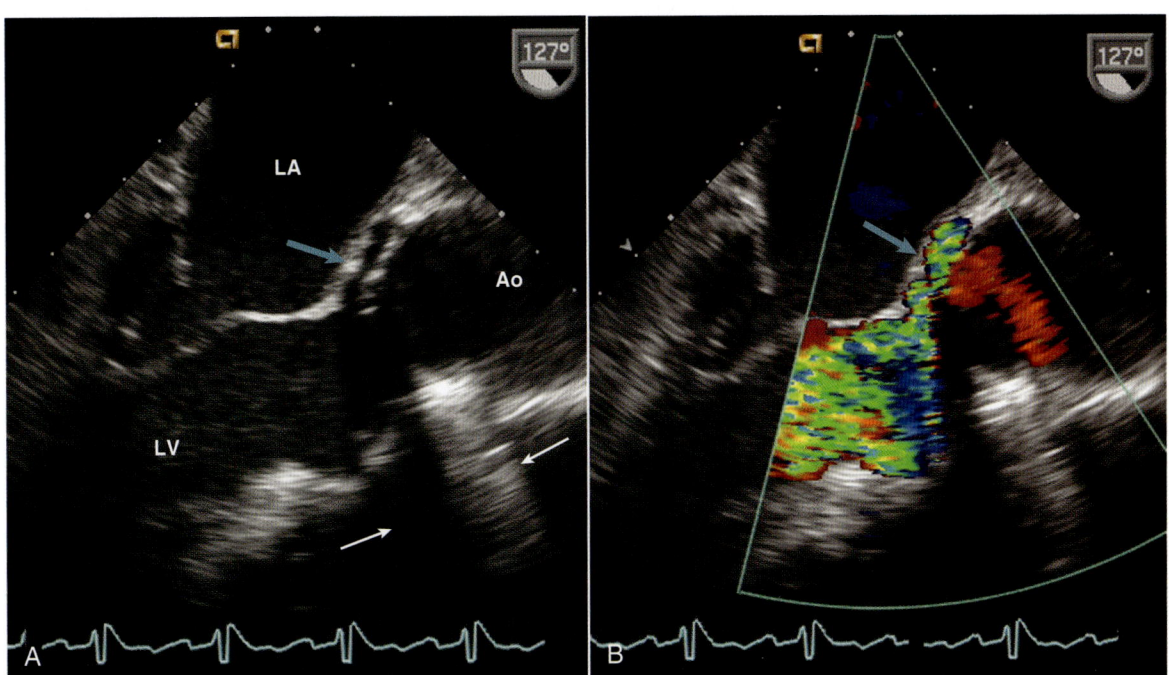

Fig. 14.19 Prosthetic valve annular abscess. TEE imaging in a patient with prosthetic valve endocarditis (A) and an echolucent space *(cyan arrow)* between the anterior mitral leaflet and the aortic sewing ring in the long-axis view. Prominent shadows and reverberations *(white arrows)* from the valve now obscure the anterior aspect of the valve. (B) ▶ Color Doppler shows diastolic flow in the abnormal echolucent area that is suggestive of paravalvular regurgitation and valve dehiscence. *Ao,* Aorta.

assessment of the *severity* of regurgitation in this situation; it is prudent to indicate the presence of regurgitation on transthoracic echocardiography with the recommendation to pursue TEE for quantitation of severity if needed. Other clues to prosthetic valve dysfunction include increased antegrade flow velocity across the prosthesis (reflecting increased antegrade volume flow due to prosthetic regurgitation) and elevated tricuspid regurgitant jet velocity due to pulmonary hypertension.

Whenever prosthetic valve endocarditis is suspected, TEE imaging should be strongly considered, given its higher sensitivity and specificity for the detection of prosthetic valve endocarditis, paravalvular abscess, and prosthetic mitral regurgitation (Figs. 14.19 and 14.20).

Endocarditis rarely can result in prosthetic valve stenosis due to impingement of the infected mass on leaflet opening or to an infected pannus on the upstream side of the valve. Visualization of the infected mass may not be possible on transthoracic imaging but is more likely on TEE or with alternate imaging approaches. Prosthetic valve stenosis is recognized by findings of an increased transvalvular pressure gradient and a decreased valve area (by pressure half-time or by continuity equation).

In an individual patient, a *change* in the appearance or flow characteristics of a prosthetic valve is more diagnostic than an observation at one point in time.

Review of previous studies (if available) performed when the patient clinically was well can improve the diagnostic yield of echocardiography.

CLINICAL UTILITY

Suspected Endocarditis

Although TEE echocardiography is more sensitive than transthoracic echocardiography for the detection of valvular vegetations, transthoracic echocardiography remains the initial procedure of choice in patients with a low pre-test likelihood of disease (the "rule out endocarditis" indication) because of the lower cost and risk of this approach (Fig. 14.21). Based on an average sensitivity of 80% and specificity of 98% for transthoracic detection of vegetations, the positive likelihood ratio of finding a vegetation is 40 (an excellent test), but the negative likelihood ratio is 0.20 (only a reasonably good test). Thus, in a patient with a pre-echo likelihood of disease of 50%, a normal transthoracic exam reduces that likelihood to 10%. In contrast, using a sensitivity of 97% and specificity of 91% for TEE diagnosis of valve vegetations, the negative likelihood ratio is 0.03, indicating that a normal TEE is reliable for excluding a diagnosis of endocarditis. A normal TEE in the patient with a pre-echo likelihood of 50% reduces the likelihood of endocarditis to 1.5%.

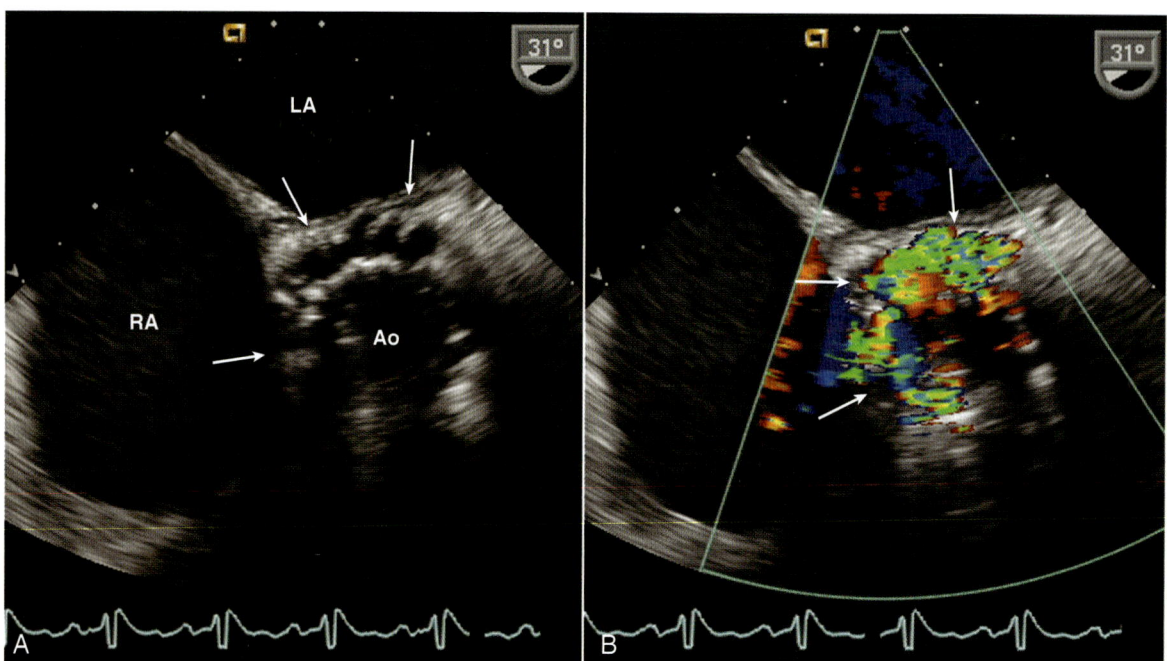

Fig. 14.20 Prosthetic valve dehiscence. (A) TEE short-axis view in the same patient as in Fig. 14.19 shows an irregular echolucent region *(arrows)* extending around the posterior aspect of the sewing ring. (B) Color Doppler confirms valve dehiscence with paravalvular regurgitation *(arrows)*. *Ao,* Aorta.

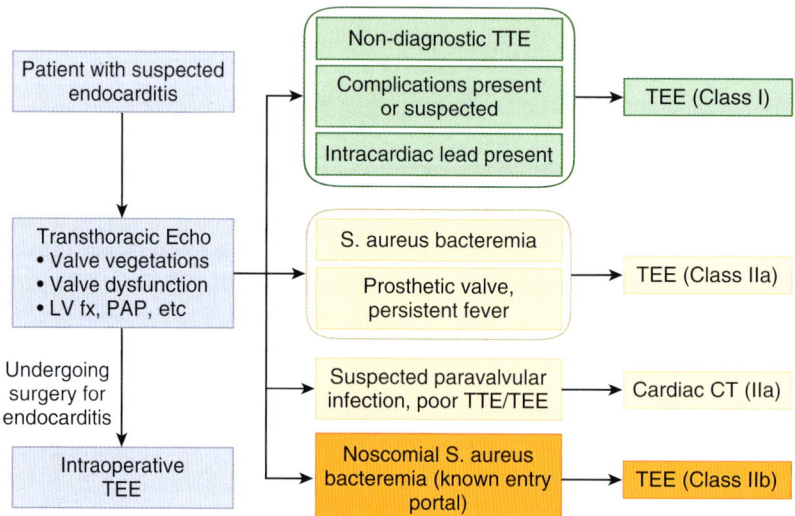

Fig. 14.21 Flow chart for the suggested role of echocardiography in the diagnosis of endocarditis. TTE is the initial step in evaluation of patients with a concern for endocarditis based on clinical or bacteriologic findings. However, TEE often is needed in addition to TTE, as indicated in this algorithm. The class of recommendation refers to the American Heart Association/American College of Cardiology 2014 and 2017 recommendations for valvular heart disease. Class I is "indicated," class IIa is "reasonable," and class IIb "may be considered." *CT,* Computed tomography; *fx,* function; *PAP,* pulmonary artery pressure.

TABLE 14.3 Diagnostic Imaging in Infective Endocarditis

	TTE	TEE	Other	AHA/ACC 2014*	ESC 2015†
Diagnosis in Patients With Suspected Infective Endocarditis (IE)					
All patients with clinically suspected IE	*†			I (B)	I (B)
Nondiagnostic TTE		*†		I (B)	I (B)
Prosthetic heart valve or intracardiac device		†			I (B)
Repeat within 5–7 days if initial study negative and clinical suspicion remains high	†	†			I (C)
Staphylococcus aureus bacteremia without known source	*†			IIa (B)	IIa (B)
Persistent fever in patient with a prosthetic valve		*		IIa (B)	
Positive TTE (except right-sided with good-quality TTE)		†			IIa (C)
Suspected paravalvular infection with suboptimal echo images			CT	IIa (B)	‡
Suspected prosthetic valve endocarditis			¹⁸F-FDG PET/CT		‡
Staphylococcus aureus bacteremia with known source (to detect possible cardiac involvement)		*		IIb (B)	
Follow-Up on Medical Therapy					
Change in signs or symptoms or concern for complications (new murmur, embolism, persisting fever, heart failure, abscess, AV block)	*†	*†		I (B)	I (B)
Routine follow-up for uncomplicated IE	†	†			IIa (B)
Perioperative Echocardiography					
Intraoperative TEE in patients undergoing valve surgery for IE		*†		I (B)	I (B)
Following Completion of Therapy					
Baseline study after treatment for IE is completed	†				I (C)

*ACC/AHA recommendation.
†ESC recommendation.
‡Added to ESC 2015 criteria for diagnosis of endocarditis as shown in Table 14.1. No specific class or level of evidence.
AHA/ACC, American Heart Association/American College of Cardiology; AV, atrioventricular; CT, Computed tomography; ESC, European Society of Cardiology; ¹⁸F-FDG, 18-fluorine–fluorodeoxyglucose; IE, infective endocarditis; PET, positron emission tomography.
Summarized from Nishimura RA, Otto CM, Bonow RO, et al. 2014 AHA/ACC guideline for the management of patients with valvular heart disease. J Am Coll Cardiol 10;63(22):e57–e185, 2014; and Habib G, Lancellotti P, Antunes MJ, et al. 2015 ESC Guidelines for the management of infective endocarditis. Eur Heart J 21;36(44):3075–3128, 2015.

TEE is appropriate in patients at high risk of endocarditis and in situations where transthoracic imaging is likely to be nondiagnostic (Table 14.3). High-risk patients include those with prosthetic valves, congenital heart disease, previous endocarditis, new heart failure, new atrioventricular block, and community-acquired staphylococcal bacteremia. Typically, transthoracic imaging also is needed in these patients to allow parallel alignment for CW Doppler evaluation of high-velocity flows, standard measurement of chamber dimensions, quantitation of LV systolic function, and measurement of pulmonary artery pressures. In addition, the combination of transthoracic imaging and TEE allows optimal visualization of both sides of the prosthetic valve because shadowing from the prosthesis occurs in opposite directions with these two approaches. TEE imaging also is reasonable when endocarditis has been detected on transthoracic echocardiogrraphy particularly when the aortic valve is involved, because of the risk of paravalvular abscess. Finally, TEE is appropriate in patients with persistent fever, recurrent bacteremia, or new atrioventricular block—all signs of paravalvular abscess formation.

Known Endocarditis

In a patient with known endocarditis, an echocardiogram is an invaluable adjunct to clinical decision making concerning potential surgical intervention and prediction

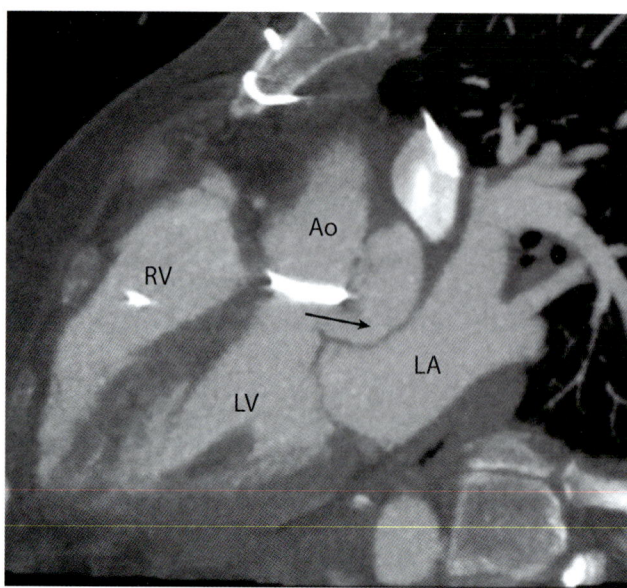

Fig. 14.22 ▶ **Computed tomographic imaging of aneurysm of aortic mitral intravalvular fibrosa.** Computed tomographic (CT) imaging in the same patient as in Fig. 14.14 demonstrates the narrow neck of the connection from the LV into the pseudoaneurysm, adjacent to the bright signal from the aortic valve prosthesis. CT imaging is helpful both for diagnosis and for surgical planning in patients with complex endocarditis. *Ao,* Aorta. *(Image courtesy James C. Lee, MD.)*

of short- and long-term prognosis. Echocardiography often allows clear definition of which (and how many) valves are affected. Echocardiographic findings are key variables in identifying indication for surgical intervention and in optimizing the timing of intervention—early (during the initial hospitalization) or at a later date.

Early surgery is indicated for patients with valve dysfunction causing heart failure, infection with resistant organisms, the presence of a paravalvular abscess or clinical heart block, and in those with persistent infection despite antibiotic therapy. Early surgery also is reasonable in patients with recurrent emboli due to persistent vegetations and may be considered when a large (>1 cm), mobile native valve vegetation is present on echocardiography, even in the absence of an embolic event. Surgery at a later date may be needed for patients with residual valve dysfunction in the absence of acute heart failure and in those with relapsing prosthetic valve endocarditis. In patients with an implanted cardiac electronic device (e.g., pacer or implanted cardiac defibrillator), evidence of infection on the leads is an indication for early device removal.

Alternate Approaches

Although echocardiography remains the primary imaging approach for diagnosis and management of infective endocarditis, both computed tomographic imaging and positron emission tomographic studies are useful in selected patients. Computed tomographic imaging allows visualization of occluder motion with mechanical valves and provides detailed information about pannus, thrombus, and masses in the paravalvular region (Fig. 14.22). The use of 18-fluorine–fluorodeoxyglucose positron emission tomographic imaging improves detection of cardiac infection in selected cases. These approaches now are incorporated into guidelines for diagnosis of endocarditis.

THE ECHO EXAM

Echo Findings in Endocarditis

Finding	Definition	TTE	TEE
Valvular vegetations	• Mass attached to leaflet with independent motion	• Sensitivity 50%–80% • Specificity 90%–100%	• Sensitivity 90%–100% • Specificity 90%–100%
Leaflet destruction	• New or worsening valve regurgitation due to loss of normal coaptation with valve closure or chordal rupture	• Accurate for detection and quantitation of regurgitation	• May better define mechanism of regurgitation
Leaflet perforation	• Disruption in leaflet tissue with a hole in the center or base	• Regurgitation detected but loss of structure difficult to identify	• 3D TEE shows discontinuity in leaflet
Abscess	• Infected area adjacent to valve, usually in the aortic or mitral annulus	• Sensitivity low • Specificity 90%–100%	• Sensitivity 90%–100% • Specificity 90%–100%
Aneurysm	• Localized dilation of a valve leaflet, aortic sinus, or aortic-mitral intervalvular fibrosa	• Distortion of aortic sinus anatomy, outpouching of mitral leaflet, space between aortic annulus and anterior mitral leaflet	• TEE more sensitive for detection of aneurysm
Pseudoaneurysm	• Contained cardiac or aortic rupture, most often around aorta or at LV base	• Abnormal echodense or echo lucent area around aorta or posterior to LV	• TEE more sensitive for diagnosis but CT imaging often needed.
Fistula	• Abnormal communication between cardiac chambers or great vessels	• Color or CW Doppler may show abnormal flow signal with timing and velocity diagnostic for location.	• TEE images allow visualization of location and size of intracardiac fistula.
Prosthetic valve dehiscence	• Detachment (partial) of the prosthetic valve from the annular tissue	• Paravalvular regurgitation is typical. Abnormal motion of valve is diagnostic but rare.	• TEE more sensitive for evaluation of prosthetic mitral valves • Combination of TTE (anterior aspect of valve) and TEE (for posterior aspect) needed for aortic prosthetic valves

SUGGESTED READING

Guidelines

1. Nishimura RA, Otto CM, Bonow RO, et al: 2017 AHA/ACC Focused Update of the 2014 AHA/ACC guideline for the management of patients with valvular heart disease: a report of the American College of Cardiology/American Heart Association Task Force on Clinical Practice Guidelines, *J Am Coll Cardiol* 70(2):252–289, 2017.
2. Nishimura RA, Otto CM, Bonow RO, et al: 2014 AHA/ACC guideline for the management of patients with valvular heart disease: executive summary: a report of the American College of Cardiology/American Heart Association Task Force on Practice Guidelines, *J Am Coll Cardiol* 63(22):2438–2488, 2014.
   The 2014 AHA/ACC valve guidelines, in conjunction with the 2017 update, provide recommendations on the use of echocardiography for diagnosis of endocarditis as summarized in Table 14.3.
3. Baddour LM, Wilson WR, Bayer AS, et al: Infective endocarditis in adults: diagnosis, antimicrobial therapy, and management of complications: a scientific statement for healthcare professionals from the American Heart Association, *Circulation* 132:1435, 2015.
   This scientific statement provides guidance for diagnosis of endocarditis, including an algorithm for integrating TTE and TEE with clinical findings. Detailed recommendations for antibiotic therapy.
4. Habib G, Lancellotti P, Antunes MJ, et al: 2015 ESC guidelines for the management of infective endocarditis: the Task Force for the Management of Infective Endocarditis of the European Society of Cardiology (ESC). Endorsed by: European Association for Cardio-Thoracic Surgery (EACTS), the European Association of Nuclear Medicine (EANM), *Eur Heart J* 36(44):3075–3128, 2015.

This document provides specific guidance on the role of echocardiography in diagnosis of infective endocarditis and includes recommendations for inclusion of newer imaging approaches as shown in Table 14.1.

Reviews and Book Chapters

5. Samad Z, Wang A: Endocarditis: the role of echocardiography in diagnosis and clinical decision making. In Otto CM, editor: *The Practice of Clinical Echocardiography*, ed 5, Philadelphia, 2017, Elsevier, pp 416–432.
   Review of the current role of echocardiography in management of the patient with suspected or known endocarditis. In addition to a review of the literature, this chapter provides useful tips on the echocardiographic approach with clear illustrations.

6. Bolger A: Infective endocarditis. In Otto CM, Bonow RO, editors: *Valvular Heart Disease*, ed 5, Philadelphia, 2018, Elsevier. In press.
   Comprehensive book chapter covering epidemiology, pathophysiology, diagnosis, complications, and treatment of infective endocarditis. In the current era, the primary cause of endocarditis is Staphylococcus, and most patients are older adults, drug users, or have implanted cardiac devices (prosthetic valve, pacer, or defibrillator). About 15% of patients with endocarditis have negative blood cultures. Diagnosis is based on echocardiography and the modified Duke criteria.

7. Oxorn DC, Otto CM: Endocarditis. In Oxorn DC, Otto CM, editors: *Intraoperative and Interventional Echocardiography: Atlas of Transesophageal Imaging*, Philadelphia, 2017, Elsevier, pp 121–148.
   This chapter presents 10 cases of endocarditis with intraoperative imaging, including pathological and surgical correlation. Numerous videos in the e-book version complement the still images.

8. Cahill TJ, Baddour LM, Habib G, et al: Challenges in infective endocarditis, *J Am Coll Cardiol* 69(3):325–344, 2017.
   State-of-the-art review article summarizing all aspects of infective endocarditis: epidemiology, prevention, diagnosis, microbiology, antibiotic therapy, and surgical intervention. Also discusses management of cardiac device infections and the role of newer imaging approaches, in addition to echocardiographic diagnosis.

9. Roldan CA: Echocardiographic findings in systemic disease characterized by immune-mediated injury. In Otto CM, editor: *The Practice of Clinical Echocardiography*, ed 5, Philadelphia, 2017, Elsevier, pp 692–793.
   Excellent summary of echocardiographic findings that could be mistaken for endocarditis, including findings in patients with systemic lupus erythematosus, rheumatoid arthritis, ankylosing spondylitis, scleroderma, and other connective tissue disorders.

Selected Clinical Studies

10. Fernández Guerrero ML, Álvarez B, Manzarbeitia F, et al: Infective endocarditis at autopsy: a review of pathologic manifestations and clinical correlates, *Medicine (Baltimore)* 91(3):152–164, 2012.
    This autopsy study reports findings from before and after the introduction of echocardiography at their institution. Comparing earlier and later time periods, mean age increased from 47 to 58 years, the frequency of comorbid conditions increased from 28% to 61%, and the frequency of rheumatic valve disease declined. Isolated aortic and mitral valve endocarditis were most common. Notably, about 25% of patients had no predisposing valve disease. This review also includes case examples with photographs of pathologic findings.

11. San Román JA, Vilacosta I, López J, et al: Role of transthoracic and transesophageal echocardiography in right-sided endocarditis: one echocardiographic modality does not fit all, *J Am Soc Echocardiogr* 25(8):807–814, 2012.
    Review of the echocardiographic approach to the evaluation of right-sided endocarditis. The authors recommend TEE in all patients with an intracardiac device and possible endocarditis. Compared with left-sided endocarditis, patients with right-sided endocarditis are more often drug users (29%), have associated pulmonary thromboembolism (25%), and have a lower in-hospital mortality rate (7% vs. 26%). Excellent anatomic and echocardiographic illustrations of normal right-sided structures that could be mistaken for endocarditis (i.e., Chiari network, crista terminalis, Eustachian valve).

12. Rasmussen RV, Høst U, Arpi M, et al: Prevalence of infective endocarditis in patients with *Staphylococcus aureus* bacteraemia: the value of screening with echocardiography, *Eur J Echocardiogr* 12(6):414–420, 2011.
    In 244 patients with S. aureus bacteremia, endocarditis was diagnosed in 22%. The prevalence of endocarditis was 38% in patients with prosthetic valves or intracardiac devices compared with 19% in those with native valves and no devices. The authors recommend echocardiography in all patients with S. aureus bacteremia because clinical findings are often nonspecific, disease prevalence is high, and the 6-month mortality rate is higher in those with versus those without (26% vs. 15%) endocarditis.

13. Grimaldi A, Ho SY, Pozzoli A, et al: Pseudoaneurysm of mitral-aortic intervalvular fibrosa, *Interact Cardiovasc Thorac Surg* 13(2):142–147, 2011.
    A pseudoaneurysm of the fibrous tissue between the aortic and mitral valves is a rare complication of valve surgery. In this series of 16 patients, the 7 patients with normal valve function and no previous history of endocarditis did well with clinical and echocardiographic follow-up. In contrast, the 9 patients with a history of endocarditis all required reintervention for residual paravalvular leak or the high risk of pseudoaneurysm rupture. Illustrations show the anatomy and echocardiographic findings.

14. Viganego F, O'Donoghue S, Eldadah Z, et al: Effect of early diagnosis and treatment with percutaneous lead extraction on survival in patients with cardiac device infections, *Am J Cardiol* 109(10):1466–1471, 2012.
    In 52 consecutive patients with cardiac device infections, percutaneous lead extraction performed within 3 days of admission was associated with a shorter duration of hospitalization and improved survival compared with those of patients with delayed lead extraction. This finding emphasizes the importance of early echocardiographic diagnosis of pacer and defibrillator lead infections.

15. Kang DH, Kim YJ, Kim SH, et al: Early surgery versus conventional treatment for infective endocarditis, *N Engl J Med* 366(26):2466–2473, 2012.
    This randomized study of early surgery (within 48 hours of diagnosis) for left-sided infective endocarditis with findings of severe valve dysfunction and large vegetations demonstrated better outcomes in patients with early intervention (n = 37) compared with those who received conventional treatment (n = 39), even though most (77%) of the patients in the conventional treatment group also underwent surgery during the initial hospitalization. The composite endpoint of death, embolic events, or recurrent endocarditis occurred in 3% of the early surgery group compared with 28% of the late surgery group (hazard ratio: 0.08; confidence interval: 0.01 to 0.65; P = .02) at 6 months.

16. Sivak JA, Vora AN, Navar AM, et al: An approach to improve the negative predictive value and clinical utility of

transthoracic echocardiography in suspected native valve infective endocarditis, *J Am Soc Echocardiogr* 29:315, 2016.

In 790 patients with a clinical suspicion of endocarditis who had undergone both TTE and TEE, use of strict criteria for a negative TTE study had a negative predictive value of 97%, a finding suggesting that TEE may not be necessary in all these patients. The strict criteria for a negative study result were normal cardiac anatomy on a moderate- or better-quality echocardiogram, no valve sclerosis or stenosis, no more than trivial valve regurgitation, no more than a trivial pericardial effusion, no implanted cardiac devices or central lines, and no evidence of vegetations.

17. Berdejo J, Shibayama K, Harada K, et al: Evaluation of vegetation size and its relationship with embolism in infective endocarditis: a real-time 3-dimensional transesophageal echocardiography study, *Circ Cardiovasc Imaging* 7:149, 2014.

In a series of 60 patients with valvular vegetations, vegetation length was longer when measured from 3D compared with 2D images, averaging 3 mm longer.

18. Miranda WR, Connolly HM, Bonnichsen CR, et al: Prosthetic pulmonary valve and pulmonary conduit endocarditis: clinical, microbiological and echocardiographic features in adults, *Eur Heart J Cardiovasc Imaging* 17(8):936–943, 2016.

A small case series of infective endocarditis in adults with a prosthetic pulmonic valve found that TTE was diagnostic in only 62% and TEE in only 56% of patients, but the combination of TTE and TEE established the presence of endocarditis in 88% of cases. Unlike typical left-sided endocarditis, patients more often presented with prosthetic valve obstruction (53%) than with regurgitation (29%).

15 Cardiac Masses and Potential Cardiac Source of Embolus

BASIC PRINCIPLES
VALVE VEGETATIONS
CARDIAC TUMORS
  Nonprimary
  Primary
    Benign Primary Cardiac Tumors
    Malignant Primary Cardiac Tumors
  Technical Considerations and Alternate
    Approaches
LEFT VENTRICULAR THROMBUS
  Predisposing Conditions
  Identification of Left Ventricular Thrombi
  Clinical Implications
  Alternate Approaches

LEFT ATRIAL THROMBUS
  Predisposing Factors
  Identification of Left Atrial Thrombi
  Prognosis and Clinical Implications
  Alternate Approaches
RIGHT-SIDED HEART THROMBI
CARDIAC SOURCE OF EMBOLUS
  Basic Principles
  Identifiable Cardiac Sources of Emboli
  Predisposing Conditions
  Indications for Echocardiography in Patients
    With Systemic Embolic Events
THE ECHO EXAM
SUGGESTED READING

A cardiac mass is defined as an abnormal structure within or immediately adjacent to the heart. The three basic types of cardiac masses are:

- Tumor
- Thrombus
- Vegetation

Abnormal mass lesions must be distinguished from the unusual appearance of a normal cardiac structure, which may be mistakenly considered an apparent "mass." Echocardiography allows dynamic evaluation of intracardiac masses with the advantage, compared with other tomographic techniques, that both the anatomic extent and the physiologic consequences of the mass can be evaluated. In addition, associated abnormalities (e.g., valvular regurgitation associated with a vegetation) and conditions that predispose to the development of a mass (e.g., apical aneurysm leading to left ventricular [LV] thrombus or rheumatic mitral stenosis resulting in left atrial [LA] thrombus) can be assessed. Disadvantages of echocardiography include suboptimal image quality in some patients, a relatively narrow field of view compared with that of computed tomography (CT) or cardiac magnetic resonance (CMR) imaging, and the possibility of mistaking an ultrasound artifact for an anatomic mass.

BASIC PRINCIPLES

The first step in assessing a possible cardiac mass is to ensure that the echocardiographic findings represent an actual mass rather than an ultrasound artifact. As discussed in detail in Chapter 1, artifacts can be caused by electrical interference, characteristics of the ultrasound transducer or system, or various physical factors influencing image formation from the reflected ultrasound signals. These include beam-width artifact, near-field "ring-down," and multipath artifact. Appropriate transducer selection, scanning technique, and evaluation from multiple examining windows will help distinguish artifacts from actual anatomic structures.

Besides ultrasound artifacts, several normal structures and normal variants may be mistaken for a cardiac mass (Table 15.1). In the ventricles, normal trabeculae, aberrant trabeculae or chordae (ventricular "webs" or false tendons) (Fig. 15.1), muscle bundles (e.g., the moderator band), or the papillary muscles may be mistaken for abnormal structures.

Valve anatomy includes a wide range of normal variation, and the appearance of a normal (but often unrecognized) structure, such as a nodule of Arantius, on the aortic valve may be considered incorrectly to

Cardiac Masses and Potential Cardiac Source of Embolus | Chapter 15

TABLE 15.1	Structures That May Be Mistaken for an Abnormal Cardiac Mass
Left atrium	Dilated coronary sinus (persistent left superior vena cava)
	Raphe between left superior pulmonary vein and LA appendage
	Atrial suture line after cardiac transplant
	Beam-width artifact from calcified aortic valve, aortic valve prosthesis, or other echogenic target adjacent to the atrium
	Interatrial septal aneurysm
Right atrium	Crista terminalis
	Chiari network (Eustachian valve remnants)
	Lipomatous hypertrophy of the interatrial septum
	Trabeculation of RA appendage
	Atrial suture line after cardiac transplant
	Pacer wire, Swan-Ganz catheter, or central venous line
Left ventricle	Papillary muscles
	LV web (aberrant chordae)
	Prominent apical trabeculations
	Prominent mitral annular calcification
Right ventricle	Moderator band
	Papillary muscles
	Swan-Ganz catheter or pacer wire
Aortic valve	Nodules of Arantius
	Lambl excrescences
	Base of valve leaflet seen en face in diastole
Mitral valve	Redundant chordae
	Myxomatous mitral valve tissue
Pulmonary artery	LA appendage (just caudal to pulmonary artery)
Pericardium	Epicardial adipose tissue
	Fibrinous debris in a chronic organized pericardial effusion

represent a cardiac mass. The belly of a valve leaflet, if cut tangentially, may appear as a "mass" when it actually is a portion of the leaflet itself seen en face. In the atrium, normal ridges adjacent to the venous entry sites (Figs. 15.2 and 15.3), normal trabeculations (Fig. 15.4), postoperative changes (see Fig. 9.31), and distortion of the free wall contour by structures adjacent to the atrium (Fig. 15.5) all may be diagnosed erroneously as a cardiac mass.

Definitive diagnosis of an intracardiac mass by echocardiography is based on:

- Excellent image quality, which requires the use of a high-frequency (5- or 7.5-MHz), short-focus transducer to evaluate the LV apex from the transthoracic (TTE) approach and the use of transesophageal (TEE) imaging to evaluate posterior cardiac structures (e.g., LA, mitral valve). Three-dimensional (3D) echocardiography often provides better definition of the location and geometry of the mass.
- Identification of the mass throughout the cardiac cycle, in the same anatomic region of the heart, from more than one acoustic window. This decreases the likelihood of an ultrasound artifact.
- Knowledge of the normal structures, normal variants, and postoperative changes that appear similar to a cardiac mass.
- Integration of other echocardiographic findings (e.g., rheumatic mitral stenosis and LA enlargement in a patient with suspected LA thrombus) and clinical data in the final echocardiographic interpretation.

Once it is clear that a cardiac mass is present, the next step is to determine whether that mass most likely is a tumor, a vegetation, or a thrombus. A definitive diagnosis generally cannot be made from the echocardiographic images alone because the microscopic

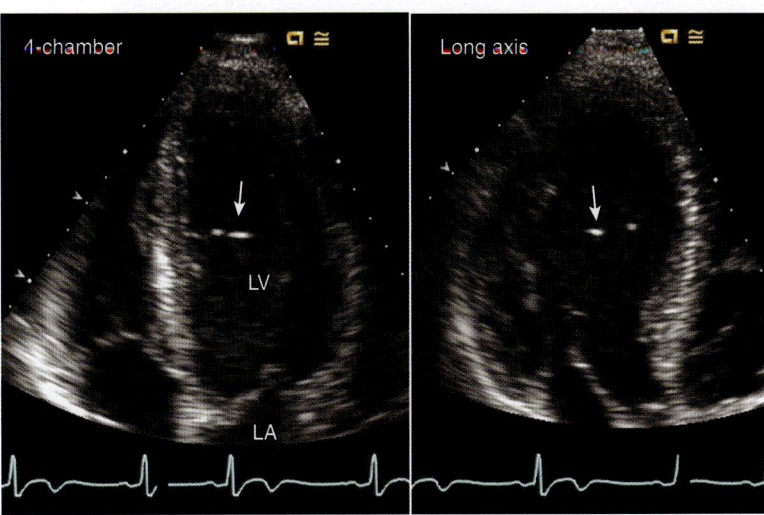

Fig. 15.1 **LV web.** Aberrant trabeculation *(arrows)* or "web" seen in an apical four-chamber view *(left)* and long-axis view appearing as bright echoes in the LV chamber with a thin structure traversing the LV chamber seen on video images.

Fig. 15.2 Christa terminalis. Normal appearance *(arrows)* in the RA in a TTE apical four-chamber view *(left)* and a TEE view *(right)*.

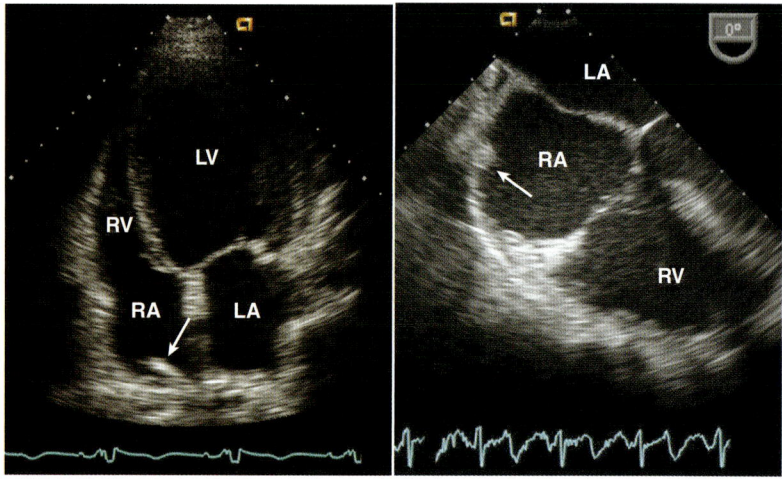

Fig. 15.3 Eustachian valve. Prominent valve *(arrows)* at the entrance of the inferior vena cava *(IVC)* into the RA seen in an apical four-chamber view *(left)* could be mistaken for a cardiac mass. A subcostal view *(right)* shows the inferior vena cava and valve more clearly.

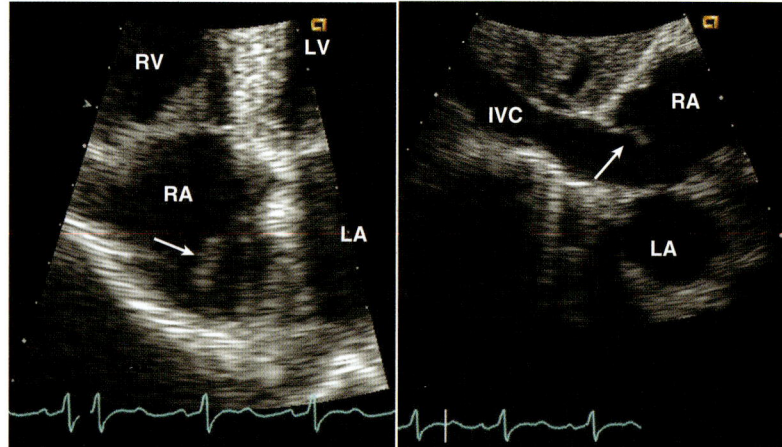

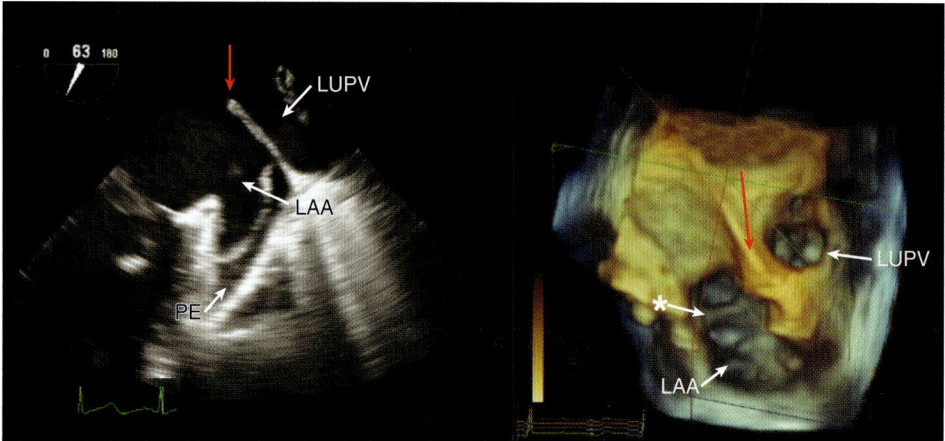

Fig. 15.4 ▶ **Normal LA appendage anatomy.** From a mid-esophageal view at about 60° of rotation *(left)*, the probe rotated to the patient's left to show the left upper pulmonary vein *(LUPV)*, as well as the prominent ridge of tissue between the appendage and left upper pulmonary vein *(red arrow)*. This ridge can be very prominent in some patients, thereby causing a reverberation artifact that could be mistaken for a thrombus in the appendage. A small pericardial effusion *(PE)* around the lateral wall of the appendage is noted. A corresponding 3D image *(right)* is seen; in the video, the appendage is noted to be fibrillating. The *asterisk* indicates a pectinate muscle. *(From Oxorn D, Otto CM. Masses. In Oxorn D, Otto CM, editors:* Intraoperative and Interventional Echocardiography: Atlas of Transesophageal Imaging, *Philadelphia, 2017, Elsevier, pp 385–414.)*

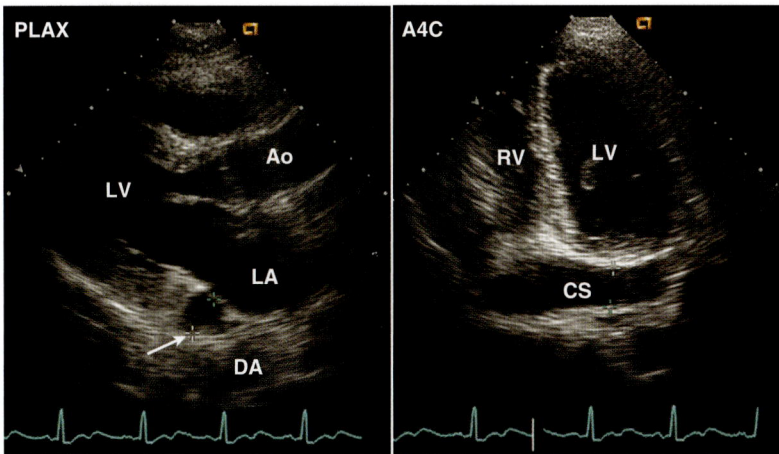

Fig. 15.5 **Persistent left superior vena cava.** Diagnosis is based on the finding of a dilated coronary sinus *(CS)* posterior to the LA *(arrow)* seen in a parasternal long-axis *(PLAX)* view (left). ▶ If ultrasound "dropout" from the wall of the coronary sinus occurs, the abnormal contour of the LA may be mistaken for a mass. In the posteriorly angulated apical four-chamber *(A4C)* view (right), the dilated coronary sinus is seen, ▶ which can be demonstrated to be connected to the RA by angulation back to a four-chamber view. *Ao,* Aorta; *DA,* descending aorta.

and bacteriologic characteristics of the structure cannot be determined. However, a reasonably secure diagnosis often can be made by integrating the clinical data, echocardiographic appearance, and associated echo Doppler findings.

VALVE VEGETATIONS

Infectious cardiac masses include valvular vegetations, which are seen in patients with endocarditis (bacterial or fungal). Noninfectious vegetations also occur in patients with nonbacterial thrombotic endocarditis (NBTE, or *marantic* endocarditis). Vegetations typically are irregularly shaped, attached to the upstream side of the valve leaflet (e.g., LA side of the mitral valve, LV side of the aortic valve), and exhibit chaotic motion that differs from that of the leaflets themselves (Fig. 15.6). Valvular regurgitation is a frequent but not invariable accompaniment of endocarditis. Valvular stenosis *due to* the vegetation is rare. Paravalvular abscess, which also manifests as a cardiac mass, often is difficult to recognize on transthoracic imaging but can be diagnosed with high sensitivity and specificity on TEE echocardiography. Infectious cardiac masses are discussed in detail in Chapter 14.

CARDIAC TUMORS

Nonprimary

Nonprimary cardiac tumors are approximately 20 times more common than primary cardiac tumors. Tumors can involve the heart by direct invasion from adjacent malignancies (lung, breast), by lymphatic spread, or by metastatic spread of distant disease (lymphoma, melanoma) (Fig. 15.7). In an autopsy series of patients with a malignant disease, cardiac involvement was present in approximately 10% of cases, although clinical recognition of cardiac involvement occurs less frequently. Melanoma has the highest rate of pericardial metastases, but because relatively few patients have melanoma, a cardiac tumor is more likely to represent a more prevalent malignant disease, as shown in Table 15.2.

Almost three fourths of cardiac metastases are due to lung, breast, or hematologic malignancies. Lymphomas associated with acquired immunodeficiency syndrome (AIDS) have frequent and extensive cardiac involvement.

Nonprimary cardiac tumors can affect the heart by:

- Invasion of the pericardium, epicardium, myocardium, or endocardium
- Production of biologically active substances
- Toxic effects of treatment on the heart (e.g., radiation or chemotherapy)

Cardiac malignancies most often involve the pericardium and epicardium (approximately 75% of metastatic cardiac disease) and manifest as a pericardial effusion, with or without tamponade physiology (Fig. 15.8). Because echocardiographic diagnosis of the *cause* of a pericardial effusion rarely is possible, the diagnosis of a pericardial effusion (and particularly tamponade) in a patient with a known malignancy should alert the clinician to the possibility of cardiac involvement. Confirmation of the diagnosis requires examination of pericardial fluid and, if necessary, pericardial biopsy. The differential diagnosis of a pericardial effusion in a patient with a known malignancy includes radiation pericarditis and idiopathic pericarditis (which is common in patients with cancer), in addition to metastatic disease. Repeat echocardiographic evaluation of patients with a malignant pericardial effusion often is needed after the initial diagnosis for assessment of therapeutic interventions and follow-up for recurrent effusion.

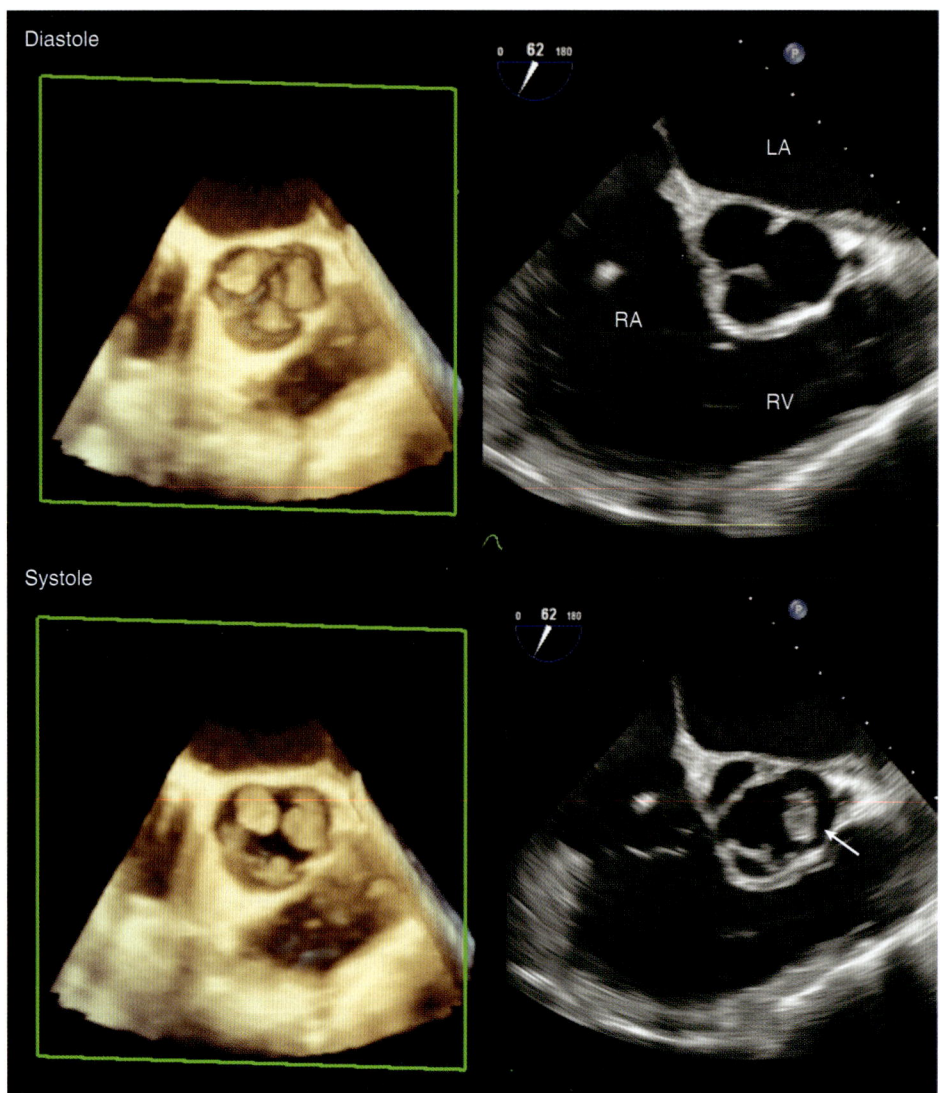

Fig. 15.6 2D and 3D images of aortic valve vegetations. TEE short-axis views of the aortic valve in diastole *(top)* ▶ and systole *(bottom)* ▶ using 3D *(left)* and 2D *(right)* imaging. 3D imaging shows three vegetations, one on each leaflet of the aortic valve. On 2D imaging only one vegetation *(arrow)* is seen in systole, with none visible on the diastolic image because the 2D image plane does not include the entire 3D height of the valve, but rather only a single image plane.

Myocardial involvement by metastatic disease is less common than pericardial involvement, but it does occur, particularly with lymphoma or melanoma. Intramyocardial masses can project into or compress cardiac chambers, with resulting hemodynamic compromise. Endocardial involvement is rarely seen.

A specific type of cardiac involvement by tumor that should be recognized by the echocardiographer is the extension of *renal cell carcinoma* up the inferior vena cava (Fig. 15.9). A "fingerlike" projection of a tumor protrudes into the right atrium (RA) from the inferior vena cava, and the tumor can be followed retrograde (from a subcostal approach) back to the kidney. Correlation with other wide-view imaging techniques is needed for full delineation of the tumor extent. *Uterine tumors* also occasionally manifest in this fashion.

Tumors also can affect the cardiac structures indirectly, as is seen in *carcinoid heart disease* (Fig. 15.10). Metastatic carcinoid tissue in the liver produces biologically active substances, including serotonin, which cause abnormalities of the right-sided cardiac valves and endocardium. Typical changes include thickening, retraction, and increased rigidity of the tricuspid and pulmonic valve leaflets, thus resulting in valvular regurgitation or, less often, valvular stenosis. Left-sided valvular involvement is rarely seen, possibly because of a lower concentration of the active molecules after passage through the lungs. Although metastatic carcinoid disease is rare, the echocardiographic

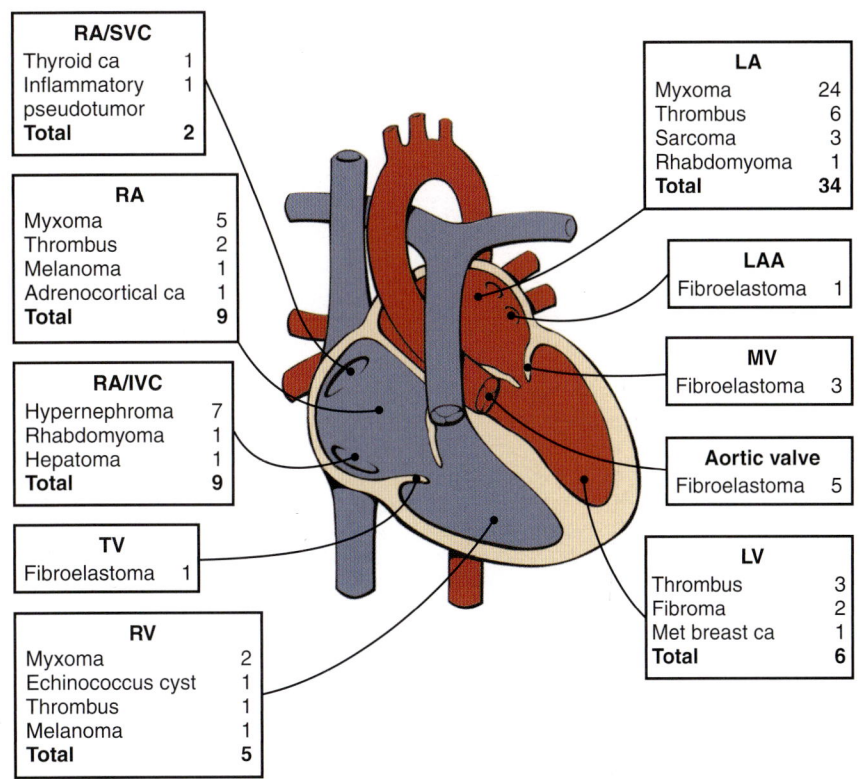

Fig. 15.7 **Distribution and pathologic characteristics of cardiac masses according to intracardiac attachment site.** In this series of 75 consecutive patients undergoing surgery for cardiac mass removal, masses were most often seen in the LA (46%), followed by the RA/inferior vena cava (IVC)/superior vena cava (SVC) (27%), LV (8%), and RV (7%); in addition, 12% were attached to a valve. The most common causes of masses requiring excision were myxomas (41%), thrombi (16%), fibroelastoma (13%), and hypernephroma (9%). The baseline or postprocedure intraoperative TEE altered management in 16% of cases. *ca,* Carcinoma; *LAA,* LA appendage; *met,* metastatic; *MV,* mitral valve; *TV,* tricuspid valve. (From Dujardin KS, Click RL, Oh JK: The role of intraoperative transesophageal echocardiography in patients undergoing cardiac mass removal, J Am Soc Echocardiogr 13:1080–1083, 2000.)

TABLE 15.2	Origin of Metastatic Cardiac Tumors in Adults (in Order of Frequency)

Lung
Lymphoma
Breast
Leukemia
Stomach
Melanoma
Liver
Colon

Data from Abraham KP, Reddy V, Gattuso P: Neoplasms metastatic to the heart: review of 3314 consecutive autopsies, *Am J Cardiovasc Pathol* 3:195–198, 1990.

Primary

As for tumors elsewhere in the body, the distinction between benign and malignant primary cardiac tumors is based on pathologic examination of tissue and its tendency to invade adjacent tissue or metastasize to distant sites (Table 15.3). Although 75% of primary cardiac tumors are benign, a pathologically benign cardiac tumor can have "malignant" hemodynamic consequences if it obstructs the normal pattern of blood flow. Thus, the echocardiographic examination includes definition of both the anatomic extent of a cardiac tumor and its physiologic consequences.

Benign Primary Cardiac Tumors

Myxomas account for 27% of primary cardiac tumors. Cardiac myxomas most often are single, arising from the fossa ovalis of the interatrial septum and protruding into the LA (in approximately 75% of cases) (Fig. 15.11). Other sites of origin include the RA (18%), the LV (4%), and the right ventricle (RV) (4%). More than one site can occur in an individual patient (5% of cases).

findings are pathognomonic and should lead to the diagnosis in a patient in whom it was not considered previously. About one third of patients with carcinoid tumors have cardiac involvement, and one half of the deaths in patients with carcinoid disease are due to heart failure resulting from severe tricuspid regurgitation.

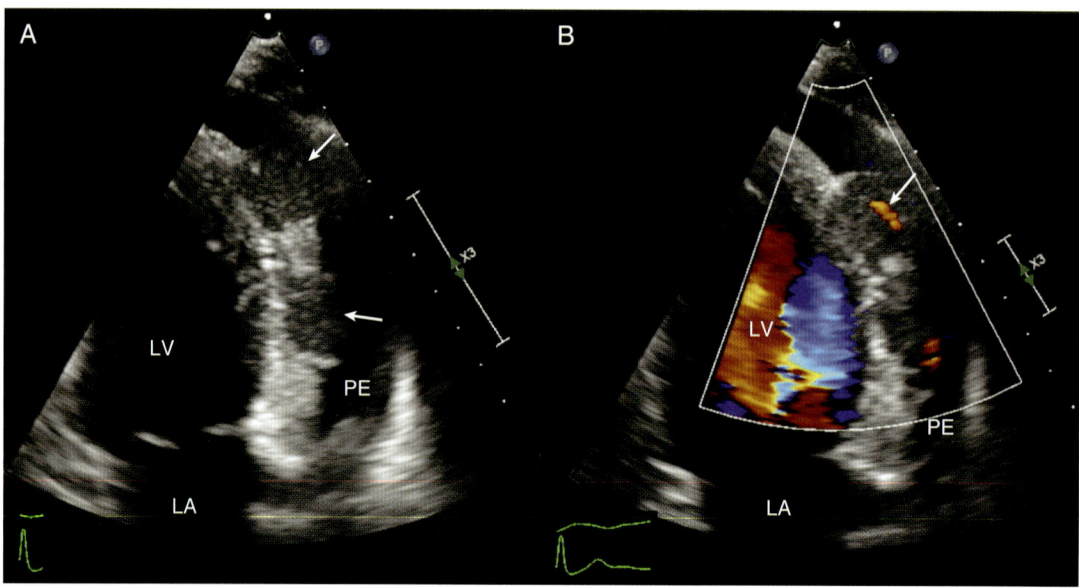

Fig. 15.8 Metastatic hepatocellular carcinoma. A mass *(arrow)* is seen involving the myocardium with marked thickening of the RV free wall and near cavity obliteration in parasternal long-axis (A) ▶ and short-axis (B) ▶ views. A pericardial effusion *(PE)* also is present.

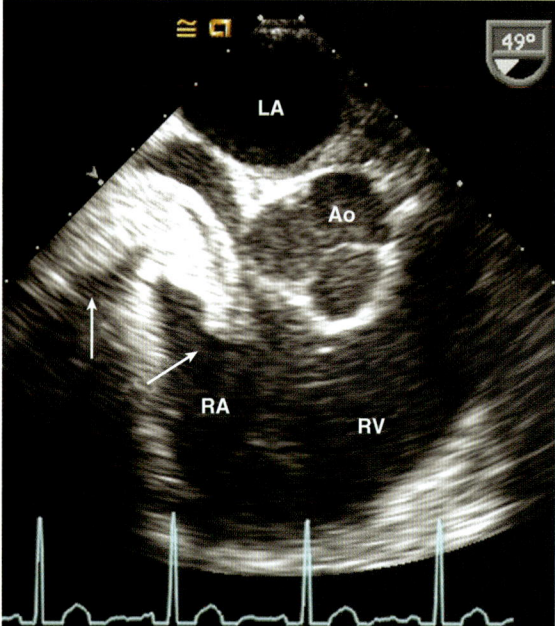

Fig. 15.9 Renal cell carcinoma. TEE imaging in a patient with renal cell carcinoma showing the extension into the RA *(arrows)* from the inferior vena cava without involvement of the atrial wall, septum, or valves. *Ao,* Aorta.

The clinical presentation of a cardiac myxoma includes constitutional symptoms (fever, malaise), clinically evident embolic events, and symptoms of mitral valve obstruction. A myxoma also may be an unexpected finding on a study requested for other clinical indications.

An LA myxoma varies in size from very small to nearly completely filling the LA chamber (Fig. 15.12), with prolapse of the tumor mass across the mitral annulus into the LV in diastole (accounting for the tumor "plop" on auscultation). The mass often has an irregular shape characterized by protruding "fronds" of tissue or a "grape cluster" appearance. The echogenicity of the mass typically is nonhomogeneous, sometimes with areas of calcification.

The degree to which the tumor causes functional obstruction to LV diastolic filling is evaluated qualitatively by color flow imaging and quantitatively by the pressure half-time method. Careful echocardiographic evaluation from multiple views, often including TEE, is needed in planning the surgical approach. Important goals of the echo examination are:

- To identify the site of tumor attachment
- To ensure that the tumor does not involve the valve leaflets themselves
- To exclude the possibility of multiple masses

Postoperatively, complete excision should be documented by echocardiography. Sequential long-term follow-up is indicated because recurrent myxomas have been reported, particularly with a familial form of this disease, with multiple myxomas, or with a less than full-thickness excision.

The echocardiographic approach to myxomas arising in other locations is similar to that described for LA myxomas, except that the imaging and Doppler examination are tailored to evaluating the specific region of tumor involvement in that patient. Again, a diagnosis based on clinical features, anatomic location, and echocardiographic appearance is only

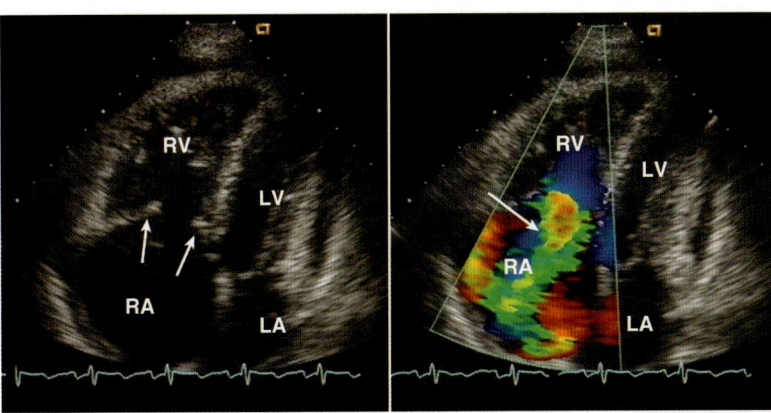

Fig. 15.10 **Carcinoid heart disease.** Thickening and shortening of the tricuspid leaflets *(arrows)* are seen in an apical four-chamber view *(left).* Mild stenosis and severe regurgitation of the tricuspid valve were present, as seen on color flow imaging *(right).*

TABLE 15.3	Primary Cardiac Tumors in Adults
Benign	
Myxoma	27%
Lipoma	10%
Papillary fibroelastoma	10%
Hemangioma	3%
Mesothelioma of the AV node	1%
Malignant	
Angiosarcoma	9%
Rhabdomyosarcoma	5%
Mesothelioma	4%
Fibrosarcoma	3%
Malignant lymphoma	2%
Extraskeletal osteosarcoma	1%
Cysts	
Pericardial	18%
Bronchogenic	2%

AV, Atrioventricular.
Data from McAllister HA, Fenoglio JJ: Tumors of the cardiovascular system. In *Atlas of tumor pathology,* fascicle 15, 2nd series, Bethesda, MD, 1978, Armed Forces Institute of Pathology.

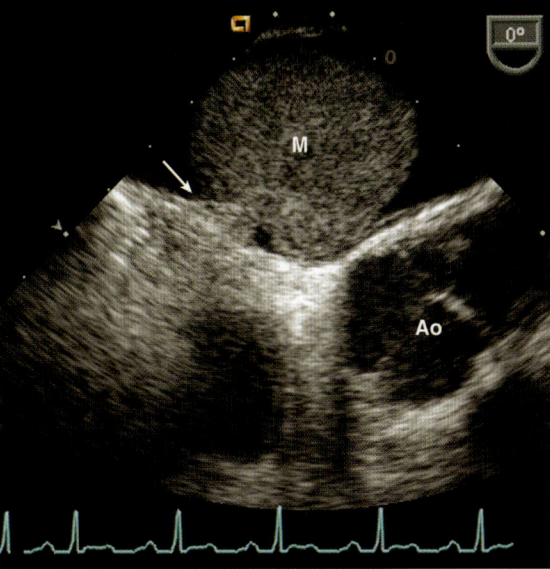

Fig. 15.11 ▶ **TEE LA myxoma.** A mass *(M)* arising from a thin stalk *(arrow)* attached to the fossa ovalis of the interatrial septum is seen in a TEE view. *Ao,* Aorta

presumptive until confirmed histologically. A "typical" myxoma may turn out to be a metastatic malignancy or a primary cardiac malignancy on pathologic examination. Hence the echocardiographic examination should be as complete as possible to exclude tissue invasion by the tumor, multiple sites of involvement, or atypical features.

A *papillary fibroelastoma* is a benign cardiac tumor that arises on valvular tissue, thus mimicking the appearance of a valvular vegetation. A papillary fibroelastoma appears as a small mass attached to the aortic or mitral valve with motion independent from the normal valve structures (Fig. 15.13). Other attachment sites for a papillary fibroelastoma include the tricuspid or pulmonic valve and nonvalvular sites. Unlike a vegetation, a fibroelastoma is more often found on the downstream side of the valve (LV side of mitral valve, aortic side of aortic valve). The histologic appearance is very similar to that of the smaller Lambl excrescences, which can be seen on normal valves in older adults. Usually a small papillary fibroelastoma is of no clinical significance; the relationship of larger benign valve tumors to embolic events is controversial. In addition, some cases of superimposed thrombus formation resulting in systemic embolic events have been described. Often these tumors are better visualized on TEE imaging.

Other benign cardiac tumors seen in adults include hemangiomas and mesotheliomas of the atrioventricular node.

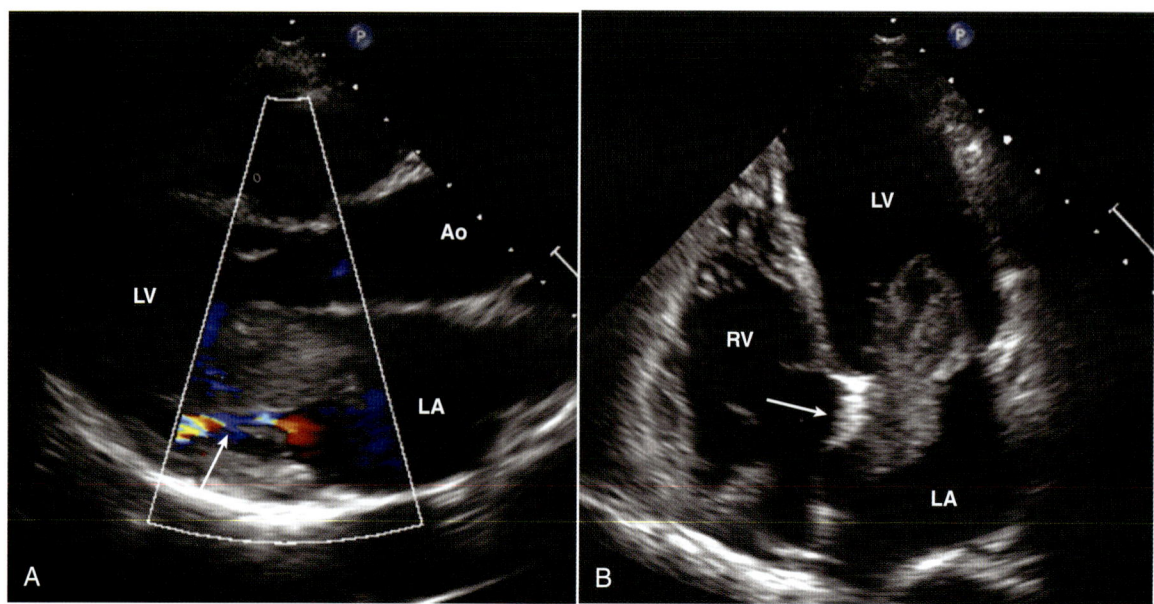

Fig. 15.12 TTE large LA myxoma. A parasternal long-axis view (A) shows the tumor prolapsing into the mitral orifice in diastole, which results in functional mitral stenosis with only a narrow flow stream seen with color Doppler. In the apical view (B), the attachment to the septum *(arrow)* and the inhomogeneous echogenicity of the myxoma are seen. *Ao,* Aorta.

Lipomatous hypertrophy of the interatrial septum manifests as a cardiac mass that is often mistaken for a tumor. Lipomatous hypertrophy typically involves the superior and inferior fatty portions of the atrial septum and spares the fossa ovalis region (Fig. 15.14). However, symmetric ellipsoid enlargements of the interatrial septum also have been described. If the cause of atrial septal hypertrophy is unclear on echocardiography, CT scanning establishes the diagnosis of lipomatous hypertrophy by showing the characteristic radiographic density of adipose tissue.

Malignant Primary Cardiac Tumors

Malignant primary cardiac tumors are rare. In adults, angiosarcomas (Fig. 15.15), rhabdomyosarcomas (Fig. 15.16), mesotheliomas, and fibrosarcomas are seen (see Table 15.1). The clinical presentation is variable, ranging from an "incidental" finding on echocardiography or nonspecific systemic symptoms (fever, malaise, fatigue) to signs and symptoms of cardiac tamponade. Because metastatic disease is far more likely than a primary cardiac origin, thorough evaluation must include a search for potential primary sites. Ultimately, the diagnosis depends on examination of tissue from the cardiac mass.

The echocardiographic examination focuses on:

- The anatomic location and extent of the tumor involvement
- The physiologic consequences of the tumor (e.g., valvular regurgitation, chamber obliteration, obstruction) (see Fig. 15.16)
- Associated findings (pericardial effusion, evidence of tamponade physiology)

Along with other imaging techniques, the echocardiographic examination helps guide therapy by determining whether the tumor is resectable or whether palliative cardiac procedures are likely to be beneficial. Specific attention also is directed toward possible involvement of the valves, coronary arteries, or conduction system.

Technical Considerations and Alternate Approaches

Although echocardiography has definite advantages for evaluating cardiac tumors, it has significant disadvantages as well. These include (1) poor acoustic access, resulting in suboptimal image quality, which limits the confidence with which tumor location and extent can be defined or results in a missed diagnosis (TEE imaging obviates this limitation in some patients); (2) the need for a careful and meticulous examination to detect and evaluate fully the cardiac tumor (as for other applications, echocardiography is operator dependent, and a significant learning curve for obtaining optimal data can be observed); and (3) the limited "field of view" inherent in echocardiography (i.e., structures adjacent to the heart in the mediastinum and lung are difficult to evaluate). Other tomographic imaging techniques, specifically CT and CMR, have the advantage of a wide field of view, so the relationship between cardiac and extracardiac tumor involvement can be evaluated. Often judicious use of both

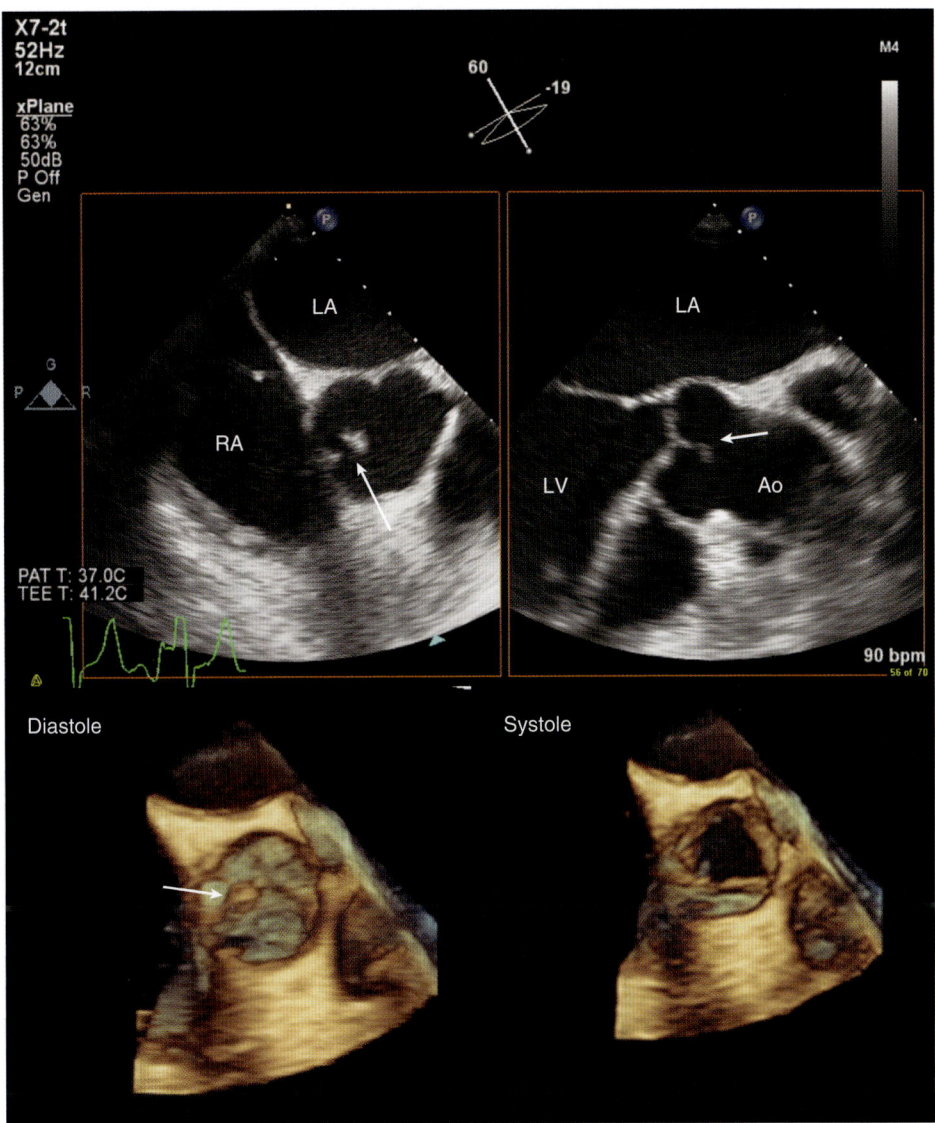

Fig. 15.13 Papillary fibroelastoma on 2D and 3D imaging. TEE imaging in this patient with an unexplained systemic embolic event shows a small, mobile echodensity *(arrows)* on the aortic side of the valve on both biplane 2D *(top)* ▶ and on 3D *(bottom)* ▶ images. This appearance is typical of a papillary fibroelastoma. *Ao,* Aorta.

echocardiographic techniques (to assess cardiac involvement in detail and to evaluate the physiologic consequences of the tumor mass) and CT or CMR (to assess potential extracardiac involvement) is needed in an individual patient for optimal clinical decision making. CT and CMR provide data on the tissue characteristics of the abnormal mass, which currently cannot be obtained with echocardiography (Fig. 15.17).

LEFT VENTRICULAR THROMBUS

Predisposing Conditions

Thrombus formation in the LV tends to occur in regions of blood stasis or low-velocity blood flow. The most familiar example of blood flow stasis in the LV is a ventricular aneurysm, in which low-velocity swirling blood flow patterns are seen. Stasis also occurs with less severe segmental wall motion abnormalities (e.g., apical akinesis) and with diffuse LV dysfunction (e.g., dilated cardiomyopathy). LV thrombus formation is extremely rare in the absence of an akinetic or dyskinetic apex or diffuse LV dysfunction. Thrombus formation also often accompanies an LV pseudoaneurysm. In this case, the thrombus lines an area of LV rupture that has been contained by the pericardium (see Figs. 8.25 and 8.26).

Even when a definite LV thrombus is not seen on echocardiographic examination, the likelihood of thrombus formation remains high in patients with

LV aneurysm, apical akinesis, or diffuse LV systolic dysfunction with an ejection fraction less than 20%. Doppler analysis of apical flow patterns has been suggested to help identify which of these patients are at the highest risk of thrombus formation. Evidence of apical flow stasis or of continuous swirling of flow around the apex is thought to identify patients at particular risk for apical thrombus.

Identification of Left Ventricular Thrombi

The sensitivity and specificity of echocardiography for detecting LV thrombi are high, about 95% and 85% to 90% respectively. A careful and thorough examination requires not only standard views but also angulated apical views and the use of higher-frequency, short-focus transducers to improve near-field resolution. It is advantageous to use a 5- or 7.5-MHz transducer from the standard apical four-chamber window and also to move the transducer slightly laterally while angulating it anteriorly to obtain an apical short-axis view. Scanning across the apex in several views usually allows for the distinction of apical thrombi from prominent apical trabeculations or false tendons, which are bright linear structures that attach to mural trabeculae. A thrombus is often (although not always) more echogenic than the underlying myocardium and has a contour distinct from the endocardial border. Contrast opacification of the LV improves the diagnosis of apical thrombus and should be considered when clinical or imaging findings raise this concern.

The diagnosis of LV thrombus is most secure when an echogenic mass is seen with a convex surface that is not a "ring-down" artifact, is clearly distinct from the endocardium, and is located in a region of abnormal wall motion (Fig. 15.18). The diagnosis of laminated thrombus is more difficult unless a clear demarcation between the thrombus and the underlying myocardium is seen, but it can be suspected when the apex appears "rounded" and akinetic, with apparent excessively thick apical myocardium.

Clinical Implications

The presence of an LV thrombus on echocardiographic examination is a strong predictor of subsequent embolic events, particularly when the thrombus protrudes into the ventricular cavity or shows independent mobility. Sessile, nonprotruding thrombi may have lower embolic potential. In some cases, apical images are suboptimal despite careful examination technique and use of left-sided contrast. In this situation, a definite exclusion of apical thrombus is not possible.

Alternate Approaches

Transthoracic echocardiography is the clinical procedure of choice for the identification of LV thrombi. TEE imaging rarely is helpful. Although specificity is high (about 96%), sensitivity is very low (only about 40%) because the apex often is missed in standard

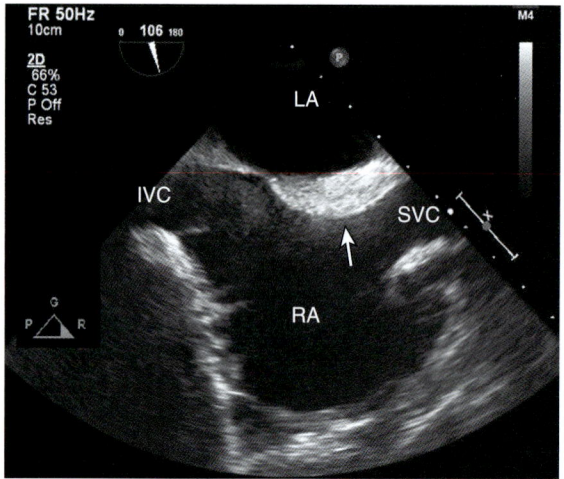

Fig. 15.14 Lipomatous hypertrophy of the interatrial septum. Thickening and increased brightness of the atrial septum *(arrow)* are seen in a TEE bicaval view with typical sparing of the thin fossa ovalis. A Eustachian valve is present at the entrance of the inferior vena cava *(IVC)* into the RA, and normal trabeculation of the atrial wall is seen. *SVC*, Superior vena cava.

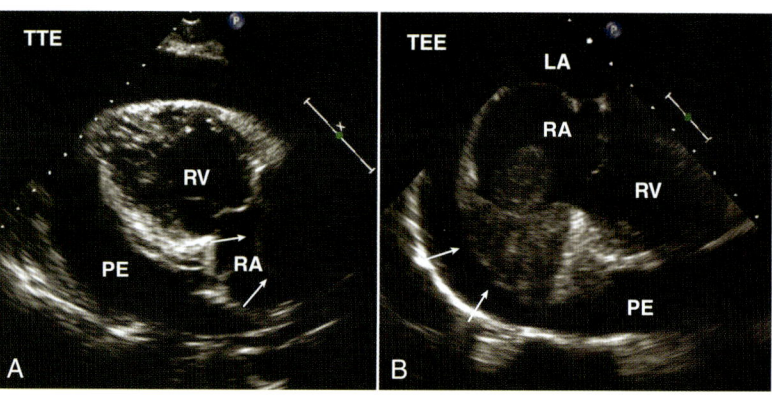

Fig. 15.15 Angiosarcoma. This 45-year-old man diagnosed with a primary cardiac angiosarcoma presented with a pericardial effusion. On a TTE RV inflow view (A), the pericardial effusion *(PE)* is seen, and a mass in the RA is faintly visualized *(arrows)*. (B) TEE images show the tumor mass in the RA and demonstrate involvement of the RA wall *(arrows)*.

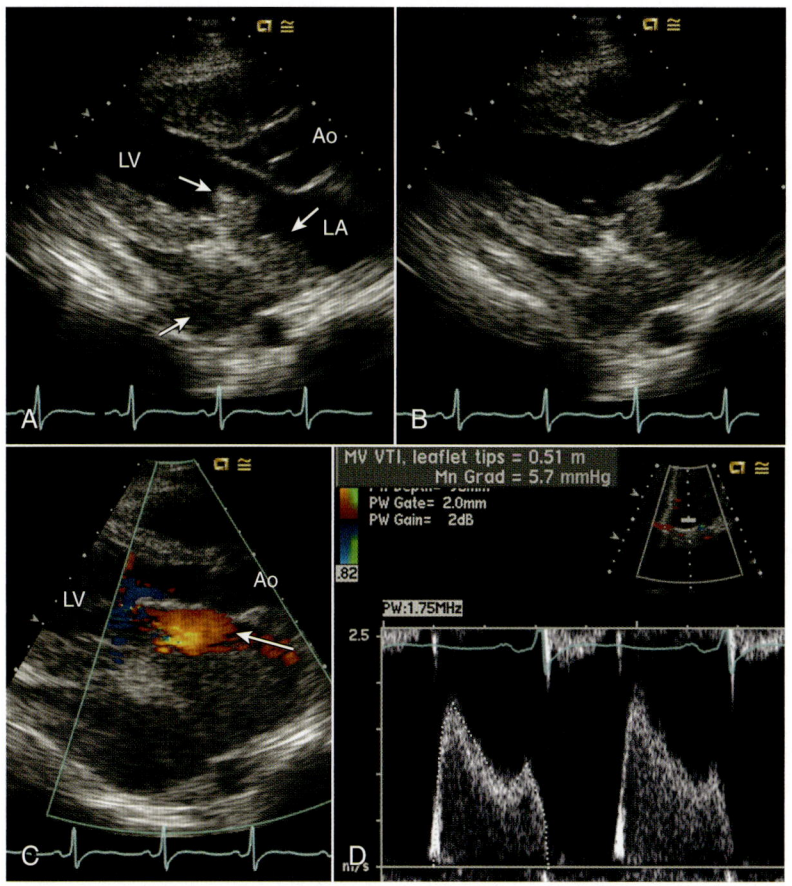

Fig. 15.16 Rhabdomyosarcoma. In the parasternal long-axis view in diastole (A), ▶ a large mass *(arrows)* is seen partly filling the left atrium with extension into the pericardial space and along the posterior mitral leaflet. In systole (B), ▶ the mitral leaflet mass prolapses into the LA. Color Doppler (C) shows only a narrow flow stream *(arrow)* from the LA to the LV in diastole, and pulsed Doppler (D) confirms mild to moderate obstruction to LV inflow with a mean gradient *(Mn Grad)* of 6 mmHg and a prolonged pressure half-time. *Ao,* Aorta.

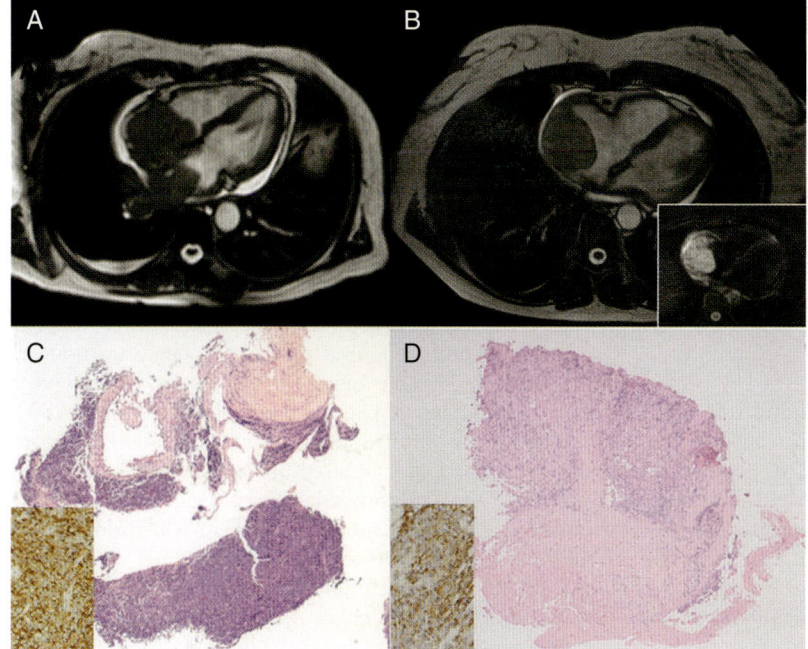

Fig. 15.17 Cardiac magnetic resonance imaging of RA masses. (A) and (B) Examples of cardiac magnetic resonance imaging for diagnosis of cardiac masses in two different patients. In (B), Note the early enhancement *(inset)*. Endomyocardial biopsy sample (C) from the patient documented in (A) shows proliferation of atypical, pleomorphic large lymphocytes. The cells stain positively for CD20 *(inset)*, in keeping with primary lymphoma. Endomyocardial biopsy sample (D) from the patient documented in (B) shows fibrous tissue and proliferation of atypical, pleomorphic spindle cells. The cells stain positively for CD31 and factor VIII *(inset)*, in keeping with angiosarcoma. *(From Basso C, Rizzo S, Valente M, Thiene G. Cardiac masses and tumours,* Heart *102[15]:1230–1245, 2016.)*

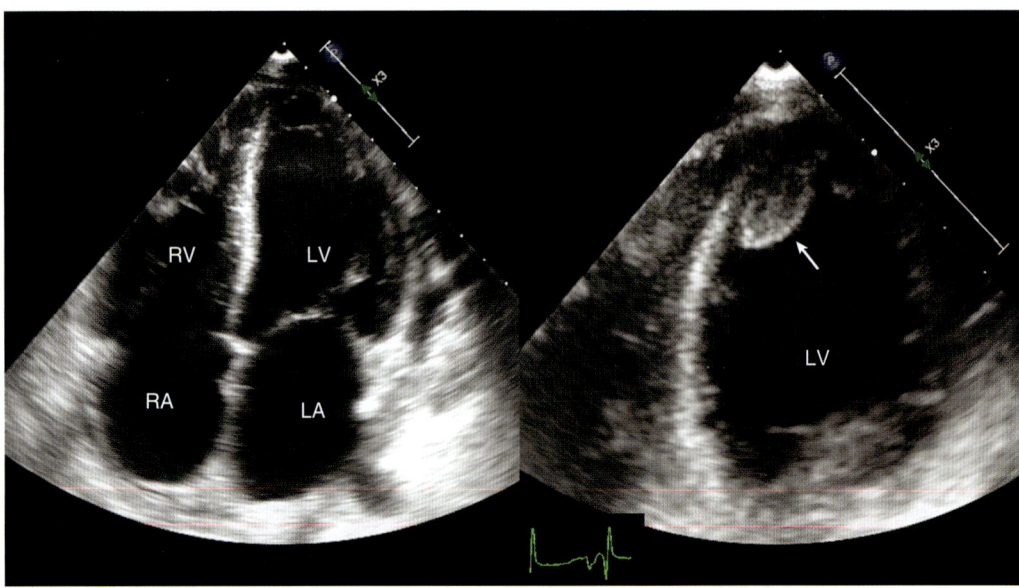

Fig. 15.18 LV apical thrombus. The standard apical four-chamber view *(left)* shows apical hypokinesis but no definite thrombus. An oblique apical view *(right)*, obtained by moving the transducer laterally and angulating anteriorly, demonstrates a protruding thrombus *(arrow)*. Left-sided echo contrast improves the sensitivity of echocardiography in patients with suspected LV thrombus.

image planes and is at a considerable distance from the transducer, thereby limiting resolution of structural detail. LV contrast angiography and radionuclide ventriculography both have low sensitivity and specificity for diagnosing LV thrombus. In the research setting, gamma-camera imaging of indium-114–labeled platelets has shown a high specificity, but this approach is not available for routine clinical use. Contrast-enhanced CMR has very high sensitivity and specificity for the detection of LV thrombus and may be appropriate in selected patients (see Appendix B, Table B.20).

LEFT ATRIAL THROMBUS

Predisposing Factors

LA thrombi tend to form in the presence of stasis of blood flow in the LA. In general, low-velocity flow in the LA is associated with:

- Atrial enlargement
- Mitral valve disease
- Atrial fibrillation

The highest incidence of LA thrombus is in patients with rheumatic mitral stenosis and atrial fibrillation. However, in the presence of mitral stenosis or poor LV function, even patients in sinus rhythm and those with only modest LA enlargement can have LA thrombi. LA thrombi are less common in patients with mitral regurgitation, presumably because the high-velocity regurgitant jet mechanically disrupts the area of blood stasis within the LA.

Identification of Left Atrial Thrombi

Visualization of LA thrombi using transthoracic echocardiography is limited by two factors:

1. The LA is in the far field of the image from both parasternal and apical windows, thus limiting resolution of LA structures and possible thrombi.
2. Large percentages of LA thrombi are found in the LA appendage, which is difficult to image from the transthoracic approach.

TEE imaging has a high sensitivity and a high negative predictive value for the diagnosis of LA thrombi. Hence, TEE evaluation is the appropriate procedure when the presence or absence of LA thrombus is important for patient management. From the TEE approach, the LA lies close to the transducer, and the appendage can be visualized using a 7.5-MHz transducer in at least two orthogonal views. Optimally, the LA appendage is evaluated by centering the appendage in the image plane at the 0° or 60° transducer position by using a small field of view and a high-frequency transducer. Then, simultaneous biplane images are acquired, and if needed, the image plane is slowly rotated through 180°, keeping the atrial appendage centered in the image, to evaluate for a possible thrombus. In addition, the body of the LA and atrial septal region are evaluated using rotational scanning from 0° to 180° from a high esophageal position (Fig. 15.19).

Stasis of blood flow appears on TEE imaging as "spontaneous" echo contrast, that is, echogenic reflections from the low-velocity blood flow look like

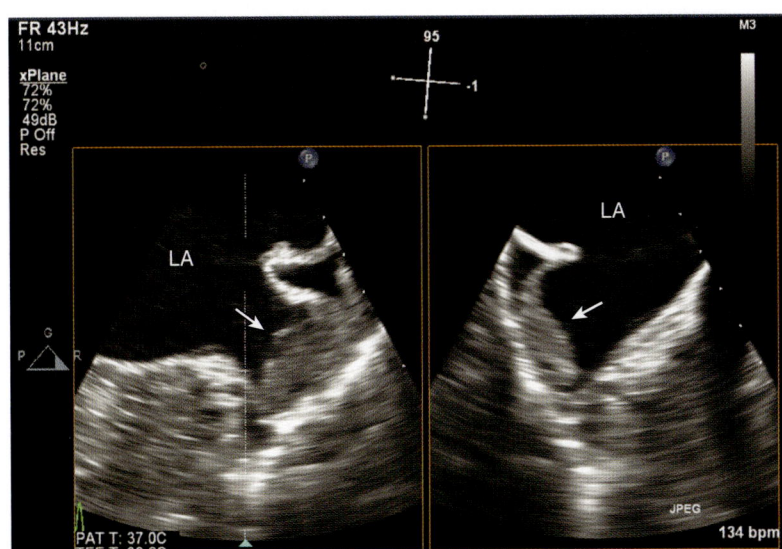

Fig. 15.19 **LA appendage thrombus.** In this 45-year-old woman with severe mitral stenosis who was referred for balloon valvotomy, orthogonal images of the LA appendage show an irregular mass *(arrows)* consistent with atrial thrombus.

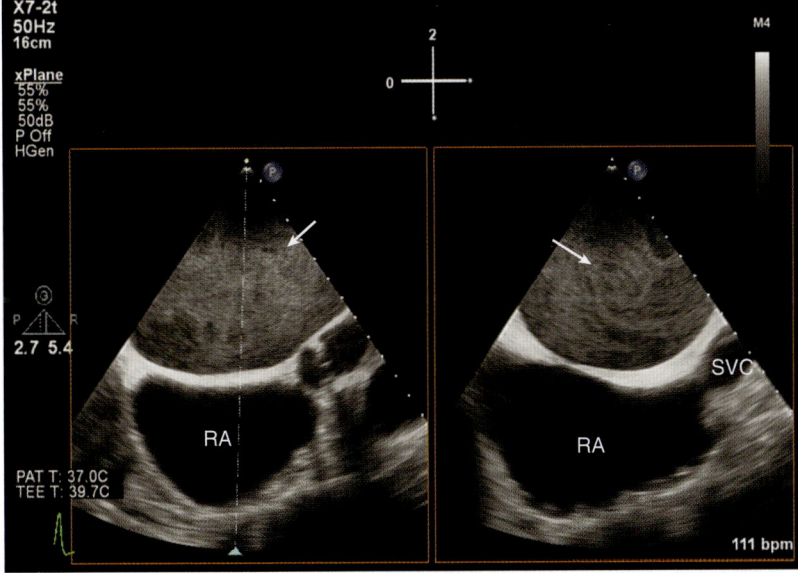

Fig. 15.20 **Spontaneous contrast in the LA.** Biplane 2D TEE images in a patient with atrial fibrillation and rheumatic mitral stenosis show swirling echodensities *(arrows)* in the LA. *SVC,* Superior vena cava.

white swirls on the echocardiographic image (Fig. 15.20). Although the appearance of "spontaneous" contrast depends on technical factors such as transducer frequency and instrument gain, in addition to the pattern of blood flow, this finding is associated with an increased risk of LA thrombus formation and embolic complications.

Doppler recordings of the pattern of blood flow in the LA appendage are helpful in identifying patients at highest risk of thrombus formation (Fig. 15.21). With a pulsed Doppler sample volume positioned approximately 1 cm from the entry of the appendage into the body of the LA, a normal contraction velocity is about 0.4 m/s; values less than this are associated with an increased risk of thrombus formation.

In some patients, the LA appendage is visualized from a transthoracic parasternal approach, starting in the short-axis view at the aortic valve level and angulating the transducer inferiorly and laterally to demonstrate the triangular appendage just inferior to the pulmonary artery. From the apical two-chamber view, the LA appendage is visualized by slight superior angulation of the transducer. If a discrete echogenic mass is seen in the LA of a patient with mitral stenosis and atrial fibrillation, the specificity of this finding for LA thrombi is high (Fig. 15.22). However, the sensitivity of transthoracic echocardiography for the detection of LA thrombus is very poor. If *no* LA thrombus is seen in a patient in whom the diagnosis is suspected, a transthoracic study certainly does *not* exclude this possibility.

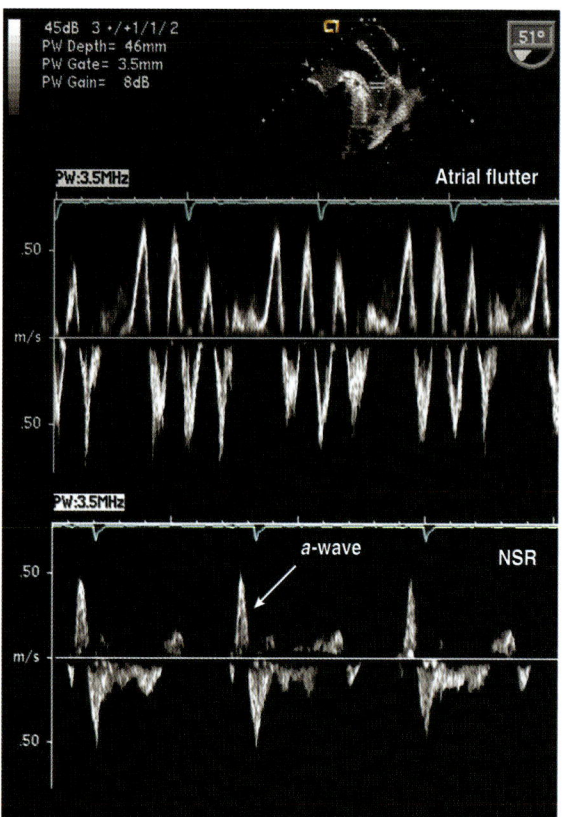

Fig. 15.21 LA appendage blood flow patterns. LA appendage flow can be recorded with a pulsed Doppler sample volume positioned about 1 cm into the appendage on TEE imaging. In a patient with atrial flutter *(top)*, flow with a velocity greater than 40 cm/s into and out of the atrial appendage is present at a rate of 300/min. In sinus rhythm *(bottom)*, normal flow shows a velocity >40 cm/s toward the transducer with atrial contraction following the electrocardiographic P wave. In contrast, when atrial fibrillation is present (see Fig. 15.23), only very low flow velocities with an irregular pattern are seen, thus leading to stasis of blood in the atrial appendage.

Prognosis and Clinical Implications

The importance of an LA thrombus depends on the clinical setting. In a patient with new atrial fibrillation and an embolic stroke, the most likely cause of the stroke is an LA thrombus whether or not one is actually imaged, and thus the demonstration of an LA thrombus would be unlikely to change clinical management. In contrast, in a patient with rheumatic mitral stenosis, the presence of an LA thrombus is a contraindication to mitral balloon valvotomy. Evaluation for LA thrombus by TEE is frequently performed before elective cardioversion and before interventional and electrophysiology procedures in which catheters or devices will be placed in the LA, for example, mitral valvuloplasty or atrial fibrillation ablation (Fig. 15.23).

Alternate Approaches

Although few direct comparisons of echocardiography versus CT or CMR have been performed, these imaging modalities also have a high sensitivity for the detection of LA thrombus. Intracardiac echocardiography is useful for evaluation of LA thrombus at the time of an invasive procedure.

RIGHT-SIDED HEART THROMBI

Formation of thrombi in the right side of the heart is rare, although it has been reported in cases of severe RV dilation and systolic dysfunction. The more likely origin of thrombi seen within the right side of the heart is a peripheral venous thrombus that has embolized and become entrapped in the tricuspid valve apparatus or RV trabeculations during passage from the peripheral veins toward the pulmonary artery (Fig. 15.24). Thrombi also frequently form on

Fig. 15.22 LA appendage thrombus on TTE imaging. TTE apical two-chamber view *(left)* showing a definite thrombus *(arrow)* in the LA appendage. The thrombus can also be seen in the atrial appendage in an anteriorly angulated apical four-chamber view *(right)*. *Ao*, Aorta; *MVR*, mitral valve replacement.

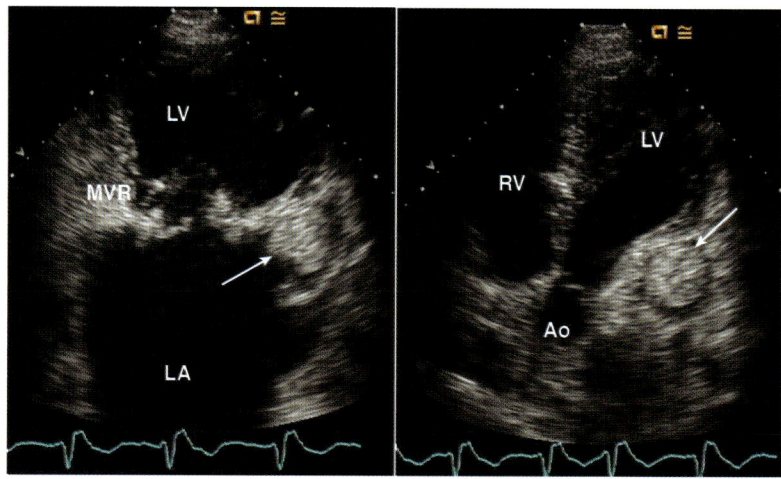

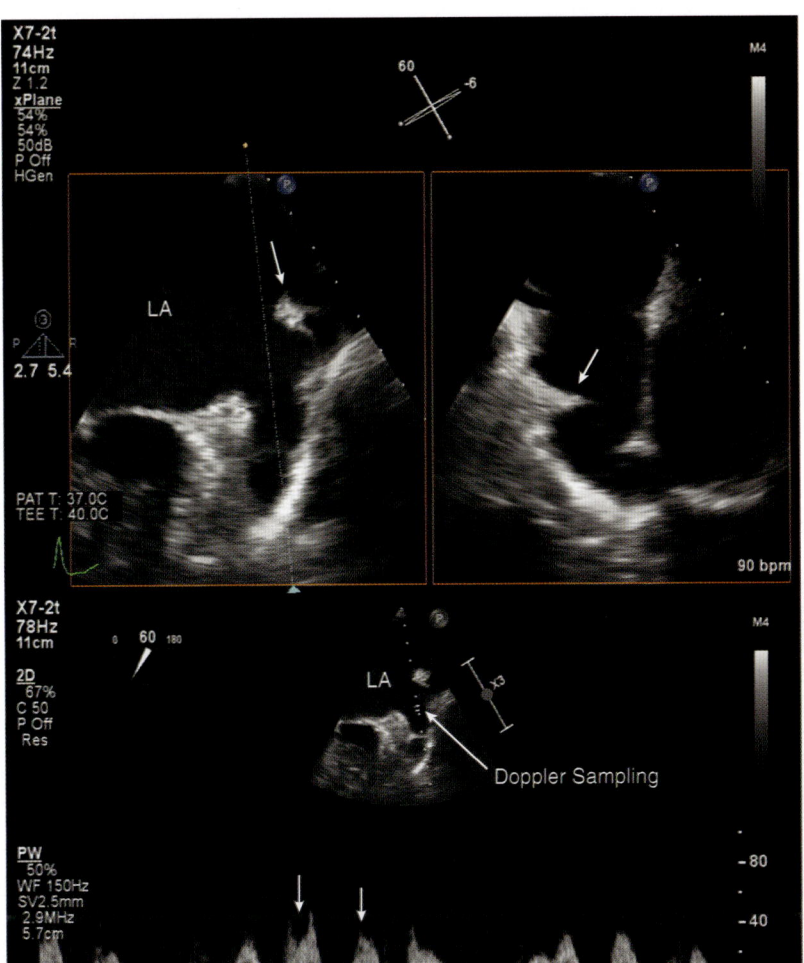

Fig. 15.23 LA appendage with atrial fibrillation. Biplane 2D TEE imaging of the left atrial appendage shows the normal ridge between the left superior pulmonary vein and atrial appendage *(upper left, arrow)* ▶ and a prominent trabeculation in the appendage *(upper right, arrow).* (Bottom) Pulsed Doppler shows low velocity irregular velocities into and out of the appendage consistent with atrial fibrillation.

indwelling catheters or pacer wires. Although thrombi in the right side of the heart are sometimes seen with meticulous transthoracic imaging (Fig. 15.25), TEE is better able to resolve the presence, extent, and attachment of right-sided heart thrombi.

When mobile echogenic targets are seen within the right heart chambers, it is important to distinguish thrombi from Eustachian valve remnants, microbubbles, or reverberation artifacts. Eustachian valve remnants, which are persistent portions of the embryologic valves of the sinus venosus, are typically mobile, thin, linear structures attached at the junction of the inferior or superior cavae and the RA cavity. A Chiari network is the term used for larger remnants that extend the length of the RA from the inferior to superior vena cava or that cross the atrium, thus attaching to the fossa ovalis. Microbubbles, which are encapsulated gas bubbles that can be seen in patients with indwelling venous access, appear as discrete echogenic targets that are usually located in different parts of the heart during successive cycles.

CARDIAC SOURCE OF EMBOLUS

Basic Principles

In a patient with a suspected cardiac origin of a systemic embolic event, echocardiographic evaluation is directed toward identification of:

- Abnormal intracardiac masses (e.g., LV thrombus, LA tumor, valvular vegetation)

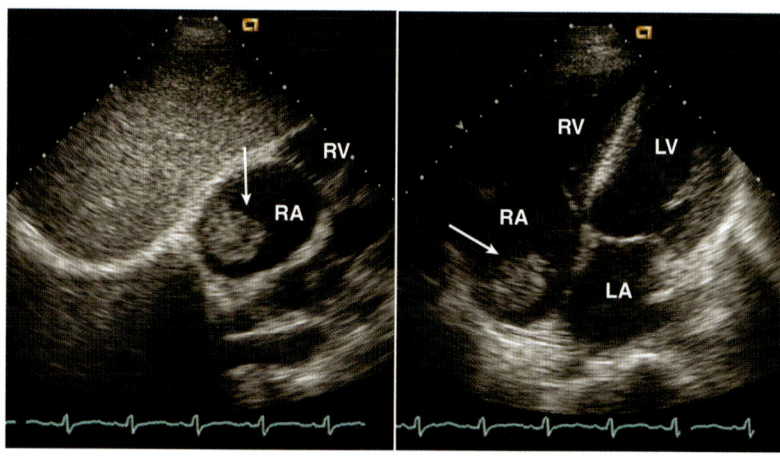

Fig. 15.24 **RA thrombus.** An echodensity *(arrows)* is seen on a subcostal view *(left)* and an apical four-chamber view *(right)*. This could be a thrombus in transit from a peripheral venous thrombosis.

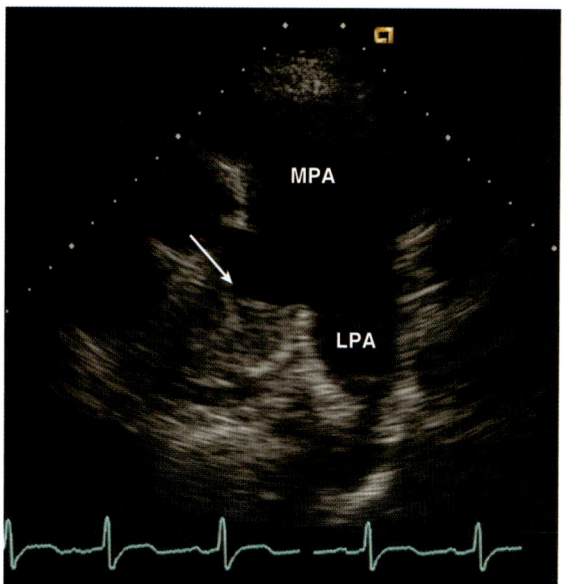

Fig. 15.25 **Pulmonary embolism.** TTE view of the main pulmonary artery *(MPA)* with bifurcation into the right pulmonary artery and left pulmonary artery *(LPA)* demonstrates an echodensity nearly filling the right pulmonary artery *(arrow)* in this 63-year-old woman with recurrent pulmonary emboli who was referred for surgical thrombectomy.

- Abnormalities that predispose the patient to the development of intracardiac thrombi (e.g., LV aneurysm, mitral stenosis, atrial flow stasis)
- Cardiac abnormalities that serve as a potential conduit for systemic embolism (e.g., patent foramen ovale, atrial septal defect)
- Aortic atheroma, with or without protruding thrombus

Note that echocardiographic evaluation *after* an index embolic event may fail to demonstrate a cardiac thrombus even if it was the cause of the clinical event because now the thrombus has embolized and is no longer in the heart. Recurrent intracardiac thrombus formation may not yet have occurred.

Identifiable Cardiac Sources of Emboli

In patients with an abnormal intracardiac mass on echocardiography in the aftermath of a recent systemic embolic event, the likelihood is very high that a portion of the mass embolized, thereby causing the clinical event. Cardiac masses known to be associated with clinical systemic embolic events include:

- Valvular vegetations
- LV and LA thrombi
- Cardiac tumors (especially LA myxomas)

In patients with suspected systemic embolic events, a definite cardiac source is documented by transthoracic echocardiography in approximately 10% to 15% of sequential cases. To some extent, the low prevalence of a definite source may relate to imaging *after* the event (when the mass is no longer in the heart). Conversely, in many patients the source of embolus was outside the heart (e.g., atheromas with or without superimposed thrombus in the carotid arteries or ascending aorta), or the intracardiac thrombi embolized soon after formation. In this latter group, it is particularly important to search for conditions that predispose the patient to intracardiac thrombus formation, even though an intracardiac thrombus is not identified at the time of the examination.

Predisposing Conditions

Apical aneurysms have a high incidence of associated thrombus formation. Other segmental wall motion abnormalities and diffuse LV systolic dysfunction also predispose to LV thrombus formation. An LV *pseudoaneurysm* is almost invariably accompanied by a thrombus lining the pseudoaneurysm cavity.

Rheumatic mitral stenosis is associated with LA thrombus formation. *Atrial fibrillation*, even when it occurs without coexisting mitral valve disease, is strongly associated with systemic embolic events, presumably because of LA thrombi. In a patient with a systemic embolic event and either paroxysmal or sustained atrial fibrillation, LA thrombus formation is so likely that even if TEE echocardiography fails to demonstrate an LA clot, it still is appropriate to treat the patient with systemic anticoagulants to prevent recurrent atrial thrombus formation.

Intracardiac thrombi occur in patients with *congenital heart disease*, particularly those with atrial dilation or ventricular dysfunction. Patients with a large atrial septal defect are at risk for "paradoxical" systemic embolization of peripheral venous thrombi. Thrombi can pass from the RA to the LA even when the shunt is predominantly left to right owing to streaming of flow or transient shifts in the RA-to-LA pressure gradient. Patients with Eisenmenger complex and a large ventricular septal defect are at risk of systemic embolization from peripheral venous thrombus formation. However, paradoxical embolization is unlikely in adults with a small ventricular septal defect because the high LV, compared with RV, pressure limits flow from right to left.

Prosthetic valves are other potential sources of embolic events; the incidence of clinical events is higher with mechanical valves compared with that of tissue valves. Demonstration of small thrombi on prosthetic valves is difficult even with TEE imaging because of shadowing and reverberations from the prosthetic leaflets and the sewing ring. Hence, the diagnosis often is presumptive when evidence exists of suboptimal anticoagulation at the time of the event or when other causes for the clinical event have been excluded even if the level of anticoagulation appears to have been adequate. In these patients, the primary goals of the echocardiographic examination are to assess prosthetic valve function (because significant thrombus often results in stenosis, regurgitation, or both) and to exclude other intracardiac sources of thrombus formation (e.g., associated LV systolic dysfunction).

TEE echocardiography provides imaging of atrial structures in more detail and has led to the recognition of other anatomic variants and disease processes that may be associated with systemic embolic events including:

- Patent foramen ovale
- Interatrial septal aneurysm
- A swirling pattern of blood flow in the LA in the absence of an exogenous "contrast" agent (thought to represent flow stasis and often called *spontaneous contrast*)
- Atherosclerosis in the aorta

A *patent foramen ovale* is present in 25% to 35% of unselected patients at autopsy. During fetal development, incomplete closure of the interatrial septum shunts oxygenated placental blood from the RA to the LA and then to the brain. This potential interatrial communication fuses within the first few days after birth in most individuals. If the flap valve covering the fossa ovalis remains unfused, usually no passage of blood occurs across the interatrial septum. The "flap" is functionally closed because LA pressure normally exceeds RA pressure. However, if RA pressure transiently exceeds LA pressure (as during a cough or the Valsalva maneuver) or if RA pressure chronically exceeds LA pressure (e.g., after pulmonary embolization or with chronic lung disease), right-to-left passage of blood (or thrombi) can occur across the interatrial septum.

An *interatrial septal aneurysm* is defined as a transient bulging of the fossa ovalis region of the interatrial septum (total excursion from the septal plane) greater than 15 mm in the absence of chronically elevated LA or RA pressure. Septal aneurysms are associated with a high likelihood (up to 90%) of associated fenestration.

Echocardiographic demonstration of a patent foramen ovale is possible with color flow Doppler imaging from a TEE approach in only about 5% to 10% of patients, with a lesser number detected by transthoracic color Doppler imaging. Detection of a patent foramen is enhanced by intravenous injection of echo-contrast material (e.g., agitated saline solution), thereby providing opacification of the right-sided heart structures (Fig. 15.26).

A saline contrast study for the detection of patent foramen ovale should:

- Use a view where contrast in the right heart will not shadow the LA
- Demonstrate contrast in the left heart within three beats of appearance in the right heart
- Record a longer digital clip to ensure correct timing of contrast appearance
- Perform at least two saline contrast injections (one at rest and one with Valsalva)
- Consider TEE whether the diagnosis could change clinical management

Using an echo-contrast agent, a patent foramen ovale is detectable at rest in approximately 5% of the general population. When maneuvers to increase RA pressure transiently are performed simultaneously with contrast injection, the prevalence of detectable patent foramen ovale by contrast TEE echocardiography increases to approximately 25%, similar to the incidence at autopsy (Fig. 15.27).

Passage of very small microbubbles through the pulmonary capillaries can occur with a peripheral injection of agitated saline; microbubbles from transpulmonary passage typically appear in the LA via the pulmonary veins late after the appearance of contrast material in the RA. With an atrial septal defect or patent foramen ovale, contrast material appears in the LA within three beats of its appearance in the right heart (Fig. 15.28).

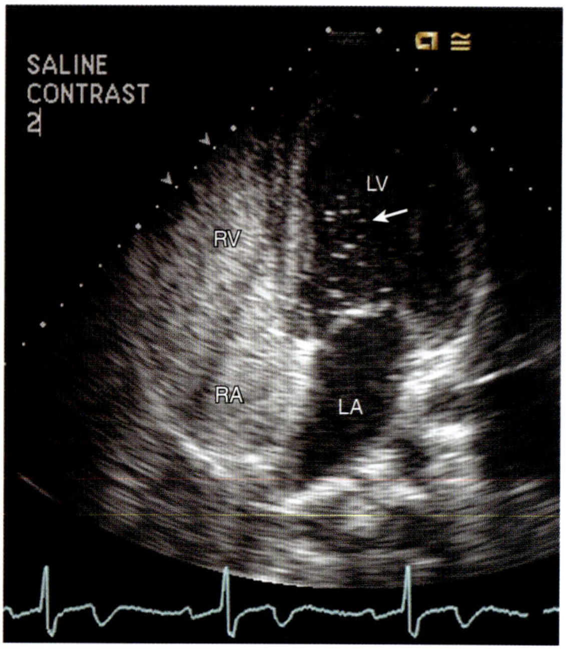

"*Spontaneous*" *contrast* is seen in the LA in the presence of stasis of blood flow. It is seen more often on TEE than on transthoracic imaging because of the higher transducer frequency and the closer proximity of the LA when interrogated from the esophagus, but it can be seen on transthoracic imaging in some patients. Spontaneous contrast is associated with LA enlargement and LA thrombus formation, and it may be a marker for a "prethrombotic" state in which definite atrial thrombi are not seen. In extreme cases of spontaneous contrast in patients with mitral stenosis, the jet of diastolic blood flow across the stenotic mitral orifice can be seen on two-dimensional (2D) imaging because of the contrast effect.

Spontaneous contrast also can be seen in the LV when stasis of blood flow is present, such as in the region of an apical aneurysm. Spontaneous contrast is observed frequently in patients with mechanical prosthetic valves. Here the mechanism of spontaneous contrast formation is different, relating to the mechanical impact of the valve occluder during closure resulting in microcavitation or the liberation of gas from solution. Of course, patients with mitral prosthetic valves also have some degree of stasis of blood flow in the LA if long-standing disease has resulted in LA enlargement and atrial fibrillation.

Fig. 15.26 ▶ **Patent foramen ovale on TTE saline contrast study.** In an apical four-chamber view, the RA and RV are opacified by saline contrast injected into an arm. A few microbubbles *(arrow)* are seen in the left side of the heart within three beats of the appearance of contrast in the right heart.

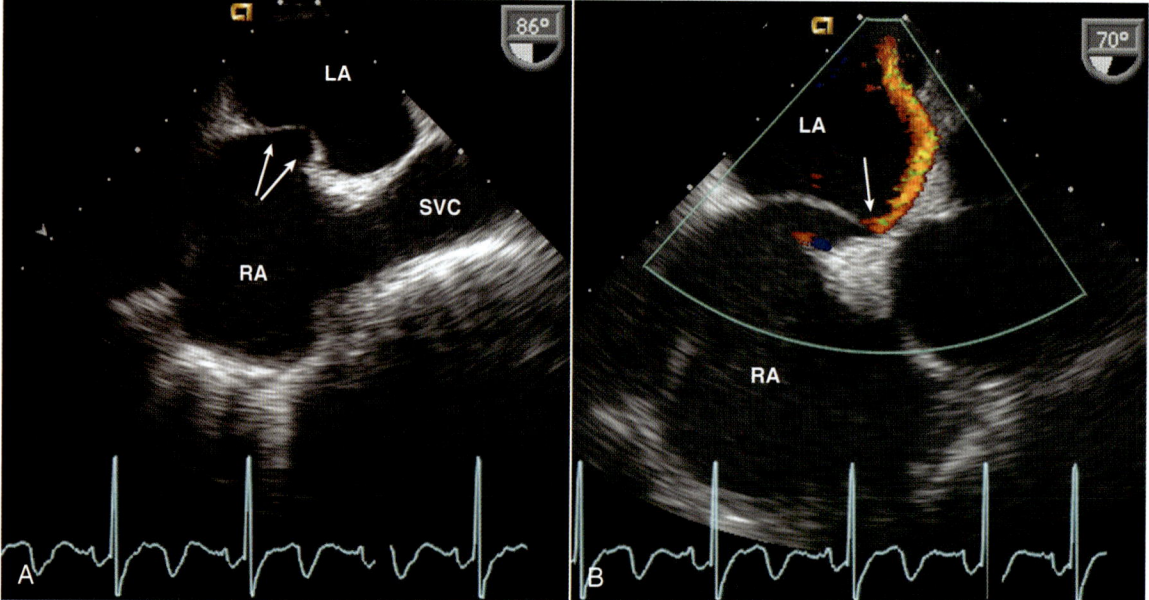

Fig. 15.27 Atrial septal aneurysm and patent foramen ovale. (A) Atrial septal aneurysm *(arrows)* seen on TEE imaging in a long-axis view of the superior vena cava *(SVC)* and RA. ▶ This is a useful view to evaluate for patent foramen ovale (B), ▶ demonstrated with color Doppler in this patient by showing a narrow jet across the patent foramen *(arrow)* from the RA to the LA.

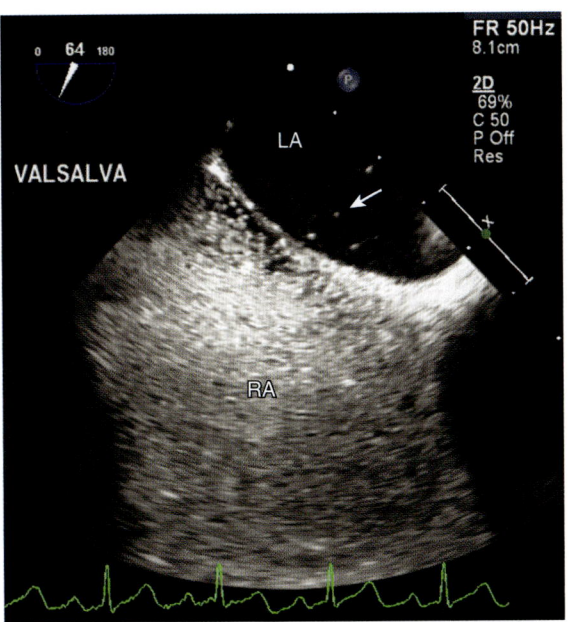

Fig. 15.28 ▶ **Patent foramen ovale on TEE saline contrast study.** The RA is opacified by saline contrast with a few microbubbles seen in the LA after Valsalva maneuver, consistent with a patent foramen ovale.

The presence of *atheroma* in the descending thoracic aorta is associated with an increased risk of stroke and transient ischemic attack. These lesions are recognized as focal areas of increased thickness in the aortic endothelium with irregular borders and nonuniform echogenicity. An atheroma is considered "complex" if thickness is greater than 4 mm, evidence of ulceration is noted, or areas of independent mobility are present.

Indications for Echocardiography in Patients With Systemic Embolic Events

Current understanding of potential cardiac causes for systemic embolism is incomplete, and considerable controversy exists about the indications for transthoracic imaging and TEE in patients with suspected systemic embolic events (Table 15.4). In patients with embolic events, the prevalence of patent foramen ovale is about 30%, compared with a prevalence of 10% in control subjects. Aortic atheromas (see Chapter 16) are seen in 20% of patients with embolic events, compared with 4% of control subjects. Other echocardiographic findings in patients with embolic events include LA

TABLE 15.4 European Association of Echocardiography Recommendations for Echocardiography in the Diagnosis and Management of Cardiac Sources of Embolism

Clinical Condition	TTE	TEE	Comments
Acute myocardial infarction	Evaluates LV and RV function and detect LV thrombus	Not useful for detection of LV thrombus	Contrast improves detection of LV thrombus on TTE.
Cardiomyopathy	Evaluates LV and RV dysfunction, detects LV thrombus	—	Contrast improves detection of LV thrombus on TTE.
Atrial fibrillation	Detects underlying structural heart disease. Used to indicate, guide, and follow-up invasive surgical procedures	Required to exclude atrial thrombus in guiding cardioversion, before ablation, in recurrent embolism, and to determine risk of future embolism	—
Detection of PFO	High sensitivity for detection of PFO with good image quality and saline contrast with Valsalva maneuver	Highest sensitivity for detection and evaluation of PFO	Factors that suggest an association between stroke and PFO include (1) a temporal relationship with a venous thrombosis, (2) younger age (<55 years) and absence of other causes, (3) associated atrial septal aneurysm, and (4) large, spontaneous, or provocable right-to-left shunt.

Continued

TABLE 15.4 European Association of Echocardiography Recommendations for Echocardiography in the Diagnosis and Management of Cardiac Sources of Embolism—cont'd

Clinical Condition	TTE	TEE	Comments
Aortic atherosclerosis	Suprasternal TTE helps identify arch atheromas.	TEE is needed when TTE images are suboptimal or when plaque characterization is needed.	—
Cardiac masses	Recommended for patients with clinical syndromes suggesting a cardiac mass or patients with conditions known to predispose them to mass formation. Recommended for follow-up after mass removal if recurrence is likely	TEE is appropriate when TTE is nondiagnostic.	—
Endocarditis	Recommended as first step in evaluation of endocarditis	Recommended when TTE findings are negative and clinical likelihood is high, with prosthetic valves or when TTE provides inadequate imaging	Repeat TTE or TEE is recommended in 7–10 days if the initial study result is negative but clinical likelihood remains high.
Prosthetic valves	TTE must be performed in patients with a prosthetic valve and embolic event.	TEE also must be performed in patients with a prosthetic valve and embolic event, even if TTE findings are negative.	Repeat TTE or TEE is recommended for follow-up after thrombolytic or anticoagulant therapy.
Intracardiac devices	TTE is recommended in patients with a device and a pulmonary embolic event or when paradoxical embolus is suspected.	TEE is also used for diagnosis of device thrombosis or infection.	Intracardiac devices include permanent pacemakers and implantable cardiac defibrillators.

PFO, Patent foramen ovale.
Summarized from Pepi M, Evangelista A, Nihoyannopoulos P, et al; European Association of Echocardiography: recommendations for echocardiography use in the diagnosis and management of cardiac sources of embolism, *Eur J Echocardiogr* 11(6):461–476, 2010.

---

thrombus in approximately 9%, spontaneous contrast in approximately 17%, and atrial septal aneurysm in 13%. The prevalence of these findings is highest in patients with cryptogenic stroke (e.g., no obvious primary cerebrovascular disease or other cause).

Current guidelines suggest that transthoracic echocardiography with a saline contrast study is appropriate in patients with neurologic or other vascular occlusive events:

- When abrupt occlusion of a major peripheral or visceral artery occurs in patients of any age
- In younger patients (<55 years) with a cerebrovascular embolic event
- In older patients with a neurologic event without other evidence of cerebrovascular disease
- In patients in whom the clinical therapeutic decision would be altered based on the echocardiographic results

The role of echocardiography in older patients with cerebrovascular disease of questionable significance or with other evident causes for the cerebrovascular event remains uncertain. If transthoracic studies are unrevealing, TEE imaging should be performed, given its higher sensitivity for diagnosis of a patent foramen ovale, LA thrombus, interatrial septal aneurysm, valvular vegetation, and small intracardiac tumors (Table 15.5).

TABLE 15.5 American Society of Echocardiography Appropriate Use Criteria for TTE and TEE in Evaluation for a Cardiac Source of Emboli

Appropriate Use	Inappropriate Use
Transthoracic Echocardiography	
<ul><li>Symptoms or conditions potentially related to a suspected cardiac etiology, including but not limited to chest pain, shortness of breath, palpitations, TIA, stroke, or peripheral embolic event</li><li>Suspected cardiac mass</li><li>Suspected cardiovascular source of embolus</li><li>Initial evaluation of suspected IE with positive blood culture results or new murmur</li><li>Reevaluation of IE at high risk for progression or complication or with a change in clinical status or cardiac examination results</li><li>Known acute pulmonary embolism, to guide therapy (e.g., thrombectomy and thrombolytic therapy)</li><li>Reevaluation of known pulmonary embolism after thrombolysis or thrombectomy for assessment of change in RV function and/or pulmonary artery pressure</li></ul>	<ul><li>Transient fever without evidence of bacteremia or new murmur</li><li>Transient bacteremia with a pathogen not typically associated with IE and/or a documented nonendovascular source of infection</li><li>Routine surveillance of uncomplicated IE when no change in management is contemplated</li><li>Suspected pulmonary embolism to establish diagnosis</li><li>Routine surveillance of prior pulmonary embolism with normal RV function and pulmonary artery systolic pressure</li></ul>
Transesophageal Echocardiography	
<ul><li>As initial or supplemental test for evaluation for cardiovascular source of embolus with no identified noncardiac source</li><li>As initial or supplemental test to diagnose IE with a moderate or high pre-test probability (e.g., Staphylococcus bacteremia, fungemia, prosthetic heart valve, or intracardiac device)</li><li>As initial test for evaluation to facilitate clinical decision making with regard to anticoagulation, cardioversion, and/or radiofrequency ablation</li><li>*Uncertain Indication: evaluation for cardiovascular source of embolus with a previously identified noncardiac source*</li></ul>	<ul><li>Evaluation for cardiovascular source of embolus with a known cardiac source in which TEE would not change management</li><li>Routine use of TEE when diagnostic TTE is reasonably anticipated to resolve all diagnostic and management concerns</li><li>Surveillance of prior TEE finding for interval change (e.g., resolution of thrombus after anticoagulation, resolution of vegetation after antibiotic therapy) when no change in therapy is anticipated</li><li>To diagnose IE with low pre-test probability (e.g., transient fever, known alternative source of infection, negative blood culture results, or atypical pathogen for endocarditis)</li><li>Evaluation when a decision has been made to anticoagulate and not to perform cardioversion</li></ul>

IE, Infective endocarditis; *TIA,* transient ischemic attack.
Data from Saric M, Armour AC, Arnaout MS, et al: Guidelines for the use of echocardiography in the evaluation of a cardiac source of embolism, *J Am Soc Echocardiogr* 29(1):1–42, 2016; and Douglas PS, Garcia MJ, Haines DE, et al: CCF/ASE/AHA/ASNC/HFSA/HRS/SCAI/SCCM/SCCT/SCMR 2011 appropriate use criteria for echocardiography. A report of the American College of Cardiology Foundation Appropriate Use Criteria Task Force, American Society of Echocardiography, American Heart Association, American Society of Nuclear Cardiology, Heart Failure Society of America, Heart Rhythm Society, Society for Cardiovascular Angiography and Interventions, Society of Critical Care Medicine, Society of Cardiovascular Computed Tomography, Society for Cardiovascular Magnetic Resonance American College of Chest Physicians, *J Am Soc Echocardiogr* 24(3):229–267, 2011.

THE ECHO EXAM

Echocardiographic Findings Associated With Systemic Embolism

Potential Embolic Source	Clinical Setting	Echocardiographic Findings	Caveats
PFO	• Cryptogenic stroke	• Saline contrast shows right-to-left shunt at the atrial level. • Best visualized in TEE	• PFO is present in 20%–30% of people.
LA thrombus	• Atrial fibrillation—before cardioversion, AF ablation, or mitral commissurotomy	• LA mass, most often located in LA appendage, often mobile	• TEE required for diagnosis of LA thrombus because of low sensitivity of TTE
Endocarditis	• Bacteremia • Clinical criteria for endocarditis	• Valve vegetations on downstream side of valve with valve destruction	• TEE often needed in addition to TTE
Prosthetic valve thrombosis	• Mechanical or bioprosthetic valve	• Mobile mass attached to leaflets or sewing ring • Valve obstruction or regurgitation	• A prosthetic valve is always a potential embolic source, even when echo findings are absent.
LV thrombus	• Apical akinesis after myocardial infarction • Global hypokinesis with dilated cardiomyopathy	• Echodense mass in LV apex	• Best seen on TTE apical views with high-frequency transducer • TEE has low sensitivity.
Aortic atherosclerosis	• Evaluation for stroke or intraoperative evaluation of aorta for graft placement	• Typical atheroma	• Aortic arch visualization suboptimal on TEE • Intraoperative direct placement of a sterile probe on the aorta is an option.
Nonbacterial thrombotic endocarditis	• Systemic inflammatory disease	• Valve masses with less independent motion than typical vegetations	• Blood cultures are needed to exclude infective endocarditis.
Lipomatous hypertrophy of the atrial septum	• Benign incidental finding	• Bright, smooth thickening of the interatrial septum with sparing of the fossa ovalis	• Echo appearance is typical, but computed tomography allows tissue characterization if diagnosis is unclear.
Papillary fibroelastoma	• Cryptogenic stroke or incidental echo finding	• Highly mobile small mass, usually attached to valve, often with a stalk	• Blood cultures are needed to exclude infective endocarditis.
Atrial myxoma	• TIA or stroke	• Well-circumscribed mass attached to atrial septum, most often in LA	• Best seen on TEE, but initial diagnosis often with TTE imaging
Secondary cardiac tumors	• Direct extension of lung or breast cancer into heart, or metastatic disease	• Pericardial effusion and tumor involvement are most common.	• Further evaluation for a specific diagnosis is needed.
Malignant primary cardiac tumors	• Rare in adults	• Intracardiac mass with invasion of chamber walls	• Imaging with cardiac magnetic resonance imaging or computed tomography provides better definition of the site and extent of tumor involvement.

AF, Atrial fibrillation; *PFO*, patent foramen ovale; *TIA*, transient ischemic attack.

Distinguishing Characteristics of Intracardiac Masses			
Characteristic	**Thrombus**	**Tumor**	**Vegetation**
Location	• LA (especially when enlarged or associated with MV disease) • LV (in setting of reduced systolic function or segmental wall abnormalities)	• LA (myxoma) • Myocardium • Pericardium • Valves	• Usually valvular • Occasionally on ventricular wall or Chiari network
Appearance	• Usually discrete and somewhat spherical *or* laminated against LV apex or LA wall	• Various: circumscribed or irregular	• Irregular shape, attached to the proximal (upstream) side of the valve with motion independent from the valve
Associated findings	• Underlying cause usually evident • LV systolic dysfunction or segmental wall motion abnormalities (exception: eosinophilic heart disease) • MV disease with LA enlargement	• Intracardiac obstruction depending on site of tumor • Clinically: fevers, systemic signs of endocarditis, positive blood culture results	• Valvular regurgitation usually present

MV, Mitral valve.

SUGGESTED READING

Cardiac Source of Embolus

1. Di Tullio M: Echocardiographic evaluation of the patient with a systemic embolic event. In Otto CM, editor: *The Practice of Clinical Echocardiography*, ed 5, Philadelphia, 2017, Elsevier, pp 802–821.
   Review of the role of echocardiography in the management of patients with systemic embolic events. Topics include LA thrombus, spontaneous echo contrast, atrial septal aneurysm, patent foramen ovale, mitral valve strands, Lambl excrescences, and aortic atheroma. Includes systematic review of the literature, examples of TTE and TEE findings, and clinical implications.

2. Pepi M, Evangelista A, Nihoyannopoulos P, et al: European Association of Echocardiography: recommendations for echocardiography use in the diagnosis and management of cardiac sources of embolism, *Eur J Echocardiogr* 11(6):461–476, 2010.
   Ischemic stroke is related to a cardiac embolic source in 15% to 30% of cases. This guideline document provides a concise overview of potential cardiac sources of embolism and provides recommendations for the use of TTE and TEE in the evaluation of patients with a stroke or transient ischemic attack..

3. Saric M, Armour AC, Arnaout MS, et al: Guidelines for the use of echocardiography in the evaluation of a cardiac source of embolism, *Am Soc Echocardiogr* 29(1):1–42, 2016.
   Comprehensive document details the echocardiographic approach to evaluation of cardiac source of embolus with recommendations for clinical use of TTE and TEE in specific clinical situations. Includes 39 illustrations, 43 online videos, and 229 references.

4. Leitman M, Tyomkin V, Peleg E, et al: Clinical significance and prevalence of valvular strands during routine echo examinations, *Eur Heart J Cardiovasc Imaging* 15(11):1226–1230, 2014.
   Valvular strands were present on about 1% of 21,000 echocardiographic studies and were most often seen on the left ventricular side of the aortic valve in men 61 to 70 years of age, often with associated leaflet thickening or calcification.

Cardiac Masses and Tumors

5. Bruce CJ: Cardiac tumors. In Otto CM, editor: *The Practice of Clinical Echocardiography*, ed 5, Philadelphia, 2017, Elsevier, pp 837–860.
   This comprehensive textbook chapter includes sections on cardiac myxomas, papillary fibroelastoma, other benign cardiac tumors, malignant primary and secondary cardiac tumors, and the differential diagnosis of a cardiac mass. Clinical management also is reviewed.

6. Auger D, Pressacco J, Marcotte F, et al: Cardiac masses: an integrative approach using echocardiography and other imaging modalities, *Heart* 97:1101–1109, 2011.
   This review presents six cases of cardiac masses and demonstrates how multimodality imaging, including echocardiography, is used for diagnosis and clinical management. Key questions imaging should address include location, size, mobility, hemodynamic effects, and extracardiac involvement. Compared with echocardiography, CT and CMR provide better assessment of extracardiac involvement and tissue characterization.

7. Bruce CJ: Cardiac tumours: Diagnosis and management, *Heart* 97:151–160, 2011.
   Detailed review of the clinical presentation, imaging features, and management of cardiac tumors. Key points are: (1) most cardiac masses are thrombi or vegetations (tumors are rare), most cardiac tumors originate outside the heart, and most primary cardiac tumors are histologically benign; (2) the diagnosis of a cardiac tumor depends on clinical history, location, age, presentation,

and histologic features, in addition to imaging characteristics; and (3) the most common benign cardiac tumor is a myxoma, the most common tumors in children are rhabdomyomas and fibromas, the most common valve-associated tumor is a fibroelastoma, and the most common malignant tumor is a sarcoma.

8. Tamin SS, Maleszewski JJ, Scott CG, et al: Prognostic and bioepidemiologic implications of papillary fibroelastomas, *J Am Coll Cardiol* 65(22):2420–2429, 2015.
   In a series of 511 patients with a papillary fibroelastoma, in the 185 patients who underwent surgical excision, recurrence was rare (1.6%), and the incidence of stroke was 2% at 1 year and 8% at 5 years. In the 326 patients with echocardiographic findings consistent with papillary fibroelastoma who did not undergo surgical excision, the risk of stroke was 6% at 1 year and 13% at 5 years. A suggested algorithm for clinical management is proposed.

9. Basso C, Rizzo S, Valente M, et al: Cardiac masses and tumours, *Heart* 102(15):1230–1245, 2016.
   Educational article reviewing the clinical presentation, imaging diagnosis, and outcomes of cardiac tumors. Includes pathologic correlation and examples of CT and CMR imaging. Detailed tables with classification of primary cardiac tumors, the prevalence of metastatic disease to the heart with noncardiac tumors, and imaging pitfalls.

Intracardiac Thrombi

10. Akoum N, Prutkin JM: The role of echocardiography in atrial fibrillation and flutter. In Otto CM, editor: *The Practice of Clinical Echocardiography*, ed 5, Philadelphia, 2017, Elsevier, pp 837–860.
    Review of the literature on LA thrombus formation and the risk of embolic events with cardioversion. Summarizes the clinical approach to the use of echocardiography in the management of patients with atrial fibrillation of prolonged or unknown duration.

11. Donal E, Ollivier R, Weillard D, et al: Left atrial function assessed by transthoracic echocardiography in patients treated by ablation for a lone paroxysmal atrial fibrillation, *Eur J Echocardiogr* 11:845, 2010.
    Echocardiographic measures of LA volume, compliance, and contractility were used to assess the effects of catheter ablation for atrial fibrillation on long-term follow-up. Although LA volumes decreased and contractility increased, at 1 year LA compliance remained abnormal, suggesting irreversible fibrosis.

12. Beigel R, Wunderlich NC, Ho SY, et al: The left atrial appendage: anatomy, function, and noninvasive evaluation, *JACC Cardiovasc Imaging* 7(12):1251–1265, 2014.
    Atrial fibrillation occurs in 0.4% to 1.0% of the entire population, with a prevalence greater than 8% in persons older than 80 years of age. Clinical scores are used to estimate the risk of embolic events in patients with atrial fibrillation, but interest has been expressed in whether anatomic or physiologic characteristics of the atrial appendage may also be useful. The shape of the LA appendage is variable, with morphology often classified as being similar in shape to a cauliflower, windsock, cactus, or chicken wing. Atrial appendage shape, contractile function, and tissue strain all are under investigation as predictors of stroke risk.

13. Alli O, Holmes D, Jr: Left atrial appendage occlusion, *Heart* 101(11):834–841, 2015.
    Review article summarizing the indications for and long-term outcomes after placement of an LA occlusion device. Echocardiographers often are asked to evaluate atrial appendage anatomy before device placement, provide imaging guidance during device placement, and assess device positioning and complications after placement.

14. Roifman I, Connelly KA, Wright GA, et al: Echocardiography vs. cardiac magnetic resonance imaging for the diagnosis of left ventricular thrombus: a systematic review, *Can J Cardiol* 31(6):785–791, 2015.
    Systematic review including 7 studies with a total of 803 patients undergoing imaging evaluation for LV thrombus. Only limited conclusions can be derived from these data because the reference standard was variable among studies, and none directly compared different imaging modalities in the same patient. CMR imaging was very accurate for diagnosis of LV thrombus, with a sensitivity of 88% and a specificity of 99%. With transthoracic imaging, the use of left-sided contrast was associated with higher sensitivity and specificity compared with noncontrast imaging.

15. Oxorn D, Otto CM: Masses. In Oxorn D, Otto CM, editors: *Intraoperative and Interventional Echocardiography: Atlas of Transesophageal Imaging*, Philadelphia, 2017, Elsevier, pp 385–414.
    This atlas chapter presents 17 cases of cardiac masses including normal variants, thrombi, and primary and secondary cardiac tumors with 2D and 3D TEE images and videos, in addition to surgical and pathologic correlation for each case.

16 Diseases of the Great Arteries

BASIC PRINCIPLES
ECHOCARDIOGRAPHIC APPROACH
   Transthoracic Approach
      Echocardiographic Imaging
      Doppler Flows
      Limitations of Transthoracic Imaging of the Aorta
   Transesophageal Approach
      Echocardiographic Imaging
      Doppler Flows
      Limitations of Transesophageal Imaging of the Aorta
AORTIC DILATION AND ANEURYSM
AORTIC DISSECTION
   Transthoracic Imaging
   Transesophageal Imaging
      Complications of Aortic Dissection
      Postoperative Evaluation After Surgery on the Ascending Aorta
AORTIC INTRAMURAL HEMATOMA
AORTIC PSEUDOANEURYSM
TRAUMATIC AORTIC DISEASE
SINUS OF VALSALVA ANEURYSM
ATHEROSCLEROTIC AORTIC DISEASE
   Aortic Atherosclerosis as a Potential Source of Embolus
   Aortic Atherosclerosis as a Marker of Coronary Artery Disease
PULMONARY ARTERY ABNORMALITIES
ALTERNATE APPROACHES
THE ECHO EXAM
SUGGESTED READING

Echocardiographic evaluation of the aorta and main pulmonary artery is a routine part of the standard echocardiographic examination. For descriptive purposes, the aorta is divided into segments, beginning at the aortic valve, including the:

- Aortic annulus
- Sinuses of Valsalva
- Sinotubular junction
- Ascending aorta
- Aortic arch
- Descending thoracic aorta
- Proximal abdominal aorta

The term *aortic root* has a variable definition that can lead to errors in communication. In studies of genetic connective tissue disorders, aortic root usually refers to the aortic sinuses, from the valve level to the sinotubular junction. However, a surgical aortic root replacement typically extends from the aortic annulus to the mid-ascending aorta. Thus, when the aorta is abnormal, more specific terms describing anatomic location are preferred.

Evaluation of the aortic annulus and sinuses is a routine component of an echocardiographic study. In addition, further evaluation of the ascending aorta, arch, and descending aorta can be performed when disease is suspected clinically. Transthoracic echocardiography (TTE) images often are suboptimal because of overlying or adjacent air-filled structures, so transesophageal echocardiography (TEE) imaging greatly enhances the diagnostic utility of echocardiography for diseases of the aorta.

BASIC PRINCIPLES

Aortic abnormalities include:

- Dilation
- Aneurysm
- Dissection
- Pseudoaneurysm
- Sinus of Valsalva aneurysm
- Atherosclerosis

The most common abnormality of the aorta is dilation, or an increase in diameter greater than expected for age and body size. When aortic dilation exceeds the expected diameter by 50% or more (>5.0 cm for the ascending aorta), the term *aneurysm* is used. Aneurysms can involve one or more segments of the aorta (ascending, arch, and descending) and may be tubular or saccular in configuration.

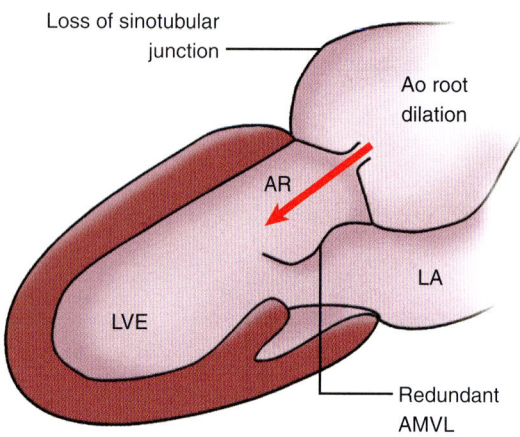

Fig. 16.1 Typical echo findings in Marfan syndrome. The proximal aorta is markedly dilated with effacement of the sinotubular junction. Aortic annular dilation results in inadequate aortic leaflet apposition with a central jet of aortic regurgitation *(AR)* and consequent LV enlargement *(LVE)*. Often, the anterior mitral leaflet *(AMVL)* is long and redundant. *Ao*, Aortic.

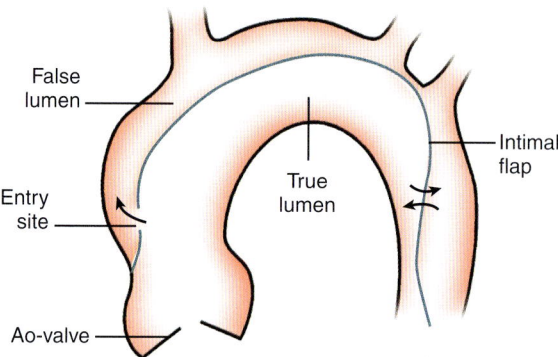

Fig. 16.2 Schematic diagram of an aortic dissection. This example shows an entry site above the sinotubular junction into a false lumen. In real time, the intimal flap shows rapid undulating motion, independent of the cardiac cycle. As indicated by the *arrows* across the intimal flap in the descending aorta, multiple flow communications between the true and false lumens may be seen with color flow imaging. *Ao-valve*, Aortic valve.

Aortic dilation associated with hypertension or atherosclerosis is characterized by normal contours of the sinuses of Valsalva and narrowing at the sinotubular junction, with enlargement primarily in the ascending aorta. A bicuspid aortic valve often is accompanied by dilation of the aortic sinuses or ascending aorta, but some narrowing at the sinotubular junction usually is preserved. Inherited connective tissue disorders that cause aneurysms of the ascending aorta, such as Marfan syndrome and Loeys-Dietz syndrome, are characterized by effacement of the sinotubular junction and enlargement of the sinuses of Valsalva, in addition to dilation of the ascending aorta, thus resulting in a "water balloon" appearance of the proximal aorta (Fig. 16.1). Systemic inflammatory diseases, such as ankylosing spondylitis, are associated with aortic aneurysms and often also affect the valve tissue. Aneurysms also may be seen in tertiary syphilis (with a characteristic pattern of calcification), aortic arteritis (such as Takayasu arteritis and giant cell arteritis), and as a result of blunt or penetrating chest trauma. Large aortic aneurysms are prone to rupture, so prophylactic repair often is recommended.

An *aortic dissection* is a life-threatening situation in which an intimal tear in the aortic wall allows passage of blood into a "false" channel between the intima and the media (Fig. 16.2). This false channel may be localized or may propagate downstream, often in a spiral fashion, because of the pressure of blood flow in the channel. Complications related to the false lumen include:

- Expansion with compression of the true aortic lumen (which supplies major branch vessels)
- Propagation down major branch vessels
- Thrombosis
- Rupture

An accurate, rapid diagnosis of the presence or absence of aortic dissection and the site of the entry tear is crucial in the treatment of patients with chest pain and suspected dissection. The most prevalent risk factors for aortic dissection are hypertension and atherosclerosis. However, patient groups with the highest risk of aortic dissection include those with Marfan syndrome and other inherited connective tissue disorders, Turner syndrome, aortitis, and vascular-type Ehlers-Danlos syndrome. Patients with a congenital bicuspid or unicuspid aortic valve also have a fivefold increased risk of aortic dissection. Dissection is more likely in patients with a preexisting aneurysm, although dissection can occur in the absence of dilation in patients with Marfan syndrome or other connective tissue disorders.

A *pseudoaneurysm* is a blood collection outside the aorta, in contrast to an aneurysm, that involves all the layers of the aortic wall. Pseudoaneurysms sometime occur due to a contained rupture after complex aortic valve or aortic surgery, as a complication of endocarditis, or following an aortic dissection.

Sinus of Valsalva aneurysms (Fig. 16.3) are congenital or due to infection, Marfan syndrome, or previous surgical procedures. A sinus of Valsalva aneurysm protrudes into adjacent chambers and sometimes is associated with a fistula. Specifically, an aneurysm of the right coronary sinus protrudes into the right ventricular (RV) outflow tract, the left coronary sinus into the left atrium (LA), and the noncoronary sinus into the right atrium (RA).

Atherosclerosis of the aorta may lead to dilation, aneurysm, or dissection. In addition, the presence of atheroma is important as a marker for coexisting coronary artery disease and as a potential source of embolic cerebrovascular events.

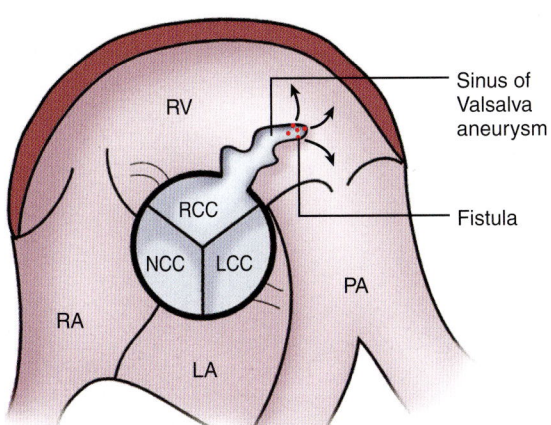

Fig. 16.3 Schematic diagram of a congenital sinus of Valsalva aneurysm. A long, "wind sock"-like membranous outpouching of the right coronary cusp *(RCC)* protrudes into the RV outflow tract. If fenestrations are present in the aneurysm, an aortic-to-RV fistula is seen. Note that an aneurysm of the left coronary cusp *(LCC)* would protrude into the LA, whereas an aneurysm of the right coronary cusp would protrude into the RA. *NCC,* Noncoronary cusp; *PA,* pulmonary artery.

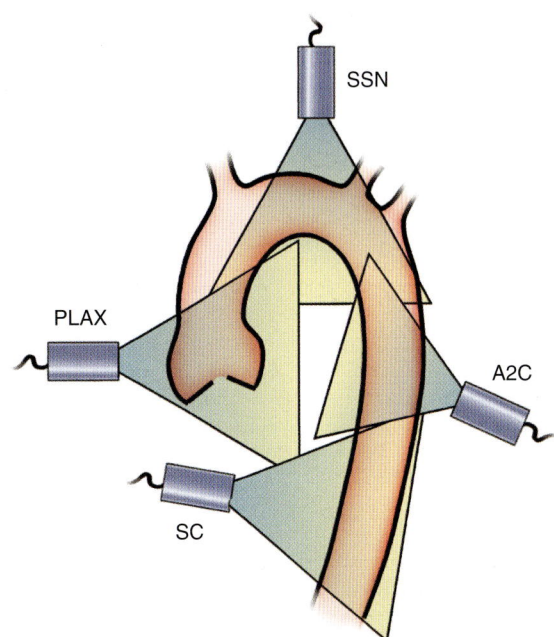

Fig. 16.4 Evaluation of the aorta from a transcutaneous approach. From a parasternal long-axis *(PLAX)* window, the sinuses and a segment of the ascending aorta are seen; from the suprasternal notch *(SSN)* window, the arch and proximal descending thoracic aorta are seen; from a posteriorly angulated apical two-chamber *(A2C)* approach, the mid-segment of the descending thoracic aorta is seen; and from a subcostal *(SC)* approach, the distal thoracic aorta and proximal abdominal aorta are seen. In some individuals, the segment of ascending aorta between the standard PLAX and SSN views can be imaged from a high parasternal position. However, in other patients, this segment of the aorta is "missed" on TTE imaging.

ECHOCARDIOGRAPHIC APPROACH

Transthoracic Approach
Echocardiographic Imaging

On transthoracic imaging, the *proximal ascending aorta* is well seen in parasternal long- and short-axis views (Fig. 16.4). Depending on ultrasound penetration, images of additional segments of the ascending aorta are obtained by moving the transducer cephalad one or more interspaces. Image quality is enhanced by positioning the patient in a steep left lateral decubitus position, thereby bringing the aorta in contact with the anterior chest wall (Figs. 16.5 and 16.6). In all adults, aortic diameter measurements should be made:

- In a two-dimensional (2D) long-axis plane through the center of the aortic sinuses and ascending aorta
- At end-diastole (onset of the QRS signal)
- From the white-black to black-white interface defining the aortic lumen
- At the aortic sinuses (maximum diameter) and mid-ascending aorta

When aortic dimensions are greater than normal or when the shape of the aortic sinuses and sinotubular junction is abnormal, additional measurements should be made as described later (Table 16.1; see also Tables A.8, A.9, and A.10 in Appendix A). Aortic sinus diameter also can be measured with an M-mode tracing at the level of the valve leaflets when a perpendicular orientation between the ultrasound beam and the aortic sinuses can be obtained. With M-mode tracings a leading edge-to-leading edge measurement convention is used. M-mode tracings may allow for more accurate identification of the aortic wall because of the high temporal sampling rate.

The *aortic arch* is imaged from a suprasternal notch or supraclavicular approach with the patient in a supine position with the neck extended. Both longitudinal (Fig. 16.7) and transverse views of the arch are obtainable in nearly all individuals. Usually, only a short segment of the ascending aorta is visible from the suprasternal notch window, but this is variable among patients. Also note that the descending aorta appears to taper because of an oblique image plane with respect to its curvature (i.e., the descending aorta is only partially in the image plane).

The *descending thoracic aorta* is seen in cross section posterior to the LA in the parasternal long-axis view. A longitudinal section of this segment of the descending aorta is obtained by clockwise rotation and lateral angulation of the transducer. From the suprasternal notch approach, a small portion of the descending thoracic aorta is seen. From the apical two-chamber view, a longitudinal section of a segment of the descending aorta is seen by lateral angulation and clockwise rotation of the transducer (Fig. 16.8).

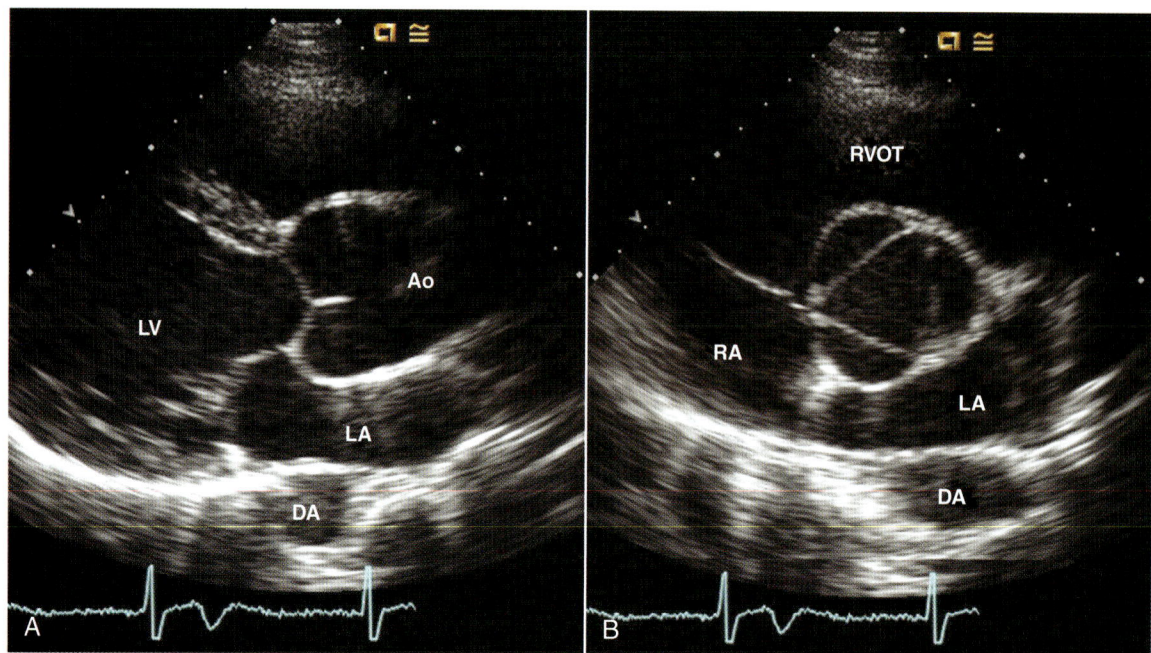

Fig. 16.5 Marfan syndrome. The parasternal long-axis view ▶ (A) shows dilated sinuses with effacement of the sinotubular junction. In a short-axis view ▶ (B), the trileaflet valve in systole is stretched so the orifice is triangular instead of the normal circular opening. *Ao*, Aorta; *DA*, descending aorta; *RVOT*, RV outflow tract.

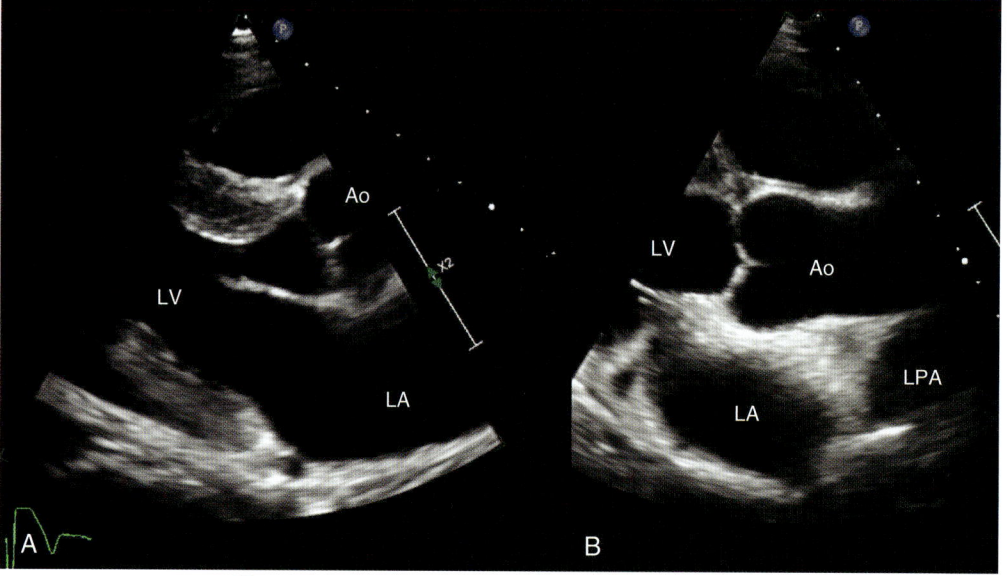

Fig. 16.6 Imaging the ascending aorta. ▶ (A) The standard parasternal long-axis view in a patient with Marfan syndrome shows only the aortic sinuses. ▶ (B) With the transducer moved up one interspace, the loss of the normal contour of the sinotubular junction *(arrow)* and more of the ascending aorta are seen. *Ao*, Aorta; *LPA*, left pulmonary artery.

From the subcostal approach, the *distal thoracic* and *proximal abdominal aorta* is seen as it traverses the diaphragm. In patients with a left pleural effusion, images of the aorta also may be obtained by imaging through the fluid from the left posterior chest (paraspinal) with the patient in a right lateral decubitus position.

Doppler Flows

Color Doppler interrogation of the ascending aorta from the parasternal approach allows for evaluation of the flow pattern in the proximal aorta and assessment of aortic regurgitation severity, with evaluation of the cause of aortic regurgitation and measurement

TABLE 16.1 Normal Aortic Root Diameters by Age

	AGE (YEARS)					
	15–29	30–39	40–49	50–59	60–69	≥70
For Men With BSA of 2.0 m²*						
Mean normal (cm)	3.3	3.4	3.5	3.6	3.7	3.8
Upper limit of normal (cm) (95% CI)	3.7	3.8	3.9	4.0	4.1	4.2
For Women With BSA of 1.7 m²†						
Mean normal (cm)	2.9	3.0	3.2	3.2	3.3	3.4
Upper limit of normal (cm)	3.3	3.4	3.6	3.6	3.7	3.9

*Add 0.5 mm per 0.1 m² BSA above 2.0 m² or subtract 0.5 mm per 0.1 m² BSA below 2.0 m².
†Add 0.5 mm per 0.1 m² BSA above 1.7 m² or subtract 0.5 mm per 0.1 m² BSA below 1.7 m².
BSA, Body surface area; CI, confidence interval.
Data from Devereux RB, de Simone G, Arnett DK, et al: Normal limits in relation to age, body size and gender of two-dimensional echocardiographic aortic root dimensions in persons≥15 years of age. Am J Cardiol 110:1189–1194, 2012.

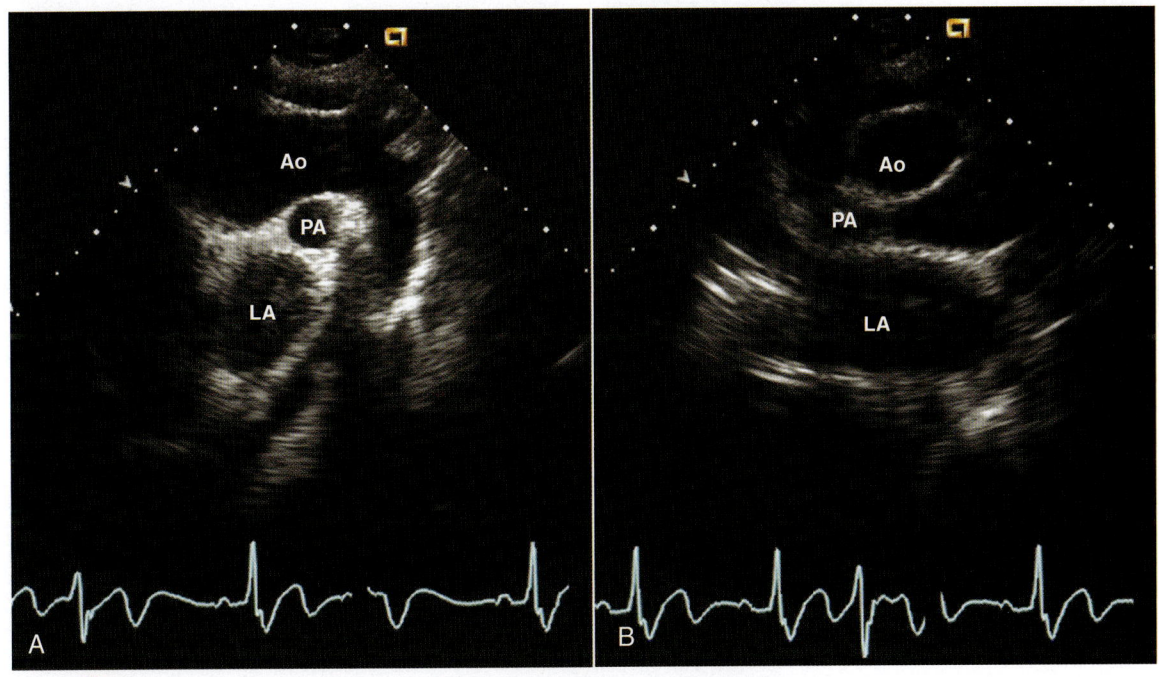

Fig. 16.7 ▶ **Suprasternal notch view of the aorta.** The long-axis view (A) shows the ascending aorta *(Ao)*, arch, and descending aorta with the right pulmonary artery *(PA)* in short axis and the LA imaged inferiorly. The short-axis suprasternal notch view (B) shows the aortic arch, pulmonary artery, and LA.

of vena contracta width. The ascending aorta also is imaged from the apical approach in an anteriorly angulated four-chamber view and in an apical long-axis view. Although 2D image quality often is suboptimal at the depth of the ascending aorta from the apical approach, this view does allow a parallel intercept angle between the Doppler beam and the direction of blood flow for spectral Doppler flow velocity measurements.

Pulsed or continuous-wave (CW) Doppler recordings of descending aortic flow from the suprasternal notch show systolic flow away from the transducer at a velocity of approximately 1 m/s. Normal flow in the descending aorta shows:

- Brief, low-velocity, early diastolic flow reversal
- Low-velocity antegrade flow in mid-diastole
- Low-velocity flow reversal at end-diastole

The use of low wall filter settings is needed to appreciate this normal flow pattern (Fig. 16.9). Flow abnormalities are seen with aortic disease (e.g., coarctation), shunts (e.g., patent ductus arteriosus), or aortic valve disease (e.g., regurgitation). Flow patterns in the proximal abdominal aorta are similar to those in the descending thoracic aorta and are easily recorded from the subcostal approach (Fig. 16.10).

Limitations of Transthoracic Imaging of the Aorta

The major limitations of the transthoracic approach to ultrasound evaluation of the aorta are acoustic access and image quality. In many individuals, acoustic access is suboptimal or minimal from one or more of the windows needed for full evaluation of the aorta, thus leaving "gaps" in the echocardiographic examination. Even when acoustic access is adequate, image quality often is poor because of beam width at the depth of the aorta, particularly the descending thoracic aorta from apical and parasternal windows. Beam-width

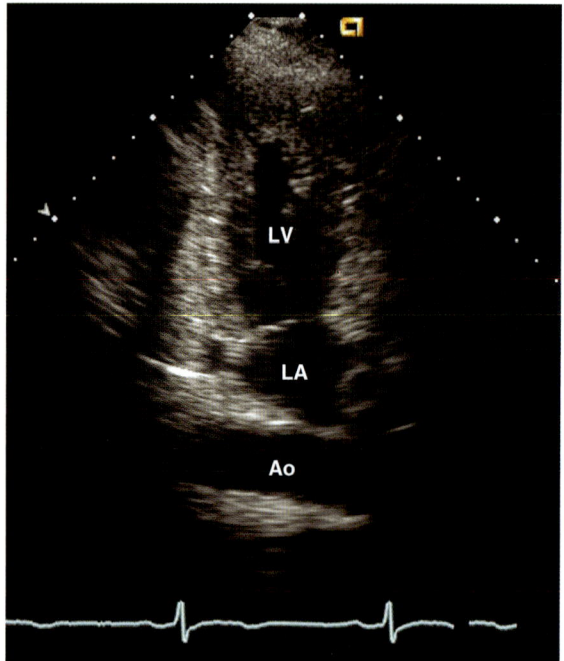

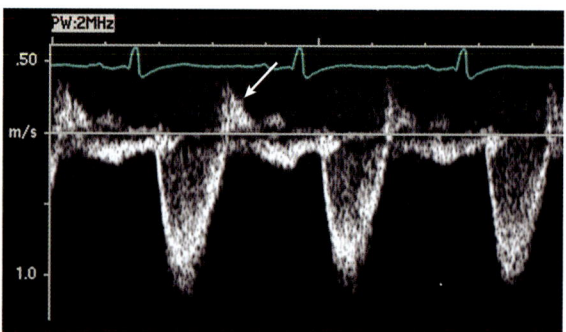

Fig. 16.8 Descending thoracic aorta. The posteriorly angulated apical two-chamber view shows the descending thoracic aorta (Ao) along its long axis in a patient with Marfan syndrome and prior aortic root replacement for type A dissection.

Fig. 16.9 Normal flow pattern in the descending thoracic aorta. Pulsed Doppler recording of flow in the descending aorta from a suprasternal notch long-axis view shows antegrade flow in systole with a maximum velocity of 1.1 m/s and a normal systolic ejection curve. In diastole, brief early diastolic flow reversal occurs, followed by low-velocity antegrade flow in mid-diastole and absence of flow (or low-velocity reversal) in end-diastole.

Fig. 16.10 Normal flow pattern in the proximal abdominal aorta. Subcostal view of the proximal abdominal aorta with color Doppler (top). The pulsed Doppler signal (bottom) shows normal antegrade flow toward the transducer in systole, followed by brief early diastolic flow reversal and slight antegrade flow in mid-diastole.

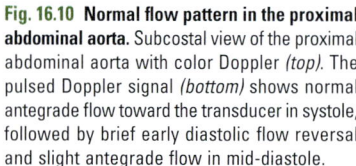
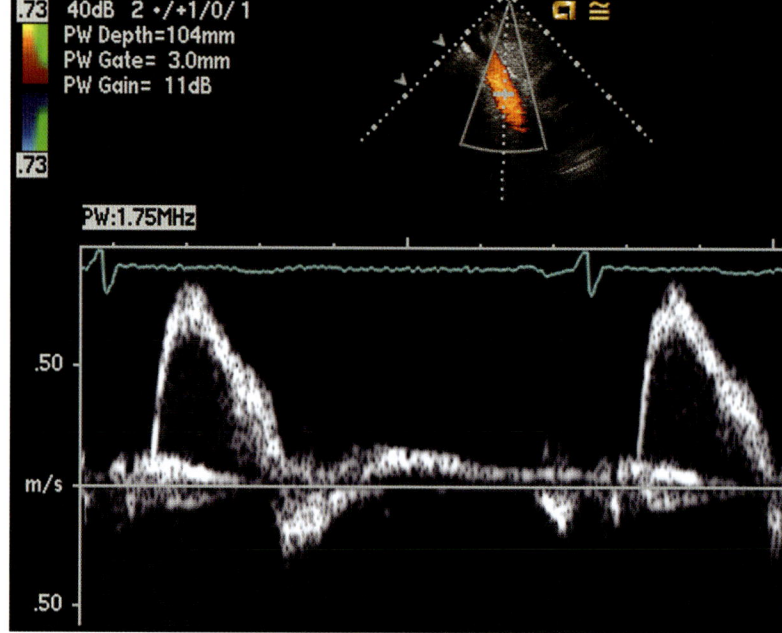

artifact, noise, and poor lateral resolution make differentiation of intraluminal defects from artifacts difficult. Because of these limitations, evaluation by TEE or other imaging modalities is appropriate in many patients with acute or chronic aortic disease.

Transesophageal Approach
Echocardiographic Imaging

From a high TEE probe position with the image plane rotated to approximately 45°, the aortic valve and *sinuses of Valsalva* are seen in short axis. Slight withdrawal of the probe in the esophagus allows short-axis imaging of the proximal ascending aorta, but more distal segments are obscured by interposition of the air-filled trachea between the esophagus (and transducer) and the ascending aorta. The long-axis view of the aortic valve, sinuses of Valsalva, and ascending aorta is obtained by rotating the image plane to approximately 120° (Fig. 16.11). In the long-axis plane, more cephalad segments of the ascending aorta are seen by slowly moving the transducer to a higher esophageal position.

The *aortic arch* is best imaged from a high esophageal position. Starting with a short-axis view of the descending thoracic aorta, the probe is withdrawn to the level of the arch, and then the entire probe is turned toward the patient's right and angulated inferiorly to obtain a long-axis view of the arch. In some patients, images of the aortic arch may be suboptimal because of the positions of the trachea and bronchi. In many cases, transthoracic suprasternal notch views of the arch provide superior image quality.

The *descending thoracic aorta* and the *proximal abdominal aorta* are well seen by the TEE approach. The descending thoracic aorta lies immediately lateral and slightly posterior to the esophagus, so posterior rotation of the probe provides excellent images in either a cross-sectional (transverse plane at 0°) or long-axis (at 90° to 120°) view (Fig. 16.12). Slight turning of the TEE probe is needed at different levels as the aorta curves relative to the esophagus. From a transgastric position, the proximal abdominal aorta is seen posterior to the stomach. Many examiners prefer to examine the length of the aorta in sequential cross-sectional views as the probe is slowly withdrawn from the stomach and esophagus, with imaging of the aortic arch just before probe removal. This ensures that the entire endothelial surface of the aorta is visualized. Any areas of abnormality can then be further examined in long-axis views, or simultaneous biplane short- and long-axis views can be recorded.

Three-dimensional (3D) TEE imaging of the aorta is not routine but is helpful when aortic pathology is present, for example, when defining the anatomy and extent of an aortic dissection flap, identifying the location and size of the dissection entry site, or quantitating total aortic atherosclerotic burden.

Doppler Flows

TEE color flow imaging of the aorta shows the normal antegrade flow pattern in the ascending aorta, arch, and descending aorta and is helpful in the evaluation of abnormal blood flow patterns when aortic dissection is present. However, quantitative evaluation of aortic

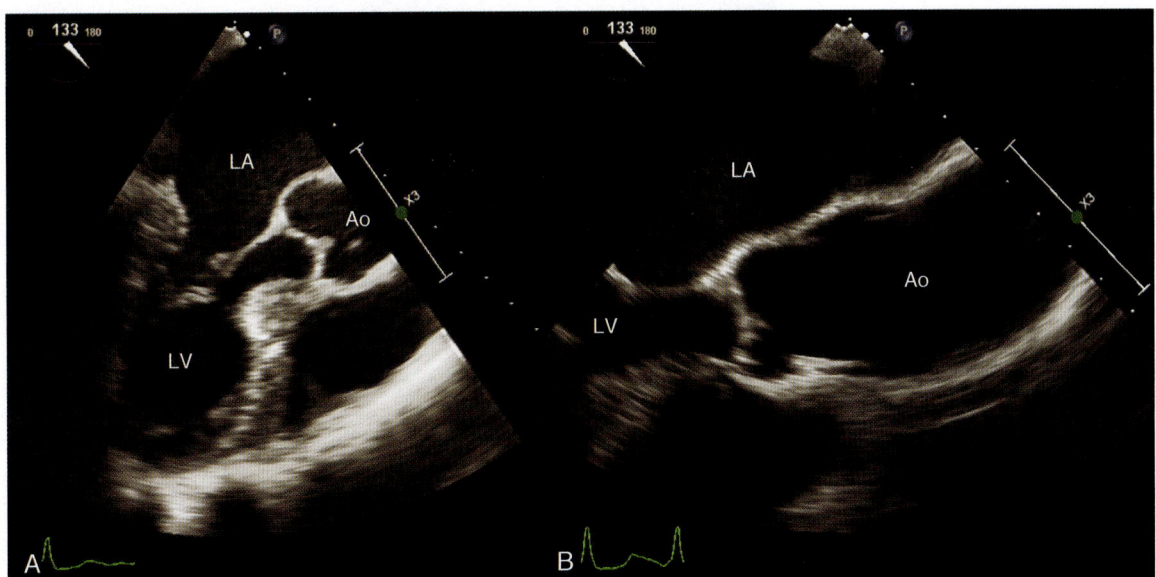

Fig. 16.11 TEE imaging of the ascending aorta. The aortic long-axis view ▶ (A) is obtained at about 120° rotation and the short-axis view ▶ (B) at about 30° to 40° rotation. Both image planes are aligned to the cardiac landmarks, analogous to TTE views, with the exact degree of rotation varying between patients. *Ao*, Aorta.

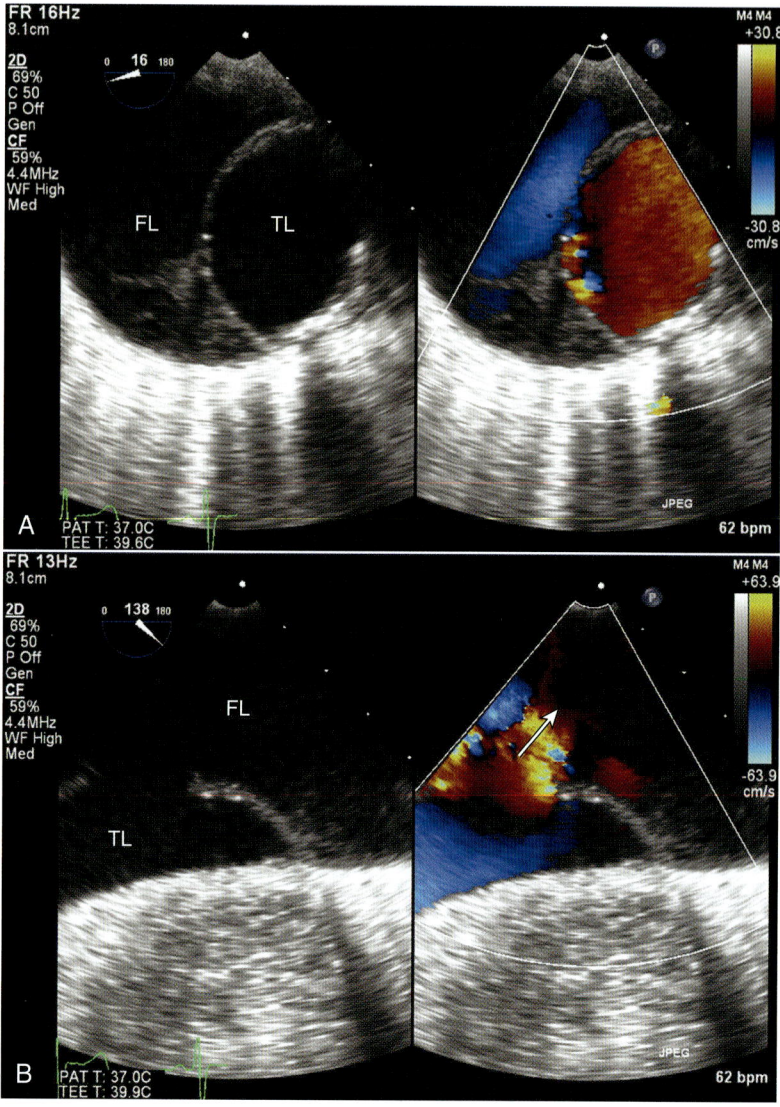

Fig. 16.12 Dissection flap with fenestration.
▶ (A) On TEE imaging, a 2D short-axis view of the descending thoracic aorta shows a dissection flap separating the smaller true lumen *(TL)*, with systolic flow in *red*, from the false lumens *(FL)*, with spontaneous contrast due to low-velocity flow. ▶ (B) In a long-axis view, a fenestration is seen with flow from the true lumen to the false lumen *(arrow)*.

flow velocities is challenging from the TEE approach. The ascending aorta is seen in a medially rotated transgastric long-axis view, although the intercept angle may not be parallel to flow, a situation that results in velocity underestimation, particularly when high velocities are present. For the descending aorta, the direction of blood flow is nearly perpendicular to the direction of the ultrasound beam, thereby limiting spectral Doppler velocity measurement, although recording Doppler flow signals in a long-axis plane with the Doppler beam aligned at the distal end of the aorta is possible. This approach likely underestimates velocity because of the nonparallel intercept angle, but it is useful to evaluate flow patterns, such as holodiastolic flow reversal with aortic regurgitation.

In addition, color Doppler evaluation of the aortic valve is a standard component of the examination because aortic valve regurgitation results from several types of aortic disease, including:

- Bicuspid aortic valve disease with eccentric regurgitation
- Annular dilation with "stretching" of the valve leaflets that results in central noncoaptation
- Dilation of the sinuses or sinotubular junction that leads to inadequate leaflet overlap
- Commissural involvement by aortic dissection that results in inadequate support of the leaflets
- A flail aortic leaflet due to extension of a dissection flap into the valve tissue
- Diffuse aortic wall and valve leaflet thickening due to an inflammatory process

Evaluation of aortic regurgitation includes the measurement of vena contracta width, identification of the origin and etiology of regurgitation, and evaluation of left ventricle (LV) size and systolic function (see Chapter 12).

Limitations of Transesophageal Imaging of the Aorta

TEE imaging provides improved image quality and allows imaging of more segments of the aorta compared with transthoracic imaging. However, the distal ascending aorta and aortic arch are not completely visualized. In addition, TEE provides little information on the major aortic branch vessels, which are better evaluated by computed tomography (CT) or magnetic resonance imaging (MRI).

AORTIC DILATION AND ANEURYSM

Aortic dilation often is first recognized on the chest radiograph or on an echocardiographic examination requested for other reasons. In specific clinical settings, such as Marfan syndrome, aortic dilation is an expected consequence of a systemic disease (Table 16.2). In these cases, echocardiography is requested to assess the presence and degree of the aortic abnormality, as well as involvement of the aortic valve. In patients with a bicuspid aortic valve, aortic dimension should be routinely measured (Fig. 16.13).

In addition to aortic dilation, the *shape* of the sinuses and sinotubular junction is altered in some disease states. Effacement of the sinotubular junction is characteristic of connective tissue disorders, with loss of the normal abrupt change in curvature between the cup-shaped sinuses and cylindrical ascending aorta. Severe effacement is easy to recognize as a smooth contour from the sinuses to the ascending aorta with no discernible transition point. Early disease is subtler, with an increased distance from the aortic valve plane to the sinotubular junction and slight straightening of the transition zone.

Measurements of aortic diameter on echocardiography are accurate and reproducible when care is taken to obtain a true diameter in the center of the vessel (nonoblique), gain settings are appropriate, and standard measurement conventions are used. In

TABLE 16.2 Aortic Disease: Clinical Echocardiographic Correlates

	Clinical Correlation	Echocardiographic Findings	Imaging Recommendations
Hypertensive heart disease	Chronic hypertension is associated with mild aortic dilation.	Dilation of the ascending aorta with normal sinuses and STJ is typical.	TTE imaging from a high interspace allows measurement of the ascending aorta.
Aortic atherosclerosis	Atherosclerosis is associated with mild aortic dilation. Aortic atheroma may cause systemic emboli, especially with large protruding atheroma with mobile thrombus.	Focal irregular thickening of the aortic wall with areas of calcification. Associated thrombus is seen as a mobile echodensity.	TEE is needed for evaluation of aortic atheroma.
Bicuspid aortic valve disease	Associated aortopathy in some patients with an increased risk of progressive dilation and dissection	Enlargement of the aortic sinuses and/or the ascending aorta, usually with a preserved STJ	CT or MRI is recommended for evaluation of the ascending aorta if not fully imaged by echocardiography.
Marfan (and Loeys-Dietz) syndrome	Aortic dilation, ectopia lentis, skeletal features, family history	Dilated sinuses with enlargement (or effacement) of the STJ. Long anterior mitral leaflet with prolapse	Aortic imaging (TTE or MRI) recommended every 6–12 months. MRI recommended annually in patients with Loeys-Dietz syndrome, from cerebrovascular circulation to pelvis. TTE recommended in first-degree relatives of patients with thoracic aneurysm or dissection or known genetic mutation

Continued

TABLE 16.2 Aortic Disease: Clinical Echocardiographic Correlates—cont'd

	Clinical Correlation	Echocardiographic Findings	Imaging Recommendations
Systemic inflammatory disease (ankylosing spondylitis, etc.)	Arthritis with systemic inflammation Aortic involvement in about 20% of patients	Dilated, thick-walled aorta with characteristic thickening extending onto base of the anterior mitral valve leaflet	TTE appropriate when aortic regurgitant murmur is present Routine surveillance not recommended
Syphilitic aortitis	Aneurysm of the ascending aorta is seen 10–25 years after initial spirochetal infection.	Dilated aorta with calcification May involve proximal coronary arteries	Rare in North America or Europe
Takayasu or giant cell arteritis	Loss of distal artery pulses in patients <40 years of age (Takayasu) or >50 years of age (giant cell) Elevated systemic inflammatory markers	Dilation of thoracic aorta and abdominal aorta	TTE and TEE show aortic dilation; aortic walls may be thickened and irregular.
Aortic dissection	Acute onset of chest pain, often described as tearing May radiate to neck or back	Intimal flap with flow in true and false lumen Type A dissection involves the ascending aorta; type B dissection is limited to the descending thoracic aorta.	TEE, MRI, or CT recommended in patients at high risk of aortic dissection Choice of procedures depends on patient variables and availability of each imaging modality.
Intramural hematoma	Acute presentation with chest or back pain	Crescent-shaped thickening of aortic wall; may be localized	Intramural hematoma may be seen on TTE, but TEE has a higher sensitivity for this diagnosis.
Aortic pseudoaneurysm	Typically seen after complex aortic valve surgery or endocarditis	Echo-free space adjacent to aorta Flow from aortic lumen in and out of the pseudoaneurysm may be seen.	TEE, CT, or MRI is needed to evaluate known or suspected aortic pseudoaneurysm.
Traumatic aortic disease	Deceleration injury can result in aortic rupture, most often at the ligamentum arteriosus (45%) or the ascending aorta (23%).	Disruption of the aorta at the junction between the arch and the descending thoracic aorta may be difficult to appreciate on TTE or TEE.	CT recommended for diagnosis Delayed diagnosis may result in pseudoaneurysm at the aortic isthmus.
Sinus of Valsalva aneurysm	Isolated congenital sinus of Valsalva aneurysms may be a smooth dilation of one sinus or may have a "wind sock" appearance. Aneurysms due to endocarditis are associated with thickening of the aortic wall and abscess formation.	Rupture may occur into the RV outflow tract from the left coronary cusp, into the RA from the right coronary cusp, or into the LA from the noncoronary cusp.	Both color and spectral Doppler images are helpful in determining which chamber is affected by a ruptured sinus of Valsalva aneurysm.

CT, Computed tomography; *MRI*, magnetic resonance imaging; *STJ*, sinotubular junction.

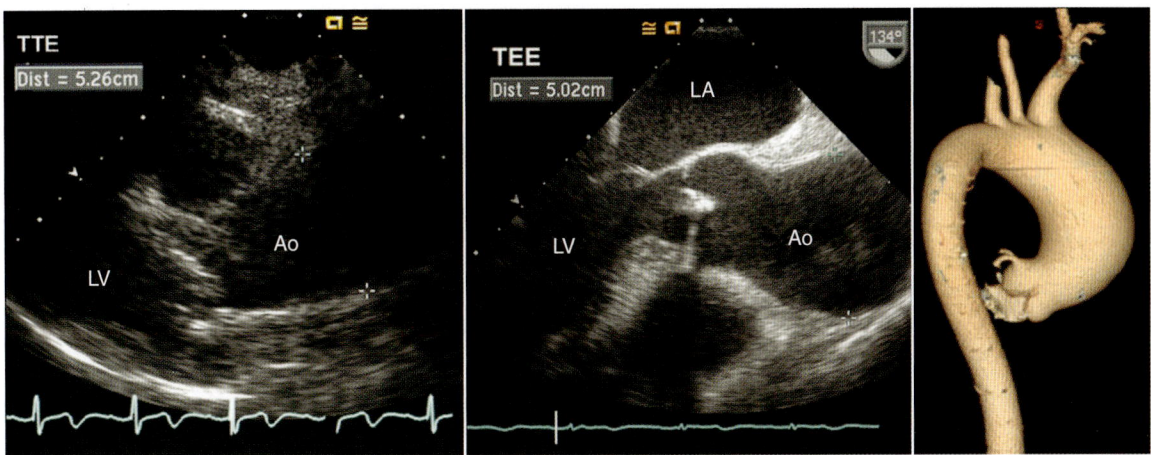

Fig. 16.13 Bicuspid aortic valve associated aortopathy. ▶ *(Left)* TTE imaging in a patient with a bicuspid aortic valve shows dilation of the ascending aorta with a maximum dimension of 5.26 cm at end-diastole. ▶ *(Center)* TEE images confirm dilation of the ascending aorta, although dimension is slightly underestimated because of a slightly oblique image plane. *(Right)* 3D reconstruction of the contrast computed tomographic images shows the location and severity of aortic dilation, but the timing of measurements during the cardiac cycle may not exactly match the echocardiographic data. *Ao,* Aorta.

patients with aortic dilation, it is important to measure aortic diameter at several locations and to specify the measurement site and timing in the cardiac cycle. The aorta is pulsatile, with the change in dimension from end-diastole to end-systole dependent on aortic compliance. Aortic compliance may be significantly altered in different disease states, but a typical normal change in aortic diameter during the cardiac cycle is 2 to 3 mm. End-systolic measurements often are used in children. However, in adults, measurements are most reliable at end-diastole because timing in the cardiac cycle (onset of the QRS) is reproducible and because end-diastolic measurements are least affected by aortic compliance or loading conditions.

Measurements (Fig. 16.14) are made at *end-diastole* at the:

- Aortic annulus (the site used for LV outflow tract diameter measurement)
- Aortic sinus leaflet tip level (the standard position of an M-mode recording of the aortic valve)
- Sinotubular junction
- Ascending aorta
- Aortic arch
- Descending thoracic aorta

Although all these measurements are not needed in every patient, quantitative evaluation of the extent and severity of aortic dilation is extremely useful in follow-up and treatment of patients with chronic, progressive aortic dilation. Each measurement is made from the black-white interface on a freeze-frame end-diastolic image, averaging several beats to ensure a consistent measurement. Aortic annulus diameter is measured at the insertion of the base of the valve leaflets in the long-axis view. The maximum aortic sinus

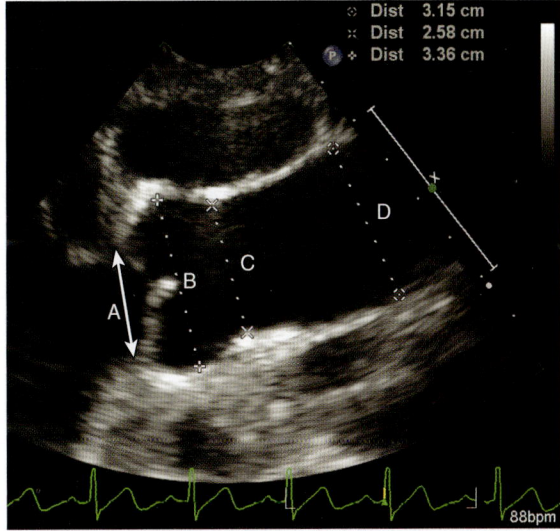

Fig. 16.14 Aortic measurements. LV outflow tract (LVOT) diameter is measured in systole *(A)* when used for transaortic stroke volume calculations or for the calculation of valve area in the continuity equation. Measurements of the aorta are made at end-diastole at the sinuses *(B)*, the sinotubular junction *(C)*, and in the mid-ascending aorta *(D)*. The site of measurement should be specified in the echocardiographic report. 2D measurements are made from inner edge to inner edge of the white-black interface. M-mode measurements of the aorta usually correspond to the sinus diameter.

dimension typically is measured in a long-axis view, but short-axis views also may be useful when anatomy is asymmetric. Note that M-mode sinus dimensions are measured at the tips of the aortic valve leaflets by using a leading edge–to–leading edge convention. The sinotubular junction is measured at the point where the curved sinus contour meets the tubular ascending aorta. The ascending aorta is measured at

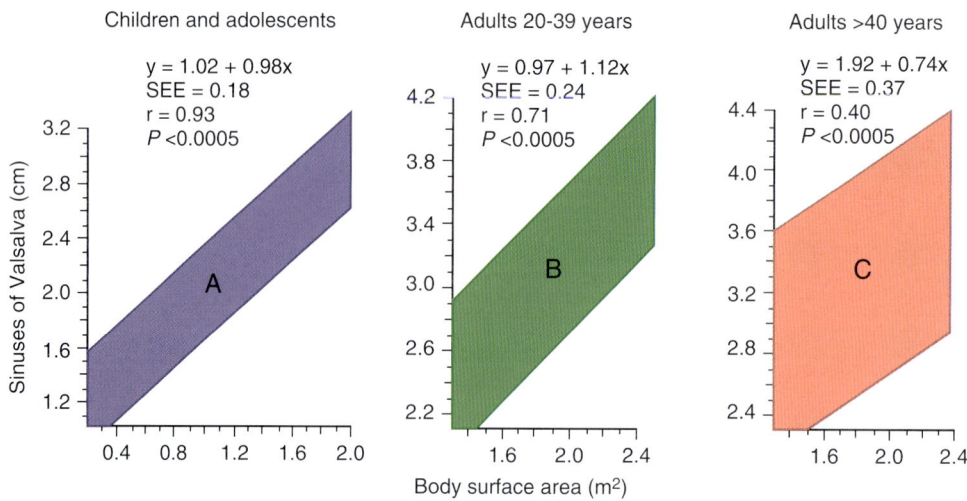

Fig. 16.15 Nomogram for normal aortic root diameter. Aortic root diameter *(vertical axis)* in relation to body surface area (horizontal axis). Normal range of aortic root dimensions for individuals <20 years of age are shown in A *(left, purple)*, between 20 and 39 years of age are shown in B *(middle, green)*, and >40 years of age are shown in C *(right, red)*. *SEE*, Standard error of estimate. *(From Roman MJ, Devereux RB, Kramer-Fox R, O'Loughlin J: Two-dimensional echocardiographic aortic root dimensions in normal children and adults,* Am J Cardiol *64[8]:507–512, 1989.)*

the maximum dimension with notation of the distance from the aortic valve. The aortic arch is measured in its mid-section, and the descending aorta is measured in the mid-thoracic region. The echo report includes the actual and expected measurements in millimeters; the ratio of the actual to the expected aortic diameter (where 1.0 is normal) may also be included (Fig. 16.15). In children, measurements are normalized for age and body size by using Z-scores, based on the standard deviation from mean normal values.

Sequential transthoracic studies of the degree of aortic dilation are used to monitor patients with Marfan syndrome or other causes of aortic aneurysm. Prophylactic ascending aorta and valve replacement may be recommended when the degree of ascending aortic dilation reaches a critical value, typically about 5.5 cm in the absence of a known genetic cause or with a bicuspid aortic valve, 5.0 cm for Marfan syndrome, 4.5 cm for Loeys-Dietz syndrome, and even lower in patients with rapid progression, a strong family history, small body size, or other contributing factors. Thus, careful measurements on sequential studies are needed to assess whether the dilation is progressive or stable over time and to determine the optimal timing of surgical intervention. Transthoracic imaging is appropriate for nonurgent serial evaluation in most patients, although additional evaluation with CT or magnetic resonance imaging (MRI) is also considered appropriate.

AORTIC DISSECTION

When transthoracic echocardiography is requested to "rule out" aortic dissection, the differential diagnosis is broad, with aortic dissection being one of many (and often the least likely) possible diagnoses. Thus, if the echocardiographic appearance of the aorta is normal, echocardiographic examination for other possible causes of chest pain is needed, including:

- Coronary artery disease (e.g., wall motion abnormalities)
- Valvular disease (e.g., aortic stenosis)
- Pulmonary embolus
- Pericarditis

When the clinical suspicion of aortic dissection is low to intermediate, a normal aorta on echocardiography further decreases the post-test likelihood of disease, so other diagnoses may be pursued. However, when the clinical suspicion is moderate to high, a "negative" transthoracic exam does *not* substantially decrease the post-test likelihood of disease, so TEE, MRI, or CT evaluation should be performed promptly.

In the patient with a possible acute aortic syndrome, the likelihood of dissection is highest in those with: (1) an underlying predisposing condition; (2) severe symptoms with an abrupt onset; (3) chest pain described as "tearing"; and (4) evidence of distal vessel compromise such as a pulse deficit, neurologic symptoms, or right-left arm blood pressure difference. Examples of patients at risk for aortic dissection include those with:

- Genetic conditions (Marfan syndrome, Turner syndrome)
- Bicuspid aortic valve disease
- Hypertension
- Atherosclerosis
- Deceleration traumatic injury

- Surgical or percutaneous procedures with aortic instrumentation
- Systemic inflammatory disorders

Transthoracic Imaging

The transthoracic examination for aortic dissection includes evaluation of the:

- Ascending aorta from the standard and high parasternal windows
- Aortic arch from the suprasternal notch window
- Descending aorta from parasternal and apical windows
- Proximal abdominal aorta from a subcostal approach

The echocardiographic diagnosis of aortic dissection (Fig. 16.16) is most secure in the presence of:

- A dilated aortic lumen
- A linear, mobile echogenic structure with a pattern of motion different from that of the aortic wall
- Different color Doppler flow patterns in the true and false lumen

When a definite, undulating intimal flap is seen, the specificity of transthoracic echocardiography for the diagnosis of dissection is high (see Appendix B, Table B.21). However, beam-width artifact and reverberations can be mistaken for intraluminal structures by an inexperienced observer; this results in a specificity of less than 100%, particularly when the images are not "classic" or when image quality is suboptimal.

Conversely, the sensitivity of transthoracic echocardiography for aortic dissection is quite low (i.e., the inability to demonstrate an internal flap does not reliably exclude the diagnosis). This low sensitivity is due to poor image quality, particularly of the segment of ascending aorta between the sinotubular junction and the aortic arch, and the poor far-field resolution of the descending thoracic aorta from the transthoracic approach.

In a patient with suspected aortic dissection, indirect signs may be present even when a flap is not identified, including:

- Aortic dilation
- Aortic regurgitation
- Pericardial effusion
- A new regional wall motion abnormality

These abnormalities do not confirm a diagnosis of dissection because many other causes for these findings are possible. However, the presence or absence of these findings should weight the clinical evidence toward or away from a diagnosis of dissection and guide the choice of additional imaging studies.

Transesophageal Imaging

TEE images of the aorta are far superior to transthoracic images in most patients because of (1) the shorter distance between the transducer and the aorta, (2) the use of a higher-frequency transducer, and (3) better ultrasound tissue penetration (higher signal-to-noise ratio). The descending thoracic aorta can be examined in its entirety from the diaphragm to the arch in both long- and short-axis planes.

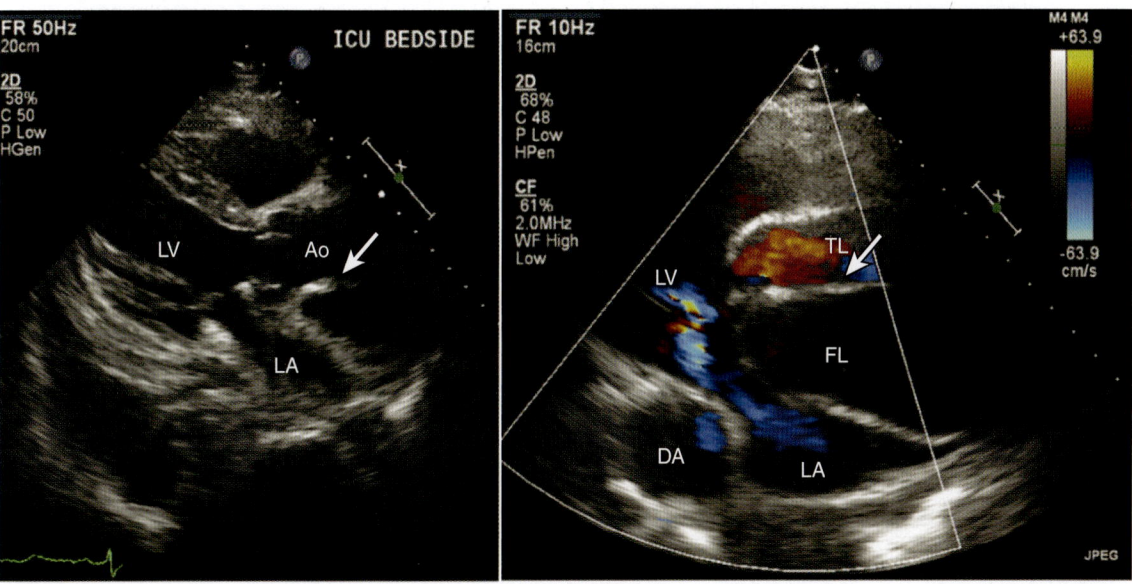

Fig. 16.16 Aortic dissection on TTE imaging. The parasternal long-axis view ▶ (left) shows a dilated ascending aorta with a linear echo (arrow), which showed motion independent of the aortic walls consistent with a dissection flap. From a higher interspace with the depth decreased, color flow Doppler ▶ (right) shows flow only in the true lumen (TL), with no flow seen in the false lumen (FL) in this view. Ao, Aorta; DA, descending aorta.

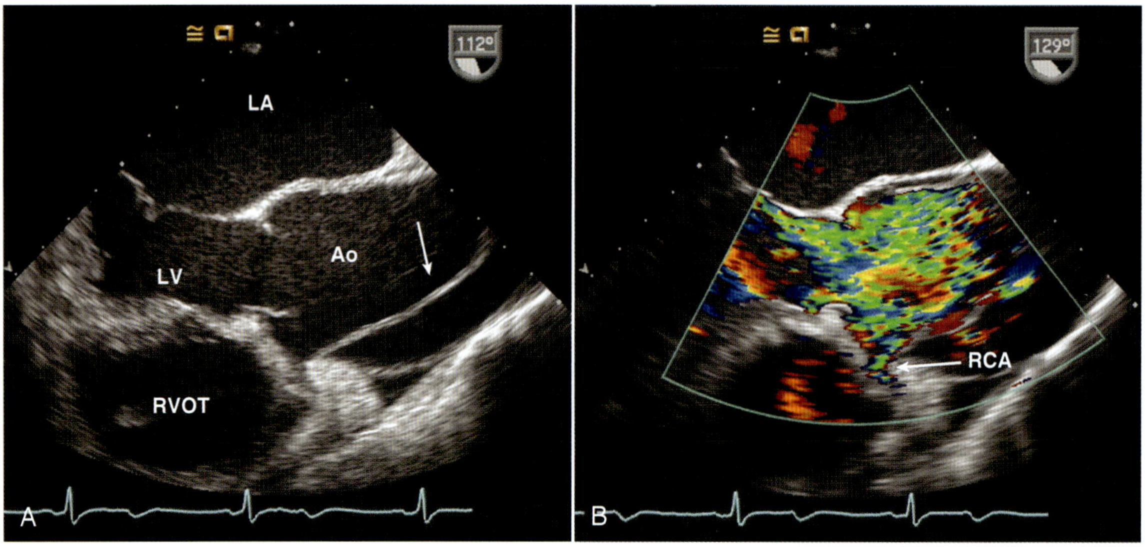

Fig. 16.17 Aortic dissection on TEE imaging. (A) A typical ascending aortic dissection with linear flap *(arrow)* originating near the ostium of the right coronary artery is shown in a TEE long-axis view. (B) Color Doppler shows disturbed systolic flow in the true lumen and indicates that the dissection flap may extend into the right coronary artery *(RCA). Ao,* Aorta; *RVOT,* RV outflow tract.

Features of aortic dissection seen on TEE imaging include any combination of:

- A dissection flap that appears as a linear, bright, echogenic structure in the aortic lumen with erratic motion compared with normal systolic pulsations (Fig. 16.17)
- Color Doppler evidence of blood flow in both the true (bounded by endothelium) lumen and the false (bounded by media) lumen
- The entry site into the false lumen
- Other communications between the two channels
- Thrombosis of the false lumen
- A hematoma in the wall of the aorta (instead of an initial flap)

The proximal segment of the ascending aorta is seen on TEE imaging in the short-axis plane at the aortic valve level. However, evaluation of the ascending aorta depends on use of a long-axis view. Evaluation of the ascending aorta is particularly important because the decision between emergency surgical intervention and medical therapy hinges on whether the dissection originates in (or involves) the ascending aorta. Note that even a localized dissection flap in the ascending aorta carries a grim prognosis and warrants surgical treatment. Color flow imaging further defines the entry site and demonstrates flow in true and false lumens. The true lumen is usually smaller than the false lumen and shows systolic expansion with systolic antegrade flow, whereas the false lumen is typically larger but shows systolic compression with reduced, absent, or retrograde flow in systole. Flow at entry sites or fenestrations usually goes from the true to the false lumen in systole.

The sensitivity of TEE for the diagnosis of aortic dissection is high (>97%). Although specificity also is high, it is less than 100% because of misinterpretation of ultrasound artifacts, such as reverberations, beam-width artifacts, and oblique imaging planes. Careful evaluation from multiple views with adjustment of instrument settings helps avoid these false-positive diagnoses.

Complications of Aortic Dissection

Complications of aortic dissection can be recognized on echocardiography and have important clinical implications both for diagnosis and therapy. Complications of aortic dissection (Fig. 16.18) include:

- Acute aortic regurgitation
- Coronary ostial occlusion
- Distal vessel obstruction
- Pericardial effusion
- Aortic rupture (pleural effusion, mediastinal hematoma)

Aortic regurgitation is nearly always present, with either chronic regurgitation due to aortic dilation or associated valve abnormalities or acute regurgitation due to further aortic dilation or to inadequate leaflet support, which results from retrograde extension of the dissection. In extreme cases, a flail aortic leaflet may be seen because of the dissection disrupting the normal attachment of the commissure to the aortic wall.

Coronary artery ostial occlusion can occur as a result of the dissection flap separating the coronary artery from normal blood flow or by compression of the vessel. The resultant wall motion abnormalities—inferior for

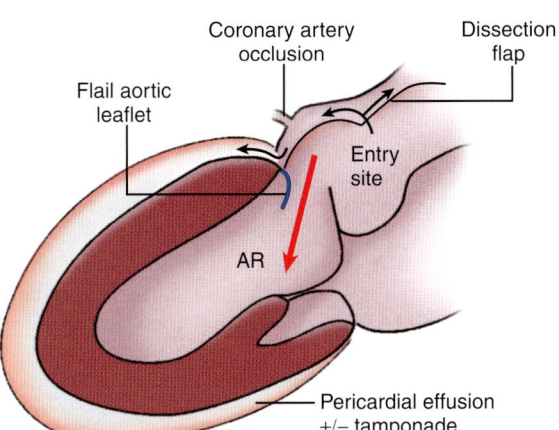

Fig. 16.18 *Potential complications of dissection of the ascending aorta.* If the dissection proceeds retrograde (as well as antegrade) from the entry site, the false lumen can cause (1) occlusion in the coronary artery ostium with resultant myocardial infarction, (2) loss of support of an aortic leaflet with consequent severe aortic regurgitation *(AR)*, or (3) rupture into the pericardium, which may result in tamponade physiology.

TABLE 16.3	Operative Uses of Transesophageal Echocardiography in Aortic Dissection
Precardiopulmonary Bypass Assessment	
Aorta	Intimal flap Entry tear* Intramural hematoma Aortic rupture Aortic pseudoaneurysm Distal extent of extension Additional tears False lumen flow patterns, including thrombus Branch vessel involvement* Coronary situs and dissection Involvement of origins of great vessels Underlying pathology Atheromatous disease Coarctation Sites of previous repairs Cannulation and cross clamp sites*
Aortic valve	Regurgitation Suitability for repair vs. replacement Sizing for allograft replacement
Mitral valve	Regurgitation Suitability for repair vs. replacement
LV and RV	Wall motion abnormalities
Pericardium	Effusion
Postcardiopulmonary Bypass Assessment	
Aorta	Confirm competency of proximal anastomosis Establish baseline for false lumen flow and distal tears
Aortic valve	Confirm competency of repaired valve
Mitral valve	Confirm competency
LV and RV	Wall motion
Intraaortic balloon	Confirm position in true lumen

*Epicardial and/or epiaortic scanning may be important in fully defining these features.
From Bolger AF: Aortic dissection and trauma: value and limitations of echocardiography. In Otto CM, editor: *The Practice of Clinical Echocardiography*, ed 4, Philadelphia, 2012, Saunders, p. 706.

right coronary obstruction, anterolateral for left main obstruction—are easily recognized on echocardiography. The diagnostic difficulty in this situation is recognizing that the wall motion abnormalities are secondary events due to aortic dissection rather than the primary event (e.g., acute myocardial infarction due to coronary thrombosis).

Distal vessel obstructions rarely are recognized during the cardiac ultrasound examination. However, the possibility of aortic dissection should be considered in patients with distal vessel obstructions who are referred for echocardiography to "rule out" a cardiac source of embolus. The correct diagnosis of distal vessel obstruction due to a dissection flap (rather than an embolus) may be made by the astute echocardiographer.

Aortic dissections can rupture in one of several ways. *External* rupture into the mediastinum or pleural space often results in exsanguination with acute hemodynamic collapse. If the rupture *thromboses*, the patient exhibits a mediastinal hematoma, a pleural effusion (more often left than right), or both. Alternatively, if the dissection ruptures at the aortic annulus into the pericardial space, the patient is likely to present with pericardial tamponade and rapid hemodynamic collapse. However, a partial rupture or a leak from the aorta into the pericardium manifests with a smaller pericardial effusion. Obviously, the presence of any amount of pericardial fluid in a patient with an aortic dissection is an alarming sign and should prompt rapid intervention.

Postoperative Evaluation After Surgery on the Ascending Aorta

In addition to the diagnosis of dissection and the evaluation of complications, TEE also is used during and after surgical repair to assess for residual dissection and aortic valve function (Table 16.3). A residual dissection flap, with flow in both true and false lumens, persists in most patients (possibly as many as 70% to 80%) following emergency surgery for acute dissection. The usual operative procedure is to close the entry site by replacing a segment of the involved aorta with a prosthetic graft. At the distal graft anastomosis, the flap may persist. Often this persistence is intentional because some branch vessels may be supplied by the false lumen and other vessels by the true lumen. Thus, the finding of a dissection flap in the aortic arch or descending aorta of a patient with a previous ascending aortic dissection and graft repair may represent stable residual disease or a second acute process. These conditions are differentiated by comparison with previous imaging studies (when available) and correlation with the operative report, clinical presentation, and other imaging modalities.

In patients with ascending aortic grafts, echocardiographic follow-up is warranted to assess for late complications. Review of the operative report is helpful in echocardiographic interpretation (Fig. 16.19). Procedures for the treatment of aortic aneurysm or dissection include:

1. Graft replacement of the ascending aorta: A tubular fabric graft is placed from above the sinotubular junction to the arch.
2. Aortic valve resuspension with replacement of the ascending aorta: The proximal anastomosis of the aortic graft is at the sinotubular junction with the aortic valve "resuspended" by attachment of the three aortic valve commissures to the proximal end of this graft. The native aortic sinuses and coronary arteries remain unchanged with this approach.
3. Valve conduit or Bentall type procedure: This is a combined replacement of the aorta and aortic valve with a composite valved conduit extending from the aortic annulus to the aortic arch with reimplantation of the native coronary artery ostia on the aortic graft. Either a mechanical or bioprosthetic valve is incorporated into the aortic graft.
4. Aortic valve reimplantation or David procedure: This is a conduit replacement of the aorta from the aortic annulus to the arch with the native valve preserved and sutured within the artificial conduit. The coronary arteries are reimplanted into the graft.
5. Additional replacement of part of the aortic arch may be done with any of these procedures. Replacement of the underside of the arch is called a hemiarch replacement.

In patients with a valved conduit, a baseline study is indicated postoperatively to allow comparison with future studies in terms of prosthetic valve function

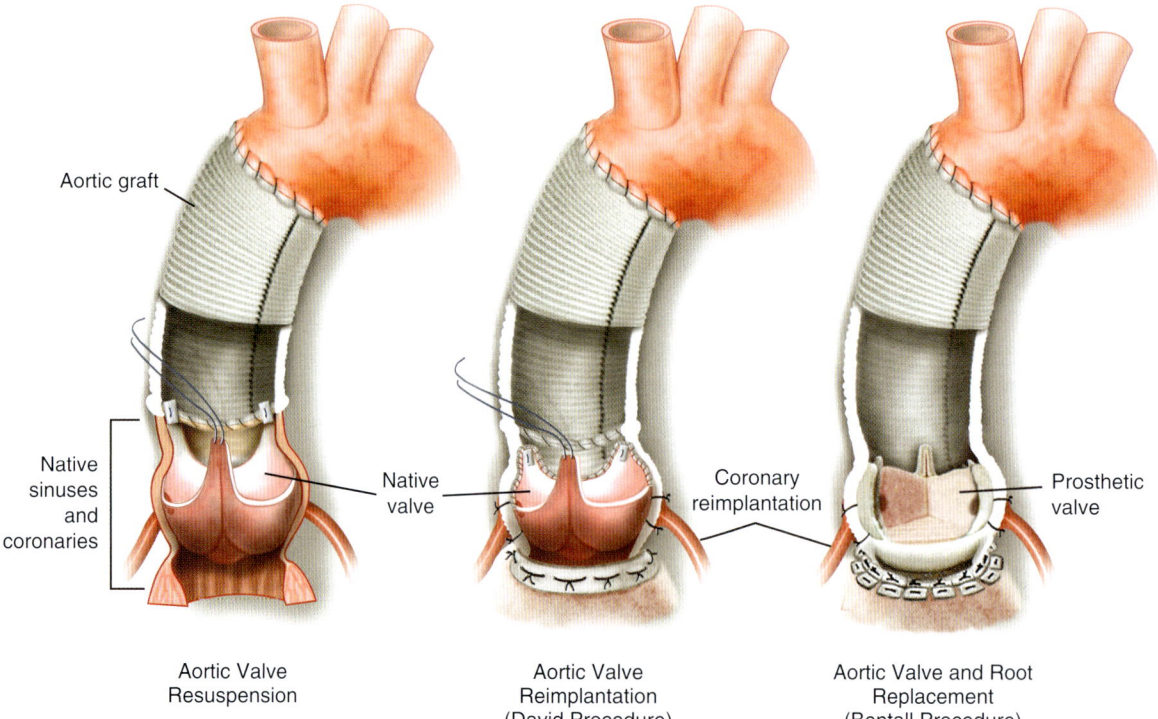

Fig. 16.19 Surgical procedures for aortic aneurysm and dissection. *(Left)* Aortic valve resuspension restores aortic valve anatomy and function by attaching the three valve commissures to the ascending aortic graft. *(Center)* Aortic valve reimplantation (i.e., David procedure) includes graft replacement of the aortic sinuses with reimplantation of the aortic valve and the coronary ostia in the sinus graft, which is then sutured to the ascending aortic graft. *(Right)* Aortic valve and root replacement (i.e., Bentall procedure) uses a combined sinus graft for the sinuses, ascending aorta, and aortic prosthetic valve (biologic or mechanical) with coronary reimplantation.

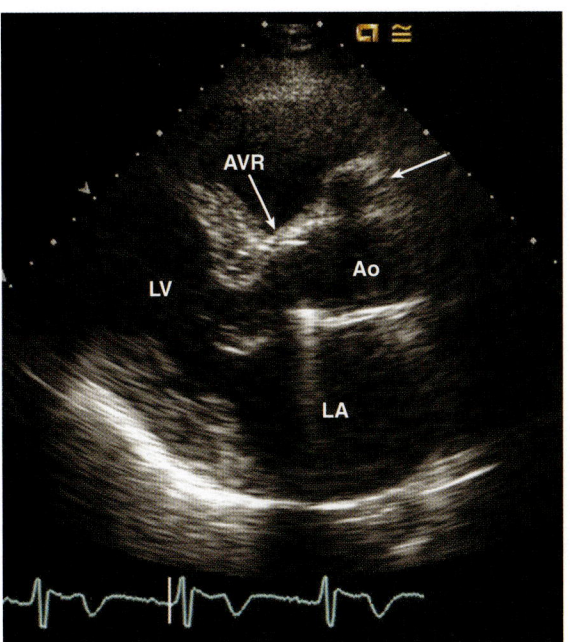

Fig. 16.20 ▶ **Ascending aortic graft and valve replacement.** This 67-year-old man with Marfan syndrome underwent composite ascending aortic graft and bileaflet mechanical valve replacement *(AVR)* 30 years ago. He has chronic stable dilation of the right coronary artery attachment to the graft *(arrow)*. *Ao,* Aorta.

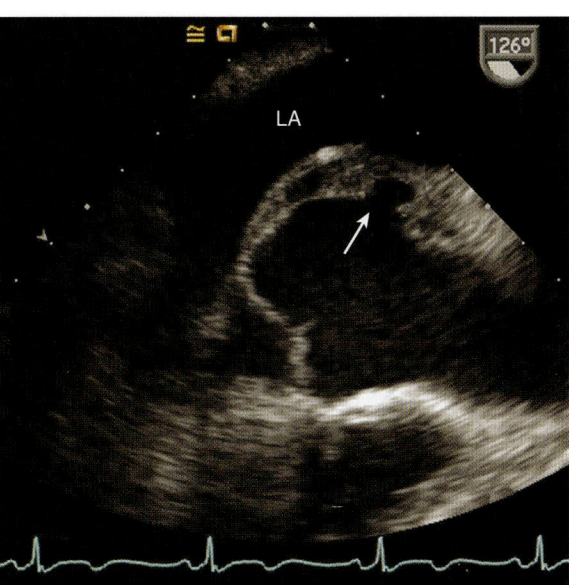

Fig. 16.21 ▶ **Aortic penetrating ulcer and intramural hematoma.** A mid-esophageal long-axis view of the ascending aorta shows a penetrating ulcer *(arrow)*, which is surrounded by hematoma. *(From Oxorn DC, Otto CM: Diseases of the great vessels. In Oxorn DC, Otto CM, editors: Intraoperative and Interventional Echocardiography: Atlas of Transesophageal Imaging, ed 2, Philadelphia, 2017, Elsevier, Fig. 10.98.)*

(see Chapter 13). The prosthetic aortic graft itself appears as an echodense, cylindrical structure with a uniform diameter (Fig. 16.20). Although most surgeons now resect the native diseased aorta, in the past the native aorta often was "wrapped around" the prosthetic graft, thus resulting in irregular areas of thickening anterior and posterior to the graft on echocardiography. Even with resection of the native aortic segment, postoperative periaortic scar tissue may be prominent. The coronary arteries retain their normal insertions if a segment of the native aorta has been preserved. In these cases, careful examination for dilation of the remaining aortic tissue and the sinuses of Valsalva is needed. When the graft extends to the aortic valve level, the right and left coronary ostia are reimplanted into the graft along with a small "button" of native aortic tissue. Dilation or loss of structural integrity of this aortic tissue or dehiscence of the coronary reimplantation suture line results in myocardial infarction due to disruption of coronary blood flow. In addition, this complication can lead to aortic rupture or pseudoaneurysm formation.

AORTIC INTRAMURAL HEMATOMA

An aortic intramural hematoma is a variant of aortic dissection with a localized collection of blood within the aortic wall, without a discrete intimal tear or false lumen, which accounts for about 5% of patients with an acute aortic syndrome. Possible mechanisms of intramural hematoma include rupture of the vasa vasorum vessels into an area of medial degeneration or a penetrating atherosclerotic ulcer without an intimal tear. About 10% to 15% of patients with an aortic intramural hematoma progress to a frank dissection with adverse clinical outcomes analogous to those seen in patients presenting initially with a clear dissection flap.

On echocardiography, an aortic intramural hematoma appears as an echogenic thickening of the aortic wall. On transthoracic imaging, intramural hematoma of the ascending aorta may be visualized, but TEE is needed for the diagnosis of other aortic segments. An intramural hematoma of the descending thoracic aorta appears on short-axis images as a crescent-shaped mass adjacent to the aortic lumen and bounded by the bright adventitial echo signal (Fig. 16.21). Long-axis imaging allows evaluation of the extent of the hematoma.

AORTIC PSEUDOANEURYSM

An aneurysm involves all the layers of the aortic wall, whereas a pseudoaneurysm is due to loss of integrity of the aortic wall, with a blood collection outside the aorta. After surgery for aortic disease, escape of blood from the graft lumen into an area contained by surrounding scar tissue or the native aorta can occur

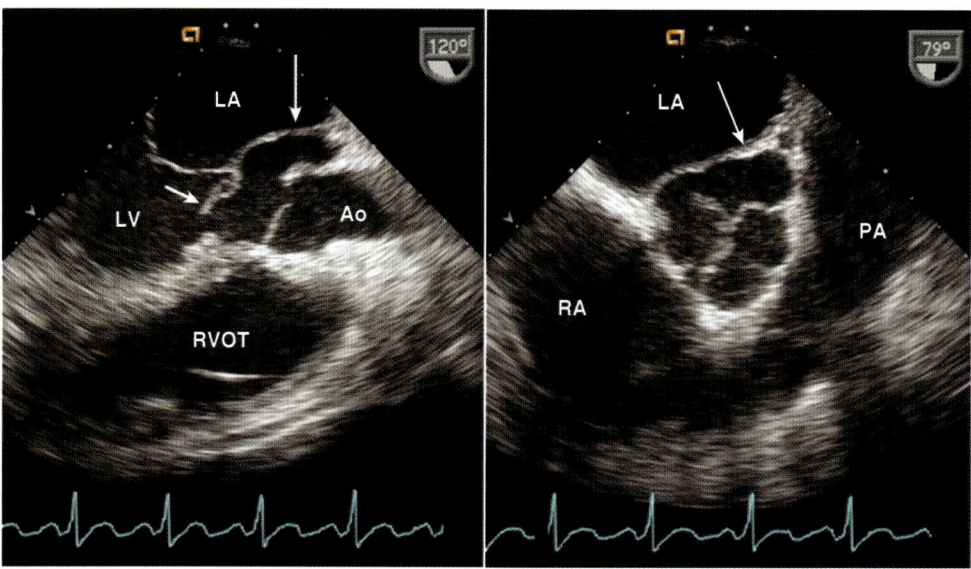

Fig. 16.22 Aortic pseudoaneurysm. Echocardiography was requested for the evaluation of cardiogenic shock in a 32-year-old man with *Pseudomonas* endocarditis. TEE imaging in a long-axis view *(left)* shows a flail noncoronary leaflet of the aortic valve *(short arrow)* in association with disruption of the posterior aortic sinus of Valsalva, resulting in a pseudoaneurysm *(long arrow)* between the aorta *(Ao)* and LA. The normal right coronary cusp of the aortic valve is seen in a closed position. On color Doppler, flow into and out of the pseudoaneurysm from the aorta and severe aortic regurgitation were seen. The short-axis view *(right)* at the level of communication between the aorta and pseudoaneurysm *(arrow)* shows the distorted appearance of the aortic valve and sinuses. *PA,* Pulmonary artery; *RVOT,* RV outflow tract.

at the proximal or distal graft anastomoses to the aorta or at the coronary reimplantation sites. Pseudoaneurysms also may occur after complex aortic valve surgery with root enlarging procedures or with endocarditis and tissue destruction.

A pseudoaneurysm appears as an echolucent area adjacent to the aortic graft (Fig. 16.22). Flow into this region can be demonstrated with color flow imaging, although a TEE study often is necessary for adequate image quality. The pseudoaneurysm may rupture into the mediastinum or pleural spaces (both of which are likely to be fatal) or back across the aortic annulus into the LV. This pseudoaortic regurgitation consists of flow from the pseudoaneurysm into the LV in diastole, with flow from the LV into the pseudoaneurysm in systole. The characteristics of this flow signal on pulsed and CW Doppler are similar to those of transvalvular aortic regurgitation. Color flow imaging shows the flow around, rather than through, the prosthetic aortic valve.

TRAUMATIC AORTIC DISEASE

Deceleration injury, from a fall or motor vehicle accident, can result in rupture of the aorta at the aortic isthmus (the junction of the arch and descending thoracic aorta adjacent to the ligamentum arteriosus). In some cases, containment of the rupture by hematoma allows diagnosis and emergency surgery. Contrast CT imaging is the optimal approach for diagnosis.

The area of disruption often is challenging to recognize on TEE; because disruption extends only a short distance, no intimal flap may be present, and demonstrating flow outside the aorta may be difficult. With delayed diagnosis, a false aneurysm may be seen at the aortic isthmus.

Aortic injury with dissection or hematoma also can be a complication of diagnostic or interventional procedures, including coronary or valve interventions, and rarely may be seen after cardiac surgery related to aortic cannulation or cross-clamping.

SINUS OF VALSALVA ANEURYSM

A sinus of Valsalva aneurysm can be due to:

- Congenital disease
- Acute infection (e.g., endocarditis)
- An inflammatory process

Echocardiographically, a dilated and distorted sinus of Valsalva is seen both in long- and short-axis views at the aortic valve level either from a TEE or transthoracic approach. A congenital aneurysm often is complex in shape, with a "wind sock" appearance of a mass of irregular, mobile echoes protruding from the aortic sinus into adjacent cardiac structures (Fig. 16.23). If the aneurysm is not fenestrated, Doppler flow examination is unremarkable. More commonly, multiple fenestrations are present, with high-velocity turbulent flow from the high-pressure aorta to the

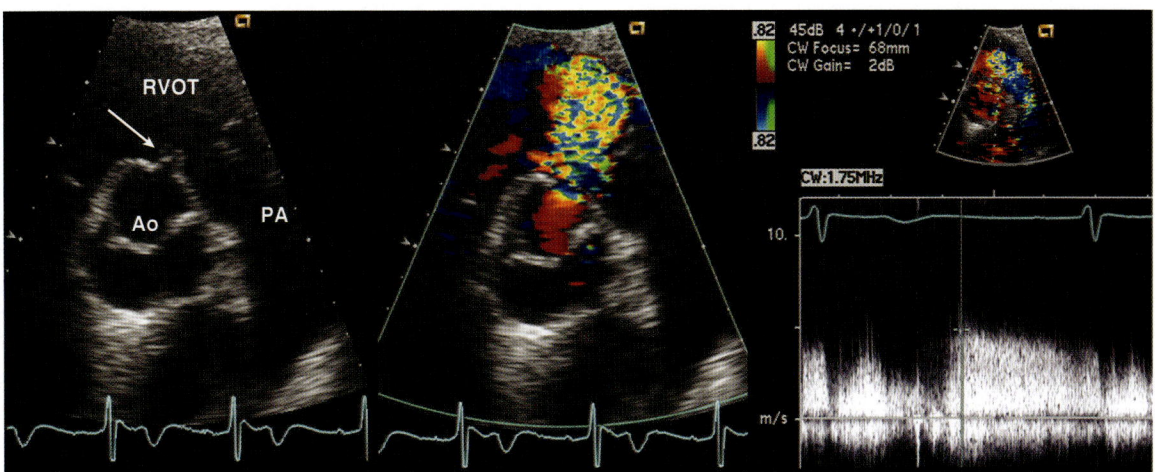

Fig. 16.23 Ruptured sinus of Valsalva aneurysm. TTE short-axis views in this 42-year-old man show *(left)* a small congenital sinus of Valsalva aneurysm of the right coronary cusp *(arrow)*, which has ruptured into the RV outflow tract *(RVOT, center)*. CW Doppler *(right)* shows high-velocity (>4 m/s) flow from the aorta into the RV in both diastole and systole, thus confirming that the communication is from the aorta, rather than the LV. *Ao,* Aorta; *PA,* pulmonary artery.

low-pressure adjacent chambers detectable by CW, pulsed wave, and color flow Doppler techniques. Note that infection of a previously competent congenital sinus of Valsalva aneurysm may result in flow across a necrotic area of infection.

Acquired sinus of Valsalva aneurysms tend to be more regular in shape. Dilation of the sinuses in Marfan syndrome symmetrically involves all three sinuses, with a rounded, smooth shape. At surgery, replacement of the ascending aorta is performed with a composite valve and graft (with reimplantation of the coronaries). If only the ascending aorta is replaced in an emergency situation, patients with Marfan syndrome are at risk of progressive dilation and rupture of the residual aortic sinus tissue. A sinus of Valsalva aneurysm due to endocarditis tends to result in a more spherical, but still irregular-appearing, dilation of the sinus and thickening of the aortic wall. Again, the aneurysm protrudes (and may rupture) into adjacent cardiac structures depending on which sinus is involved.

ATHEROSCLEROTIC AORTIC DISEASE

Aortic Atherosclerosis as a Potential Source of Embolus

The excellent-quality images of the aorta obtained by TEE imaging have led to the observation of extensive atherosclerotic plaque in many individuals, with mobile thrombi attached to the atheroma in some cases. These observations have generated the hypothesis that atherosclerosis of the ascending aorta and arch may serve as a nidus for embolic material, resulting in cerebrovascular events. These areas of atherosclerosis rarely are seen on transthoracic imaging because of poor image quality related to acoustic access, the depth of the aorta from the transthoracic approach, and the use of a lower-frequency transducer. Echocardiographic evaluation of the extent and severity of atheroma correlates well with histologic examination, and TEE echocardiography is both sensitive and specific for the detection of atheroma-related thrombus formation.

Intraoperative evaluation of the ascending aorta for atheroma to avoid entering the aorta at a site of atherosclerotic disease now is routine before placement of aortic cannula or bypass grafting surgery. Either TEE imaging or direct sterile epiaortic imaging may be used for this evaluation.

Aortic Atherosclerosis as a Marker of Coronary Artery Disease

The presence of detectable atherosclerotic plaques in the descending aorta on TEE (Fig. 16.24) indicates the presence of atherosclerosis and thus is a marker of coronary artery disease, with a sensitivity of 90%. Conversely, the absence of detectable atherosclerosis in the descending thoracic aorta suggests that significant coronary artery disease is not present, with a specificity of 90%.

PULMONARY ARTERY ABNORMALITIES

Most abnormalities of the pulmonary artery are congenital, including poststenotic dilation, branch pulmonary artery stenosis, and an abnormal position of the pulmonary artery, as in transposition of the great vessels. However, the pulmonary artery may

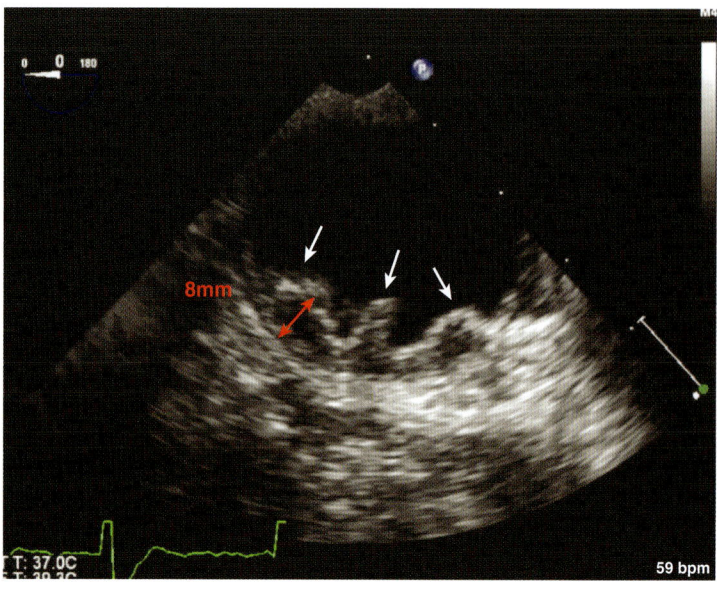

Fig. 16.24 ▶ **Aortic atheroma.** In this patient undergoing transcatheter aortic valve implantation, TEE views of the descending aorta show a complex protruding atheroma *(white arrows)*. Thickness of atheroma shown by *red arrow*. (From Oxorn DC, Otto CM: Diseases of the great vessels. In Oxorn DC, Otto CM, editors: Intraoperative and Interventional Echocardiography: Atlas of Transesophageal Imaging, ed 2, Philadelphia, 2017, Elsevier, Fig. 10.91.)

be involved by systemic diseases that affect the aorta, such as Takayasu arteritis. Pulmonary artery dissection is rare but has been reported in patients with chronic pulmonary hypertension.

The finding of a dilated pulmonary artery in the absence of complex congenital heart disease raises the possibility of:

- Right-sided volume overload (e.g., atrial septal defect)
- Pulmonary hypertension
- Idiopathic dilation of the pulmonary artery

The finding of a dilated main pulmonary artery mandates a careful evaluation for right-sided pressure or volume overload. Idiopathic dilation of the pulmonary artery is a rare diagnosis and should be considered only if no other cause exists for pulmonary artery dilation.

The pulmonary artery can be depicted on TTE in a parasternal short-axis view at the aortic valve level or in an RV outflow view. In adults, it is difficult to visualize the anterior pulmonary artery wall because of overlying lung tissue. In younger patients, the pulmonary artery can be demonstrated from the anteriorly angulated apical four-chamber view by further anterior angulation. The subcostal short-axis view allows an alternate approach to depict the pulmonary artery in most patients. From the suprasternal notch window, the right pulmonary artery is seen in cross section in the long-axis view of the aortic arch and in its long axis in the orthogonal view (see Fig. 16.7). The left pulmonary artery can be imaged by slight lateral angulation and posterior rotation from the standard long-axis suprasternal notch view.

TEE images of the pulmonary artery are obtained in a 0° image plane by slowly withdrawing the probe to an esophageal level superior to the LA. This view shows the long axis of the pulmonary artery and its bifurcation, but cannot be obtained in all patients because of interposition of the air-filled bronchus (Fig. 16.25). The pulmonary artery also is imaged in the 90° plane (analogous to the transthoracic RV outflow view) by turning the transducer to the patient's right from the LV long-axis view. However, image quality often is suboptimal because of the distance of the pulmonary artery from the transducer in this view.

ALTERNATE APPROACHES

Although TEE has high sensitivity and specificity for diagnosis of acute aortic dissection and can be performed quickly at the patient's bedside (Table 16.4), alternate imaging approaches often are preferred, depending on the clinical setting. The choice of imaging procedure depends on the urgency of the clinical presentation, the frequency of imaging, and the additional information needed. In the acute setting, CT angiography is the primary diagnostic modality because radiologists are on site at all times, whereas echocardiographers typically need to travel to the medical center. For long-term serial monitoring of patients with aortic disease, either CT or MRI imaging is appropriate, with MRI preferred to avoid repetitive (albeit low-dose) radiation exposure. Alternatively, the choice of imaging procedures may be driven by the specific additional information needed in an individual patient. Examples include distal vessel anatomy (angiography), adjacent mediastinal

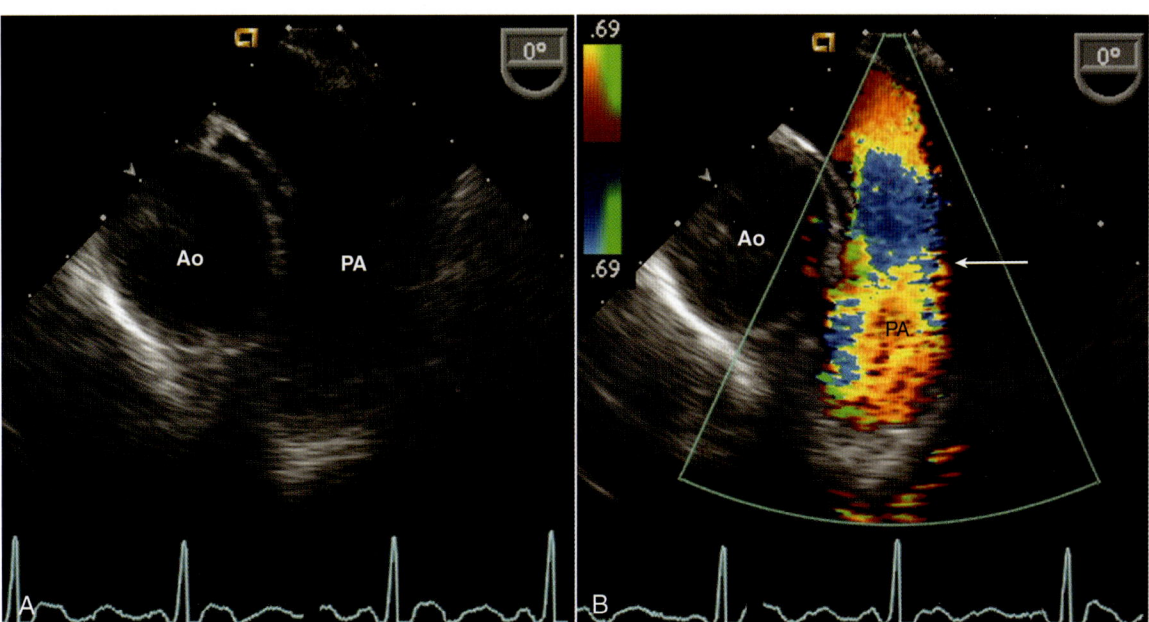

Fig. 16.25 Pulmonary artery on TEE imaging. (A) The pulmonary artery is seen in long axis from a high esophageal position in the 0° image plane orientation. This view cannot be obtained in all patients because of interposition of the air-filled bronchus. (B) Color Doppler shows flow in the pulmonary artery *(PA)* directed toward the transducer. Aliasing from red to blue *(arrow)* occurs because the antegrade velocity exceeds the Nyquist limit of 69 cm/s. *Ao*, Aorta.

TABLE 16.4 Diagnostic Imaging Procedures in Aortic Disease

Imaging Approach	Advantages	Caveats
Transthoracic echocardiography	Portable, rapid Inexpensive Evaluation of LV function, valve function, and PE Aortic measurements at end-diastole at multiple sites	Moderate sensitivity and specificity for dissection due to poor acoustic access and suboptimal image resolution Aortic lumen diameters are measured at end-diastole perpendicular to the long axis of the aorta.
Transesophogeal echocardiography	High sensitivity and specificity for aortic dissection Portable, rapid Evaluation of LV function, valve function, PE Aortic measurements at end-diastole at multiple sites	TEE procedure has some risk. Cannot evaluate coronary or branch vessel anatomy Aortic lumen diameters are measured at end-diastole perpendicular to the long axis of the aorta.
Computed tomography	High sensitivity and specificity for aortic dissection Wide field of view Coronary and distal vessel anatomy 3D reconstruction of aorta	Not portable Ionizing radiation Few data on LV and aortic valve External diameter of aorta is measured perpendicular to long axis of aorta. It may be slightly larger than echo measurement.
Cardiac magnetic resonance imaging	High sensitivity and specificity for aortic dissection Wide field of view Distal branch vessel anatomy 3D reconstruction of aorta	High cost, not portable Can evaluate proximal coronary anatomy only. Limited evaluation of coronary involvement with dissection External diameter of aorta is measured perpendicular to long axis of aorta. It may be slightly larger than echo measurement.

PE, Pericardial effusion.

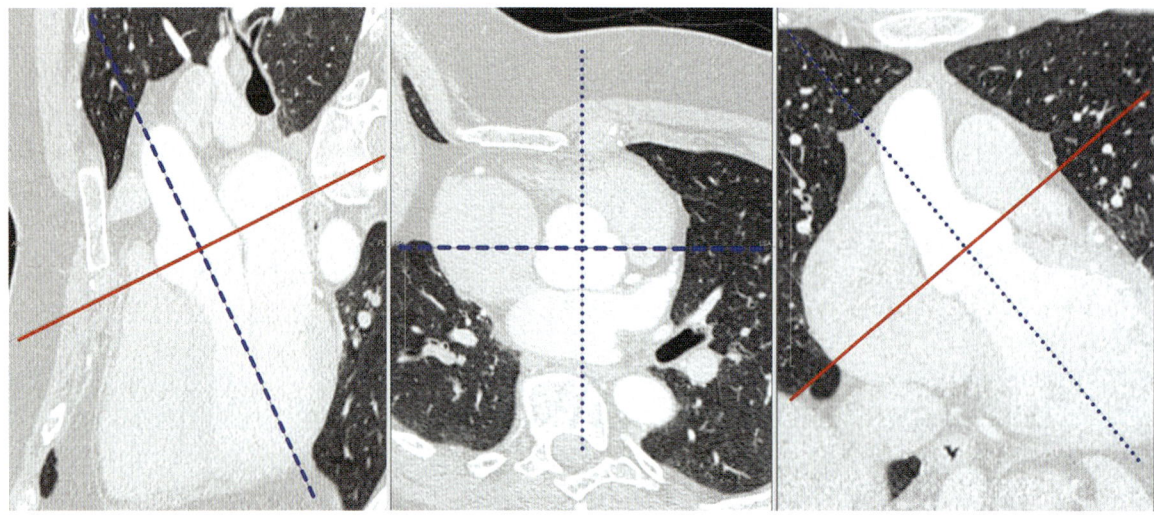

Fig. 16.26 Computed tomographic imaging of the aorta. Example of double-oblique measurements. After 3D reconstruction of computed tomographic data, two orthogonal planes *(left and right images)* are adjusted to go through the axis of the structure to be measured (in this case the aortic root). A third plane *(center image)* orthogonal to the first and second is used to measure an exact cross section of the structure of interest. All segments of the aorta should be measured in this fashion to avoid skewed slices and false results. *(From Radke RM, Baumgartner H: Diagnosis and treatment of Marfan syndrome: an update,* Heart *100[17]:1382–1391, 2014, Fig. 3.)*

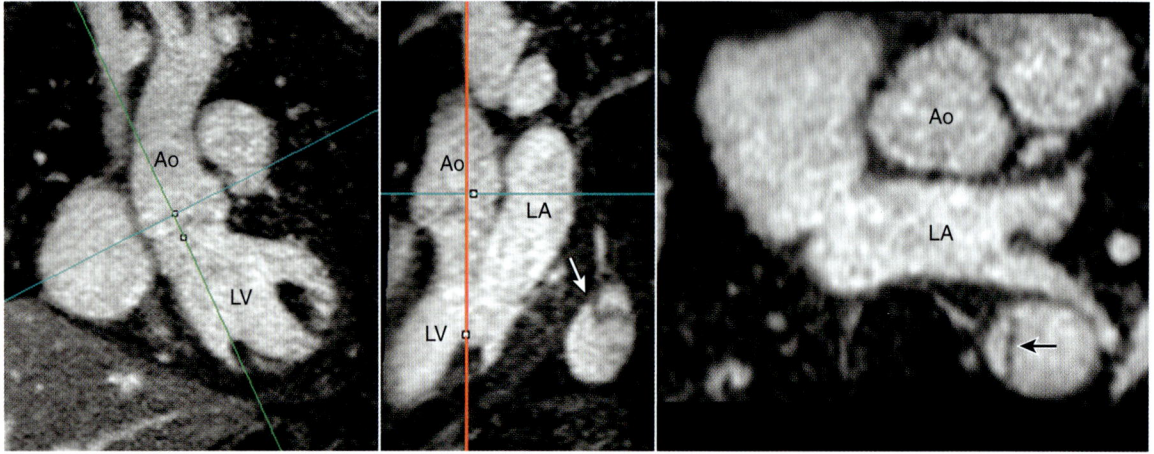

Fig. 16.27 Magnetic resonance angiography. Magnetic resonance imaging with gadolinium enhancement allows acquisition of a full-volume dataset to include the entire aorta *(Ao)*. As shown in the *left* and *center* images, the image plane can be aligned with the long axis of the aorta in two orthogonal views, with measurements made from the correctly oriented short-axis image on the *right*. The dissection flap in the descending aorta *(arrow)* again is seen in this patient. *(Images courtesy Eric Krieger, MD.)*

disease (CT or MRI imaging), or valvular function (echocardiography).

Both CT angiography and MRI imaging provide excellent-quality images of the aorta with sensitivities and specificities for the diagnosis of aortic dissection as high as or higher than TEE (Figs. 16.26 and 16.27). Chest CT can be used to evaluate aortic disease with the advantages of a wide field of view, high accuracy, and wide availability. Chest CT may identify associated pericardial effusion but is of limited value in the evaluation of LV or aortic valve function. 3D reconstructions of CT scans enhance the ability to relate anatomic findings to one another. Disadvantages include the use of contrast, ionizing radiation, and the nonportable nature of the study.

MRI imaging of the aorta has the advantages of high resolution, high diagnostic accuracy, a wide field of view, and the ability to orient the images along the long axis of the aorta. As with chest CT, MRI imaging equipment is not portable, but contrast is not required for aortic imaging, and no exposure to ionizing radiation occurs. MRI imaging also allows evaluation for aortic regurgitation, pericardial effusion, and LV function. Both chest CT and MRI imaging provide data on branch vessel involvement, information that rarely is obtainable with echocardiography.

THE ECHO EXAM

Examination of the Aorta

Aortic Segment	Modality	View	Recording	Limitations
Aortic sinuses	TTE	Parasternal long-axis	Images of sinuses of Valsalva, aortic annulus, and sinotubular junction	Shadowing of posterior aortic sinuses
	TEE	High esophageal long-axis	Standard long-axis plane by rotating to about 120°–130°	
Ascending	TTE	Parasternal long-axis	Move transducer superiorly to image sinotubular junction and ascending aorta.	Only limited segments visualized, variable among patients
	TTE Doppler	Apical	LVOT and ascending aorta flow recorded with pulsed or CW Doppler from an anteriorly angulated four-chamber view	Velocity underestimation if the angle between the Doppler beam and flow is not parallel
	TEE	High esophageal long-axis	From long-axis view, move transducer superiorly to image ascending aorta.	The distal ascending aorta may not be visualized.
Arch	TTE	Suprasternal	Long- and short-axis views of aortic arch	Descending aorta appears to taper as it leaves the image plane.
	TEE	High esophageal	From the short-axis view of the initial segment of the descending thoracic aorta, turn the probe toward the patient's right side, and angulate inferiorly.	View is not obtained in all patients. The aortic segment at the junction of the ascending aorta and arch may not be visualized.
Descending thoracic	TTE	Parasternal and modified apical views	Rotate from long-axis view to image thoracic aorta in long axis posterior to LV. From apical 2-chamber view, use lateral angulation and counterclockwise rotation to image aorta.	Depth of thoracic aorta on TTE limits image quality. TEE is usually needed for diagnosis.
	TTE Doppler	Suprasternal	Descending aorta flow recorded with pulsed Doppler from SSN view	Low wall filters needed to evaluate for holodiastolic flow reversal
	TEE	Short-axis aorta	Sequential short-axis views of the aorta from the level of the diaphragm to the arch with the image plane turned posteriorly and the transducer slowly withdrawn	Long-axis views allow further evaluation of abnormal findings.
Proximal abdominal	TTE	Subcostal	Long axis of proximal abdominal aorta	Only the proximal segment is visualized.
	TTE Doppler	Transgastric	Proximal abdominal aorta flow recorded with pulsed Doppler	Low wall filters needed to evaluate for holodiastolic flow reversal
	TEE	Transgastric	From the transgastric position, portions of the abdominal aorta may be seen posteriorly.	Does not allow evaluation of entire abdominal aorta

LVOT, LV outflow tract; *SSN,* suprasternal notch.

Continued

Key Features of Aortic Diseases

Aortic Dissection	Key Features	Associated Findings
Dissection flap	In aortic lumen True and false lumen	Independent motion Entry sites Thrombosis of false lumen
Intramural hematoma	Crescent-shaped thickening of aortic wall	
Indirect findings	Aortic dilation Aortic regurgitation Coronary ostial involvement Pericardial effusion	
Complications of Aortic Dissection		
Aortic regurgitation	Due to aortic root dilation Due to leaflet flail	
Coronary artery occlusion	Ventricular fibrillation Acute myocardial infarction	
Distal vessel obstruction	Carotid (stroke) Subclavian (upper limb ischemia)	
Aortic rupture	Into the pericardium	Pericardial effusion Pericardial tamponade
	Into the mediastinum Into the pleural space	Pleural effusion Exsanguination
Sinus of Valsalva Aneurysm		
Congenital	Complex shape Protrusion into RV outflow tract Fenestrations	
Acquired	Infection or inflammation Symmetric shape Communication with aorta Potential for rupture	
Aortic Atheroma		
	Complex (≥4 mm or mobile) Associated with:	Coronary artery disease Cerebroembolic events

SUGGESTED READING

Guidelines

1. Goldstein SA, Evangelista A, Abbara S, et al: Multimodality imaging of diseases of the thoracic aorta in adults: from the American Society of Echocardiography and the European Association of Cardiovascular Imaging: endorsed by the Society of Cardiovascular Computed Tomography and Society for Cardiovascular Magnetic Resonance, *J Am Soc Echocardiogr* 28(2):119–182, 2015.
   Recommendations for imaging the aorta with details of image acquisition, strengths, and limitations of each modality. Normal aortic size is related to age, body size, and sex. In children, aortic size is normalized to height, but indexing aortic size in adults is more problematic. The regressions equations in Fig. 16.5 and upper limits of normal in Tables A.9 and A.10 are recommended as benchmarks. All imaging modalities are subject to physiologic and measurement variability, so small changes on serial studies should be interpreted with caution.

2. Evangelista A, Flachskampf FA, Erbel R, et al: European Association of Echocardiography; Pepi M, Breithardt OA, Plonska-Gosciniak E (document reviewers): Echocardiography in aortic diseases: EAE recommendations for clinical practice, *Eur J Echocardiogr* 11(8):645–658, 2010. Erratum in: *Eur J Echocardiogr* 12(8):642, 2011.
   This guideline recommends TEE as the ultrasound procedure of choice for the evaluation of the thoracic aorta. The relationships among age, body size, and aortic diameter should be considered in the diagnosis of aortic enlargement. Echocardiography also allows evaluation of aortic elastic properties, detection of atheroma, and diagnosis of aortic dissection. However, CT and MRI imaging are more reliable for evaluation of the arch and descending aorta. Provides details and examples of image acquisition and measurement.

3. Hiratzka LF, Bakris GL, Beckman JA, et al: 2010 ACCF/AHA/AATS/ACR/ASA/SCA/SCAI/SIR/STS/SVM guidelines for the diagnosis and management of patients with thoracic aortic disease: a report of the American College of Cardiology Foundation/American Heart

Association Task Force on Practice Guidelines, American Association for Thoracic Surgery, American College of Radiology, American Stroke Association, Society of Cardiovascular Anesthesiologists, Society for Cardiovascular Angiography and Interventions, Society of Interventional Radiology, Society of Thoracic Surgeons, and Society for Vascular Medicine, *Circulation* 121:e266–e369, 2010.
Comprehensive guideline document including normal values for aortic dimensions, a review of multimodality imaging for aortic disease, and recommendations for the diagnosis and management of aortic disease.

Aortic Aneurysm and Dissection

4. Bolger AF: Aortic dissection and trauma: value and limitations of echocardiography. In Otto CM, editor: *The Practice of Clinical Echocardiography*, ed 5, Philadelphia, 2017, Elsevier, pp 677–691.
Review of the pathophysiologic and clinical presentation of aortic dissection and the role of echocardiography for the initial diagnosis, management at the time of surgery, and long-term follow-up.

5. Tan CN, Fraser AG: Perioperative transesophageal echocardiography for aortic dissection, *Can J Anaesth* 61:362–378, 2014.
Review article with nice illustrations of aortic dissection types, echo findings and approaches to surgical repair. Numerous online videos.

6. Wang CJ, Rodriguez Diaz CA, Trinh MA: Use of real-time three-dimensional transesophageal echocardiography in type A aortic dissections: advantages of 3D TEE illustrated in three cases, *Ann Card Anaesth* 18(1):83–86, 2015.
Short article highlighting the role with 3D imaging in aortic dissection.

7. Devereux RB, de Simone G, Arnett DK, et al: Normal limits in relation to age, body size and gender of two-dimensional echocardiographic aortic root dimensions in persons ≥15 years of age, *Am J Cardiol* 110:1189–1194, 2012.
Based on data in 1207 apparently normal subjects, nomograms are proposed for normal aortic diameters in men and women. Using height, expected aortic diameter is calculated as:

$1.519 + (age\ [years] \times 0.010)$
$+ (height\ [centimeters] \times 0.010)$
$- (sex\ [1 = man, 2 = woman] \times 0.247)$

Z-score then is calculated as the difference between the measured and predicted aortic diameter divided by 0.215. A Z-score over 1.97 to 3.0 indicates mild, 3.01 to 4.0 moderate, and >4.0 severe aortic dilation.

8. Evangelista A: Imaging aortic aneurysmal disease, *Heart* 100(12):909–915, 2014.
Review of multimodality imaging for evaluation of aortic aneurysmal disease with useful figures and online videos.

9. Pape LA, Awais M, Woznicki EM, et al: Presentation, diagnosis, and outcomes of acute aortic dissection: 17-year trends from the International Registry of Acute Aortic Dissection, *J Am Coll Cardiol* 66(4):350–358, 2015.
This registry includes data on 4428 patients with aortic dissection enrolled at 28 centers over an 18-year period. Most patients (83%) with an ascending aorta dissection present with chest pain, described as severe or worst-ever in 93%. Over this time period, the use of CT for the initial diagnosis increased from 46% to 73% of cases. In contrast, the use of TEE as the initial diagnostic test decreased from 50% to 23%. Early mortality for ascending aortic dissection decreased from 31% to 22%.

Aortic Intramural Hemorrhage

10. Chou AS, Ziganshin BA, Charilaou P, et al: Long-term behavior of aortic intramural hematomas and penetrating ulcers, *J Thorac Cardiovasc Surg* 151(2):361–372, 2016.
In 55 patients with an aortic intramural hematoma, the initial presentation consisted of symptoms of aortic rupture (18%), with aortic dissection being less common. Over 9 months of follow-up, 57% had progressive disease, with 43% requiring late surgery. In 53 patients with penetrating atherosclerotic ulcer, 32% presented with rupture symptoms, and 30% underwent late surgery.

11. Matsushita A, Fukui T, Tabata M, et al: Preoperative characteristics and surgical outcomes of acute intramural hematoma involving the ascending aorta: a propensity score-matched analysis, *J Thorac Cardiovasc Surg* 151(2):351–358, 2016.
Based on a series of 460 patients with acute aortic syndromes involving the ascending aorta, compared with patients with a typical dissection, the 121 patients with aortic intramural hematoma were characterized by older age, female sex, history of hypertension and hyperlipidemia, and presentation with cardiac tamponade. However, operative mortality was lower and long-term survival was higher in those with an intramural hematoma.

Inherited Connective Tissue Disorders

12. Cheng A, Lewin M, Olson A: Echocardiography in patients with inherited connective tissue disorders. In Otto CM, editor: *The Practice of Clinical Echocardiography*, ed 5, Philadelphia, 2017, Elsevier, pp 677–691.
This chapter summarizes the different types of inherited connective tissue disorders, echocardiography findings, and clinical outcomes.

13. Detaint D, Michelena HI, Nkomo VT, et al: Aortic dilatation patterns and rates in adults with bicuspid aortic valves: a comparative study with Marfan syndrome and degenerative aortopathy, *Heart* 100(2):126–134, 2014.
The degree and rate of aortic dilation in 353 patients with a bicuspid aortic valve were compared with 50 patients with Marfan syndrome and 51 patients with a degenerative aortopathy, matched for sex, blood pressure, and follow-up duration. Aortic dilation was present in 87% of patients with bicuspid aortic valve, with the largest diameter in the ascending aorta (60%) or sinuses (27%). Progressive aortic dilation occurred in most patients with bicuspid aortic valve, but 43% had no change over time. In contrast, progressive aortic dilation was seen in 80% of the patients with Marfan syndrome.

14. Radke RM, Baumgartner H: Diagnosis and treatment of Marfan syndrome: an update, *Heart* 100(17):1382–1391, 2014.
Review of the diagnostic criteria for Marfan syndrome and the imaging approach. TTE is the primary imaging modality for diagnosis, follow-up, and family screening. In addition, CT and MRI are used to image the entire aorta on sequential studies. The authors recommend using Z-score indexed for height (not body surface area) for normalizing aortic diameters with an absolute threshold over 40 mm in adults considered abnormal.

15. Kuijpers JM, Mulder BJ: Aortopathies in adult congenital heart disease and genetic aortopathy syndromes: management strategies and indications for surgery, *Heart* 103(12):952–966, 2017.
Educational review article summarizes inherited aortopathies from a clinical point of view. Sections include appropriate imaging strategies for diagnosis and follow-up, pharmacological therapy, indications for surgery, pregnancy considerations, and sports participation.

Aortic Atheroma

16. Weissler-Snir A, Greenberg G, Shapira Y, et al: Transoesophageal echocardiography of aortic atherosclerosis: the additive value of three-dimensional over two-dimensional imaging, *Eur Heart J Cardiovasc Imaging* 16(4):389–394, 2015.
In 67 patients, 3D imaging of 100 aortic atherosclerotic plaques provided useful information on atheroma thickness and irregularity of contour.

17. Denny JT, Pantin E, Chiricolo A, et al: Increasing severity of aortic atherosclerosis in coronary artery bypass grafting patients evaluated by transesophageal echocardiography, *J Clin Med Res* 7(1):13–17, 2015.
The extent of atheroma visualized on intraoperative TEE in 124 patients undergoing coronary artery bypass grafting surgery increased significantly from 2002 to 2009. The presence of atheroma is important in optimizing the surgical approach to reduce the risk of stroke.

Aortic Surgery

18. Malaisrie SC, McCarthy PM: Surgical approach to diseases of the aortic valve and the aortic root. In Otto CM, Bonow RO, editors: *Valvular Heart Disease: A Companion to Braunwald's Heart Disease*, ed 5, Philadelphia, 2018, Elsevier. In press.
Summary of the surgical approach to both the aortic valve and aortic disease. Illustrations are helpful in understanding the echocardiographic anatomy of the Bentall procedure (combined aortic valve and root replacement with coronary reimplantation) and the David procedure (root replacement with preservation of the native aortic valve within the graft).

19. Oxorn DC, Otto CM: Diseases of the great vessels. In Oxorn DC, Otto CM, editors: *Intraoperative and Interventional Echocardiography: Atlas of Transesophageal Imaging*, ed 2, Philadelphia, 2017, Elsevier.
This atlas chapter presents images and videos for 16 patients with aortic disease who were undergoing operative intervention.

17 The Adult With Congenital Heart Disease

BASIC PRINCIPLES
  Stenosis
  Regurgitation
  Shunts
  Connections

CONGENITAL STENOTIC LESIONS
  Congenital Aortic Valve Stenosis
  Subaortic Stenosis
  Congenital Obstructions to Right Ventricular Outflow

CONGENIITAL ABNORMALITES OF THE AORTA AND CORONARY ARTERIES
  Aortic Coarctation
  Sinus of Valsalva Aneurysm
  Coronary Arteriovenous Fistula
  Anomalous Origins of the Coronary Arteries

CONGENITAL REGURGITANT LESIONS
  Ebstein Anomaly of the Tricuspid Valve
  Cleft Mitral Valve

INTRACARDIAC SHUNTS
  Atrial Septal Defects
    Anatomy
    Transthoracic Imaging
    Contrast Echocardiography
    Transesophageal Imaging

  Ventricular Septal Defects
    Anatomy
    Imaging
    Doppler Findings
  Patent Ductus Arteriosus

OTHER CONDITIONS MANIFESTING IN ADULTHOOD
  Corrected Transposition of the Great Arteries
  "Incidental" Congenital Anomalies

COMMON TYPES OF PALLIATED ADULT CONGENITAL HEART DISEASE
  Classification of Types of Procedures
  Tetralogy of Fallot
  Complete Transposition of the Great Arteries
  Fontan Physiology

LIMITATIONS OF ECHOCARDIOGRAPHY AND ALTERNATE APPROACHES
  Measurement of RV Volumes and Ejection Fraction
  Calculations of Shunt Ratios
  Imaging Cardiac Anatomy
  Intracardiac Hemodynamics

INTEGRATING THE DIAGNOSTIC APPROACH

THE ECHO EXAM

SUGGESTED READING

ongenital heart disease in adults has two basic categories:

- The initial clinical presentation of previously undiagnosed and untreated congenital defects
- Survival into adulthood of patients with known congenital heart disease and previous surgical procedures

In adult patients with no previous diagnosis of heart disease, a congenital defect often is not considered as a potential cause of symptoms, and thus the initial diagnosis may be made at the echocardiographic examination. In these patients, the diagnostic challenge is to recognize and correctly evaluate the congenital abnormality. In contrast, in patients with known congenital disease and previous surgical procedures, the goals are to identify the postoperative anatomy and assess the physiologic consequences of residual defects in each patient. With "corrective" surgery, as with "palliative" procedures, many patients have significant residual or progressive abnormalities.

Both these challenges can be met by a logical and methodical approach to the echocardiographic examination with the application of the basic principles of ultrasound imaging and Doppler data described throughout this text. In addition to careful integration of imaging and Doppler data, evaluation with other imaging modalities, such as cardiac magnetic resonance (CMR) imaging or computed tomography (CT), often is needed for complete assessment of congenital heart disease.

A comprehensive discussion of the echocardiographic findings in adult congenital heart disease is beyond the scope of this text. Instead, an overview of the echocardiographic approach to these patients and examples of the more common abnormalities are presented. The reader is referred to the specialized

473

references listed at the end of the chapter for more detailed information. The goal of this chapter is to allow preliminary diagnosis of congenital heart disease; advanced training is recommended for definitive imaging and diagnosis of congenital heart disease.

BASIC PRINCIPLES

Congenital heart diseases in adults include (Table 17.1):

- Stenotic lesions
- Abnormalities of the aorta and coronary arteries
- Regurgitant lesions
- Intracardiac shunts
- Abnormal connections
- Combinations or complex congenital disease

Stenosis

Congenital stenotic lesions, including obstruction to right ventricular (RV) or left ventricular (LV) outflow (either subvalvular, valvular, or supravalvular), obstruction to LV inflow (congenital mitral stenosis, cor triatriatum), and narrowings in the great vessels (aortic coarctation, branch pulmonary artery [PA] stenosis), are common.

The anatomy of a congenital stenotic lesion differs from that seen in acquired valve disease, but the physiology and fluid dynamics are similar, with normal velocity flow upstream and a flow disturbance downstream from the narrowing. In the narrowed region itself, a high-velocity laminar jet of flow is present, with velocity (V, in m/s) related to the pressure difference (ΔP, in mmHg) across the narrowing, as stated in the simplified Bernoulli equation:

$$\Delta P = 4V^2 \quad \text{(Eq. 17.1)}$$

When a parallel intercept angle is obtained between the jet and the ultrasound beam, quantitative data on stenosis severity and intracardiac hemodynamics are reliable. For example, if the maximum velocity across a subpulmonic membrane is 4.5 m/s, then the maximum RV-to-PA systolic pressure difference is approximately 80 mmHg. Quantitative evaluation of stenosis severity for a congenitally stenotic lesion includes the calculation of maximum and mean pressure gradients as for acquired valve stenosis. Similarly, when possible, valve area calculations are performed using either the continuity equation (aortic valve) or the pressure half-time method (mitral valve).

Several significant differences between congenital and acquired stenosis should be noted. First, congenital stenosis of ventricular outflow, for both the RV and the LV, may involve the subvalvular or the supravalvular region rather than (or in addition to) stenosis of the valve itself (Fig. 17.1). Careful evaluation with conventional pulsed Doppler or color flow imaging to identify the poststenotic flow disturbance is helpful in determining the exact site of obstruction. Second, when serial stenoses are present, quantitation of the contribution of each level of obstruction to the overall degree of stenosis is difficult using Doppler echo methods. Third, the proximal flow pattern in congenital stenosis often is characterized by a greater increase in velocity because of anatomic tapering of the proximal flow region (e.g., in aortic coarctation or with congenital pulmonic stenosis). In these situations, accurate pressure gradient calculations should include the proximal velocity (V_{prox}), as well as the maximum a jet velocity (V_{jet}) in the Bernoulli equation:

$$\Delta P = 4(V^2_{\text{jet}} - V^2_{\text{prox}}) \quad \text{(Eq. 17.2)}$$

Otherwise, the evaluation of congenital stenosis is similar to the evaluation of acquired stenosis in adults, and the methods described in detail in Chapter 11 are applied in this patient group.

Regurgitation

Careful imaging of a congenitally regurgitant valve usually reveals the specific mechanism of regurgitation in that patient. For the atrioventricular valves, particular attention is focused on the number and position of papillary muscles; the chordal attachments (especially aberrant ones); leaflet size, shape, thickness, redundancy, and motion; and annulus size and shape. Malformations include myxomatous changes of the leaflets, abnormal leaflet position (Ebstein anomaly), and abnormal chordal attachments (atrioventricular canal defect) (Fig. 17.2). The semilunar valves may be regurgitant because of great vessel dilation or leaflet fenestration. Three-dimensional (3D) imaging is helpful in the evaluation of leaflet anatomy and the mechanism of regurgitation.

The physiology of congenital regurgitation is no different from that of acquired regurgitation. A flow disturbance occurs in the chamber receiving the regurgitant flow with progressive dilation (and eventual dysfunction) of the volume-overloaded cardiac chambers. The evaluation of congenital regurgitation is similar to the evaluation of acquired regurgitation, as detailed in Chapter 12.

Shunts

An abnormal intracardiac communication is characterized by blood flow across the defect, with the direction, timing, and volume of flow determined by the size of the orifice, the pressure gradient across the defect, and the relative resistance to flow of the vascular beds on each side of the defect. If left-sided heart pressures exceed right-sided pressures (pulmonary vascular resistance is low), left-to-right flow across the defect predominates. In addition, small degrees of

TABLE 17.1 Unoperated Congenital Heart Disease Seen in Adults

Congenital Defect	Anatomic Findings	Doppler Findings
Bicuspid aortic valve	Bicuspid valve identified in systole (raphe seen in diastole)	Mild stenosis and/or regurgitation
Unicuspid aortic valve	Abnormal, deformed aortic valve with systolic doming; the unicuspid orifice is best seen on 3D imaging.	Aortic stenosis (ranging from mild to severe) and/or aortic regurgitation
Subaortic membrane	Membrane from anterior MV leaflet to ventricular septum; TEE often needed for visualization	High-velocity signal just proximal to aortic valve; AR due to valve degeneration from high-velocity jet
Pulmonic stenosis	Subvalvular or valvular pulmonic stenosis. When valvular, the pulmonic valve leaflets are thickened with systolic doming.	Mild pulmonic stenosis (more severe stenosis is recognized and treated in childhood)
Congenital mitral valve disease	Cleft anterior leaflet (often associated with primum ASD), supramitral ring, parachute mitral valve, or double-orifice mitral valve	Regurgitation with anterior leaflet cleft Congenital mitral stenosis
Aortic coarctation	Coarctation is not be easy to visualize because the descending thoracic aorta goes out of the image plane from the SSN; about 50% have an associated bicuspid aortic valve, highly pulsatile ascending aorta, and hypokinetic abdominal aorta.	High-velocity systolic flow in descending thoracic aorta with holodiastolic antegrade flow with severe obstruction; nonparallel intercept angle limits quantitation of severity in unoperated patients
Sinus of Valsalva aneurysm	Dilated, thin sinus with "wind sock" type of projection into adjacent cardiac structures, depending on sinus involved	May have fistula from aorta into RA, LA, RV, or LV, depending on cusp involved
Coronary arteriovenous fistula	Difficult to visualize the fistula, but coronary sinus and proximal coronary artery often dilated	Disturbed flow in coronary sinus or in abnormal epicardial echolucent structures
Coronary anomalies	Coronary artery arising from opposite sinus of Valsalva Anomalous left coronary artery arising from PA (ALCAPA) Anomalous right coronary artery arising from PA (ARCAPA)	When coronary artery arises from PA, flow goes retrograde from the coronary artery into the PA. LV dysfunction due to myocardial ischemia is common.
Ebstein anomaly	Septal tricuspid valve leaflet is adherent to septum, appearing "apically displaced"; apparent RA enlargement (part of anatomic RV is physiologically part of RA).	Tricuspid regurgitation, ASD
Atrial septal defects	RV and RA volume overload with RVE, RAE, and paradoxical ventricular septal motion TEE shows 3D septal anatomy	$Q_p:Q_s$ is calculated from Doppler stroke volume measurements in LVOT (or Ao) versus PA
	Secundum: Absence of IAS in fossa ovalis region best seen on parasternal short-axis views or subcostal 4-chamber view.	Color flow imaging of left-to-right flow across IAS; IV echo contrast shows some right-to-left shunting or "negative contrast" from left-to-right shunt
	Primum: Defect in IAS adjacent to central fibrous body; associated with atrioventricular valve abnormalities (cleft anterior MV leaflet) and inlet VSD. Best seen in 4-chamber view	Color flow imaging of left-to-right flow across IAS; often with associated mitral regurgitation
	Sinus venosus: Defect at vena cava–RA junction (often associated with anomalous PVR) TEE helpful for imaging defect Suspect when $Q_p:Q_s$ is elevated without clear evidence of secundum or primum ASD.	TEE to visualize site of defect and left-to-right flow with color imaging. It may be associated with anomalous pulmonary venous return. CMR imaging often helpful
Partial anomalous pulmonary venous return	RVE, RAE, and paradoxical septal motion reflecting right-sided volume overload (often associated with ASD)	Suspect when $Q_p:Q_s$ >1 with no evidence for flow across IAS.

Continued

TABLE 17.1 Unoperated Congenital Heart Disease Seen in Adults—cont'd

Congenital Defect	Anatomic Findings	Doppler Findings
Ventricular septal defects	*Small VSD*: membranous, muscular, or outlet defects are difficult to image; membranous defects are usually partially or completely closed (ventricular septal aneurysm) by the septal leaflet of the tricuspid valve.	High-velocity jet from left to right in systole with pulsed or CW Doppler; color flow imaging shows flow disturbance on RV side of the defect; normal PA pressures.
	Eisenmenger VSD: Large defect with equal size and wall thickness of LV and RV	Low-velocity bidirectional flow across the ventricular defect; severe pulmonary hypertension
Patent ductus arteriosus	Mild LV and LA enlargement; duct itself rarely visualized in adults	Diastolic flow reversal in the PA (typically along the anterior PA wall); diastolic flow reversal in the descending thoracic aorta
Congenitally corrected transposition of the great arteries (cc-TGA)	Atrioventricular discordance and ventriculoarterial discordance. Because of the double discordance, the blood flow path is physiologically normal: RA to LV to PA; LA to RV to Ao. Associated defects are common, including pulmonic stenosis, VSD, heart block, and Ebstein-type anomaly of the (systemic) tricuspid valve with systemic atrioventricular valve regurgitation.	Normal physiology in absence of associated defects; Doppler findings of pulmonic stenosis, VSD, atrioventricular valve regurgitation when present
Persistent left superior vena cava	Dilated coronary sinus; absence of innominate vein on SSN view	Contrast injection from left arm opacifies coronary sinus first, then the RA
Tetralogy of Fallot	Large, overriding aorta, VSD, subvalvular or valvular pulmonic stenosis	High-velocity flow in RVOT and/or across pulmonic valve; bidirectional flow across VSD

Ao, Aorta; *AR*, aortic regurgitation; *ASD*, atrial septal defect; *CMR*, cardiac magnetic resonance; *IAS*, interatrial septum; *IV*, intravenous; *LVOT*, LV outflow tract; *MV*, mitral valve; *PA*, pulmonary artery; *PVR*, pulmonary venous return; $Q_p:Q_s$, pulmonic-to-systemic shunt ratio; *RAE*, RA enlargement; *RVE*, RV enlargement; *RVOT*, RV outflow tract; *SSN*, suprasternal notch; *VSD*, ventricular septal defect.

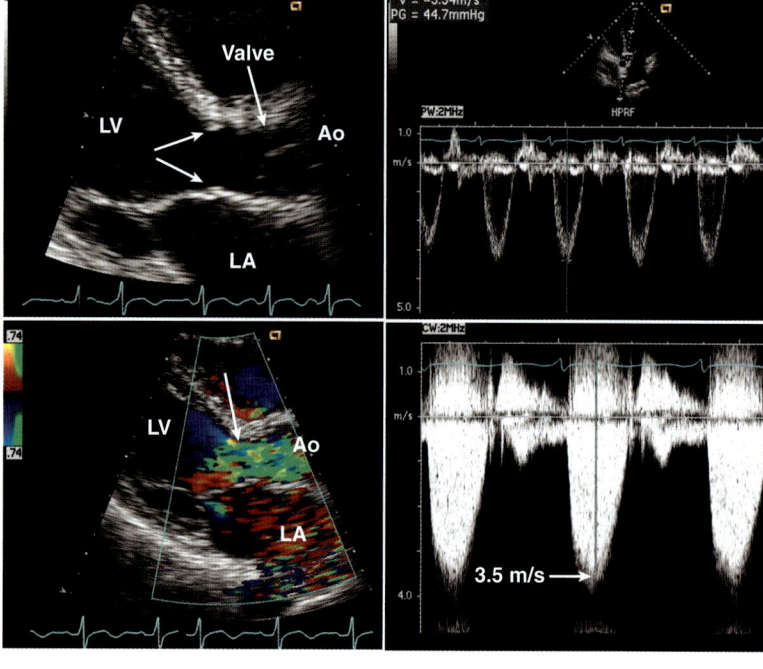

Fig. 17.1 Subaortic stenosis. Parasternal long-axis 2D view *(top left)* in a patient with a systolic murmur showing a subtle ridge *(arrows)* in the LV outflow tract. Color Doppler *(bottom left)* shows an increased flow velocity in this region that suggests the possibility of a subaortic membrane *(arrows)*. High-pulse repetition frequency Doppler *(top right)* shows an increase in velocity to at least 3.3 m/s at this location, and CW Doppler *(bottom right)* shows a maximum outflow velocity of 3.5 m/s. *Ao*, Aorta.

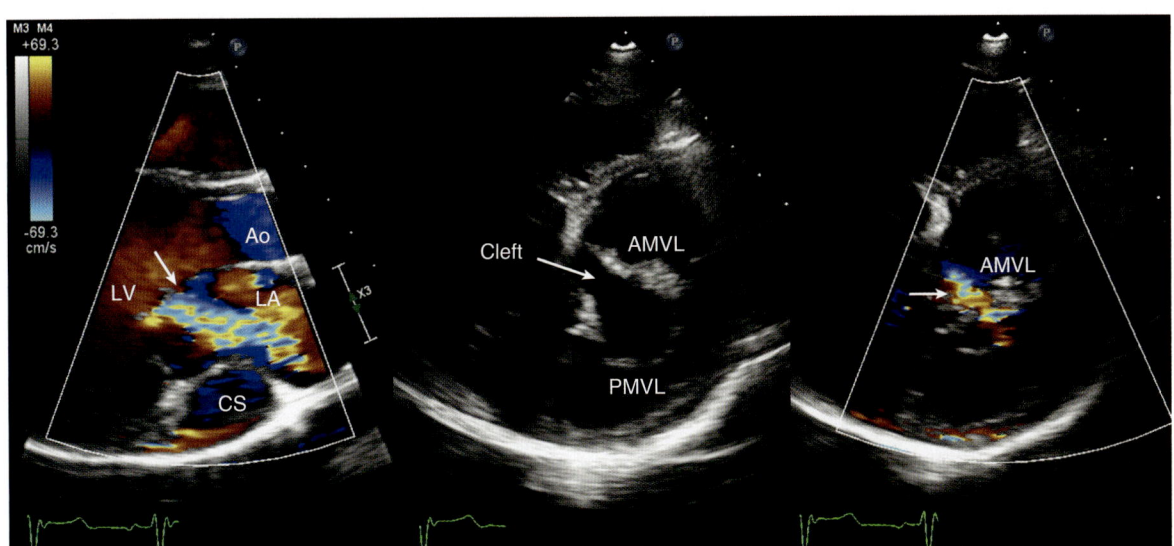

Fig. 17.2 Cleft anterior mitral valve leaflet. The TTE parasternal long-axis view *(left)* shows a jet of mitral regurgitation *(arrow)* that appears to originate in the center of the anterior mitral valve leaflet *(AMVL)*. An incidental finding of a dilated coronary sinus *(CS)* consistent with a persistent left superior vena cava also is seen. The short-axis view at the mitral valve level show the cleft in the anterior leaflet on 2D imaging *(center)* with color Doppler demonstrating that regurgitation originates at the cleft *(right)*. *Ao,* Aorta; *PMVL,* posterior mitral valve leaflet.

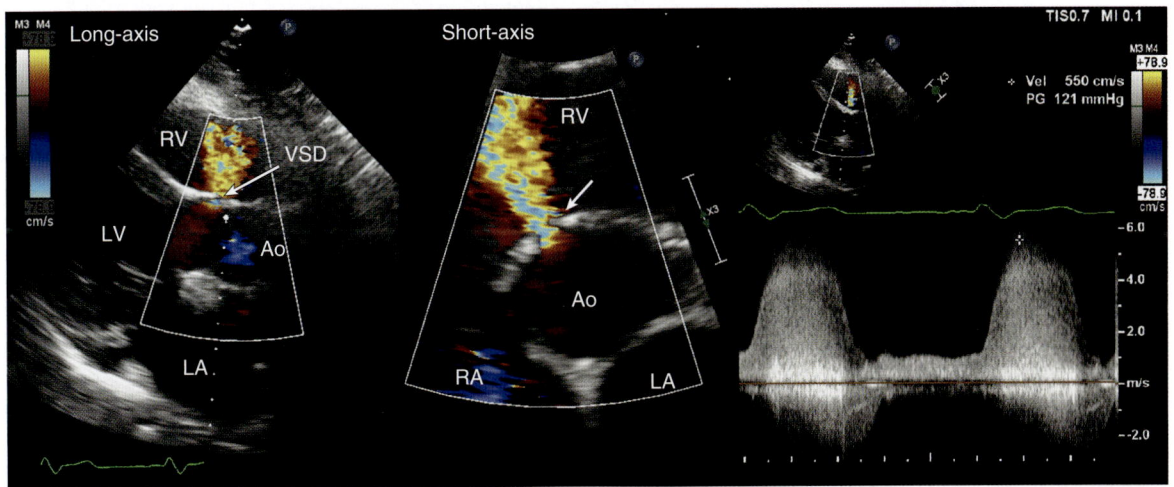

Fig. 17.3 Small, membranous ventricular septal defect. In the parasternal long-axis view *(left)*, color flow Doppler shows a systolic flow disturbance in the RV outflow tract from flow through the small ventricular septal defect *(VSD)*. The short-axis view *(center)* demonstrates the exact site of the defect just on the LV side of the aortic valve in a position typical for a membranous VSD. CW Doppler *(center)* from the parasternal window demonstrates a high-velocity (5.5 m/s) signal toward the transducer (with some channel cross-talk) corresponding to the large difference in pressure between the LV and the RV in systole. Because LV diastolic pressure is slightly higher than RV diastolic pressure, low-velocity flow from left to right also is seen in diastole. *Ao,* Aorta.

right-to-left shunting are present briefly during the cardiac cycle because right-sided pressures transiently exceed left-sided pressures.

With conventional pulsed Doppler ultrasound or with color flow imaging, a flow disturbance is found downstream from the defect: on the right side of the interventricular septum for a ventricular septal defect (VSD), in the right atrium (RA) for an atrial septal defect (ASD), and in the PA for a patent ductus arteriosus.

Analogous to a stenotic or regurgitant orifice, the velocity of blood flow through the shunt orifice is related to the pressure gradient across the defect, as stated in the Bernoulli equation. Thus, a small VSD results in a high-velocity systolic flow signal (approximately 5 m/s) because LV systolic pressure greatly exceeds RV systolic pressure (by approximately 100 mmHg) (Fig. 17.3). Conversely, flow across an ASD typically is low in velocity because only a modest left atrial (LA)–to–RA pressure difference is present.

A left-to-right intracardiac shunt imposes chronic volume overload on the receiving chamber(s) with consequent dilation of the affected chamber(s). With

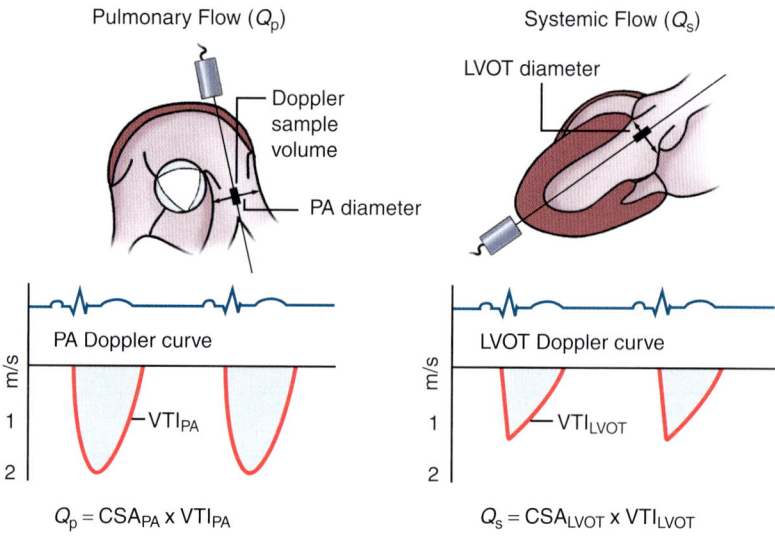

Fig. 17.4 Doppler shunt ratio calculation. Pulmonary flow (Q_p) is calculated from transpulmonic stroke volume calculation using pulmonary artery *(PA)* diameter measured at the site of the Doppler sample position and the velocity-time integral *(VTI)* of PA flow. A circular cross-sectional area *(CSA)* is assumed. Similarly, systemic flow (Q_s) is calculated from LV outflow tract *(LVOT)* diameter and the velocity-time integral of the LV outflow tract.

an ASD, both RA and RV dilation, along with paradoxical septal motion, are seen. With a patent ductus arteriosus, the volume overload is imposed on the LA and LV. Although it could seem that a VSD would cause RV volume overload, in fact, RV size usually is normal because the LV effectively ejects the shunt flow directly into the PA via the septal defect in systole. Instead, LA and LV dilation is seen because these chambers receive the increased pulmonary blood flow as it returns to the left side of the heart via the pulmonary veins.

The volume of blood flow (Q) across an intracardiac shunt—the ratio of pulmonary to systemic blood flow ($Q_p:Q_s$)—is determined by Doppler echo measurements of stroke volume at two intracardiac sites (Fig. 17.4). In the case of an ASD, transpulmonic volume flow (Q_p) is calculated from the PA cross-sectional area (CSA) and velocity-time integral (VTI), whereas systemic volume flow (Q_s) is calculated from measurements of LV outflow tract (LVOT) cross-sectional area and velocity-time integral:

$$Q_p = CSA_{PA} \times VTI_{PA} \quad \text{(Eq. 17.3)}$$

$$Q_s = CSA_{LVOT} \times VTI_{LVOT} \quad \text{(Eq. 17.4)}$$

so that:

$$Q_p:Q_s = \frac{CSA_{PA} \times VTI_{PA}}{CSA_{LVOT} \times VTI_{LVOT}} \quad \text{(Eq. 17.5)}$$

This approach is accurate when two-dimensional (2D) images are of adequate quality for precise diameter measurements (for calculation of a circular cross-sectional area) and when Doppler velocity data are recorded at a parallel intercept angle to flow. Potential errors in estimation of the $Q_p:Q_s$ ratio are the same as for any Doppler echo stroke volume measurement (see Chapter 6).

ECHO MATH: Calculation of Shunt Ratio

Example

A 26-year-old woman undergoes echocardiography for symptoms of decreased exercise tolerance. She is found to have an enlarged RA and RV with paradoxical septal motion and the following Doppler data:

RV outflow velocity	1.8 m/s
Velocity-time integral (VTI_{RVOT})	32 cm
Diameter	2.6 cm
LV outflow velocity	1.1 m/s
Velocity-time integral (VTI_{LVOT})	16 cm
Diameter	2.4 cm

The right heart enlargement suggests that an ASD may be present. The shunt ratio is calculated from the ratio of pulmonary flow (Q_p), measured in the RV outflow tract (RVOT), and systemic flow (Q_s), measured in the LV outflow tract (LVOT). At each site, cross-sectional area (CSA) is calculated as the area of a circle:

$$CSA_{RVOT} = \pi (D/2)^2 = 3.14(2.6/2)^2 = 5.3 \text{ cm}^2$$

$$CSA_{LVOT} = \pi (D/2)^2 = 3.14(2.4/2)^2 = 4.5 \text{ cm}^2$$

Flow (stroke volume) at each site then is calculated:

$$Q_p = CSA_{RVOT} \times VTI_{RVOT} = 5.3 \text{ cm}^2 \times 32 \text{ cm} = 170 \text{ cm}^3$$

$$Q_s = CSA_{LVOT} \times VTI_{LVOT} = 4.5 \text{ cm}^2 \times 16 \text{ cm} = 72 \text{ cm}^3$$

so that

$$Q_p/Q_s = 170/72 = 2.4$$

These calculations are consistent with a significant shunt that is likely to cause progressive right heart dysfunction unless the defect is closed.

With significant left-to-right shunting, pulmonary pressures become elevated, and irreversible pulmonary hypertension develops over time. When pulmonary vascular resistance equals or exceeds systemic vascular resistance, the direction of shunt flow reverses, resulting in decreased systemic oxygen saturation and cyanosis. Irreversible pulmonary hypertension with equalization of pulmonary and systemic pressures due to an intracardiac shunt is known as *Eisenmenger physiology*. This can occur in infancy, particularly with a large VSD, but it also can occur later in life when the pulmonary-to-systemic shunt ratio chronically exceeds about 2:1.

Connections

Echocardiographic diagnosis is more difficult when abnormal connections exist between the atrium and the ventricles, between the ventricles and great vessels, or both. In adults, poor acoustic access further compromises the examination; but with a systematic approach, a correct anatomic evaluation usually is possible.

Because the position of the heart in the chest often is abnormal, the echocardiographer cannot rely on the intrathoracic position of the chambers for correct identification of cardiac anatomy. *Dextroposition* is a rightward shift in the cardiac position with otherwise normal anatomy; for example, due to decreased right lung volume or severe scoliosis. Acoustic windows are shifted rightward, but image planes are similar to normal. With *dextroversion*, the cardiac apex points to the right, but the right and left heart chambers are otherwise normally related. Long-axis views are obtained with the image plane aligned from the left shoulder to the right hip, and the apical window is mid-line or right of the sternum. In contrast, with mirror image *dextrocardia*, cardiac anatomy is a mirror image of normal (the right-sided chambers are left of the left-sided chambers), and the heart is located in the right hemithorax with the apex in the right mid-clavicular line. Thus, acoustic windows are on the right chest with image planes mirror images of normal. The term *situs inversus* refers to right-to-left reversal of thoracic and abdominal viscera.

Atrial situs refers to the position of the RA and LA in the chest. The inferior vena cava nearly always drains into the RA, thereby allowing correct identification of this chamber by imaging the inferior vena cava from a subcostal approach and following it into the RA. Thus, the subcostal window often is a useful starting point for the examination of a patient with complex congenital heart disease. The LA, then, is the "other" atrial chamber because although the pulmonary veins normally drain into the LA, this is not always the case (e.g., partial or total anomalous pulmonary venous return).

The anatomic RV and LV are distinguished from each other by several features (Fig. 17.5). The anatomic RV has:

- Prominent trabeculation
- A moderator band
- An infundibular region
- A more apical atrioventricular annulus than the LV
- A tricuspid valve

Fibrous continuity of the anterior mitral valve leaflet and the aortic valve occurs only with a normally related LV and aortic root. When the anatomic RV connects to the aortic root, a band of myocardium is seen between the base of the atrioventricular valve leaflet and the great vessel. When abnormal connections of the anatomic ventricles are present, the ventricle pumping blood to the pulmonary bed is called the *subpulmonic ventricle* and the ventricle pumping blood into the aorta is called the *systemic ventricle*.

The atrioventricular valves develop with the appropriate anatomic ventricle, so identification of the mitral valve is another feature that differentiates the LV from the RV. Caution is needed if a cleft anterior mitral valve leaflet is present because it may superficially resemble the tricuspid valve. In addition to the number of atrioventricular valve leaflets, the relative positions of the atrioventricular valve annuli are helpful because the tricuspid valve annulus lies slightly closer to the apex than the mitral valve annulus. Note that ventricular size, shape, and/or wall thickness do not distinguish the two ventricles because congenital lesions can result in dilation and hypertrophy of either chamber.

After identifying the atrium and ventricles, attention is directed toward the great vessels. The aortic root is best identified by following the vessel downstream to image the arch and head and neck vessels. Visualization of the origins of the coronary arteries is helpful, but anomalous origin of the coronary arteries from the PA must be considered. The PA is identified by its bifurcation into right and left branches.

The position of the great vessels within the thorax and relative to one another often is altered in congenital disease. Normally, the PA lies anterior and slightly medial to the aortic root at its origin and then courses posteriorly and laterally, with the right PA lying posterior to the ascending aorta. The aortic annulus normally lies posterior to the RV outflow tract, with the aortic root extending medially and anteriorly before turning posterolaterally to form the aortic arch. The normal relationship of the aortic and pulmonic valve planes is approximately perpendicular to each other, with the pulmonary valve slightly more superior within the chest than the aortic valve. With transpositions of the great vessels, these relationships are altered, so the semilunar valves lie in the same tomographic plane, and the aorta and the PA lie parallel to each other instead of in their normal "crisscross" positions. If the aorta is anterior and to the left, *L* (for levo) transposition is present. An anterior and medial (rightward) aorta is termed *D* (for dextro) transposition.

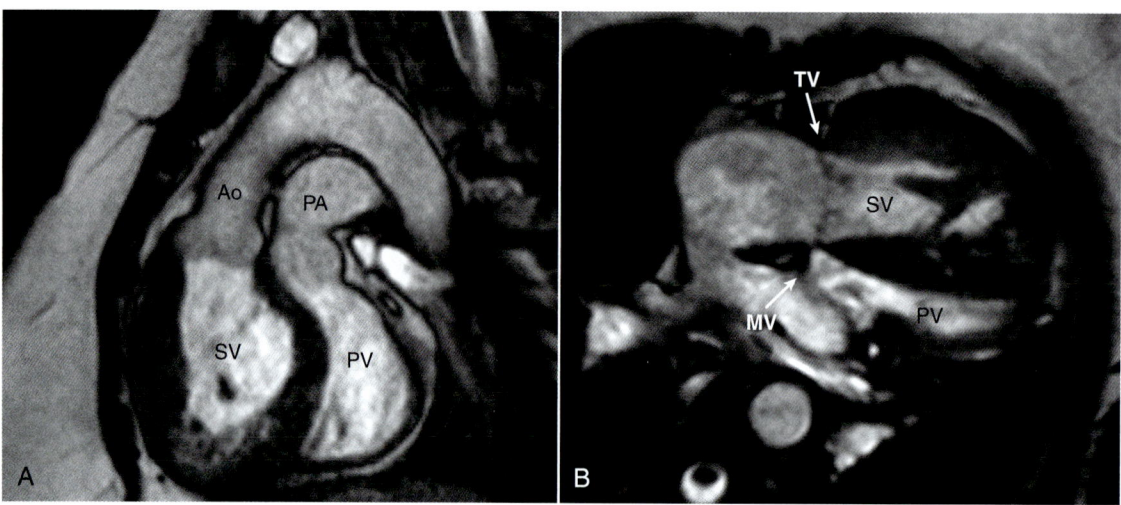

Fig. 17.5 Transposition of the great arteries. CMR images demonstrate the anatomic relationships of the great arteries and ventricles. (A) The longitudinal view shows the side-by-side orientation of the great arteries and the systemic ventricle *(SV)* and pulmonary ventricle *(PV)*. The aorta *(Ao)* is anterior to the pulmonary artery *(PA)*. (B) In a four-chamber view, the systemic ventricle is an anatomic RV, as demonstrated by the presence of a moderator band, prominent trabeculation, and the slightly more apical insertion of the tricuspid valve *(TV)* compared with the mitral valve *(MV)*. The systemic ventricle is appropriately hypertrophied. The pulmonary ventricle is an anatomic LV.

Most patients with abnormal connections between the cardiac chambers and great vessels have associated abnormalities that require echocardiographic evaluation. These include intracardiac shunts, stenotic and regurgitant lesions, pulmonary hypertension, and ventricular dysfunction. The echocardiographic examination in these patients is facilitated by:

- Knowledge of the patient's clinical history, including previous surgical procedures and diagnostic tests
- Formulation of specific clinical questions to be answered by the echocardiographic examination

During the examination, the physician and the sonographer work together to identify:

- Cardiac chambers, great vessels, and their connections
- Associated defects
- Physiologic consequences of each lesion
- Clinical questions that remain unanswered at the end of examination

In addition, the echocardiographer should suggest other appropriate imaging modalities to address any areas of uncertainty.

CONGENITAL STENOTIC LESIONS

Congenital Aortic Valve Stenosis

Although a congenital bicuspid aortic valve is the most common type of congenital heart disease (reported to occur in 1% to 2% of the general population), the bicuspid valve often is functionally normal until about age 50 years or later, when superimposed fibrocalcific changes lead to aortic valve stenosis. Significant regurgitation of a congenital bicuspid valve occurs somewhat less commonly but manifests in young adulthood with a diastolic murmur and symptoms of exercise intolerance.

The presentation of significant LV outflow obstruction in a young adult should prompt consideration of abnormalities other than a bicuspid valve, specifically a unicuspid aortic valve, a subaortic membrane, or hypertrophic cardiomyopathy. A unicuspid aortic valve appears as a thickened, deformed valve with systolic bowing of the valve on ultrasound imaging. A high parasternal short-axis view shows the eccentric unicuspid opening in systole. 3D transthoracic echocardiography (TTE) or transesophageal echocardiography (TEE) further defines valve anatomy. Doppler echocardiography allows measurement of the transvalvular gradient and valve area as for any type of aortic valve stenosis. Restenosis of the aortic valve in patients who previously underwent surgical valvotomy in childhood or adolescence is common. Restenosis occurs in up to 40% of patients a mean of 13 years after open surgical valvotomy.

Subaortic Stenosis

Congenital subaortic obstruction ranges anatomically from a muscular ridge to a thin membrane. Although typically located 1 to 1.5 cm apically from the aortic valve plane, the membrane sometimes is located immediately adjacent to the aortic valve. In either case, a subaortic membrane is difficult to see in adults because of poor acoustic access. The possibility of a subaortic membrane should be considered when high-velocity flow is recorded in the LV outflow tract, but the aortic valve leaflets appear normal. TEE allows direct imaging of the subaortic membrane, especially if multiple image planes or 3D images are used to identify this thin structure. Conventional pulsed Doppler, high-pulse repetition frequency Doppler, and color flow imaging are helpful from either TTE or TEE approaches in demonstrating that, in contrast to valvular aortic stenosis, the increase in antegrade velocity and poststenotic flow disturbance occurs on the LV side of the aortic valve and indicates that subaortic obstruction is present. Coexisting aortic regurgitation occurs because of chronic exposure of the aortic valve leaflets to the high-velocity subaortic flow, resulting in a "jet lesion" on the aortic valve, or (rarely) because of fibrous attachments from the subaortic membrane to the aortic valve leaflets.

Congenital Obstructions to Right Ventricular Outflow

The level of RV outflow obstruction ranges from subvalvular (in the muscular outflow tract), valvular to supravalvular (either in the main PA or its major branches). Pulmonic stenosis sometimes occurs as an isolated anomaly but more often is part of a complex of defects (e.g., tetralogy of Fallot) or is associated with other abnormalities (e.g., corrected transposition). The level of outflow obstruction is determined using pulsed Doppler and color flow to identify the anatomic site at which the flow velocity increases and the poststenotic flow disturbance appears. The obstruction itself is seen on 2D or 3D imaging as a muscular subpulmonic ridge; as deformed, doming pulmonic valve leaflets; or as a narrowing in the PA. If significant obstruction is present, compensatory RV hypertrophy typically is seen.

The degree of obstruction is measured by Doppler ultrasound by using the Bernoulli equation (Fig. 17.6), with the proviso that only an estimate of the total obstruction is possible if serial stenoses are present. Note that in the presence of pulmonic stenosis, the tricuspid regurgitant jet velocity remains an accurate reflection of the RV to RA systolic pressure difference but no longer indicates PA systolic pressure. Instead, PA systolic pressure (PAP) is estimated by calculating the:

(1) RV systolic pressure (RVSP) based on the tricuspid regurgitant jet velocity (V_{TR}) and RA pressure (RAP) estimated from the inferior vena cava size and respiratory variation:

$$RSVP = 4V_{TR}^2 + RAP \quad \text{(Eq. 17.6)}$$

(2) RV-to-PA gradient ($\Delta P_{RV\text{-}PA}$) from the pulmonic stenosis jet velocity (V_{PS}):

$$\Delta P_{RV-PA} = 4V_{PS}^2 \quad \text{(Eq. 17.7)}$$

(3) PA systolic pressure (PAP) by subtracting the transpulmonic gradient from the estimated RV systolic pressure:

$$PAP = (\Delta P_{RV-RA} + P_{RA}) - \Delta P_{RV-PA} \quad \text{(Eq.17.8)}$$

The end-diastolic velocity in the pulmonic regurgitation jet also provides useful data on PA pressures because it reflects the diastolic pressure difference between the PA and the RV (high in patients with pulmonary hypertension, low in patients with pulmonic stenosis, and normal PA diastolic pressures).

ECHO MATH: Calculation of Pulmonary Pressures With Pulmonic Valve Disease

Example
A 24-year-old with a history of a cardiac murmur has an echocardiogram which shows:

RV outflow velocity	1.6 m/s
PA velocity	3.1 m/s
Tricuspid regurgitant jet	3.4 m/s
Estimated RA pressure	5 mmHg (small inferior vena cava with normal respiratory variation)

Because the RV outflow velocity is elevated, the maximum pulmonic valve gradient should be calculated using the proximal velocity (V_{prox}^2) in the Bernoulli equation:

$$\Delta P = 4(V_{jet}^2 - V_{prox}^2)$$

$$\Delta P = 4[(3.1)^2 - (1.6)^2] = 4[9.6 - 2.6] = 28 \text{ mmHg}$$

If the proximal velocity is not included, the gradient would be overestimated at 38 mmHg.

Estimated pulmonary systolic pressure (PAP) is calculated by subtracting the pulmonic valve gradient from the estimated RV pressure because pulmonic stenosis is present:

$$PAP = (\Delta P_{RV-RA} + P_{RA}) - \Delta P_{RV-PA}$$
$$PAP = (4V_{TR}^2 + P_{RA}) - \Delta P_{RV-PA}$$
$$= [4(3.4)^2 + 5] - 28 = 23 \text{ mmHg}$$

Thus, estimated PA systolic pressure is normal even though the tricuspid regurgitant jet indicates an RV systolic pressure of 51 mmHg.

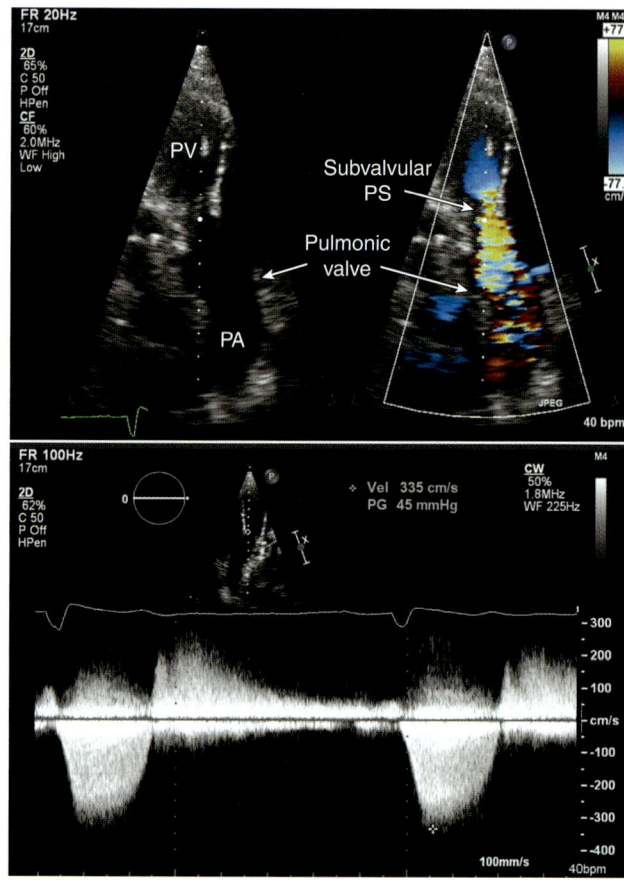

Fig. 17.6 Subpulmonic stenosis. ▶ In an anteriorly angulated four-chamber view *(top)*, color Doppler shows an increase in velocity proximal to the pulmonic valve in this patient with complete transposition. CW Doppler *(bottom)* demonstrates a velocity of 3.4 m/s and a diastolic signal consistent with moderate to severe pulmonic regurgitation. *PA,* Pulmonary artery; *PS,* pulmonic stenosis; *PV,* pulmonary ventricle.

CONGENITAL ABNORMALITIES OF THE AORTA AND CORONARY ARTERIES

Aortic Coarctation

A congenital narrowing in the proximal descending thoracic aorta most often is located just upstream from the entry site of the ductus arteriosus. Less often, postductal coarctation is seen. The coarctation usually is relatively discreet, with involvement of only a short segment of the aorta, but sometimes is a long, tubular narrowing. Imaging the coarctation site is difficult from a TTE suprasternal notch window in adults. Even in normal individuals, the descending thoracic aorta appears to taper because the tomographic view cuts the aorta obliquely as it leaves the image plane. Restenosis manifests at variable ages in adults with previous surgical coarctation repair, depending on the specific surgical procedure and the patient's age at the time of repair. For both operated and unoperated coarctations, TEE imaging with a long-axis view of the descending aorta can be helpful, although CT and CMR imaging now are the standard clinical approaches.

Doppler examination shows an increased velocity across the coarctation and, if the obstruction is severe, persistent antegrade flow into diastole (Fig. 17.7) sometimes called *diastolic run-off*. If the velocity proximal to the coarctation is elevated, the proximal velocity should be included in the Bernoulli equation for pressure gradient estimation. The jet direction in an unoperated coarctation is very eccentric, so it rarely is possible to achieve a parallel alignment between the ultrasound beam and the jet direction, a situation that leads to underestimation of the severity of the obstruction. In restenosis of a previously operated coarctation, the jet orientation tends to be more symmetric, and a parallel intercept angle with correct estimation of the pressure gradient is more likely. In either case, other clinical methods for assessing the severity of the coarctation are available (e.g., upper versus lower extremity blood pressure).

Sinus of Valsalva Aneurysm

A congenital aneurysm of the aortic sinuses of Valsalva appears as a thin, dilated area that projects into adjacent cardiac structures, often with a fistulous communication, depending on which sinus is involved. On echocardiographic imaging, a congenital aneurysm often has a "wind sock" appearance with a long, convoluted, mobile sac of tissue extending from the

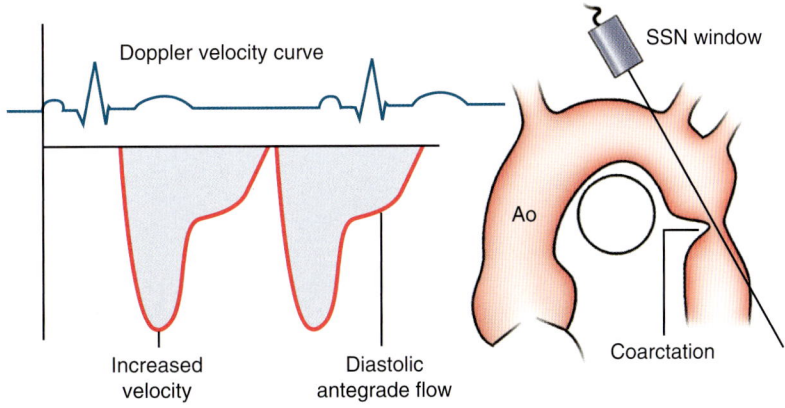

Fig. 17.7 Aortic coarctation. From a suprasternal notch *(SSN)* window, CW Doppler of the coarctation shows an increased velocity in systole, with persistent antegrade flow into diastole. Imaging of the coarctation often is suboptimal in adults. *Ao,* Aorta.

aortic sinus into adjacent cardiac structures (see Fig. 16.3). This appearance contrasts with the more symmetric dilation seen in aneurysms due to endocarditis. An aneurysm of the noncoronary sinus projects into the RA, the left coronary cusp into the LA, and the right coronary cusp into the RV outflow tract. If a fistula is present, pulsed and color Doppler flow images demonstrate a left-to-right shunt with a flow disturbance in the receiving chamber. Continuous-wave (CW) Doppler shows a high-velocity systolic and diastolic flow signal.

Coronary Arteriovenous Fistula

A coronary arteriovenous fistula is a rare congenital anomaly that manifests in young adults as a continuous murmur. The abnormal communication typically arises from a coronary artery and empties into the coronary sinus or RA. A coronary arteriovenous fistula is recognized echocardiographically as an abnormal area of dilation with diastolic or continuous flow in addition to a flow disturbance at the site of entry into the cardiac chamber (Fig. 17.8).

Anomalous Origins of the Coronary Arteries

Other coronary artery abnormalities diagnosed on echocardiography, particularly when TTE or TEE images are of high quality, include an anomalous circumflex coronary artery arising from the right sinus of Valsalva, an anomalous right coronary artery arising from the left sinus of Valsalva, or the left main coronary arising from the right sinus of Valsalva.

An anomalous coronary artery arising from the PA only occasionally is diagnosed initially in adulthood because the resulting myocardial ischemia usually leads to significant clinical manifestations at a younger age. With an anomalous left coronary (ALCAPA) or right coronary artery arising from the pulmonary artery (ARCAPA), the flow direction from the aorta is antegrade in the coronary artery that comes off the aorta and then retrograde in the anomalous coronary artery, which then drains into the pulmonary artery. Thus, these rare lesions are diagnosed on echocardiography based on a diastolic flow disturbance in the main pulmonary artery.

CONGENITAL REGURGITANT LESIONS

Ebstein Anomaly of the Tricuspid Valve

Ebstein anomaly is characterized by adherence of the basal segments of one (most often the septal) or more of the leaflets of the tricuspid valve to the RV endocardium that results in the appearance of apical displacement of the tricuspid valve attachment (Fig. 17.9). In Ebstein anomaly, the distance between the tricuspid and mitral annulus exceeds the normal 10-mm difference. In severe cases, the tricuspid valve is displaced nearly to the RV apex. In addition, the tricuspid valve leaflets are thickened and malformed. Functionally, tricuspid regurgitation nearly always is present, ranging from mild to severe. Typically, no antegrade obstruction to RV diastolic filling is present (Fig. 17.10).

Owing to the apical displacement of the tricuspid leaflet insertion, a portion of the anatomic RV physiologically serves as part of the RA. This "atrialized" ventricle adds to the appearance of RA enlargement, which is augmented by chronic atrial volume overload from tricuspid regurgitation. Ebstein anomaly occurs as an isolated anatomic defect or in association with an aberrant atrioventricular conduction bypass tract (Wolff-Parkinson-White syndrome), an ASD, or other congenital anomalies (e.g., ventricular inversion). Ebstein anomaly of the anatomic tricuspid valve in a patient with corrected transposition results in systemic atrioventricular valve regurgitation and chronic volume overload of the systemic ventricle.

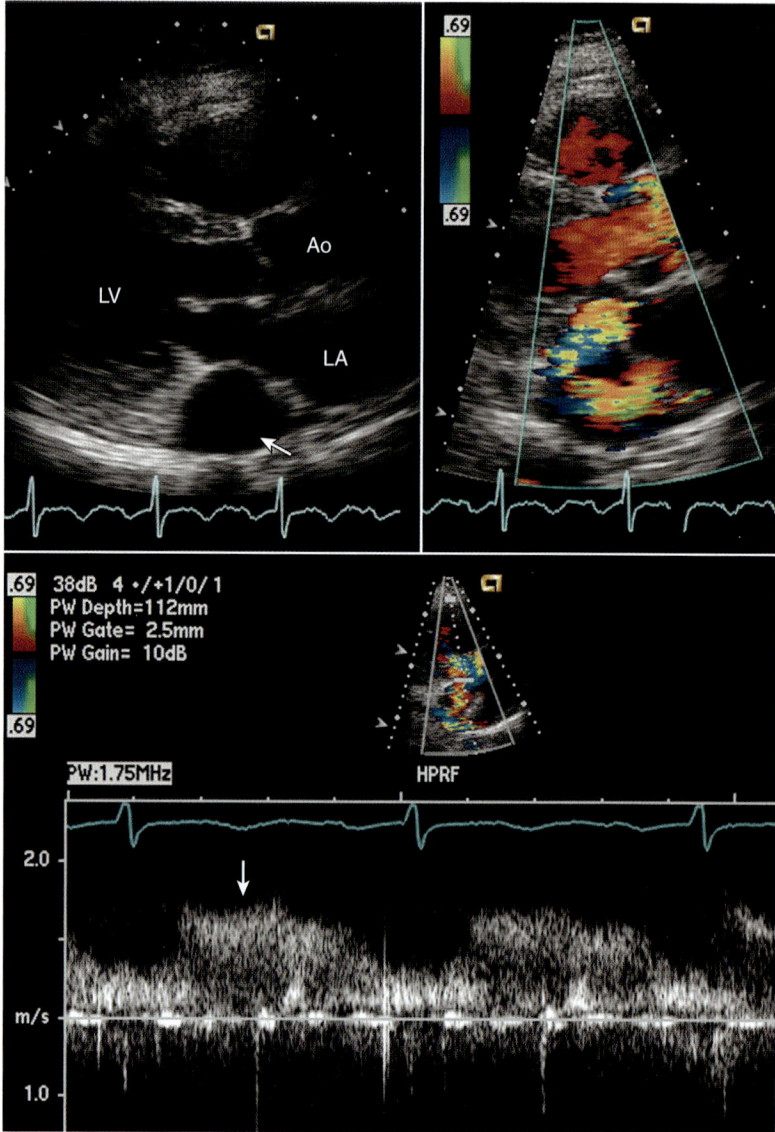

Fig. 17.8 **Coronary arteriovenous fistula.** In this 24-year-old woman with a continuous murmur, the 2D long-axis view (upper left) ▶ shows a large, echo-free space in the region of the coronary sinus (arrow). Color Doppler (upper right) ▶ shows a swirling flow pattern from the aorta into this space. In combination with other image planes, this finding was consistent with a right coronary–to–coronary sinus atrioventricular fistula. Pulsed Doppler recordings (bottom) confirmed low-velocity flow, predominantly in diastole (arrow) but extending into systole, consistent with a coronary fistula. Ao, Aorta.

Cleft Mitral Valve

Congenital abnormalities of the mitral valve include congenital mitral stenosis due to a parachute mitral valve (one papillary muscle), a double orifice mitral valve, a supramitral ring, or other abnormalities of the leaflets or papillary muscles. The lesion most often diagnosed in adults is a cleft anterior mitral valve leaflet, frequently in association with an atrioventricular canal defect or primum ASD but sometimes as an isolated finding resulting in mitral regurgitation. The cleft in the anterior leaflet is seen best in the parasternal short-axis view, whereas lateral-to-medial angulation in the long-axis image plane shows the differing patterns of motion of the medial and lateral leaflet segments (see Fig. 17.2). A cleft mitral valve with adequate systolic apposition of leaflet segments is functionally normal but more often results in significant mitral regurgitation due to inadequate leaflet closure. In adults with myxomatous mitral valve disease, 3D imaging often demonstrates deep clefts in either the anterior or posterior mitral leaflet, but this phenotype is distinct from a congenital cleft anterior mitral valve leaflet.

INTRACARDIAC SHUNTS

Atrial Septal Defects

Anatomy

Three basic anatomic types of ASDs are recognized (Fig. 17.11). The most common is a secundum defect, in which the central section of the atrial septum (the fossa ovalis) is absent because of failure of the secundum atrial septum to cover the foramen secundum during development. A secundum ASD typically is an ovale defect in the center of the septum with a diameter of 1 to 2 cm.

A primum ASD is the absence of the section of the interatrial septum adjacent to the central fibrous body. Developmentally, abnormal formation of the septum primum occurs with failure of closure of the foramen primum, which often is associated with abnormalities of the atrioventricular valves, especially a cleft anterior mitral leaflet. In a more severe developmental abnormality—called an *atrioventricular canal* or *endocardial cushion defect*—the entire central fibrous body is absent, resulting in a primum ASD, a VSD, and abnormalities of the atrioventricular valves (Figs. 17.12 and 17.13).

The third type of ASD is the sinus venosus defect. This abnormal communication between the RA and the LA is developmentally related to abnormal fusion between the embryologic sinus venosus and the atrium and thus is located near the junction of the atrium with either the superior or inferior vena cava. Partial

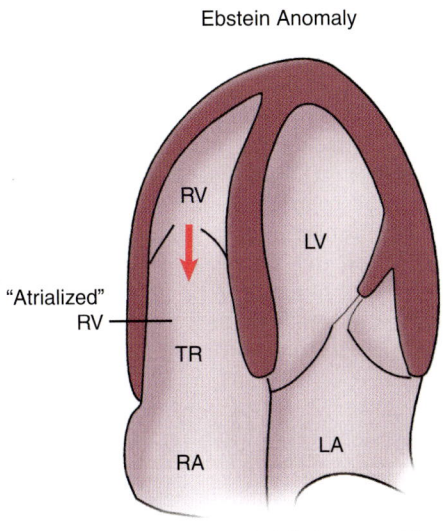

Fig. 17.9 Ebstein anomaly. Noted are apical displacement of the tricuspid valve and "atrialization" of the base of the RV. Tricuspid regurgitation *(TR)* with RV and RA enlargement typically is present.

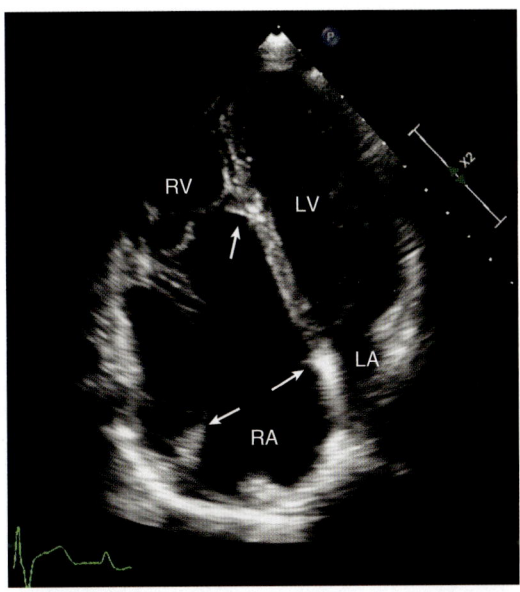

Fig. 17.10 Imaging in patient with Ebstein anomaly. In this apical four-chamber view, the tricuspid valve insertion is apically displaced *(upper arrow)*, compared with the tricuspid annulus *(lower arrows)*, with RV and RA enlargement. The portion of the RV between the leaflet insertion and annulus often is termed the "atrialized" RV.

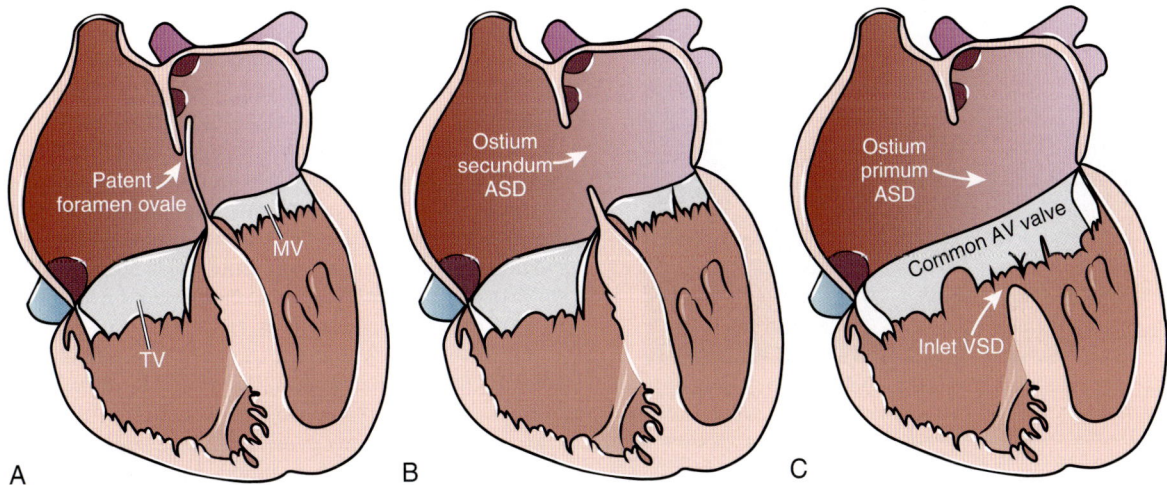

Fig. 17.11 Schematic of atrial level shunts. (A) Patent foramen ovale. (B) Ostium secundum atrial septal defect *(ASD)*. (C) Ostium primum ASD with a common atrioventricular *(AV)* valve and associated inlet ventricular septal defect *(VSD)*. *MV,* Mitral valve; *TV,* tricuspid valve. (From Lin J, Aboulhosn JA: Contgenital shunts. In Otto CM, editor: The Practice of Clinical Echocardiography, ed 5, Philadelphia, 2017, Elsevier, p 881, Fig. 44.2.)

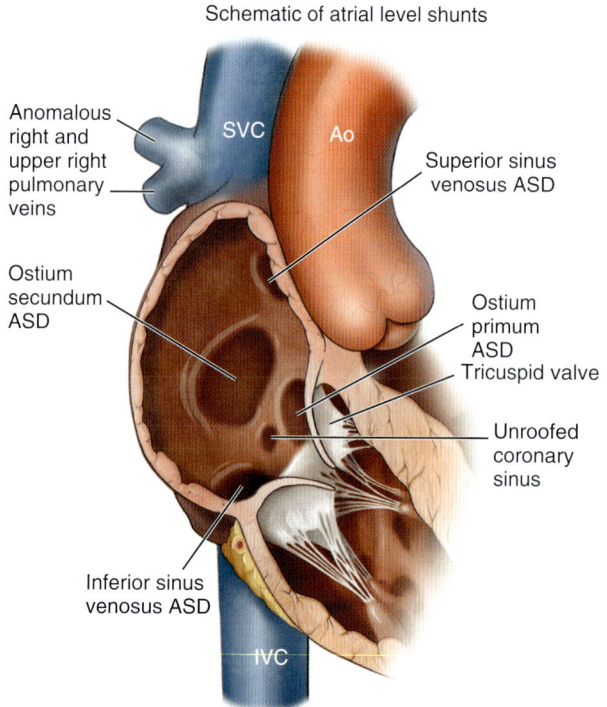

Fig. 17.12 Anatomy of atrial septal defects. Right atrial view of the interatrial septum demonstrating the location of different types of atrial septal defect (ASD). *Ao,* Aorta; *IVC,* inferior vena cava; *SVC,* superior vena cava. (From Lin J, Aboulhosn JA: Contgenital shunts. In Otto CM, editor: The Practice of Clinical Echocardiography, ed 5, Philadelphia, 2017, Elsevier, p 883, Fig. 44.3.)

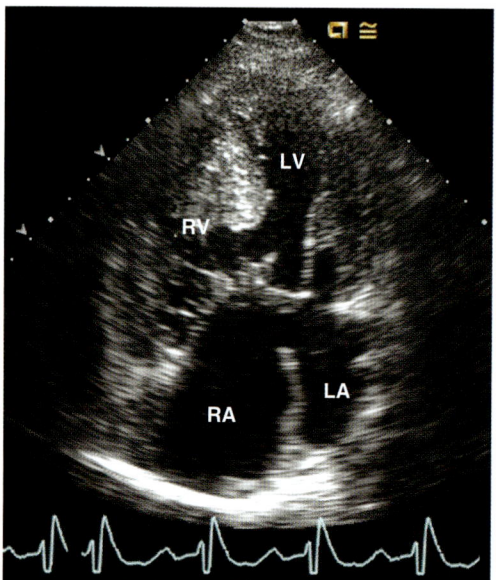

Fig. 17.13 Example of atrioventricular canal defect. Ostium primum atrial septal defect (ASD) with an accompanying ventricular septal defect (VSD)—also called an atrioventricular canal—in a young woman with Down syndrome. This apical four-chamber view in systole shows the ASD, VSD, and common atrioventricular valve. RV and LV pressures are equal in systole, and pressure in all four chambers is equal in diastole. These findings are consistent with Eisenmenger physiology unless severe pulmonic stenosis is present.

anomalous pulmonary venous return often is associated with a sinus venosus defect but also occurs as an isolated defect, which often is not diagnosed until adulthood. Anomalous pulmonary veins drain directly into the RA or into the superior or inferior vena cava.

Transthoracic Imaging

TTE has a sensitivity of 89% for the detection of a secundum ASD and 100% for a primum defect, but only 44% for a sinus venosus defect. TTE imaging of an ASD is most reliable from a subcostal approach so that the ultrasound beam is perpendicular to the plane of the interatrial septum. From apical or parasternal windows, apparent loss of signal from the atrial septum is due to a parallel alignment between the ultrasound beam and the structures of interest (i.e., no ultrasound is reflected back to the transducer). Secundum ASDs are seen in the central portion of the atrial septum (Fig. 17.14), and primum defects are seen adjacent to the annuli of the atrioventricular valves. TTE imaging of a sinus venosus defect is challenging, so this diagnosis should be considered in patients with unexplained right heart enlargement or paradoxical septal motion.

If an ASD is associated with a significant left-to-right shunt, RA enlargement, RV enlargement, and paradoxical septal motion consistent with right-sided volume overload (Fig. 17.15) are uniformly present. In fact, evidence for right-sided heart volume overload often is the first abnormality noted during the echocardiographic examination. Shunt flow is quantitated by measuring stroke volume in the PA (pulmonary blood flow) and in the LV outflow tract (systemic blood flow) (Fig. 17.16).

The subcostal window is optimal for color imaging of flow across the ASD, because the direction of flow is parallel to the ultrasound beam. Color flow imaging from other windows (including parasternal and apical) also is helpful because it is the location and timing of the flow disturbance—rather than the absolute velocity of flow—that are diagnostic of the defect in the atrial septum. Color flow imaging shows a broad flowstream from LA to RA in both diastole and systole, with a more prominent diastolic component. With large shunts, the flow across the atrial septum extends across the open tricuspid valve into the RV in diastole. Proximal flow acceleration on the LA side of the septum usually is evident.

However, in some cases, the diastolic-systolic low-velocity flow signal across the ASD is difficult to distinguish from other venous flow signals in the RA. Care must be taken to avoid mistaking superior vena cava flow into the RA, which often streams along the interatrial septum, for ASD flow. This appearance can be particularly misleading in high-volume flow states, such as pregnancy. Occasionally, a tricuspid

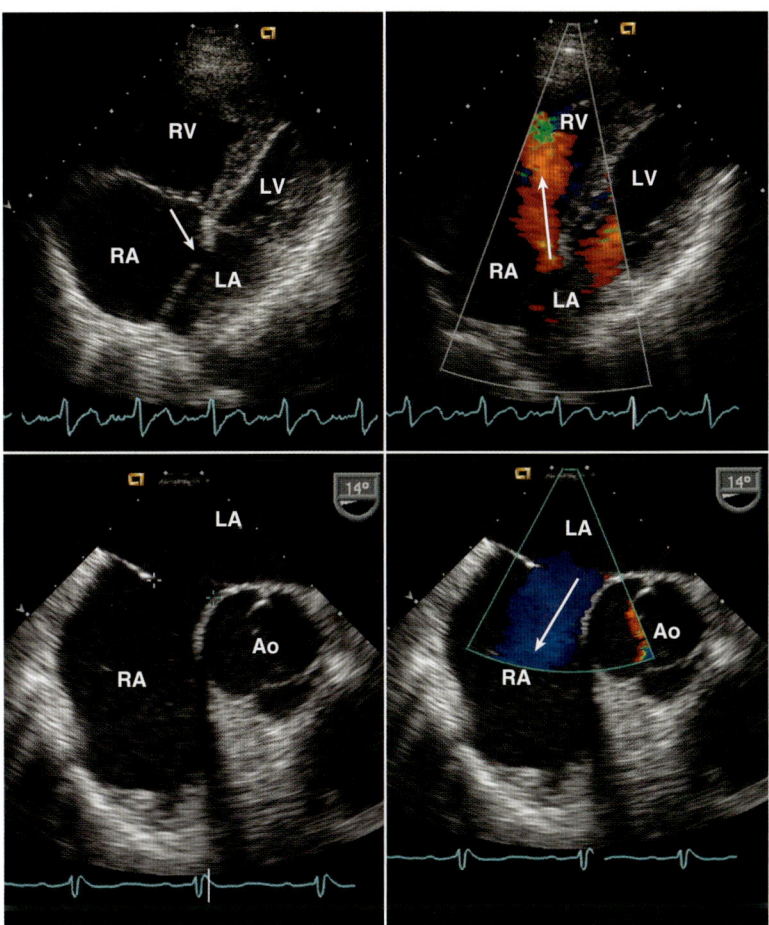

Fig. 17.14 **Secundum atrial septal defect.** A foreshortened TTE apical four-chamber view *(top left)* shows the atrial defect *(arrow)* in association with marked RA and RV enlargement due to the left-to-right shunt seen on color flow imaging *(top right)*. TEE imaging allows more precise localization and measurement of the septal defect *(bottom left)*. Left-to-right flow across the defect is low in velocity, because the pressure difference is small, so a uniform color signal is seen *(bottom right)*. *Ao,* Aorta.

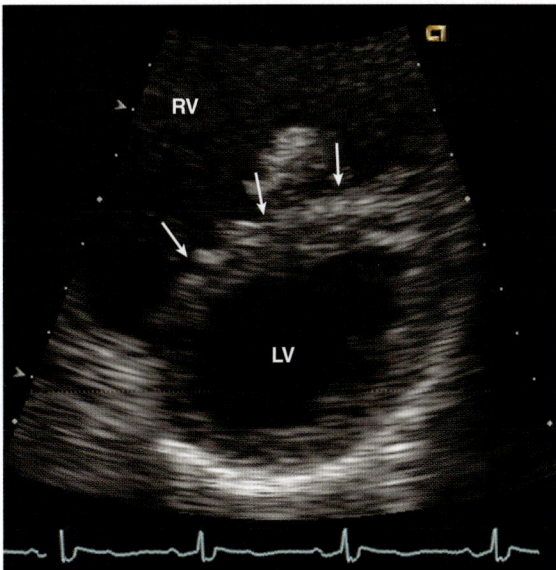

Fig. 17.15 **RV enlargement due to a secundum atrial septal defect.** This parasternal short-axis view in diastole shows the flattened septal curvature *(arrows),* consistent with RV volume overload.

regurgitant jet directed along the interatrial septum also results in a confusing flow pattern.

Contrast Echocardiography

In a patient with a primum or secundum ASD, peripheral venous injection of agitated saline shows passage of microbubbles across the interatrial septum, even when the shunt is predominantly left to right in direction. The explanation for this observation is that RA pressure transiently and briefly exceeds LA pressure, thus allowing passage of a small volume of blood (and microbubbles) from right to left across the atrial septum. Dense contrast in the RA also allows demonstration of a "negative" contrast jet across the ASD; that is, the blood flow from the LA into the RA appears as an area with no echo contrast.

Contrast echo studies are rarely needed for the diagnosis of an ASD when typical imaging, Doppler, and color flow imaging findings are present. The principle of using echo contrast to identify very small degrees of right-to-left shunting also is used to detect a patent foramen ovale as a potential source of a systemic embolic event (see Chapter 15).

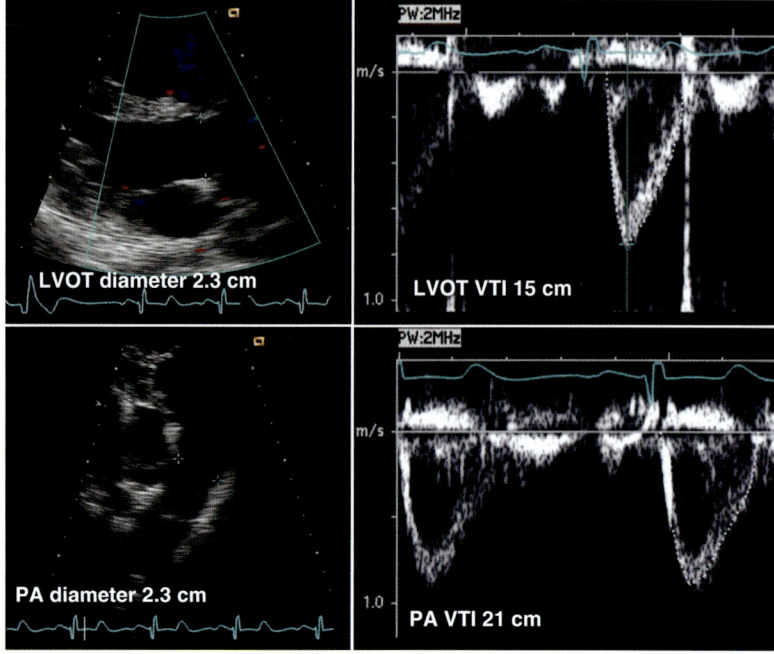

Fig. 17.16 Calculation of the shunt ratio in a patient with an atrial septal defect. Systemic flow (Q_s) is calculated from the LV outflow tract (LVOT) diameter (2.2 cm) and Doppler velocity-time integral (VTI; 15 cm) (top), whereas pulmonary blood flow is calculated from the pulmonary artery (PA) diameter (2.3 cm) and Doppler velocity-time integral (21 cm) (bottom). In this example, Q_p is 87, and Q_s is 57 mL, so Q_p:Q_s is only 1.5, a value of borderline significance.

Transesophageal Imaging

TEE is recommended for preprocedural evaluation of adults with an ASD, guidance of transcatheter closure of the defect, and intraoperative assessment in patients undergoing surgical repair. In addition, when evidence for right-sided volume overload is present in the absence of a visualized ASD or other definable cause for volume overload (e.g., tricuspid regurgitation), TEE imaging should be performed to evaluate for the possibility of a sinus venosus defect or partial anomalous pulmonary venous return (Fig. 17.17).

The TEE approach (Fig. 17.18) to the evaluation of an ASD is:

- Center the atrial septum in a four-chamber view to show the fossa ovalis region.
- Rotate the TEE image plane in 20° to 30° increments from 0° to 90° to examine the entire surface of the atrial septum and the size of the rim available for anchoring a transcatheter closure device.
- Be sure to include the entry of the superior and inferior vena cavae into the RA in the views of the atrial septum to avoid missing a sinus venosus defect.
- Acquire real-time and full-volume 3D images of the atrial septum to provide better assessment of the size and shape of the defect (Fig. 17.19).
- Use color Doppler to visualize flow across the defect, either simultaneously with or subsequent to imaging.
- Identify the entry of all four pulmonary veins into the atrium and document expected flow patterns in each vein with color and pulsed Doppler modalities.

TEE imaging also is useful for the guidance of transcatheter closure of the ASD (Fig. 17.20).

Ventricular Septal Defects

Anatomy

Four anatomically different types of VSDs are recognized (Fig. 17.21). The most common type is a *perimembranous VSD* located in the region of the membranous septum immediately inferomedial to the aortic valve and lateral to the septal leaflet of the tricuspid valve. Small membranous VSDs often close spontaneously during childhood by approximation of the tricuspid valve septal leaflet across the defect. A completely closed defect usually is undetectable in adulthood, but a residual anatomic abnormality—a ventricular septal aneurysm—sometimes is visualized at the closure site without evidence of blood flow from the LV to the RV. Incomplete closure leads to a persistent, albeit smaller, VSD, which is difficult to distinguish from a septal aneurysm on 2D imaging. However, color flow and CW Doppler images show typical evidence for an abnormal flow communication between the LV and the RV, even when the defect is small.

Muscular VSDs occur at any location in the muscular portion of the septum and often are multiple. When they are small, imaging the defect is not possible with a tomographic imaging technique (e.g.,

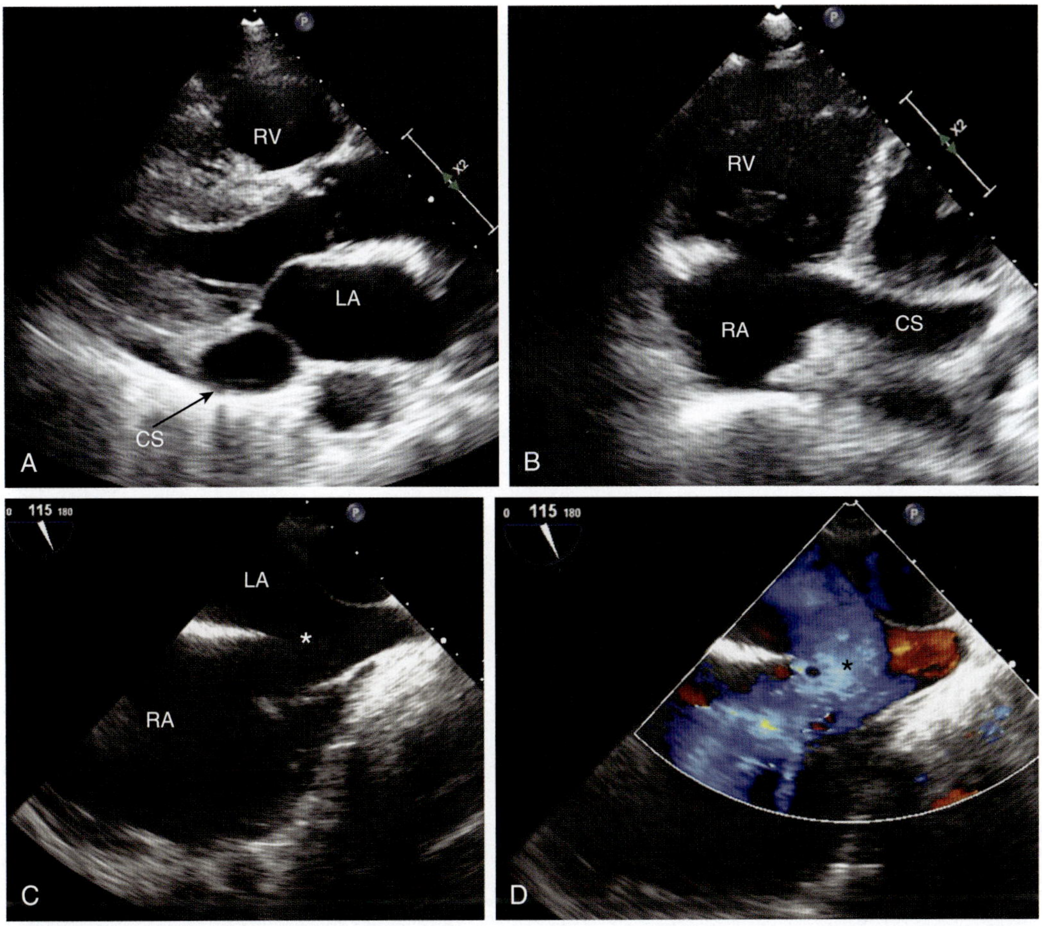

The Adult With Congenital Heart Disease | Chapter 17 | 489

Fig. 17.17 Sinus venosus atrial septal defect. Patient with a superior sinus venosus atrial septal defect, persistent left superior vena cava (SVC) to the coronary sinus *(CS)*, and partial anomalous pulmonary venous return of the right upper pulmonary vein. (A) Parasternal long-axis view, with a severely dilated coronary sinus. (B) Apical four-chamber view. The RA and RV are severely dilated, and the dilated coronary sinus is visualized draining into the RA. (C) TEE mid-esophageal bicaval view. The SVC overrides the interatrial septum, and the sinus venosus defect is apparent *(asterisk)*. The dilated right pulmonary artery is visualized posteriorly. (D) TEE mid-esophageal bicaval view with color Doppler demonstrating left-to-right shunting across the sinus venosus defect *(asterisk)*. *(From Lin J, Aboulhosn JA: Contgenital shunts. In Otto CM, editor: The Practice of Clinical Echocardiography, ed 5, Philadelphia, 2017, Elsevier, p 889, Fig. 44.9.)*

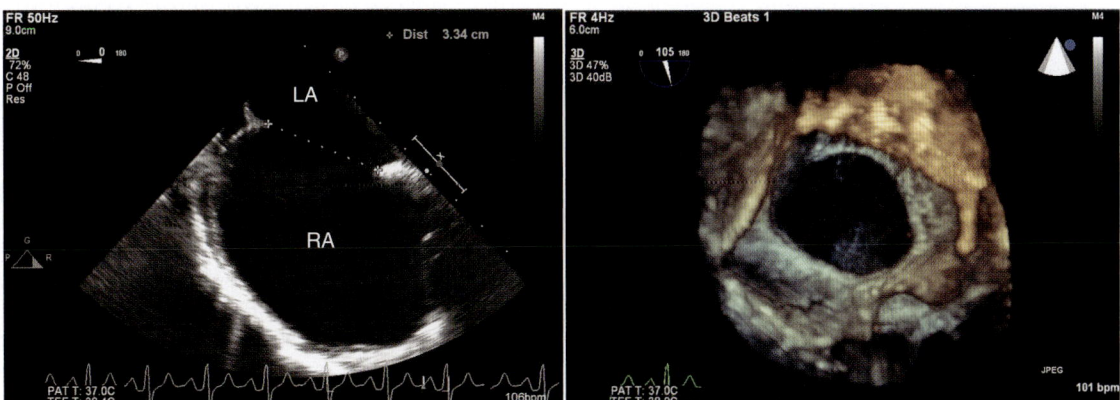

Fig. 17.18 TEE 3D imaging of a secundum atrial septal defect. TEE imaging demonstrates a large secundum atrial septal defect on 2D imaging in a standard view at 0° rotation *(left)*. With a full-volume 3D image looking from the LA side of the septum, the shape and size of the defect are better seen *(right)*.

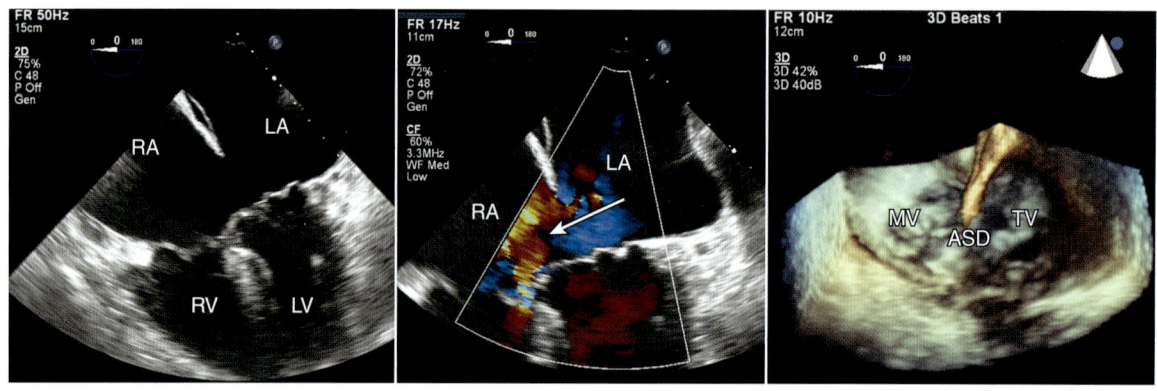

Fig. 17.19 Ostium primum atrial septal defect. In this 64-year-old man, the TEE four-chamber view *(left)* ▶ shows an ostium primum atrial septal defect *(ASD)*, with color Doppler *(center)* ▶ showing left-to-right flow across the large defect *(arrow)*. 3D imaging *(right)* ▶ shows the relationship between the ASD and the mitral valve *(MV)* and tricuspid *(TV)* valve.

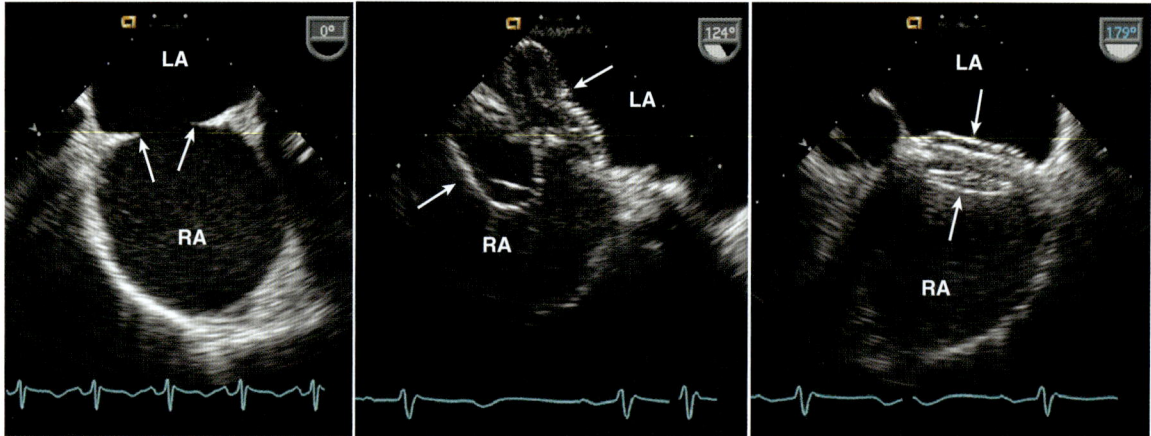

Fig. 17.20 Transcatheter secundum atrial septal defect closure. TEE echocardiography during placement of a percutaneous atrial septal device (ASD) closure device shows: (1) the secundum ASD *(left)*, ▶ (2) the device across the defect with the LA side being pulled into position *(arrow)* and the RA side being deployed *(center)*, ▶ and (3) closure of the defect with full deployment of both the LA and RA sides of the device *(right)*. ▶

echocardiography), even when multiple image planes are examined. Again, Doppler data are diagnostic in this situation.

Inlet VSDs are the result of failure of complete formation of the central fibrous body. This defect is located inferior to the aortic valve plane, adjacent to the mitral and tricuspid valve annuli. Inlet defects often are associated with other anomalies of the central fibrous body such as a primum ASD, atrioventricular valve abnormalities, or a complete atrioventricular canal defect.

Supracristal VSDs are located in the RV outflow portion of the septum (above the crista ventricularis), lateral and just inferior to the aortic valve. These defects are rarely initially diagnosed in adulthood.

Imaging

Large defects are visualized easily with 2D echocardiography, but small defects are difficult to demonstrate.

Perimembranous VSDs are imaged best in a parasternal long-axis view angulated slightly medially (see Fig. 17.3). In the short-axis view just below the aortic valve level, the VSD is seen in a 10 o'clock position inferior to the right coronary cusp of the aortic valve and adjacent to the septal leaflet of the tricuspid valve. In this view, a supracristal VSD is located at the 2 o'clock position, inferior to the left coronary leaflet of the aortic valve and adjacent to the pulmonic valve. A supracristal VSD is imaged in the long-axis plane by lateral angulation of the transducer from the standard long-axis view. Muscular VSDs are best seen in sequential basal-to-apical short-axis views of the LV, in the apical four-chamber view, or using 3D imaging with a view of the entire septal surface. Inlet VSDs are best imaged in the apical four-chamber view or from the parasternal window in a short-axis view at the mitral valve level.

Most VSDs seen in adults are associated with a very small flow volume, so chamber sizes and

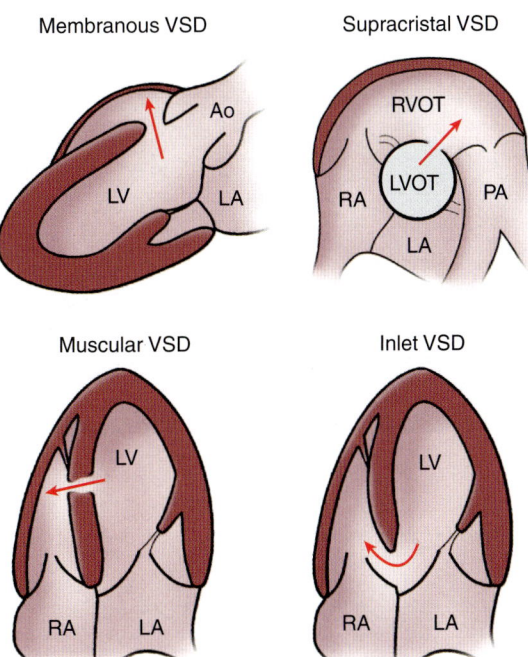

Fig. 17.21 Ventricular septal defect anatomy. A membranous ventricular septal defect *(VSD)* is seen in a medially angulated parasternal long-axis view, immediately adjacent to the aortic valve. A supracristal VSD is seen well in a short-axis view just below the aortic valve with flow from the LV outflow tract *(LVOT)* into the outflow region of the RV. A muscular VSD can be located anywhere in the muscular portion of the ventricular septum and may be multiple. An inlet VSD is seen in the apical four-chamber view, often associated with an atrioventricular canal defect. *Ao,* Aorta; *RVOT,* RV outflow tract.

ventricular function are normal. When a significant volume of left-to-right flow is present across a VSD, dilation of the LV and LA occurs because of volume overload of these chambers. RV size usually is normal because the systolic flow across the defect is ejected directly into the PA, and LV systolic function typically is preserved because the shunt flow is ejected into the low-impedance pulmonary vascular bed. With large shunts, pulmonary vascular hypertension supervenes, resulting in Eisenmenger physiology with RV hypertrophy and dilation (Fig. 17.22).

Doppler Findings

Color Doppler flow imaging shows a flow disturbance on the right side of the ventricular septum (with a left-to-right shunt). The presence and location of this flow disturbance are diagnostic for a VSD, even in the absence of a demonstrable defect on imaging. The flow disturbance is detectable in the defect itself, with proximal acceleration on the left side of the septum, immediately adjacent to the defect. Doppler ultrasound has a sensitivity of 90% and a specificity of 98% for the detection of a VSD.

CW Doppler ultrasound shows a high-velocity left-to-right signal, with the shape of the velocity curve similar to that of mitral regurgitation, as determined by the instantaneous LV-to-RV pressure differences (see Fig. 14.16). In diastole, left-to-right shunting persists at a lower velocity (proportional to the diastolic LV-to-RV pressure differences), with the shape of the time-velocity curve similar to that of mitral stenosis. Brief reversal of flow may be, but is not always, present during isovolumic relaxation and contraction phases. Both the diastolic flow and brief reversals during the isovolumic periods are low velocity and thus are not appreciated except at low high-pass filter settings on the Doppler spectral recording. Because this reversal of flow does not always occur, intravenous injection of echo-contrast material is less sensitive for the detection of an intracardiac shunt at the ventricular level than at the atrial level.

Calculation of a pulmonic-to-systemic shunt ratio rarely is needed in adults with VSDs because either (1) the defect is small with a small volume of left-to-right shunt, or (2) a large defect with a significant shunt in childhood now has resulted in Eisenmenger physiology with equalization of RV and LV pressures. If calculation of a shunt ratio is needed, systemic flow is calculated in the aorta, and pulmonary flow is calculated either in the PA (if not disturbed by the septal defect flow) or across the mitral valve (pulmonary venous return).

Patent Ductus Arteriosus

A patent ductus arteriosus often is difficult to image in adults because of limited acoustic access. However, the chronic volume overload of the LA and LV is manifested as dilation of these chambers. Left-to-right flow through the ductus is detectable with either conventional pulsed or color Doppler flow imaging using both parasternal short-axis and RV outflow views of the PA (Figs. 17.23 and 17.24). Diastolic ductal flow in the PA, typically seen along the lateral wall of this vessel, has a sensitivity of 96% and a specificity of 100% for the diagnosis of a patent ductus arteriosus. Recording of flow in the descending aorta, from a suprasternal notch approach, shows holodiastolic flow reversal due to antegrade flow into the ductus in diastole. This finding must be distinguished from diastolic flow reversal due to aortic regurgitation because the two conditions sometimes coexist in adult patients.

OTHER CONDITIONS MANIFESTING IN ADULTHOOD

Corrected Transposition of the Great Arteries

Congenitally corrected transposition of the great arteries is variously termed and abbreviated cc-TGA

Fig. 17.22 Large ventricular septal defect. In this 26-year-old woman with Eisenmenger physiology, a large ventricular septal defect *(between arrows)* is seen in a parasternal long-axis view *(left)* and an apical four-chamber view *(right)*. Severe RV hypertrophy is present. Doppler examination will show low-velocity bidirectional flow across the defect due to equalization of RV and LV pressures. *Ao*, Aorta.

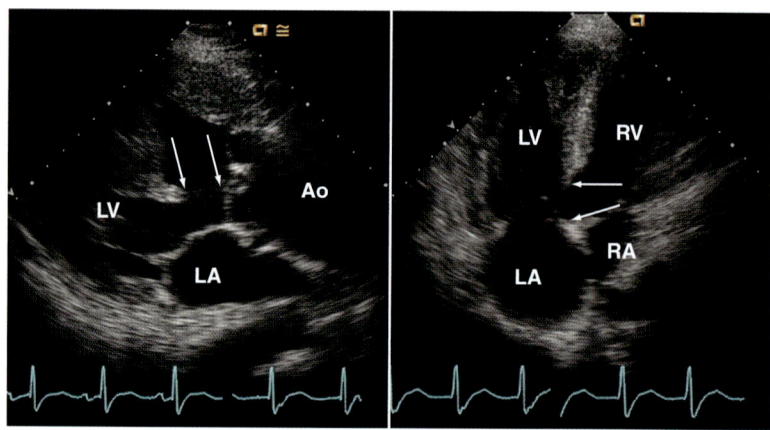

Fig. 17.23 Patent ductus arteriosus. Flow *(arrow)* from the descending aorta *(DA)* into the pulmonary artery *(PA)* often streams along the lateral wall of the PA on color flow imaging. Pulsed or CW Doppler shows holodiastolic flow reversal in the PA. Systolic flow typically is also abnormal, because aortic pressure exceeds PA pressure throughout the cardiac cycle (giving rise to a continuous murmur on auscultation). *RVOT*, RV outflow tract.

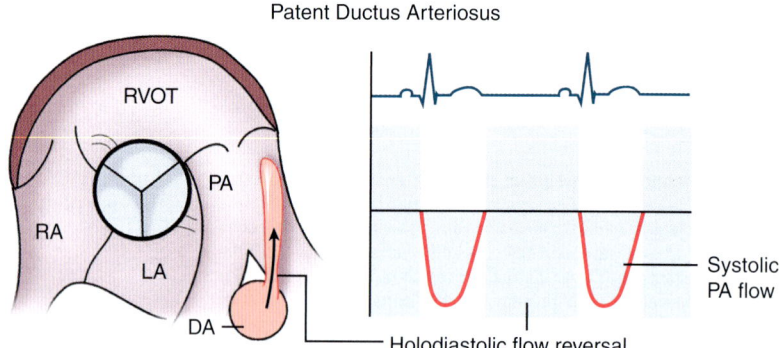

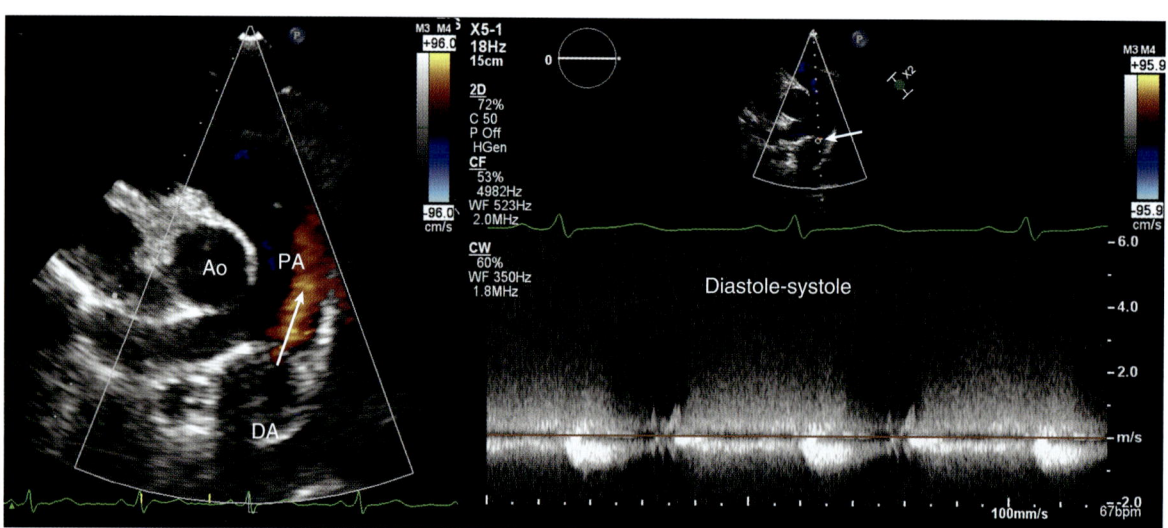

Fig. 17.24 Echocardiographic findings of patent ductus arteriosus. The parasternal short-axis view *(left)* shows the pulmonary artery *(PA)* with a color jet *(arrow)* in diastole distal to the pulmonic valve arising from the descending aorta *(DA)*. CW Doppler *(right)* of the patent ductus flow shows characteristic high-velocity flow toward the transducer in both diastole and systole because aortic pressure is higher than PA pressure throughout the cardiac cycle. Flow that occurs without a break from diastole to systole is termed *continuous*. *Ao*, Aorta.

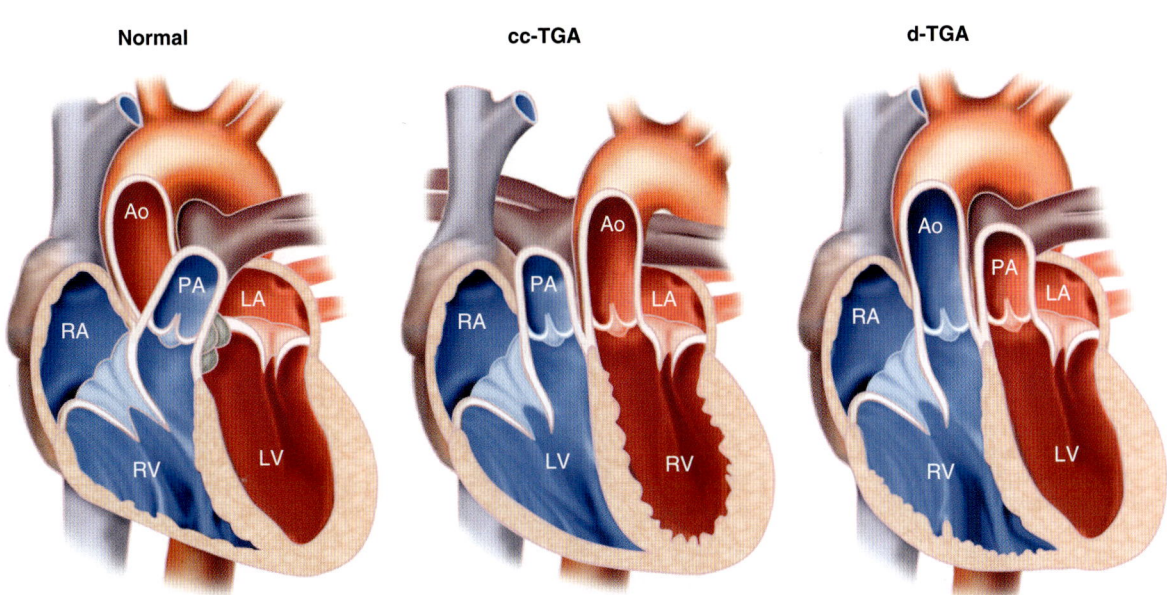

Fig. 17.25 Transposition of the great arteries. Basic anatomy of a normal heart, a heart with congenitally corrected transposition of the great arteries (cc-TGA), and a heart with complete transposition of the great arteries (d-TGA). In patients with cc-TGA, systemic venous blood returns to the RA, passes across the mitral valve into an anatomic LV (the pulmonary ventricle), and is ejected into the pulmonary artery *(PA)*. Pulmonary venous return into the LA is directed across the tricuspid valve into an anatomic RV (the systemic ventricle) and from there into the aorta *(Ao)*. Common associated abnormalities are an Ebstein-type malformation of the tricuspid valve resulting in systemic atrioventricular valve regurgitation, pulmonic stenosis, ventricular septal defect(VSD), and complete heart block. The aorta is anterior on the patient's left side, and the aorta and the PA are parallel to each other. With d-TGA, the aorta arises from the RV, and the PA arises from the LV. Before corrective surgery, delivery of oxygenated blood to the systemic circulation depends on intracardiac shunting via an atrial septal defect (ASD) or a VSD.

("congenitally corrected"); l-TGA (because the aorta is to the left of the transposed PA); or ventricular inversion, because the anatomic RV serves as the systemic ventricle, and the anatomic LV serves as the pulmonic ventricle. With corrected transposition, the physiologic pathway of oxygenated and unoxygenated blood flow through the heart is normal: systemic venous blood returns to the RA, crosses the mitral valve into an anatomic LV, and then is ejected into the PA; pulmonary venous return to the LA crosses the tricuspid valve into an anatomic RV and then is ejected into the aorta (Fig. 17.25). In the absence of associated defects, the diagnosis often is made "incidentally" in adulthood (Fig. 17.26). However, associated defects, including VSDs, pulmonic stenosis, complete heart block, and Ebstein anomaly of the "inverted" tricuspid valve, are common. Dilation and eventual systolic dysfunction of the systemic ventricle are common, although it is unclear whether this is due to the anatomy of the RV being less suited to performing as the systemic ventricle, to inadequate coronary blood flow via the right coronary artery, or to associated systemic atrioventricular valve regurgitation.

On echocardiographic examination, corrected transposition is recognized by identifying the anatomic ventricles in a side-by-side orientation and demonstrating the pathway of blood flow. Associated defects have 2D echo and Doppler findings as described for each abnormality. In addition, the position of the great vessels is abnormal, with the two semilunar valves lying in the same image plane—best seen in parasternal short-axis views—and with the great vessels parallel to one another—best seen in parasternal long-axis views. Typically, the aortic annulus is anterior and to the left of the pulmonic valve (hence the "l" in l-TGA). Corrected transposition also is associated with dextroversion (apex points toward the right), which makes the echocardiographic examination technically more difficult because the cardiac structures lie directly behind the sternum, limiting acoustic access.

"Incidental" Congenital Anomalies

A few congenital anomalies have no known adverse clinical effects but are important in that, if not recognized, they may be mistaken for pathologic conditions and prompt other (possibly harmful) diagnostic tests. A persistent left superior vena cava is seen in a small percentage (0.3% to 0.5%) of otherwise normal individuals and in a higher percentage (3% to 10%) of patients with other congenital heart abnormalities. Because this vein drains into the coronary sinus, dilation of the coronary sinus is seen on parasternal long- and short-axis views and on an apical

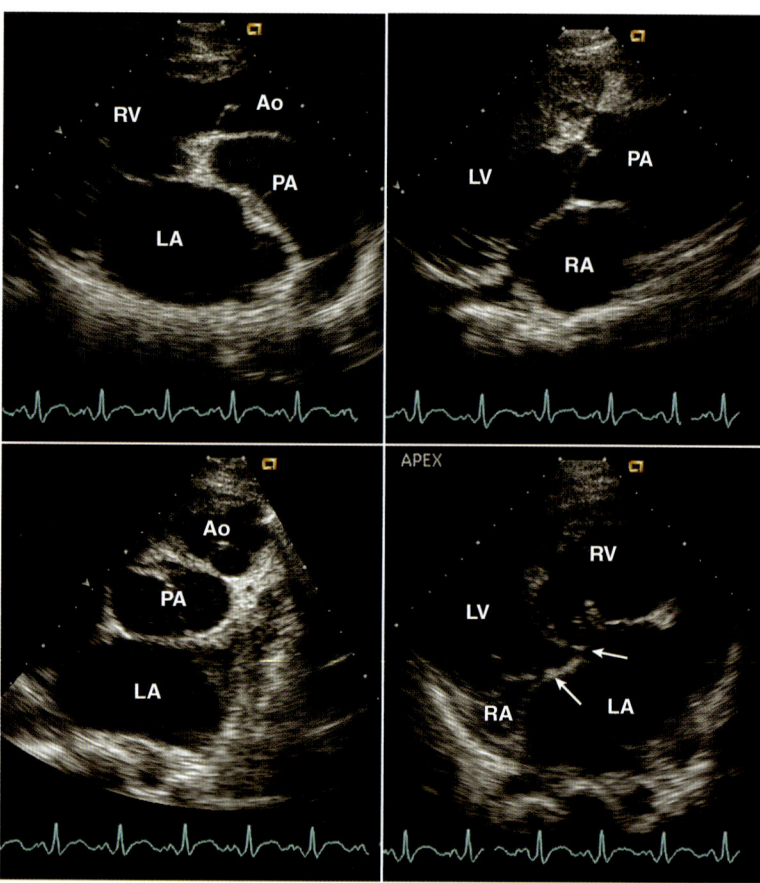

Fig. 17.26 Congenitally corrected transposition of the great arteries. Two long-axis images are obtained from a parasternal position with the aorta (Ao) and the pulmonary artery (PA) in a side-by-side orientation. The systemic RV and anteriorly located aorta are seen *(upper left)*, ▶ with the muscular separation between the atrioventricular valve and semilunar valve evident. This anterior great vessel was identified as the aorta by following it superiorly to the arch and head and neck vessels. With slight lateral angulation, a long-axis view of the venous LV and posteriorly located (and dilated) PA is seen *(upper right)*. ▶ Note the fibrous continuity between the atrioventricular and semilunar valve. In the short-axis view *(lower left)*, ▶ the aortic and pulmonic valves are both seen in cross section, with the aortic valve located anterior to the pulmonic valve. The apical four-chamber view in the standard display format *(lower right)* ▶ demonstrates the anatomic RV on the patient's left, which serves as the systemic ventricle. Note apical displacement of the tricuspid valve septal leaflet compared with the mitral leaflet insertion *(arrows)*. This patient has significant regurgitation of the systemic (anatomic tricuspid) atrioventricular valve resulting in LA enlargement.

four-chamber view angulated posteriorly (see Fig. 15.5). This last view nicely illustrates the entry of the dilated coronary sinus into the RA. The diagnosis can be confirmed (if questions remain) by injection of echo-contrast material, which will first opacify the coronary sinus and then the RA, into the left arm. Injection of echo-contrast material into the right arm will opacify only the RA. The dilated coronary sinus often protrudes into the LA, particularly on the parasternal long-axis view, and is sometimes mistaken for an LA mass.

Idiopathic dilation of the PA is another uncommon benign abnormality. The diagnosis is made when the PA is enlarged, but no evidence of pulmonic stenosis (which could result in poststenotic dilation) or other congenital abnormalities is present.

A Chiari network is a prominent inferior vena cava valve with fibrous extensions to the crista terminalis, coronary sinus valve, or both; it is seen in 2% of patients undergoing TEE echocardiography. These fibrous connections are fenestrated and lax, forming a "network" that shows rapid, chaotic motion during the cardiac cycle. On 2D imaging, the appearance of small, echogenic targets moving rapidly in the RA suggests this diagnosis. Although the Chiari network itself is benign, the likelihood of an associated atrial septal aneurysm or patent foramen ovale is high (see Fig. 15.27).

COMMON TYPES OF PALLIATED ADULT CONGENITAL HEART DISEASE

Classification of Types of Procedures

Numerous palliative and corrective surgical treatments for congenital heart disease have been developed since the first closure of a patent ductus arteriosus in 1938. These procedures are grouped into several categories, as indicated in Table 17.2 and as listed here:

- Relief of stenosis
- Closures
- Shunts
- Pulmonary banding
- Atrial switch
- Arterial switch
- Conduits

The approximate years during which each procedure was performed are shown in Table 17.2 to indicate which are likely to be encountered in a patient of a given age and to provide a historical

TABLE 17.2 Common Operations for Congenital Heart Disease Seen in Surviving Adults

Type	Procedure	Defects Treated	Description	Years
Shunts	Blalock-Taussig	Reduced pulmonary blood flow (TOF, pulmonary atresia, tricuspid atresia)	Classic: Anastomosis of subclavian artery to PA (with or without modification)	1945–1990s
			Interposition tube graft (subclavian remains intact)	1945–present
	Potts	Alternate to Blalock-Taussig	Descending aorta to left PA	1946–mid-1960s
	Waterston	Alternate to Blalock-Taussig	Ascending aorta to right PA	1962–1980s
	Glenn	Single-ventricle anatomy before Fontan procedure	Classic Glenn: SVC to divided right PA only	1959–1980s
			Bidirectional Glenn: SVC to right PA without isolation from left PA	1985–1990s
Atrial mixing	Surgical atrial septostomy	TGA (early palliation), mitral atresia, complex congenital heart disease	Also called Blalock-Hanlon procedure	1950–early 1980s
	Balloon atrial septostomy (BAS)	TGA, tricuspid atresia, hypoplastic left heart syndrome with restrictive PFO	Percutaneous atrial septostomy, also called Rashkind procedure	1966–present
Closures	ASD closure	ASD with significant shunt	Primary or patch closure	1954–present
			Transcatheter closure	1990–present
	VSD closure	Isolated VSD or with other anomalies (TOF)	Primary or patch closure	1954–present
	PDA ligation	PDA	Ligation ± division of PDA	1938–present
			Transcatheter closure	1981–present
	Endocardial cushion defect repair	Endocardial cushion defect (also called atrioventricular canal defect)	Closure of ASD and VSD, repair of atrioventricular valve abnormalities (e.g., cleft mitral leaflet)	1955–present
PA banding	Surgical reduction in flow area of PA	Large left-to-right shunt lesions	PA band to decrease PA flow and pressure	1952–present
Atrial baffles	Mustard/Senning	TGA (replaced by arterial switch procedure)	Atrial baffle directs systemic venous return to PA via anatomic LV and pulmonary venous return to aorta via anatomic RV.	1959–1990s
Relief of stenosis	Aortic coarctation repair	Aortic coarctation	End-to-end anastomosis, patch enlargement, interposition graft, subclavian flap repair	1944–present
			Balloon dilation for recoarctation	1983–present
	Pulmonic valvuloplasty	TOF, pulmonic stenosis	Surgical relief of pulmonary stenosis or	1948–present
			Transcatheter balloon dilation of pulmonic stenosis	1982–present
	Transcatheter pulmonic valve implantation.	Residual pulmonic regurgitation or restenosis after pulmonic valve surgery	Transcatheter bioprosthetic valve placed within a surgical conduit or previous bioprosthetic valve	2010–present
	Aortic valvotomy	Congenital aortic stenosis	Direct surgical valvotomy or percutaneous balloon dilation	1954–present
	Mitral repair	Congenital mitral stenosis	Surgical commissurotomy—initially a "closed" procedure without cardiopulmonary bypass	1949–1990s (closed) 1960s–present (open)
	Konno procedure	LV outflow obstruction not amenable to valvotomy and LVOT too small for an adequate-size prosthetic valve	LVOT enlargement by creation of a VSD, which is then patched, plus aortic valve replacement	1976–present

Continued

TABLE 17.2 Common Operations for Congenital Heart Disease Seen in Surviving Adults—cont'd

Type	Procedure	Defects Treated	Description	Years
Complex repairs	Arterial switch	d-TGA (compete transposition)	Switch of ascending aorta and main PA; coronaries transposed to neoaorta (also called Jatene procedure)	1988–present
	Fontan procedure	Single-ventricle anatomy, tricuspid atresia, double-inlet ventricle, hypoplastic left heart syndrome	Direct connection of systemic venous return to PA with no intervening RV via: (1) RA-to-PA anastomosis (no longer performed), (2) intracardiac conduit, or (3) lateral tunnel (see Fig. 17.34)	1971–present
	Rastelli procedure	d-TGA + VSD + subvalvular pulmonic stenosis, truncus arteriosus, double-outlet RV	Conduit from RV to PA, LV directed to aorta via VSD patch (see Fig. 17.31)	1968–present
	Double-switch procedure	cc-TGA (physiologically corrected transposition)	Interatrial baffle (Mustard or Senning) plus arterial switch	2000–present
	TOF repair	TOF	VSD patch closure. Relief of pulmonic stenosis, often with transannular patch or bioprosthetic valve	1954–present
	Hypoplastic left heart syndrome repair	Hypoplastic left heart syndrome	Three-stage procedure: Stage I: The PA is used to augment the hypoplastic ascending aorta (Damus-Kaye-Stansel anastomosis), and a Blalock-Taussig shunt provides pulmonary blood flow. Together these are called a Norwood procedure. Stage II: A Glenn procedure is performed, and the Blalock-Taussig shunt is taken down. Stage III: The Fontan procedure is completed.	1981–present

ASD, Atrial septal defect; *cc-TGA*, congenitally corrected transposition of the great arteries; *d-TGA*, complete transposition of the great arteries *LVOT*, LV outflow tract; *PA*, pulmonary artery; *PDA*, patent ductus arteriosus; *PFO*, patent foramen ovale; *SVC*, superior vena cava; *TGA*, transposition of the great arteries; *TOF*, tetralogy of Fallot; *VSD*, ventricular septal defect.

explanation of why a patient had a particular procedure. Current surgical and interventional approaches provide a more complete anatomic and physiologic correction than earlier procedures. However, many patients with older surgical procedures continue to be seen as they survive longer in adulthood.

Procedures to relieve congenital stenotic lesions include aortic coarctation repair; pulmonic, aortic, or mitral valvotomy either with direct surgical inspection or with a percutaneous balloon; and the Konno procedure to relieve LV outflow obstruction. A residual gradient usually is present after these procedures, and valvular regurgitation is common.

Procedures to close congenital intracardiac shunts—ASDs, VSDs, patent ductus arteriosus—are conceptually straightforward and use approaches that include suturing the edges of the defect together (primary closure), using a surgical pericardial or synthetic patch to cover the defect, or closing the shunt with a percutaneous device. The most common long-term complication of shunt closure is a residual shunt.

In conditions with low pulmonary blood flow (e.g., tetralogy of Fallot, complete transposition of the great arteries, pulmonary atresia, or tricuspid atresia), an intracardiac shunt can be created to increase pulmonary blood flow. Shunts redirect flow from a systemic artery to a PA (Blalock-Taussig, Potts, Waterston), from a systemic vein to the PA (Glenn), or at the atrial level (Blalock-Hanlon or balloon atrial septostomy). In some cases, these shunts are removed ("taken down") at the time of subsequent corrective surgery. Complications of surgical shunts include:

- Inadequate pulmonary blood flow due to kinking or closure of the shunt
- Excessive pulmonary blood flow resulting in pulmonary hypertension
- Thrombus formation

Pulmonary banding is a palliative procedure that creates functional pulmonic stenosis to reduce pulmonary blood flow and "protect" the pulmonary vasculature from irreversible pulmonary hypertension. Banding is performed in patients with a large left-to-right shunt when definitive repair is not possible or must be delayed. If the degree of banding is not adequate, pulmonary hypertension still ensues. Distal migration of the band results in unequal right versus left PA obstruction.

Other intracardiac repairs include the Fontan procedure, which directs systemic venous return to the PA without an intervening RV in patients with an absent right heart (e.g., tricuspid atresia) and other more complex repairs, as indicated in Table 17.2. When patients with previous surgical procedures for congenital heart disease are referred for echocardiographic evaluation, more detailed references on congenital heart disease are helpful in planning, performing, and interpreting the echocardiographic examination.

Tetralogy of Fallot

The three primary characteristics of tetralogy of Fallot (Figs. 17.27 and 17.28) are:

- Membranous VSD
- Large aorta positioned across ("overriding") the VSD
- RV outflow obstruction—subvalvular, supravalvular, or valvular

The fourth feature of this tetralogy is RV hypertrophy secondary to outflow obstruction. Adults with an untreated tetralogy of Fallot are rarely seen because of the high mortality rate of this condition without surgical intervention. In adults with a repaired tetralogy of Fallot, the VSD patch is evident, the aortic root is enlarged, and some degree of residual RV outflow obstruction usually persists. However, the major long-term issue in adults with surgically treated tetralogy of Fallot is late pulmonic regurgitation (Fig. 17.29).

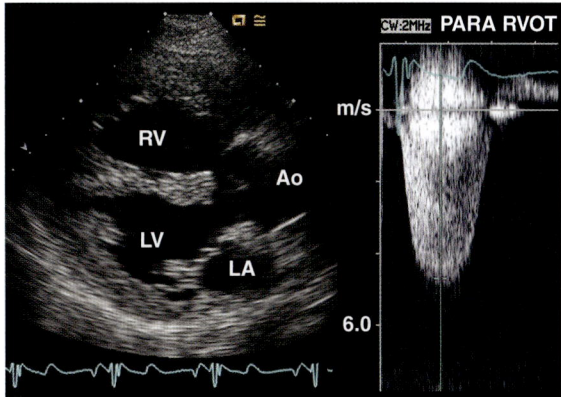

Fig. 17.28 Unrepaired tetralogy of Fallot. In this 23-year-old man, the overriding aorta and ventricular septal defect are seen in the parasternal long-axis view *(left)*. The CW Doppler signal across the stenotic pulmonic valve has a maximum velocity of 5 m/s, consistent with severe pulmonic stenosis and low pulmonary pressures *(right)*. *Ao*, Aorta; *PARA*, parasternal, *RVOT*, RV outflow tract.

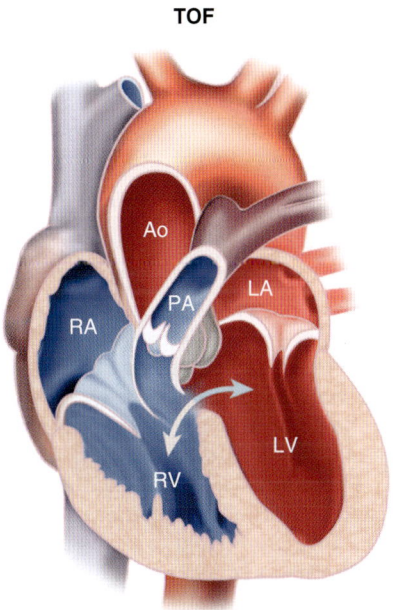

Fig. 17.27 Tetralogy of Fallot. Schematic diagram of tetralogy of Fallot *(TOF)* shows a large ventricular septal defect with an enlarged aorta *(Ao)* that spans (or overrides) the defect. Also noted are pulmonic stenosis (subpulmonic or valvular) and compensatory RV hypertrophy. *PA*, Pulmonary artery.

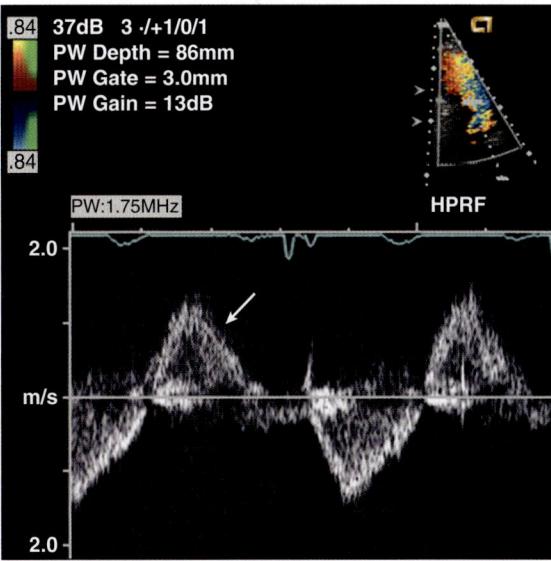

Fig. 17.29 Severe pulmonic regurgitation after tetralogy of Fallot repair. In a 34-year-old woman with a repaired tetralogy of Fallot and progressive RV enlargement, the CW Doppler signal across the pulmonic valve shows laminar forward and reverse low-velocity flow *(arrow)* consistent with severe pulmonic regurgitation. Because the flow velocity is low, this finding often is missed on real-time viewing of the images, thus emphasizing the importance of frame-by-frame review when this diagnosis is suspected.

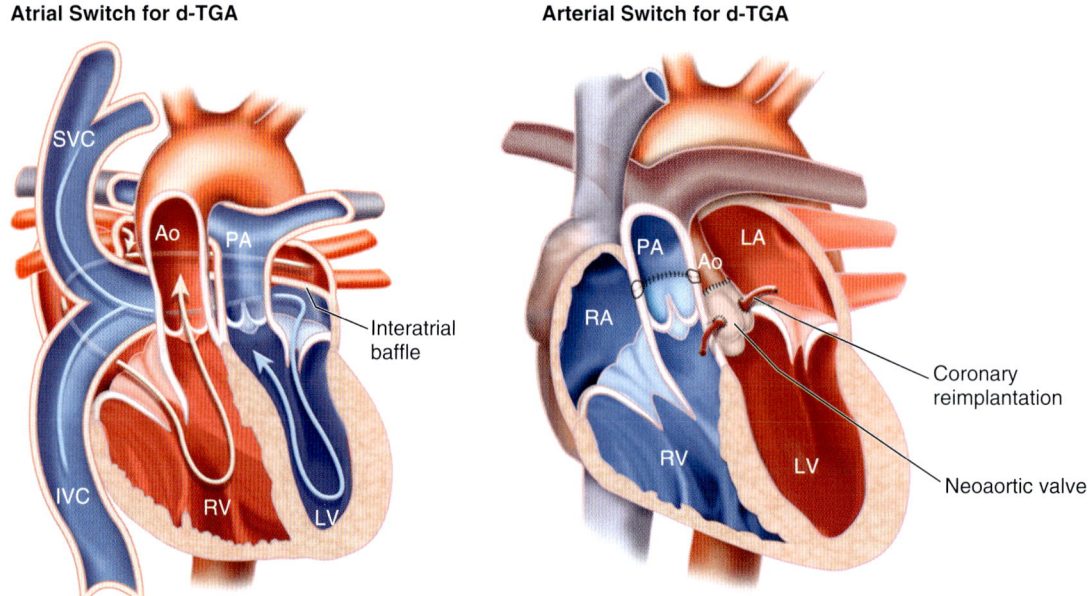

Fig. 17.30 **Atrial and arterial switch procedures for complete transposition of the great arteries.** *(Left)* With an atrial switch operation, such as a Mustard or Senning procedure, an interatrial baffle directs systemic venous return to the anatomic LV (and then to the pulmonary artery *[PA]*) and pulmonary venous return to the anatomic RV (and then aorta *[Ao]*). Adequate visualization of the interatrial baffle usually requires TEE imaging in adults *(right)*. With the arterial switch procedure, the PA and aorta are transected and reconnected to the correct ventricle. The coronary artery ostia are reimplanted into the neoaorta (the native pulmonic sinuses that are now connected to the aorta). In some patients, dilation of the neo-aorta and aortic regurgitation are late complications. *d-TGA*, Complete transposition of the great arteries; *IVC*, inferior vena cava; *SVC*, superior vena cava.

With severe pulmonic regurgitation, color Doppler imaging is unimpressive because diastolic reverse flow is laminar and low in velocity. The pulsed or CW Doppler signal is diagnostic with diastolic reversal of flow equal in signal strength to antegrade flow, with the signal reaching the zero baseline before end-diastole, because of the equalization of pulmonic and RV diastolic pressures. Evaluation of RV size and systolic function on serial studies is particularly important, although quantitative CMR measurement of RV volumes and ejection fraction now is considered the optimal approach.

Complete Transposition of the Great Arteries

With complete transposition of the great arteries (often abbreviated *d-TGA*), at birth pulmonary venous flow returning to the anatomic left ventricle is ejected into the pulmonary artery, whereas systemic venous return into the anatomic right ventricle is ejected into the aorta. Survival initially depends on mixing of blood via an ASD or VSD to provide oxygenated blood to the systemic circulation, followed by a surgical repair that redirects systemic venous return to the pulmonary artery and pulmonary venous return to the aorta via a "switch" at either the atrial or arterial level.

Older adults with complete transposition of the great arteries most likely had an atrial switch procedure, whereas younger adults more likely underwent an arterial switch or Rastelli procedure (Figs. 17.30 and 17.31). Atrial switch (Mustard or Senning) procedures for complete transposition are designed to redirect systemic venous return to the PA (via the anatomic LV) and pulmonary venous return to the aorta (via the anatomic RV). The 3D anatomy of these baffles is complex and is difficult to demonstrate on a TTE study because of poor ultrasound penetration at that depth (Fig. 17.32). A TEE approach improves image quality, but an experienced examiner and multiple tomographic planes are needed to assess the interatrial baffle fully. Late complications of this procedure include baffle obstruction, baffle leaks, systolic dysfunction of the systemic (anatomic right) ventricle, and arrhythmias.

The arterial switch procedure has replaced the interatrial baffle repair for complete transposition. The aorta and the PA are transected and reconnected to the correct ventricular chambers, thereby resulting in a physiologic normal flow pattern. Complications of this procedure are related to reimplantation of the coronary arteries and supravalvular great vessel obstruction at the anastomotic sites. Long term, dilation of the "aortic sinuses" with aortic regurgitation (the anatomic pulmonary root and valve) also is seen (Fig. 17.33). The transposed positions of the aorta and the PA are seen on echocardiography, and with other imaging approaches in patients with complete

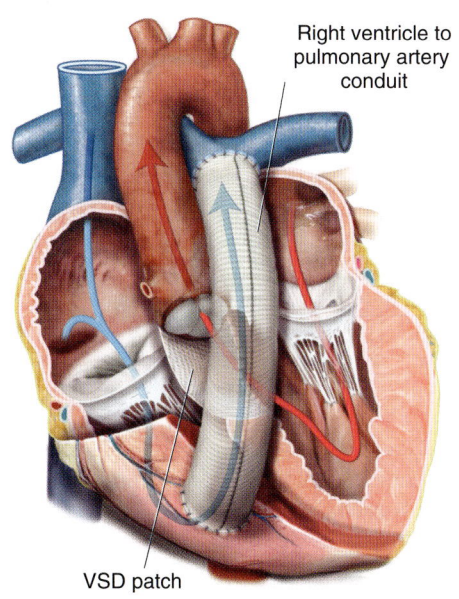

Fig. 17.31 Rastelli repair. When transposition of the great arteries TGA is accompanied by a ventricular septal defect *(VSD)* and pulmonic stenosis, the Rastelli procedure includes a patch to direct flow from the LV across the VSD into the aorta. A valved conduit connects the RV to the pulmonary artery. *(From Deen JF, Krieger EV: Transposition of the great arteries. In Otto CM, editor:* The Practice of Clinical Echocardiography, *ed 5, Philadelphia, 2017, Elsevier, p 951, Table 48.2.)*

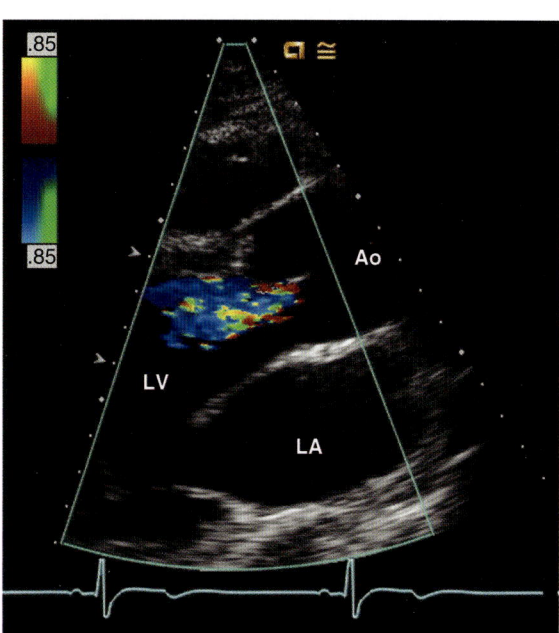

Fig. 17.33 Aortic regurgitation after an arterial switch for complete transposition of the great arteries. Parasternal long-axis view of the neoaortic valve (originally the pulmonic valve) in a 24-year-old man with complete transposition of the great arteries and a great vessel switch procedure as a child. Moderate aortic regurgitation now is present, and the aortic sinuses are dilated. *Ao,* Aorta.

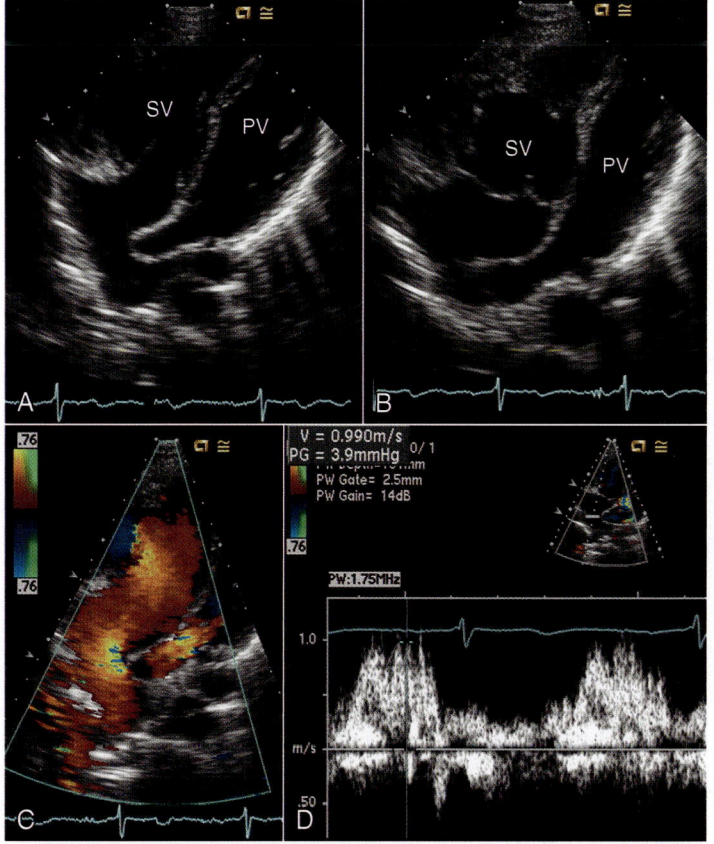

Fig. 17.32 Interatrial baffle repair for complete transposition of the great arteries. In this 38-year-old man who underwent intraatrial baffle repair in childhood, the apical views (A and B) show that the systemic ventricle *(SV)* is an anatomic RV with prominent trabeculation, a moderate band, and a tricuspid valve. The pulmonic ventricle *(PV)* is an anatomic LV. With the image plane angled posteriorly ▶ (A), the pulmonary venous return channel of the baffle is well seen. Color Doppler ▶ (C) shows normal inflow, which is confirmed by pulsed Doppler recordings (D) showing low-velocity diastolic flow. With the apical view angled anteriorly ▶ (B), the systemic venous return limb of the baffle is seen. Further anterior angulation showed the side-by-side aorta and pulmonary artery.

transposition, even after an atrial or arterial switch procedure.

Fontan Physiology

In patients with tricuspid atresia or other types of complex congenital heart disease with only one functional ventricle (single-ventricle physiology), various approaches are used to ensure adequate flow to the pulmonary circulation to allow oxygenation of blood. The Fontan procedure connects systemic venous return to the PA without an intervening ventricular chamber. This connection currently is made directly from the inferior vena cava to the PA (lateral tunnel or extracardiac) with the superior vena cava connected to the PA (a bidirectional Glenn connection) (Fig. 17.34). An RA-to-PA connection, with severe RA enlargement, still is occasionally seen in patients with an older Fontan procedure. Evaluation of patients with a Fontan procedure is complicated by the numerous variations of the surgical approach in the method of connecting systemic venous return to the PA, broadly categorized as interatrial versus lateral tunnel. TEE imaging often is required for adequate visualization, although TTE may be adequate for evaluation of Doppler flow patterns. (Fig. 17.35). Late complications of the Fontan procedure include baffle obstruction, interatrial shunts, and thrombus formation.

LIMITATIONS OF ECHOCARDIOGRAPHY AND ALTERNATE APPROACHES

Measurement of RV Volumes and Ejection Fraction

Accurate quantitative measures of RV size and function are needed for clinical decision making in adults with congenital heart disease; for example, in patients with repaired tetralogy of Fallot and pulmonic regurgitation. Echocardiography allows categorization of RV size as normal versus mild, moderate, or severe dilation and allows a similar qualitative estimate of systolic function. CMR imaging now allows accurate measurement of RV size and volume and currently is recommended, in conjunction with periodic echocardiography, for patient management (Fig. 17.36).

Calculations of Shunt Ratios

Accurate calculation of shunt ratios by Doppler echocardiography depends on accurate stroke volume determinations at two intracardiac sites. Each of these stroke volume determinations is affected by several factors, as discussed in Chapter 6. Alternate methods for calculation of pulmonary-to-systemic shunt ratios include: (1) cardiac catheterization with measurement

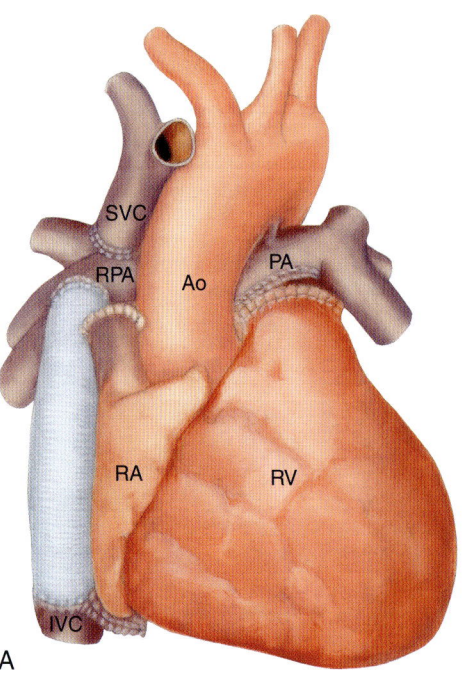 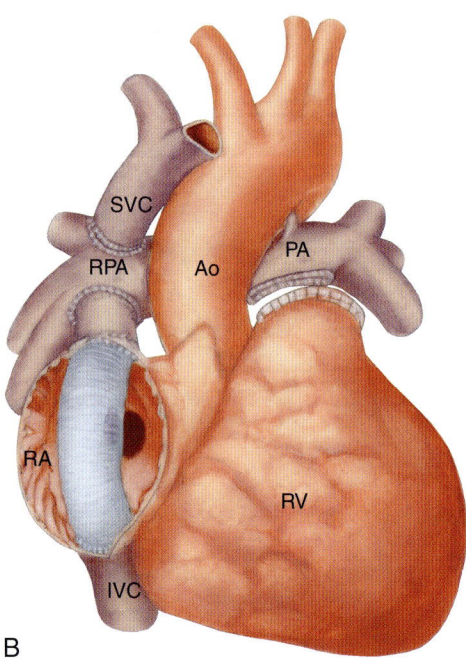

Fig. 17.34 Fontan procedure. The Fontan conduit directs systemic venous return to the pulmonary artery *(PA)* using (A) an extracardiac tube from the inferior vena cava *(IVC)* plus a superior vena cava *(SVC)* anastomosis to the right PA *(RPA)* in a patient with tricuspid atresia or (B) an internal lateral tunnel from the IVC to the reconnected SVC. The early Fontan repair connected the RA directly to the PA. These patients often have severe RA enlargement at long-term follow-up. *Ao*, Aorta. *(From Child J: Echocardiographic evaluation of the adult with postoperative congenital heart disease. In Otto CM, editor:* The Practice of Clinical Echocardiography, *ed 3, Philadelphia, 2007, Saunders, Fig. 44.15.)*

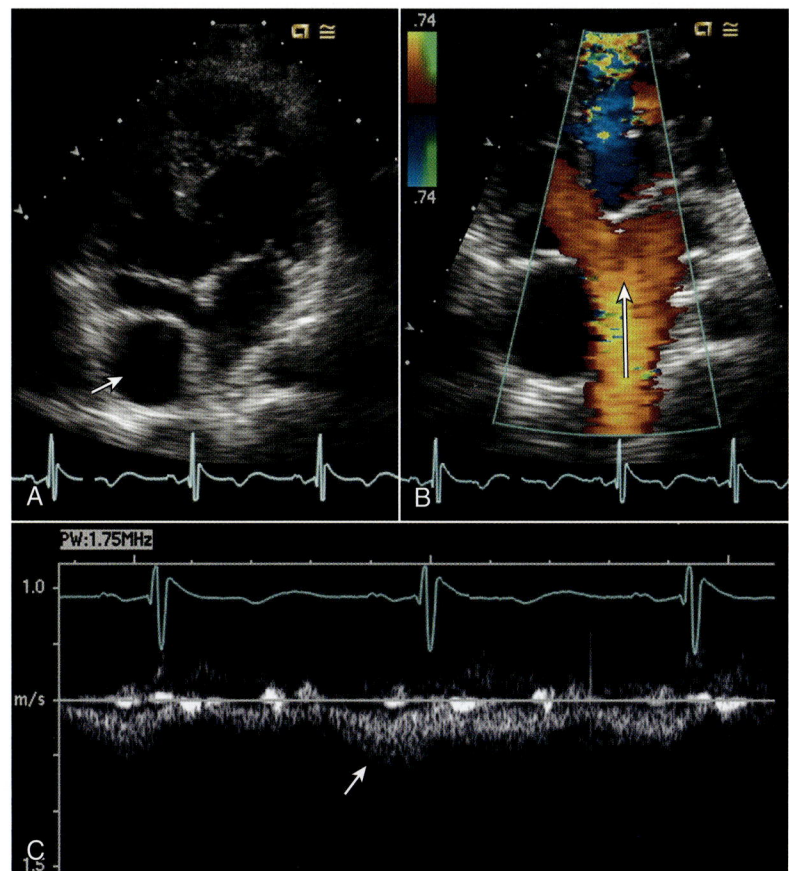

Fig. 17.35 Fontan conduit on TTE imaging. Apical "four-chamber" view (A) ▶ in a patient with single-ventricle anatomy shows a large ventricular septal defect, two atrioventricular valves, and an atrial septal defect. The Fontan conduit is seen as a circular structure *(arrow)* adjacent to the LA. Color Doppler (B) ▶ shows pulmonary venous inflow into the ventricle *(arrow)*; no color is seen in the Fontan because flow is low in velocity and perpendicular to the ultrasound beam. Pulsed Doppler (C) shows low-velocity continuous flow in the conduit *(arrow)*. Often, TEE or CMR imaging is needed for better visualization of the Fontan conduit.

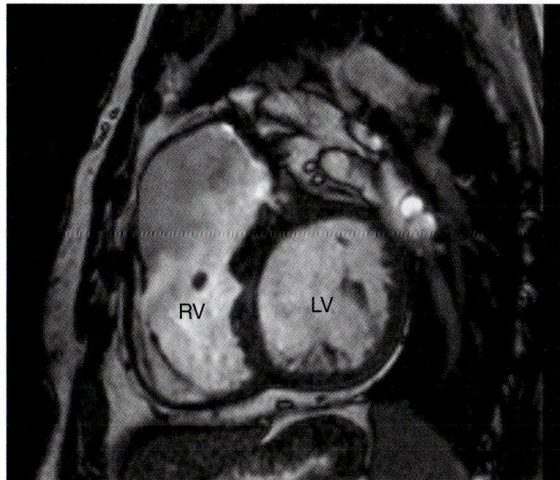

Fig. 17.36 Right ventricular volumes on cardiac magnetic resonance imaging. CMR image showing severe dilation of the RV in a patient with severe pulmonic regurgitation after childhood repair of tetralogy of Fallot. Quantitative RV volumes and ejection fraction are measured by tracing the end-diastolic and end-systolic borders on a series of parallel slices that encompass the RV chamber.

of intracardiac oxygen saturations and total body oxygen consumption and (2) first-pass radionuclide estimation from the early recirculation pattern of the time-activity curve.

Imaging Cardiac Anatomy

TTE imaging in adult patients with congenital heart disease is limited by poor acoustic access (Table 17.3). Even when image quality is acceptable, lateral resolution at the depth of interest on TTE limits evaluation of posterior conduits, interatrial baffle repair procedures, sinus venous ASDs, or anomalous pulmonary venous return. TEE offers improved image quality, particularly of posterior structures, and is a useful adjunct to TTE imaging in this patient population. Although 3D imaging is helpful in selected cases, the limitations of acoustic access and ultrasound artifacts are still present. In adults with congenital heart disease, 3D imaging is most helpful for evaluation of ASDs, 3D visualization of atrioventricular valve anatomy, and quantitation of ventricular function. In addition, 3D imaging is essential during transcatheter interventions to guide the procedure, immediately detect

TABLE 17.3 Alternate Diagnostic Imaging Procedures in Congenital Heart Disease

Diagnostic Test	Strengths	Weaknesses
Echocardiography (TTE, including Doppler)	• Detailed 2D anatomy allowing identification of anatomic chambers, valves, and great vessels; blood flow pathway; structural abnormalities • Assessment of stenotic and regurgitant lesions by Doppler • Detection of intracardiac shunts • Assessment of ventricular size and systolic function • $Q_p:Q_s$ calculations • Estimate of PA pressure • Noninvasive, no discomfort	• Poor acoustic access limits image quality in some individuals. • Definition of posterior structures is suboptimal. • $Q_p:Q_s$ calculation depends on accurate diameter measurements. • No direct measures of intracardiac pressures • Limited quantitation of RV size and function
Echocardiography (TEE)	• Excellent image quality, especially of posterior structures • Detailed Doppler evaluation of pulmonary veins, interatrial septum, and atrioventricular valves is possible. • Planning and guidance for transcatheter intervention	• Anterior cardiac structures now in far field of ultrasound image • Apex often cannot be visualized. • Oblique image planes limit quantitative measurements of chamber size. • Some risk of procedure, plus discomfort to patient
Computed tomography (CT)	• Detailed anatomic images on gated to cardiac cycle • Excellent for aortic anatomy and dimension, coronary artery anatomy, extracardiac abnormalities, and exact position of cardiac structures in the chest	• Intravenous contrast injection • Radiation exposure • Few physiologic data
Cardiac magnetic resonance (CMR) imaging	• Detailed anatomic images • Excellent for posterior structures, extracardiac vascular abnormalities, and position related to chest wall • Blood has intrinsic "contrast" using different magnetic resonance imaging sequences. • Images are realigned to cardiac major and minor axes. • Cine-CMR images allow reproducible quantification of right and LV function. • Valve stenosis and regurgitation can be measured. • Quantification of $Q_p:Q_s$	• Expensive, not portable • Challenging in patients with pacemaker or defibrillator • Some patients are claustrophobic.
Cardiac catheterization	• Direct measurement of intracardiac pressures • Detection and quantitation of intracardiac shunts • Assessment of ventricular size and systolic function • Coronary anatomy • Calculation of pulmonary vascular resistance	• Invasive (risks and discomfort) • Expensive • Requires contrast injection for visualization of structures

PA, Pulmonary artery; $Q_p:Q_s$, pulmonary-to-systemic shunt ratio.

complications, and assess anatomy and blood flow at the completion of the procedure.

Evaluation of extracardiac anatomy by echocardiography limits evaluation of the PA branches, systemic arterial or venous shunts to the PA, and abnormalities of the ascending aorta and aortic arch. Other tomographic imaging techniques are especially helpful in assessing the position of the cardiac structures in the chest and in evaluating mediastinal abnormalities not accessible by ultrasound. Both CT and CMR imaging are helpful, with the advantage of a wide field of view for both techniques (Fig. 17.37). With both CT and CMR imaging, data are reformatted, in an orientation based on the long axis of the LV, into standard long- and short-axis views facilitating identification of abnormal structures.

Other limitations of echocardiography are due to the use of a tomographic approach. For example,

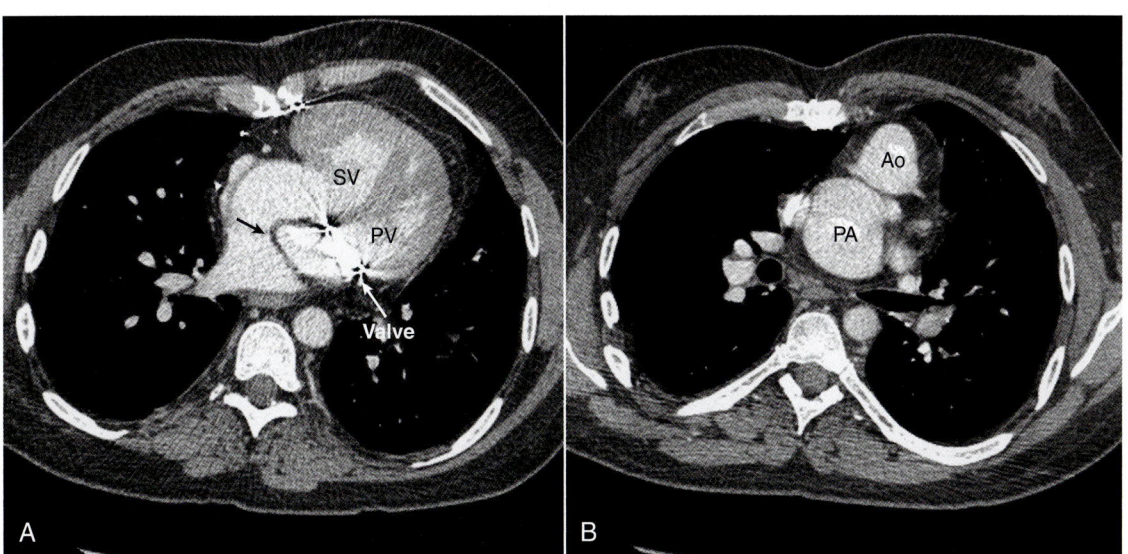

Fig. 17.37 Computed tomography imaging with contrast in a patient with complete transposition of the great arteries. (A) The interatrial baffle repair *(arrow)* directing pulmonary venous return to the systemic ventricle *(SV)* is seen. This patient also has a mechanical pulmonary atrioventricular valve replacement. (B) At the level of the great arteries, the aorta *(Ao)* is anterior and slightly leftward to the pulmonary artery *(PA)*. *PV*, Pulmonary ventricle.

coronary anatomy cannot be assessed adequately with tomographic techniques. CT or direct coronary angiography is needed. Another example of potential shortcomings of echocardiography is that multiple VSDs may be missed unless careful evaluation in numerous tomographic planes is performed, although 3D imaging is helpful when image quality is adequate. A silhouette technique, such as ventriculography from an angle at which the septum forms one of the borders of the ventricular chamber, has a high reliability for detection of multiple VSDs. Limitations of angiography include the risks of contrast dye injection and its cost and invasive nature.

Intracardiac Hemodynamics

Although the definitive method for the assessment of intracardiac hemodynamics remains cardiac catheterization with direct pressure measurement, much indirect information on intracardiac hemodynamics is derived from the CW Doppler signal. PA pressure is approximated by the evaluation of pulmonic regurgitation, the tricuspid regurgitant jet, or both. Maximum and mean pressure gradients across stenotic valves are measured accurately with Doppler techniques. Inferences about the chronicity of regurgitation and the presence or absence of *v*-waves are possible based on the shape of the regurgitant velocity curve. Estimates of LV end-diastolic pressure are possible based on aortic regurgitant velocity at end-diastole, the pattern of LV diastolic filling, or pulmonary venous flow patterns. However, invasive pressure measurements still are often needed for appropriate clinical decision making in adults with congenital heart disease. In particular, evaluation of pulmonary vascular resistance, which requires invasive data, is an essential factor in patient treatment.

INTEGRATING THE DIAGNOSTIC APPROACH

Whichever diagnostic imaging procedure is performed first in an individual patient—be it echocardiography, catheterization, CT, or CMR imaging—the next step should be to consider the data acquired in terms of both the anatomic and physiologic diagnoses and the certainty that each of these diagnoses are correct. Then, the remaining important clinical questions should be formulated, and the most appropriate study to answer those questions should be performed next. When this approach is used, the echocardiogram usually is the initial test to assess cardiac anatomy and physiology, or is performed only to answer a specific clinical question.

THE ECHO EXAM

Categories of Congenital Heart Disease

Congenital Stenotic Lesions

Subvalvular
Valvular
Supravalvular
Great vessels (e.g., aortic coarctation)

Congenital Regurgitant Lesions

Ebstein anomaly
Cleft mitral valve

Abnormal Intracardiac Communications

Atrial septal defect
Ventricular septal defect
Patent ductus arteriosus

Abnormal Chamber and Great Vessel Connections

Transposition of the great arteries (d-TGA)
Congenitally corrected transposition (l-TGA or cc-TGA)
Tetralogy of Fallot
Tricuspid atresia
Truncus arteriosus

Approach to the Echocardiographic Examination in Adults With Congenital Heart Disease

Before the Examination

Review the clinical history.
Obtain details of any prior surgical procedures.
Review results of prior diagnostic tests.
Formulate specific questions.

Sequence of Examination

Identify cardiac chambers, great vessels, and their connections.
Identify associated defects, and evaluate the physiology of each lesion.

Regurgitation and/or stenosis (quantitate as per Chapters 11 and 12)
Shunts (calculate $Q_p:Q_s$)
Pulmonary hypertension (calculate pulmonary pressure)
Ventricular dysfunction (measure ejection fraction if anatomy allows)

After the Examination

Integrate echo and Doppler findings with clinical data.
Summarize findings.
Identify which clinical questions remain unanswered, and suggest appropriate subsequent diagnostic tests.

Clues to the Identification of Cardiac Structures in Adults With Congenital Heart Disease

Structure	Anatomic Feature	Echo Approach
Right atrium	• Inferior vena cava enters RA	• Start with subcostal approach to identify RA
Right ventricle	• Prominent trabeculation • Moderator band • Infundibulum • Tricuspid valve • Apical location of annulus	• Apical 4-chamber view to compare annular insertions of 2 ventricles • Parasternal view for valve anatomy and infundibulum
Pulmonary artery	• Bifurcates	• Parasternal long-axis view or apical 4-chamber view angulated very anteriorly
Left atrium	• Pulmonary veins usually enter LA.	• TEE imaging for pulmonary vein anatomy
Left ventricle	• Mitral valve • Basal location of annulus • Fibrous continuity between anterior mitral leaflet and semilunar valve	• Apical 4-chamber view and parasternal long- and short-axis views
Aorta	• Gives rise to aortic arch and arterial branches	• Start with parasternal long-axis view and move transducer superiorly to follow vessel to its branches.

SUGGESTED READING

1. Otto CM, editor: *The Practice of Clinical Echocardiography*, ed 5, Philadelphia, 2017, Elsevier. Section on Adult Congenital Heart Disease (Stout K, section editor).
   This textbook provides only a basic introduction to echocardiography in adults with congenital heart disease. Health care providers who plan to perform or interpret echocardiographic studies in these patients are encouraged to read the following additional chapters:
   Lin J, Aboulhosn J: Chapter 44: Congenital Shunts
   Bhatt A, DeFaria Yeh D: Chapter 45: Left Heart Abnormalities
   Kim Y: Chapter 46: Right Heart Abnormalities
   Valente AM, Sanders SP: Chapter 47: Complex Conotruncal Abnormalities
   Deen JF, Krieger KV: Chapter 48: Transposition of the Great Arteries
   Burchill LJ, Wald RM, Mertens L: Chapter 49: Single Ventricles: Echocardiographic Assessment After the Fontan operation

2. Lewin MB, Stout K: *Echocardiography in Congenital Heart Disease*, Philadelphia, 2012, Elsevier.
   This Otto Practical Echocardiography Series book provides a concise and practical approach to the evaluation of the pediatric or adult patient with congenital heart disease. Bulleted text is amply illustrated, and online cases with videos provide further examples.

3. Silvestry FE, Cohen MS, Armsby LB, et al; American Society of Echocardiography; Society for Cardiac Angiography and Interventions: Guidelines for the echocardiographic assessment of atrial septal defect and patent foramen ovale: from the American Society of Echocardiography and Society for Cardiac Angiography and Interventions, *J Am Soc Echocardiogr* 28(8):910–958, 2015.
   Review of the anatomy of the interatrial septum and types of atrial septal defects followed by detailed descriptions of the imaging views and protocols recommended for TTE or TEE evaluation of the atrial septum. The role of echo monitoring during transcatheter closure also is summarized. 55 figures, 28 videos, 159 references.

4. Valente AM, Cook S, Festa P, et al: Multimodality imaging guidelines for patients with repaired tetralogy of Fallot: a report from the American Society of Echocardiography: developed in collaboration with the Society for Cardiovascular Magnetic Resonance and the Society for Pediatric Radiology, *J Am Soc Echocardiogr* 27(2):111–141, 2014.
   This comprehensive document summarizes the use of multimodality imaging in management of patients with tetralogy of Fallot. Echocardiography is recommended for serial follow-up of cardiac function; however, CMR now is the reference standard for measurement of RV size and function, as well as severity of pulmonic regurgitation in adults with repaired tetralogy of Fallot. CT is an alternative when CMR is not possible; nuclear scintigraphy is useful for measurement of pulmonary perfusion. Invasive hemodynamic study and angiography are needed in some cases and are essential during catheter-based interventions. Detailed scanning protocols and recommended reporting elements are provided. 18 figures, 7 tables, 195 references.

5. Cohen MS, Eidem BW, Cetta F, et al: Multimodality imaging guidelines of patients with transposition of the great arteries: a report from the American Society of Echocardiography developed in collaboration with the Society for Cardiovascular Magnetic Resonance and the Society of Cardiovascular Computed Tomography, *J Am Soc Echocardiogr* 29(7):571–621, 2016.
   Review and recommendations for multimodality imaging in patient with transposition of the great arteries. Echocardiography is the primary diagnostic imaging modality for periodic evaluation, including before and after surgical or transcatheter intervention. TTE may need to be supplemented by TEE, depending on image quality and the clinical situation. CMR is primarily useful after surgical intervention for evaluation of baffles, conduits, and extracardiac structures, including branch PAs and the aortic arch. CT is an alternate approach when CMR is not possible. Nuclear scintigraphy is used to asses myocardial viability or pulmonary blood flow. Stress imaging is helpful after the arterial switch operation when coronary ischemia is a clinical concern. Cardiac catheterization and angiography are needed in selected cases and are essential during interventional procedures. 51 figures, 24 videos, 227 references.

6. Hornung TS, Calder L: Congenitally corrected transposition of the great arteries, *Heart* 96:1154–1161, 2010.
   Review of the anatomy, clinical presentation, and diagnostic approach to the adult with congenitally corrected transposition of the great arteries. Medical and surgical treatment options are discussed. In some patients, a "double-switch" surgical repair may be considered, with both an interatrial baffle to direct systemic and pulmonary venous return to the correct anatomic ventricle and an arterial switch to connect the aorta and PA to the correct ventricles.

7. Kochar A, Kiefer T: Coronary artery anomalies: when you need to worry, *Curr Cardiol Rep* 19(5):39, 2017.
   Coronary artery anomalies include coronary arteries arising from the opposite sinus of Valsalva, coronary fistula, and congenital coronary aneurysms. Multimodality imaging with CT angiography and magnetic resonance imaging provide a definitive diagnosis, but these patients are often first identified with TTE.

8. Sreedhar R: Acyanotic congenital heart disease and transesophageal echocardiography, *Ann Card Anaesth* 20(Suppl):S36–S42, 2017.
   Concise review article describing TEE finding with ASDs, VSDs, atrioventricular canal defects, patent ductus arteriosus, coarctation of the aorta, pulmonic stenosis, and cor triatriatum.

9. Dijkema EJ, Leiner T, Grotenhuis HB: Diagnosis, imaging and clinical management of aortic coarctation, *Heart* 103(15):1148–1155, 2017.
   Review article on clinical presentation, diagnosis, and management of aortic coarctation. Often echocardiography provides the initial clues to the diagnosis, but CMR now is considered the preferred imaging modality for definitive diagnosis and clinical follow-up. Excellent illustrations of multimodality imaging.

10. Khraiche D, Ben Moussa N: Assessment of right ventricular systolic function by echocardiography after surgical repair of congenital heart defects, *Arch Cardiovasc Dis* 109(2):113–119, 2016.
    Right ventricular dilation and systolic dysfunction are common in adults with previous interventions for congenital heart disease, such as tetralogy of Fallot with residual postoperative pulmonic valve regurgitation. CMR is the reference standard for evaluation of the RV in these patients. Newer approaches such as 2D strain and 3D echo quantitation of RV volumes and ejection fraction also show promise and may be more widely used in the future.

11. Biglino G, Capelli C, Bruse J, et al: Computational modelling for congenital heart disease: how far are we from clinical translation?, *Heart* 103(2):98–103, 2017.

Introduction to the concept and methodology for computation modeling of the complex anatomy and intracardiac flow dynamics seen in patients with congenital heart disease. Patient-specific simulations allow preprocedure planning in complex cases with the ability to assess the likely impact of a specific intervention.

12. Vettukattil JJ: Three dimensional echocardiography in congenital heart disease, *Heart* 98:79–88, 2012.
    Review of 3D echocardiographic applications in congenital heart disease with several illustrations. Practical points for 3D image acquisition include starting from a probe position perpendicular to the structure of interest, using high gain settings to provide uniform echogenicity, centering the image with an appropriate sector width and elevation, synchronization of full volumes with the electrocardiogram and respiration to avoid artifacts, and using 3D zoom on TEE imaging.

13. Simpson J, Lopez L, Acar P, et al: Three-dimensional echocardiography in congenital heart disease: an expert consensus document from the European Association of Cardiovascular Imaging and the American Society of Echocardiography, *J Am Soc Echocardiogr* 30(1):1–27, 2017.
    The document reviews 3D echocardiographic imaging in patients with congenital heart disease. 3D imaging complements 2D imaging for assessment of congenital shunts, stenotic and regurgitant valve lesions, and evaluation of abnormal cardiac connections. The strength of recommendation for 3D imaging is high for evaluation of the atrial or ventricular septum; tricuspid, mitral, or aortic valve; and LV outflow tract when subaortic obstruction is present. 3D imaging is less useful for evaluation of the aortic arch, RV outflow tract, pulmonic valve, or branch PAs. 3D imaging is particularly important for guidance of transcatheter procedures.

18. Intraoperative and Interventional Echocardiography

BASIC PRINCIPLES
   Indications
   Preoperative Diagnosis
   Hemodynamics
   Surgical Manipulation and Instrumentation
   Time Constraints
ECHOCARDIOGRAPHIC APPROACH
   Views
   Sequence
   Reporting and Image Storage
LIMITATIONS AND TECHNICAL CONSIDERATIONS
   Image Plane Orientation
   Doppler Interrogation Angle
   Technical Issues in the Operating Room and Interventional Suite
   Optimization of Instrument Settings
CLINICAL UTILITY OF INTRAOPERATIVE TEE
   Monitoring Ventricular Function
   Valvular Heart Disease
   Mitral Valve Repair
   Valve Stenosis
   Endocarditis
   Prosthetic Valve Dysfunction
   Aortic Disease
      Aortic Dissection
      Aortic Atheroma
   Cardiomyopathies
      Hypertrophic Cardiomyopathy
      Ventricular Assist Devices
      Heart Transplantation
   Congenital Heart Disease
CLINICAL UTILITY IN TRANSCATHETER AND HYBRID PROCEDURES
   Atrial Septal Defect Closure
   Transcatheter Valve Implantation
   Transcatheter Mitral Valve Repair
   Other Transcatheter Interventions
THE ECHO EXAM
SUGGESTED READING

Echocardiography plays a key role in the management of patients undergoing cardiac procedures in the operating room, cardiac catheterization laboratory, and hybrid procedure suites. Echocardiographic approaches include transthoracic echocardiography (TTE), transesophageal echocardiography (TEE), epicardial imaging, or intracardiac echocardiography, depending on the specific procedure and monitoring needs. TTE imaging typically is performed by a cardiac sonographer or noninvasive cardiologist, epicardial imaging by the cardiac surgeon, and intracardiac echocardiography is performed by the interventional cardiologist. Intraoperative or intraprocedural TEE typically is performed by appropriately trained cardiovascular anesthesiologists or cardiologists.

The principles of diagnostic TEE and intraoperative TEE are identical in terms of image plane orientation, anatomic findings, and Doppler flow patterns (see Chapter 3). In addition, standard methods for the evaluation of ventricular systolic and diastolic function, valve dysfunction, congenital heart disease, and so on, as described in previous chapters, are also used for intraoperative TEE. Three-dimensional (3D) echocardiography is particularly important during monitoring of procedures in the operating room and is essential for guidance during some transcatheter procedures.

Typically, baseline TEE data are recorded after the induction of anesthesia but before cardiopulmonary bypass or beginning the interventional procedure. TEE data are again recorded after the surgical or transcatheter intervention and weaning from cardiopulmonary bypass. As with diagnostic TEE, intraprocedural TEE provides images of great clarity and diagnostic value. However, intraprocedural TEE differs from standard diagnostic TEE in several respects:

- Time constraints often require a focused examination.
- Altered loading conditions affect the evaluation of valve and ventricular dysfunction.

TABLE 18.1 Recommendations for Training in Basic and Advanced Perioperative Echocardiography*

Qualifications	Basic	Advanced	Maintenance of Competence
TEE studies interpreted and reported (supervised)	150	300	50 exams/year (25 personally performed)
TEE studies performed (supervised)	50	150	15 Category I CME hours every 3 years
Program director	Advanced perioperative training	Advanced training plus 150 additional exams	Participation in a CQI program
Program (perioperative exam volume and diversity)	Wide variety	Full spectrum	
Documentation of training	NBE certification or verification by training director		

*This table shows the minimum number of procedures recommended to achieve and maintain competency.
CME, Continuing medical education in echocardiography; CQI, continuous quality improvement; NBE, National Board of Echocardiography. Summarized from Mathew JP, Glas K, Troianos CA, et al: American Society of Echocardiography; Society of Cardiovascular Anesthesiologists. American Society of Echocardiography/Society of Cardiovascular Anesthesiologists recommendations and guidelines for continuous quality improvement in perioperative echocardiography, *J Am Soc Echocardiogr* 19(11):1303–1313, 2006. The specific cognitive and technical skills needed for competency are listed in that reference.

- Baseline and postintervention evaluations should have matched loading conditions.
- Urgent decision making based on imaging information may be necessary.
- Any limitations of the TEE information must be promptly recognized.
- Clear communication between the echocardiographer and surgeon or interventional cardiologist is essential.

This chapter provides an introduction to the basic principles and major clinical applications of intraoperative TEE. Echocardiographers who practice intraprocedural TEE should review training guidelines and refer to the additional books and articles included in the Suggested Reading at the end of this chapter (Table 18.1). In addition, other imaging modalities often are used in the operating room (e.g., epicardial echocardiography) and in the interventional laboratory (e.g., fluoroscopy or intracardiac echocardiography) for procedural guidance (see Chapter 4).

BASIC PRINCIPLES

Indications

The indications for intraprocedural TEE range from basic monitoring of cardiovascular function to evaluation of function after complex intracardiac surgical repairs (Table 18.2). In addition to traditional surgical approaches in the operating room with full cardiopulmonary bypass, TEE now also is used with alternate surgical and transcatheter approaches. The role of TEE has become more important as imaging replaces direct visualization of cardiac structure and function.

Preoperative Diagnosis

For elective surgical and transcatheter procedures, the diagnosis and surgical plan should be determined before the operative date (Fig. 18.1). Often, diagnostic TEE is performed as part of surgical planning in addition to other diagnostic imaging studies, such as coronary angiography, cardiac magnetic resonance (CMR) imaging, or computed tomography (CT). This allows time to review and discuss the diagnostic data, resolve any apparent discrepancies, and obtain additional data, as needed. In addition, the surgical options can be reviewed and discussed with the patient.

Preoperative assessment is particularly important for valvular and congenital heart disease, both for technical and physiologic reasons. From a technical point of view, valve stenosis is best evaluated by TTE imaging, which allows multiple interrogation angles to ensure that the maximum jet velocity is recorded. On TEE, the constraints in transducer position often result in underestimation of stenosis severity. From a physiologic point of view, the altered loading conditions during anesthesia frequently result in underestimation of regurgitant severity, for example, if afterload is reduced.

Even when the preoperative diagnostic evaluation is complete, baseline intraprocedural TEE is important to:

- Confirm the diagnosis
- Provide additional information on valve repairability
- Serve as a baseline comparison for the postprocedure study
- Check for other abnormalities
- Monitor left ventricular (LV) function

TABLE 18.2 Indications for Intraoperative or Intraprocedural TEE

Clinical Setting	Procedure	Timing and Goals
Monitoring ventricular function	Before and after cardiopulmonary bypass in high-risk patients	LV volumes, global and regional function
	During noncardiac surgery in high-risk patients	LV volumes, global and regional function
Cardiac surgical procedures	Mitral valve repair	Mechanism and severity of MR Residual MR and complications after mitral valve repair
	Prosthetic valve replacement	Evaluation after valve implantation Detection of complications
	Complex surgical valve procedures	Aortic valve resuspension and aortic root repair Coronary artery reimplantation
	Endocarditis	Valve involvement and dysfunction Assessment after repair or valve replacement
	Hypertrophic cardiomyopathy	LV outflow anatomy before and after myectomy Evidence of subaortic obstruction
	Aortic dissection repair	Dissection flap location and flow Residual dissection after repair
	Congenital heart disease	Complex anatomy and function before and after surgical repair
Transcatheter interventions	Transcatheter aortic valve implantation (TAVI)	Aortic valve anatomy and function before and after valve implantation
	Transcatheter mitral valve procedures (balloon valvotomy, mitral clip placement, transcatheter mitral valve implantation)	Mitral valve function before and after procedure Guidance during procedure
	Prosthetic valve dysfunction	Guide and monitor transcatheter closure of paravalvular regurgitation Guide valve-in-valve implantation
	Atrial septal defect or patent foramen ovale closure	Baseline size and anatomy of defect Residual shunt post-procedure Assess for complications
	Septal ablation for hypertrophic cardiomyopathy	Baseline and post-procedure LV outflow obstruction Determine optimal site for ablation
Placement of intracardiac devices	Cannula placement Ventricular assist devices Aortic cannulation (avoid atheroma)	Guide positioning during placement
General surgical complications	Loculated pericardial effusion after surgical or transcatheter procedures	Detection, size, and hemodynamic consequences
	Intracardiac air after surgical procedures	Recognition and treatment

In elective cases, when unexpected findings are present on the baseline intraprocedural TEE, management is individualized based on the specific findings and the urgency of the procedure. Usually, the surgical procedure can be modified as needed; for example, closure of an incidental patent foramen ovale at the time of mitral valve repair. However, major unexpected findings may require consultation with the patient's primary cardiologist or rescheduling of the procedure.

In emergency cases, the intraprocedural TEE recorded before cardiopulmonary bypass sometimes is the primary diagnostic study. For example, with an acute aortic dissection, promptly transferring the patient to the operating room and obtaining TEE images quickly after the induction of anesthesia may be optimal. In these situations, the echocardiographer should ensure that the diagnosis is correct, evaluate for complications, and promptly communicate this information to the surgeon.

Hemodynamics

Assessment of cardiac hemodynamics and ventricular function in the operating room is affected by:

- Positive pressure mechanical ventilation
- Volume status
- Myocardial "stunning" secondary to aortic cross-clamping
- Effects of cardiopulmonary bypass
- Pharmacologic therapy

Typically, general anesthesia is provided by inhalational agents with supplemental opioids and muscle relaxants, all of which alter preload and afterload. Many agents impair myocardial contractility, decrease systemic vascular resistance, or both. During weaning from cardiopulmonary bypass, vasodilators or vasopressors may be used to maintain a normal systemic vascular resistance, and inotropic agents may be used if ventricular systolic function is impaired. Positive pressure ventilation at baseline and after cardiopulmonary bypass reduces systemic venous return because of the increase in intrathoracic pressure; this effect is most pronounced when ventricular filling volumes are low. The combination of changes in preload, afterload, and contractility result in variation in the severity of valve regurgitation (Fig. 18.2). Antegrade velocities and pressures gradients also vary with volume flow rates.

TEE images and Doppler data optimally are recorded at loading conditions similar to those in the patient's baseline state and with matched loading conditions on the baseline and post–cardiopulmonary bypass studies. Basic parameters, such as heart rate and blood pressure, should be recorded on the echocardiographic images to ensure comparable loading conditions, with measures of systemic vascular resistance, filling pressures, and cardiac output also noted, when possible. After the patient is weaned from cardiopulmonary bypass, preload on the post-bypass study is optimized with volume infusion, often by using TEE images of LV size as a measure of LV filling status, and afterload is adjusted using pharmacologic agents as needed, to match the baseline study.

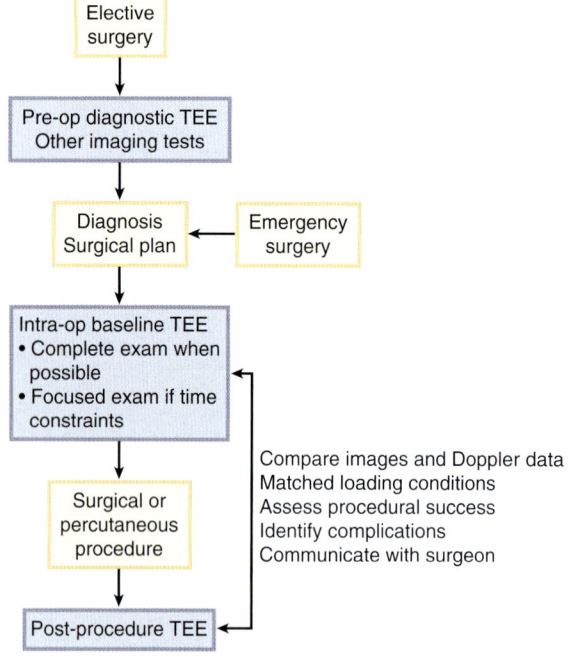

Fig. 18.1 Flow chart illustrating integration of intraoperative transesophageal echocardiography into clinical decision making.

Surgical Manipulation and Instrumentation

During an open cardiac surgical procedure, the effects of surgical manipulation are directly observable on the TEE images (Fig. 18.3). For example, if the left atrial (LA) appendage was inverted during a mitral valve repair procedure, the inverted appendage sometimes appears as a "mass" in the LA that disappears when the appendage resumes its normal shape. Cannulas for cardiopulmonary bypass are visualized to confirm correct positioning but also result in shadowing and reverberations that limit the evaluation of cardiac function. Infusion of cardioplegia results

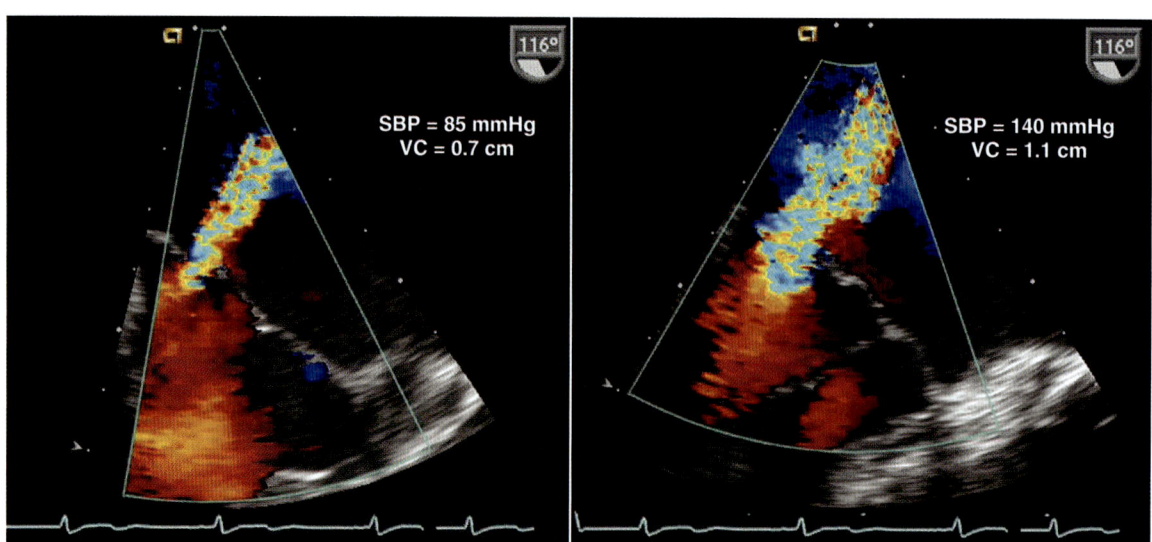

Fig. 18.2 **Effect of loading conditions on mitral regurgitant severity.** Color Doppler flow imaging shows a vena contracta *(VC)* width of 0.7 cm when the systolic blood pressure *(SBP)* is 85 mmHg compared with VC width of 1.1 cm at an SBP of 140 mmHg on images taken a few minutes apart with no other intervention. *(Courtesy Donald C. Oxorn, MD.)*

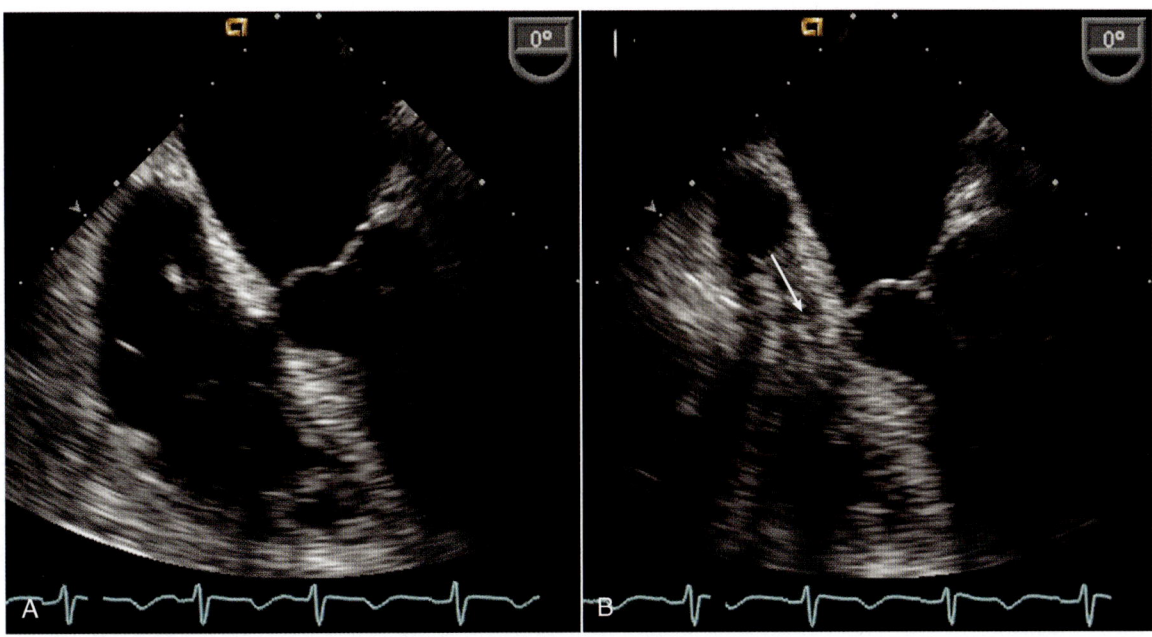

Fig. 18.3 External cardiac compression on intraoperative transesophageal echocardiography. Comparison of the normal baseline TEE four-chamber view (A) with the same view (B) when the surgeon's hand is compressing the right heart *(arrow)*. *(Courtesy Donald C. Oxorn, MD.)*

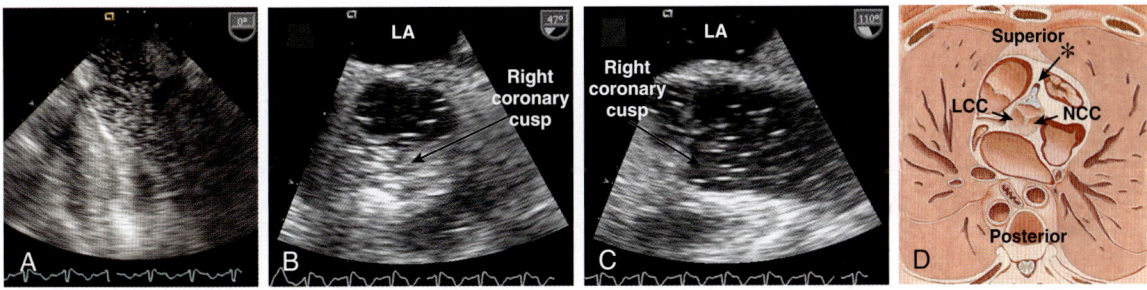

Fig. 18.4 Air emboli: right coronary artery. (A) The LV and LA cavities are full of bubbles following release of the aortic cross-clamp. ▶ Short-axis (B) ▶ and long-axis (C) views of the aortic valve show the bubbles coalescing in the vicinity of the right coronary cusp. The cross-sectional figure (D), with the patient supine, shows that the right coronary cusp *(asterisk)* is most superior, so that bubbles collect in the right coronary sinus of Valsalva and may embolize down the right coronary artery. *LCC,* Left coronary cusp; *NCC,* noncoronary cusp. (From Oxorn DC: Intraoperative and procedural echocardiography: basic principles. In Otto CM, editor: The Practice of Clinical Echocardiography, ed 5, Philadelphia, 2017, Elsevier, Fig. 4.7.)

in a contrast effect with increased echogenicity of the perfused myocardium. Intracardiac air related to the open surgical procedure has a characteristic bright appearance, so that TEE imaging helps ensure that no residual intracardiac air is present at the end of the procedure (Fig. 18.4). Electronic interference from electrocautery creates an artifact on TEE images and disrupts the color Doppler signal.

Time Constraints

A complete systematic TEE examination is recommended during intraprocedural evaluation whenever possible. However, when clinical urgency limits the time available for imaging, the data needed are prioritized, and the most important images and Doppler data are recorded first, with care taken to ensure that adequate data are recorded for any clinical decision making. Most patients have had a complete diagnostic study before entering the operating room so that the baseline intraprocedural TEE focuses on the views needed for comparison to the postprocedure images.

Quantitative approaches that are simple and fast are preferred over more complex methods, when possible. For example, valve regurgitation quantitation by measurement of vena contracta width is similar and faster than optimizing the proximal isovelocity signal or comparing volume flow rates across the regurgitant valve and a normal valve. LV ejection fraction most often is visually estimated, rather than tracing end-diastolic and end-systolic borders for a biplane ejection fraction calculation. 3D image acquisition with semiautomated border detection facilitates

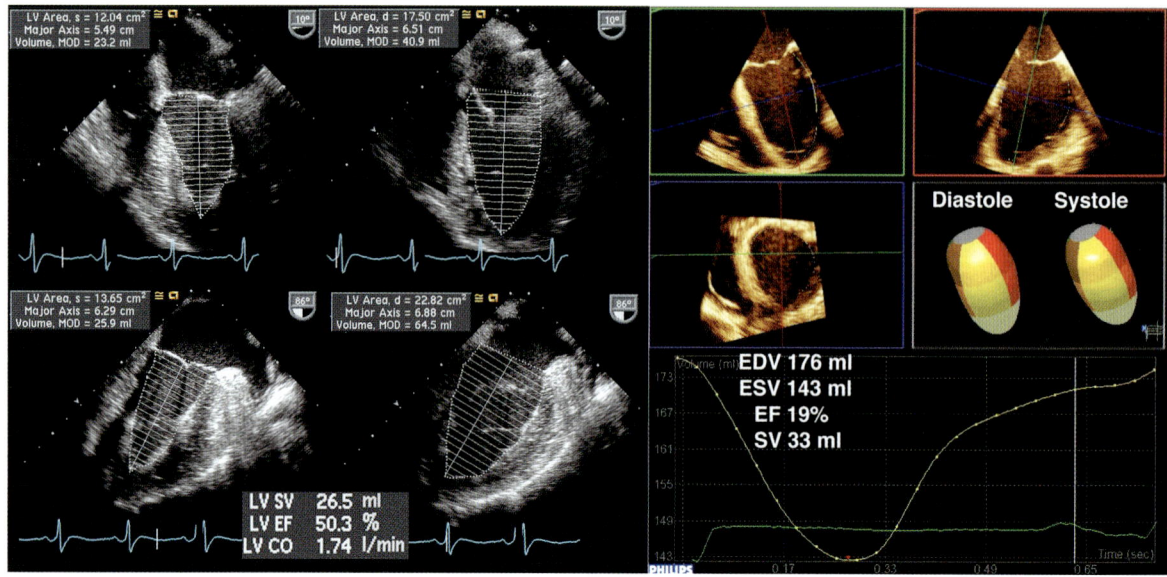

Fig. 18.5 2D and 3D transesophageal echocardiography calculation of ejection fraction. ▶ Measurements of systolic *(s, left in left image)* and diastolic *(d, right in left image)* area made in the four-chamber *(top in left image)* and two-chamber *(bottom in left image)* views are used to obtain volumetric data by the method of disks *(MOD)*. *(Left image)* From these measurements, stroke volume *(SV)*, ejection fraction *(EF)*, and cardiac output *(CO)* can be calculated. *(Right image)* 3D TEE is used to calculate ejection fraction in a patient with cardiomyopathy. *EDV*, End-diastolic volume; *ESV*, end-systolic volume. (Data from Oxorn DC: Intraoperative and procedural echocardiography: basic principles. In Otto CM, editor: The Practice of Clinical Echocardiography, ed 5, Philadelphia, 2017, Elsevier, Fig. 4.5.)

quantitative evaluation of LV function. The use of simultaneous imaging in two planes (Fig. 18.5) and the use of simultaneous two-dimensional (2D) imaging and color Doppler helps minimize the exam time while enabling the echocardiographer to acquire a complete image set. Once images are obtained, the echocardiographer also needs to be cognizant of any limitations in the data and communicate those issues to the surgeon. If the echocardiographic data are essential for decision making, adequate time for imaging without electronic artifacts needs to be provided.

ECHOCARDIOGRAPHIC APPROACH

Views

The primary goal of an intraprocedural TEE exam is to address the specific clinical issue in that patient, so a focused examination is appropriate in many situations. However, a complete examination requires only a few minutes and is recommended whenever possible (Table 18.3). The American Society of Echocardiography and the Society of Cardiovascular Anesthesiologists recommend a standard series of 20 2D views that are supplemented by 3D imaging (Fig. 18.6) and Doppler data. Each view is recorded as a 2-second cine loop, so all these images can be recorded within 10 minutes by an experienced operator, even assuming an average of 30 seconds to obtain each view. Additional time is needed for the evaluation of abnormal findings, color and Doppler spectral recordings, and discussions among the anesthesiologist, surgeon, and cardiologist.

Quantitation of LV systolic function using the biplane apical approach with 2D imaging or 3D LV volumes is recommended when time allows (Fig. 18.7). In addition, 3D volumetric imaging now is routine in views appropriate for the specific diagnosis and procedure, for example, 3D imaging of the interatrial septum in a patient undergoing atrial septal defect closure or 3D imaging of the mitral valve in patient with mitral regurgitation who is undergoing a transcatheter valve procedure.

In addition to imaging data, a screening Doppler study is recommended. A basic intraprocedural TEE includes color Doppler evaluation for regurgitation of the aortic, mitral, and tricuspid valves in at least two orthogonal views. Evaluation of the pulmonic valve is more difficult and is needed only in specific situations, such as congenital pulmonic valve disease, after cardiac transplantation, or with right ventricular (RV) assist device placement. Additional Doppler data recordings are tailored to the specific clinical indication. For example, when significant regurgitation is present, additional color Doppler data, such as vena contracta, are recorded. Color Doppler also allows detection of intracardiac shunts, including a patent foramen ovale. Continuous-wave (CW) Doppler recordings are helpful for the evaluation of valve stenosis and regurgitation and for the estimation of pulmonary pressures, if a pulmonary artery catheter has not been placed. Pulsed

TABLE 18.3 Comprehensive TEE Exam Components and Sequence

View	Comments
Mid-esophageal Views	
Evaluate primary study indication	Endocarditis evaluation, cardiac source of embolus, acute aortic syndrome, etc.
LV size and function	Depth to include entire LV. Transducer angle 0°–130°. Global and regional function, 3D LV volumes, and EF
RV size and function	Depth to include entire RV. Transducer angle 0°–70°
Left atrium	Decrease depth to below MV. Sweep across the atrium at transducer angles between 0° and 90°.
LA appendage	Biplane imaging. Adjust position to decrease artifact from ridge between LUPV and LAA. Pulsed-wave Doppler of velocities for atrial fibrillation
Right atrium	Decrease depth to just below mitral valve. Sweep across the atrium at transducer angles between 0° and 90°.
Mitral valve	2D imaging and color Doppler from multiple views, transducer angle 0°–130°. Quantitation of regurgitation severity, vena contracta, and PISA EROA calculation for more than mild regurgitation. Mitral inflow gradient for stenosis. 3D en face view of valve rotated to aortic valve at top of display
Aortic valve	2D imaging and color Doppler from multiple views, transducer angle 0°–130°. Vena contracta for more than mild regurgitation. 3D en face view of valve rotated to right coronary cusp at bottom of display
Ascending aorta (upper esophageal)	Transducer angle 100°. Measure if dilated (sinuses, sinotubular junction, mid-ascending aorta).
Tricuspid valve	2D imaging and color Doppler from multiple views, transducer angle 0°–60°
Pulmonic valve	2D imaging and color Doppler, transducer angle 70°
Interatrial septum and bicaval view	2D imaging and color Doppler at lower Nyquist setting, transducer angle 100°. If shunt suspected, 3D en face view and agitated saline contrast study. If present, evaluate.
Pulmonary veins	2D imaging and color Doppler, transducer angle 0° and 100° for left and right pulmonary veins. Pulsed-wave Doppler if significant MR, to evaluate for flow reversal
Pericardial space	Sweep across the heart at a transducer angle of 0°.
Transgastric Views	
Ventricular function	Evaluate biventricular size and function, transducer angle 0° and 120°. Rotate probe tip rightward for RV and tricuspid valve. En face view of MV with color Doppler if significant MR
Deep transgastric view	Advance probe from transgastric view. Visualize LV outflow for Doppler interrogation if needed.
Aorta View	
Descending thoracic aorta	Image from the diaphragm to the aortic arch. Biplane imaging, 0° and 90°. Pulsed-wave Doppler if significant AR, to evaluate for flow reversal. Image atherosclerotic plaque.

AR, Aortic regurgitation; *EF*, ejection fraction; *EROA*, estimated regurgitant orifice area; *LAA*, LA appendage; *LUPV*, left upper pulmonary vein; *MR*, mitral regurgitation; *MV*, mitral valve; *PISA*, proximal isovelocity surface area.
From Freeman RV: The comprehensive diagnostic transesophageal echocardiogram: integrating 2D and 3D imaging, Doppler quantitation and advanced approaches, In Otto CM, editor: *The Practice of Clinical Echocardiography*, ed 5, Philadelphia, 2017, Elsevier, pp 56–57.

Doppler recordings are used to evaluate LA filling via the pulmonary veins, LV diastolic filling, and atrial appendage function.

Sequence

Several sequences of image acquisition are possible, and all are appropriate as long as the needed diagnostic images are obtained. Some echocardiographers prefer to obtain all the views from each transducer position:

- Mid-esophageal
- Transgastric
- Upper esophageal

This approach minimizes the time needed for acquisition and is easy to remember.

Protocol for Three-Dimensional Transesophageal Echocardiography Image Acquisition	
Left Ventricle	1. Obtain a view of the left ventricle from the 0°, 60° or 120° mid-esophageal positions 2. Use the biplane mode to check that the left ventricle is centered in a second view 90° to the original. 3. Acquire using wide-angle, multibeat mode 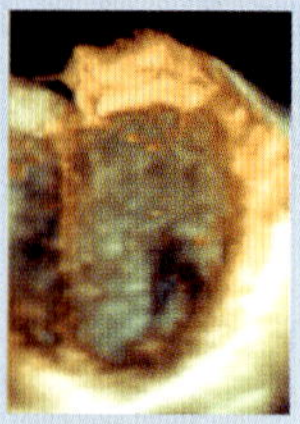
Right Ventricle	1. Obtain a view of the right ventricle from the 0° mid-esophageal position with the right ventricle tilted so that it is in the center of the image. 2. Acquire using wide-angle, multibeat mode 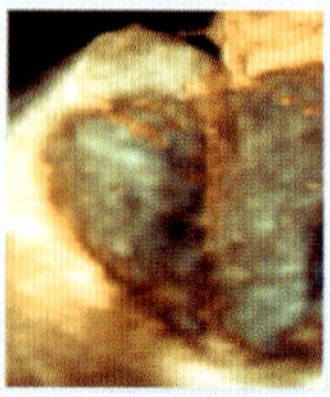
Interatrial Septum	1. 0° with the probe rotated to the interatrial septum 2. Acquire using narrow-angle, single-beat or wide-angle, multibeat modes 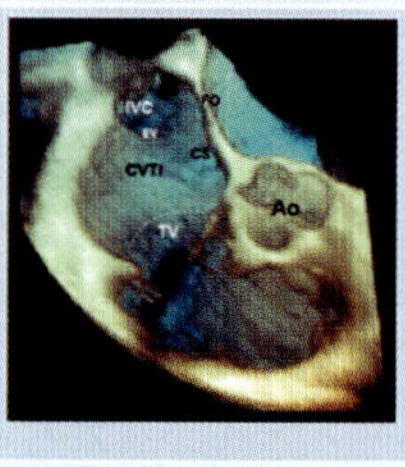
Aortic Valve	1. Obtain a view of the aortic valve from either the 60° mid-esophageal, short-axis view on the 120° mid-esophageal, long-axis view. 2. Acquire using either the narrow-angle, single-beat or the wide-angle, multibeat modes 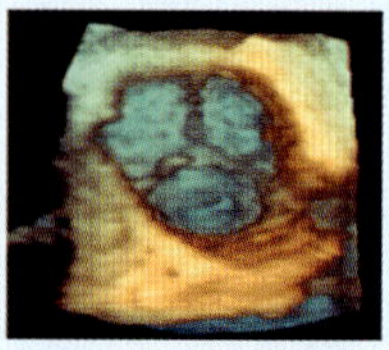
Mitral Valve	1. Obtain a view of the mitral valve from the 0°, 60°, 90° or 120° mid-esophageal views 2. Use the biplane mode to check that the mitral valve annulus is centered with the acquisition plane in a second view 90° to the original. 3. Acquire using narrow-angle, single-beat mode 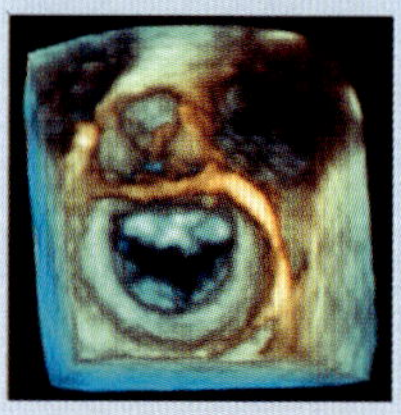
Pulmonic Valve	1. Obtain a view of the pulmonic valve from either the 90° high-esophageal view or the 120° mid-esophageal, 3-chamber view rotated to center the pulmonic valve 2. Acquire using narrow-angle, single-beat mode 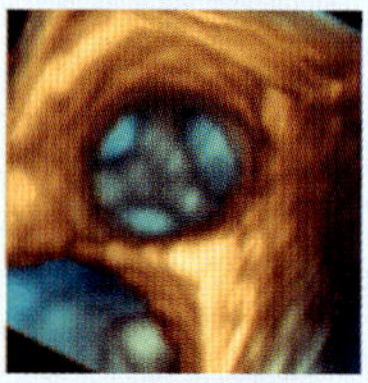
Tricuspid Valve	1. Obtain a view of the tricuspid valve from either the 0° to 30° mid-esophageal, 4-chamber view tilted so that the valve is centered in the imaging plane or the 40° transgastric view with anteflexion 2. Acquire using narrow-angle, single-beat mode 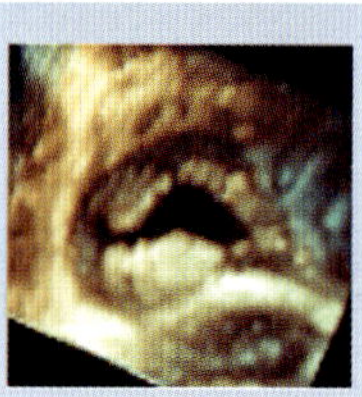

Fig. 18.6 Summary of 3D transesophageal acquisition views. *(From Hahn RT, Abraham T, Adams MS, et al: Guidelines for performing a comprehensive transesophageal echocardiographic examination: recommendations from the American Society of Echocardiography and the Society of Cardiovascular Anesthesiologists, J Am Soc Echocardiogr 26(9):921–964, 2013.)*

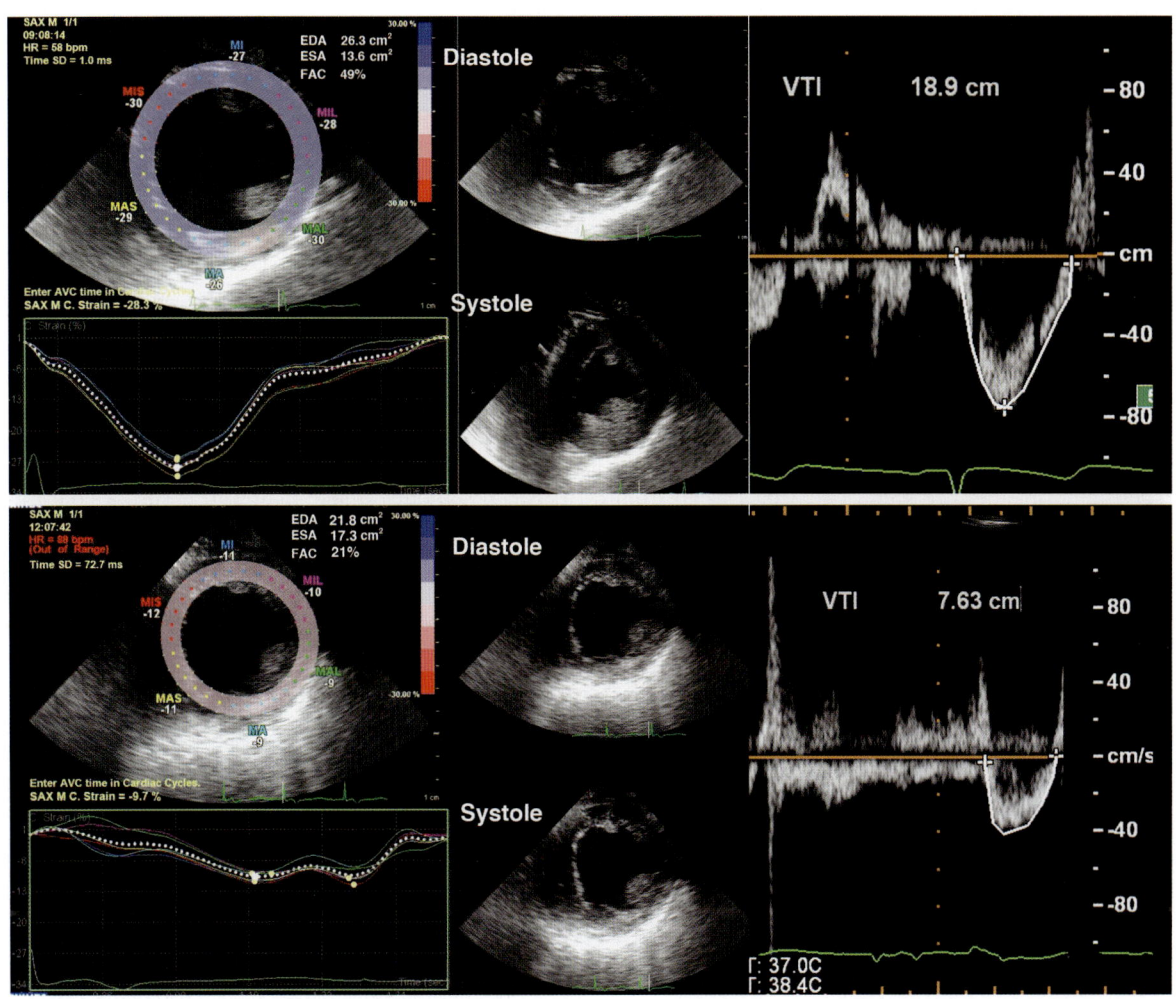

Fig. 18.7 **Assessment of left ventricular function.** Surrogates for LV function are presented in a patient before and after cardiopulmonary bypass. In the *top three panels*, circumferential strain *(left)*, ▶ end-diastolic area *(EDA)* and end-systolic area *(ESA; center)* ▶ and LV outflow tract velocity-time integral *(VTI; right)* are obtained before bypass in a patient undergoing mitral valve replacement. ▶ In the *lower three panels*, ▶ the same measurements are made following a long pump run and aortic cross-clamp time. Decrements in all three parameters are seen. These returned toward baseline with time and following institution of resuscitative measures. *EDA*, End-diastolic area; *ESA*, end-systolic area; *FAC*, fractional area of change. (From Oxorn DC: Intraoperative and procedural echocardiography: basic principles. In Otto CM, editor: The Practice of Clinical Echocardiography, ed 5, Philadelphia, 2017, Elsevier, Fig. 4.6.)

In this sequence, starting in a mid-esophageal four-chamber view with depth adjusted to show the entire LV, the image plane is rotated toward the two-chamber view and then the long-axis view (see Figs. 3.3, 3.7, and 3.9). The "mitral commissural" view describes a two-chamber plane in which both the medial and lateral commissures are seen, similar to the standard two-chamber view at about 60° rotation. An additional "two-chamber" view at about 90° rotation provides visualization of additional segments of the mitral valve and the LA appendage. These views also allow sequential evaluation of regional wall motion in the four-chamber view (inferior septum and lateral wall), the two-chamber view (inferior wall and anterior wall), and the long-axis view (posterior wall and anterior septum). A full-volume 3D acquisition allows measurement of LV ejection fraction, assessment of regional wall motion, and evaluation of global and regional longitudinal strain.

From the long-axis view, depth is decreased to focus on the aortic and mitral valves. Then the transducer is moved superiorly in the esophagus to visualize the ascending aorta, first in long axis (see Fig. 3.10), followed by rotation of the image plane to a short-axis view of the ascending aorta, with the pulmonary artery seen in long axis. The probe is advanced to a short-axis view of the aortic valve (see Fig. 3.13) and then the tricuspid and pulmonic valves. Turning the probe to the right with further rotation of the image plane yields the bicaval view of the right atrium (RA) (see Fig. 3.12). 3D real-time and multibeat volumetric images of the aortic and mitral valve are obtained from this probe position.

From the transgastric position, standard views include the short-axis views at the mid-LV and mitral valve levels, followed by rotation of the image plane to about 90° to show the two-chamber view (see Figs. 3.16 and 3.18). The probe is then turned rightward for a long-axis view, which includes the aorta, and an RV inflow view. From the deep transgastric position, an anteriorly angulated four-chamber view is obtained in some patients. The descending thoracic aorta is examined in sequential short-axis views from the level of the diaphragm to the arch, as the probe is slowly withdrawn in the esophagus. These short-axis views are supplemented with long-axis views at 90° rotation when abnormalities are seen. The arch is seen from an upper esophageal position by turning the image plane rightward, with a short-axis view obtained by rotation of the image plane.

Another approach is to evaluate each structure of interest in at least two orthogonal views, combining imaging, color, and spectral Doppler evaluations of each structure. With this approach, a complete examination includes:

- All four cardiac chambers (LV, RV, LA, RA)
- All four valves (aortic, mitral, tricuspid, pulmonic)
- Both great arteries (aorta, pulmonary artery)
- Systemic and pulmonary venous return (inferior vena cava, superior vena cava, four pulmonary veins)
- Atrial septum and LA appendage

This approach is useful with a focused examination, starting with the primary structures of interest and continuing on to evaluate other structures as time allows. Even when a different sequence of imaging is used, the anatomic approach also provides a quick checklist to ensure that every structure has been evaluated before the examination is completed. 3D imaging is integrated into the 2D imaging sequence with the 3D examination focused on the specific structure of interest, such as the mitral valve in patients undergoing mitral valve repair.

Reporting and Image Storage

Intraprocedural TEE results are communicated directly to the surgeon at the time of data acquisition to facilitate prompt decision making. Intraprocedural TEE results should be available throughout the surgical procedure, verbally or in written format. In addition, a permanent written or electronic report that includes indications, a description of the procedure, and diagnostic findings should be included in the medical record. The report should indicate whether a comprehensive examination (most of the 20 recommended views) was recorded or whether it was a focused or limited examination to address a specific clinical issue. Intraprocedural TEE images and reports should be stored at each medical center in digital format with other echocardiographic images and reports to allow later review and comparison with subsequent studies.

LIMITATIONS AND TECHNICAL CONSIDERATIONS

Image Plane Orientation

As with any echocardiographic study, intraprocedural 2D TEE images should be aligned in standard image planes corresponding to long-axis, short-axis, four-chamber, and two-chamber views, with scanning between standard image planes to ensure a comprehensive study. 3D views also are recorded in standard orientations (see Chapter 4). Internal anatomic landmarks are used to define correct image alignment. The rotation angles provided in tables serve only as a guide to the typical angle needed for a given view; the actual rotation angle varies from patient to patient. In addition, individual variability in the anatomic relationship between the esophagus and the heart results in variability in image plane orientation, so correct alignment of views is not always possible.

Doppler Interrogation Angle

A parallel alignment between the Doppler beam and blood flow of interest is not always possible on TEE imaging. The probe position is constrained by the anatomic relationship between the esophagus and the heart, so even with careful adjustment of transducer position and rotation of the image plane, the interrogation angle is typically still nonparallel, with potential underestimation of flow velocities. Intercept angle has a limited impact on the diagnostic value of color Doppler because the color Doppler flow image corresponds to the spatial pattern of the flow disturbance, even though exact velocities cannot be accurately measured. For spectral Doppler recordings, a near-parallel alignment is easily obtained by TEE for antegrade and regurgitant flow across the mitral valve (Fig. 18.8) and for LA appendage and pulmonary vein flow. From a high esophageal position, flow in the pulmonary artery also can be recorded at a near-parallel intercept angle. However, alignment of the Doppler beam with the LV outflow tract and transaortic flow is problematic. On mid-esophageal views, parallel alignment is not possible. Sometimes better alignment can be obtained from a transgastric long-axis view or a deep transgastric anteriorly angulated four-chamber view. However, underestimation of velocity is likely and should be considered, particularly with TEE evaluation of aortic stenosis severity.

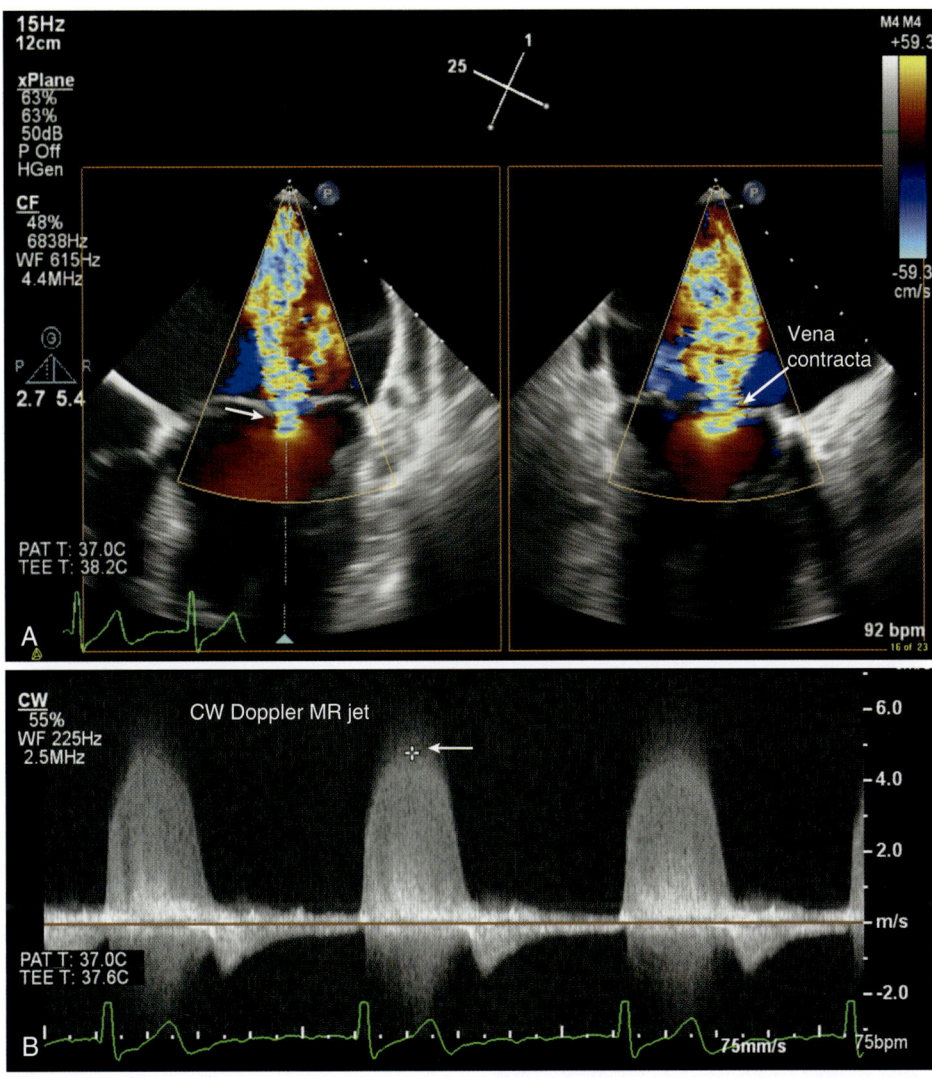

Fig. 18.8 Transesophageal echocardiography quantitation of mitral regurgitation. The orientation of the mitral regurgitant *(MR)* jet allows a parallel intercept angle between the ultrasound beam and the direction of blood flow. (A) Vena contracta width *(arrow)* is 2.6 mm for this central jet of functional regurgitation. ▶ (B) The CW Doppler regurgitant signal *(arrow)* is less dense than antegrade flow, which is also consistent with mild to moderate regurgitation.

Technical Issues in the Operating Room and Interventional Suite

During intraoperative or intraprocedural TEE, the echocardiographer needs to be alert to interference or technical artifacts. Cannulas, catheters, and other devices cause acoustic shadows or reverberations, obscuring the structure or flow of interest (Fig. 18.9). Electronic interference from electrocautery or other procedures precludes diagnostic images or Doppler data (Fig. 18.10). If reverberations and shadowing cannot be avoided by repositioning the probe, alternate approaches, such as epicardial scanning with a sterile transducer, need to be considered. Electronic devices should be paused when possible to allow recording of echocardiographic data without interference artifacts.

Optimization of Instrument Settings

Intraprocedural TEE is facilitated by presetting the instrument settings to optimize image recording with minimal additional adjustment of parameters during the examination. Images are recorded using one- or two-beat cine-loop image acquisition triggered to the QRS signal or by setting a fixed recording time (if the electrocardiogram signal is not adequate for consistent triggering).

Typically, the study is started with standard transducer frequency, depth, gain, processing, and

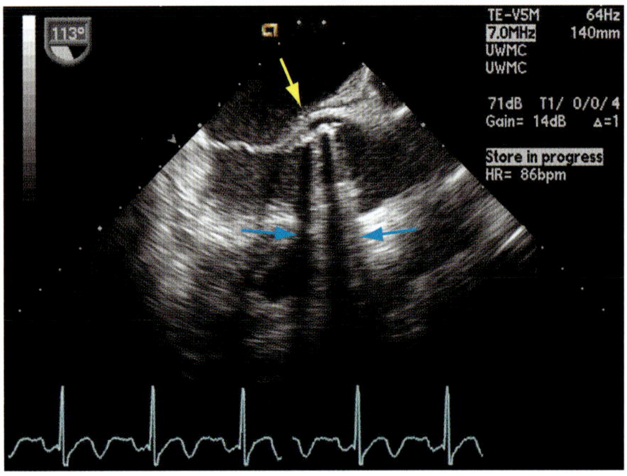

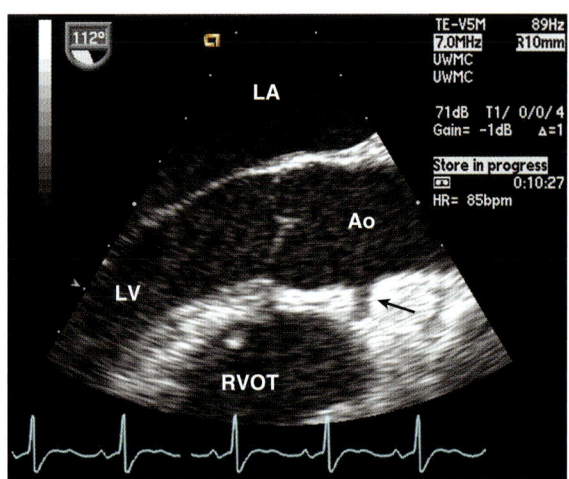

Fig. 18.9 Shadowing and reverberations on transesophageal echocardiography. ▶ The long-axis TEE view in a patient with endocarditis in a mechanical aortic valve prosthesis shows shadows and reverberations originating from the posterior aspect of the prosthetic valve *(yellow arrow)* extending in alternating bands *(between blue arrows)* of dark (shadows) and white (reverberations) to obscure more distal structures, including the anterior aspect of the valve and the LV outflow tract. *HR,* Heart rate.

Fig. 18.11 Aortic valve in long axis. ▶ The aortic valve and aortic sinuses are evaluated in a long-axis view using a shallow depth and zoom mode with a high transducer frequency to optimize image resolution. The origin of the right coronary artery *(RCA)* is seen *(arrow)*. *Ao,* Aorta; *HR,* heart rate.

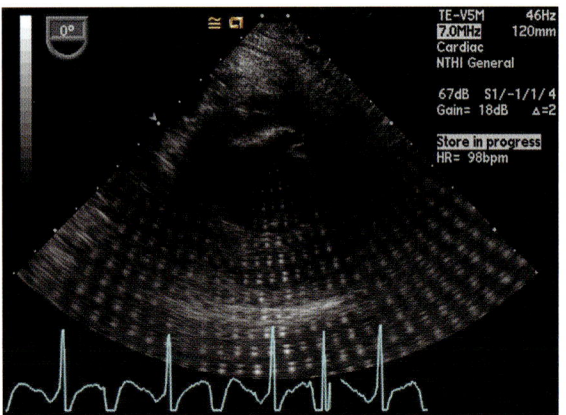

Fig. 18.10 Electronic artifact. In a transgastric short-axis view, electronic artifact from the surgical cautery system not only creates a geometric artifact pattern but also obscures the 2D image. Doppler flow data are not reliable when electronic artifact is present. *HR,* Heart rate.

sector width settings. However, each of these parameters should be adjusted for optimal image recording during the TEE study. A higher transducer frequency (7 MHz) should be used to optimize resolution of near structures, such as the LA appendage, whereas lower frequencies (5 or 3.5 MHz) are needed for optimal penetration to visualize the LV apex in the four-chamber view or on transgastric views. Depth should be adjusted to show the structure of interest: for example, starting with a depth of 15 to 16 cm in the four-chamber view for ventricular function and then decreasing depth to just beyond the mitral valve for the examination of valve function (Fig. 18.11). Zoom mode provides improved image resolution and frame rate when examining the atrial appendage, the aortic valve, or the mitral valve. Gain should be adjusted as needed based on image quality.

3D echocardiographic views are tailored to the specific clinical situation. Many operators find it helpful to begin with real-time 3D imaging, using a narrow sector and zoom mode to optimize frame rate. Gain settings are increased to fill in the structures of interest, and the image is rotated and cropped to show the pathology of interest. Additional acquisition of a four-beat full-volume dataset allows further cropping and analysis with higher-density image data.

With color Doppler imaging, the color sector is adjusted so that depth just includes the flows of interest, which allows a higher frame rate because of the shorter pulse-repetition frequency at a lesser depth. However, the color sector should always extend to the top of the image because frame rate is not improved by excluding this section of the image. Usually, color flow data are recorded initially with a relatively wide sector width to ensure that the spatial extent of the flow disturbance is visualized, with the sector width then narrowed to allow a higher frame rate. For vena contracta or proximal isovelocity surface area calculations, the color scale baseline and Nyquist limit also are adjusted to provide clear definition of the jet width and the proximal acceleration zone (Fig. 18.12).

Spectral Doppler is recorded using the same principles as those used for any Doppler recording. Gray-scale gain and low-pass ("wall") filters are adjusted to optimize the flow signal, the velocity scale is adjusted so the flow signal fits within but nearly fills the velocity range, the zero baseline is adjusted up or down depending on the flow of interest, and data are recorded with the time scale at 50 to 100 mm/s.

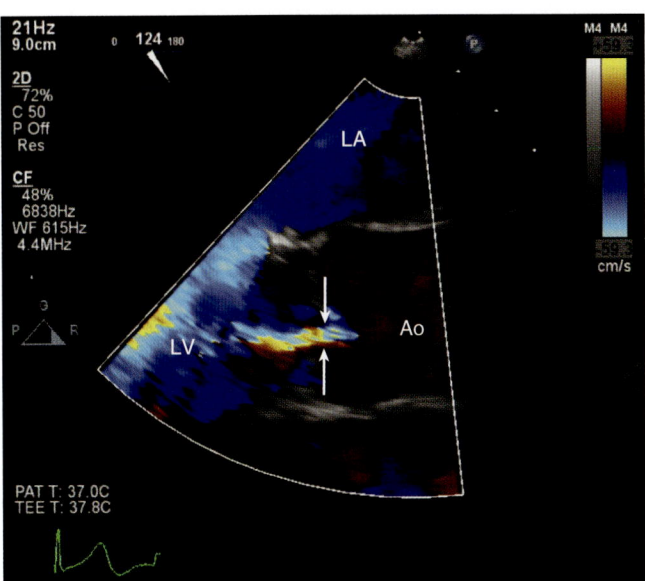

Fig. 18.12 Aortic regurgitation vena contracta. ▶ Measurement of vena contracta width *(arrows)* is most accurate using zoom mode to enlarge the area of interest. The image plane and color parameters are adjusted to show the proximal flow acceleration, the narrow vena contracta, and distal jet expansion. In this example, vena contracta width is 3 mm consistent with mild regurgitation. *Ao,* Aorta.

CLINICAL UTILITY OF INTRAOPERATIVE TEE

Clinical applications of intraoperative and intraprocedural TEE continue to evolve as new surgical and percutaneous approaches are developed. Some of the current established indications are briefly discussed here as examples of the clinical utility of this approach. Echocardiographers performing TEE during surgical or percutaneous procedures should obtain additional training and consult reference sources as appropriate.

Monitoring Ventricular Function

Intraoperative TEE is useful in high-risk patients undergoing cardiac or noncardiac surgical procedures (Table 18.4). Images of the LV provide continuous monitoring of:

- Ventricular preload (LV volume)
- Overall LV systolic function
- Regional LV function
- RV function

In general, the size of the ventricular chamber is a direct reflection of filling volume and can be used to optimize preload. Typically, ventricular size is evaluated qualitatively during the procedure, although a quick measurement of end-diastolic and end-systolic dimensions provides a useful scale factor at baseline. In most patients, increases in filling volumes and pressures correlate with increases in ventricular volumes. Conversely, ventricular size is small, despite adequate filling pressures, in patients with restrictive cardiomyopathy, pericardial constraint, and severe right heart dysfunction or in high contractility states.

Overall systolic function is usually estimated visually in the transgastric short-axis view. The area change in ventricular size provides a quick and accurate visual correlate of ejection fraction (see Chapter 6). Although 2D or 3D measurements of ejection fraction are well validated and recommended at baseline, repeated measurements are not always feasible given the rapid time course of hemodynamic changes in the operating room. Similarly, although Doppler cardiac output measurements in the aorta or pulmonary artery can be reliably made, time factors make these approaches unrealistic. In addition, cardiac output typically is continuously monitored by right heart catheter techniques.

The transgastric short-axis view is also useful for monitoring regional ventricular function because it includes myocardium supplied by all three major coronary arteries (Fig. 18.13). An acute change in regional ventricular function suggests coronary ischemia, although changes in regional wall motion are not always due to epicardial coronary disease. Other causes of regional dysfunction include hypovolemia, conduction defects, and myocardial stunning after cardiopulmonary bypass. TEE monitoring of ventricular function during interventions to reverse ischemia allow assessment of the effects of therapy. Evaluation of RV systolic function is important because dysfunction may occur due to inadequate cardioplegia or air embolism, which preferentially affects the right coronary artery when separating from cardiopulmonary bypass. Coronary ischemia in the distribution of a coronary bypass graft may also be due to mechanical occlusion or a kink in a vein graft or spasm of an internal mammary graft.

TABLE 18.4 Basic Principles for Intraoperative or Intraprocedural TEE

Parameter	View	Additional Imaging	Clinical Pointers
LV Function			
LV volumes	• Image LV in mid-esophageal 4-chamber and 2-chamber views; trace at end-systole and end-diastole for LV volume calculation.	• Acquire multibeat full volume for 3D measurements.	
Cardiac output	• Calculate LV outflow tract circular CSA using diameter in mid-esophageal long-axis view. • Record pulsed Doppler VTI from transgastric long-axis or apical view.	• Alternatively use 3D zoom or full-volume mode to allow multiplanar reconstruction of the LV outflow tract and planimetry to measure its area.	• Measurements should be made in systole. • Calculate stroke volume as LV outflow CSA times VTI. Multiply by heart rate for cardiac output.
Ejection fraction	• 3D or 2D biplane LV volumes and EF from a high TEE 4-chamber and 2-chamber view	• Calculate fractional area change using planimetry of mid-papillary transgastric short-axis views of the LV in systole and diastole.	• Use 3D software to calculate volumes and EF.
Other measures of global systolic function	• Visual assessment of endocardial and myocardial thickening in each myocardial segment	• Image mitral valve in mid-esophageal 4-chamber to facilitate tissue Doppler imaging of lateral mitral annulus with measurement of S'.	
Strain	• Measure strain using speckle tracking in the mid-esophageal views and the transgastric midpapillary view.	• Recognize that properly identifying the region of interest is of paramount importance.	• Global longitudinal strain is an alternate measure of global LV systolic function. Target diagrams display regional function.
Diastolic function	• Image mitral valve in mid-esophageal 4-chamber view to acquire pulsed-wave Doppler inflow. • Image pulmonary vein to acquire pulsed-wave Doppler flow.	• Image mitral valve in mid-esophageal 4-chamber view to facilitate tissue Doppler imaging of lateral mitral annulus.	• Measure E, A, and DT from mitral inflow. • Measure E' and A' on tissue Doppler. • Calculate E/E'.
RV Function			
Global RV systolic function	• Using the transgastric window, align M-mode parallel to the lateral tricuspid annulus for TAPSE.	• Using the transgastric window, align tissue Doppler gate parallel to the lateral tricuspid annulus to assess S'.	• Measure TAPSE and S'.
Regional wall motion	• Visual assessment of endocardial and myocardial thickening	• Measure strain using speckle tracking.	• Acquire 3D volumes.
Position and Function of Intracardiac Devices			
Position of IABP	• Image the descending thoracic aorta.	• Identify the tip of the balloon (suspending its inflation temporarily may help).	• Image the left subclavian artery. • Assess the distance between balloon tip and left subclavian artery.
LVAD inflow cannulae	• Image LV in mid-esophageal 4-chamber and 2-chamber views.	• Assess position of the cannula tip relative to the ventricular walls.	• Also consider 3D to assess cannula position. • Color Doppler to assess velocities

TABLE 18.4 Basic Principles for Intraoperative or Intraprocedural TEE—cont'd

Parameter	View	Additional Imaging	Clinical Pointers
LVAD outflow cannula	• Image the mid-esophageal long axis and look for cannula entering the ascending aorta.	• Use color Doppler to assess velocities.	
Percutaneous transaortic LV assist device	• Image the mid-esophageal long axis.	• Assess aortic valve pathology.	• Asses depth of device into LV. • Assess mitral valve function.
Total artificial heart	• Use mid-esophageal 4-chamber view to assess mechanical atrioventricular valves. • Also visualize atria and adjacent pericardial or pleural fluid.	• Mid-esophageal long-axis views to look at aortic and pulmonic prosthetic valves.	• Look for central "cleaning" jets with this type of mechanical valve. • Be vigilant for atrial compression from effusions.
V-V ECMO	• Image the venae cavae and the tricuspid valve using a bicaval view. • Obtain a transgastric long-axis view of the right heart.	• Use color Doppler to ensure that outflow from the device goes through tricuspid valve into the RV.	
Coronary sinus cannula	• View in low mid-esophageal 4-chamber view with retroflexion.	• View in bicaval with medial turn of probe.	
Femoral venous cannula	• Bicaval view		

CSA, Cross-sectional area; *DT*, deceleration time; *EF*, ejection fraction; *IABP*, intraaortic balloon pump; *LVAD*, LV assist device; *TAPSE*, tricuspid annular plane systolic excursion; *V-V ECMO*, venovenous extracorporeal membrane oxygenation; *VTI*, velocity-time integral.
Modified from Hall MT, Oxorn DC: Intraoperative and procedure echocardiography: basic principles. In Otto CM, editor: *The Practice of Clinical Echocardiography*, ed 5, Philadelphia, 2017, Elsevier.

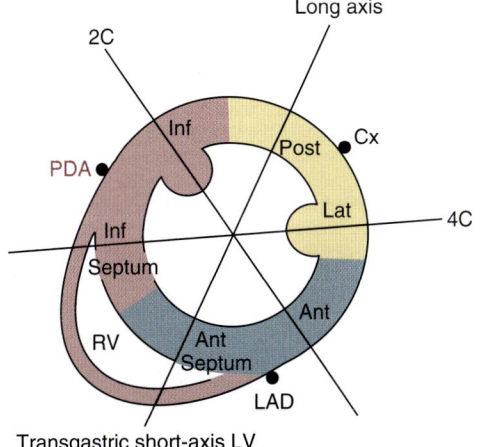

Fig. 18.13 Schematic transgastric short-axis view showing the relationship between regional wall motion and coronary anatomy. The intersecting lines show which myocardial segments are seen in the mid-esophageal four-chamber *(4C)*, two-chamber *(2C)*, and long-axis views. Typically, the inferior *(Inf)* septum and inferior wall are perfused by the posterior descending coronary artery *(PDA)*; the anterior *(Ant)* septum and anterior wall by the left anterior descending *(LAD)* coronary artery; and the lateral *(Lat)* and posterior *(Post)* walls by branches of the circumflex *(Cx)* coronary artery.

Valvular Heart Disease

Mitral Valve Repair

In patients undergoing elective mitral valve repair, the baseline intraoperative TEE provides additional detailed 2D and 3D information on mitral valve anatomy and the mechanism and severity of regurgitation (Fig. 18.14). If needed, annular size is measured in four-chamber and long-axis views or with 3D imaging.

Even when a comprehensive preoperative examination has been done, the echocardiographer in the operating room needs to be familiar with, and record, images demonstrating the baseline pathology for comparison with the postrepair study. Standard terminology for mitral valve anatomy facilitates communication between the echocardiographer and the surgeon. The anterior and posterior leaflets meet at the medial and lateral valve commissures, with the posterior leaflet extending around more of the annulus than the anterior leaflet. The posterior mitral leaflet typically has three distinct scallops, which are labeled from the perspective of a surgeon looking at the valve from the LA side. Thus, posterior leaflet scallops are

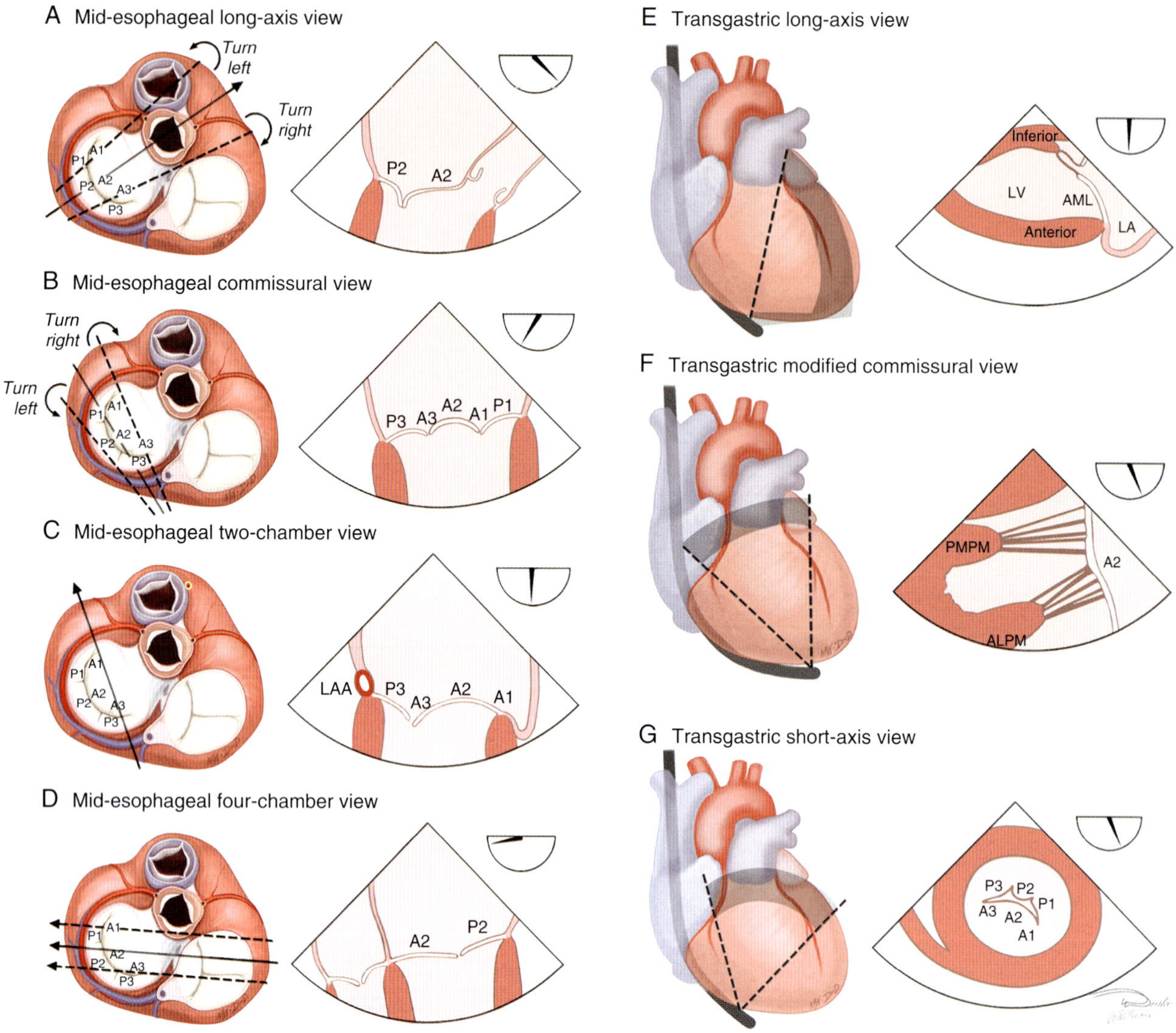

Fig. 18.14 Standard 2D transesophageal views for assessing the mitral valve. *Lines* indicate the expected positions of the scan planes in different views. In the mid-esophageal long-axis and commissural positions, *dashed lines* indicate the effect of turning the probe left (counterclockwise) or right (clockwise) from the standard positions. Using the annulus diameter and position of the LV apex as landmarks ensures that the long-axis view reliably visualizes the A2/P2 coaptive surface and the commissural view visualizes the A1/A2 and A3/P3 coaptive surfaces. In the mid-esophageal four-chamber view, *dashed lines* indicate the effect of withdrawing/anteflexing or advancing/retroflexing the probe from the standard position. *ALPM*, Anterolateral papillary muscle; *AML*, anterior mitral leaflet; *LAA*, LA appendage; *PMPM*, posteromedial papillary muscle. *(From Drake DH, Zimmerman KG, Sidebotham DA: Transesophageal echocardiography for surgical repair of mitral regurgitation. In Otto CM, editor:* The Practice of Clinical Echocardiography, *ed 5, Philadelphia, 2017, Elsevier, Fig. 19.4.)*

numbered from lateral (P1) to medial (P3), with central (P2) in the middle, with corresponding terms for the anterior leaflet.

Using rotational scanning from a mid-esophageal transducer position, both the four-chamber and long-axis views show the central (A2 and P2) scallops of both leaflets. As the image plane is rotated from 0° to 45°, first A3 and P1 are seen, and then, with further rotation, both P3 and P1 are seen in the "bicommissural view," typically at a rotation angle of 60° to 90°. In this view, both the medial and lateral commissures are seen, with the P3 and P1 posterior leaflet scallops at their attachments to the annulus. The central (A2) anterior leaflet scallop fills the center section of the annulus, and it moves in and out of the image during the cardiac cycle.

Another approach to the visualization of the mitral leaflet scallops is to start in the four-chamber view and then either tilt the image plane superiorly or slightly withdraw the probe, to show the more anterior or lateral scallops (A1 and P1), then tilt posteriorly or advance the probe to show the posterior or medial segments (A3 and P3). From the two-chamber or bicommissural plane, turning the image plane toward

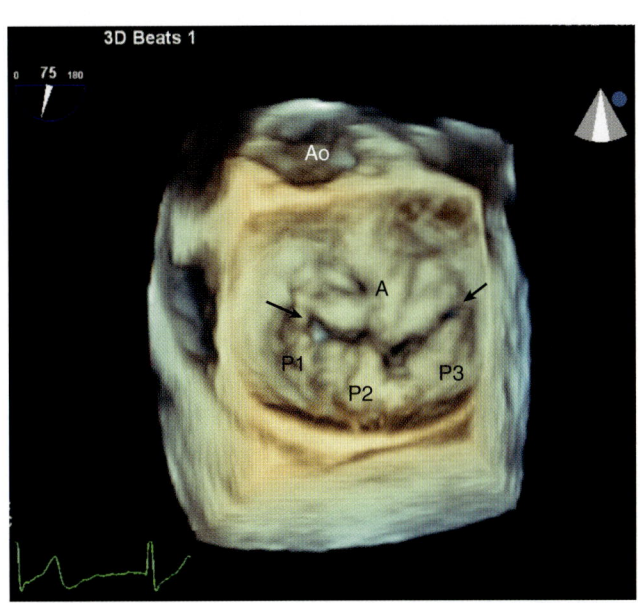

Fig. 18.15 **3D TEE imaging of the mitral valve.** ▶ Standard procedural 3D view of the mitral valve viewed from the LA side with the anterior leaflet *(A)* on top and the posterior leaflet with three segments from lateral *(P1)* to medial *(P3)* as indicated. This patient with mild diffuse leaflet thickening and prolapse also has inadequate coaptation at the lateral and medical commissures *(arrow)*. Ao, Aorta.

the patient's right side shows all three scallops of the anterior leaflet, and turning leftward shows all three scallops of the posterior leaflet. Transgastric short-axis views at the mitral valve level also are helpful.

Mitral valve anatomy in patients undergoing surgical repair for mitral regurgitation is well visualized by 3D echocardiography (Fig. 18.15). The position of the TEE transducer posterior to the mitral valve, with the ultrasound imaging beam relatively perpendicular to the surface of the closed valve, results in excellent image quality and the ability to include the entire valve in the image field. As 3D imaging becomes widely available in formats that allow real-time or rapid image reconstruction, 3D imaging of the mitral valve likely will become the standard approach to evaluation in the operating room.

The mechanism of regurgitation in patients undergoing mitral valve repair most often is myxomatous disease, with fewer cases of rheumatic valve disease. With primary leaflet disease, anatomy is described for each leaflet segment in terms of thickness, redundancy, and motion, and any areas of calcification or chordal fusion and shortening are described. Prolapse describes motion of the leaflet into the LA in systole, with a curved shape in systole due to intact chordal attachments (Fig. 18.16). A flail segment indicates chordal rupture with the tip of the disrupted segment directed toward the LA in systole. Secondary mitral regurgitation often is due to ischemic disease. With secondary mitral regurgitation, leaflet motion typically is restricted with a tethering effect due to LV dilation and regional wall motion, which results in inadequate systolic leaflet coaptation. Restricted leaflet motion also is seen with rheumatic valve disease or with dilated cardiomyopathy.

Color Doppler imaging is helpful for determining the mechanism of mitral regurgitation. The origin of the regurgitant jet as it crosses the valve indicates the area of inadequate coaptation. The direction of the regurgitant jet in the atrium tends to be anterior with posterior leaflet dysfunction, posterior with anterior leaflet dysfunction, and central with functional regurgitation. Complex or multiple jets are seen when more than one mechanism of regurgitation is present.

Regurgitant severity is best evaluated before the patient is anesthetized in the operating room because of the potential effects of altered loading conditions. However, baseline measures of regurgitant severity are needed for comparison with the postrepair images. Jet size and shape are not reliable indicators of regurgitant severity because they are affected by many other factors, including driving pressure, chamber size and compliance, and cardiac rhythm. The recommended basic measurements of mitral regurgitant severity in the operating room are:

- Vena contracta width
- CW Doppler signal intensity relative to antegrade flow
- Pulmonary vein systolic flow reversal

A simple, reliable measure of regurgitant severity is vena contracta width, with the echocardiographer taking care to measure the narrowest diameter between the proximal jet acceleration on the ventricular side of the valve and the area of jet expansion in the LA. Accuracy is enhanced by using zoom images, a fast frame rate, and careful image alignment (see Chapter 12). The CW Doppler signal density compared with antegrade flow also provides a quick qualitative measure of regurgitant severity. Pulmonary vein systolic flow reversal indicates severe regurgitation in patients

I	II	IIIa	IIIb

Fig. 18.16 Carpentier classification for leaflet dysfunction. Type I dysfunction is defined as mitral regurgitation in the presence of normal leaflet motion. Examples include annular dilatation, leaflet perforation, and leaflet cleft. Type I dysfunction can also result from the combination of degenerative and secondary disease. Type II dysfunction refers to excessive leaflet motion. Examples include leaflet prolapse and flail due to degenerative disease. Type III dysfunction refers to restricted leaflet motion. Type IIIa is leaflet restriction that occurs predominantly in diastole. Examples include rheumatic disease, radiation-induced valvulopathy, and dystrophic calcification. Type IIIb is leaflet restriction that occurs predominantly in systole. Type IIIb may be symmetric or asymmetric. Examples include dilated cardiomyopathy (symmetric) and myocardial infarction (asymmetric). *(From Drake DH, Zimmerman KG, Sidebotham DA: Transesophageal echocardiography for surgical repair of mitral regurgitation. In Otto CM, editor: The Practice of Clinical Echocardiography, ed 5, Philadelphia, 2017, Elsevier, Fig. 19.2.)*

in sinus rhythm, although interrogation of all four pulmonary veins is needed with eccentric jets. In nonsinus rhythms, the pulmonary vein flow pattern is altered because of the rhythm and is not an accurate reflection of regurgitant severity. If further quantitation is needed, the proximal isovelocity surface area approach can be applied in the operating room.

After the surgical valve repair and weaning from cardiopulmonary bypass, imaging and Doppler studies of the mitral valve are repeated. Loading conditions should be adjusted to match conditions at the time of the baseline study as much as possible, and the same image planes and Doppler flows should be recorded with the same instrument settings (Fig. 18.17). The most common mitral valve repair is quadrangular resection of a posterior leaflet scallop (usually P2), with reapproximation and suturing of the resected edges and placement of an annuloplasty ring. The exact repair varies from patient to patient; more complex repairs include modifications to the anterior leaflets, use of artificial chords, and chordal transfer or shortening. Knowledge of the exact repair is needed for the postpump TEE evaluation to ensure that expected postoperative changes are distinguished from abnormal findings. The use of intraprocedural TEE is associated with a higher rate of successful mitral valve repair at both academic and community medical centers.

Complications of mitral valve repair detectable by TEE include:

- Persistent mitral regurgitation
- Systolic anterior mitral leaflet motion
- Mitral stenosis
- Ventricular systolic dysfunction
- Injury of the circumflex artery
- Tricuspid regurgitation

With a successful mitral valve repair, no or minimal residual mitral regurgitation occurs. More than trivial mitral regurgitation, after optimization of loading conditions, should prompt consideration of an additional repair or valve replacement. Excessive reduction in mitral annular size is associated with systolic anterior motion of the mitral leaflet with resultant LV outflow obstruction and mitral regurgitation, although this complication is infrequent with current surgical techniques. Functional mitral stenosis can occur with some repairs and is easily detected by recording the antegrade mitral flow velocity after valve repair. Ventricular dysfunction often is transient because of cardioplegia; persistent dysfunction suggests preoperative dysfunction that is more evident with a competent mitral valve or a complication of the procedure, such as coronary artery air embolism. Tricuspid regurgitation often accompanies mitral valve disease and should be evaluated both at baseline and on the postrepair study.

Valve Stenosis

Whenever possible, aortic stenosis should be fully evaluated before the patient is in the operating room (see Chapter 11). TEE calculation of continuity equation valve area is possible in some cases if the LV outflow and aortic flow velocities can be recorded

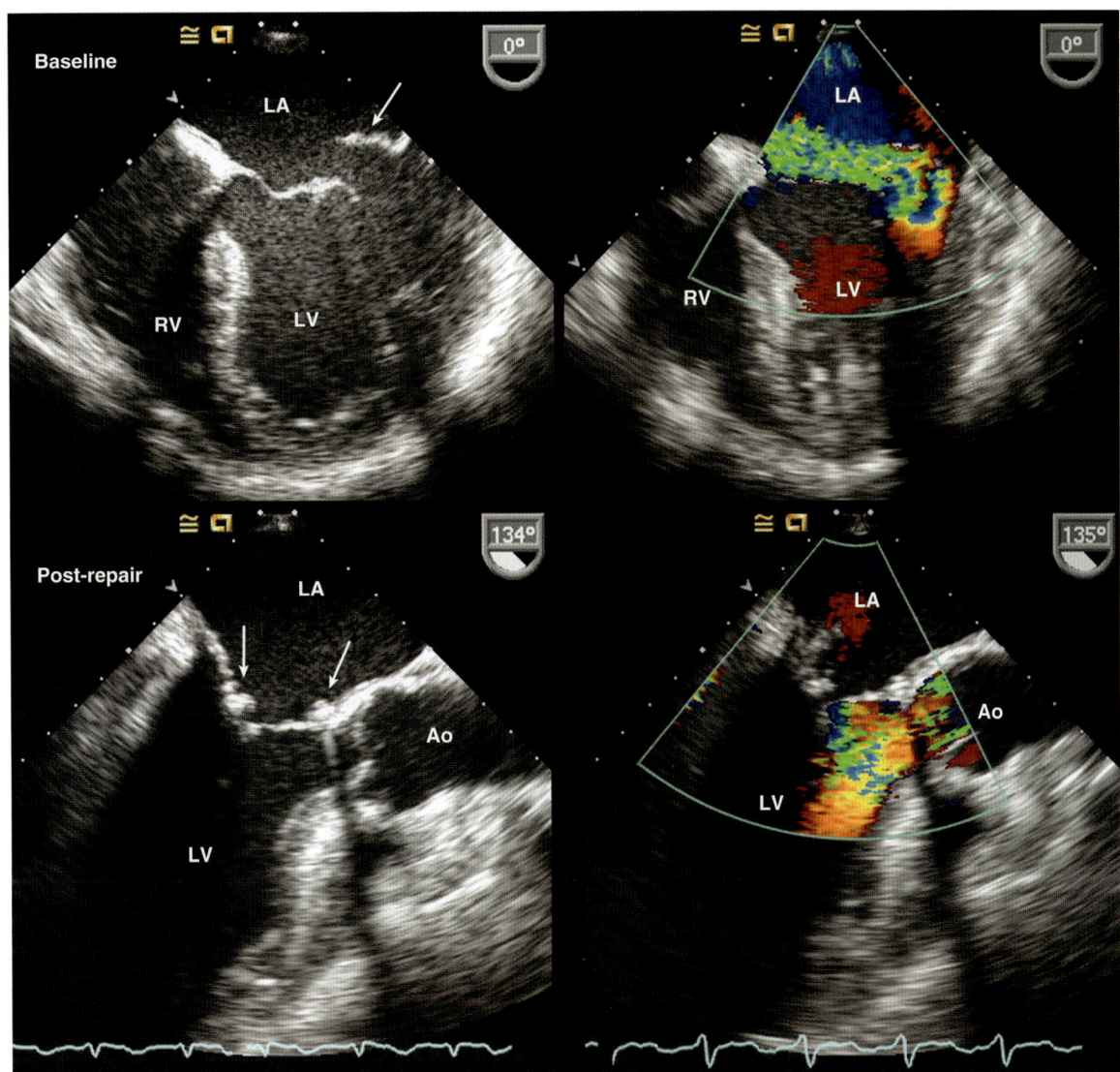

Fig. 18.17 Mitral valve repair. 2D *(left)* and color Doppler *(right)* intraoperative TEE images were taken in a patient with myxomatous mitral valve disease before *(top)* and after *(bottom)* mitral valve repair. Before repair, severe mitral prolapse with a partial flail leaflet segment and moderate to severe mitral regurgitation is seen in the four-chamber view. After repair, the long-axis view shows the annuloplasty ring *(arrows)*. Regurgitation was not detected at loading conditions similar to those of the baseline study. *Ao,* Aorta.

from transgastric long-axis planes. Unfortunately, this approach may significantly underestimate stenosis severity because of the inability to align the Doppler beam parallel to flow from a TEE approach, which results in inaccurate velocity data. TEE short-axis views of the valve are accurate for the determination of valve anatomy, and planimetry of valve area is possible in many cases. In other cases, the complex 3D geometry of the orifice and distortion of aortic valve anatomy are challenging; ensuring measurement at the minimal orifice is facilitated with 3D imaging (see Fig. 11.6). Reverberations and shadowing by valve calcification affect the accuracy of planimetry with either 2D or 3D approaches.

Some specific circumstances in which intraprocedural TEE evaluation is especially helpful are:

- Detection of bicuspid valve
- Degree of valve calcification
- Aortic sinus and ascending aorta dilation

For example, in the patient undergoing coronary bypass grafting, aortic valve replacement is appropriate with moderate or severe asymptomatic stenosis. In equivocal cases, the finding of a bicuspid aortic valve or extensive valve calcification on TEE tips the balance toward valve replacement. Conversely, a trileaflet valve with minimal calcification and only mild to moderate aortic stenosis does not need intervention. Bicuspid

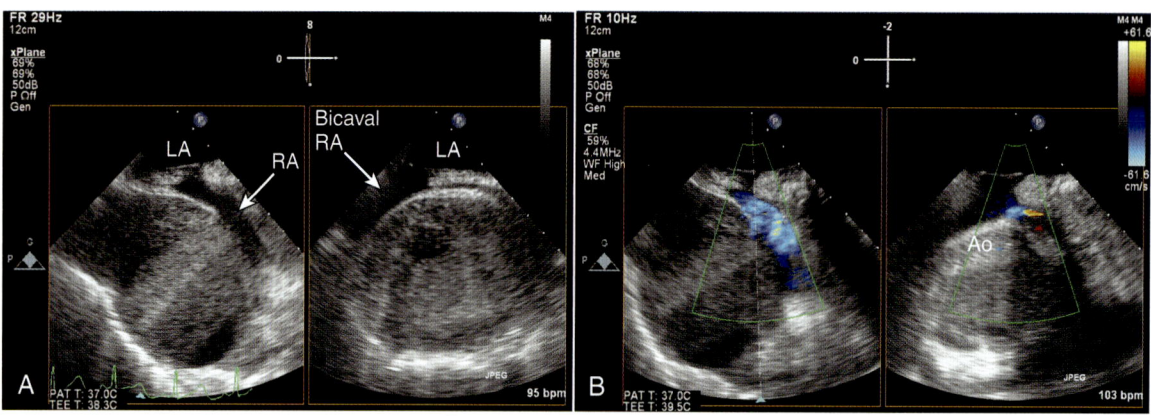

Fig. 18.18 Localized tamponade after aortic surgery. (A) ▶ In a patient with a complex aortic valve and root replacement with coronary reimplantation, hypotension in the early postoperative period was due to localized compression of the RA by pericardial thrombus, as seen in a simultaneous four-chamber and bicaval view using 3D TEE. (B) ▶ Color Doppler demonstrates a narrow flowstream in the compressed, slitlike RA.

aortic valve disease often is accompanied by aortic dilation. Intraprocedural TEE often provides improved images and measurements of the aortic sinuses and ascending aorta. The surgical approach may be modified to include aortic root replacement if significant aortic dilation is present that was not recognized preoperatively. With percutaneous or hybrid approaches to aortic valve replacement, intraprocedural TEE is used to monitor the procedure, ensure correct placement of the valve, provide immediate assessment of valve function, and detect any complications of the procedure (Fig. 18.18).

Endocarditis

Intraprocedural TEE is essential in patients undergoing valve surgery for endocarditis (see Chapter 14). The TEE study should include assessment of:

- Presence and location of vegetations
- Mechanisms of valve dysfunction
- Severity of regurgitation
- Paravalvular abscess
- Other complications such as fistulas, pseudoaneurysms

Given the complex patterns of valve destruction with endocarditis, careful review of the images with the surgeon is essential for planning the operative repair. Even with a complete presurgical evaluation, additional changes may occur between the time of that study and the surgical procedure, so the echocardiographer should perform a complete study. The baseline intraprocedural study also provides a comparison with the postprocedure images.

Prosthetic Valve Dysfunction

After implantation of a prosthetic valve, TEE evaluation is helpful to confirm normal function. In addition to the normal patterns of mild regurgitation for prosthetic valves, a small amount of paravalvular regurgitation is not unusual immediately after implantation. However, a significant paravalvular leak suggests suture dehiscence that may require immediate intervention. The orientation and function of a mechanical valve are easily visualized (Fig. 18.19). Occasionally, mechanical valve disk motion is impaired by excessive retained mitral leaflet tissue or other anatomic factors.

Aortic Disease

Aortic Dissection

Intraprocedural TEE is accurate for the diagnosis of the presence and extent of an aortic dissection. Often, these patients are promptly transferred to the operating room after a CT scan showing an ascending aortic dissection, with no prior TEE imaging. The intraprocedural study confirms the presence and origin of the dissection flap and provides assessment of aortic valve function (Fig. 18.20). It is particularly important to determine whether the dissection involves the ascending aorta (type A), requiring surgical intervention, or whether it affects only the descending aorta (type B), often managed medically.

A complete examination of the aorta includes mid-esophageal views of the sinuses and the ascending aorta in both short- and long-axis views, thereby ensuring that the aorta is examined from the annulus level as far superiorly as possible with slow withdrawal of the probe (see Chapter 16). Aortic diameters are measured at end-diastole, from the inner edge to inner edge of the black-white interface, at the annulus, sinuses, sinotubular junction, and mid-ascending aorta. The descending thoracic aorta is imaged from the transgastric position to a very high esophageal position with slow withdrawal of the probe in the esophagus. Sequential short-axis views ensure that the entire

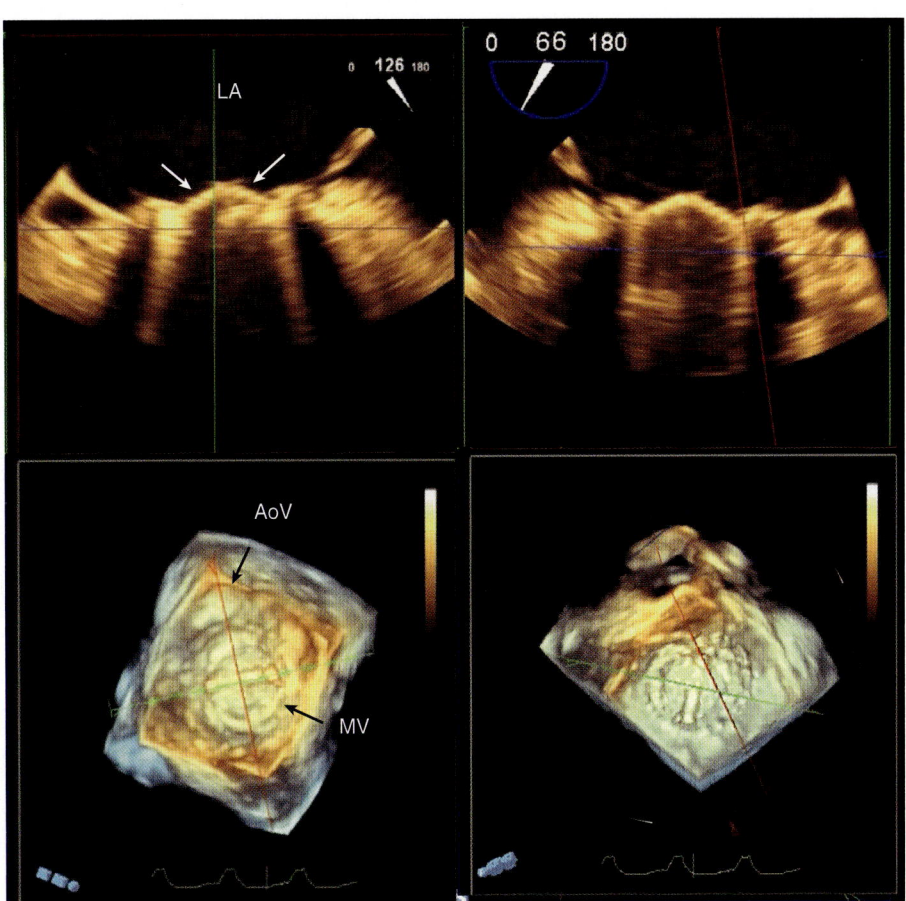

Fig. 18.19 Intraoperative transesophageal echocardiography after mechanical mitral valve replacement. In the patient on the *left*, the mitral valve *(MV)* has been implanted in the "anatomic" position, with the location of the two prosthetic valve occluders matching the normal positions of the native anterior and posterior mitral valve leaflets. The *bottom left* shows the "surgeon's view" (the view the surgeon would have from the right side of the operating table with the LA open), with the *red line* intersecting the valve, resulting in the reconstructed 2D mid-esophageal long-axis view seen in the *top left* image. The leaflets close symmetrically and are indicated by *white arrows*. In the patient on the *right*, the valve has been implanted in the "antianatomic position" with the prosthetic valve occluders oriented at about 90° from the positions of the native valve leaflets. In the 3D image *(lower right)*, the *green line* intersects the valve, resulting in a reconstructed 2D image plane similar to a bicommissural view *(top right)*. The leaflets again close symmetrically. *AoV*, Aortic valve. *(From Oxorn DC, Otto CM: Surgical prosthetic valves. In Oxorn DC, Otto CM, editors: Intraoperative and Interventional Echocardiography: Atlas of Transesophageal Imaging, ed 2, Philadelphia, 2017, Elsevier, Fig. 5.25.)*

endocardial surface is visualized. Supplemented long-axis views at each level are appropriate, especially when abnormal findings are present; however, abnormalities medial or lateral to the long-axis plane are missed with this approach. Descending aortic diameter is measured in the distal, mid-, and proximal descending aorta. The aortic arch is seen from a high TEE position with the image plane turned and tilted to show the length of the arch. In each view, depth and gain settings are adjusted to optimize visualization of a dissection flap, intramural hematoma, or atheroma. Color Doppler is helpful in showing flow patterns in the true and false lumens when a dissection is present. The spectral Doppler pattern, recorded in a long-axis view of the descending aorta, shows holodiastolic flow reversal when severe aortic regurgitation is present.

Other key findings are regional wall motion abnormalities, resulting from involvement of the right coronary artery, and pericardial effusion, resulting from impending rupture. After the repair, a dissection flap typically persists in the descending aorta, and the postrepair TEE images serve as a baseline for future follow-up studies. If the aortic valve has been resuspended, postrepair imaging of leaflet opening and Doppler evaluation for regurgitation are essential.

Aortic Atheroma

Cardiac surgery usually involves cannulation or manipulation of the aorta, which is associated with adverse neurologic events because of embolization of aortic atheromas (Fig. 18.21). Detection of a

Fig. 18.20 Intraoperative transesophageal aortic dissection. (A) ▶ In this mid-esophageal short-axis view, a fenestrated dissection flap is seen during systole *(arrow, left)*. In diastole *(top right)*, the right coronary artery is seen *(arrow)*. (B) ▶ In the long-axis view, the *left* image clearly shows the dissection flap *(arrow)*. In addition, the aortic diameter at the level of the sinuses of Valsalva is enlarged at 5 cm. On the *bottom right*, the arrow indicates trace aortic regurgitation. *AoV*, Aortic valve; *RVOT*, RV outflow tract. (From Oxorn DC: Intraoperative and procedural echocardiography: basic principles. In Otto CM, editor: The Practice of Clinical Echocardiography, ed 5, Philadelphia, 2017, Elsevier, Figs. 10.23 and 10.24.)

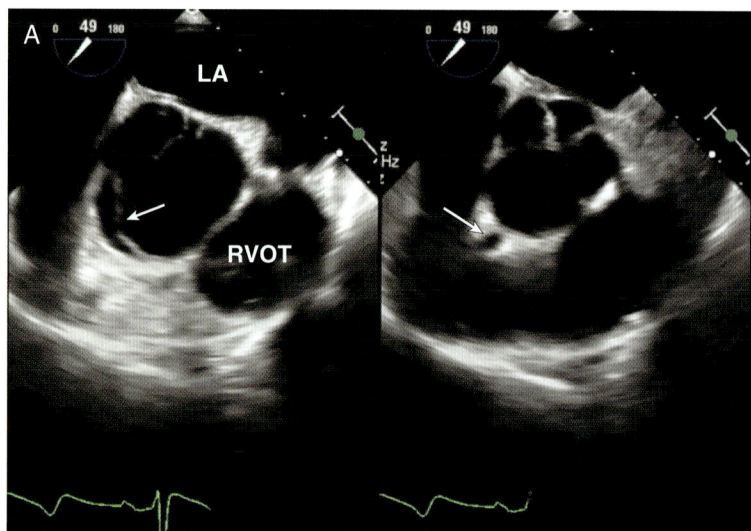

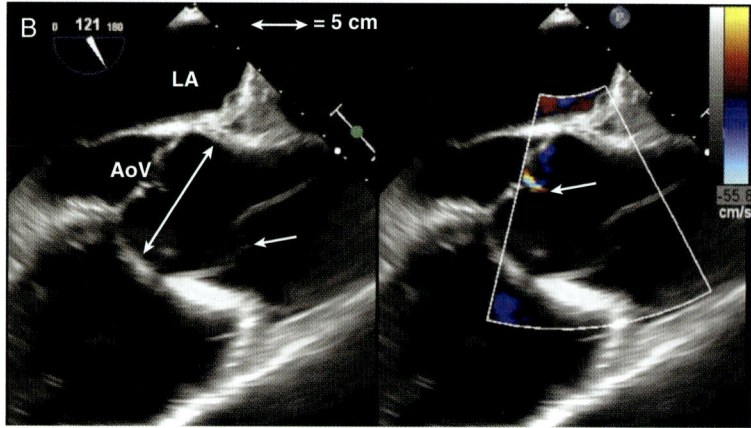

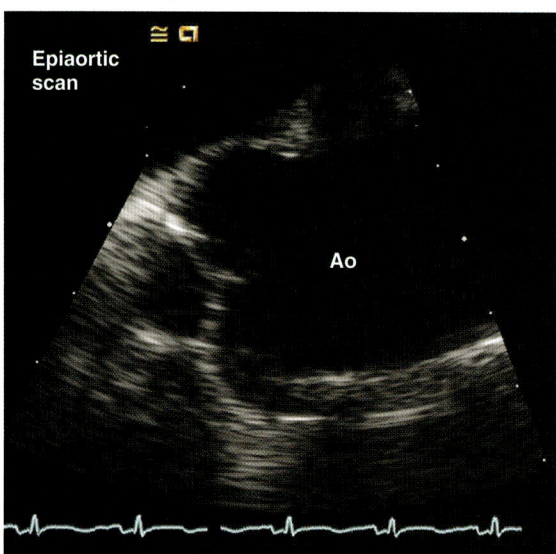

Fig. 18.21 Epiaortic scan. Long-axis view of the aortic valve, aortic sinuses, and proximal ascending aorta *(Ao)* on an epiaortic scan with the transducer in a sterile sleeve placed directly on the anterior surface of the heart during the cardiac surgical procedure. No significant atheromas are seen in this example.

protruding, mobile, or large (>3 mm) atheroma is a marker of increased risk. Atheroma can be detected by TEE, although epiaortic scanning provides higher accuracy because it allows for more complete imaging of the entire endothelial surface of the ascending aorta. The recommended minimum epiaortic examination consists of three short-axis views of the ascending aorta (proximal, mid-, and distal) and two long-axis views (proximal and distal). The location of any plaques should be described with measurement of plaque thickness and notation of any mobile components.

Cardiomyopathies

Hypertrophic Cardiomyopathy

Intraprocedural TEE is used to guide the extent of myectomy in patients with LV outflow obstruction resulting from hypertrophic cardiomyopathy to assess:

- Severity and location of septal hypertrophy
- Immediate hemodynamic results
- Complications of the procedure

Careful evaluation of the degree and location of hypertrophy in terms of distance from the aortic valve and by myocardial segment allows for tailoring of the depth, width, and length of the myomectomy (see Chapter 9). Imaging is performed from both midesophageal and transgastric transducer positions, using multiple image planes to assess septal anatomy fully. Color Doppler localizes the level of obstruction at the site of flow acceleration in the LV outflow tract and is useful for the detection and evaluation of associated mitral regurgitation. The LV outflow gradient may be recorded with CW Doppler from a deep transgastric view or the transgastric long-axis view, although underestimation is likely because of a nonparallel intercept angle.

After the procedure, TEE allows assessment of residual outflow obstruction and detection of complications, such as a ventricular septal defect. Often, LV outflow obstruction caused by systolic anterior motion of the mitral valve is accompanied by significant mitral regurgitation, which resolves when normal mitral leaflet motion is restored. Postoperative TEE results in additional surgical procedures in about 4% of cases.

Ventricular Assist Devices

When placement of a ventricular assist device is considered, intraprocedural TEE ensures that the patient has no preexisting contraindications to this procedure, for example, significant aortic regurgitation would result in an inability to unload the LV. Another example is a patent foramen ovale, which allows right-to-left shunting when left-sided pressure is reduced, leading to arterial oxygen desaturation or paradoxical embolism. The presence of an aortic atheroma also influences the exact site for placement of the aortic inflow cannula. LV or LA clot also should be excluded.

In addition, intraprocedural TEE assists with the placement of ventricular assist devices by assessment of (see Table 18.4):

- Placement of inflow and outflow cannula
- Ventricular volumes and systolic function
- Doppler inflow and outflow velocities
- De-airing of the pump before activation

LV assist devices include extracorporeal devices that use cannulas and an external pump to direct blood from the LV apex into the aorta. Some pumps provide pulsatile flow, whereas others provide nonpulsatile axial (continuous) flow. Some devices are placed percutaneously, directing blood from the LA (via a transseptal cannula) into the aorta. In addition, some intracorporeal devices fit inside the heart. Because these devices are currently in development, frequent changes in technology occur, so the echocardiographer needs information on each specific device, including information on the use of cannulas, optimal device or cannula placement, and expected flow patterns

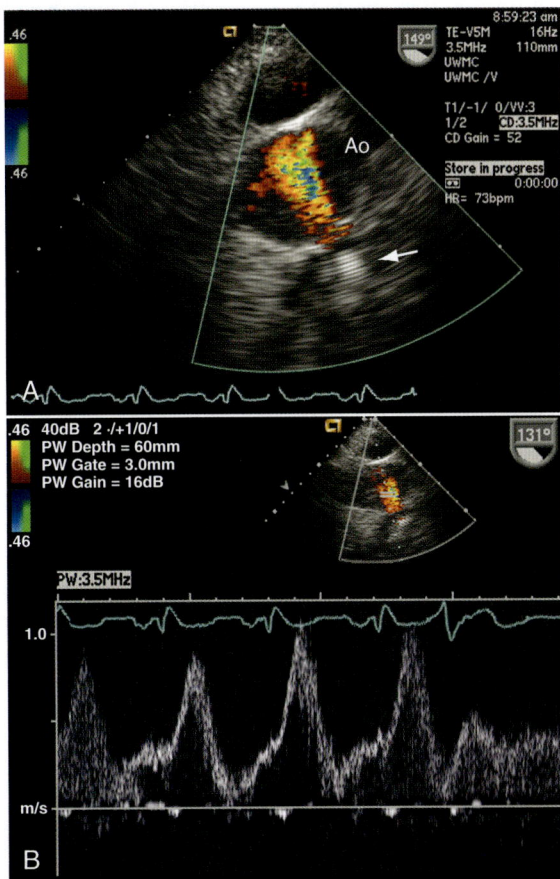

Fig. 18.22 Left ventricular assist device. ▶ (A) TEE in a patient with an LV assist device shows the color Doppler signal of flow from the outflow cannula *(arrow)* into the ascending aorta *(Ao)*. (B) Pulsed *(PW)* Doppler interrogation of this flow shows predominant systolic flow about 1 m/s in velocity, with persistent antegrade flow in diastole.

(Fig. 18.22). Complications of ventricular assist devices include intracardiac thrombus formation, obstruction of inflow or outflow cannula as a result of positioning or thrombus formation, regurgitation of the pump valves, and inadequate flow volumes. Nonpulsatile devices are challenging to evaluate by TEE, but ventricular size is one factor in adjusting flow rates for these devices. With continuous flow devices, excessive LV drainage results in collapse of the ventricular chamber that leads to obstruction of the inflow cannula and a drop in flow rates.

Heart Transplantation

After heart transplantation, intraprocedural TEE is used to evaluate the anastomoses to the aorta and the pulmonary artery. The RA and LA anastomoses also are evaluated to ensure that no obstruction to systemic or pulmonary venous return exists and to serve as a baseline for atrial anatomy on subsequent diagnostic studies. With lung transplantation, all four pulmonary veins are imaged with recording of Doppler flow to ensure normal flow patterns. Evaluation of RV size and systolic function is particularly important after either heart or lung transplantation.

Congenital Heart Disease

Intraprocedural TEE is essential in the surgical and percutaneous management of patients with congenital heart disease (see Chapter 17). Postprocedure evaluation ensures complete closure of ventricular and atrial septal defects, functional status of repaired or replacement valves, and patency of conduits. Except for simple defects, such as closure of an isolated atrial septal defect, intraprocedural TEE for congenital heart disease should be performed by echocardiographers with additional training and experience in pediatric or adult congenital heart disease.

CLINICAL UTILITY IN TRANSCATHETER AND HYBRID PROCEDURES

The approach to echocardiographic imaging in patients undergoing transcatheter procedures for structural heart disease parallels the basic approach to intraoperative TEE. A complete diagnostic transthoracic study is performed before the procedure, along with other imaging tests as needed for decision making about the timing and type of intervention. A preprocedure TEE also is appropriate in many cases to allow optimal visualization of the anatomy and to aid in planning the procedure. During the procedure, views that show the anatomy and allow guidance of the procedure are used for monitoring; 3D imaging is particularly helpful for transcatheter intervention (Table 18.5). After the procedure, images and Doppler data are acquired to evaluate procedural results and detect complications.

Echocardiographic imaging is used to guide interventions for several types of structural heart disease (Fig. 18.23). Rapid advances in interventional procedures for structural heart disease will require the echocardiographer to work closely with the interventional team to provide useful imaging data.

TEE monitoring during interventional procedures typically requires general anesthesia because patients do not tolerate having the probe in position for a long period while awake. When general anesthesia is needed for the procedure itself, this is not an issue, but in other cases, alternate echocardiographic approaches, such as TTE or intracardiac echocardiography, may be more appropriate.

TABLE 18.5 Echocardiography in Transcatheter Interventions for Valve Disease

Procedures	Preprocedural Evaluation	Procedural Monitoring	Evaluation of Complications
Transcatheter aortic valve implantation	Aortic stenosis severity Leaflet number and calcification Annulus diameter (2D TTE or TEE)	Aortic cusp length (<annular-coronary ostial distance) LV outflow tract shape (avoid subaortic septal bulge) Assess for aortic atheroma. Positioning and function of prosthetic valve	Paraprosthetic regurgitation Mitral regurgitation Coronary ostial occlusion (LV wall motion abnormalities) Cardiac tamponade Aortic dissection or rupture
Balloon mitral valvotomy	Mitral stenosis severity Mitral valve morphology Commissural fusion and calcification Coexisting mitral regurgitation LA thrombus	Transseptal puncture Position of dilating balloon Changes in ΔP and MVA Mitral regurgitation severity	Worsening mitral regurgitation Atrial septal defect
Transcatheter mitral valve repair	Valve anatomy Severity of mitral regurgitation Mechanism of mitral regurgitation Mitral coaptation length and depth Flail leaflet gap and width	Transseptal puncture Position of delivery system Residual regurgitation	Leaflet or chordal tears Pericardial effusion Suboptimal position of device
Closure of prosthetic paravalvular regurgitation	Presence and severity of paraprosthetic mitral regurgitation Prosthetic valve function LA thrombus	Location and size of paravalvular defects (3D TEE) Catheter placement Seating of device	Residual regurgitation Device dislodgment Pericardial effusion/tamponade

MVA, Mitral valve area; *ΔP*, pressure gradient.

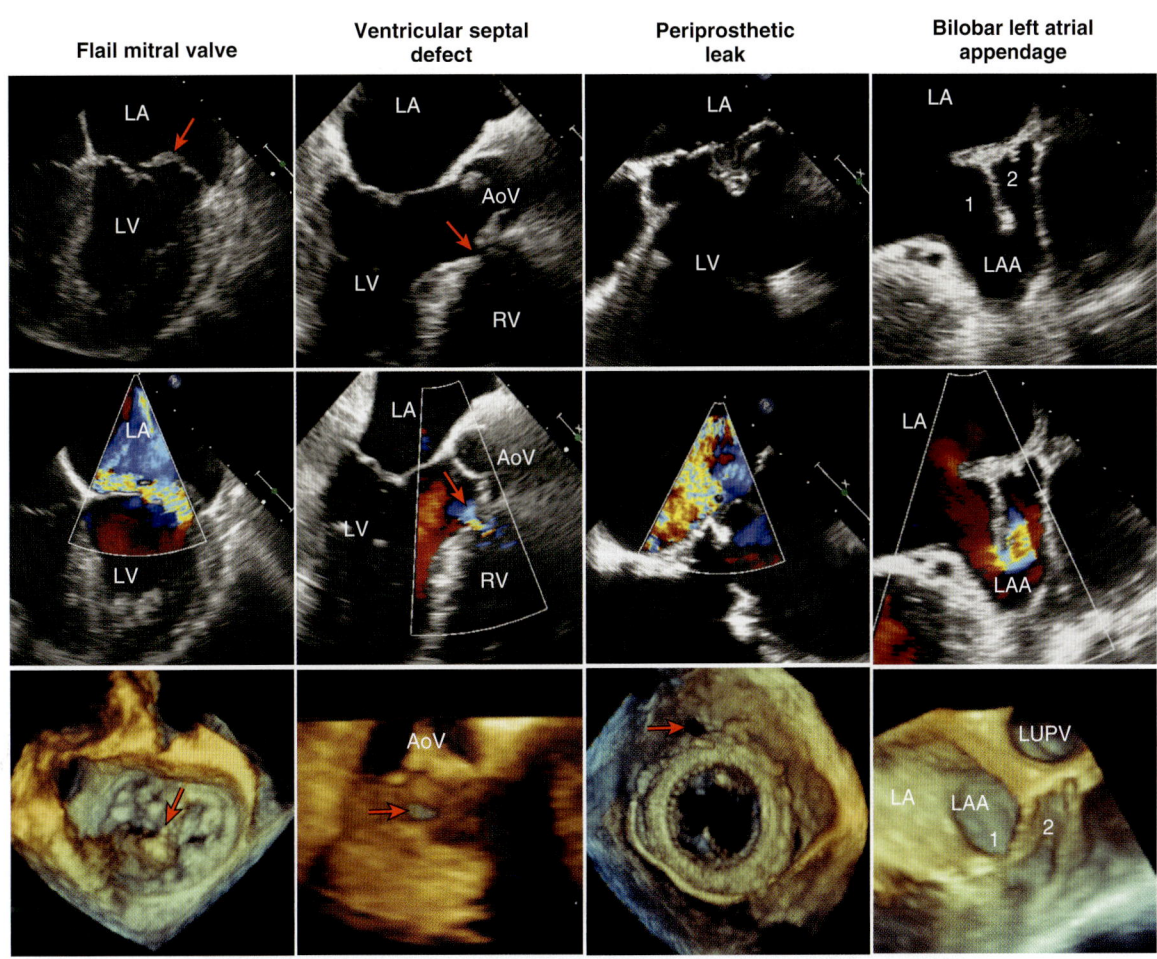

Fig. 18.23 **Intraprocedural echocardiographic evaluation of structural heart disease.** Typical examples of patients with structural heart disease referred for percutaneous interventions. The first patient has a flail posterior mitral leaflet *(arrow)* and was referred for mitral clip repair. The second patient has a membranous ventricular septal defect *(arrow)* and was referred for percutaneous repair of the defect. The third patient has a periprosthetic mitral valve leak *(arrow)* and two prior open heart operations and was referred for percutaneous repair. The fourth patient illustrates an anatomic variant of the LA appendage *(LAA)*, in this case bilobar, an important consideration for use of an LA appendage occluder. *AoV,* Aortic valve; *LUPV,* left upper pulmonary vein. (From Salcedo EE, Carroll JD: Echocardiographic guidance of structural heart disease interventions. In Otto CM, editor: The Practice of Clinical Echocardiography, ed 4, Philadelphia, 2012, Saunders.)

Atrial Septal Defect Closure

Transcatheter closure of a patent foramen ovale or secundum atrial septal defect typically is performed using echocardiographic guidance. Most often, both 2D and 3D TEE images are used (Fig. 18.24). Alternatively, the interventional cardiologist my use intracardiac echocardiography for procedural guidance (see Fig. 4.19).

Transcatheter Valve Implantation

In the patient with severe aortic stenosis who is being considered for transcatheter aortic valve implantation (TAVI), baseline TTE imaging provides visualization of valve anatomy and the degree of leaflet calcification, quantitation of stenosis severity, and evaluation of LV geometry and function (Table 18.6). Multimodality imaging is recommended before the procedure. TAVI valve size is determined from gated contrast-enhanced CT angiography, which allows visualization and measurement of the 3D shape of the annulus and sinuses, as well as measurement of the distance from the valve leaflets to the coronary ostia.

The role of TEE during the TAVI procedure has evolved as this technology has matured. Initially, most TAVI procedures were performed using general anesthesia with continuous TEE guidance to position the valve, assess function immediately after implantation, and detect complications (Fig. 18.25). Increasingly, TAVI procedures are performed with sedation using only fluoroscopic images to guide valve placement. TTE imaging after the procedure is used to detect complications and assess valve function. Long term, echocardiography is used to monitor valve function; the presence of paravalvular aortic regurgitation is a poor prognostic sign and should be monitored closely.

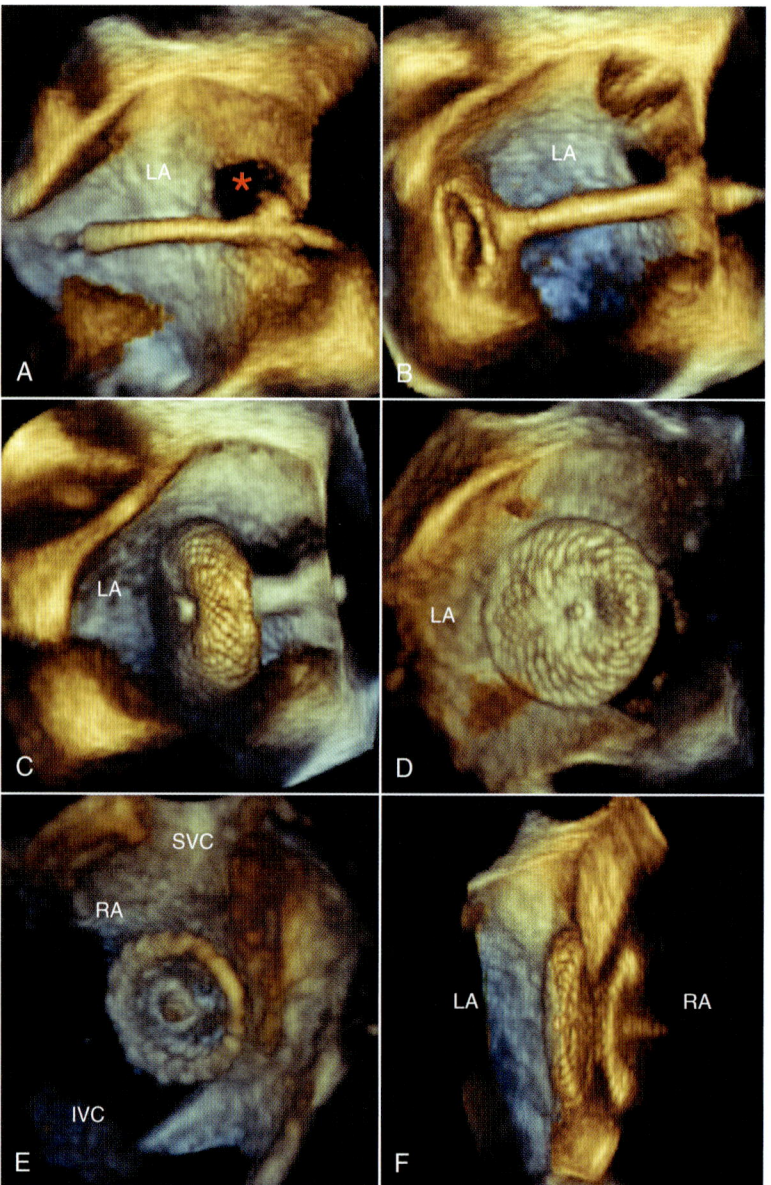

Fig. 18.24 **3D transesophageal echocardiography guidance of Amplatzer (St Jude Medical, Minneapolis, Minn.) atrial septal defect closure device.** (A) to (F) All views are zoom 3D images of the interatrial septum as seen from the LA (A, B, C, and D), from the RA (E), or from an anteroposterior perspective (F). (A) The delivery catheter is seen in the LA entering through the atrial septal defect *(asterisk)*. (B) The LA disk is being deployed. (C) The LA disk is fully deployed, and the catheter is pulled back. (D) The catheter is pulled back until the left hemidisk abuts the interatrial septum. (E) The right hemidisk is deployed and sits in the RA inferior to the superior vena cava *(SVC)* and superior and anterior to the inferior vena *(IVC)*. (F) The device is seen in profile with one hemidisk in the LA and the other in the RA. *(From Salcedo EE, Carroll JD: Echocardiographic guidance of structural heart disease interventions. In Otto CM, editor:* The Practice of Clinical Echocardiography, *ed 4, Philadelphia, 2012, Saunders.)*

TABLE 18.6 Checklist for TAVI Imaging Assessment

PREPROCEDURE

Region of Interest	Recommended Approach and Key Measures	Additional Comments
Aortic valve morphology	☐ TTE • Trileaflet, bicuspid, or unicuspid • Valve calcification • Leaflet motion • Annular size and shape	☐ TEE particularly useful for subaortic membranes ☐ Cardiac MRI if echocardiography nondiagnostic ☐ ECG-gated thoracic CTA if MRI contraindicated
Aortic valve function	☐ TTE • Maximum aortic velocity • Mean aortic valve gradient • Aortic valve area • Stroke volume index • Presence and severity of AR	☐ Additional parameters • Dimensionless index • AVA by planimetry (echo, CT, MRI) • Dobutamine stress echocardiography for LFLG AS-reduced EF • Aortic valve calcium score if LFLG AS diagnosis in question
LV geometry and other cardiac findings	☐ TTE • LVEF, regional wall motion • Hypertrophy, diastolic fx • Pulmonary pressure estimate • Mitral valve (MR, MS, MAC) • Aortic sinus anatomy and size	☐ CMR: identification of cardiomyopathies ☐ Myocardial ischemia and scar: CMR, PET, DSE, thallium ☐ CMR imaging for myocardial fibrosis and scar
Annular sizing	☐ TAVI CTA-gated contrast enhanced CT thorax with multiphasic acquisition. Typically reconstructed in systole 30%–40% of the R-R window.	☐ Major/minor annulus dimension ☐ Major/minor average ☐ Annular area ☐ Circumference/perimeter
Aortic root measurements	☐ Gated contrast-enhanced CT thorax with multiphasic acquisition. Typically reconstructed in diastole 60%–80%.	☐ Coronary ostia heights ☐ Mid-sinus of Valsalva (sinus to commissure, sinus to sinus) ☐ Sinotubular junction ☐ Ascending aorta (40 cm above valve plane, widest dimension, at level of PA) ☐ Aortic root and ascending aorta calcification ☐ For additional measurement, see Table 18.1
Coronary disease and thoracic anatomy	☐ Coronary angiography ☐ Nongated thoracic CTA	☐ Coronary artery disease severity ☐ Bypass grafts: number/location ☐ RV-to–chest wall distance ☐ Aorta-to–chest wall relationship
Noncardiac imaging	☐ Carotid ultrasound ☐ Cerebrovascular MRI	☐ Consider depending on clinical history.
Vascular Access (Imaging Dependent on Renal Function)	**Recommended Approach**	**Key Parameters**
Normal renal function (GFR >60) or ESRD not expected to recover	☐ TAVI CTA*	☐ Aorta, great vessel, and abdominal aorta ☐ Dissection; atheroma; stenosis; calcification ☐ Iliac/subclavian/femoral luminal dimensions, calcification, and tortuosity

Continued

TABLE 18.6 Checklist for TAVI Imaging Assessment—cont'd

Vascular Access (Imaging Dependent on Renal Function)	Recommended Approach	Key Parameters
Borderline renal function	☐ Contrast MRA ☐ Direct femoral angiography (low contrast)	☐ Institutional dependent protocols ☐ Luminal dimensions and tortuosity of peripheral vasculature
Acute kidney injury or ESRD with expected recovery	☐ Noncontrast CT of chest, abdomen, and pelvis ☐ Noncontrast MRA ☐ Consider TEE if balancing risk and benefits.	☐ Degree of calcification and tortuosity of peripheral vasculature

PERIPROCEDURE

Imaging Goals	Recommended Approach	Additional Details
Interventional planning	☐ TAVI CTA	☐ Predict optimal fluoroscopy angles for valve deployment.
Confirmation of annular sizing	☐ Preprocedure MDCT	☐ Consider contrast aortic root injection if needed. ☐ 3D TEE to confirm annular size[†]
Valve placement	☐ Fluoroscopy using general anesthesia	☐ TEE (if using general anesthesia)
Paravalvular leak	☐ Direct aortic root angiography	☐ TEE (if using general anesthesia)
Procedural complications	☐ TTE ☐ TEE (if using general anesthesia) ☐ Intracardiac echocardiography (alternative)	☐ See Suggested Reading 18.

LONG-TERM POSTPROCEDURE

Imaging Goals	Recommended Approach	Additional Details
Evaluate valve function	☐ TTE (see Suggested Reading 18 for frequency)	☐ Key elements of echocardiography • Maximum aortic velocity • Mean aortic valve gradient • Aortic valve area • Paravalvular and valvular AR
LV geometry and other cardiac findings	☐ TTE • LVEF, regional wall motion • Hypertrophy, diastolic fx • Pulmonary pressure estimate • Mitral valve (MR, MS, MAC)	

*TAVI CTA: Unless otherwise noted, this refers to single arterial-phase CTA of the chest, abdomen, and pelvis. Typically, the thorax is acquired using ECG-gated multiphase acquisition. At minimum, acquisition and reconstruction should include end-systole, usually between 30% and 40% of the R-R window.
[†]TEE: Given the use of CT, the role in annular sizing before TAVI with TEE is limited. Periprocedural use of TEE is limited to cases performed.
AR, Aortic regurgitation; *AS*, aortic stenosis; *AVA*, aortic valve area; *CMR*, cardiovascular magnetic resonance; *CT*, computed tomography; *CTA*, computed tomography angiography; *DSE*, dobutamine stress echocardiography; *ECG*, electrocardiogram; *EF*, ejection fraction; *ESRD*, end-stage renal disease; *fx*, function; *GFR*, glomerular filtration rate; *LFLG*, low flow low gradient; *LVEF*, LV ejection fraction; *MAC*, mitral annular calcification; *MDCT*, multidetector computed tomography; *MR*, mitral regurgitation; *MRA*, magnetic resonance angiogram; *MRI*, magnetic resonance imaging; *MS*, mitral stenosis; *PA*, pulmonary artery; *PET*, positron emission tomography; *TAVI*, transcatheter aortic valve implantation.
From Otto CM, Kumbhani DJ, Alexander KP, et al: 2017 ACC expert consensus decision pathway for transcatheter aortic valve replacement in the management of adults with aortic stenosis: a report of the American College of Cardiology Task Force on Clinical Expert Consensus Documents, *J Am Coll Cardiol* 69(10):1313–1346, 2017.

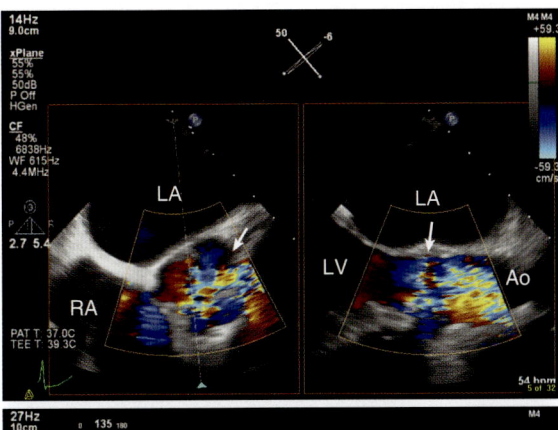

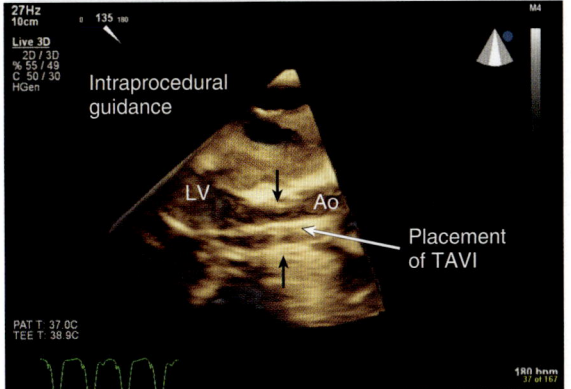

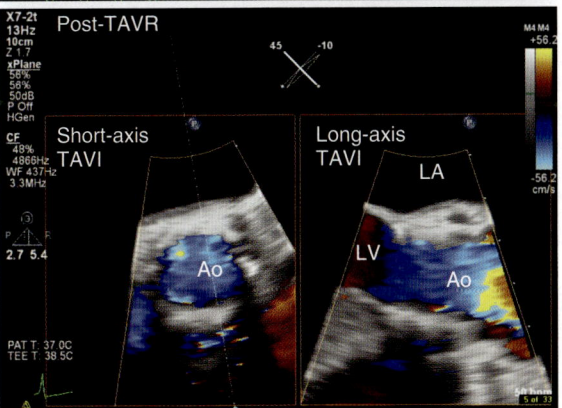

Fig. 18.25 Transesophageal echocardiography guidance of transcatheter aortic valve implantation. TEE can be used during transcatheter aortic valve implantation (TAVI) in patients receiving general anesthesia. This example shows baseline *(top)* ▶ color Doppler imaging in short- and long-axis views in a patient with severe aortic stenosis. 3D imaging helps guide positioning of the valve *(middle)*, ▶ with the guidewire seen as a linear bright echo extending from the aorta *(Ao)* into the LV. The position of the valve is shown by the *black arrows* with reverberation artifacts distal to the valve. After valve implantation *(bottom)*, ▶ short- and long-axis views now show normal velocity laminar flow across the valve.

Transcatheter Mitral Valve Repair

Based on the complex anatomy of the mitral valve apparatus, several approaches to transcatheter reduction of mitral regurgitation severity are in various stages of study or approval. Currently, the most common

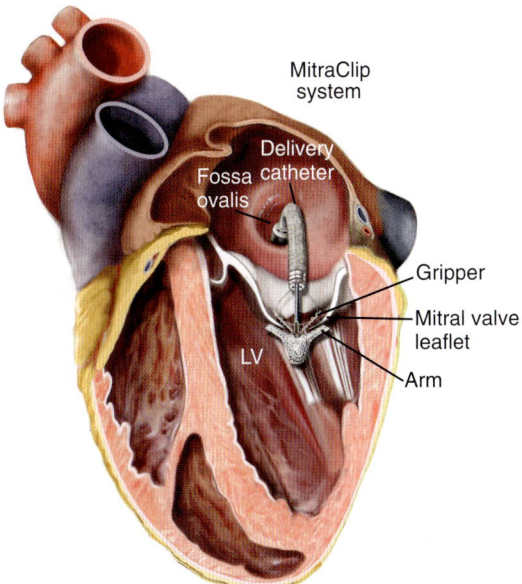

Fig. 18.26 Transcatheter mitral valve repair. The MitraClip system (Abbott Laboratories, Abbot Park, Ill.) with the delivery catheter entering the LA through the fossa ovalis area and the clip with open arms in the LV near the tip of the mitral valve leaflets. *(From Salcedo EE, Quaife RA, Kim MS, Carroll JD: Transcatheter mitral valve repair: role of echocardiography in patient selection, procedural guidance and evaluation of outcomes. In Otto CM, editor: The Practice of Clinical Echocardiography, ed 5, Philadelphia, 2017, Elsevier, Fig. 20.2.)*

transcatheter mitral valve procedure is placement of a clip that connects the center of the anterior and posterior leaflet tips to improve leaflet coaptation (Fig. 18.26). Others are similar to annuloplasty ring placement with changes in shape and size of the annulus, for example, with a device in the coronary sinus that lies immediately adjacent to the annulus. These procedures require a detailed baseline evaluation of mitral valve anatomy, with measurements specific to each procedure, such as annulus diameters or leaflet coaptation and tenting distances. For guidance of transcatheter mitral procedures, a real-time 3D view that clearly demonstrates the area of interest is obtained; this view is then used to guide the procedure (Fig. 18.27). TEE during the procedure allows measurement of transmitral diastolic gradients and assessment of residual regurgitation at each step of the procedure (Fig. 18.28). Long term, TEE is used to assess for residual mitral valve dysfunction.

Other Transcatheter Interventions

Echocardiography also is used to guide catheter septal ablation for hypertrophic cardiomyopathy (see Chapter 9), closure of prosthetic valve paravalvular leaks (Fig. 18.29), closure of post–myocardial infarction ventricular septal defects, or procedures to occlude the LA appendage (Fig. 18.30).

Fig. 18.27 Procedural transesophageal echocardiography guidance of mitral valve clip placement. TEE is essential for correct placement of a mitral valve clip to reduce regurgitant severity. A combination of 3D and 2D imaging is used to guide the clip *(arrow)* from the LA to the correct position on the LA size of the mitral valve, as shown in biplane images *(top)* ▶. The open arms of the clip can be seen in the *top right* image. Imaging then is used to guide grasping of the leaflets and to assess the degree of residual mitral regurgitation. 3D imaging after placement of two clips *(bottom)* ▶ shows clips *(arrows)* in the mid-section of the leaflets with the resultant dual orifices *(asterisks)*. *BP,* Blood pressure.

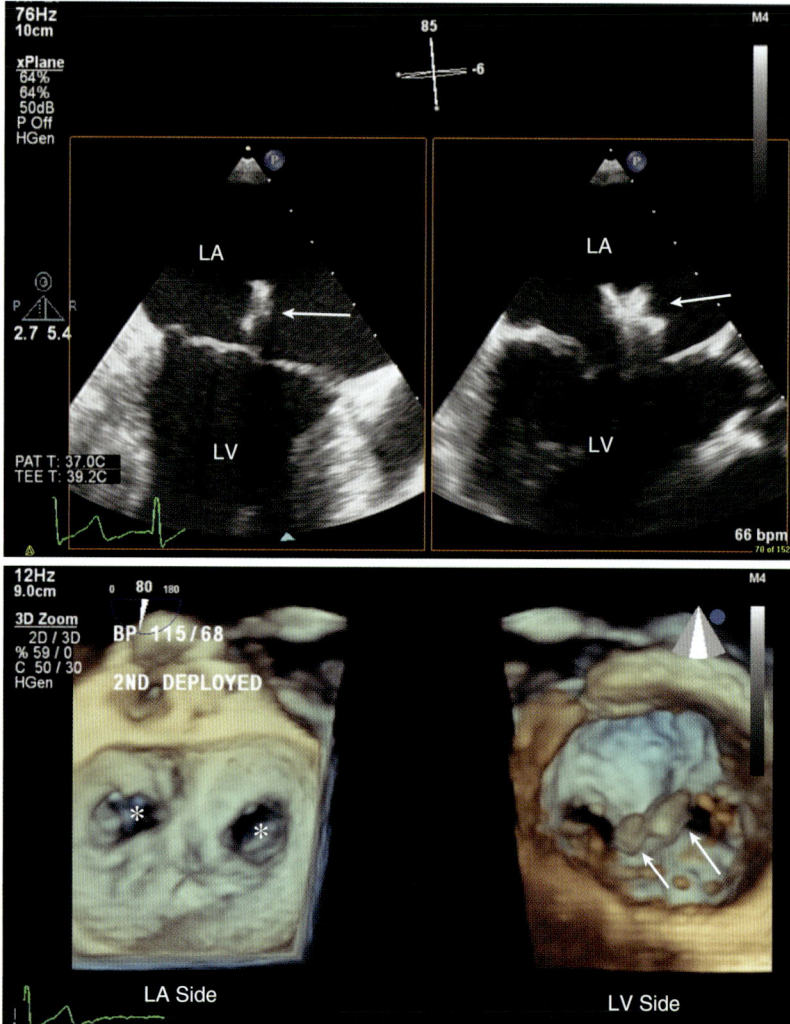

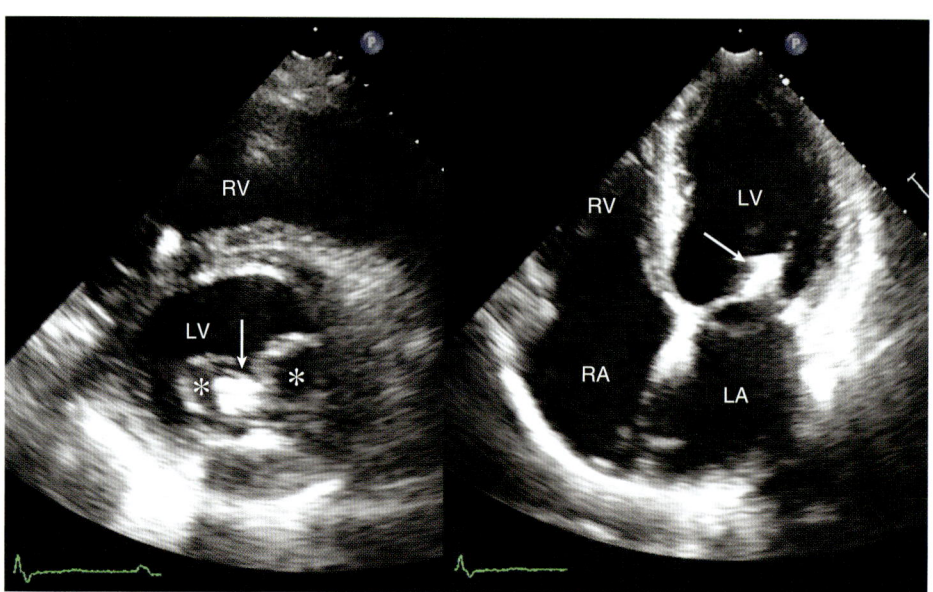

Fig. 18.28 Transthoracic echocardiography after mitral valve clip placement. The typical appearance of the mitral valve on TTE imaging after placement of a mitral valve clip *(arrows)* shows the double orifice mitral valve *(asterisks)* in the parasternal long-axis view *(left)* ▶ and the altered leaflet motion in the apical four-chamber view *(right)*. ▶

Intraoperative and Interventional Echocardiography | Chapter 18

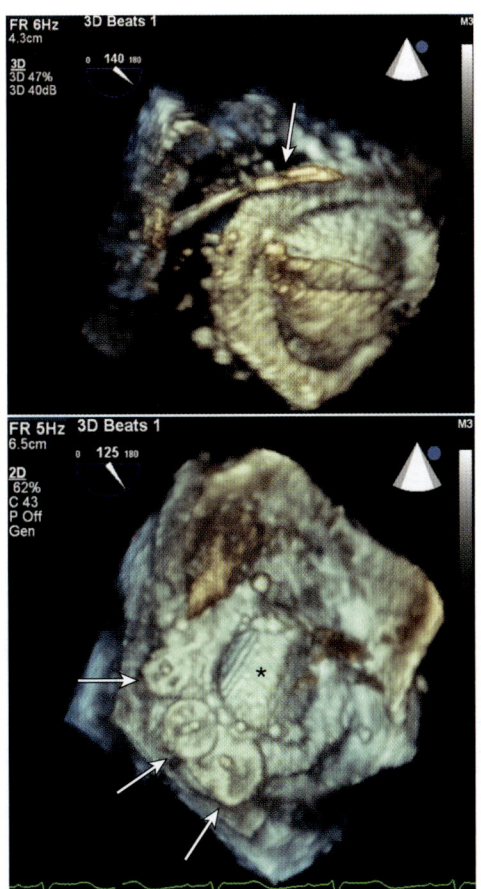

Fig. 18.29 ▶ ▶ **Closure of paravalvular leak.** In this patient with severe paravalvular regurgitation around a mitral valve prosthetic valve *(asterisk)*, several transcatheter closure devices *(arrows)* have been placed around the annulus to reduce regurgitant severity.

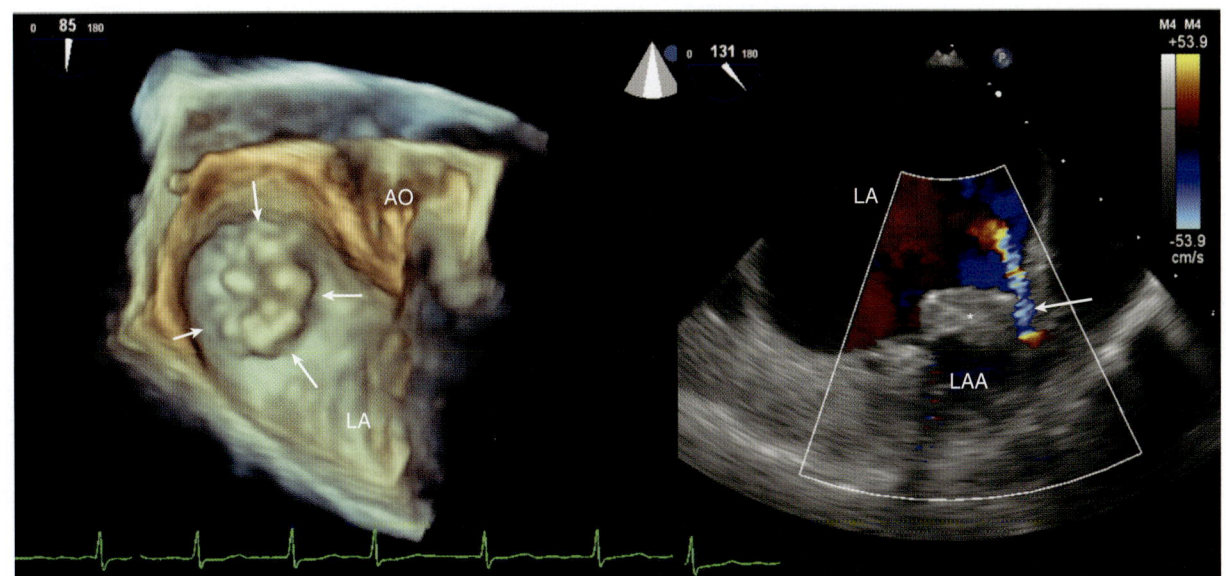

Fig. 18.30 ▶ ▶ **Transesophageal echocardiography after LA appendage occluder device placement.** 3D TEE imaging shows the LA appendage (LAA) occluder device *(arrows)* blocking the orifice of the LA appendage into the LA. 2D color Doppler shows a small residual leak around the device *(asterisk)*. Ao, Aorta.

THE ECHO EXAM

Basic Principles of Intraprocedural TEE

- Establish diagnosis preprocedure when possible.
- The goals of the baseline TEE are to:
  - Confirm the diagnosis.
  - Provide additional information on repairability.
  - Serve as a comparison with postprocedure studies.
  - Assess LV and RV function.
  - Check for other abnormalities.
- Perform a complete study unless there are clinical or time constraints.
- Record postprocedure images at similar loading conditions to those of baseline.
- Communicate and discuss findings at time of study.
- Report TEE findings in medical record, and store TEE images.

Factors That Affect Cardiac Hemodynamics During Surgical or Transcatheter Procedures

Heart rate and blood pressure
Positive pressure mechanical ventilation
Volume status
Myocardial "stunning" secondary to aortic cross-clamping
Effects of cardiopulmonary bypass
Pharmacologic therapy

Imaging for Transcatheter Interventions

Procedure	Procedural Planning	Procedural Guidance*	Postprocedure Evaluation
Transcatheter aortic valve replacement	TTE, CT	TEE optional	TTE
Transcatheter mitral valve repair procedures	TTE, 3D TEE	3D TEE essential	TTE, TEE
Balloon mitral valvotomy	TTE and TEE	TEE or ICE	TTE
Transcatheter closure for paravalvular regurgitation	3D TEE	3D TEE essential	TTE, TEE
Atrial septal defect or patent foramen ovale closure	TTE, 3D TEE	TEE or ICE	TTE, TEE
Septal ablation for hypertrophic cardiomyopathy	TTE	TTE or TEE	TTE
Transcatheter pulmonic valve replacement	TTE, CT	TEE optional	TTE
LA appendage occlusion	TEE, CT	TEE essential	TEE

*In addition to fluoroscopy.
ICE, Intracardiac echocardiography.

Key Data for Intraoperative TEE			
Procedure	**Before Procedure**	**During Procedure**	**After Procedure**
Mitral valve repair	• Valve anatomy • Repairability • Regurgitation 　• Mechanism 　• Severity	• Baseline anatomy and regurgitation pre-CPB • Residual MR post-CPB	• Assess for complications 　• Persistent MR 　• Mitral SAM 　• Functional mitral stenosis 　• Tricuspid regurgitation 　• Circumflex artery injury • LV function
Valve stenosis	• Valve anatomy and calcification • Severity of stenosis • LV function • PA pressures	• Baseline LV function • Baseline valve anatomy and function • Post-CPB assess repaired or prosthetic valve	• Paravalvular regurgitation • LV function
Endocarditis	• Vegetations • Abscess formation • Valve function • LV function • PA pressures	• Baseline valve anatomy and function • Post-CPB valve function	• Baseline postsurgery valve function • LV function
Prosthetic valve dysfunction	• Valve thrombosis • Pannus formation • Paravalvular regurgitation	• Baseline study to guide surgical intervention • Post-CPB assessment of new prosthetic valve	• Baseline prosthetic valve function • Follow-up depends on residual lesions and valve type.
Aortic dissection	• Confirm diagnosis. • Extent of dissection distally • Coronary ostial involvement • Aortic valve function • Pericardial effusion	• Post-CPB documentation of residual dissection flap distal to repair • Assess flow in true and false lumen. • Aortic valve function • LV function	• Long-term follow-up of aortic valve and LV function • Residual dissection flap distally
Hypertrophic cardiomyopathy	• Location and severity of septal thickening • Severity of subaortic dynamic obstruction • MR	• Residual subaortic obstruction • Ventricular septal defect • Residual MR	• Long-term hemodynamic results • LV systolic and diastolic function
Congenital heart disease	• Diagnosis of complex anatomy • Surgical planning • Integration with data from other imaging modalities	• Baseline evaluation of each lesion anatomy and hemodynamics • Residual lesions after CPB	• Long-term anatomic and functional results • Ventricular function • Pulmonary pressures

CPB, Cardiopulmonary bypass; *MR*, mitral regurgitation, *PA*, pulmonary artery; *SAM*, systolic anterior motion.

SUGGESTED READING

General

1. Oxorn DC: Intraoperative and procedural echocardiography: basic Principles. In Otto CM, editor: *The Practice of Clinical Echocardiography*, ed 5, Philadelphia, 2017, Elsevier.
   This atlas (print, online, and smartdevice) uses a case-based format to show cine and still-frame echocardiographic and Doppler images with correlation between the clinical presentation and outcome, radiologic studies, and surgical findings. Suggested readings are provided for each case. Includes 154 cases, spanning the full range of intraoperative TEE studies, including coronary disease, mitral and aortic valve disease, endocarditis, prosthetic valves, right-sided valve disease, adult congenital heart disease, hypertrophic cardiomyopathy, pericardial disease, disease of the great vessels, and cardiac masses.

2. Hahn RT, Abraham T, Adams MS, et al: Guidelines for performing a comprehensive transesophageal echocardiographic examination: recommendations from the American Society of Echocardiography and the Society of Cardiovascular Anesthesiologists, *J Am Soc Echocardiogr* 26(9):921–964, 2013.
   Consensus statement on the approach to a comprehensive TEE study both for diagnostic studies in the pre- and postprocedure setting and for intraprocedural monitoring. Sections include training and certification, indications, patient sedation, instrument controls and manipulation, and views for specific cardiac

structures. Detailed tables provide excellent summaries of the TEE exam. An essential reference for procedural echocardiography. 172 references.

3. Oxorn D, editor: *Intraoperative Echocardiography*, Philadelphia, 2012, Saunders.
   This book in the four-volume Practical Echocardiography Series (series editor: Otto CM), provides a comprehensive overview of intraoperative TEE. Information is presented in a concise, bulleted text format with key points and numerous illustrations. Chapters include mitral and aortic valve disease, prosthetic valves, ventricular function, aortic disease, and congenital heart disease.

4. Thys DM, Brooker RF, Cahalan MK, et al: Practice guidelines for perioperative transesophageal echocardiography: an updated report by the American Society of Anesthesiologists and the Society of Cardiovascular Anesthesiologists Task Force on Transesophageal Echocardiography, *Anesthesiology* 112(5):1084–1096, 2010.
   TEE is recommended for all valvular heart disease surgical procedures and should be considered in coronary bypass grafting surgery. The goals of the TEE exam are to: (1) confirm and provide additional detail about the preoperative diagnosis, (2) evaluate for unsuspected pathology, (3) adjust the anesthesia and surgical plan as indicated, and (4) evaluate the results of surgical intervention. TEE or intracardiac echocardiography also should be used during catheter-based interventions for structural heart disease. In patients undergoing noncardiac surgery, TEE is recommended in patients with suspected or known heart disease that may result in clinical deterioration during the procedure, and it should be used in patients with unexplained hypotension or hypoxemia. Table 1 in this reference provides sensitivity and specificity data for diagnosis of numerous conditions by perioperative TEE

Monitoring Ventricular Function and Noncardiac Surgery

5. Oxorn DC: Intraoperative and procedural echocardiography: basic principles. In Otto CM, editor: *The Practice of Clinical Echocardiography*, ed 5, Philadelphia, 2017, Elsevier.
   Review of the use of TEE by a cardiac anesthesiologist for monitoring ventricular function in the operating room. This chapter also has detailed sections on special situations, including separation from cardiopulmonary bypass, off-pump coronary bypass surgery, positioning of intravascular devices, and transplant surgery.

6. Gouveia V, Marcelino P, Reuter DA: The role of transesophageal echocardiography in the intraoperative period, *Curr Cardiol Rev* 7(3):184–196, 2011.
   In patients undergoing noncardiac surgery, TEE provides data on cardiac output and ventricular preload. Using TEE to optimize loading conditions leads to decreased perioperative mortality and morbidity. A practical approach to TEE evaluation in noncardiac surgery is presented.

7. Sidebotham S, Merry A, Leggett M, et al: *Practical Perioperative Transesophageal Echocardiography: Text with DVD*, ed 2, Oxford, 2011, Butterworth-Heinemann.
   This 384-page book with DVD provides a concise overview of TEE that is helpful for TEE imaging in all clinical settings, with a focus on perioperative TEE and critical care echocardiography.

Cardiac Surgery

8. Drake DH, Zimmerman KG, Sidebotham DA: Transesophageal echocardiography for surgical repair of mitral regurgitation. In Otto CM, editor: *The Practice of Clinical Echocardiography*, ed 5, Philadelphia, 2017, Elsevier, pp 343–374.
   Comprehensive book chapter with beautiful illustrations and online videos detailing the role of echocardiography in patients undergoing surgical mitral valve repair.

9. Woo A: Hypertrophic cardiomyopathy: echocardiography in diagnosis and management of patients. In Otto CM, editor: *The Practice of Clinical Echocardiography*, ed 5, Philadelphia, 2017, Elsevier, pp 505–533.
   This chapter on all aspects of echocardiography in patients with hypertrophic cardiomyopathy includes a section on intraoperative echocardiography and on outcomes following myectomy. It has several figures on intraoperative evaluation and more than 20 references in this section.

10. Sidebotham DA, Allen SJ, Gerber IL, et al: Intraoperative transesophageal echocardiography for surgical repair of mitral regurgitation, *J Am Soc Echocardiogr* 27(4):345–366, 2014.
    Review article providing a practical approach, with an example, to TEE evaluation in patients undergoing surgical mitral valve repair.

Ventricular Assist Devices

11. Kirkpatrick JN: Echocardiography in mechanical circulatory support: normal findings, complications and speed changes. In Otto CM, editor: *The Practice of Clinical Echocardiography*, ed 5, Philadelphia, 2017, Elsevier, pp 596–618.
    This chapter details echocardiographic evaluation of ventricular assist devices. The types of devices and changes in cardiac structure after device implantation are also summarized. Approaches to diagnosing assist device malfunction and effect of changes in pump speed on cardiac output and function are also presented.

Transcatheter Procedures

12. Salcedo EE, Quaife RA, Kim MS, et al: Transcatheter mitral valve repair: role of echocardiography in patient selection, procedural guidance and evaluation of outcomes. In Otto CM, editor: *The Practice of Clinical Echocardiography*, ed 5, Philadelphia, 2017, Elsevier, pp 374–394.
    Advanced textbook chapter on TEE evaluation and procedural guidance in patients undergoing transcatheter mitral valve repair. Artist-drawn illustrations show how each type of transcatheter mitral repair works, with 2D and 3D echo images and videos showing typical findings, results and complications.

13. Zamorano JL, Badano LP, Bruce C, et al: EAE/ASE recommendations for the use of echocardiography in new transcatheter interventions for valvular heart disease, *Eur J Echocardiogr* 12(8):557–584, 2011.
    Detailed review of current transcatheter interventions with recommendations for echocardiographic evaluation before, during, and after the procedure. Illustrations show examples of procedural complications and how measurements should be made. Procedures included are TAVI, closure of prosthetic paravalvular regurgitation, and transcatheter mitral valve repair procedures.

14. Tsang W, Lang RM, Kronzon I: Role of real-time three dimensional echocardiography in cardiovascular interventions, *Heart* 97(10):850–857, 2011.
    Practical guide to 3D TEE imaging for transcatheter interventions, including mitral valvotomy, mitral regurgitation procedures, LA appendage device occlusion, closure of atrial septal defects and patent foramen ovale, TAVI, and transcatheter occlusion of paravalvular leaks.

Percutaneous Valve Implantation

15. Bloomfield GS, Gillam LD, Hahn RT, et al: A practical guide to multimodality imaging of transcatheter aortic valve replacement,

JACC Cardiovasc Imaging 5(4):441–455, 2012.

Clear and well-illustrated summary of the role of imaging in transcatheter valve implantation, including patient selection, detailed evaluation of valve anatomy, procedural guidance, and postprocedure follow-up. The importance of correct measurement of aortic annulus diameter and measurement of leaflet length versus annular-coronary ostial distance is emphasized. Other imaging modalities are also needed in patient evaluation and should be integrated with the echocardiographic data.

16. Zamorano JL, Badano LP, Bruce C, et al: EAE/ASE recommendations for the use of echocardiography in new transcatheter interventions for valvular heart disease, *J Am Soc Echocardiogr* 24(9):937–965, 2011.

This European Association of Echocardiography and American Society of Echocardiography consensus statement reviews the indications and procedural aspects of TAVI. The key elements in echocardiographic evaluation are delineated, with clear illustrations for each measurement. Periprocedural complications detectable by echocardiography include deployment of the valve toward the aorta or LV, aortic regurgitation (central or paravalvular), mitral regurgitation or distortion of mitral anatomy by the delivery system, coronary ostial occlusion, tamponade, and aortic dissection.

17. Hahn RT, Kodali S, Tuzcu EM, et al: Echocardiographic imaging of procedural complications during balloon-expandable transcatheter aortic valve replacement, *JACC Cardiovasc Imaging.* 8(3):288–318, 2015.

This compendium of examples from a large clinical trial shows potential complications associated with TAVI and approaches for prevention. Includes 35 figures and 42 online videos.

18. Otto CM, Kumbhani DJ, Alexander KP, et al: 2017 ACC expert consensus decision pathway for transcatheter aortic valve replacement in the management of adults with aortic stenosis: a report of the American College of Cardiology Task Force on Clinical Expert Consensus Documents, *J Am Coll Cardiol* 69(10):1313–1346, 2017.

Practical clinical approach with simple checklists for implementation into practice detailing recommended multimodality imaging approach in patients being considered for TAVI.

APPENDIX A

Normal Values for Echocardiographic Measurements

TABLE A.1 Reference Values for Echocardiographic Chamber Quantification

Chamber	Measurement	Normal Range (Women)	Normal Range (Men)	Units
Left ventricle	Diastolic diameter	3.8–5.2	4.2–5.8	cm
	Systolic diameter	2.2–3.5	2.5–4.0	cm
	2D diastolic volume	46–106	62–150	mL
	(indexed to BSA)	*29–61*	*34–74*	*mL/m^2*
	2D systolic volume	14–42	21–61	mL
	(indexed to BSA)	*8–24*	*11–31*	*mL/m^2*
	Ejection fraction	54–74	52–72	%
	Septal wall thickness	0.6–0.9	0.6–1.0	cm
	Posterior wall thickness	0.6–0.9	0.6–1.0	cm
	LV mass (2D method)	66–150	96–200	g
	(indexed to BSA)	*44–88*	*50–102*	*g/m^2*
	Relative wall thickness	0.22–0.42	0.24–0.42	
Left atrium	AP diameter	2.7–3.8	3.0–4.0	cm
	(indexed to BSA)	*1.5–2.3*	*1.5–2.3*	*cm/m^2*
	LA volume	22–52	18–52	mL
	(indexed to BSA)	*16–34*	*16–34*	*mL/m^2*
Right atrium	RA major dimension	1.9–3.1	1.8–3.0	cm
	RA minor dimension	1.3–2.5	1.3–2.5	cm
	2D echo RA volume	9–33	11–39	mL/m^2
		Normal Range (Women and Men)		
Right ventricle	RV basal diameter	2.5–4.1		cm
	RV subcostal wall thickness	0.1–0.5		cm
	RVOT proximal diameter	2.1–3.5		cm
	RVOT distal diameter	1.7–2.7		cm
	Fractional area change	35–63		%
	TAPSE	1.7–3.1		cm

AP, Anterior-posterior diameter in long-axis view; *BSA,* body surface area; *RVOT,* RV outflow tract; *TAPSE,* tricuspid annular plane systolic excursion.
Data from Lang RM, Badano LP, Mor-Avi V, et al: Recommendations for cardiac chamber quantification by echocardiography in adults: an update from the American Society of Echocardiography and the European Association of Cardiovascular Imaging, *J Am Soc Echocardiogr* 28(1):1–39.e14, 2015.
Ranges were calculated from the mean value plus or minus 2 standard deviations.

TABLE A.2   Normal Ranges and Severity Partition Cutoff Values for 2D-Derived LV Ejection Fraction and LA Volume

	MEN				WOMEN			
	Normal Range	Mildly Abnormal	Moderately Abnormal	Severely Abnormal	Normal Range	Mildly Abnormal	Moderately Abnormal	Severely Abnormal
LV EF (%)	52–72	41–51	30–40	<30	54–74	41–53	30–40	<30
Maximum LA volume/BSA (mL/m^2)	16–34	35–41	42–48	>48	16–34	35–41	42–48	>48

BSA, Body surface area; EF, ejection fraction.
From Lang RM, Badano LP, Mor-Avi V, et al: Recommendations for cardiac chamber quantification by echocardiography in adults: an update from the American Society of Echocardiography and the European Association of Cardiovascular Imaging, J Am Soc Echocardiogr 28(1):1–39.e14, 2015.

TABLE A.3   Normal Echocardiographic Valve Annulus and Great Vessel Dimensions in Adults

	Range (cm)	RANGE (cm/m^2)	
		Indexed to BSA	Upper Limit of Normal*
Aorta (End-Diastole)*			
Annulus diameter	1.4–2.6	1.3 ± 0.1 cm/m^2	<1.6 cm/m^2
Diameter at leaflet tips	2.2–3.6	1.7 ± 0.2 cm/m^2	<2.1 cm/m^2
Ascending aorta diameter	2.1–3.4	1.5 ± 0.2 cm/m^2	
Arch diameter	2.0–3.6		
Mitral Annulus			
End-diastole	2.7 ± 0.4		
End-systole	2.9 ± 0.3		
Pulmonary Artery			
Annulus diameter	1.5–2.1		
Main PA	0.9–2.9		
Inferior Vena Cava Diameters			
1–2 cm from RA junction	Normal <1.7		

*See Chapter 16 for a more detailed approach to normalization of aortic dimensions for age and body size.
BSA, Body surface area; PA, pulmonary artery.
Data from Roman et al: Am J Cardiol 64:507, 1989; Pini et al: Circulation 80:915, 1989; Schnittger et al: J Am Coll Cardiol 2:934, 1983; Kircher et al: Am J Cardiol 66:493, 1990.

Appendix A | Normal Values for Echocardiographic Measurements

TABLE A.4 Normal Antegrade Doppler Flow Velocities

Normal Range	(m/s)
Ascending aorta	1.0–1.7
LV outflow tract	0.7–1.1
LV inflow	
E-velocity	0.6–1.3 (0.72 ± 0.14)
Deceleration slope	5.0 ± 1.4 m/s
A-velocity	0.2–0.7 (0.47 ± 0.4)
Pulmonary artery	0.5–1.3
RV inflow	
E-velocity	0.3–0.7
RA filling (SVC, HV)	
Systole	0.32–0.69 (0.46 ± 0.08) m/s
Diastole	0.06–0.45 (0.27 ± 0.08) m/s
LA filling (pulmonary vein)	
Systole	0.56 ± 0.13 m/s
Diastole	0.44 ± 0.16 m/s
Atrial reversal	0.32 ± 0.07 m/s

A, Late (atrial) diastolic peak; *E*, early diastolic peak; *HV*, hepatic vein; *SVC*, superior vena cava.
Data from Wilson et al: *Br Heart J* 53:451, 1985; Hatle, Angelsen: *Doppler ultrasound in cardiology*, ed 2, Philadelphia, 1985, Lea & Febiger; Van Dam et al: *Eur Heart J* 8:1221, 1987; 9:165, 1988; Jaffe et al: *Am J Cardiol* 68:550, 1991; Appleton et al: *J Am Coll Cardiol* 10:1032, 1987.

TABLE A.5 Effect of Aging on Parameters of LV Diastolic Filling in Normal Subjects

Parameter	Age 21–49 yr* Mean (95% CI)	Age >50 yr* Mean (95% CI)	Age >70 yr[†] Mean (95% CI)
E velocity (m/s)	0.72 (0.44–1.0)	0.62 (0.34–0.9)	0.44 (0.25–0.76)
A velocity (m/s)	0.4 (0.2–0.6)	0.59 (0.31–0.87)	59 (0.38–0.84)
E/A ratio	1.9 (0.7–3.1)	1.1 (0.5–1.7)	0.8 (0.5–1.2)
Deceleration time (ms)	179 (139–219)	210 (138–282)	140 (90–230)
IVRT (ms)	76 (54–98)	90 (56–124)	—

CI, Confidence interval; *IVRT*, isovolumic relaxation time.
*Data from Cohen GI, Pietrolungo JF, Thomas JD, Klein AL: A practical guide to assessment of ventricular diastolic function using Doppler echocardiography, *J Am Coll Cardiol* 27:1753–1760, 1996. Normal reference values were derived from 61 subjects 21 to 49 years of age and 56 subjects older than 50 years.
[†]Data from Sagie A, Benjamin EJ, Galdersisi M, et al: Reference values for Doppler indexes of left ventricular diastolic filling in the elderly, *J Am Soc Echocardiogr* 6:570–576, 1993. Reference values were derived from 114 healthy older adult subjects in the Framingham Heart Study.

TABLE A.6 Normal Doppler Parameters for Selected Mechanical and Bioprosthetic Aortic Valves*

Valve	Size	Peak Gradient (mmHg)	Mean Gradient (mmHg)	Peak Velocity (m/s)	Effective Orifice Area (cm^2)
Mechanical					
St. Jude Medical	19	35.17 ± 11.16	18.96 ± 6.27	2.86 ± 0.48	1.01 ± 0.24
Bileaflet	21	28.34 ± 9.94	15.82 ± 5.67	2.63 ± 0.48	1.33 ± 0.32
	23	25.28 ± 7.89	13.77 ± 5.33	2.57 ± 0.44	1.6 ± 0.43
	25	22.57 ± 7.68	12.65 ± 5.14	2.4 ± 0.45	1.93 ± 0.45
	27	19.85 ± 7.55	11.18 ± 4.82	2.24 ± 0.42	2.35 ± 0.59
	29	17.72 ± 6.42	9.86 ± 2.9	2 ± 0.1	2.81 ± 0.57
	31	16.0	10 ± 6	2.1 ± 0.6	3.08 ± 1.09
Medtronic-Hall	20	34.37 ± 13.06	17.08 ± 5.28	2.9 ± 0.4	1.21 ± 0.45
Tilting-disk	21	26.86 ± 10.54	14.1 ± 5.93	2.42 ± 0.36	1.08 ± 0.17
	23	26.85 ± 8.85	13.5 ± 4.79	2.43 ± 0.59	1.36 ± 0.39
	25	17.13 ± 7.04	9.53 ± 4.26	2.29 ± 0.5	1.9 ± 0.47
	27	18.66 ± 9.71	8.66 ± 5.56	2.07 ± 0.53	1.9 ± 0.16
ATS Open Pivot	16	47.7 ± 12	27 ± 7.3	3.44 ± 0.47	0.61 ± 0.09
Bileaflet	19	47 ± 12.6	26.2 ± 7.9	3.41 ± 0.43	0.96 ± 0.18
	21	25.5 ± 6.1	14.4 ± 3.5	2.4 ± 0.39	1.58 ± 0.37
	23	19 ± 7	12 ± 4	—	1.8 ± 0.2
	25	17 ± 8	11 ± 4	—	2.2 ± 0.4
	27	14 ± 4	9 ± 2	—	2.5 ± 0.3
	29	11 ± 3	8 ± 2	—	3.1 ± 0.3
Björk-Shiley	17	—	—	4.1	—
Tilting-disk	19	27.0	—	3.8	1.1
	21	38.94 ± 11.93	21.8 ± 3.4	2.92 ± 0.88	1.1 ± 0.25
	23	33.86 ± 11	17.34 ± 6.86	2.42 ± 0.4	1.22 ± 0.23
	25	20.39 ± 7.07	11.5 ± 4.55	2.06 ± 0.28	1.8 ± 0.32
	27	19.44 ± 7.99	10.67 ± 4.31	1.77 ± 0.12	2.6
	29	21.1 ± 7.1	—	1.87 ± 0.18	2.52 ± 0.69
	31	—	—	2.1 ± 0.14	—
Carbomedics	17	33.4 ± 13.2	20.1 ± 7.1	—	1.02 ± 0.2
Bileaflet	19	33.3 ± 11.19	11.61 ± 5.08	3.09 ± 0.38	1.25 ± 0.36
	21	26.31 ± 10.25	12.68 ± 4.29	2.61 ± 0.51	1.42 ± 0.36
	23	24.61 ± 6.93	11.33 ± 3.8	2.42 ± 0.37	1.69 ± 0.29
	25	20.25 ± 8.69	9.34 ± 4.65	2.25 ± 0.34	2.04 ± 0.37
	27	19.05 ± 7.04	8.41 ± 2.83	2.18 ± 0.36	2.55 ± 0.34
	29	12.53 ± 4.69	5.8 ± 3.2	1.93 ± 0.25	2.63 ± 0.38
Bioprosthetic					
Carpentier-Edwards	19	43.48 ± 12.72	25.6 ± 8.02	—	0.85 ± 0.17
Stented bioprosthesis	21	27.73 ± 7.6	17.25 ± 6.24	2.37 ± 0.54	1.48 ± 0.3
	23	28.93 ± 7.49	15.92 ± 6.43	2.76 ± 0.4	1.69 ± 0.45
	25	23.95 ± 7.05	12.76 ± 4.43	2.38 ± 0.47	1.94 ± 0.45
	27	22.14 ± 8.24	12.33 ± 5.59	2.31 ± 0.39	2.25 ± 0.55
	29	22.0	9.92 ± 2.9	2.44 ± 0.43	2.84 ± 0.51
	31	—	—	2.41 ± 0.13	—

Continued

TABLE A.6 Normal Doppler Parameters for Selected Mechanical and Bioprosthetic Aortic Valves—cont'd

Valve	Size	Peak Gradient (mmHg)	Mean Gradient (mmHg)	Peak Velocity (m/s)	Effective Orifice Area (cm²)
Carpentier-Edwards pericardial	19	32.13 ± 3.35	24.19 ± 8.6	2.83 ± 0.14	1.21 ± 0.31
Stented bioprosthesis	21	25.69 ± 9.9	20.3 ± 9.08	2.59 ± 0.42	1.47 ± 0.36
	23	21.72 ± 8.57	13.01 ± 5.27	2.29 ± 0.45	1.75 ± 0.28
	25	16.46 ± 5.41	9.04 ± 2.27	2.02 ± 0.31	—
	27	19.2 ± 0	5.6	1.6	—
	29	17.6 ± 0	11.6	2.1	—
CryoLife-O'Brien stentless	19		12 ± 4.8		1.25 ± 0.1
Stentless bioprosthesis	21		10.33 ± 2		1.57 ± 0.6
	23		8.5		2.2
	25		7.9		2.3
	27		7.4		2.7
Edwards Prima stentless	19	30.9 ± 11.7	15.4 ± 7.4	—	1 ± 0.3
Stentless bioprosthesis	21	31.22 ± 17.35	16.36 ± 11.36	—	1.25 ± 0.29
	23	23.39 ± 10.17	11.52 ± 5.26	2.8 ± 0.4	1.49 ± 0.46
	25	19.74 ± 10.36	10.77 ± 9.32	2.7 ± 0.3	1.7 ± 0.55
	27	15.9 ± 7.3	7.1 ± 3.7	—	2 ± 0.6
	29	11.21 ± 8.6	5.03 ± 4.53	—	2.49 ± 0.52
Medtronic Freestyle stentless	19		13.0		
Stentless bioprosthesis	21		7.99 ± 2.6		1.6 ± 0.32
	23		7.24 ± 2.5		1.9 ± 0.5
	25		5.35 ± 1.5		2.03 ± 0.41
	27		4.72 ± 1.6		2.5 ± 0.47
Medtronic Mosaic Porcine	21		12.43 ± 7.3		2.1 ± 0.8
Stented bioprosthesis	23		12.47 ± 7.4		2.1 ± 0.8
	25		10.08 ± 5.1		2.1 ± 1.6
	27		9.0		—
	29		9.0		—

*Data on additional valve types and references for this data are available in the original publication.
Data from Rosenhek R, Binder T, Maurer G, et al: Normal values for Doppler echocardiographic assessment of heart valve prostheses, J Am Soc Echocardiogr 16:1116–1127, 2003.

Normal Values for Echocardiographic Measurements | Appendix A

TABLE A.7 Normal Doppler Parameters for Selected Mechanical and Bioprosthetic Mitral Valves*

Valve	Size	Peak Gradient (mmHg)	Mean Gradient (mmHg)	Peak Velocity (m/s)	Pressure Half-Time (ms)	Effective Orifice Area (cm^2)
Mechanical						
Carbomedics	23	—	—	1.9 ± 0.1	126 ± 7	—
Bileaflet	25	10.3 ± 2.3	3.6 ± 0.6	1.3 ± 0.1	93 ± 8	2.9 ± 0.8
	27	8.79 ± 3.46	3.46 ± 1.03	1.61 ± 0.3	89 ± 20	2.9 ± 0.75
	29	8.78 ± 2.9	3.39 ± 0.97	1.52 ± 0.3	88 ± 17	2.3 ± 0.4
	31	8.87 ± 2.34	3.32 ± 0.87	1.61 ± 0.29	92 ± 24	2.8 ± 1.14
	33	8.8 ± 2.2	4.8 ± 2.5	1.5 ± 0.2	93 ± 12	—
St Jude Medical	23		4.0	1.5	160	1.0
Bileaflet	25	—	2.5 ± 1	1.34 ± 1.12	75 ± 4	1.35 ± 0.17
	27	11 ± 4	5 ± 1.82	1.61 ± 0.29	75 ± 10	1.67 ± 0.17
	29	10 ± 3	4.15 ± 1.8	1.57 ± 0.29	85 ± 10	1.75 ± 0.24
	31	12 ± 6	4.46 ± 2.22	1.59 ± 0.33	74 ± 13	2.03 ± 0.32
Medtronic-Hall	27			1.4	78	
Tilting-disk	29			1.57 ± 0.1	69 ± 15	
	31			1.45 ± 0.12	77 ± 17	
Bioprosthetic						
Carpentier-Edwards	27		6 ± 2	1.7 ± 0.3	98 ± 28	
Stented bioprosthesis	29		4.7 ± 2	1.76 ± 0.27	92 ± 14	
	31		4.4 ± 2	1.54 ± 0.15	92 ± 19	
	33		6 ± 3		93 ± 12	
Carpentier-Edwards pericardial	27		3.6	1.6	100	
Stented bioprosthesis	29		5.25 ± 2.36	1.67 ± 0.3	110 ± 15	
	31		4.05 ± 0.83	1.53 ± 0.1	90 ± 11	
	33		1.0	0.8	80	
Medtronic Intact Porcine	29		3.5 ± 0.51	1.6 ± 0.22		
Stented bioprosthesis	31		4.2 ± 1.44	1.6 ± 0.26		
	33		4 ± 1.3	1.4 ± 0.24		
	35		3.2 ± 1.77	1.3 ± 0.5		

*Data on additional valve types and references for this data are available in the original publication.
Data from Rosenhek R, Binder T, Maurer G, et al: Normal values for Doppler echocardiographic assessment of heart valve prostheses, *J Am Soc Echocardiogr* 16:1116–1127, 2003.

TABLE A.8 Equations for Calculation of Expected Aortic Sinus Dimension Based on Body Size

Patient's Age (yr)	Expected Sinus Dimension (cm) (BSA)
<20	1.02 + 0.98
20–39	0.97 + 1.12
≥40	1.92 + 0.74

BSA, Body surface area.
Data from Roman MJ, Devereux RB, Kramer-Fox R, O'Loughlin J: Two-dimensional echocardiographic aortic root dimensions in normal children and adults, *Am J Cardiol* 64:507–512, 1989.

TABLE A.9 Normal Aortic Root Diameter by Age for Men With a Body Surface Area of 2.0 m²*

	AGE (YR)					
	15–29	30–39	40–49	50–59	60–69	≥70
Mean normal (cm)	3.3	3.4	3.5	3.6	3.7	3.8
Upper limit of normal (cm) (95% CI)	3.7	3.8	3.9	4.0	4.1	4.2

*Add 0.5 mm per 0.1 m² BSA greater than 2.0 m² or subtract 0.5 mm per 0.1 m² BSA less than 2.0 m².
BSA, Body surface area; CI, confidence interval.
From Goldstein SA, Evangelista A, Abbara S, et al: Multimodality imaging of diseases of the thoracic aorta in adults: from the American Society of Echocardiography and the European Association of Cardiovascular Imaging: endorsed by the Society of Cardiovascular Computed Tomography and Society for Cardiovascular Magnetic Resonance, *J Am Soc Echocardiogr* 28(2):119–182, 2015.

TABLE A.10 Normal Aortic Root Diameter by Age for Women With a Body Surface Area of 1.7 m²*

	AGE (YR)					
	15–29	30–39	40–49	50–59	60–69	≥70
Mean normal (cm)	2.9	3.0	3.2	3.2	3.3	3.4
Upper limit of normal (cm)	3.3	3.4	3.6	3.6	3.7	3.9

*Add 0.5 mm per 0.1 m² BSA greater than 1.7 m² or subtract 0.5 mm per 0.1 m² BSA less than 1.7 m².
From Goldstein SA, Evangelista A, Abbara S, et al: Multimodality imaging of diseases of the thoracic aorta in adults: from the American Society of Echocardiography and the European Association of Cardiovascular Imaging: endorsed by the Society of Cardiovascular Computed Tomography and Society for Cardiovascular Magnetic Resonance, *J Am Soc Echocardiogr* 28(2):119–182, 2015.

APPENDIX B

Evidence Tables

Table B.1 Selected Studies Validating 2D-Echocardiographic LV Volume Measurements

First Author and Year	Volume/Method	n	r	Regression Equation	SEE	Standard of Reference
Schiller 1979	Modified Simpson's rule Diastolic volume Systolic volume Ejection fraction	30	0.80 0.90 0.87	Echo = 0.7 angio − 1 mL Echo = 0.7 angio − 2 mL Echo = angio + 5%	15 mL 8.5 mL 7.6%	
Folland 1979	Modified Simpson's rule Ejection fraction Ejection fraction	35	0.78 0.75	Angio = 1.01 echo + 0.04 Radionuclide = 0.75 echo + 0.07	9.7% 8.7%	Single-plane angio Radionuclide
Parisi 1979	Modified Simpson's rule Diastolic volume Systolic volume Ejection fraction	50	0.82 0.90 0.80	Angio = 1.08 echo + 30 mL	39 mL 29 mL 9%	Single-plane angio
Silverman 1980	Biplane area-length Diastolic volume Systolic volume Ejection fraction	20	0.96 0.91 0.82	Echo = 1.05 angio − 3.64 Echo = 1.37 angio − 1.37 Echo = 9.87 angio + 0		Biplane angio
Starling 1981	Simpson's rule Diastolic volume Systolic volume Ejection fraction	70	0.80 0.88 0.90	Echo = 0.66 angio + 42 mL Echo = 0.72 angio + 18 mL Echo = 0.76 angio + 12%	34 mL 27 mL 7%	Single or biplane (n = 30) LV angio
Quinones 1981	Simplified method Ejection fraction	55	0.93 0.91		6.7% 7.4%	Radionuclide Angio
Tortoledo 1983	Simplified method Diastolic volume Systolic volume Ejection fraction	52	0.88 0.94 0.92	Angio = 1.07 echo − 7.3 mL Angio = 1.0 echo + 1.3 mL Angio = 0.93 echo + 3.5 mL	28 mL 19 mL 7%	Single-plane angio
Erbel 1983	Simpson's rule Diastolic volume Systolic volume Ejection fraction	46	0.91 0.94 0.80	Echo = 0.66 angio + 0.8 mL Echo = 0.57 angio + 18 mL Echo = 0.61 angio + 13%	26 mL 19 mL 9%	Single-plane LV angio
Zoghbi 1990	Echo-tilt method Diastolic volume Systolic volume Ejection fraction	24	0.92 0.96 0.82	Angio = 0.80 echo + 37 mL Angio = 0.97 echo − 1 mL Angio = 1.17 echo − 4%	23 mL 16 mL 10%	Biplane angio
Smith 1992	TEE Simpson's rule Diastolic volume Systolic volume Ejection fraction	36	0.85 0.94 0.85	Echo = 0.75 angio + 0.2 mL Echo = 0.78 angio − 3.5 mL Echo = 0.82 angio + 9.0 mL	42 mL 22 mL 8%	LV angio (single-plane)

Angio, Angiography; *SEE*, standard error of the estimate.
Data from Schiller et al: *Circulation* 60:547–555, 1979; Folland et al: *Circulation* 60:760–766, 1979; Parisi et al: *Clin Cardiol* 2:257–263, 1979; Silverman et al: *Circulation* 62:548–557, 1980; Starling et al: *Circulation* 63:1075–1084, 1981; Quinones et al: *Circulation* 64:744–753, 1981; Tortoledo et al: *Circulation* 67:579–584, 1983; Erbel et al: *Circulation* 67:205–215, 1983; Zoghbi et al: *J Am Coll Cardiol* 15:610–617, 1990; Smith et al: *J Am Coll Cardiol* 19:1213–1222, 1992.

Table B.2 Selected Clinical Studies Validating 3D Echocardiographic LV Volume Measurements

First Author and Year	Method	n	r	Limits of Agreement	Standard of Reference
				SEE	
Gopal 1993	Normal adults	15	EDV 0.92 ESV 0.81	7 mL 4 mL	CMR
Sapin 1994	Patients (mean age 48 yr)	35	EDV 0.97 ESV 0.98	11.0 mL 10.2 mL	LV angio
Gopal 1997	Patients with abnormal LV	30	EDV 0.90 ESV 0.93	31.8 mL 24.1 mL	CMR
Kuehl 1998	Patients	24	EDV 0.9 ESV 0.94 EF 0.93	23.9 17.2 7.0 mL	LV angio
Mele 1998	Patients	50	EDV 0.95 ESV 0.96 EF 0.92	15.2 11.4 6.2 mL	LV angio, RN, CMR
Qin 2000	Patients (13 with LV aneurysms)	29	LV volumes r = 0.97	−28 mL (mean difference)	CMR
Lee 2001	Patients	25	EDV 0.99 ESV 0.99 EF 0.92	11.3 mL 10.2 mL 6%	CMR
Kawai 2003	Patients	15	EDV 0.94 ESV 0.96 EF 0.93	EDV 21.6 mL ESV 14.8 mL EF 7.6%	CT
				Bland-Altman Analysis*	
Jenkins 2004	RT 3D	50	EDV 0.98 ESV 0.99 EF 0.92 LV mass 0.87	0 ± 5 mL 1 ± 4 mL 0 ± 2% 0 ± 13 g	CMR
Jenkins 2006	RT 3D	110	Online analysis EDV 0.78 ESV 0.86 EF 0.64 Offline analysis EDV 0.86 ESV 0.91 EF 0.81	 −44 ± 35 ml −21 ± 28 mL −2 ± 10% −15 ± 28 mL 10 ± 22 mL −1 ± 8%	CMR
Soliman 2008	RT 3D	24	EDV 0.98 ESV 0.98 EF 0.97 LV mass 0.98	−0.1 ± 19.8 mL −4.2 ± 8.3 mL 0.2 ± 6.2% −5.8 ± 15.4 mL	CMR
Muraru 2010	RT 3D	23	EDV 0.98 ESV 0.98 EF 0.95	−2.7 (−14.9 + 9.5) mL −1.7 (−9.8 + 6.4) mL −0.1 −4.8 + 5.1)	CMR
Macron 2010	RT 3D (2-beats)	66	EDV 0.94 ESV 0.96 EF 0.92	−17 ± 21 mL −9 ± 16 ml 1 ± 6%	CMR
Marsan 2011	RT 3D in patients with LV aneurysm	52	EDV 0.97 ESV 0.98 EF 0.97	21.6 ± 40.4 mL 19.8 ± 40.1 mL −0.9 ± 4.5%	CMR
Chang 2011	RT 3D (single beat)	109	EDV 0.91 ESV 0.94 EF 0.91	41.4 ± 36.5 mL −7.91 ± 33.1 mL −8.26 ± 12.8%	CMR
Aurich 2014	RT 3D	47	EF 0.74 (2D auto-EF) EF 0.73 (3D)	9 ± 17% 9 ± 17%	CMR
Yang 2016	RT 3D (single beat)	34	EDV 0.93 ESV 0.95 EF 0.91	−31.8 ± 25.8 mL −28.5 ± 28.2 mL 6.4 ± 6.3%; Y	CMR (same day)

TABLE B.2 Selected Clinical Studies Validating 3D Echocardiographic LV Volume Measurements—cont'd

*Bias and limits of agreement by Bland-Altman.
angio, Angiography; CMR, cardiac magnetic resonance imaging; CT, computed tomography; DOP, Doppler; EDV, end-diastolic volume; ESV, end-systolic volume; RN, radionuclide angiography; RT, real-time; SEE, standard error of the estimate.
Data from Gopal et al: *J Am Coll Cardiol* 22:258–270, 1993; Sapin et al: *J Am Coll Cardiol* 24:1054, 1994; Gopal et al: *J Am Soc Echocardiogr* 10:853, 1997; Kuehl et al: *J Am Soc Echocardiogr* 11: 1113–1124, 1998; Mele et al: 11:1001, 1998; Qin et al: *J Am Coll Cardiol* 36:900–907, 2000; Lee et al: *J Am Soc Echocardiogr* 14:1001–1009, 2001; Kawai et al: *J Am Soc Echocardiogr* 16:11011–11015, 2003; Jenkins et al: *J Am Coll Cardiol* 18:878–886, 2004; Jenkins et al: *J Am Soc Echocardiogr* 19:1119–1128, 2006; Soliman et al: *Am J Cardiol* 15:778–783, 2008; Muraru et al: *Eur J Echocardiogr* 11:359–368, 2010; Macron et al: *Circ Cardiovasc Imaging* 3:450–455, 2010; Marson et al: *Ann Thorac Surg* 91:113–121, 2011; Chang et al: *J Am Soc Echocardiogr* 24:853–859, 2011;Aurich et al: *J Am Soc Echocardiogr* 27(10):1017–1024, 2014; Yang et al: *J Am Soc Echocardiogr* 29(9):853–860, 2016. See also Dorosz JL, Lezotte DC, Weitzenkamp DA, et al: Performance of 3-dimensional echocardiography in measuring left ventricular volumes and ejection fraction: a systematic review and meta-analysis, *J Am Coll Cardiol* 59(20):1799–1808, 2012.

Table B.3 Selected Studies Validating Doppler Volume Flow Measurement

First Author and Year	Volume Flow Site and Method	n	r	Regression Equation	SEE	Standard of Reference
Huntsman 1983	Ascending aorta	100	0.94	DOP = 0.95x + 0.38	0.58 L/min	TD CO
Fisher 1983	Mitral leaflets	52	0.97	DOP = 0.98x + 0.02	0.23 L/min	Roller pump
Meijboom 1983	Mitral leaflets	26	0.99	DOP = 0.97x + 0.07	0.13 L/min	EM flow and roller pump
	RVOT	26	0.99	DOP = 0.96x + 0.11	0.16 L/min	Roller pump
Lewis 1984	Mitral annulus	35	0.96	TD = 0.91x + 5.1	5.9 mL	TD SV
	LVOT	39	0.95	TD = 0.91x + 7.8	6.4 mL	TD SV
Stewart 1985	Mitral leaflets	29	0.97	DOP = 0.98x + 0.3	0.3 L/min	Roller pump
	Aortic annulus	33	0.98	DOP = 1.06x + 0.2	0.3 L/min	Roller pump
	Pulmonary annulus	30	0.93	DOP = 0.89x + 0.4	0.5 L/min	Roller pump
Bouchard 1987	Aortic leaflets	41	0.95	DOP = 0.97x + 1.7	7 mL	TD SV
Dittmann 1987	Mitral annulus	40	0.86	DOP = 0.88 + 1.75	0.80 L/min	TD CO
	LVOT (M-mode)	40	0.93	DOP = 0.94x + 0.44	0.59 L/min	TD CO
DeZuttere 1988	Mitral orifice(instantaneous)	30	0.91	DOP = 0.92x + 0.35	0.53 L/min	TD CO
Hoit 1988	Mitral leaflets	48	0.93	DOP = 1.1x − 0.45	0.36 L/min	TD CO
Otto 1988	LVOT (proximal to aortic stenosis)	52	0.91	DOP = 1.0x + 0.03	0.25 L/min	EM flow and timed collection
Burwash 1993	LVOT (proximal to aortic stenosis)	75	0.86	Flow probe CO = 0.92 DOP + 0.26	0.50 L/min	Transit-time flow probe
Lefrant 2000	Ascending aorta	58 patients (314 paired data)	0.84	DOP = 0.84 TD + 1.39		TD CO
Gentles 2001	Ascending aorta	20 children with complex CHD	0.96	DOP = 0.98 Fick − 0.08 mL		Fick CO
Chandraratna 2002	Pulmonary artery (continuous)	50 ICU patients	0.92	DOP = 0.93 TD + 0.60	0.7 L/min	TD CO

CHD, Congenital heart disease; CO, cardiac output; DOP, Doppler; EM, electromagnetic flow meter; ICU, intensive care unit; LVOT, left ventricular outflow tract; RVOT, RV outflow tract; SEE, standard error of the estimate; SV, stroke volume; TD, thermodilution.
Data from Huntsman et al: *Circulation* 67:593–601, 1983; Fisher et al: *Circulation* 67:872–877, 1983; Meijboom et al: *Circulation* 68:437–445, 1983; Lewis et al: *Circulation* 70:425–431, 1984; Stewart et al: *J Am Coll Cardiol* 6:653–662, 1985; Bouchard et al: *J Am Coll Cardiol* 9:75–83, 1987; Dittman et al: *J Am Coll Cardiol* 10:818–823, 1987; DeZuttere et al: *J Am Coll Cardiol* 11:343–350, 1988; Hoit et al: *Am J Cardiol* 62:131–135, 1988; Otto et al: *Circulation* 78:435–441, 1988; Burwash et al: *Am J Physiol* 265:H1734–H1743, 1993; Lefrant et al: *Intensive Care Med* 26:693–697, 2000; Gentles et al: *J Ultrasound Med* 20:365-370, 2001; Chandraratna et al: *J Am Soc Echocardiogr* 15:1381–1386, 2002.

TABLE B.4 Selected Studies Validating Noninvasive Pulmonary Artery Pressure Measurement Compared With Direct Measurement by Right Heart Catheterization

First Author and Year	Method	n	r	Regression Equation	SEE
Pulmonary Artery Pressure					
Kitabatake 1983	Time to peak flow (RVOT)	33	−0.88	Log(mean PAP) = 0.0068 (AcT) + 2.1 mmHg	—
Stevenson 1989	TR-jet Time to peak flow (PA) IVRT PR	50	0.96 0.63 0.97 0.96	—	6.9 mmHg 16.4 mmHg 5.4 mmHg 4.5 mmHg
Yock 1984	TR jet	62	0.95	Doppler ΔP_{RV-RA} = 1.03 ΔP + 0.71 mmHg	7 mmHg
Berger 1985	TR jet	69	0.97	$PAP_{Systolic}$ = 1.23 (DOP ΔP) − 0.09 mmHg	4.9 mmHg
Currie 1985	TR jet	127	0.96	DOP ΔP_{RV-RA} = 0.88 ΔP + 2.2 mmHg	7 mmHg
Pepi 1994	TR jet with RA pressure based on IVC	110	0.99	—	5.4 mmHg
Lee 1989	PR	29	0.94	DOP $PAP_{Diastolic}$ = 0.95 (cath) − 1.0 mmHg	Mean difference: 3.3 ± 2.2 mmHg
Chandraratna 2002	PR	50	0.91	DOP $PAP_{Diastolic}$ = 0.82 (cath) + 0.96	3.3 mmHg
Aduen 2009*	Mean PAP by TR jet TR mean ΔP Peak PR velocity	102		Bland Altman −1.5 (−1.2 to 4.3) mmHg 6.1 (4.0 to 8.1) mmHg −5.6 (−7.8 to −3.4) mmHg	Median % difference 17% 21% 28%
Er 2010	Mean PAP by TR mean ΔP	164	0.93	Bland Altman 0.3 (+12 to −12) mmHg	PAP_{mean} ≥25.5 mmHg 98% accurate for pulmonary hypertension
Aduen 2011	Mean PAP by TR mean ΔP	117		Doppler versus catheter mean PAP mean difference −1.6 ± 7.7 mmHg	Accuracy (calculated PAP_{mean} within 10 mmHg) was 81%
Nagueh 2011	PASP, PADP, RAP, LV SV in patients with heart failure	79		Stroke volume: r = 0.83 (P < 0.001) PA systolic pressure (TR jet): r = 0.83 (P < 0.001) PA diastolic pressure (PR jet): r = 0.51 (P = 0.009) RA pressure (IVC method): r = 0.85 (P < 0.001)	
Pulmonary Vascular Resistance					
Gurudevan 2007	Systolic velocity tricuspid annulus (tS_m)	50	−0.71	PVR = 3698 − 1227 × ln(tS_m) dyne-s-cm^{-5}	tS_m >10 has a sensitivity of 80% and specificity of 100% for PVR >1000 dyne-s-cm^{-5}
Abbas 2003	V_{TR}/VTI_{RVOT}	44	0.93	PVR = (V_{TR}/VTI_{RVOT}) × 10 + 0.16	SD 0.0 ± 0.41 Wood units
Farzaneh-Far 2008	V_{TR}/VTI_{RVOT}	22	0.70	(V_{TR}/VTI_{RVOT}) > 0.12 predicts PVR >1.5 Wood units	Sensitivity 100% Specificity 86%

AcT, Acceleration time; *DOP*, Doppler; *IVC*, inferior vena cava; *IVRT*, isovolumic relaxation time; *ΔP*, pressure gradient; *PA*, pulmonary artery; *PADP*, pulmonary artery diastolic pressure; *PAP*, pulmonary artery pressure; *PASP*, pulmonary artery systolic pressure; *PR*, pulmonic regurgitation; *PVR*, pulmonary vascular resistance; *RAP*, right atrial pressure; *SEE*, standard error of the estimate; *SV*, stroke volume; *TR*, tricuspid regurgitation; *V*, velocity; *VTI*, velocity-time integral.
*Contrast enhanced Doppler signals, Bland Altman shown as mean difference (95% limits of agreement).
Data from Kitabatake et al: *Circulation* 68:302-309, 1983; Stevenson et al: *J Am Soc Echocardiogr* 2:157–171, 1989; Yock et al: *Circulation* 70:657–662, 1984; Berger et al: *J Am Coll Cardiol* 6:359–365, 1985; Currie et al: *J Am Coll Cardiol* 6:750–756, 1985; Pepi et al: *J Am Soc Echocardiogr* 7(1):20–26, 1994; Lee et al: *Am J Cardiol* 64:1366–1370, 1989; Chandraratna et al: *J Am Soc Echocardiogr* 15:1381–1386, 2002; Aduen et al: *J Am Soc Echocardiogr* 22: 814–819, 2009; Er et al: *PLoS One* 5(12):e15670, 2010; Aduen et al: *Chest* 139:347–532, 2011; Nagueh et al: *Circ Cardiovasc Imaging* 4:220–227, 2011; Gurudevan et al: *J Am Soc Echocardiogr* 20:1167–1171, 2007; Abbas et al: *J Am Coll Cardiol* 41 1021-1027, 2003; Farzaneh-Far et al: *Am J Cardiol* 101:259–262, 2008.

Table B.5 Selected Studies Validating Doppler Measures of LV Filling Pressures

Echo Parameter	Reference Standard	r	Breakpoints	Sensitivity (%)	Specificity (%)	Reference
Transmitral Flow						
E/A	PAWP	0.72	E/A >1.1 predicts PAWP >12 mmHg			Appleton 1993
E/A	LVEDP		E/A >2.0 associated with LVEDP >20 mmHg	100	100	Channer 1986
DT	PAWP	−0.90	DT ≤120 ms predicts PAWP ≥20 mmHg	100	99	Giannuzzi 1994
DT	LVEDP	−0.74	DT <140 ms predicts LVEDP ≥20 mmHg	90	99	Cecconi 1996
DT	LAP	0.73	DT <180 ms predicts LAP ≥20 mmHg	100	100	Nishimura 1996
ΔA-velocity with Valsalva	LVEDP	0.85	↓A-wave by 21 ± 15 cm/s with LVEDP <15 mmHg ↑A-wave by 18 ± 13 cm/s with LVEDP >25 mmHg			Schwammenthal 2000
Pulmonary Vein Flow						
a_{dur}	LVEDP		a_{dur} >0.35 m/s predicts LVEDP >15 mmHg			Nishimura 1990
a_{dur}	LVEDP		a_{dur} > A_{dur} predicts LVEDP >15 mmHg	85	79	Rossvold 1993
a_{dur}	LVEDP		a_{dur} > A_{dur} + 20 ms predicts LVEDP >12 mmHg	71	95	Appleton 1993
A_{dur}/a_{dur}	LVEDP	−0.70	A_{dur}/a_{dur} ≤0.9 predicts LVEDP ≥20 mmHg	90	90	Cecconi 1996
$PV_S/(PV_S + PV_D)$	LAP	−0.88	$PV_S/(PV_S + PV_D)$ <55% indicates LAP ≥15 mmHg	91	87	Kuecherer 1990
$PV_D DT$	LAP	−0.92	DT of PV_D <175 ms predicts LAP >17 mmHg	100	94	Kinnaird 2001
Tissue Doppler						
E/E′	PAWP	0.87	PAWP = 1.24 (E/E′) + 1.9 mmHg			Nagueh 1997
E/E′	Mean LVDP	0.64	E/E′ <8 predicts normal LVDP E/E′ >15 predicts mean LVDP >15 mmHg		86	Ommen 2000
E/E′	LVDP (pre-a wave)	0.74	E/E′ ≥9 predicts elevated LVDP (>12 mmHg)	81	80	Kim 2000
E/E′	BNP levels and clinical outcome in HFrEF		Septal E/E′ correlated with BNP levels (r = 0.38) and adverse cardiac events (HR: 1.91; CI: 1.25–2.96).			Tang 2011
E/E′	Direct LA pressure in HFrEF	0.46	Septal E/E′ ≥15 was the most accurate predictor of LAP ≥15 mmHg with ROC area >0.9	84	91	Ritzema 2011
E/E′	PAWP in HRrEF	0.61	Average E/E′ >15 predicted PAWP >15 mmHg with ROC area 0.92. Accuracy higher without LBBB or CRT	89	91	Nagueh 2011

A_{dur}, Time duration of transmitral A-velocity; a_{dur}, time duration of pulmonary venous a-velocity; *BNP*, B-type natriuretic peptide; *CI*, confidence interval; *CRT*, cardiac resynchronization therapy; *DT*, deceleration time (of E-wave); *E*, early diastolic transmitral flow velocity; *E′*, early diastolic myocardial Doppler tissue velocity; *E/A*, ratio of early to late diastolic filling velocity; *HFrEF*, heart failure with reduced ejection fraction; *HR*, hazard ratio; *LAP*, left atrial pressure; *LBBB*, left bundle branch block; *LVDP*, LV diastolic pressure; *LVEDP*, LV end-diastolic pressure; *PAWP*, pulmonary artery wedge pressure; PV_D, diastolic pulmonary vein velocity; PV_S, systolic pulmonary vein velocity; $PV_D DT$, deceleration time of PV_D; *PWP*, pulmonary wedge pressure; *ROC*, receiver-operator curve.

Data from Appleton et al: *J Am Coll Cardiol* 22:1972–1982, 1993; Channer et al: *Lancet* 1:1005–1007, 1986; Giannuzzi et al: *J Am Coll Cardiol* 23:1630–1637, 1994; Cecconi et al: *J Am Soc Echocardiogr* 9:241–250, 1996; Nishimura et al: *J Am Coll Cardiol* 28:1226–1233, 1996; Schwammenthal et al: *Am J Cardiol* 86:169–174, 2000; Nishimura et al: *Circulation* 8:1488–1497, 1990; Rossvold et al: *J Am Coll Cardiol* 21:1007, 1993; Kuecherer et al: *Circulation* 82:1127–1139, 1990; Kinnaird et al: *J Am Coll Cardiol* 37:2025–2030, 2001; Nagueh et al: *J Am Coll Cardiol* 15:1527–1533, 1997; Ommen et al: *Circulation* 102:1788–1794, 2000; Kim et al: *J Am Soc Echocardiogr* 13:980–985, 2000; Tang et al: *J Card Fail* 17(2):128–134, 2011; Ritzema et al: *JACC Cardiovasc Imaging* 4(9):927–934, 2011; Nagueh et al: *Circ Cardiovasc Imaging* 4(3):220–227, 2011. For E/E′ also see: Sharifov OF, Schiros CG, Aban I, et al: Diagnostic accuracy of tissue Doppler index e/e′ for evaluating left ventricular filling pressure and diastolic dysfunction/heart failure with preserved ejection fraction: a systematic review and meta-analysis, *J Am Heart Assoc* 5(1):e002530, 2016.

TABLE B.6 Selected Studies on the Diagnostic Accuracy of Exercise Echocardiography Compared With Coronary Angiography*

First Author and Year	n	Exercise Type	Sensitivity (%)	Specificity (%)	Accuracy (%)
Armstrong 1987	123	TME	87	86	88
Ryan 1988	64	TME	78	100	86
Marwick 1992	179	TME	84	86	85
Quinones 1992	112	TME	74	88	78
Ryan 1993	309	UBE	91	78*	87
Marwick 1995	161	TME/UBE	80	81	81
Luotolahti 1996	118	UBE	94	72	92
Roger 1997	340	TME	78	41	69

*In all studies, significant coronary artery disease was defined as a 50% stenosis in an epicardial vessel.
TME, Treadmill exercise treadmill testing; UBE, upright bicycle exercise.
Data from Armstrong et al: J Am Coll Cardiol 10:531–538, 1987; Ryan et al: J Am Coll Cardiol 11:993–999, 1988; Marwick et al: J Am Coll Cardiol 19:74–81, 1992; Quinones et al: Circulation 85:1026–1031, 1992; Ryan: J Am Soc Echocardiogr 6: 186–197, 1993; Marwick et al: J Am Coll Cardiol 26:335–341, 1995; Luotolahti et al: Ann Med 28:73–77, 1996; Roger et al: Circulation 95: 405–410, 1997. See also Ashley EA, Myers J, Froelicher V: Exercise testing in clinical medicine, Lancet 356(9241):1592–1597, 2000; and Dowsley T, Al-Mallah M, Ananthasubramaniam K, et al: The role of noninvasive imaging in coronary artery disease detection, prognosis, and clinical decision making. Can J Cardiol 29(3):285–296, 2013.

TABLE B.7 Selected Studies on Diagnostic Accuracy of Dobutamine Stress Echocardiography Compared With Coronary Angiography

First Author and Year	n	% With CAD	% Stenosis Considered Significant	Sensitivity (%)	Specificity (%)
Cohen and 1991	70	27	70	86	95
Sawada and 1991	103	44	50	89	85
Mazeika and 1992	50	26	70	78	93
Martin and 1992	40	35	50	76	60
Segar and 1992	85	—	50	95	82
Marcovitz and 1992	141	21	50	96	66
Marwick and 1993	217	65	50	72	83
Lewis 1999*	92	27	50	50	81
Eroglu 2006[†]	36	78	50	93	75
Nedelijkovic 2006	166	42	50	96	92

*All subjects in this study were women.
[†]Sensitivity and specificity were the same for 2D and real-time 3D imaging, but acquisition time was shorter with 3D imaging.
CAD, Coronary heart disease.
Data from Cohen et al: Am J Cardiol 67:1311–1318, 1991; Sawada et al: Circulation 83:1602–1614, 1991; Mazeika et al: J Am Coll Cardiol 19:1203–1211, 1992; Martin et al: Ann Intern Med 116:190–196, 1992; Segar et al: J Am Coll Cardiol 19:1197–1202, 1992; Marcovitz et al: Am J Cardiol 69:1269–1273, 1992; Marwick et al: J Am Coll Cardiol 22:159–167, 1993; Lewis et al: J Am Coll Cardiol 33(6):1462–1468, 1999; Eroglu et al: Eur Heart J 27(14):1719–1724, 2006; Nedelijkovic et al: Cardiovasc Ultrasound 4:22, 2006. See also: Heijenbrok-Kal MH, Fleischmann KE, Hunink MG. Stress echocardiography, stress single-photon-emission computed tomography and electron beam computed tomography for the assessment of coronary artery disease: a meta-analysis of diagnostic performance. Am Heart J. 2007 Sep;154(3):415-23.

Table B.8 Selected Studies on the Prognostic Value of Exercise Stress Echocardiography

First Author and Year	n	Female (%)	Study Group	Outcomes (Event Rate)	Median Follow-Up (yr)	Multivariate Predictors of Outcome*
Arruda-Olson 2002	5798	43	CAD	Cardiac death/MI (4.4%)	3.2	• Exercise workload (METs) • Exercise WMSI
Marwick 2001	5375	37	CAD	All deaths (12%)	5.5	• Duke treadmill score • Resting wall motion (scar) • Exercise wall motion (ischemia)
Elhendy 2002	4347	49	CAD	Cardiac death/MI (3.1%)	3.0	• Resting EF • Exercise wall motion (ischemia)
Bergeron 2004	3260	55	Chest pain and/or dyspnea	Cardiac death/MI (3.3%)	3.1	• Previous MI • Ejection fraction • Rest to exercise ΔWMSI
Shaw 2005[†]	4234 women 6898 men			Cardiac death 2.4% in women 3.3% in men	5	• LV function and extent of ischemia • Risk-adjusted 5-year survival was 99.4, 97.6, and 95% for exercising women with no, single-vessel, and multivessel ischemia ($P < 0.0001$). • Exercising men had a 2.0-fold higher risk at every level of worsening ischemia ($P < 0.0001$).
Peteiro 2010	2947	395	CAD	Mortality (5.6%), MACE (12.8%)	1.9 ± 1.6	• Peak exercise WMSI predicted MACE (HR 2.19, 95% CI 1.30-3.69, $P = 0.003$) and mortality (HR 1.58, 95% CI 1.07-2.35, $P = 0.02$).
Arruda 2001a	2632	44	CAD age ≥65 yr	Cardiac death/MI (5.6%)	2.9	• Exercise workload • Exercise ΔEF • Rest to exercise ΔESV
Arruda 2001b	718	18	Previous CABG	Cardiac death/MI (10.6%)	2.9	• Exercise workload • Exercise ΔEF
Elhendy 2001	563	40	Diabetes and CAD	Cardiac death/MI (8.9%)	3.0	• Exercise workload • Resting EF • Extent of ischemia
Elhendy 2003	483	42	CAD and LVH on ECG	Cardiac death/MI (12.4%)	3.0	• Exercise workload • Resting WMSI • Rest to exercise ΔEF
McCully 1998	1325	52	Normal exercise echo	Overall and cardiac event-free survival	1.9	• Overall survival of study group significantly better than an age- and sex-matched group obtained from life tables ($P < 0.0001$). • Cardiac event-free survival rates at 1, 2, and 3 years were 99.2%, 97.8%, and 97.4%, respectively. • The cardiac event rate per person-year of follow-up was 0.9%.
Bouzas-Mosquera 2009	4004	41	Normal ECG stress	Death (7.8%), MACE (4.6%)	4.5 ± 3.4	• Change in WMSI from rest to exercise predicted mortality (HR: 2.73, CI 1.40 to 5.32, $P = 0.003$) and MACE (HR: 3.59, CI: 1.42 to 9.07, $P = 0.007$).

*In addition to clinical factors including male sex, age, diabetes, hypertension, smoking, and previous CABG.
[†]Included both treadmill and dobutamine stress echo.
Δ, Change; CABG, coronary artery bypass graft; CAD, suspected or known coronary artery disease, CI, 95% confidence interval; ECG, electrocardiogram; EF, ejection fraction; ESV, end-systolic volume; LVH, LV hypertrophy; MACE, major adverse cardiac events; METs, metabolic equivalents; MI, myocardial infarction; WMSI, wall motion score index.
Data from Arruda et al: J Am Coll Cardiol 37:1036–1041, 2001a; Arruda et al: Am J Cardiol 87:1069–1073, 2001b; Arruda-Olson et al: J Am Coll Cardiol 39.625–631, 2002, Bergeron et al. J Am Coll Cardiol 43.2242–2246, 2004; Bouzas-Mosquera. J Am Coll Cardiol 53(21):1981–1990; 2009; Elhendy et al: J Am Coll Cardiol 20:1623–1629, 2002; Elhendy et al: J Am Coll Cardiol 37:1551–1557, 2001; Elhendy et al: J Am Coll Cardiol 41:129–135, 2003; Marwick et al: Circulation 103:2566-2571, 2001; McCully et al: J Am Coll Cardiol 31(1):144–149, 1998; Peteiro et al: Eur Heart J 31(2):187–195, 2010; Shaw et al: Eur Heart J 26(5):447–456, 2005.

Table B.9 Selected Studies on the Prognostic Value of Pharmacologic Stress Echocardiography

First Author and Year	n	Female (%)	Study Group	Outcomes (Event Rate)	Median Follow-Up (yr)	Multivariate Predictors of Outcome*
Biagini 2005a	3381	33	CAD	Cardiac death, MI (30%)	7 ± 3.4	• Resting WMA • Ischemia
Marwick 2001	3156	43	CAD	Cardiac death (8%)	3.8 ± 1.9	• Resting WMA • Ischemia
Chaowalit 2006	2349	43	Diabetes	Death, MI, late coronary revascularization (57%)	5.4 ± 2.2	• Extent of ischemia • Ventricular function • Failure to reach target heart rate
Poldermans 1999	1659	29	DSE for suspected CAD	Cardiac death (6.5%), MI (7.7%), revascularization (12%0	3.0	• Stress-induced ischemia (hazard ratio: 3.3; 95% CI: 2.4 to 4.4) • Extensive rest WMA (hazard ratio: 1.9; 95% CI: 1.3 to 2.6)
Biagini 2005b	1434	33	CAD ≥65 yr	Cardiac death/MI (40%)	6.5	• Resting WMA • Ischemia
Chuah 1998	860	44	CAD	Cardiac death/MI (10%)	2 ± 0.8	• Stress WMA • Rest to exercise ΔESV

*In addition to clinical factors including male sex, age, diabetes, smoking, history of heart failure, and previous coronary artery bypass graft.
CAD, Known or suspected coronary artery disease; CI, confidence interval; DSE, dobutamine stress echocardiography; ΔESV, change in end-systolic volume; MI, myocardial infarction; WMA, wall motion abnormalities.
From Biagini et al: *J Am Coll Cardiol* 45:93–97, 2005a; Marwick et al: *J Am Coll Cardiol* 37:754–760, 2001; Chaowalit et al: *J Am Coll Cardiol* 47:1029–1036, 2006; Biagini et al: *Gerontol A Biol Sci Med Sci* 60:1333–1338, 2005b; Chuah et al: *Circulation* 97:1474–1480, 1998; Poldermans et al: *Circulation* 99:757–762, 1999.

Table B.10 Test Performance Characteristics for Echocardiographic Findings in Tamponade

Characteristic	Sensitivity (%)	Specificity (%)
Any collapse	90	65
RA collapse	68	66
RV collapse	60	90
RA + RV collapse	45	92
Abnormal venous flow*	75	91
Abnormal venous flow + 1 collapse	67	91
Abnormal venous flow + 2 collapses	37	98

*Abnormal venous (hepatic vein or superior vena cava) flow defined as: marked systolic over diastolic component, expiratory accentuation of this difference, and expiratory reversal of diastolic flow.
From Merce J, Sagrista-Sauleda J, Permanyer-Miralda G, et al: Correlation between clinical and Doppler echocardiographic findings in patients with moderate and large pericardial effusion: implications for the diagnosis of cardiac tamponade, *Am Heart J* 138(4):759–764, 1999.

TABLE B.11 Test Performance Characteristics for Five Principal Echocardiographic Findings in Constrictive Pericarditis

Variable*	Sensitivity (%)	Specificity (%)	Positive Predictive Value (%)	Negative Predictive Value (%)
Individual Variables				
#1 ventricular septal shift	93	69	92	74
#2 change in mitral E velocity ≥14.6%[†]	84	73	92	55
#3 medial e velocity ≥9 cm/s	83	81	94	57
#4 medial e′/lateral e′ ≥0.91	75	85	95	50
#5 HV ratio in expiration ≥0.79	76	88	96	49
Combinations Among #s 1, 3, and 5[‡]				
#1 (with or without #s 3 and/or 5)	93	69	92	74
#1 and #3 (with or without #5)	80	92	97	56
#1 with #s 3 and/or 5	87	91	97	65
#1 with both #s 3 and 5	64	97	99	42

*Cutpoints for continuous variables were selected from receiver-operator curve analysis.
[†]Based on [(expiratory velocity − inspiratory velocity)/inspiratory velocity × 100]; value will be slightly lower if the currently recommended [(expiratory velocity − inspiratory velocity)/expiratory velocity × 100] is used.
[‡]Limited to echocardiographic findings (in **bold**) that were independently associated with the diagnosis of constrictive pericarditis.
HV, Hepatic vein (HV ratio = diastolic reversal velocity/forward velocity).
From Welch TD, Ling LH, Espinosa RE, et al: Echocardiographic diagnosis of constrictive pericarditis: Mayo Clinic criteria, *Circ Cardiovasc Imaging* 7(3):526–534, 2014.

TABLE B.12 Selected Studies Validating Doppler Pressure Gradients in Valvular Stenosis (In Vivo Simultaneous Data)

First Author and Year	n	Study Group/Model	r	Range (mmHg)	SEE (mmHg)
Callahan 1985	120	Supravalvular constriction (canines)	0.99 (ΔP_{max}) 0.98 (ΔP_{mean})	7179 N/A	5.2 4.3
Smith 1985	88	Supravalvular constriction (canines)	0.98 (ΔP_{max}) 0.98 (ΔP_{mean})	5–166 5–116	5.3 3.3
Currie 1985	100	Adults with valvular aortic stenosis	0.92 (ΔP_{max}) 0.92 (ΔP_{mean})	2–180 0–112	15 10
Smith 1986	33	Adults with valvular aortic stenosis	0.85 (ΔP_{max})	27–138	N/A
Simpson 1985	24	Adults with valvular aortic stenosis	0.98 (ΔP_{max})	0–120	N/A
Burwash 1993	98	Chronic valvular aortic stenosis (canines)	0.95 (ΔP_{max}) 0.91 (ΔP_{mean})	10–128 5–77	8.4 5.3

N/A, Not available; *ΔP*, pressure gradient; *SEE*, standard error of the estimate.
Data from Callahan et al: *Am J Cardiol* 56:989–993, 1985; Smith et al: *J Am Coll Cardiol* 6:1306–1314, 1985; Currie et al: *Circulation* 71:1162–1169, 1985; Smith et al: *Am Heart J* 111:245–252, 1986; Simpson et al: *Br Heart J* 53:636–639, 1985; Burwash et al: *Am J Physiol* 265:H734–H1743, 1993.

TABLE B.13 Selected Studies of Aortic Valve Area Determination

First Author and Year	Comparison	n	Study Group	r*	Range (cm²)	SEE* (cm²)
Hakki 1981	Simplified vs. original Gorlin formula	60	Aortic stenosis	0.96	0.2–2.0	0.10
Zoghbi 1986	Cont eq vs. Gorlin	39	Aortic stenosis	0.95	0.4–2.0	0.15
Otto 1986	Cont eq vs. Gorlin	48	Aortic stenosis	0.71	0.2–3.7	0.32
Oh 1988	Cont eq vs. Gorlin	100	Aortic stenosis	0.83	0.2–1.8	0.19
Danielson 1989	Cont eq vs. Gorlin	100	Aortic stenosis	0.96	0.4–2.0	—
Cannon 1985	Gorlin vs. videotape of valve opening	42	Porcine valves in pulsatile flow model	0.87	0.6–2.5	0.28
	New formula vs. actual orifice area	42	Porcine valves in pulsatile flow model	0.98	0.6–2.5	0.11
Segal 1987	Cont eq vs. actual valve area		In vitro pulsatile flow with orifice plates	0.99	0.05–0.5	0.016
	Gorlin formula vs. actual valve area			0.87		0.047
Cannon 1988	Gorlin vs. known valve area	135	Prosthetic aortic valves	0.39	0.6–2.3	—
Nishimura 1988	Cont eq vs. Gorlin	55	Pre-BAV Post-BAV	0.72 0.61	0.2–0.9 0.5–1.3	0.10 0.17
Desnoyers 1988	Cont eq vs. Gorlin	42	Pre-BAV	0.74	0.3–1.3	—
Tribouilloy 1994	TEE vs. cont eqTEE vs. Gorlin	54	Aortic stenosis	0.96 0.90	0.3–2.0	0.11 0.12
Kim 1997	TEE vs. Gorlin	81	Aortic stenosis	0.89	0.4–2.0	0.04
Bland Altman Mean Difference						
Goland 2007	3D TEE AVA vs. 2D TTE AVA	33	Aortic stenosis	0.99	0.45–1.98	0.00 (−0.15 to 0.15) cm²
	3D TEE AVA vs. Gorlin AVA	15		0.86	0.4–1.4	0.01 (−0.20 to 0.22) cm²
De la Morena 2009	3D TEE AVA vs. TTE 2D AVA	59	Aortic stenosis	0.72†	0.3–1.3	4.04 (0.37–0.45) cm²
Furukawa 2012	TEE 3D AVA vs. TEE 2D AVA	25	Aortic stenosis	0.95	0.4–1.1	−0.14 (range −0.41 to 0.12) cm²

*If not stated in the publication, statistics were calculated from the raw data provided in tables. A blank indicates that data for this calculation were not available.
†Interclass correlation coefficient.
AVA, Aortic valve area *BAV*, balloon aortic valvuloplasty; *Cont eq*, continuity equation; *Gorlin*, Gorlin formula valve area; *SEE*, standard error of the estimate; *TEE*, planimetered 2D valve area on TEE; *3D AVA*, planimetry of aortic valve area on 3D imaging.
Data from Hakki et al: *Circulation* 63:1050–1055, 1981; Zoghbi et al: *Circulation* 73:452–459, 1986; Otto et al: *J Am Coll Cardiol* 7:509–517, 1986; Oh et al: *J Am Coll Cardiol* 11:1227–1234, 1988; Danielson et al: *Am J Cardiol* 63:1107–1111, 1989; Cannon et al: *Circulation* 71:1170–1178, 1985; Segal et al: *J Am Coll Cardiol* 9:1294–1305, 1987; Cannon et al: *Am J Cardiol* 62:113–116, 1988; Nishimura et al: *Circulation* 78:791–799, 1988; Desnoyers et al: *Am J Cardiol* 62:1078–1084, 1988; Tribouilloy et al: *Am Heart J* 128:526–532, 1994; Kim et al: *Am J Cardiol* 79:436–441, 1997; Goland et al: *Heart* 93(7):801–807, 2007; de la Morena et al: *Eur J Echocardiogr* 11(1):9–13, 2010; Furukawa et al: *J Cardiol* 59(3):337–343, 2012.

TABLE B.14 Selected Studies of Mitral Valve Area Determination

First Author and Year	Comparison	n	Study Group	r	Range (cm^2)	SEE (cm^2)
Gorlin 1951	MVA by Gorlin formula vs. direct autopsy or surgery	11	MS	0.89	0.5–1.5	0.15
Libanoff 1968	T½ at rest vs. exercise	20	Mitral valve disease	0.98	20–340 ms	21 ms
Henry 1975	2D echo vs. direct measurement at surgery	20	MS patients undergoing surgery	0.92	0.5–3.5	—
Holen 1977	MVA by Doppler vs. Gorlin	10	MS	0.98	0.6–.4	0.18
Hatle 1979	T½ vs. Gorlin MVA	32	MS	0.74	0.4–3.5	—
Smith 1986	2D echo vs. Gorlin	37	MS alone	0.83	0.4–2.3	0.26
		35	Prior commissurotomy	0.58		0.28
	T½ MVA vs. Gorlin	(37)	MS alone	0.85		0.22
		(35)	Prior commissurotomy	0.90		0.14
Come 1988	T½ MVA vs. Gorlin	37	Pre-MBC	0.51	0.6–1.3	—
			Post-MBC	0.47	1.2–3.8	—
	Gorlin vs. Gorlin		Repeat catheter	0.74	0.4–1.4	—
Thomas 1988	Predicted vs. actual T½	18	Pre-MBC		0.93–0.96	
			Post-MBC		0.52–0.66	
Chen 1989	T½ MVA vs. Gorlin	18	Pre-MBC	0.81	0.4–1.2	0.11
			Immediately post-MBC	0.84	1.3–2.6	0.20
			24–48 hr post-MBC	0.72	1.3–2.6	0.49
Faletra 1996	2D echo vs. direct measurement	30	MS undergoing surgical mitral valve replacement	0.95	0.6–2.0	0.06
	T½ vs. direct measurement	30		0.80		0.09
	Cont eq vs. direct measurement	30		0.87		0.09
	Flow area vs. direct measurement	30		0.54		0.10
Bland Altman Mean Difference						
Dreyfus 2011	3D MVA on TEE vs. 2D MVA on TTE	80	MS	0.79	0.45–2.20	0.0004 ± 0.22 cm^2
Schlosshan 2011	3D MVA on TEE vs. 2D MVA	43	MS	0.87	0.5–2.5	−0.16 ± 0.22 cm^2
	3D MVA on TEE vs. T½ MVA			0.73		−0.23 ± 0.28 cm^2
	3D MVA on TEE vs. Cont. eq MVA			0.83		0.05 ± 0.22 cm^2

Cont eq, Continuity equation; *Gorlin*, Gorlin formula valve area; *MBC*, mitral balloon commissurotomy; *MS*, mitral stenosis; *MVA*, mitral valve area; *SEE*, standard error of the estimate; *T½*, pressure half-time.
Data from Gorlin et al: *Am Heart J* 41:1–29, 1951; Libanoff et al: *Circulation* 38:144–150, 1968; Henry et al: *Circulation* 51:827–831, 1975; Holen et al: *Acta Med Scand* 201:83–88, 1977; Hatle et al: *Circulation* 60:1096–1104, 1979; Smith et al: *Circulation* 73:100–107, 1986; Come et al: *Am J Cardiol* 61:817–825, 1988; Thomas et al: *Circulation* 78:980–993, 1988; Chen et al: *J Am Coll Cardiol* 13:1309–1313, 1989; Faletra et al: *J Am Coll Cardiol* 28:1190–1197, 1996; Dreyfus J et al: *Eur J Echocardiogr* 12(10):750–755, 2011; Schlosshan D et al: *JACC Cardiovasc Imaging* 4(6):580–588, 2011.

TABLE B.15 Selected Studies Validating Quantitative Evaluation of Regurgitant Severity Using Doppler Echocardiography

First Author and Year	Method	Standard of Reference	n	r	SEE
Color Jet Area					
Spain 1989	Color jet area	Angio LV, TD-CO	15 patients with MR	0.62 (RF)	—
Tribouilloy 1992	Regurgitant jet width at origin	Angio LV, TD-CO	31 patients with MR	0.85 (RSV)	—
Enriquez-Sarano 1993	Color jet area	Doppler SV at two sites	80 patients with MR	0.69 (RF)	4.4 cm^2
Vena Contracta					
Tribouilloy 2000	Vena contracta width	Doppler EROA and RV	79 patients with AR	0.89 (EROA)	0.08 cm^2
				0.90 (RV)	18 mL
Hall 1997	Vena contracta width	Doppler EROA and RV	80 patients with MR	0.86 (EROA)	0.15 cm^2
				0.85 (RV)	20 mL
PISA					
Recusani 1991	PISA (hemispherical)	Rotometer	In vitro, constant flow	0.94–0.99 (flow rate)	1.0–1.6 L/min
Utsunomiya 1991	PISA (hemispherical)	Actual flow rate stopwatch and cylinder	In vitro, pulsatile flow	0.99 (flow rate)	0.53 L/min
Vandervoort 1993	PISA	Actual flow rate	In vitro, steady flow	0.98–0.99 (flow rate)	—
Giesler 1993	PISA	LV angio, Fick CO	16 patients with MR	0.88 (RSV)	17 mL
Chen 1993	PISA	Doppler SV at two sites	46 patients with MR	0.94 (RSV)	18 mL
CW Doppler					
Teague 1986	AR half-time	Angio LV, Fick CO	32 patients with AR	~0.88 (RF)	11%
Masuyama 1986	AR half-time	Angio LV, ID-CO	20 patients with AR	~0.89 (RF)	—
Volume Flow at Two Sites					
Ascah 1985	Transmitral vs. transaortic SV	EM-flow	30 flow rates in canine model	0.83 (RF)	—
Kitabatake 1985	Transaortic vs. transpulmonic SV	Angio LV, TD-CO	20 patients with AR	0.94 (RF)	—
Rokey 1986	Transmitral vs. transaortic SV	Angio LV, TD-CO	19 patients with MR and 6 with AR	0.91 (RF)	7%
Distal Flow Reversals					
Boughner 1975	Diastolic flow reversal in descending Ao	Angio LV, Fick CO	15 patients with AR	0.91 (RF)	—
Touche 1985	Diastolic flow reversal in descending Ao	Angio LV, TD-CO	30 patients with AR	0.92 (RF)	8.8%

TABLE B.15 Selected Studies Validating Quantitative Evaluation of Regurgitant Severity Using Doppler Echocardiography—cont'd

First Author and Year	Method	Standard of Reference	n	r	SEE
3D Doppler Color Flow Imaging					
Marsan 2009	3D vena contracta	CMR	64 patients with functional MR	0.94	−0.08 (−7.7 to −7.6) mL/beat*
Zeng 2011	3D vena contracta	Quantitative Doppler	49 patients with MR	$r^2 = 0.86$	0.02 cm^2
Perez de Isla 2012	3D vena contracta	CMR	32 patients with AR	0.88	—

*Bland-Altman mean difference and limits of agreement.
Angio, Angiography; Ao, aorta; AR, aortic regurgitation; CMR, cardiac magnetic resonance imaging; CO, cardiac output; EM-flow, volume flow rate measured by electromagnetic flowmeter; EROA, effective regurgitant orifice area; ID, indicator dilation; MR, mitral regurgitation; PISA, proximal isovelocity surface area method; RF, regurgitant fraction; RSV, regurgitant stroke volume; SEE, standard error of the estimate; SV, stroke volume; TD, thermodilution.
Data from Spain et al: J Am Coll Cardiol 13:585–590, 1989; Tribouilloy et al: Circulation 85:1248–1253, 1992; Enriquez-Sarano et al: J Am Coll Cardiol 21:1211–1219, 1993; Tribouilloy et al: Circulation 102:558–564, 2000; Hall et al: Circulation 95: 636–642, 1997; Rescusani et al: Circulation 83:594–604, 1991; Utsunomiya et al: J Am Soc Echocardiogr 4:338–348, 1991; Vandervoort et al: J Am Coll Cardiol 22:535–541, 1993; Giesler et al: Am J Cardiol 71:217–224, 1993; Chen et al: J Am Coll Cardiol 21:374–383, 1993; Teague et al: J Am Coll Cardiol 8:592–599, 1986; Masuyama et al: Circulation 73:460–466, 1986; Ascah et al: Circulation 72:377–383, 1985; Kitabatake et al: Circulation 72:523–529, 1985; Rokey et al: J Am Coll Cardiol 7:1273–1278, 1986; Bougher et al: Circulation 52:874–879, 1975; Touche et al: Circulation 72:819–824, 1985; Marsan et al: JACC Cardiovasc Imaging 2(11):1245–1252, 2009; Zeng et al: Circ Cardiovasc Imaging 4(5):506–513, 2011; Perez de Isla et al: Int J Cardiol 166(3):640-645, 2011.

TABLE B.16 Validation of Doppler Echo Prosthetic Mean Valve Gradients Compared With Invasive Data (Selected Series)

First Author and Year	Valve Type (Position)	n	r	SEE (mmHg)	Mean Difference
Sagar 1986	Hancock and B-S (mitral)	19	0.93	2.5	—
Sagar 1986	Hancock and B-S (aortic)	11	0.94	7.4	—
Wilkins 1986	Starr-Edwards, B-S porcine (mitral)	11	0.96	—	—
Burstow 1989	Mixed (aortic)	20	0.94	3	—
	Mixed (mitral)	20	0.97	1.2	—
Baumgartner 1990	St. Jude	In vitro	0.98	1.9	10 ± 3 mmHg
	Hancock	In vitro	0.98	1.4	2 ± 1 mmHg
Stewart 1991	Bioprosthetic (aortic)	In vitro	0.78-0.98	—	Overestimation by Doppler
Baumgartner 1992	St. Jude	In vitro	0.98	2.0	13 ± 8 mmHg
	Medtronic-Hall	In vitro	0.99	0.5	0.8 ± 0.6 mmHg
	Starr-Edwards	In vitro	0.97	2.0	8 ± 4 mmHg
	Hancock	In vitro	0.99	1.5	1.9 ± 1.6 mmHg

B-S, Björk-Shiley tilting-disk mechanical valve; SEE, standard error of the estimate.
From Sager KB, et al: J Am Coll Cardiol 7:681–687, 1986; Wilkins GT, et al: Circulation 74:786–795, 1986; Burstow DJ, et al: Circulation 80:504–514, 1989; Baumgartner H, et al: Circulation 82:1467–1475, 1990; Stewart SF, et al: J Am Coll Cardiol 18:769–779, 1991; Baumgartner H, et al: J Am Coll Cardiol 19:324–332, 1992.

Table B.17 Validation of Doppler Echo Prosthetic Valve Areas (Selected Series)

First Author and Year	Valve Type (Position)	n	Comparison	r	SEE	Mean Difference
Sagar 1986	Hancock and B-S (mitral)	12	T½ vs. Gorlin	0.98	0.1 cm^2	—
Wilkins 1986	Porcine (mitral)	8	T½ vs. Gorlin	0.65	—	—
Rothbart 1990	Bioprosthetic (aortic)	22	Cont eq vs. Gorlin at catheterization	0.93	—	—
Chafizadeh 1991	St. Jude (aortic)	67	Cont eq vs. actual orifice area	0.83	—	Doppler effective orifice area less than actual orifice area
Baumgartner 1992	St. Jude Medtronic-Hall Hancock aortic	In vitro In vitro In vitro	Cont eq vs. Gorlin	0.99 0.97 0.93	0.08 0.10 0.10	0.4–0.6 cm^2 0–0.25 cm^2 0–0.25 cm^2

B-S, Björk-Shiley tilting-disk mechanical valve; *Cont eq*, continuity equation valve area with Doppler and 2D echo data; *Gorlin*, Gorlin formula valve area using invasive data; *SEE*, standard error of the estimate; *T ½*, Doppler pressure half-time method.
From Sager KB, et al: *J Am Coll Cardiol* 7:681–687, 1986; Wilkins GT, et al: *Circulation* 74:786–795, 1986: Rothbart R, et al: *J Am Coll Cardiol* 15:817–824, 1990; Chafizadeh ER, Zoghbi WA: *Circulation* 83:213–223, 1991; Baumgartner H, et al: *J Am Coll Cardiol* 19:324–332, 1992.

Table B.18 Accuracy of Echocardiographic Diagnosis of Valvular Vegetations (Selected Studies)

First Author and Year	Study Entry Criteria (Standard of Reference)	No. of Valves	Percent Prosthetic (%)	TTE Sensitivity	TTE Specificity	TEE Sensitivity	TEE Specificity
Mugge 1989	Definite endocarditis *plus* surgery or autopsy	91	23	53/91 (58%)	—	82/91 (90%)	—
Jaffe 1990	Definite endocarditis *plus* surgery or autopsy	38	16	38/44 (86%)	—	—	—
Burger 1991	Suspected endocarditis and clinical outcome	101	—	35/39 (90%)	61/62 (98%)	—	—
Shively 1991	Suspected endocarditis and clinical outcome	6	18	7/16 (44%)	49/50 (98%)	15/16 (94%)	50/50 (100%)
Pedersen 1991	Suspected endocarditis and clinical outcome	24	42	5/10 (50%)	13/14 (93%)	10/10 (100%)	14/14 (100%)
Daniel 1993	Prosthetic valve with surgically confirmed endocarditis	33	100	12/33 (36%)	—	27/33 (82%)	—
Sochowski 1993	Suspected endocarditis with initially negative TTE study	65	12	—	—	Negative predictive value = 56/65 (86%)	
Shapiro 1994	Suspected endocarditis	68	—	23/34 (68%)	31/34 (91%)	33/34 (97%)	31/34 (91%)

Data from Mugge et al: *J Am Coll Cardiol* 14:631–638, 1989; Jaffe et al: *J Am Coll Cardiol* 15:1227–1233, 1990; Burger et al: *Angiology* 42:552–560, 1991; Shiveley et al: *J Am Coll Cardiol* 18:391–397, 1991; Pedersen et al: *Chest* 100:351–356, 1991; Daniel et al: *Am J Cardiol* 71:210-215, 1993; Sochowski, et al: *J Am Coll Cardiol* 21:216–221, 1993; Shapiro et al: *Chest* 105:377, 1994.

Table B.19 Accuracy of Echocardiographic Diagnosis of Paravalvular Abscess (Selected Series)

First Author and Year	Study Entry Criteria	No. of Valves	Percentage Prosthetic (%)	TTE Sensitivity	TTE Specificity	TEE Sensitivity	TEE Specificity
Daniel 1991	Endocarditis with surgery or autopsy	137	25	13/46 (28%)	90/91 (99%)	40/46 (87%)	87/91 (96%)
Jaffe 1990	Endocarditis with surgery or autopsy	7	—	5/7 (71%)	—	—	—
Karalis 1992	Endocarditis with surgery or autopsy	55	46	13/24 (54%)	—	24/24 (100%)	—

Data from Daniel et al: *N Engl J Med* 324:795–800, 1991; Jaffe et al: *J Am Coll Cardiol* 15:1227–1233, 1990; Karalis et al: *Circulation* 86:353–362, 1992.

Table B.20 Sensitivity and Specificity of Diagnostic Tests for Intracardiac Thrombus Formation

Test	Sensitivity (%)	Specificity (%)
LA Thrombus		
TTE*	53–63	95–99
TEE[†]	99	100
CT with contrast[‡]	36–100	72–94
Contrast angiography[‡]	70	88
CMR[§]	100	94
LV Thrombus		
TTE[ǀ]	92–95	86–88
TEE[¶]	40 ± 14	96 ± 3.6
LV Angiography[#]	26–31	—
Contrast-enhanced CMR[¶]	88–93	85–99

CMR, Cardiac magnetic resonance imaging; CT, computed tomographic imaging.
*Shrestha et al: *Am J Cardiol* 48:954–960, 1981; Chiang et al: *J Ultrasound Med* 6:525–529, 1987; Bansal et al: *Am J Cardiol* 64:243–246, 1989.
[†]Aschenberg et al: *J Am Coll Cardiol* 7:163–166, 1986; Olson et al: *J Am Soc Echocardiogr* 5:52–56, 1992; Hwang et al: *Am J Cardiol* 72:677, 1993.
[‡]Tang et al: *J Interv Card Electrophysiol* 22:199, 2008; Patel et al: *Heart Rhythm* 5:253, 2008; Gottlieb et al: *J Cardiovasc Electrophysiol* 19:247, 2008.
[§]Ohyama et al: *Stroke* 34:2436, 2003.
[ǀ]Visser et al: *Chest* 83:228–232, 1983; Stratton et al: *Circulation* 66:156–165, 1982.
[¶]Srichai et al: *Am Heart J* 152:75, 2006.
[#]Reeder et al: *Mayo Clin Proc* 56:77, 1981.

Table B.21 Diagnosis of Aortic Dissection

First Author and Year	n	Approach	Sensitivity (%)	Specificity (%)	Prevalence of Dissection (%)	Standard of Reference
Victor 1981	42	TTE	80	96	36	Angiography
Erbel 1987	21	TTE TEE	29 100	—	100	Surgery or angiography
Hashimoto 1989	22	TTE TEE CT	71 100 100	—	100	Angiography (17) and/or surgery (12)
Ballal 1991	61	TEE CT	97 67	100 100	56	Angiography, surgery, or autopsy
Nienaber 1992	53	TTE TEE CMR	83 100 100	63 66 100	58	Surgery, autopsy, or angiography
Nienaber 1993	110	TTE TEE CMR CT	59 98 98 94	83 98 87 83	56	Surgery (62), autopsy (7), and/or angiography (64)
Chirillo 1994	70	TEE	98	97	57	Surgery
Keren 1996	112	TEE	98	95	40	CT, CMR, aortography, surgery or autopsy
Evangelista 1996	13	TEE	99	100	49	Surgery, autopsy, and CMR
Silverman 2000	78	CMR	100	100	65	Surgery
Yoshida 2003	45	CT	100	100	78	Surgery

		Sensitivity (%)	Specificity (%)	LIKELIHOOD RATIO*	
				Positive	Negative
Shiga 2006	1139 (meta-analysis) TEE CT CMR	 98 (95-99) 100 (96-100) 98 (95-99)	 95 (92-97) 98 (87-99) 98 (95-100)	 14.1 (6.0–33.2) 13.9 (4.2–46.0) 25.3 (11.1–57.1)	 0.04 (0.02–0.08) 0.02 (0.01–0.11) 0.05 (0.03–0.10)

*Likelihood ratios greater than 10 and less than 0.1 are considered strong evidence for confirming or ruling out a diagnosis in most clinical settings.
CMR, Cardiac magnetic resonance imaging; CT, computed tomography.
Data from Victor et al: *Am J Cardiol* 48:1155–1159, 1981; Erbel et al: *Br Heart J* 58:45–51, 1987; Hashimoto et al: *J Am Coll Cardiol* 14:1253–1262, 1989; Ballal et al: Circulation 84:1903–1914, 1991; Neinaber et al: *Circulation* 85:434–447, 1992; Neinaber et al: N Engl J Med 328:1–9, 1993; Chirillo et al: *Am J Cardiol* 74:590–595, 1994; Keren et al: *J Am Coll Cardiol* 28:627–636, 1996; Evangelista et al: J Am Coll Cardiol 27:102–107, 1996; Silverman et al: *Int J Card* Imaging 16:461–470, 2000; Yoshida et al: *Radiology* 22:8430–8435, 2003; Shiga et al: *Arch Intern Med* 10:166(13):1350–1356, 2006.

INDEX

A

Abscess, paravalvular, 403t, 410–413, 410f, 419t
  echocardiographic diagnosis of, 563t
Accreditation, quality assurance and, 135
Accuracy
  of diagnostic testing, 122–123
  of left ventricle imaging, 157–158
  of POCUS, 134–135
Acoustic impedance, 4, 4t
Acoustic intensity, 4
Acoustic shadowing, 14, 14f, 14t
Acoustic window
  transducer, 35
  for transthoracic tomographic views, 49
Advanced heart failure therapies, 257–259
  cardiac resynchronization therapy, 257
  cardiac transplantation, 258–259
    acute rejection in, 259
    allograft in, 258–259, 259f
    post-transplant monitoring in, 259
  left ventricular assist devices, 257–258, 257f
  limitations, technical considerations, and alternate approaches in, 259
Advanced perioperative echocardiography, recommendations for, 508t
Afterload, 145
  definition of, 146, 146f
Aging
  changes, echocardiography and, 61
  left ventricular diastolic filling and, 544t
  left ventricular diastolic function and, 191, 192f
ALARA (As Low As Reasonably Achievable), 29
Allograft, cardiac, 258–259, 259f
Amplitude (dB), 2t
Anatomic valve relationships, 43f
Aneurysms
  aortic dilation and, 455–458, 455t–456t, 457f–458f
  atypical, 438
  in endocarditis, 403t, 419t
  interatrial septal, 439, 440f
  left ventricular, 228, 228f
  sinus of Valsalva, 455t–456t, 464–465, 465f, 475t–476t, 482–483
    transesophageal approach in, 453
    transthoracic approach in, 448, 449f
  ventricular, 431
Angina, indications for transthoracic echocardiography, 139t–141t
Angiosarcoma, 432f

Annular calcification, mitral, 345
Annular dilation
  aortic regurgitation and, 336–338
  tricuspid regurgitation secondary to, 359
Anomalous pulmonary venous return, 475t–476t
Antegrade Doppler flow velocities, 544t
Antegrade intracardiac flows, normal, 55–59
  in descending aorta, 59
  left atrial filling, 58
  left ventricular inflow, 56–57
  left ventricular outflow, 56
  right atrial filling, 59
  right ventricular inflow, 58
  right ventricular outflow, 56
  transthoracic views for, 55t
Aorta
  abnormalities of, aortic regurgitation and, 336–338
  ascending, TEE view of, 74f
  congenital abnormalities of, 482–483
    aortic coarctation, 482, 483f
    sinus of Valsalva aneurysms, 482–483
  descending, in normal antegrade intracardiac flows, 59
  examination of, 469t
  view, in comprehensive TEE exam, 513t
Aortic arch
  transesophageal approach in, 453
  transthoracic approach in, 449
Aortic atheroma, intraoperative TEE for, 527–528, 528f
Aortic atherosclerosis, 455t–456t
  cardiac sources of embolism and, 441t–442t, 444t
Aortic coarctation, 475t–476t, 482, 483f
Aortic dilation, 448
Aortic diseases
  diagnostic imaging procedures for, 466–468, 467t
  indications for transthoracic echocardiography, 132t, 139t–141t
  intraoperative TEE for, 526–528
  key features of, 470t
Aortic dissection, 448, 448f, 455t–456t, 458–463
  aortic regurgitation and, 336–338
  ascending aorta, postoperative evaluation after surgery on, 461–463, 461t, 463f
  complications of, 460–461, 461f
  diagnosis of, 564t
  intraoperative TEE for, 526–527, 528f, 539t
  surgical procedure for, 462, 462f
  transesophageal imaging for, 459–463, 460f
  transthoracic imaging for, 459, 459f
Aortic intramural hematoma, 463, 463f

Aortic leaflet coaptation point, 51
Aortic pseudoaneurysm, 455t–456t, 463–464, 464f
Aortic regurgitation (AR), 336–345, 338f
  aortic flow reversal in, 341, 342f
  aortic valve vegetation and, 404, 405f
  chronic
    asymptomatic, timing of surgical intervention for, 345
    stages of, 344t
  clinical echocardiographic correlation of, 337t
  clinical utility for, 345
  CW Doppler for, 341–343, 342f
  diagnostic utility for, 345
  echo approach to, 365t
  indirect signs of, 339, 340f
  left ventricular response in, 339, 339f
  regurgitant volume and fraction in, 343
  screening examination for, 340–341, 340f–341f
  severity of
    evaluation of, 340–343, 343b
    quantitation of, 365t
  valve apparatus in, diagnostic imaging of, 336–338
  vena contracta and, 341
"Aortic root", 36–37
Aortic sinuses, 36–37
  dimension, calculation of, 547t
  3D echocardiography of, 105t
Aortic stenosis (AS), 291–305, 320t
  bicuspid aortic valve, 292–294, 293f
  calcific, 292, 292f
  causes of, 291f
  clinical applications in, 301–304
  coexisting valvular disease, 300–301
  congenital, 294
  diagnostic imaging of, 291–294
  differential diagnosis of, 294, 295f
  discrepancies in measures of, 299t
  disease progression and prognosis of, 303–304
  left ventricular response to, 301
  low flow, evaluation of, 304–305
  pitfalls in, 299t
  rheumatic, 294
  severity of, quantitation of, 294–300, 301b
    continuity equation valve area, 297–300, 298f
    maximum aortic jet velocity in, 296f, 296t
    pressure gradients in, 296–297, 297f
  stages of, 302t
  timing of intervention in, 301–303, 303f
  valve, congenital, 480
Aortic valve
  anatomy of, 39f
  visualization of, 73
  area determination, 558t

Page number followed by *t* indicates table; by *f* figure; and by *b* box.

565

Aortic valve *(Continued)*
  long-axis images of, 38, 83*f*
  M-mode recording, 52*f*
  recommendations for systematic 3D study, 102*t*
  short-axis view of, 42, 42*f*
  three-dimensional TEE image acquisition in, 514*f*
  3D echocardiography of, 83*f*, 105*t*
  transesophageal echocardiography of, 77*f*, 81–82, 82*t*, 84*f*
  volume-rendered 3D image displays for, 101, 103*f*
Aortic valve vegetations
  transesophageal echocardiography of, 407–408, 407*f*
  transthoracic echocardiography of, 402–404, 402*f*, 404*f*–405*f*
Aortitis, syphilitic, aortic regurgitation and, 336–338
Aperture, 8*t*
Apical image planes, 45*f*
Apical window, for transthoracic tomographic views, 44–47
  four-chamber view, 44–47
  long-axis view, 47, 49*f*
  other, 47
  two-chamber view, 47, 48*f*
AR. *see* Aortic regurgitation
Arrhythmogenic right ventricular dysplasia, 242*t*–243*t*, 256, 256*f*
Artificial heart, 258
AS. *see* Aortic stenosis
Ascending aorta, in comprehensive TEE exam, 513*t*
ASDs. *see* Atrial septal defects
Asymmetric left ventricular hypertrophy, hypertrophic cardiomyopathy and, 246–248, 247*f*
Atheroma, 441
Atherosclerosis, of aorta, 448
  cardiac sources of embolism and, 441*t*–442*t*, 444*t*
Atherosclerotic aortic disease, 465
  as marker of coronary artery disease, 465, 466*f*
  as potential source of embolus, 465
Athlete's heart, features of, 265*t*
Atrial contractile function, left ventricular diastolic function and, 193
Atrial contraction (*A*-wave), 56–57
Atrial fibrillation, with thrombus formation, 437*f*, 439
Atrial filling, left, 182, 187–188
  Doppler data recording in, 188, 188*f*
  nomenclature and measurements in, 187–188, 188*f*
Atrial inflow patterns, of normal color Doppler flow patterns, 61
Atrial septal defects (ASDs), 475*t*–476*t*, 484–488
  anatomy of, 484–486, 485*f*–486*f*
  closure devices, placement of, 531, 532*f*
  contrast echocardiography for, 487
  echocardiography for, 105
  transesophageal imaging for, 488, 489*f*–490*f*
  transthoracic imaging for, 486–487, 487*f*–488*f*
Atrial septum
  recommendations for systematic 3D study, 102*t*
  transesophageal views for evaluation of, 87*t*–88*t*

Atrial situs, 479
Atrioventricular canal defect, 485, 486*f*
Atrium
  left. *see* Left atrium
  right. *see* Right atrium
Attenuation, 4*t*, 5–6
A-wave. *see* Atrial contraction

B
Bacteremia
  in endocarditis, 417, 417*t*
  indications for echocardiography, 130*f*
Ball-cage mechanical valve, 373
Balloon mitral commissurotomy, mitral stenosis and, 314–315, 317*f*–318*f*
Balloon mitral valvotomy, for valve disease, 530*t*
Bandwidth, 8*t*
Basal chordae, 43
Baseline TEE data, 507–508
Basic perioperative echocardiography, recommendations for, 508*t*
Bayesian analysis, 124, 125*f*
Beam shape, focusing and, 7–8, 9*f*–10*f*
Beam width, 23
  effect on 2D imaging, 11*f*
Beam-width artifacts, 14, 14*t*, 15*f*, 405
Bicuspid aortic valve, 292–294, 293*f*, 475*t*–476*t*
Bicuspid aortic valve disease, 455*t*–456*t*
  aortic regurgitation and, 336–338
Bioeffects, 27–28, 29*f*
Bioprosthetic valves, 370–371, 372*f*–373*f*, 376*f*
  aortic, Doppler parameters for, 545*t*–546*t*
  failure of, 373–374
  imaging of, 375–377
  longevity of, 375–377
  mitral, Doppler parameters for, 547*t*
Biplane ejection fraction, 70
Burst length, 24
  color Doppler flow imaging and, 25*f*

C
CAD. *see* Coronary artery disease
Calcific aortic stenosis, 292, 292*f*
Carcinoid heart disease, 426–427, 429*f*
  tricuspid regurgitation and, 359
Cardiac chambers, transesophageal views for evaluation of, 87*t*–88*t*
Cardiac cycle, 144–145, 145*f*
Cardiac Doppler applications, 18
Cardiac hemodynamics, factors affecting, 538*t*
Cardiac masses, 422–446
  cardiac sources of embolism and, 441*t*–442*t*
  characteristics of, 445*t*
  echocardiography for, basic principles of, 422–425, 423*t*, 424*f*
  indications for transthoracic echocardiography, 132*t*
  thrombus as
    left atrial, 434–436, 444*t*
      alternate approaches to, 436
      identification of, 434–435, 435*f*–436*f*
      predisposing factors of, 434
      prognosis and clinical implications of, 436, 437*f*

Cardiac masses *(Continued)*
  left ventricular, 431–434, 444*t*
    alternate approaches to, 432–434
    clinical implications of, 432
    identification of, 432, 434*f*
    predisposing conditions of, 431–432
  right-sided heart, 436–437, 438*f*
  tumors as, 425–431
    nonprimary, 425–427, 427*f*–428*f*, 427*t*
    primary, 427–430, 429*t*
      benign, 427–430
      lipomatous hypertrophy as, 430, 432*f*, 444*t*
      malignant, 430, 444*t*
      myxomas as, 427, 429*f*–430*f*, 444*t*
      papillary fibroelastoma as, 429, 431*f*, 444*t*
      secondary, 427–430
      technical considerations and alternate approaches to, 430–431, 433*f*
    valve vegetations in, 425, 426*f*
Cardiac output, 147
  in intraoperative or intraprocedural TEE, 520*t*–521*t*
Cardiac resynchronization therapy, 257
Cardiac rhythm, left ventricular diastolic function and, 193, 193*f*
Cardiac transplantation, 258–259
  acute rejection in, 259
  allograft in, 258–259, 259*f*
  post-transplant monitoring in, 259
Cardiac tumors, 425–431
  indications for transthoracic echocardiography, 139*t*–141*t*
  nonprimary, 425–427, 427*f*–428*f*, 427*t*
  primary, 427–430, 429*t*
    benign, 427–430
    lipomatous hypertrophy as, 430, 432*f*, 444*t*
    malignant, 430, 444*t*
    myxomas as, 427, 429*f*–430*f*, 444*t*
    papillary fibroelastoma as, 429, 431*f*, 444*t*
  secondary, 427–430
  technical considerations and alternate approaches to, 430–431, 433*f*
Cardiac valves, transesophageal imaging and Doppler assessment of, 82*t*
Cardiomyopathies, 235–267
  arrhythmogenic right ventricular dysplasia, 242*t*–243*t*, 256, 256*f*
  cardiac sources of embolism and, 441*t*–442*t*
  dilated, 236–245
    alternate approaches for, 241–245
    basic principles in, 236, 236*f*, 236*t*
    clinical utility for, 241, 242*t*–243*t*, 244*f*
    echocardiographic approach in, 236–240, 237*f*–241*f*
    features of, 265*t*
    limitations and technical considerations in, 240–241
  echo approach to, 266*t*
  features of, 265*t*
  hypertrophic, 245–252
    alternate approaches for, 252
    basic principles in, 236*t*, 245–252, 245*f*–247*f*
    clinical utility for, 242*t*–243*t*, 251–252

Index

Cardiomyopathies *(Continued)*
   indications for transthoracic echocardiography, 131t, 139t–141t
   intraoperative TEE for, 528–530
   left ventricular noncompaction, 242t–243t, 256, 256f
   restrictive, 252–255
      alternate approaches for, 255
      basic principles in, 236t, 252–255, 253f
      clinical utility for, 242t–243t, 255
      echocardiographic approach in, 253–255
   tako-tsubo, 239, 240f
Carpentier classification, for leaflet dysfunction, 524f
Categorical variables, 122
Cavitation, 27–28
Certification, quality assurance and, 135
Chagas disease, dilated cardiomyopathy in, 239, 239f
CHD. *see* Congenital heart disease
Chest pain
   echocardiographic approach to, 129f
   POCUS for, 134
Chiari network, 494
Chordal elongation, mitral regurgitation and, 345–346, 347f
Cleft mitral valve, 477f, 484
Clinical data, integration of, 124–126
Clinical quantitative Doppler methods, 54–55
   measurement of volume flow in, 54
   spatial pattern of flow of, 55
   velocity-pressure relationships of, 54
Color Doppler flow imaging, 23–27, 24f, 25t
   artifacts, 25–27, 26f, 26t
   instrument controls, 24–25
   normal patterns, 59–61
      atrial inflow patterns, 61
      impact of physics, 59–60
      LV inflow patterns, 60f
      LV outflow, 59f
      physiologic valvular regurgitation, 61
      signal aliasing, 60f
      ventricular inflow, 61
      ventricular outflow, 60–61
   principles of, 23–24
   signal aliasing and, 27f
   for valvular regurgitation, 329–332
      limitations and alternate approaches to, 335–336, 336f
Color Doppler frame rate, 26f
Color Doppler physics, impact of, 59–60
Color flow map, 24
Comprehensive TEE exam, components and sequence of, 513t
Concentric hypertrophy, 156
Conduits, valved, 373
Congenital aortic stenosis, 294
Congenital heart disease (CHD), 473–506
   aorta and coronary arteries, congenital abnormalities of, 482–483
      anomalous origins of, 483
      aortic coarctation, 482, 483f
      coronary arteriovenous fistula, 483, 484f
      sinus of Valsalva aneurysms, 482–483

Congenital heart disease (CHD) *(Continued)*
   basic principles of, 474–480, 475t–476t
      connections, 479–480, 480f
      regurgitation, 474, 477f
      shunts, 474–479, 477f–478f, 478b, 478t
      stenosis, 474, 476f
   cardiac structures in, identification of, 504t
   categories of, 504t
   congenital regurgitant lesions, 483–484
      cleft mitral valve, 477f, 484
      Ebstein anomaly, of tricuspid valve, 483, 485f
   congenital stenotic lesions, 480–481
      congenital aortic valve stenosis, 480
      congenital obstructions, to right ventricular outflow, 481, 481b, 481t, 482f
      subaortic stenosis, 480–481
   diagnostic approach, integrating, 503
   echocardiography and alternate approaches in, limitations of, 500–503, 501f, 504t
      imaging cardiac anatomy, 501–503, 502t, 503f
      intracardiac hemodynamics, 503
      RV volumes and ejection fraction measurement, 500
      shunt ratios calculations, 500–501
   indications for transthoracic echocardiography, 132t, 139t–141t
   intracardiac shunts, 484–491
      atrial septal defects, 484–488
      patent ductus arteriosus, 491, 492f
      ventricular septal defects, 488–491
   intraoperative TEE for, 530, 539t
   other conditions manifesting in, 491–494
      corrected transposition of the great arteries, 491–493, 493f–494f
      "incidental" congenital anomalies, 493–494
   palliated, types of, 494–500
      classification of, 494–497, 495t–496t
      complete transposition of the great arteries, 498–500, 498f–499f
      Fontan physiology, 500, 500f–501f
      tetralogy of Fallot, 497–498, 497f
   with thrombus formation, 439
Congenital obstructions, to right ventricular outflow, 481, 481b, 481t, 482f
Congenital regurgitant lesions, in adults, 474, 477f, 483–484
   cleft mitral valve, 477f, 484
   Ebstein anomaly, of tricuspid valve, 483, 485f
Congenital stenotic lesions, in adults, 474, 476f, 480–481
   congenital aortic valve stenosis, 480
   congenital obstructions, to right ventricular outflow, 481, 481b, 481t, 482f
   subaortic stenosis, 480–481
Congenitally corrected transposition of the great arteries (CC TGA), 475t–476t, 491–493, 493f–494f
Constrictive pericarditis, echocardiographic findings in, 557t

Continuity equation
   for mechanical aortic valves, 381
   for mitral prosthesis, 382–383
   prosthetic valve stenosis and, 387
   valve area, of aortic stenosis, 297–300, 298f
Continuous wave Doppler, 17t, 19
   of prosthetic valve regurgitation, 383–384, 383f–384f
   recordings, 512–513
   of mitral regurgitation, 86f
Contractility, 145, 146f
Contrast echocardiography, 112–115
   applications of, 112–114, 114f, 118t
   in atrial septal defects, 487
   contrast agents in, 112, 113f
   indications for, 114t
   limitations of, 114–115
   safety in, 114–115
Core diagnostic echocardiographic elements, 62
Coronary angiography
   dobutamine stress echocardiography *vs.*, 554t
   exercise echocardiography *vs.*, 554t
Coronary anomalies, 475t–476t
Coronary arteries
   anatomy of, 204–207, 205f–206f, 231t
   congenital abnormalities of
      anomalous origins of, 483
      coronary arteriovenous fistula, 483, 484f
   left, 73f
Coronary arteriovenous fistula, 475t–476t, 483, 484f
Coronary artery disease (CAD), 204–234
   aortic atherosclerosis as marker of, 465, 466f
   basic principles in, 204–211
      coronary artery anatomy in, 204–207, 205f–206f, 231t
      left ventricular wall motion and, evaluation of, 207–210
      sequence of events in ischemia, 210, 210f
      ventricular function, global and regional, evaluation of, 211, 211t, 212f
   diagnosis of, 220
   echocardiographic diagnosis of, 230t
   end-stage ischemic cardiac disease, 228–229
      echocardiographic approach to, 229
      left ventricular systolic dysfunction and, differentiation from other causes of, 228, 229f, 232t
      limitations and alternate approaches to, 229
   indications for transthoracic echocardiography, 139t–141t
   myocardial infarction, 221–228
      basic principles in, 221
      clinical utility for, 222–228
      echocardiographic imaging in, 221, 222f–223f
      limitations and alternate approaches in, 222
      mechanical complications of, 224–228, 224f, 225t, 226f–228f, 231t–232t
   myocardial ischemia, 211–221, 212t
      alternate approaches for, 217–219, 218t, 219f
      clinical utility for, 219–221, 220t

Coronary artery disease (CAD) (*Continued*)
  dobutamine stress echocardiography in, 214–217
  exercise echocardiography in, 213–214, 214*f*
  limitations and technical aspects in, 217
  stress echocardiography in, basic principles of, 211–213, 213*f*
  vasodilators and, 217
Coronary sinus, 90
  dilation of, 39
Coronary sinus cannula, in intraoperative or intraprocedural TEE, 520*t*–521*t*
Cost-effectiveness, of diagnostic testing, 126
Credentialing, quality assurance and, 136
Crista terminalis, 41, 424*f*
Cystic medial necrosis, aortic regurgitation and, 336–338

D

DCM. *see* Dilated cardiomyopathy
Decibels (dB), 3, 3*b*, 3*f*
Deep transgastric view, in comprehensive TEE exam, 513*t*
Descending thoracic aorta
  transesophageal approach in, 453, 513*t*
  transthoracic approach in, 449, 452*f*
Dextrocardia, 479
Dextroposition, 479
Dextroversion, 479
Diagnostic echocardiography, 120
  indications for, 127–133
Diagnostic testing
  basic principles of, 122–126
  clinical outcomes of, 126, 126*f*
  cost-effectiveness of, 126
  integration of clinical data and test results, 124–126
  receiver-operator curve for, 123*f*
Diagnostic transesophageal echocardiography
  intraprocedural and, 507–508
  principles of, 507
Diastole, phases of, 179, 179*f*
Diastolic dysfunction
  causes of, 182, 182*t*
  clinical classification of, 194–198, 194*t*, 195*f*
    estimates of diastolic filling pressures, 194–195
    mild, 195, 196*f*
    moderate, 195–196, 197*f*
    severe, 196–198, 197*f*
    examples of, 199*t*
Diastolic filling curves, 179*f*, 180–181
Diastolic filling rate, early, 181
Diastolic function
  echocardiographic techniques in assessment of, 202*t*
  in hypertensive heart disease, 260, 260*f*
  imaging parameters in, 182–183
    left atrial volumes, 183
    left ventricular changes, 182–183
  in intraoperative or intraprocedural TEE, 520*t*–521*t*
  parameters of, 179–182, 185*t*
    atrial pressures and filling curves, 181–182, 182*f*
    ventricular compliance, 180, 181*f*

Diastolic function (*Continued*)
  ventricular diastolic filling (volume) curves, 180–181
  ventricular diastolic pressures, 180
  ventricular relaxation, 180, 180*f*
  quantitation of, 184*t*
  reporting of, 200
  in restrictive cardiomyopathy, 254–255, 254*f*
Diastolic pressures
  curves, 179*f*
  ventricular, 180
Diastolic run-off, 482
Diffuse effusion, in pericardial effusion, 272–273, 273*f*–274*f*
Dilated cardiomyopathy (DCM), 236–245
  alternate approaches for, 241–245
  basic principles in, 236, 236*f*, 236*t*
  clinical utility for, 241, 242*t*–243*t*, 244*f*
  echocardiographic approach in, 236–240, 237*f*–241*f*
  features of, 265*t*
  limitations and technical considerations in, 240–241
Displacement, myocardial mechanics, 106
Distal flow disturbance in, valvular stenosis, 290, 290*f*
Distal thoracic aorta, transthoracic approach in, 450
Dobutamine stress echocardiography, 214–217
  compared with coronary angiography, 554*t*
  in ischemia, 214–215, 215*f*–216*f*
  in myocardial viability, 215–217
Doppler analysis, principles of, 1–32
Doppler beam width artifact, 23*f*
Doppler echocardiography, 16–27
  color. *see* Color Doppler flow imaging
  regurgitant severity and, 560*t*–561*t*
  tissue. *see* Tissue Doppler imaging
  velocity data, 16–23
Doppler effect, 17*t*, 18*f*
Doppler equation, 16–18, 18*f*
Doppler evaluation
  of hypertrophic cardiomyopathy, 249, 249*f*
  of left ventricular systolic function, 158–163
    ejection acceleration times, 161–162
    limitations of, 162–163
    stroke volume calculation, 158–159, 158*b*, 158*f*
    transvalvular volume flow rates, differences in, 160–161
    ventricular pressure rise, 162, 162*b*, 162*f*
Doppler interrogation angle, in intraoperative and interventional echocardiography, 516, 517*f*
Doppler methods, clinical quantitative, 54–55
  measurement of volume flow in, 54
  spatial pattern of flow of, 55
  velocity-pressure relationships of, 54
Doppler physics, 17*t*
Doppler quantitation, principles of, 65*t*
Doppler recordings, optimization of, 31*t*
Doppler velocities, 84
  data, 16–23
    artifacts, 22–23, 22*t*, 23*f*
    instrument controls, 21–22

Doppler volume flow measurement, 551*t*
Duroziez sign, 341
Duty factor, 8*t*
Dyssynchrony, 107*t*, 111–112, 118*t*

E

Early-diastolic peak velocity (*E*-wave), 56–57
Ebstein anomaly, 475*t*–476*t*, 483, 485*f*
  tricuspid regurgitation and, 359
Echocardiographic anatomy, normal, terminology for, 37*t*
Echocardiographic chamber quantification, reference values for, 542*t*
Echocardiographic image acquisition, 1–32
  bioeffects and safety of, 27–29, 28*t*, 29*f*
  optimization of, 30*t*–31*t*
  transducers, 6–10, 8*t*
  ultrasound imaging modalities, 10–16
  ultrasound tissue interaction, 4–6, 4*t*, 5*f*
  interpretation, 36
Echocardiography
  aging changes on, 61
  for aortic regurgitation, 345
  appropriateness criteria of, 126–127, 127*f*
  in constrictive pericarditis, 557*t*
  in coronary artery disease, 221, 222*f*–223*f*
  diagnostic, 36, 61–62, 120, 127–133
    additional components of, 62
    core elements of, 61–62, 63*t*
  in dilated cardiomyopathy, 236–240, 237*f*–241*f*
  diseases of great arteries, 449–455
  Doppler. *see* Doppler echocardiography
  in end-stage ischemic cardiac disease, 229
  evaluation of, technical aspects of, 375, 376*f*
  in hypertrophic cardiomyopathy, 246–250
  indications for, 126–127
  intracardiac. *see* Intracardiac echocardiography
  laboratory structure of, 137–138, 138*t*
  measurements, 16
    normal values for, 542
  physician and, 136, 137*t*
  prosthetic valve evaluation by, 375
  in pulmonary heart disease, 262–263
  quality assurance in, 135*f*
  reporting in, 137
  in restrictive cardiomyopathy, 253–255
  sonographer and, 136
  stress. *see* Stress echocardiography
  in tamponade, 556*t*
  three-dimensional. *see* Three-dimensional echocardiography
  transesophageal. *see* Transesophageal echocardiography
  transthoracic. *see* Transthoracic echocardiography
  two-dimensional. *see* Two-dimensional echocardiography
Effusion, pericardial. *see* Pericardial effusion
Eisenmenger physiology, 479

Index

Ejection acceleration times
　systolic function and, 161–162
　ventricular pressure rise, rate of, 162, 162b
Ejection fraction, 147b
　in intraoperative or intraprocedural TEE, 520t–521t
　2D and 3D echocardiographic measurement of, 151t, 153t
Electrocardiographic (ECG) electrodes, 36
Electrodes, electrocardiographic, 36
Electronic interference band, 23
　on color flow, 27
Electronic processing artifacts, 14t, 16
Embolus, cardiac source of, 437–442
　basic principles of, 437–438
　echocardiography for
　　findings of, 444t
　　indications for, 441–442, 441t–443t
　identification of, 438
　predisposing conditions of, 438–441
End-stage ischemic cardiac disease, 228–229
　echocardiographic approach to, 229
　left ventricular systolic dysfunction and, differentiation from other causes of, 228, 229f, 232t
　limitations and alternate approaches to, 229
Endocardial cushion defect, 485
Endocarditis, 400–421
　aortic regurgitation and, 336, 338f
　cardiac sources of embolism and, 441t–442t, 444t
　diagnosis of, 403t
　echocardiographic approach to, 401t, 402–413
　　alternate approaches to, 418, 418f
　　clinical utility of, 415–418
　　findings in, 419t
　　intracardiac fistula in, 403t, 410–413, 412f, 419t
　　limitations of, 413–415
　　paravalvular abscess in, 403t, 410–413, 410f, 419t
　　technical considerations to, 413–415
　　valve dysfunction in, 409
　　valvular vegetations in, 402–409, 403t, 419t
　fungal, 408f
　indications for transthoracic echocardiography, 131t, 139t–141t
　intraoperative TEE for, 526, 539t
　known, 417–418
　mitral regurgitation and, 347
　nonbacterial thrombotic, 413, 413f
　prosthetic valves and, 392–394, 395f, 414–415, 414f–416f
　　dysfunction of, 375
　suspected, 415–417, 416f
　tricuspid regurgitation and, 359
　with underlying valve disease, 413–414
Endocardium
　in left ventricle imaging, 156–157
　posterior wall, 51–52
Epiaortic scan, 527–528, 528f
E-point septal separation (EPSS), 51
　aortic regurgitation and, 339
EPSS. see E-point septal separation
Equipment, in echocardiography laboratory structure, 138t

Esophageal position, of transesophageal echocardiography, 70–75
　four-chamber plane, 70–71, 70f–72f
　long-axis plane, 73, 74f
　short-axis plane, 73–75
　two-chamber plane, 71–73, 72f
Esophageal trauma, risk of TEE, 68
Eustachian valve, 424f
E-wave. see Early-diastolic peak velocity
Exercise, systolic function and, 147
Exercise echocardiography. see also Stress echocardiography
　compared with coronary angiography, 554t
　in myocardial ischemia, 213–214, 214f
　prognostic value of, 555t
Expertise, of diagnostic testing, 123

F

Fabry disease, restrictive cardiomyopathy and, 254, 254f
Fast Fourier transform (FFT), 18
Femoral venous cannula, in intraoperative or intraprocedural TEE, 520t–521t
Fever, indications for echocardiography, 130f
Fibroelastoma, papillary, 429, 431f, 444t
Fistula, in endocarditis, 403t, 410–413, 412f, 419t
Flow-velocity profiles, 53–54, 54f
Fluid dynamics
　of valvular regurgitation, 325–326, 325f, 325t
　of valvular stenosis, 289–291
　　distal flow disturbance in, 290, 290f
　　high-velocity jet in, 289, 289f
　　pressure gradient and velocity, relationship between, 289–290
　　proximal flow patterns in, 290–291, 291f
Focal depth, 8t
Four-chamber plane
　of esophageal position, 70–71, 70f–72f
　standard image and, 35
　of transgastric position, 78
Four-chamber view, 44–47, 46f
Frequency bandwidth, 7
Frequency (f), 2, 2t
Full-volume gated acquisition volume-rendered images, 98, 98t

G

Geometry, ventricular, 145–147
　classification of, 156
　left, 155–156
Giant cell arteritis, 455t–456t
Global systolic function, in intraoperative or intraprocedural TEE, 520t–521t
Grating lobes, 8
Great arteries, diseases of, 447–472
　alternate approaches in, 466–468, 467t, 468f
　aortic dilation and aneurysm, 455–458, 455t–456t, 457f–458f
　aortic dissection, 458–463
　aortic intramural hematoma, 463, 463f
　aortic pseudoaneurysm, 463–464, 464f
　atherosclerotic aortic disease, 465
　basic principles of, 447–448
　echocardiographic approach in, 449–455
　　transesophageal approach in, 453–455
　　transthoracic approach in, 449–453

Great arteries, diseases of (Continued)
　pulmonary artery abnormalities, 451f, 465–466, 467f
　sinus of Valsalva aneurysm, 464–465, 465f
　traumatic aortic disease, 464
Great vessels
　dimension, in adults, 543t
　transesophageal views for evaluation of, 87t–88t

H

Handheld ultrasound, features of, 134t
HCM. see Hypertrophic cardiomyopathy
Heart, enlarged, 128f
Heart disease
　carcinoid, tricuspid regurgitation and, 359
　congenital. see Congenital heart disease
Heart failure (HF)
　diagnoses in, 265t
　indications for transthoracic echocardiography, 129f, 131t
　symptoms with hypertension, 261
Heart rate, left ventricular diastolic function and, 191f
Heart transplantation, intraoperative TEE for, 529–530
Hemodynamics, in intraoperative and interventional echocardiography, 509–510, 510f
Hepatocellular carcinoma, metastatic, 428f
HF. see Heart failure
Hibernating myocardium, 223
High-PRF Doppler, 21, 21f
　example of, 22f
High-velocity jet, in valvular stenosis, 289, 289f
Homograft valves, 372
　aortic, 375
Hybrid procedures, intraoperative and interventional echocardiography in, 530–535, 530t, 531f
　atrial septal defect closure devices, placement of, 531, 532f, 533t–534t, 535f
　other transcatheter interventions, 535, 537f
　transcatheter mitral valve repair, 535, 535f–536f
Hypertension
　chronic, aortic regurgitation and, 336–338
　heart failure symptoms and, 261
　indications for transthoracic echocardiography, 131t, 139t–141t
　pulmonary. see Pulmonary hypertension
Hypertensive heart disease, 260–262, 455t–456t
　alternate approaches for, 261–262
　basic principles in, 260
　clinical utility for, 261
　　diagnosis and prognosis, 261
　　evaluation of heart failure symptoms in patient with hypertension, 261
　echocardiographic approach in, 260–261
　　diastolic function, 260, 260f
　　other echocardiographic findings in, 261

Hypertensive heart disease *(Continued)*
    systolic function, 261
    ventricular hypertrophy, 260, 260f
  limitations and technical considerations in, 261
Hypertrophic cardiomyopathy (HCM), 245–252
  alternate approaches for, 252
  basic principles in, 236t, 245–252, 245f–247f
  echocardiographic approach for, 246–250
  features of, 265t
  limitations and technical considerations in, 250–251, 250f–251f
  clinical utility for, 242t–243t, 251–252
    diagnosis and screening, 251
    evaluation of medical therapy, 251
    monitoring of percutaneous septal ablation, 251–252, 252f
    patient selection for implanted cardiac defibrillators, 251
    surgical therapy, 252
  echocardiographic approach for, 246–250
    asymmetric left ventricular hypertrophy, 246–248, 247f
    dynamic subaortic LV outflow tract obstruction, 248–249, 248f–250f
    left ventricular diastolic function, 248
    mitral valve abnormalities, 250
  intraoperative TEE for, 528–529, 539t

I

ICE. *see* Intracardiac echocardiography
Image acquisition, in 3D echocardiography, 96–99, 97f, 98t, 99f–100f
Image plane orientation, in intraoperative and interventional echocardiography, 516
Impella device, in intraoperative or intraprocedural TEE, 520t–521t
Implanted cardiac defibrillators, hypertrophic cardiomyopathy and, 251
"Incidental" congenital anomalies, 493–494
Increased wall thickness, cause of, 265t
Inferior vena cava, 42
Inferior vena cava dilation, in pericardial tamponade, 278
Inlet ventricular septal defects, 490
Instrument settings, in intraoperative and interventional echocardiography, 517–518, 518f–519f
Instrumentation, surgical, in intraoperative and interventional echocardiography, 510–511, 511f
Interatrial septum
  comprehensive TEE exam of, 513t
  three-dimensional TEE image acquisition of, 514f
  volume-rendered 3D image displays of, 101, 103f
Interatrial septum view, 72f
Intercept angle, 17t
Intermediate ultrasound, features of, 134t

Interventional echocardiography, 507–541
  approach of, 512–516
    reporting and image storage in, 516
    sequence in, 513–516
    views in, 512–513, 513t, 514f–515f
  basic principles of, 508–512
    hemodynamics in, 509–510, 510f
    indications for, 508, 509t
    preoperative diagnosis of, 508–509, 510f
    surgical manipulation and instrumentation of, 510–511, 511f
    time constraints in, 511–512, 512f
  limitations and technical considerations for, 516–518
    Doppler interrogation angle in, 516
    image plane orientation in, 516
    instrument settings, optimization of, 517–518, 518f–519f
    operating room and interventional suite, technical issues in, 517, 518f
  transcatheter and hybrid procedures, clinical utility in, 530–535, 530t, 531f
    atrial septal defect closure devices, placement of, 531, 532f, 533t–534t, 535f
    other transcatheter interventions, 535, 537f
    transcatheter mitral valve repair, 535, 535f–536f
Interventional suite, intraoperative and interventional echocardiography in, 517, 518f
Intraaortic balloon pump (IABP), in intraoperative or intraprocedural TEE, 520t–521t
Intracardiac devices, 414–415
  cardiac sources of embolism and, 441t–442t
  in intraoperative or intraprocedural TEE, 520t–521t
Intracardiac echocardiography (ICE), 115–116
  applications for, 116, 116t, 117f, 118t
  instrumentation, 115, 115f
  technique in, 115–116
Intracardiac flows
  antegrade, 55–59
    in descending aorta, 59
    left atrial filling, 58
    left ventricular inflow, 56–57
    left ventricular outflow, 56
    right atrial filling, 59
    right ventricular inflow, 58
    right ventricular outflow, 56
    transthoracic views for, 55t
  blood, 54f
  normal, 52–61
Intracardiac shunts, in adults, 484–491
Intracardiac tumors. *see* Cardiac tumors
Intramural hematoma, 455t–456t
Intraoperative echocardiography, 507–541
  approach of, 512–516
    reporting and image storage in, 516
    sequence in, 513–516
    views in, 512–513, 513t, 514f–515f
  limitations and technical considerations for, 516–518
    Doppler interrogation angle in, 516, 517f

Intraoperative echocardiography *(Continued)*
    image plane orientation in, 516
    instrument settings in, optimization of, 517–518, 518f–519f
    operating room and interventional suite, technical issue in, 517, 518f
  principles of, 508–512
    hemodynamics in, 509–510, 510f
    indications for, 508, 509t
    preoperative diagnosis of, 508–509, 510f
    surgical manipulation and instrumentation, 510–511, 511f
    time constraints in, 511–512, 512f
  transcatheter and hybrid procedures, clinical utility in, 530–535, 530t, 531f
    atrial septal defect closure devices, placement of, 531, 532f
    other transcatheter interventions, 535, 537f
    transcatheter mitral valve repair, 535, 535f–536f
    transcatheter valve implantation, 531, 533t–534t, 535f
Intraoperative transesophageal echocardiography
  clinical utility of, 519–530
    in aortic disease, 526–528
    in cardiomyopathies, 528–530
    in congenital heart disease, 530
    in monitoring ventricular function, 519, 520t–521t, 521f
    in valvular heart disease, 521–526
  external cardiac compression on, 510–511, 511f
  indications for, 509t
  key data for, 539t
  principles of, 507, 520t–521t, 538t
Intraprocedural transesophageal echocardiography
  diagnostic and, 507–508
  indications for, 508, 509t
  instrument settings in, 517
  principles for, 520t–521t
  reporting and image storage in, 516
Ischemia
  dobutamine stress echocardiography in, 214–215, 215f–216f
  sequence of events in, 210, 210f
Ischemic cardiac disease, end-stage, 228–229
  echocardiographic approach to, 229
  indications for transthoracic echocardiography, 139t–141t
  left ventricular systolic dysfunction and, differentiation from other causes of, 228, 229f, 232t
  limitations and alternate approaches to, 229
Isovolumic relaxation, 179
  time, 189, 189f

L

Lambl excrescence, 404, 404f
Laminar flow, 52–53
Lateral resolution artifact, 14t
Leaflet destruction, in endocarditis, 403t, 409, 419t
Leaflet dysfunction, 523, 524f
Leaflet perforation, 419t
  mitral, 408, 409f

Left atrial enlargement, in mitral stenosis, 312–313, 313f
Left atrial filling, 58, 182, 187–188
  Doppler data recording in, 188, 188f
  nomenclature and measurements in, 187–188, 188f
Left atrium
  appendage, volume-rendered 3D image displays for, 101, 103f
  in mitral regurgitation, 350–351
  3D echocardiography of, 105t
  transesophageal echocardiography of, 89, 513t
  volume, normal ranges, 543t
Left coronary artery, 73f
Left ventricle (LV)
  ejection fraction
    normal ranges of, 543t
    TEE measurement of, 89f
  function of
    in intraoperative or intraprocedural TEE, 520t–521t
    quantitation of, 512, 515f
  geometry of, 155–156
  imaging of, 147–158
    accuracy of, 157–158
    biplane, 88f
    dimension of, 148–149, 149t, 151f
    endocardial definition in, 156–157
    geometric assumptions, 157
    limitations of, 156–158
    qualitative evaluation of, systolic function, 147–148
    quantitative evaluation of, systolic function, 148–155
    reproducibility of, 157–158
    speckle tracking strain, 155, 156f
    strain rate imaging, 153–155
    three-dimensional echocardiography, 105t, 149–152, 153t, 155f
    transesophageal echocardiography, 87–89, 147, 149t, 513t
    transthoracic echocardiography, 149t
    two-dimensional echocardiography, 148–152, 152f, 153t, 154f
    2D guided M-mode, 148–149, 149t, 150f
    wall stress, 153–155
  mass of, 155–156
  in mitral regurgitation, 350–351, 351f
  in M-mode recording, 51–52, 53f
  recommendations for systematic 3D study, 102t
  three-dimensional TEE image acquisition in, 514f
  volume-rendered 3D image displays for, 101, 103f
  volumes, 150–152, 154f
    in intraoperative or intraprocedural TEE, 520t–521t
    measurement for
      2D-echocardiographic, 549t
      3D-echocardiographic, 550t–551t
Left ventricular assist device (LVAD), 257–258, 257f, 529, 529f
  in intraoperative or intraprocedural TEE, 520t–521t
Left ventricular diastolic function
  factors affecting Doppler evaluation of, 190–193
  pathophysiology, 192–193
    cardiac rhythm and atrial contractile function, 193, 193f

Left ventricular diastolic function (Continued)
    left ventricular systolic function, 192
    mitral valve disease, 192–193, 193f
  physiologic factors, 190–192
    age, 191, 192f
    preload, 191–192, 192f
    respiration, heart rate, and PR interval, 191, 191f
  hypertrophic cardiomyopathy and, 248
Left ventricular filling, Doppler evaluation of, 183–185
  Doppler data recording in, 185
  nomenclature and measurements in, 183, 186f
  pressure, 553t
  volumetric flow rates in, 183–185, 186f–187f
Left ventricular inflow, 56–57, 86f
Left ventricular noncompaction, 242t–243t, 256, 256f
Left ventricular outflow, 56, 57f, 71f, 159–160, 160f
Left ventricular outflow tract obstruction, dynamic subaortic, hypertrophic cardiomyopathy and, 248–249, 248f–250f
Left ventricular relaxation, rate of, 189–190, 190f
Left ventricular response
  in aortic regurgitation, 339, 339f
  in aortic stenosis, 301
  in mitral stenosis, 312
Left ventricular systolic dysfunction
  aortic stenosis with, 304–305, 304f–305f
  differentiation from other causes of, 228, 229f, 232t
Left ventricular systolic function
  Doppler evaluation of, 158–163
    ejection acceleration times, 161–162
    limitations of, 162–163
    stroke volume calculation, 158–159, 158b, 158f
    transvalvular volume flow rates, differences in, 160–161
    ventricular pressure rise, 162, 162b, 162f
  left ventricular diastolic function and, 192
Left ventricular wall motion, evaluation of, 207–210
  transesophageal imaging in, 209–210
  transthoracic imaging in, 207–209, 207f–209f
Left ventricular web, 423f
Likelihood ratio, 124
Linear dimensions, in systolic function, 148–149
Lipomatous hypertrophy, 430, 432f, 444t
Loculated effusion, in pericardial effusion, 273, 274f
Long-axis plane
  of aortic valve, 83f
  of esophageal position, 73, 74f
  image, 73, 75f
  standard image and, 35
  of transgastric position, 78–79, 80f
  volume measurement, 47f

Low flow aortic stenosis, with normal LV ejection fraction, 305
LVAD. see Left ventricular assist device

M

Marfan syndrome, 450f, 455t–456t
  aortic regurgitation and, 336–338
  echo findings in, 448, 448f
  mitral regurgitation and, 347
Marginal chordae, 43
Maximum aortic jet velocity, of aortic stenosis, 296f, 296t
Mechanical valve, 372f, 373, 374f
  aortic
    continuity equation for, 381
    Doppler parameters for, 545t–546t
  ball-cage, 373
  imaging of, 377, 377f
  mitral, Doppler parameters for, 547t
Medical therapy, hypertrophic cardiomyopathy and, 251
Men, aortic root diameter for, 548t
Method of disks, 150–152
MI. see Myocardial infarction
Microcavitation, in prosthetic valves, 377
Mid-esophageal views, in comprehensive TEE exam, 513t
Mirror-image artifact, 23, 24f
Mitral annular calcification, 306, 308f, 345
Mitral-aortic intervalvular fibrosa, aneurysm of, 410, 411f
Mitral leaflet perforation, transesophageal echocardiography of, 408, 409f
Mitral regurgitation (MR), 345–359
  clinical echocardiographic correlation of, 353t
  clinical follow-up for, 356
  clinical utility of, 356–359
  CW Doppler recording of, 86f
  echo approach to, 366t
  functional, 349, 350f
  intervention for
    decision making concerning type of, 359
    timing of, 356
  ischemic, 347–348, 349f
  left atrium response to, 350–351
  left ventricular response to, 350–351, 351f
  mitral stenosis and, 313–314
  myocardial infarction and, 224, 224f
  proximal isovelocity surface area and, 354, 354f–355f
  pulmonary vasculature response to, 350–351
  pulmonary vein flow reversal and, 354–356
  regurgitation volume and orifice area and, 354
  rheumatic, 347
  screening examination for, 351–352
  severity of
    diagnosis and, 356
    evaluation of, 351–356, 352f, 356b
    quantitation of, 355f, 366t
  stages of
    primary, 357t
    secondary, 358t
  transesophageal echocardiography for, 516, 517f
  valve apparatus in, diagnostic imaging of, 345–349, 345f–348f
  vena contracta and, 352

Mitral stenosis (MS), 305–315, 321t
  coexisting valvular disease, 314
  consequences of, 312–314
  diagnostic imaging of mitral valve, 306–307
  differential diagnosis of, 306–307
  The French Three-Group grading of, 316t
  mitral annular calcification in, 306, 308f
  rheumatic disease in, 306, 306f–307f
  severity, quantitation of, 307–312, 314b
    mitral valve area in, 307–309
    pressure gradients in, 307, 308f
    technical considerations and potential pitfalls in, 309–312, 312t
  stages of, 315t
Mitral valve, 51
  abnormalities, hypertrophic cardiomyopathy and, 250
  anatomy of, 39f
  anterior and posterior, 38–39
  area
    determination of, 559t
    in mitral stenosis, 307–309
  direct imaging of, 307, 309f–310f
  disease. see also Mitral regurgitation; Mitral stenosis
    congenital, 475t–476t
  left ventricular diastolic function and, 192–193, 193f
  imaging of, 85f
  M-mode recording, 52f
  recommendations for systematic 3D study, 102t
  in short-axis plane, 43, 44f
  stroke volume calculations, 160, 161f
  three-dimensional TEE image acquisition in, 514f
  3D echocardiography of, 105t
  transesophageal echocardiography of, 82–84, 82t, 513t
  transgastric position of, 79f
  2D echocardiography of, 316t
  vegetations, transthoracic echocardiography of, 402f, 404–405, 405f–406f
  volume-rendered 3D image displays for, 101, 103f
Mitral valve repair, intraoperative TEE for, 521–524, 522f–525f, 539t
M-mode, 10–11, 12f
  2D guided, of left ventricle, 148–149, 149t, 150f
M-mode echocardiography, 111–112
  patterns of septal motion on, 168, 171f
M-mode recordings, 49–52
  aortic valve, 52f
  and left atrium of, 50–51
  clinical quantitative Doppler methods of, 54–55
  mitral valve, 52f
  normal antegrade intracardiac flows of, 55–59
  normal color Doppler flow patterns of, 59–61
  other, 52
MR. see Mitral regurgitation
MS. see Mitral stenosis
Multiple simultaneous 2D image planes, 100–101, 101f

Murmur, echocardiographic approach to, 129f
Muscular right ventricular outflow tract, 39–40
Muscular ventricular septal defects, 488–490
Myocardial infarction (MI), 221–228
  acute
    cardiac sources of embolism and, 441t–442t
    indications for transthoracic echocardiography, 139t–141t
  basic principles in, 221
  clinical utility for, 222–228
    diagnosis in emergency department, 222–223
    evaluation of interventional therapy, 223
    myocardial viability, 223–224
  echocardiographic imaging in, 221, 222f–223f
  limitations and alternate approaches in, 222
  mechanical complications of, 224–228, 224f, 225t, 226f–228f, 231t–232t
Myocardial ischemia, 211–221, 212t
  alternate approaches for, 217–219, 218t, 219f
  clinical utility for, 219–221, 220t
    diagnosis of coronary artery disease, 220
    extent and location of ischemic areas, 220
    prognostic implications, 221
  dobutamine stress echocardiography in, 214–217
  exercise echocardiography in, 213–214, 214f
  limitations and technical aspects in, 217
  stress echocardiography in, 211–213, 213f
  vasodilators and, 217
Myocardial mechanics, 106–112
  clinical utility, 110–111
  dyssynchrony, 111–112
  LV and LA, 190
  strain and strain rate in
    by speckle tracking, 109–110, 111f, 118t
    by tissue Doppler, 106–109, 107f–110f, 118t
  torsion, 111–112
  twist, 111–112
Myxomas, cardiac, 427, 429f–430f, 444t
Myxomatous mitral valve disease
  echocardiography for, 105
  mitral regurgitation and, 345–346

N
Native valves, prosthetic valves and, differences between, 383
Nyquist limit, 17t

O
Oblique sinus, in pericardium, 268
Operating room, intraoperative and interventional echocardiography in, 517, 518f
Outflow obstruction, in hypertrophic cardiomyopathy, 249, 250f

Outflow tract diameter, aortic stenosis and, 299–300
Outflow tract velocity, aortic stenosis and, 300

P
Pacer lead infections
  transesophageal echocardiography of, 409f
  transthoracic echocardiography of, 406
Palliated adult congenital heart disease, types of, 494–500
  classification of, 494–497, 495t–496t
  complete transposition of the great arteries, 498–500, 498f–499f
  Fontan physiology, 500, 500f–501f
  tetralogy of Fallot, 497–498, 497f
Papillary fibroelastoma, 429, 431f, 444t
Papillary muscle
  rupture
    mitral regurgitation and, 348
    myocardial infarction and, 224, 224f
  in short-axis plane, 43, 45f
Paradoxical septal motion, 166–167, 169f, 359
Parasternal window, for transthoracic tomographic views, 36–44
  long-axis, 36–40, 38f
  outflow view, 36–40
  right ventricular inflow, 36–40, 40f
  short-axis, 42–44
Paravalvular abscess, 403t, 410–413, 410f, 419t
  echocardiographic diagnosis of, 563t
Parietal pericardium, 268
Patent ductus arteriosus, 475t–476t, 491, 492f
Patent foramen ovale, 439, 440f–441f, 441t–442t, 444t
Patient-prosthesis mismatch, 379, 391
Percutaneous septal ablation, hypertrophic cardiomyopathy and, 251–252, 252f
Pericardial adipose tissue, 274
Pericardial constriction, 278–284, 283t
  basic principles of, 278–279, 279f–280f
  clinical utility in, 282–284
  echocardiographic approach to, 279–282
    Doppler examination for, 280–281, 282f–283f
    imaging for, 280, 281f
    restrictive cardiomyopathy vs., 281–282, 284f
Pericardial disease, 268–287, 285t
  causes of, 270t
  clinical-echocardiographic correlates, 271t
  echocardiographic approach to, 272t
  indications for transthoracic echocardiography, 132t, 139t–141t
  pericardial constriction, 278–284
    basic principles of, 278–279, 279f–280f
    clinical utility in, 282–284
    echocardiographic approach to, 279–282
  pericardial effusion, 271–275
    basic principles of, 270t, 271, 271f–272f
    clinical utility in, 274–275, 276f
    diagnosis of, 272–274

Pericardial disease *(Continued)*
  pericardial tamponade, 275–278
    clinical utility in, 278
    diagnosis of, 278
    echocardiographic approach to, 275–278, 276f
  pericarditis, 268–269
    acute, 271t
    basic principles of, 268–269
    clinical utility in, 269
    echocardiographic approach to, 269, 270f
Pericardial effusion, 271–275
  basic principles of, 270t, 271, 271f–272f
  clinical utility in, 274–275, 276f
  diagnosis of, 272–274
    diffuse effusion, 272–273, 273f–274f
    distinguishing from pleural fluid, 273–274, 274f–275f
    loculated effusion, 273, 274f
  myocardial infarction and, 227
Pericardial reflections, 268
Pericardial space, 268
  in comprehensive TEE exam, 513t
Pericardial tamponade, 275–278, 283t
  clinical utility in, 278
  diagnosis of, 278
  echocardiographic approach to, 275–278, 276f
    inferior vena cava dilation, 278
    reciprocal changes in ventricular volumes, 276–277
    respiratory variation in diastolic filling, 277–278, 277f–278f
    right atrial systolic collapse, 275, 276f
    right ventricular diastolic collapse, 275–276, 277f
    tissue Doppler early diastolic velocity, 278
Pericardial thickening, 269, 270f, 284f
Pericardiocentesis, echo-guided, for pericardial tamponade, 278, 279f
Pericarditis, 268–269
  basic principles of, 268–269
  clinical utility in, 269
  echocardiographic approach to, 269, 270f
Pericardium
  anatomy and physiology of, 268, 269f
  cysts of, 270f, 274
Perimembranous ventricular septal defect, 488
Perioperative echocardiography, recommendations for, 508t
Persistent left superior vena cava, 425f
Pharmacologic stress echocardiography, 556t
Physical laboratory, in echocardiography laboratory structure, 138t
Physician
  in echocardiography laboratory structure, 138t
  education and training of, 136, 137t
Physiologic valvular regurgitation, of normal color Doppler flow patterns, 61
Piezoelectric crystal, 6–7, 6f
Point of care cardiac ultrasound (POCUS), 118t, 120–122, 133–135
  indications for, 135t
  instrumentation, 133
  providers for, 134–135, 135f
  safety and limitations in, 135

Post-test probability, 124–126, 125f
Power output, 8t
PR interval, left ventricular diastolic function and, 191
Pre-test probability, 124–126, 125f
Precision, of diagnostic testing, 123
Predictive value, 124
Preload, 145–146, 146f
  left ventricular diastolic function and, 191–192, 192f
Pressure curves, diastolic, 179f
Pressure gradients
  in aortic stenosis, 296–297, 297f
  in mitral stenosis, 307, 308f
  in prosthetic valve stenosis, 380
  and velocity, relationship between, in valvular stenosis, 289–290
Pressure half-time valve area, in mitral stenosis, 307–309, 311f
Pressure-volume loop, 145, 145f
PRF. *see* Pulse repetition frequency
Primum atrial septal defect, 485, 490f
Probability, pre-test and post-test, 124–126, 125f
Probe angulation, of transesophageal echocardiography, 71f
Propagation velocity, 189, 189f
Prosthetic paravalvular regurgitation, closure of, 530t
Prosthetic valve dysfunction
  intraoperative TEE for, 526, 527f, 539t
  mechanisms of, 373–375
    endocarditis as, 375
    primary structural failure as, 373–374
    thromboembolic complications as, 375
Prosthetic valve endocarditis, 414–415, 414f–416f
Prosthetic valves, 370–399
  basic principles of, 370–375
  bioprosthetic, 370–371, 372f–373f, 376f
  cardiac sources of embolism and, 441t–442t
  clinical echocardiographic correlates of, 371f
  clinical utility of, 387–396
  Doppler echocardiography of, 378–380
    antegrade flow patterns and velocities in, 378–379, 379f
    areas, 562t
    clicks in, 378, 378f
    mean gradients, 561t
    normal regurgitation in, 379–380
  echo evaluation in, technical aspects of, 375, 376f
  echocardiography of, 375–387
  endocarditis, 392–394, 395f
  homograft, 372
  imaging of, 375–378
  implantation of, baseline function of, 387
  indications for transthoracic echocardiography, 131t, 139t–141t
  limitations and alternate approaches to, 387
  mechanical, 373, 374f, 377f
  microcavitation in, 377
  native valves and, differences between, 383
  patient-prosthesis mismatch, 391

Prosthetic valves *(Continued)*
  regurgitation in, 383–386, 392, 394f
    detection of, 383–384, 383f–385f
    severity and etiology of, 384–386
  stenosis, 380–383, 387–389, 388f–390f
    aortic, 380–382, 381f
    findings of significant valve dysfunction with, 382t
    mitral, 382–383
    pressure gradients and, 380
    valve areas in, 380–383
  TEE evaluation of, 397t–398t
  thrombosis in, 394–396, 396f
    with thrombus formation, 439, 444t
  transcatheter valve implantation and, 389, 391f–392f, 393t
  TTE evaluation of, 397t
  types of, 370–373
  valved conduits, 373
Proximal abdominal aorta
  transesophageal approach in, 453
  transthoracic approach in, 450
Proximal ascending aorta, transthoracic approach in, 449, 450f
Proximal flow convergence, valvular regurgitation and, 331–332, 332f
Proximal flow patterns, in valvular stenosis, 290–291, 291f
Proximal isovelocity surface area (PISA), 325, 331, 332f–334f
  mitral regurgitation and, 354, 354f–355f
  velocity of, 331
Pseudoaneurysm, 226–227, 227f, 275, 448
  in endocarditis, 403t, 419t
  with thrombus formation, 438
Pulmonary artery
  abnormalities, 451f, 465–466, 467f
  flow, 86f
  3D echocardiography of, 105t
  velocity curve, 171–172
Pulmonary artery pressure measurement, noninvasive, *vs.* measurement by right heart catheterization, 552t
Pulmonary artery velocities
  normal, 58f
    LV inflow and, 58f
    RV outflow tract and, 56
Pulmonary embolism, 438f
Pulmonary heart disease, 262–264
  alternate approaches for, 264
  chronic *vs.* acute, 262, 262f
  clinical utility for, 264
  echocardiographic approach in, 262–263
    pulmonary pressures, 262, 263f
    right ventricular pressure overload, 262–263, 264f
    secondary tricuspid regurgitation, 263
  limitations and technical considerations in, 263–264
Pulmonary hypertension
  indications for transthoracic echocardiography, 139t–141t
  in mitral stenosis, 313
Pulmonary pressures
  pulmonary heart disease and, 262, 263f
  with pulmonic valve disease, calculation of, 481b, 481t
Pulmonary systolic pressure, 168–171, 170b, 170t, 171f

Pulmonary vasculature, 168–174
  limitations of, 174
  pulmonary systolic pressure estimates, 168–171, 170b, 170t, 171f
  resistance, 171–174
    calculation of, 172–174
  right atrial pressure, estimation of, 171, 173f, 173t
Pulmonary veins, 77f
  anatomy of, 90f
  in comprehensive TEE exam, 513t
  flow of, 90f
Pulmonary venous inflow, measures of, 188
Pulmonary venous return, anomalous, 475t–476t
Pulmonary regurgitant velocity, 171, 172f
Pulmonic regurgitation, 363–364, 363f–364f, 367t
Pulmonic stenosis, 316–318, 319f, 475t–476t
Pulmonic valve
  recommendations for systematic 3D study, 102t
  three-dimensional TEE image acquisition in, 514f
  3D echocardiography of, 105t
  transesophageal echocardiography of, 82t, 84, 513t
  volume-rendered 3D image displays for, 101, 103f
Pulmonic valve disease, pulmonary pressures with, calculation of, 481b, 481t
Pulmonic valve motion, patterns of, 53f
Pulse (or burst) length, 8t
Pulse repetition frequency (PRF), 6–7, 8t, 17t, 19–20
Pulsed Doppler, 17t
  signal aliasing, 21f
Pulsed-wave Doppler ultrasound, 19–21, 20f

R

Range ambiguity, 14t, 15, 22–23
Real-time narrow 3D section, 96
Real-time 3D-zoom volume-rendered images, 96, 98t, 99f
Reciprocal changes, in ventricular volumes, in pericardial tamponade, 276–277
Reflection, 4t, 5
Refraction, 4t, 5, 14t, 15, 16f
Regional wall motion, in intraoperative or intraprocedural TEE, 520t–521t
Regurgitant fraction (RF), 329
  aortic regurgitation and, 343
Regurgitant orifice area (ROA), 329
  mitral regurgitation and, 354
Regurgitant volume (RVol), 326, 328
  aortic regurgitation and, 343
  calculation of, 335
  mitral regurgitation and, 354
Regurgitation
  aortic, 336–345, 338f
    aortic flow reversal in, 341, 342f
    chronic, stages of, 344t
    chronic asymptomatic, timing of surgical intervention for, 345
    clinical echocardiographic correlation of, 337t
    clinical utility for, 345
    CW Doppler for, 341 343, 342f
    diagnostic utility for, 345
    echo approach to, 365t

Regurgitation (Continued)
    indirect signs of, 339, 340f
    left ventricular response in, 339, 339f
    regurgitant volume and fraction in, 343
    screening examination for, 340–341, 340f–341f
    severity of, evaluation of, 340–343, 343b, 365t
    valve apparatus in, diagnostic imaging of, 336–338
    vena contracta and, 341
  mitral, 345–359
    clinical echocardiographic correlation of, 353t
    clinical follow-up for, 356
    clinical utility of, 356–359
    echo approach to, 366t
    functional, 349, 350f
    intervention for, timing of, 356
    ischemic, 347–348, 349f
    left atrium response to, 350–351
    left ventricular response to, 350–351, 351f
    in mitral stenosis, 313–314
    primary, stages of, 357t
    proximal isovelocity surface area and, 354, 354f–355f
    pulmonary vasculature response to, 350–351
    pulmonary vein flow reversal and, 354–356
    regurgitation volume and orifice area and, 354
    rheumatic, 347
    screening examination for, 351–352
    secondary, stages of, 358t
    severity of, evaluation of, 351–356, 352f, 355f, 356b, 366t
    valve apparatus in, diagnostic imaging of, 345–349, 345f–348f
    vena contracta and, 352
  paraprosthetic, 385, 386f
  pathologic, 379–380
  in prosthetic valves, 383–386, 392, 394f
    detection of, 383–384, 383f–385f
    normal, 379–380
    severity and etiology of, 384–386
  tricuspid, 359–363
    clinical utility of, 361–363
    diagnostic imaging of, 359
    echo approach to, 367t
    right ventricular and right atrial dilation and, 359
    severity of, evaluation of, 359–361, 360f–361f
    stages of, 362t
  valvular, 324–369
    basic principles of, 324–327
    color Doppler imaging in, 329–332
      jet size and shape, 329–330, 329f–330f
      limitations and alternate approaches to, 335–336, 336f
    detection of, 327, 327f
    distal flow reversals in, 334, 335f
    Doppler evaluation of, 328t
    etiology of, 324–325
    fluid dynamics of, 325–326, 325f, 325t
    jet in, 325–326, 326t
    in normal individuals, 327, 328f

Regurgitation (Continued)
    proximal flow convergence and, 331–332, 332f–334f
    pulmonic, 363–364, 363f–364f
      echo approach to, 367t
    severity of, approaches to quantitation of, 327–336
    vena contracta and, 330–331, 331f–332f
    volume flow at two intracardiac sites and, 334–335, 335f
    volume overload in, 326, 326f
Relative wall thickness, 156
Relaxation, ventricular, 180, 180f
Renal cell carcinoma, 426, 428f
Reproducibility, of left ventricle imaging, 157–158
Resolution, 4t
Respiration, left ventricular diastolic function and, 191
Respiratory variation, in diastolic filling, in pericardial tamponade, 277–278, 277f–278f
Restrictive cardiomyopathy, 252–255
  alternate approaches for, 255
  basic principles in, 236t, 252–255, 253f
  features of, 265t
  limitations and technical considerations in, 255
  clinical utility for, 242t–243t, 255
  echocardiographic approach in, 253–255
    anatomic features, 253–254, 253f–254f
    diastolic function, 254–255, 254f
Revascularization, indications for transthoracic echocardiography, 139t–141t
Reverberations, 14, 14t, 15f
Reverse doming, 339
Reynolds number (R_e), 53
Rhabdomyosarcoma, 433f
Rheumatic aortic stenosis, 294
Rheumatic disease
  in mitral stenosis, 306, 306f–307f
  tricuspid regurgitation and, 359
Rheumatic mitral stenosis, with thrombus formation, 439
Right atrial filling, 59, 181
Right atrial pressure, estimation of, 171, 173f, 173t
Right atrial systolic collapse, in pericardial tamponade, 275, 276f
Right atrium
  anatomy of, 41f
  3D echocardiography of, 105t
  transesophageal echocardiography of, 90, 513t
Right heart
  catheterization, vs. noninvasive pulmonary artery pressure measurement, 552t
  stroke volume calculations, 160, 161f
Right ventricle (RV)
  function of, in intraoperative or intraprocedural TEE, 520t–521t
  imaging of, 163f
  recommendations for systematic 3D study, 102t
  size of, 163–164, 164f
  three-dimensional TEE image acquisition in, 514f
  3D echocardiography of, 105t

Right ventricle (RV) *(Continued)*
 transesophageal echocardiography of, 89, 513*t*
 volume-rendered 3D image displays for, 101, 103*f*
Right ventricular diastolic collapse, in pericardial tamponade, 275–276, 277*f*
Right ventricular diastolic function, 198–200
 Doppler data recording in, 198
 physiologic factors that affect right ventricular filling in, 198
 right atrial filling and, 198–200, 200*f*
 right ventricular filling and, 198, 200*f*
Right ventricular infarction, myocardial infarction and, 227
Right ventricular inflow, 36–40, 40*f*, 58
 anatomy of, 41*f*
Right ventricular outflow, 56
 congenital obstructions to, 481, 481*b*, 481*t*, 482*f*
 transesophageal echocardiography of, 75*f*
Right ventricular pressure overload, pulmonary heart disease and, 262–263, 264*f*
Right ventricular systolic function, 164–166, 167*f*–168*f*
 echo approach to, 163–168
 limitations of, 168
 right ventricle imaging, 163*f*
 right ventricle size, 163–164, 164*f*
 ventricular septal motion, patterns of, 166–168
Rotation, myocardial mechanics, 106, 107*t*
RV index of myocardial performance (RIMP), 166*b*

S

Sample volume, Doppler physics, 17*t*
Scattering, 4*t*, 5
Secondary tricuspid regurgitation, pulmonary heart disease and, 263
Secundum atrial septal defect, 484–485, 489*f*–490*f*
Sensitivity, of diagnostic testing, 122, 122*f*
Short-axis plane
 of aortic valve, 81–82, 84*f*
 of esophageal position, 73–75
 standard image and, 35
 of transgastric position, 76
Shunts
 congenital, 474–479, 477*f*–478*f*
 intracardiac, 484–491
  atrial septal defects, 484–488
  patent ductus arteriosus, 491, 492*f*
  ventricular septal defects, 488–491
 ratios, calculations of, 478*b*, 478*t*, 500–501
Signal aliasing, 17*t*, 20, 56
 of normal color Doppler flow patterns, 60, 60*f*
 principle of, 20*f*
 pulsed Doppler, 21*f*
Simpson's rule, 150–152
Simultaneous multiplane mode, 98
Sinus of Valsalva aneurysms, 410, 455*t*–456*t*, 464–465, 465*f*, 475*t*–476*t*, 482–483
 transesophageal approach in, 453
 transthoracic approach in, 448, 449*f*

Sinus venosus defect, 485–486, 489*f*
Situs inversus, 479
Sonographer
 in echocardiography laboratory structure, 138*t*
 education and training of, 136
Sound waves, 1
Spatial peak pulse average (SPPA), 28
Spatial peak temporal average (SPTA) intensity, 28
Specificity, of diagnostic testing, 122, 122*f*
Speckle tracking strain (STE)
 imaging, 109–110, 111*f*, 118*t*
 left ventricular, 155, 156*f*
 myocardial, 107*t*
Spectral analysis, 17*t*, 18–19, 19*f*
Spectral Doppler, recording of, 518
Spontaneous contrast, 377, 440
Standard image planes, 34–35
Standard three orthogonal echocardiographic image planes, 34–35
Standard views, nomenclature of, 34–35, 35*f*
State-of-the-art ultrasound, features of, 134*t*
Stenosis
 aortic, 291–305, 320*t*
  bicuspid aortic valve, 292–294, 293*f*
  calcific, 292, 292*f*
  causes of, 291*f*
  clinical applications in, 301–304
  coexisting valvular disease, 300–301
  congenital, 294
  diagnostic imaging of, 291–294
  differential diagnosis of, 294, 295*f*
  left ventricular response to, 301
  low flow, evaluation of, 304–305
  rheumatic, 294
  severity of, quantitation of, 294–300, 301*b*
  stages of, 302*t*
 mitral, 305–315, 321*t*
  consequences of, 312–314
  diagnostic imaging of mitral valve, 306–307
  differential diagnosis of, 306–307
  The French Three-Group grading of, 316*t*
  mitral annular calcification in, 306, 308*f*
  rheumatic disease in, 306, 306*f*–307*f*
  severity, quantitation of, 307–312, 314*b*
  stages of, 315*t*
 prosthetic valve, 380–383, 387–389, 388*f*–390*f*
  findings of significant valve dysfunction with, 382*t*
  mitral, 382–383
  pressure gradients and, 380
  valve areas in, 380–383
 pulmonic, 316–318, 319*f*
  pulmonary systolic pressure and, 170
 tricuspid, 315–316, 319*f*
 valvular, 288–323
  approach to the evaluation of, 288
  fluid dynamics of, 289–291

Stenosis *(Continued)*
 distal flow disturbance in, 290, 290*f*
 high-velocity jet in, 289, 289*f*
 pressure gradient and velocity, relationship between, 289–290
 proximal flow patterns in, 290–291, 291*f*
Strain
 in intraoperative or intraprocedural TEE, 520*t*–521*t*
 left ventricular wall, 153–155
 myocardial mechanics, 106, 107*t*, 108, 110*f*
Strain rate, myocardial mechanics, 106
Strain rate imaging, 107*t*, 108, 108*f*
 left ventricular wall, 153–155
Stress, left ventricular wall, 153–155
Stress echocardiography, 132–133, 133*t*
 dobutamine, 214–217
  in ischemia, 214–215, 215*f*–216*f*
  in myocardial viability, 215–217
 dobutamine, compared with coronary angiography, 554*t*
 indications for, 132–133, 133*t*
 myocardial ischemia and, 211–213, 213*f*
 pharmacologic, 556*t*
 3D, 105*t*
Stroke volume, 147*b*, 326*f*
 left ventricular systolic function, 158–159, 158*b*, 158*f*
 mitral valve in, 160, 161*f*
 right heart in, 160, 161*f*
 sites for measurement, 159–160
 transaortic, calculation of, 334–335
Strut chordae, 43
Subaortic membrane, 475*t*–476*t*
Subaortic stenosis, 480–481
Subcostal window, for transthoracic tomographic views, 47–48
 four-chamber view of, 50*f*
Suboptimal image quality, 13–14, 14*t*
Subpulmonic ventricle, 479
Superior vena cava, persistent left, 475*t*–476*t*
Supracristal ventricular septal defects, 490
Suprasternal notch window, for transthoracic tomographic views, 48–49, 51*f*
Surface-rendered volumetric imaging, 100, 100*f*
Surgical manipulation, in intraoperative and interventional echocardiography, 510–511, 511*f*
Surgical therapy, hypertrophic cardiomyopathy and, 252
Syphilitic aortitis, 455*t*–456*t*
 aortic regurgitation and, 336–338
Systemic inflammatory disease, 455*t*–456*t*
Systemic ventricle, 479
Systole, definition of, 144–145
Systolic function
 ejection acceleration times and, 161–162
 in hypertensive heart disease, 261
 left ventricular
  Doppler evaluation of, 158–163
  qualitative evaluation of, 147–148
  quantitative evaluation of, 148–155
  ventricular pressure rise and, 162, 162*b*, 162*f*

Systolic function (Continued)
  physiology of, 145–146
  right ventricular, 164–166, 167f–168f
    echo approach to, 163–168

T

Takayasu arteritis, 455t–456t
Tako-tsubo cardiomyopathy, 239, 240f, 242t–243t
Tamponade
  echocardiographic findings in, 556t
  physiology, in pericardial effusion, 271
TAPSE. see Tricuspid annular plane systolic excursion
TDI. see Tissue Doppler imaging
TEE. see Transesophageal echocardiography
Testing zone, 125, 125f
Tetralogy of Fallot, 475t–476t, 497–498, 497f
TGA. see Transposition of the great arteries
Thoracic aorta, descending
  long-axis view of, 39
  transesophageal echocardiography and, 79–80, 81f
Three-dimensional color Doppler imaging, 98
Three-dimensional echocardiography (3DE), 16, 96–106, 507
  applications of, 118t
  clinical utility, 103–106, 105t
  endocardial definition, 157
  examination protocol in, 101, 102t, 103f
  image acquisition in, 96–99, 97f, 98t
  image display in, 99–101, 100f–101f
  limitations of, 106
  quantitation from, 101–103, 104f
  techniques, 69
  ventricular volumes, calculation of, 149–152, 153t, 155f
Three-dimensional TEE imaging, 67
  image acquisition of, 514f
Thrombosis, prosthetic valves and, 394–396, 396f
Thrombotic endocarditis, nonbacterial, 444t
Thrombus
  formation
    intracardiac, diagnostic tests for, 563t
    prosthetic valve dysfunction and, 375
  indications for transthoracic echocardiography, 139t–141t
  left atrial, 434–436, 444t
    alternate approaches to, 436
    identification of, 434–435, 435f–436f
    predisposing factors of, 434
    prognosis and clinical implications of, 436, 437f
  left ventricular, 431–434, 444t
    alternate approaches to, 432–434
    clinical implications of, 432
    identification of, 432, 434f
    myocardial infarction and, 228
    predisposing conditions of, 431–432
  in mitral stenosis, 312–313
  right-sided heart, 436–437, 438f
Time constraints, in intraoperative and interventional echocardiography, 511–512
Tissue Doppler early diastolic velocity, in pericardial tamponade, 278

Tissue Doppler imaging (TDI), 27, 107t
  strain and strain rate, 106–109, 107f–110f, 118t
  velocities, 106, 108f
Tissue Doppler myocardial imaging, 185–187, 187f
Tissue harmonic imaging (THI), 12
Tissue valves, 370–371, 372f
  stented, 370–371, 375
  stentless, 370–371, 375
Tomographic imaging, in transthoracic echocardiography, 33–34
Torsion, myocardial mechanics, 106, 107t, 111–112
Total artificial heart, 258
  in intraoperative or intraprocedural TEE, 520t–521t
Total stroke volume, 326
TR. see Tricuspid regurgitation
Transcatheter aortic valve implantation (TAVI), 531, 533t–534t, 535f
  for valve disease, 530t
Transcatheter aortic valve replacement (TAVR), 531
  imaging assessment, checklist for, 533t–534t
  TEE guidance of, 535f
Transcatheter mitral valve repair
  intraoperative and interventional echocardiography in, 535, 535f–536f
  for valve disease, 530t
Transcatheter procedures
  echocardiography for, 105
  imaging for, 538t
  intraoperative and interventional echocardiography in, 530–535, 530t, 531f
    atrial septal defect closure devices, placement of, 531, 532f, 533t–534t, 535f
    other transcatheter interventions, 535, 537f
    transcatheter mitral valve repair, 535, 535f–536f
Transcatheter valves, 375
  implantation of
    echo evaluation after, 393t
    prosthetic valves and, 389, 391f–392f
Transducers, 6–10, 8t, 96–99, 97f
  beam shape and focusing of, 7–8, 10f
  motion, 35f
  resolution of, 9–10, 10t, 11f, 13f
  schematic diagram of, 6f
  types of, 7
Transesophageal echocardiography (TEE), 35–36, 67–95, 130–132, 131f, 132t, 507
  aortic valve of, 81–82, 84f
    short-axis view, 77f
  in atrial septal defects, 488, 489f–490f
  basic exam sequence of, 92t–93t
  bicaval view of, 76f
  for cardiac sources of emboli, 443t
  chamber anatomy and filling patterns of, 87–90
  contraindications for, 68t
  of descending thoracic aorta, 79–80, 81f
  esophageal position of, 70–75
    four-chamber plane, 70–71, 70f–72f
    long-axis plane, 73, 74f
    short-axis plane, 73–75
    two-chamber plane, 71–73, 72f

Transesophageal echocardiography (TEE) (Continued)
  exam, components and sequence of, 513t
  examination of, 90–91
  in great artery diseases, 453–455
    Doppler flows in, 453–455
    echocardiographic imaging in, 453, 453f–454f
    limitations of, 455
  image plane rotation of, 69f
  indications for, 67, 130–132, 131f, 132t
  of left ventricle, 147, 149t
  in left ventricular wall motion, 209–210
  probe angulation, 71f
  protocols of, 67–68
  risk of complications for, 67–68, 69t
  RV outflow tract view of, 75f
  shadowing and reverberations on, 517, 518f
  three-dimensional, image acquisition of, 514f
  tomographic views of, 68–80
  transducer motions in, 69, 70f
  transgastric position of, 76–79
    four-chamber plane, 78
    image planes, 77f
    long-axis plane, 78–79
    short-axis plane, 76, 78f
  valve anatomy and function of, 80–84
  for valvular regurgitation, 325
  ventricular systolic function, 175t
Transgastric image planes, 77f
Transgastric position, of transesophageal echocardiography, 76–79, 513t
  four-chamber plane, 78
  image planes, 77f
  long-axis plane, 78–79, 80f
  short-axis plane, 76, 78f
  two-chamber plane, 76–78
Transit time effect, 23
Transmission frequency, 8t
Transplantation, cardiac, 258–259
  acute rejection in, 259
  allograft in, 258–259, 259f
  post-transplant monitoring in, 259
Transposition of the great arteries (TGA)
  complete, 498–500, 498f–499f
  congenitally corrected, 475t–476t, 491–493, 493f–494f
Transthoracic echo image orientation nomenclature, 34t
Transthoracic echocardiography (TTE)
  aging changes, 61
  in atrial septal defects, 486–487, 487f–488f
  basic image planes used in, 34f
  for cardiac sources of emboli, 443t
  diagnostic, 61–62
    additional components, 64t–65t
    core elements of, 64t
  in great artery diseases, 449–453
    Doppler flows in, 450–452, 452f
    echocardiographic imaging in, 449–450, 449f, 451f, 451t
    limitations of, 452–453
  indications for, 36, 127–130, 128t–130f, 130t–132t, 139t–141t
  of left ventricle, 149t
  in left ventricular wall motion, 207–209, 207f–209f

Transthoracic echocardiography (TTE) (Continued)
  M-mode recordings of, 49–52
  normal anatomy and flow patterns on, 33–66
    basic imaging principles of, 33–36
    echocardiographic image interpretation, 36
    examination technique of, 36
    image orientation of, 35–36
    technical quality of, 36
  normal intracardiac flow patterns of, 52–61
  for specific cardiac structures, 37t
  tomographic views of, 36–49
  for valvular regurgitation, 325
  ventricular systolic function, 175t
Transvalvular velocity, in aortic stenosis, 296f
Transvalvular volume flow rates, differences in, 160–161
Transverse sinus, in pericardium, 268
Trauma, esophageal, risk of TEE, 68
Traumatic aortic disease, 455t–456t
Tricuspid annular plane systolic excursion (TAPSE), 52
  right ventricular systolic function and, 165–166, 166f
Tricuspid regurgitant jet, 84
Tricuspid regurgitant velocity, 168–171, 172f
Tricuspid regurgitation (TR), 359–363
  clinical utility of, 361–363
  diagnostic imaging of, 359
  echo approach to, 367t
  right ventricular and right atrial dilation and, 359
  severity of, evaluation of, 359–361, 360f–361f
  stages of, 362t
Tricuspid stenosis (TS), 315–316, 319f
Tricuspid valve
  disease. see Tricuspid regurgitation; Tricuspid stenosis
  Ebstein anomaly of, 483, 485f
  recommendations for systematic 3D study, 102t
  three-dimensional TEE image acquisition in, 514f
  3D echocardiography of, 105t
  transesophageal echocardiography of, 82t, 84, 513t
  volume-rendered 3D image displays for, 101, 103f
Tricuspid valve vegetation, 405–406, 407f
TS. see Tricuspid stenosis
TTE. see Transthoracic echocardiography
Twist, myocardial mechanics, 106, 107t, 111–112
Two-chamber plane
  as esophageal position, 71–73, 72f
  standard image planes, 35
  as transgastric position, 76–78
Two-dimensional echocardiography, 11–16, 33
  endocardial definition, 157
  image production of, 11–13, 13f
  imaging artifacts of, 13–16, 14f
  instrument settings of, 13
  of left ventricle, 148
  of right ventricle, 163, 164f, 165t
  ventricular volumes, calculation of, 149–152, 152f, 153t, 154f

U
Ultrasound, 2
  cardiac, 120
    examination types, 121t
  features of, 134t
  imaging modalities, 10–16
    echocardiographic imaging measurements of, 16
    M-mode, 10–11, 12f
    three-dimensional echocardiography of, 16
    two-dimensional echocardiography of, 11–16
  intensity of, 28
Ultrasound tissue interaction, 4–6, 4t, 5f
  attenuation of, 5–6
  reflection in, 5
  refraction of, 5
  scattering in, 5
Ultrasound waves, 1–4, 2t
  schematic diagram of, 2f
Unicuspid aortic valve, 475t–476t
Uterine tumors, 426

V
Valve annulus dimension, in adults, 543t
Valve dehiscence, prosthetic, in endocarditis, 403t, 416f, 419t
Valve regurgitation, indications for transthoracic echocardiography, 131t, 139t–141t
Valve stenosis
  due to endocarditis, 409
  indications for transthoracic echocardiography, 131t, 139t–141t
  intraoperative TEE for, 524–526, 526f, 539t
Valve vegetations, in cardiac masses, 425, 426f
Valved conduits, 373
  imaging of, 377–378
Valvular heart disease
  indications for transthoracic echocardiography, 139t–141t
  intraoperative TEE for, 521–526
    endocarditis, 526
    mitral valve repair, 521–524, 522f–525f
    prosthetic valve dysfunction, 526, 527f
    valve stenosis, 524–526, 526f
  POCUS for, 134
Valvular regurgitation, 324–369
  aortic, 336–345, 338f
    aortic flow reversal in, 341, 342f
    chronic, stages of, 344t
    chronic asymptomatic, timing of surgical intervention for, 345
    clinical echocardiographic correlation of, 337t
    clinical utility for, 345
    CW Doppler for, 341–343, 342f
    diagnostic utility for, 345
    echo approach to, 365t
    indirect signs of, 339, 340f
    left ventricular response in, 339, 339f
    regurgitant volume and fraction in, 343
    screening examination for, 340–341, 340f–341f
    severity of, evaluation of, 340–343, 343b, 365t

Valvular regurgitation (Continued)
    valve apparatus in, diagnostic imaging of, 336–338
    vena contracta and, 341
  basic principles of, 324–327
  color Doppler imaging in, 329–332
    jet size and shape, 329–330, 329f–330f
    limitations and alternate approaches to, 335–336, 336f
  detection of, 327, 327f
  distal flow reversals in, 334, 335f
  Doppler evaluation of, 328t
  etiology of, 324–325
  fluid dynamics of, 325–326, 325f, 325t
  jet in, 325–326, 326t
  mitral, 345–359
    clinical echocardiographic correlation of, 353t
    clinical follow-up for, 356
    clinical utility of, 356–359
    echo approach to, 366t
    functional, 349, 350f
    intervention for, timing of, 356
    ischemic, 347–348, 349f
    left atrium response to, 350–351
    left ventricular response to, 350–351, 351f
    primary, stages of, 357t
    proximal isovelocity surface area and, 354, 354f–355f
    pulmonary vasculature response to, 350–351
    pulmonary vein flow reversal and, 354–356
    regurgitation volume and orifice area and, 354
    rheumatic, 347
    screening examination for, 351–352
    secondary, stages of, 358t
    severity of, evaluation of, 351–356, 352f, 355f, 356b, 366t
    valve apparatus in, diagnostic imaging of, 345–349, 345f–348f
    vena contracta and, 352
  in normal individuals, 327, 328f
  proximal flow convergence and, 331–332, 332f–334f
  pulmonic, 363–364, 363f–364f
    echo approach to, 367t
  severity of, approaches to quantitation of, 327–336
  tricuspid, 359–363
    clinical utility of, 361–363
    diagnostic imaging of, 359
    echo approach to, 367t
    right ventricular and right atrial dilation and, 359
    severity of, evaluation of, 359–361, 360f–361f
    stages of, 362t
  vena contracta and, 330–331, 331f–332f
  volume flow at two intracardiac sites and, 334–335, 335f
  volume overload in, 326, 326f
Valvular stenosis, 288–323
  aortic stenosis, 291–305, 320t
    bicuspid aortic valve, 292–294, 293f
    calcific, 292, 292f
    causes of, 291f
    clinical applications in, 301–304
    coexisting valvular disease, 300–301
    congenital, 294
    diagnostic imaging of, 291–294

Valvular stenosis (Continued)
  differential diagnosis of, 294, 295f
  left ventricular response to, 301
  low flow, evaluation of, 304–305
  rheumatic, 294
  severity of, quantitation of, 294–300, 301b
  stages of, 302t
 approach to the evaluation of, 288
 Doppler pressure gradients in, 557t
 fluid dynamics of, 289–291
  distal flow disturbance in, 290, 290f
  high-velocity jet in, 289, 289f
  pressure gradient and velocity, relationship between, 289–290
  proximal flow patterns in, 290–291, 291f
 mitral stenosis, 305–315, 321t
  consequences of, 312–314
  diagnostic imaging of mitral valve, 306–307
  differential diagnosis of, 306–307
  The French Three-Group grading of, 316t
  mitral annular calcification in, 306, 308f
  rheumatic disease in, 306, 306f–307f
  severity, quantitation of, 307–312, 314b
  stages of, 315t
 pulmonic stenosis, 316–318, 319f
 tricuspid stenosis, 315–316, 319f
Valvular vegetations
 aortic, 402–404, 402f, 404f–405f, 407–408, 407f
 echocardiographic diagnosis of, 562t
 in endocarditis, echocardiography for, 402–409, 403t
  diagnostic accuracy of, 408–409
  transesophageal, 407–408, 407f
  transthoracic, 402–406, 403t
 mitral, 402f, 404–405, 405f–406f
 tricuspid, 405–406, 407f
Vasodilators, myocardial ischemia and, 217
Vegetations, valvular
 active vs. healed, 413
 aortic, 402–404, 402f, 404f–405f, 407–408, 407f
 in cardiac masses, 425, 426f
 in endocarditis, echocardiography for, 402–409, 403t
  diagnostic accuracy of, 408–409
  transesophageal, 407–408, 407f
  transthoracic, 402–406, 403t
 mitral, 402f, 404–405, 405f–406f
 tricuspid, 405–406, 407f

Veins, pulmonary, 77f
 anatomy of, 90f
 flow of, 90f
Velocity
 myocardial mechanics, 106
 pressure gradient and, relationship between, in valvular stenosis, 289–290
Velocity of propagation (c), 2, 2t
Velocity-pressure relationships, 54, 55b
Velocity ratio, 382
Vena contracta
 aortic regurgitation and, 341
 mitral regurgitation and, 352
 valvular regurgitation and, 330–331, 331f–332f
Venovenous extracorporeal membrane oxygenation (V-V ECMO), in intraoperative or intraprocedural TEE, 520t–521t
Ventricular assist devices, intraoperative TEE for, 529, 529f
Ventricular compliance, 180, 181f
Ventricular diastolic filling and function, 178–203
 approaches to, 189–190, 200, 201f
 basic principles in, 179–182
  causes of diastolic dysfunction, 182, 182t
  normal respiratory changes, 182
  parameters of diastolic function, 179–182
  phases of diastole, 179, 179f
 diastolic dysfunction and, clinical classification of, 194–198, 194t, 195f
  estimates of diastolic filling pressures, 194–195
  mild diastolic dysfunction, 195, 196f
  moderate diastolic dysfunction, 195–196, 197f
  severe diastolic dysfunction, 196–198, 197f
 diastolic function reporting in, 200
 imaging diastolic function parameters in, 182–183
 left atrial filling and, 187–188
 left ventricular diastolic function and, factors affecting Doppler evaluation of, 190–193
  pathophysiology, 192–193
  physiologic factors, 190–192
 left ventricular filling and, Doppler evaluation of, 183–185
  Doppler data recording in, 185
  nomenclature and measurements in, 183, 186f
  volumetric flow rates in, 183–185, 186f–187f

Ventricular diastolic filling and function (Continued)
  right ventricular diastolic function and, 198–200
  tissue Doppler myocardial imaging in, 185–187, 187f
Ventricular diastolic filling (volume) curves, 180–181
Ventricular diastolic pressures, 180
Ventricular function
 in comprehensive TEE exam, 513t
 global and regional, evaluation of, 211, 211t, 212f
 monitoring, intraoperative TEE for, 519, 520t–521t, 521f
 regional, evaluation of, 148, 175t
Ventricular geometry, 145–147
 classification of, 156
 left, 155–156
Ventricular hypertrophy, in hypertensive heart disease, 260, 260f
Ventricular inflow patterns, of normal color Doppler flow patterns, 61
Ventricular outflow patterns, of normal color Doppler flow patterns, 60–61
Ventricular pressure rise, systolic function and, 162, 162b, 162f
Ventricular relaxation, 180, 180f
Ventricular rupture, myocardial infarction and, 226, 227f
Ventricular septal defects (VSDs), 475t–476t, 488–491
 anatomy of, 488–491, 491f
 Doppler findings in, 491
 imaging in, 477f, 490–491, 492f
 myocardial infarction and, 224–226, 226f
Ventricular septal motion, patterns of, 166–168
Ventricular volumes, 146–147
 left, 150–152, 154f
 3D echocardiographic calculation of, 149–152, 153t, 155f
 2D echocardiographic calculation of, 149–152, 152f, 153t, 154f
Visceral pericardium, 268
Volume flow, measurement of, 54, 54b
VSDs. see Ventricular septal defects
V-V ECMO. see Venovenous extracorporeal membrane oxygenation
V-wave, 351–352

W
Wall motion score index, 211
Wavelength (λ), 2b, 2t, 3, 3f
Women, aortic root diameter for, 548t